volume 3

Fundamentals of Nursing

COLLABORATING FOR OPTIMAL HEALTH

SECOND EDITION

Edited By

Karen J. Berger, RN, MS, EdD
Member, Board of Directors
Institute for the Advancement of Leadership
San Diego, California
Formerly Professor and Assistant Director
Department of Nursing Education
Grossmont College
El Cajon, California

Marilyn Brinkman Williams, RN, MN
Professor, Department of Nursing Education
Grossmont College
El Cajon, California

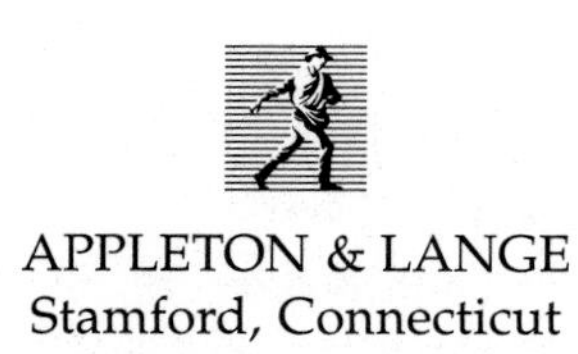

APPLETON & LANGE
Stamford, Connecticut

Notice: The authors and the publisher of this volume have taken care to make certain that the doses of drugs and schedules of treatment are correct and compatible with the standards generally accepted at the time of publication. Nevertheless, as new information becomes available, changes in treatment and in the use of drugs become necessary. The reader is advised to carefully consult the instruction and information material included in the package insert of each drug or therapeutic agent before administration. This advice is especially important when using, administering, or recommending new or infrequently used drugs. The authors and publisher disclaim all responsibility for any liability, loss, injury, or damage incurred as a consequence, directly or indirectly, of the use and application of any of the contents of the volume.

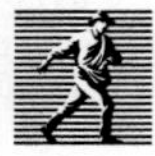

Copyright © 1999 by Appleton & Lange
A Simon & Schuster Company

All rights reserved. This book, or any parts thereof, may not be used or reproduced in any manner without written permission. For information, address Appleton & Lange, Four Stamford Plaza, PO Box 120041, Stamford, Connecticut 06912-0041
www.appletonlange.com

99 00 00 01 02 03 / 10 9 8 7 6 5 4 3 2 1

Prentice Hall International (UK) Limited, *London*
Prentice Hall of Australia Pty. Limited, *Sydney*
Prentice Hall Canada, Inc., *Toronto*
Prentice Hall Hispanoamericana, S.A., *Mexico*
Prentice Hall of India Private Limited, *New Delhi*
Prentice Hall of Japan, Inc., *Tokyo*
Simon & Schuster Asia Pte. Ltd., *Singapore*
Editora Prentice Hall do Brasil Ltda., *Rio de Janeiro*
Prentice Hall, *Upper Saddle River, New Jersey*

Library of Congress Cataloging-in-Publication Data
Fundamentals of nursing : collaborating for optimal health / edited by
Karen J. Berger, Marilyn Brinkman Williams.—2nd ed.
p. cm.
Includes bibliographical references and index.
ISBN 0-8385-2594-6 (pbk. : alk. paper)
1. Nursing. 2. Nurse and patient. I. Berger, Karen J.
II. Williams, Marilyn Brinkman.
[DNLM: 1. Nursing Care. 2. Nurse-Patient Relations. 3. Patient Participation. WY 100 F97983 1998]
RT41.B37 1998
610.73—dc21
DNLM/DLC
for Library of Congress 97-37909
CIP

Acquisitions Editor: David P. Carroll
Editor-in-Chief: Sally J. Barhydt
Senior Production Editor: Karen W. Davis
Associate Production Editor: Angela Dion
Designer: Janice Barsevich Bielawa
Art Coordinator: Eve Siegel
Manufacturing Buyers: Shirley Dahlgren, Lynne Vail-Nagle
Photographer, Chapter and Unit Openers: George D. Dodson

PRINTED IN THE UNITED STATES OF AMERICA

ISBN 0-8385-2594-6
90000
9 780838 525944

Contents in Detail

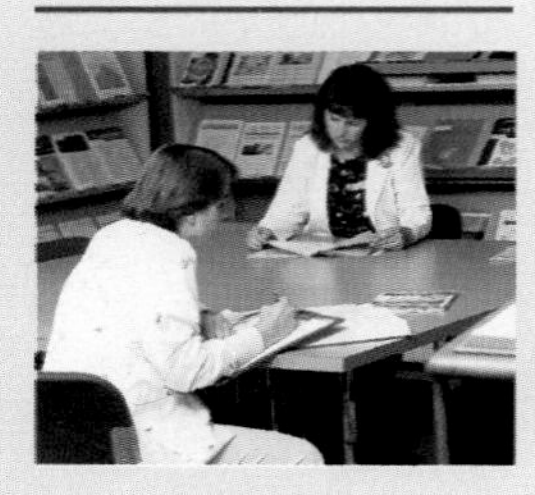

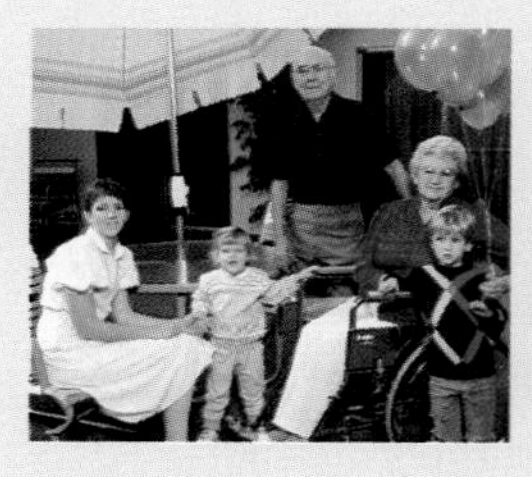

VOLUME II NURSING COLLABORATION AND HEALTH CARE

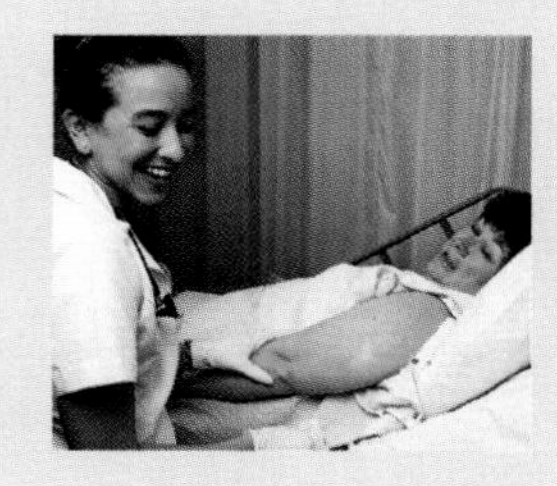

Concepts Directory

Roman numerals in **boldface** type indicate volume numbers.

Skills Directory

Roman numerals in **boldface** type indicate volume numbers.

W

Procedure Directory

UNIT VIII

Collaborative Nursing Assessment and Management

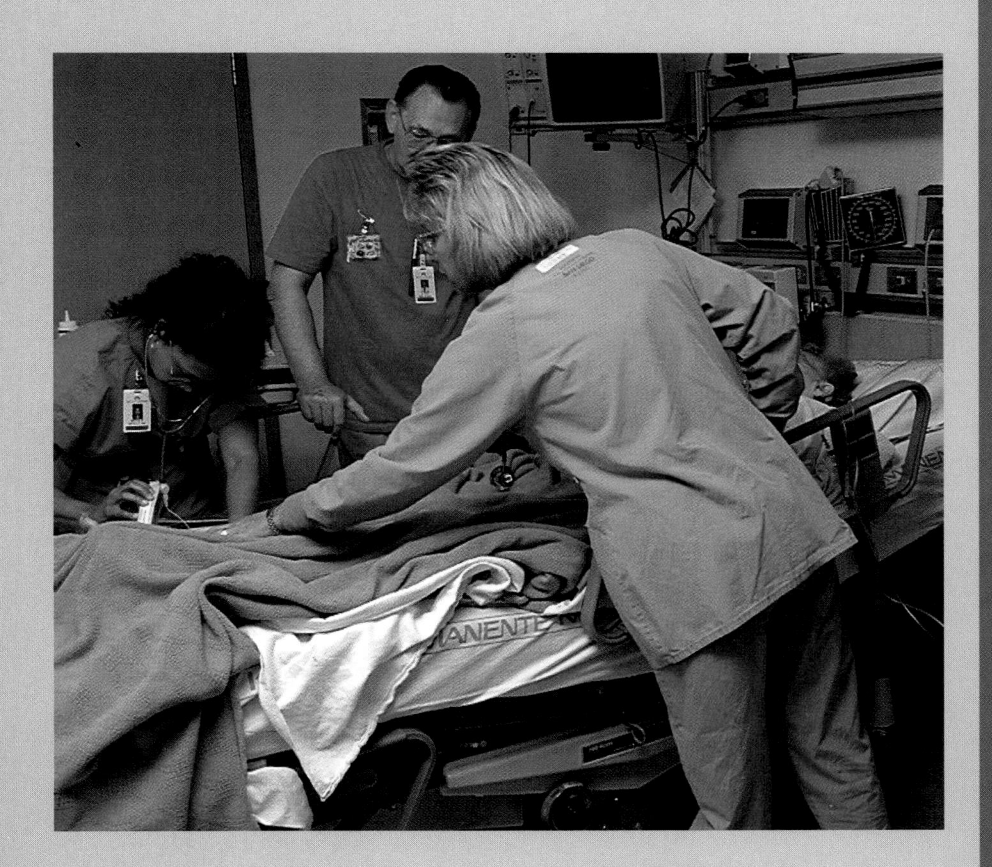

25

Wellness and Well-being

Marilyn Brinkman Williams and Ruth Ann Benfield

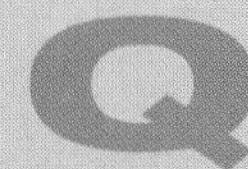

Barbara McMaster, 78 years old, lives alone in a one-bedroom, second-floor apartment in a retirement community. She belongs to a Bridge club and a current events discussion group that meet each week at the retirement community. She views her overall health as excellent. Barbara had not seen a health care professional for several years until she developed a cyst on her back. It was removed 3 weeks ago, but the incision has not healed well. A home health nurse visits Barbara twice a week to do wound care. Barbara says, "I have always felt well and been able to take care of myself, but I don't know what to think about this healing problem."

Is Barbara well or ill?

What factors impact on her level of wellness and well-being?

What lifestyle practices should the nurse assess as she evaluates Barbara's health status?

What health-promotion activities should the nurse include in the plan of care?

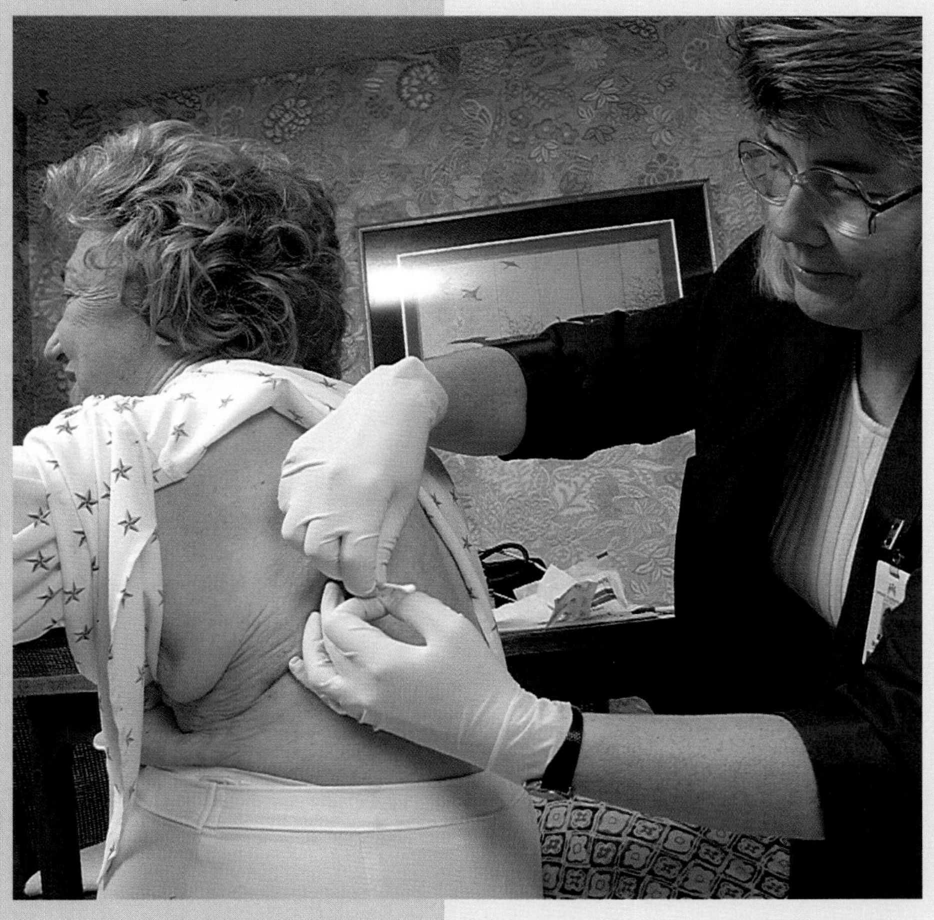

CHAPTER OUTLINE

Nursing practice extends far beyond the care of physiologic conditions. In recent decades, changing patterns of morbidity and mortality, coupled with the skyrocketing costs of medical care, have focused increasing attention by many in health care on measures to promote health and prevent disease and disability. Most of the major threats to health no longer come from disease-producing bacterial or viral agents. Chronic conditions, many related to lifestyle factors or environmental hazards, and injuries resulting from accidents and violence are the basis for the majority of health problems today.[1] Therefore, it is increasingly widely accepted that the scope of health care encompasses physiologic, psychological, social, and environmental factors that influence and determine an individual's level of health.

As Chap. 7 emphasized, the concepts of wellness and well-being are integral to a focus on health promotion and disease prevention. Active self-responsibility—personal action to protect and promote one's own health—is embedded in the concept of wellness. Within this context, individuals are active participants and determinants of their own level of wellness rather than just passive recipients of health-related care. The goal of high-level wellness is achieved through a collaborative effort between individuals and nurses or other health care providers. When patients are full participants in health care decision making, nurses are educators and facilitators. Nursing practice focuses on cultivating self-care, educating patients about health maintenance and health promotion, and motivating them to actively apply that knowledge to develop lifestyles and behaviors that are conducive to health, yet reflect their own needs and preferences.

For individuals faced with illness or disability, nurses provide aspects of care that patients cannot accomplish for themselves; however, the ultimate goal is still to empower patients for self-determination and self-management so that they will be able to attain their own level of optimal health and well-being.[2]

The concepts of wellness and well-being were introduced in Chap. 7. They are integral to all aspects of nursing practice and provide a foundation for the development of a collaborative approach to patient care. In this chapter, these concepts are further developed. Circumstances that interfere with wellness and well-being, including those related to receiving health (or illness) care

are explored. Nursing approaches to assess wellness and well-being, and maximize patients' potential for both are discussed.

SECTION 1

UNDERSTANDING WELLNESS

This section is intended to develop readers' understanding of wellness and its implications for nursing practice. Incorporating the concepts of wellness and well-being into daily nursing practice begins with an application of the basic principles that constitute the wellness framework found in Chap. 7. Concepts from social and behavioral sciences that enhance nurses' abilities to use wellness/well-being principles more effectively in patient care are presented here. This section also examines alterations in wellness that occur in the course of daily living and within the context of the health care experience.

OPTIMAL WELLNESS

ELEMENTS OF A WELLNESS LIFESTYLE

Two classic studies that demonstrated the significant affects of personal behavior on health are the Framingham Heart Study and the Alameda County Study.

The Framingham Heart Study, a long-term study of 5000 residents of Framingham, Massachusetts was begun in 1949. The purpose of the study was to identify factors contributing to the development of coronary heart disease and high blood pressure. The researchers found that heart disease is more prevalent among individuals who smoke, have high blood pressure and high cholesterol levels, and who exercise infrequently. Obesity was also identified as a significant contributor to hypertension and elevated cholesterol levels.

The Alameda County Study of 7000 adults, which examined the relationship of personal habits to individual health, showed a positive correlation between adhering to seven basic health practices and life expectancy and physical well-being. The seven basic practices have been the basis of health teaching in schools and many other settings for many years. They include (1) sleeping 7 to 8 hours each night, (2) eating three meals a day at regular intervals with little snacking, (3) eating breakfast every day, (4) maintaining desirable body weight, (5) avoiding excessive alcohol consumption, (6) getting regular exercise, and (7) not smoking. Social factors also have an important influence on health. Other studies have shown that social support contributes to individuals' deciding to adopt positive health behaviors and to psychological well-being.[3–6]

As these studies have indicated, developing a personal lifestyle that focuses on achieving high-level wellness can have a significant impact on health. Carolyn Chambers Clark has described a concept of "wellness nursing," examined through six elements: (1) eating well, (2) being fit, (3) feeling good, (4) caring for self and others, (5) fitting in, and (6) being responsible (Chap. 7). These dimensions of wellness and the concept of a collaborative nurse–patient relationship are the foundation on which this and subsequent chapters are based.

Eating Well

Eating well means ingesting foods that are satisfying and provide balanced nourishment. Good nutrition provides the essential nutrients needed for normal growth and development and contributes to maintaining the alertness and energy that are needed for full and productive living.[2]

Food choices have important health implications. Dietary intake can increase or decrease a person's risk for heart disease, adult-onset diabetes, hypertension, dental caries, cardiovascular disease, and cancer. Choosing healthy foods begins with a basic understanding of food composition and the use of various nutrients in the body.

Eating provides far more than daily nutrient requirements, however. Many psychological, emotional, and social needs are met in the act of eating. People engage in eating for the pleasurable sensations and enjoyment. Eating can provide an opportunity for social interaction. Ethnic and cultural backgrounds mandate rituals, customs, and beliefs that influence food choices, the manner of serving and eating food, and the meaning that food has for an individual.[8]

Eating habits based on moderation, variety, and sound nutritional practices are an important part of an integrated wellness lifestyle. A detailed discussion of nutrition and specific recommendations for dietary choices that support wellness and well-being can be found in Chap. 28.

Being Fit

Fitness is a state in which body systems function optimally. Many positive physiologic benefits result from a combination of sound nutritional practices and a regular exercise program, including improved cardiovascular endurance; increased muscle strength; lower blood pressure and pulse rate; and reduced percentage of body fat, blood cholesterol, and triglyceride levels. Exercise is also known to improve digestion, nutrient use, and elimination.

In addition to physiologic benefits, regular exercise contributes to a positive sense of well-being through increased energy, reduced fatigue, fewer bodily aches and pains, fewer colds and increased resistance to disease, improved self-esteem and self-regard, improved sleep, increased self-confidence and assertiveness, and increased libido and enhanced sexual vitality.[9] Regular exercise has also been shown to be an effective stress reduction technique.

Although the traditional view of "being fit" focuses on cardiac fitness, a wellness perspective is more comprehensive and includes (1) muscle strength and endurance, (2) flexibility, (3) cardiorespiratory fitness, and (4) body composition.[9] An exercise program that enhances fitness in all four areas is desirable. Fitness and the benefits of exercise are discussed further in Chap. 33.

Feeling Good

Feeling good evolves from functioning with a sense of purpose, successfully meeting life's challenges, and maintaining a sense of personal control over life circumstances. It relates to an individual's ability to reduce or manage stress, to rest and relax, and to maintain a positive outlook on life in general. For some people, the concept of feeling good refers primarily to *physical* wellness. They enthusiastically focus their attention on exercising regularly and eating properly, but disregard the mental, emotional, spiritual, and social dimensions of wellness. Optimal health and wellness are achieved only when harmony exists among all the parts of the whole.

The spiritual dimension of life is a unifying force that integrates all other dimensions of human beings—physical, mental, psychological, and social.[10] Spirit gives meaning and direction to an individual's life. It is the basis for a sense of satisfaction or dissatisfaction with living. Important signs of spiritual health include a sense of inner tranquillity and feelings of being at peace with nature, fellow humans, and for some, with God.

Feeling good as an aspect of wellness also encompasses a balanced response to stress (see also Chap. 8). In society today, stress comes not so much from physical threats as from the by-products of modern civilization. These include physical factors such as noise, polluted air and water, and rushed schedules; emotional stressors such as financial worries, frustrations at work, marital strife, and sexual dysfunctions; and spiritual problems such as inner emptiness, chronic boredom, and lack of fulfillment. These pressures can cause prolonged, excessive stress that accelerates the aging process, consumes vitality, and increases susceptibility to disease.[9] The emotional consequences of excessive stress may be even more harmful than the physiologic effects because they inhibit effective coping practices and reinforce the initial stress response.

Individuals who maintain well-being develop stress reduction strategies that meet their unique needs and lifestyle. Stress management techniques include active and passive types of relaxation. Active methods include physical activities ranging from walking, jogging, and swimming, to yoga and dancing or quiet activities, such as reading and needlework. Passive relaxation can be achieved via massage or spas that relax the muscles as well as the mind, or through the use of psychological relaxation techniques.[11] A discussion of various relaxation techniques can be found in Section 3 of this chapter.

Caring for Self and Others

Caring for self refers to activities an individual performs to achieve, maintain, or promote optimal health and well-being. Maintaining adequate sleep and rest patterns, engaging in recreational activities, and sustaining an ability to laugh and enjoy life are critical components of physical and psychological wellness. Perhaps even more important, however, are actions directed toward self-nurturance, self-improvement, and personal growth.[1]

Although wellness emphasizes individual potential, an important component of wellness is developing and maintaining positive social relationships with others. Research supports the importance of a social support system for physical and emotional health.[3–7] A social support system is the set of interpersonal relationships through which an individual maintains a social identity; gives and receives emotional support, material aid, and information; and makes new social contacts.

Social wellness requires a balance between receiving support from others to meet one's own needs and being able to offer support and assistance to others. Maintaining a balance between one's own needs and the needs of others requires an ability to say no when others' demands exceed one's capabilities and to assertively seek assistance when needed.

Fitting In

Fitting in refers to the ability to live in harmony with the environment. In recent years increased attention has been focused on the health consequences of environmental factors such as smog, water pollution, noise, and overcrowding. The effect of human lifestyles and choices on the environment is a related issue. Although some view these problems as too monumental for personal action to influence, this perspective is a denial of the power and responsibility we all bear. Individual choices can become collective action. Personal behavior can improve the immediate environment and the community environment and thereby enhance one's wellness and well-being.

Increasing one's sensitivity to the impact that personal choices have on the environment and becoming more aware of the influences that home, work, and social surroundings have on self are important steps toward creating positive environmental conditions. "Fitting in" includes taking responsibility for protecting the environment and protecting oneself from harmful environmental elements. Choosing to live and work in smoke-free areas; following basic safety practices; minimizing exposure to known pollutants, infectious agents, carcinogens, and excessive noise; and providing for personal space and privacy for self and family are ways of enhancing one's personal environment to protect health and promote wellness.

Optimal well-being also requires attention to the emotional and spiritual elements in the environment. If social interactions create a stressful climate, individuals expend physical and emotional energy attempting to adapt, leaving them continually exhausted and irritable. Conversely, a work or home environment that allows opportunities for continued self-development and expression, provides frequent positive "rewards" and support for accomplishments, and allows people to fulfill meaningful roles contributes to individuals' psychological and emotional well-being. Individuals who recognize that their home or work environments are stress filled can initiate change. First, they can examine the extent to which their own behavior or their responses to the behavior of others contributes to the problem; then they can make a conscious effort to discontinue those actions. Often one person's efforts can be a catalyst for others to make positive changes as well.

Being Responsible

Self-responsibility is the key element in developing and practicing a wellness lifestyle. Each of the dimensions of wellness depends on individuals accepting personal accountability for using their inner resources and decision-making skills. Being responsible requires self-awareness—an ability to recognize one's limitations as well as one's strengths. It also demands that individuals become active, knowledgeable, and informed participants in matters related to health and well-being.

Active self-responsibility does not eliminate or discount the need for intervention or treatment by health care professionals.

COLLABORATIVE STRATEGY
SELF-RESPONSIBILITY

Self-responsibility has been a central theme in the wellness movement as it has evolved in both the United States and Canada. It is also a key value of the collaborative philosophy of patient care. In a collaborative relationship, nurses and patients make health care decisions jointly. This fosters patients' responsibility even while their capacity for self-care (the ability to carry out the activities of daily living independently) may be diminished.

Rather, in seeking the assistance of a physician or nurse, individuals are exercising responsibility for their health. The extent to which individuals are able to meet their health needs determines the appropriate level of assistance from professionals. The goal of professional intervention should be to maintain, restore, or increase individuals' ability to provide their own self-care. Nurses can best facilitate self-responsibility through patient education and mutual goal setting and decision making. Increased knowledge promotes self-confidence, self-reliance, and motivation—all important determinants of self-care behaviors.

THE EXPERIENCE AND MANIFESTATIONS OF WELLNESS

What does it feel like to experience wellness? How can one recognize wellness in other individuals? Because the concept of wellness is multifaceted and encompasses all aspects of human existence, a description of the characteristics of wellness covers a variety of areas.

- *Self-esteem/self-acceptance.* Self-awareness characterizes those who maintain high-level wellness. These individuals understand and respect themselves. They accept their personal accomplishments, strengths, and limitations. They can deal with difficulties and learn from them. They exhibit a sense of confidence. A positive body image is an element of their self-esteem. It is exhibited in the way they dress, their posture, and the way they express themselves.
- *Satisfying interpersonal relationships.* Persons who like themselves can develop and maintain relationships based on mutual trust, loyalty, and caring. They can reveal personal feelings and accept them from others. They are generally outgoing and interesting to be with. They can meet others' needs without disregarding their own.
- *Fitness and energy.* Individuals experiencing high-level wellness are physically fit, active, and energetic. They engage in daily activities with zeal and enthusiasm. They sleep well and wake refreshed and energized.
- *Positive outlook.* A sense of optimism and happiness is a prominent manifestation of high-level wellness. Well individuals have positive expectations for the future and a healthy sense of humor. They feel good about self, relationships, and life in general.
- *Inner harmony.* Individuals experiencing high-level wellness report feelings of deep inner happiness and joy. This inner satisfaction comes from self-discovery and a strong sense of belonging. It is manifested by a sense of peace, hope, and the ability to love and be loved.
- *Focus and sense of purpose.* Wellness is demonstrated by a clear sense of purpose in life that is determined but flexible. This attitude facilitates setting and pursuing reasonable life goals. A well individual deterred from achieving a particular goal will explore new options rather than become discouraged or give up.

FACTORS AFFECTING WELLNESS

VALUES, PHILOSOPHY, AND SPIRITUALITY

Individual values are personal standards that provide direction and define what is "good" or moral. Values provide the basis for making decisions or choices and largely determine how individuals react to various life situations. Values are shaped by family and life experiences. While they evolve as a result of maturation, they are relatively consistent over time.

Closely related to values are the concepts of spirituality and personal philosophy. Spirituality emanates from an individual's sense of values and is a quality that gives meaning to life. Personal philosophy embodies one's value system. It is the way in which personal values relate to one another, guide personal choices, and shape one's concept of how to live.

Often, values, spirituality, and personal philosophy are expressed in an individual's religious preference. For others, spirituality is experienced through the process of self-actualization and developing a personal connection to a greater reality in the form of nature, history, or whatever has particular meaning for an individual.

LIFESTYLE

An individual's choice of lifestyle directly reflects personal values. Lifestyle is an individual's unique way of living. It encompasses everything from communication style and self-expression to career choices, recreational activities, eating habits, and interpersonal relationships. Lifestyle choices can promote wellness or compromise health. Pender and colleagues note that lifestyle restructuring

INSIGHTS FROM NURSING LITERATURE
MOTIVATION AS A FACTOR IN WELLNESS

Fleury J. Wellness motivation theory: an exploration of theoretical relevance. Nurs Res. *1996;45:277–283.*

The researcher in this study explored the motivational processes inherent in health behavior change used by older, rural African Americans to initiate and sustain health-related behaviors over time. The sample consisted of 10 women and 4 men, a majority of whom were being treated for cardiovascular risk factors such as diabetes, high blood pressure, obesity, and elevated cholesterol. The researcher interviewed the subjects in a community center setting over a period of 5 months.

The findings showed the determinants of motivation to be embedded in the subjects' cultural context, which included family, community, and church. Participants relied more on their support networks and informal health care system for dealing with symptoms of illness than on outside medical providers. Religion was a primary factor in all aspects of subjects' lives, including health. Health was viewed as a gift from God, achieved through leading a "good" life. Thus, subjects stressed that they could not predict future health outcomes, but felt secure God would provide for them. They felt a lack of understanding from health care providers who recommended treatment beyond their capacity to understand or realistically incorporate into their lives.

is central to health promotion. They stress the importance of creating an environment in which health-promoting lifestyles can be acquired and sustained. This ideal can be attained if health promotion and disease prevention are made an integral part of all health professionals' practice. This shift in emphasis will empower individuals, families, and communities to develop their health promotion potential.[12]

LOCUS OF CONTROL, SELF-EFFICACY, AND SELF-CONCEPT

An individual's personal sense of mastery and control in large part determines the extent to which he or she engages in wellness behaviors. **Locus of control** refers to the extent to which individuals believe that events in their lives are self-controlled (an internal orientation), or are determined by forces outside themselves such as fate, luck, or chance (an external orientation).[9] Studies indicate that individuals with an external orientation do not engage in health promotion activities, while internally controlled individuals are more self-directed, more assertive in seeking assistance and information, and more likely to change behavior patterns.[13–15] Scales to assess locus of control have been developed by psychologists.[16,17] One example appears in Section 3 of this chapter.

Another factor that influences health decisions is **self-efficacy**—an individual's belief that he or she can successfully execute a behavior necessary to produce a desired result.[18] Self-efficacy is presumed to develop through personal experience with an activity, observing another person perform a task, and verbal persuasion. In difficult situations, people who have doubts about their capabilities often decrease their efforts and give up, while those with a strong sense of efficacy exert greater effort to master the problem.[19] Nursing interventions that promote self-efficacy can assist patients in initiating or maintaining health promoting behaviors.

Self-concept is directly related to an individual's locus of control and sense of self-efficacy. It refers to an individual's unique perception of his or her own body (appearance and functions) and nonbody (spiritual, emotional, and intellectual makeup) images. Self-concept forms the foundation for a person's perception and interpretation of daily events. It determines attitudes, levels of aspiration, and motivation. Individuals with poor self-concepts are likely to feel they have little personal control over life events and low self-efficacy. Often they will neglect illness prevention or health promotion activities. Self-concept and self-expression are discussed in more detail in Chaps. 11 and 26.

HARDINESS AND RESILIENCE

Hardiness and resilience are personality characteristics that researchers have found to positively influence individuals' responses to stress in their lives.[20,21] **Hardiness,** as defined by Kobasa and colleagues, encompasses control (a belief that one can influence life events), commitment (a sense of purpose that promotes a desire to be actively involved in life events), and challenge (a belief that change is to be expected in life and provides opportunities for growth).[20] **Resilience** implies courage, adaptability, emotional stamina, and a positive outlook in spite of tragedy and personal losses.[21]

Individuals having these qualities do not necessarily experience less stress or illness than others, but their response to misfortune modifies their risk. Hardy, resilient individuals use more effective coping strategies; thus, loss and change are less likely to overwhelm them.

Nurses can make inferences about hardiness and resiliency from verbalizations, expressions of emotion, and psychological responses to stress. Some researchers have suggested that a hardiness training program that teaches strategies to develop control over one's life, to become more committed to oneself, and to choose to perceive unexpected events as a challenge could help vulnerable individuals develop increased resistance to stress.[22,23] This kind of teaching may benefit all individuals facing long-term stressors such as chronic disease.

COLLABORATIVE STRATEGY

SELF-EFFICACY AND SELF-CONFIDENCE

Self-efficacy, a personal belief that one can do something, is closely allied to self-confidence. Self-confidence is a consciousness of one's own power. A collaborative nurse–patient relationship facilitates both self-efficacy and self-confidence through endorsement of patients' participation as full partners in decision making. A decision-making partnership implicitly acknowledges patients' personal strengths and knowledge and creates opportunities for explicitly reinforcing their skills.

CULTURE AND SOCIOECONOMIC STATUS

Cultural background strongly influences health beliefs and participation in activities that have impact on wellness and well-being. Health values, attitudes, and behaviors are learned within the context of the family beginning at an early age. Culture, therefore, often determines the traditional ways its members cope with illness.[24] The strength of persons' ties to their culture of origin influences their use of outside health care providers, the roles of familial and community support systems, and healing rituals (Chap. 10).

Socioeconomic status profoundly affects an individual's lifestyle, health practices, and level of wellness. In general, poor people get sick more often and stay sick longer because of inadequate health maintenance, lack of prevention, poor nutrition, and limited access to health services. The poor are more vulnerable to disease and less able to cope with it than those in higher socioeconomic populations.[25] There is also evidence that low-income groups are less likely to have effective social networks to call upon for support during illness.[26]

Poverty may also exert a negative influence on an individual's motivation to engage in health-promoting activities. Physiologic essentials, such as food, shelter, and safety, must be met before individuals can devote energy to activities that meet security, belonging, self-esteem, and other higher-order needs related to high-level wellness.

AGE

Sound knowledge and application of principles and theories of growth and development enable nurses to consider expected physical growth and psychosocial and cognitive development and to anticipate potential stage-related hazards to wellness when providing patient care. These concepts are presented in Chaps. 11 and

12. Chapter 11 presents a discussion of theories of individual development. Chapter 12 discusses the principles of growth and development, major milestones for each age group, and the application of those concepts to the care of patients from birth through late adulthood.

Many lifestyle and personal health habits are learned throughout the developmental process.[27] Children's health practices fall largely under their parents' control. Adolescents, too, may follow parents' examples. Role-modeling, whether exemplifying behaviors that promote health and wellness or behaviors that undermine them, is a powerful influence. Emphasizing self-responsibility at an early age and reinforcing its importance through young adulthood provides a foundation for positive lifestyle habits throughout life. Table 25–1 summarizes wellness tasks by age and developmental stage.

ALTERED WELLNESS

LIFESTYLE CHOICES THAT ALTER WELLNESS

Each person adapts and reacts to the stresses and demands of daily life in a unique way. In some cases, the choices are behaviors or personal habits that diminish wellness and contribute to serious health problems. Lifestyle choices, such as smoking, lack of exercise, and excessive calorie intake are responsible for 6.5 percent of cancers in the United States.[28] Many other health problems have been linked to unhealthy behaviors. These unhealthy behaviors represent the converse of the dimensions of wellness described earlier in this chapter.

Eating Poorly

Unfortunately, for many Americans unhealthy nutrition is a way of life. More than 40 percent of the American food dollar is spent on eating in restaurants. With increasing numbers of women employed outside the home, the use of convenience foods to prepare meals at home has become increasingly attractive. Both of these trends contribute to meals high in fat, sugar, salt, and calories, and low in complex carbohydrates.[29] Convenience foods are often highly refined, processed, colored, preserved, and artificially sweetened. These eating trends have made obesity the most frequent nutritional disorder in the United States. The latest US government statistics reveal that 59 percent of men and 49 percent of women are obese.[30] Obesity has been linked to cardiovascular disorders, hypertension, diabetes, and breast and colon cancers. Two thirds of Americans die of diseases linked to diet.[31] Chapter 28 contains a more comprehensive discussion of nutrition.

Lack of Fitness

For many Americans a basically sedentary lifestyle is coupled with unhealthy nutritional habits. Inactivity is a serious health hazard that has been linked to conditions such as osteoporosis, hypertension, chronic fatigue, premature aging, poor muscular tone, and limited flexibility. These conditions, in turn, are major contributors to lower back pain, injury, tension, obesity, and coronary heart disease.[32,33] A sedentary lifestyle may also encourage other harmful lifestyle practices such as overeating, smoking, and alcohol ingestion and has serious implications for emotional and psychological well-being. Additional information related to physical activity and fitness can be found in Chap. 33.

Feeling Stressed

Stress is an unavoidable element in modern society that can produce health-damaging effects. Stress-linked diseases affect every body system. Hypertension, one of many stress-linked diseases, affects more than 50 million Americans and predisposes its victims to other life-threatening consequences such as arteriosclerosis, congestive heart failure, and stroke.[34]

Stressors inherent in contemporary life make it difficult to avoid stress-related symptoms, but certain types of individuals are at increased risk. Research by Friedman and Rosenmann indicated that people with "striving personalities" (Type A) are prime candidates for stress-related health problems.[35] Type A individuals live their lives according to the calendar and the clock. They are extremely competitive and are classic "workaholics."

Although Type A personality is certainly a potent risk factor for the development of stress-related disorders, other responses to stressors also result in altered wellness. Ineffective coping leaves anyone, regardless of personality type, "feeling stressed" and susceptible to unhealthy personal habits and stress-related disease. Stress, stressors, and coping are discussed further in Chap. 8.

Ceasing to Care for Self or Others

Individuals may choose, consciously or unconsciously, not to participate in self-care activities for a variety of reasons such as lack of knowledge, poor motivation, lack of financial resources, or poor self-concept. Neglecting basic health maintenance activities can have serious negative effects on wellness. Even for well individuals, failure to engage in regular dental care or screening procedures such as breast self-examination may permit diseases to reach an advanced state before they are detected. Those with health problems such as hypertension or diabetes that can be controlled by prudent care and treatment measures may suffer irreversible damage if self-care practices are not routinely performed.

Loss of the desire or ability to care for others implies diminished wellness. Persistence of this state can severely threaten wellness and well-being. For many people, periods of solitude are valued interludes that support self-awareness and inner tranquility. Humans are by nature social, however. When seclusion and withdrawal from social interaction becomes a usual pattern, there is a loss of shared experiences, exchange of ideas, and regard for and from others. Often loss of regard for self underlies or results from this situation.

In some cases, inability to care for self or others is manifested in violence against others (see *Carelessness and Violence* which follows). Concepts related to self, self-concept, and self expression are addressed in Chap. 26.

Difficulty Fitting in With the Environment

A multitude of stressors, most created by human civilization and "progress," have a negative influence on wellness. Some of these stressors are linked to human impact on the global environment. Others stem from conditions or events in one's immediate environment: home, school, or work place. Individuals and societies whose approach to the global environment is to exploit it are, in fact, contributing to its degradation. Examples are overpopulation, depletion of natural resources, and global warming. These phenomena have an impact on the health, wellness, and well-being of all of us.

TABLE 25-1. WELLNESS TASKS FOR AGE/DEVELOPMENTAL GROUPS

Age/Developmental Stage	Wellness Tasks
Infancy: Birth to 1 year	Developing attachment and trust Meeting nutritional needs Maintaining physical safety Developing identity: me vs. not me Learning social and emotional responses Establishing health assessment routine
Toddler: 1–3 years	Forming emerging self-concept Developing autonomy Expanding social interactive skills Maintaining physical safety Expanding mobility Learning about basic hygiene Maintaining health assessment routines

Preschool: 3–5 years	Expanding self-concept
	Learning to take initiative
	Developing a conscience
	Learning basic health habits:
	  Healthy foods
	  Adequate rest
	  Independent toileting
	  Safe play
	Establishing preventive health routines

School Age: 5–12 years	Increasing physical and emotional independence Refining psychomotor and cognitive skills Developing positive self-concept Learning cooperation and competition Learning about social and moral responsibilities Learning risk taking and its consequences Learning healthy stress management Continuing regular preventive health care

Often accidents are associated with hazards in the immediate environment. Accidents threaten health in all age groups, especially the young and the elderly. Accidents are the leading cause of death among children and adolescents under age 19. For the elderly, falls related to altered visual, auditory, and tactile acuity or decreased mobility and coordination are the most debilitating type of accidents. In this age group, complications of the original injury are often life threatening.

Lack of Self-responsibility

The fact that not all people develop self-responsibility is evident from the large number who engage in harmful or potentially harmful activities. Behaviors such as smoking, drug and alcohol abuse, unsafe sexual practices, and violence often begin in adolescence and continue into adulthood.

Smoking. Smoking is recognized to be the single most preventable cause of death in the United States. It accounts for more than 400,000 deaths each year, or about one death in every five.[36] This includes about 30 percent of all cancer deaths. Cigarette smoking is also the leading cause of chronic lung disease and cardiovascular disease.[37]

Although there has been a dramatic shift in the smoking behavior of Americans over the past 20 years, roughly 25 percent of adult Americans smoke.[38] Tobacco use among teens continues to increase. The CDC estimates that more than 5 million people now under age 18 will die prematurely because of smoking if current patterns of smoking behavior persist.[39] Recent information on the hazards of "secondhand" smoke indicates that nonsmokers suffer ill effects because of others' irresponsible choices. Although many public areas are now "smoke-free," family members living with smokers are still at risk.

TABLE 25-1. CONTINUED

Age/Developmental Stage	Wellness Tasks
Adolescence: 12–18 years	Developing a positive self-concept/body image Refining individual identity: gender, social, cultural, personal values Taking responsibility for own behavior Developing healthful lifestyle habits Making social and emotional commitments to others Considering life goals; acquiring skills to attain them Continuing regular preventive health care
Young Adult: 18–35 years	Selecting and pursuing a career Establishing home separate from parents Becoming part of a community Maintaining healthful lifestyle Making commitment to a life partner Taking responsibility for nurturing a family Maintaining satisfying friendships Seeking regular health assessment/screening
Middle Adult: 35–65 years	Accepting changes relating to aging in self and parents Resolving disparity between personal goals and actual accomplishments Discovering new aspirations and activities Maintaining mature relationships with adult children Nurturing grandchildren Maintaining healthful lifestyle
Late Adulthood: 65+ years	Accepting life's achievements Adapting to end of career, retirement Adjusting lifestyle: coping with declining function while maximizing participation in activities Coping with the loss of friends, family through death Adapting living arrangements Coping with increasing dependency Continuing regular health assessment/screening Preparing for one's own death

Source: Adapted from Bruhn JG, Cordova FD, Williams JA, Fuentes RG. The wellness process. Commun Health. *1977;2:209–221.*

Alcohol and Drug Abuse. Alcohol is the cause of 100,000 deaths each year in the United States.[37] Alcohol abuse is also directly related to cirrhosis of the liver, cerebrovascular disease, and various cancers.

Another 20,000 deaths are caused by other drugs.[37] Drugs such as marijuana, cocaine, hallucinogens, and misuse of some prescription medications also pose risks. Many of these drugs create physical and psychological dependency, which leads to physical, psychological, and social problems for individuals, families, and communities. The "war on drugs" is now a national and international concern.

Unsafe Sexual Activity. Unsafe sexual practices have serious implications for wellness. Having sexual intercourse with multiple partners and failing to use precautions to block transmission of infection and undesired pregnancy with either primary or casual partners is unsafe. The consequences, unplanned pregnancies and sexually transmitted diseases (STDs), have negative physical, psychological, and social ramifications. The most serious outcome of unsafe sexual activity is acquired immunodeficiency syndrome (AIDS). Nationally, AIDS is the leading cause of death among 25- to 44-year-olds (19 percent of deaths) and the eighth leading cause of death overall (2 percent of deaths).[40] Although AIDS is often considered a disease of homosexual males, infection and death rates among women and heterosexuals is rising.[40] Sexuality and sexual expression are explained further in Chap. 26.

Carelessness and Violence. Irresponsible use of potentially lethal force or weapons is resulting in increasing numbers of injuries and deaths. Automobile accidents, many caused by reckless

INSIGHTS FROM NURSING LITERATURE

A FOCUS ON GENDER AS A FACTOR IN HEALTH INTERVENTION PROGRAMS

Tiedje LB, Starn JR. Intervention model for substance-using women. Image. *1996;28:113–118.*

The authors point out that society has a double standard for its toleration of substance use and has always dealt more harshly with women than men who abuse alcohol and other substances. Indeed, they stress, treatment programs are designed for male users. Consequently, they note, women may avoid seeking treatment.

The authors stress the importance of designing treatment programs from a feminist perspective. A feminist perspective, they state, recognizes connectedness to others as the foundation of women's self-concepts. Thus, they advise that substance-abuse treatment programs for women focus on relationships. They recommend treatment of women be offered in the context of a nurturing environment and a caring, healing relationship with a professional. Emphasis on "relational" treatment approaches equip women with the skills for managing and maintaining healthy relationships. Such treatment, which addresses the root cause of female substance abuse, may involve helping women to remember and heal the childhood pain of abuse or neglect, undo previous socialization patterns that cause women to remain silent about their needs, or reform broken relationships.

driving and or driving under the influence of alcohol or drugs, are responsible for over half of the yearly deaths among children and adolescents[41] and nearly 40 percent of those among 15- to 24-year-olds.[37]

Violence of all types is on the rise in the United States as well. Family violence in the form of battering and rape is becoming increasingly pervasive. Although there are male victims of domestic violence, well over 90 percent of the victims are female.[42,43] The National Crime Victimization Survey (NCVS) report estimates that more than 2.5 million women experience some form of violence each year and that nearly 2 of every 3 of these are attacked by a relative or a person they know.[44] A national survey on domestic violence indicates that 14 percent of American women reported having experienced battering from a husband or boyfriend.[43] Sometimes the violence is sexual. The NCVS indicates that over 133,000 women are raped annually, but estimates that only 53 percent of rapes are actually reported. In over half of the rapes reported to police, the perpetrator was known to the victim.[44] Unfortunately, some women have responded to fears of becoming victims of violence by purchasing guns. Whereas around 12 million women owned guns in 1989,[45] 20 million possessed guns in 1995.[46] Some attribute the increase to advertising campaigns by gun manufacturers and the National Rifle Association.[47] If this is so, it represents collective irresponsibility on the part of these organizations. In fact, having a gun in one's home increases the risk for homicide, rather than providing protection from it.[48]

Child abuse and maltreatment are serious and common problems on our society as well. Approximately 4 percent of children under 17 years old are abused annually in the United States.[49] Some experts believe that child abuse is underreported. Reporting standards vary from state to state and in some cases health professionals fail to recognize abuse.[50] There are many theories that attempt to explain causes of child abuse. Although abusive parents are often found to abuse drugs or alcohol, this factor by no means accounts for all cases.[51] It is a complex problem and a significant public health challenge to prevent and treat.

Elder abuse is a form of family violence that is coming under increasing investigation. Although there is agreement that there are no reliable national estimates of prevalence, reports range from 4 to 10 percent.[52]

Gun violence has become a national emergency. In 1992, firearms killed nearly 40,000 people in the United States.[47] This figure includes homicides, suicides, and unintentional shootings. Most of those killed by guns are males: the death rate for men is 4 times that of women and black men are nearly 7 times more likely to be killed by a gun than white men.[31] Increasing gun use among children and adolescents is a growing concern. Surveys report that many high school students either carry guns or have easy access to them.[53]

These examples of lack of self-responsibility are disturbing on several levels. Whereas some may believe informed adults have a right to make choices about their own behavior regardless of the effect on their own health or wellness, many of the behaviors discussed above create a danger to others. Moreover, there is no evidence that all of the choices are informed and not all of them involve adults. In some cases, there is evidence that the information needed to make informed decisions is lacking. For example, a survey investigating use of contraceptive method and condom use among women at risk for HIV infection revealed that up to 15 percent of them believed that contraceptives such as Norplant and surgical sterilization also protected them against STDs.[54] Recent publicity about the tobacco industry implies that it withheld important information about the addicting properties of cigarettes from the general public. The implications for health professionals must not be overlooked. We must expand our efforts to inform the public about health and wellness promotion and disease prevention so adults can make responsible, informed choices and look for creative solutions for threats to public health that result from individual behavior.

CIRCUMSTANCES THAT THREATEN WELLNESS AND WELL-BEING

Research by Holmes and Rahe revealed a marked correlation between multiple life changes (eg, marriage, birth, illness, or death of a loved one) and an abrupt and serious change in emotional and/or physical health. This effect was consistent whether the change was negative or positive. They also found that even a few

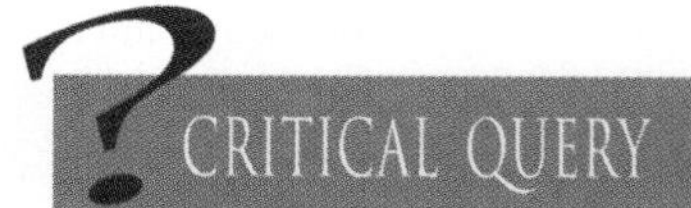

Violence is becoming more prevalent in our society.[44,47,52,53] Is this a health problem? A social problem? Is it a problem within the domain of nursing to treat? If so, what assessments and implementations are appropriate?

days of stress and change can result in minor illnesses such as headaches, stomachaches, and colds.[55]

A life event that is so stressful that it overwhelms one's ability to cope is a crisis. Some crises are developmental: periods of transition that every person experiences during life that are accompanied by changes in thoughts, feelings, and abilities. Situational crises are external events that occur suddenly or unexpectedly (eg, natural disasters, death of parent or spouse). Crisis carries with it a profound sense of helplessness and powerlessness. Disorganization of all aspects of life may occur in response to the acute level of emotional and psychological distress. Although crisis is characteristically of relatively short duration, the impact on well-being is devastating. Additional information related to crisis can be found in Chap. 8.

Disease

As discussed in Chap. 7, disease is a pathologic condition of altered functioning, or malfunctioning. Often, having a disease causes feelings of suffering and distress. Disease is a threat, not only because it may bring discomfort, but also because it can interfere with participating in one's usual role activities and social interactions. If prolonged, disease often jeopardizes economic security. The disruptions related to disease sometimes result in negative changes in self-concept.

Change in Self-concept

A positive self-concept usually contributes to adopting a wellness lifestyle and feelings of well-being. Self-concept may be negatively altered by many different life events. Loss of valued roles (wife, father, professional) or permanent changes in body appearance or functioning are examples. The ensuing feelings of inferiority interfere with social interactions and commitment to a healthful lifestyle. The mental, emotional, and physical harmony that characterizes wellness and the sense of feeling good and satisfied with life are often lost as well. To make the effort required to maintain wellness and well-being, one must value oneself.

Change in Social Relationships

As discussed earlier in the chapter, social support is important to wellness and well-being. Healthy adult relationships are reciprocal; they involve mutual exchanges. Giving and receiving positive regard, pleasure, help, and emotional support is part of the human need for love and belonging. Loss of reciprocity in valued relationships threatens one's system of social support. When instead one person in a relationship becomes overly dependent on the other, or overly controlling, that relationship becomes a source of stress. Losing a valued relationship is even more threatening. Depression, withdrawal from usual activities, and even ceasing to carry out basic self-care tasks are typical reactions.

Health Care Experiences

Being a recipient of health care is not a universally positive experience. This is particularly true if the reason for seeking care is to determine whether the symptoms one is experiencing are indicators of disease. The following sections identify some experiences associated with health care that can threaten wellness and well-being and address common responses to health care experiences.

Becoming a Patient. A person can be a patient of a health care provider or facility for health assessment, health maintenance, or diagnosis and treatment of disease. As discussed in Chap. 13, even the decision to seek health care can be stressful and take some time to accomplish. If the outcome of the health care experience is learning that one has a disease needing treatment, this may add still more stress, as discussed above.

Fear and Anxiety. Fear and anxiety, are typical immediate responses to new health care experiences. When seeking health care, anxiety about what is unknown is common. Is something wrong with me? Is it serious? What will they have to do to correct it? Will there be pain and disfigurement? These concerns may dominate a patient's thought processes. Often, anxiety subsides when unknowns are replaced by concrete information, even if it is confirmation that disease is present. Discussing treatment options, risks, and benefits in a straightforward way facilitates effective coping for most people. Some also desire information about sensations associated with tests or procedures or hospital routines, if hospitalization is required as part of treatment.

Even with information of this kind, however, fear is a natural response to certain therapies. The need for surgery often generates fear of dying, pain, or disfigurement or that a malignant tumor is present. Many people fear the uncomfortable side effects of chemotherapeutic drugs. Effective nursing implementation can reduce levels of anxiety and fear associated with health care experiences. Specific strategies are presented later in the chapter.

Exposure to Pain and Discomfort. For many patients, being a recipient of health care includes undergoing a variety of diagnostic and therapeutic treatments, tests, and invasive procedures that subject them to varying degrees of pain and discomfort.

Pain is a subjective experience that can significantly alter wellness. Pain is a direct barrier to usual activities that most individuals consider part of being well. Margo McCaffery, a recognized authority in the nursing care of patients in pain, states that "pain is whatever the person experiencing it says it is, existing whenever the person says it does."[56] Pain is comprised of two components: physiologic stimuli and emotional responses. The integration of these two components produces a unique pain experience for each individual. Unless there is neurologic pathology, all individuals have the same basic physiologic makeup, but show differences in pain tolerance. Individuals' responses to pain are swayed by variables such as the degree of powerlessness they experience, the presence and attitudes of other people, the amount of information they are given, the degree of threat the pain imposes, personal and past experiences with pain, cognitive level, and the extent to which they have used pain for secondary gains.[56] *Secondary gains* are advantages such as attention or other desired responses that some people derive from illness or its symptoms.

Any of these variables affect the personal meaning of a particular painful event and therefore influence how individuals

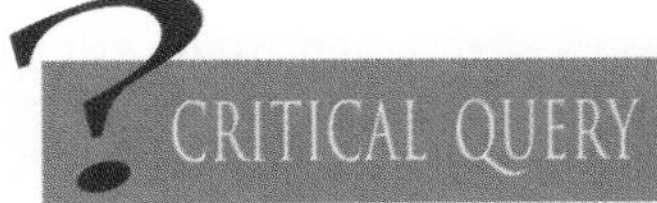

Pain is a subjective phenomenon and is sometimes used for secondary gains.[56] Does this mean that nurses should base their implementations for pain relief on objective data (eg, increased heart rate and BP or grimacing) only? What might be the risks associated with this approach?

express or react to pain. Patients undergoing an acutely painful experience may withstand the pain surprisingly well if they view the experience as beneficial. For example, a woman giving birth to a healthy infant may require no medicine for pain relief, but the same woman may be unable to tolerate dental work without local anesthetic. In the latter situation she may view the pain as serving no useful purpose or experience anxiety or fear, which serves to exacerbate the pain sensation.

Adequate pain management is vital to patient well-being. Unrelieved pain taxes patients' coping abilities both physically and emotionally. It directs patients' attention inward and drains emotional and physical energy. Patients may feel powerless and controlled by the pain and may react with depression, irritability, withdrawal, or hostility. Nurses can use many pain control measures to assist patients to maintain an acceptable level of comfort. The relaxation techniques presented later in this chapter are often effective pain relief measures. A detailed discussion of pain and other pain control measures is presented in Chap. 32.

Disturbance in Body Image and Self-Esteem. Emotional adjustment to many of the therapeutic treatments used in health care may be a difficult task for patients. Invasive procedures are procedures in which a body cavity is entered through the use of a tube, needle, or other device. They are an integral part of today's high-tech health care. Chemical dyes, radioactive substances, and a host of other materials may be injected into the body for diagnostic purposes. Tubes and other devices may be inserted through the skin or any number of natural or surgical openings in the body. Aside from the obvious physiologic hazards these procedures may present, invasive procedures can significantly affect an individual's sense of control, personal space, and body boundaries. Even "common" tubes, such as intravenous lines, urinary catheters, or nasogastric tubes, may be viewed as threatening by patients. More dramatic invasions of one's body such as surgery or endoscopy (use of a viewing device to observe the inside of a body cavity) are often deeply disturbing.

Treatments need not be invasive, however, to pose a threat to body image and self-esteem. Even requirements to restrict one's diet or activity or the need to use medications on a long-term basis to maintain normal functioning imply inferiority or vulnerability to some patients. Therefore, they can disturb one's image of an intact body even though no changes may be visible. Nurses can assist patients' adaptation to treatments through patient education and support, and through encouraging their active involvement in the therapeutic regimen. Careful attention to each patient's unique needs and responses enables individuals to receive maximum benefits from the treatments while minimizing stressful effects. A more detailed focus on body image and self-esteem in illness/disease appears in Chap. 26.

Admission to the Hospital. Hospital admission has been compared to the culture shock experienced when arriving in a foreign country. The language, dress, food, and daily routines have little in common with those of the person entering this "new world." The "rules" for acceptable behavior are unclear. The anxiety that accompanies a hospital admission makes coping with these feelings of strangeness more difficult. Moreover, hospitalized patients are subjected to loss of privacy and personal space, social isolation, altered sensory stimulation, and other risks to well-being. The following sections elaborate on some of these stressors. Refer also to Chap. 13.

SOCIAL ISOLATION. A health crisis often precipitates modifications in usual social interaction patterns. Hospital rules and routines limit the amount and type of contact permitted with family and other loved ones. Unpredictable intrusions by hospital personnel preclude emotional and physical intimacy. These actual and perceived barriers between patient and family cause stress and frustration. Interactions with care providers, even when supportive and nurturing, cannot replace a person's primary social support system.

ALTERED SENSORY STIMULATION. Restrictions in meaningful contact with loved ones, stark surroundings, limited mobility, and losing the sense of order afforded by one's usual daily routines creates sensory deprivation for many patients in a hospital. Some patients are dependent on prostheses such as dentures, hearing aids, eyeglasses, or contact lenses to compensate for sensory deficits. For these patients, sensory input is severely impaired when they are hospitalized unless special efforts are made to assure that these devices are in reach or in place.

The opposite condition, sensory overload, is more common on busy units and intensive care areas. In these settings, bright lights may be in use around the clock. Monitoring equipment emits loud warning noises to alert personnel of malfunction or change in patient condition. Admission or transfer of patients occurs at any hour of the day or night. Treatments to oneself or others interrupt sleep–wake cycles. Pain, fear, or other internal sensations magnify the impact of these stimuli. The negative impact on healing or progressing toward wellness can be significant.

LOSS OF AUTONOMY. Autonomy is the power to choose one's actions. It is part of wellness: feeling good and being responsible. Recognition of patients' rights to be involved in decisions that affect their well-being has resulted in a collaborative approach to health care becoming more common, even in inpatient settings. Nevertheless, many choices available to well individuals living in their own space cannot be accommodated in a hospital. There may be some restrictions necessary to maintain efficient operation of the hospital, others to treat the disease that caused the patient to be admitted. No matter how reasonable such limitations may seem to health care providers and even to patients, the loss of autonomy often creates stress and diminishes well-being.

EXPOSURE TO RISKS. Risks threaten wellness because of their potential for harm and because of the stress associated with threat. Health care facilities strive to maintain a safe and comfortable environment for all patients. Nevertheless, there are risks, including exposure to nosociomial infections, undesirable effects of medications, and negative effects associated with surgical procedures. Nursing

COLLABORATIVE STRATEGY

LOSS OF AUTONOMY

Whenever a person is hospitalized, an automatic loss of autonomy occurs. Just by entering the hospital—a world characterized by formal rules, policies, and informal behavior norms that are the creation of others—patients give up power to make personal choices. A collaborative nurse–patient relationship is particularly beneficial in this context because it promotes preserving patients' self-determination by encouraging their active participation in health care decision making.

measures to maintain a physically safe environment for hospitalized patients are discussed in Section 3.

Nosocomial infections are hospital acquired, which means that exposure to the causative organism occurred while a person was hospitalized. Nosocomial infections are not present or incubating on admission to the hospital. A hospital is one of the most likely places to acquire an infection. Microorganisms that may be antibiotic resistant and more virulent than microorganisms normally found in the community are present in the hospital environment. Hospital-acquired infections affect over 2 million patients each year in the United States or approximately 6 percent of all people admitted to acute care facilities. Surgical patients have the highest incidence of infection. Nearly 70 percent of all nosocomial infections develop in postoperative patients.[57]

Factors that predispose individuals to acquiring a nosocomial infection include extremes of age, compromised body defenses, exposure to invasive procedures, and long-term hospitalization. The major sites affected by nosocomial infections are the urinary tract, surgical wounds, respiratory system, and the bloodstream.[57] A detailed discussion of epidemiology and the chain of transmission of infection can be found in Chap. 9. A discussion of infection control measures is included later, in Section 3.

A *medication* is any substance that is used therapeutically in the diagnosis, treatment, or prevention of disease. Most people admitted to hospitals receive medications as part of their treatment. Although medications are also used in all other levels of care, patients in a hospital are likely to have less control over the medications they are given. At times, hospital patients are unaware of what medications they are receiving. Proper use of medications promotes a sense of well-being through their intended therapeutic actions. For example, analgesics ease the pain of a surgical incision and antibiotics combat infection.

Unfortunately, medications also have unintended effects called *side effects,* which may be harmless or potentially harmful. For example, some analgesics, such as morphine, are effective in relieving pain, but may also produce nausea and diffuse itching. The side effects are tolerated in order to receive the beneficial action of the drug. Drug interactions are a related concern. Many hospitalized patients receive multiple medications. The combined effects of these medications is usually a stronger therapeutic action, but unpleasant effects are also common.

Some people are concerned about taking medications because they view them as undesirable chemicals. They feel that using what they consider to be unnatural substances carries inherent risks of disrupting balance and function within the body. Another concern that makes some people hesitant about taking some medications is the fear of becoming addicted. Providing accurate information about drugs and their effects, while being sensitive to patient concerns, can reduce the stress associated with fears such as these. Fear of pain or distress related to invasion of body boundaries from medications administered via injection or intravenously is another common stressor related to receiving medications, even among adult patients.

Nurses are sometimes insensitive to these kinds of concerns, feeling that they are juvenile or insignificant in light of the overall disease process or its therapy. Also, because administering medications is so much a part of nurses' daily routines, they may forget having had similar feelings themselves. These kinds of responses are not helpful to patients. Accepting the genuineness and intensity of whatever concerns patients may have about receiving medications and empathically working with them to resolve their feelings is more effective.

Any medication has the potential to harm a patient if administered improperly. It is the responsibility of nurses to ensure that patients receive safe and therapeutic doses of prescribed medications. Medication errors can be avoided by applying basic principles of medication administration and sound nursing judgment. Nurses must understand a patient's drug's action, administer it properly, and monitor the patient's response. In addition, knowledge of a patient's condition and previous responses assists nurses in determining whether a particular drug or dosage is appropriate and should be given. The principles of safe medication administration are presented later in this chapter.

Surgery exposes patients to numerous risks. Several have been identified in previous sections. A detailed discussion about surgery and associated nursing responsibilities can be found in a later section of this chapter, *Restorative Care.*

THE EXPERIENCE AND MANIFESTATIONS OF ALTERED WELLNESS

A variety of signs and symptoms can indicate altered wellness. Many of these conditions are normal reactions to everyday events, but their persistence generally implies a problem.

- *Anxiety and fear.* Individuals faced with unfamiliar or threatening situations often experience anxiety and fear. People who are anxious or fearful exhibit increased heart rate, respirations, and agitation or withdrawal. These two concepts differ in that anxiety is dread of the unknown while fear is linked to an identifiable source.[58]
- *Depression.* Depression triggers changes in feelings and thought content. It is characterized by sadness, apathy, lack of energy, and withdrawal from social contact. Depressed individuals express feelings of failure and lack of a sense of personal worth or value to others.[58]
- *Signs and symptoms of stress.* Each individual's response to stress is unique, creating a highly personalized range of behaviors. Some of the most common behaviors including overeating or lack of appetite; excessive smoking or drinking; headaches; irritability; sleep disorders; fatigue; depression; sweating; muscle tension; heart palpitations; or altered elimination.
- *Pain.* This is the number one symptom causing an individual to seek health care. Pain is a major threat to well-being. It is a private, individual experience. Persons with acute pain often exhibit increased pulse, respiration, and blood pressure; diaphoresis; holding affected body parts; grimacing; lying listlessly, afraid to move; crying or moaning. Because of adaptive changes over time, these manifestations may not be present in a person suffering with chronic pain.
- *Fatigue.* Symptoms of fatigue include dark circles under the eyes; ptosis (drooping) of the eyelids; an expressionless face; and frequent yawning. Severe fatigue results in increased irritability; disorientation; listlessness; and an inability to concentrate or think clearly.
- *Powerlessness.* Powerlessness is individual's perceived lack of control over a current situation. Individuals who feel powerless appear passive or apathetic. They may express dissatisfaction or frustration with their present situation and express doubt regarding their role performance. Sometimes powerlessness progresses to depression.

- *Loneliness.* This is an emotional response to lack of intimacy or human contact. Loneliness may be hidden or expressed through withdrawal, depression, or a profound sense of powerlessness. Attention-seeking behaviors, such as complaints of vague physical symptoms or displays of hostility or anger toward others, sometimes are indicators of loneliness.[59]
- *Internal conflict and dissatisfaction.* Altered states of wellness are often characterized by internal conflict and personal dissatisfaction with life in general. They often present themselves as inappropriate coping mechanisms such as overeating; excessive drinking or smoking; use of recreational drugs; or other self-destructive behaviors.

SECTION 2

ASSESSMENT OF WELLNESS AND WELL-BEING

WELLNESS AND WELL-BEING DATA COLLECTION

The general elements of wellness—in particular, the personal, social, and stress and coping aspects—are described in this discussion of assessment. The details of assessing other aspects of wellness are presented in each of the following chapters in this unit.

Wellness and well-being assessments are important because they provide an overall understanding of patients as individuals and present a picture of the context in which their health problems evolved and in which they will be resolved. Patients' strengths and resources become apparent in a wellness assessment. They are as significant in collaborative planning for health promotion and disease prevention as the factors creating health problems.

Thorough and accurate wellness assessments depend on full, open exchanges between nurse and patient during the health history and examination. The level of rapport a nurse establishes with patients in the opening moments of the health interview is usually a significant factor in putting them at ease and may enhance or detract from the interaction that occurs thereafter. Given that the assessment of wellness and well-being often involves issues that are of a personal nature, such as lifestyle and coping patterns, skill in enlisting patients' participation is of paramount importance. Generally patients are responsive to caring, concern, spontaneity, and openness. A clear invitation to the patient to become a partner in the decision-making process is also an extremely important factor. It supports patients' sense of control in the situation and conveys to patients that they are not alone, a message that builds trust.

WELLNESS AND WELL-BEING HISTORY

Much of the data on which a wellness assessment is based cannot be measured or directly verified for the following reasons:

1. Psychological and emotional functioning is difficult to quantify and measure and thus assessment of these aspects is heavily reliant on a patient's self-report.
2. Patients' assessment of their own functioning is subjective. Individuals may feel that they are coping well when others, including health care professionals, would not agree.
3. Assessment by family members is subjective. Although they may have more intimate knowledge of a patient than nurses, they are only reporting their perceptions of a patient's well-being.
4. Some elements of nurses' assessments of patients involve subjectivity and may be influenced by personal values, experiences, and psychological state.
5. Dissimilar perceptions resulting from different values and cultural beliefs held by patients and nurses may contribute to a misinterpretation of assessment data.[58]

Thus, while patients' self-reports are vital to a wellness and well-being assessment, validation that the messages conveyed are the messages intended is necessary to ensure that nurses understand patients' and family members' points of view (see Chap. 15). To validate, nurses can paraphrase or summarize their understanding of patients' statements and ask patients to provide clarifying feedback.

Further, self-report data must be augmented by nurses' observations to evaluate whether patients' self-reports correspond to their behavior. Does a patient report feeling good but look dejected, sad, or depressed? Such inconsistencies suggest the need to obtain more information.

The tone, that is, the quality or character, of the communication during history taking is another relevant cue. Just as there are awkward moments in everyday social exchanges when the tension level rises inexplicably, there also may be tension as nurses and patients are getting to know one another. Nurses should look upon these moments as important clues; they sometimes signal that a patient has underlying feelings about the topic. When such moments occur, follow up either immediately or later to determine their significance. Establishing their meaning may help a nurse to better understand a patient's experience.

Primary Concern

A patient's primary concern is the aspect of the health problem about which he or she is most distressed. Nurses can obtain those data by asking, "What about your problem bothers you the most?"

Patients differ in their awareness of the links between their life situation and their health problems. Some patients will recognize that their health problem is related to life stressors, lifestyle, or health habits. They may actually identify being "overstressed" as their primary concern. Patients with the same chief complaint (reason for seeking health care) can have very different primary concerns. Such differences can have an important impact on the selection of caregiving strategies. This is illustrated by the two examples presented below.

> Brian Berry is a 36-year-old single man admitted to the hospital for back pain. When asked, "What about this problem bothers you the most?" Brian responds "I've never had pain like this before. I'm not sure if I can stand it much longer." Brian's primary concern is his ability to tolerate severe pain.
>
> Melissa Landon, on the other hand, a 25-year-old single woman, is also admitted with back pain. When asked the same question, she responds "Well, the pain is terrible, but the thing is that I've already missed too much work, and my boss said that if I miss any more, he'd fire me. I've got a brand new condo with payments to make!" Melissa's primary concern is the potential threat her illness poses to her financial security and lifestyle.

Care strategies would differ in each case. In both situations the primary concern represents a threat to patient well-being and provides valuable information for developing strategies to enhance wellness.

Current Understanding

Patients' beliefs about a health problem affect their response to it. The perceived causes of the problem and the impact of the problem on daily living are key variables. The perceived cause of the problem influences patients' confidence in their ability to correct the problem. Motivation to make changes increases if the impact on a patient's daily living is significant. The following example demonstrates a nurse's use of current understanding data.

> Mr. Jones has had a cough and hoarseness for the past 3 months. He has smoked for 10 years and recently increased his smoking from one to two packs a day. When asked what stimulates or aggravates his cough, Mr. Jones links it to his increased smoking, which he says is because of stress at work. Knowing this, the nurse is able to direct the assessment to factors contributing to stress at work.

Past Health Problems/Experiences

Information about a patient's response to past illnesses and previous health care experiences predicts possible responses to the present situation. Some patients bring fears and anxieties associated with previous hospitalizations. Consequently, they may approach the current situation with a lack of confidence in themselves and others. Other patients have successfully weathered intense pain or other effects of illness and grown from them. The following example illustrates the value of data about past health care experiences.

> Mrs. Bertini is admitted to the hospital for an appendectomy. The nurse asks about previous surgeries and finds out she had an operation as a child. Mrs. Bertini volunteers that she remembers having had unbearable pain and is worried about repeating that negative experience. The nurse notes this information and Mrs. Bertini's need for preoperative teaching regarding patient-controlled pain relief measures.

Personal, Family, and Social History

The personal, family, and social history (PFSH) is one of the most important elements of the wellness/well-being assessment. This part of the history deals with lifestyle habits, social and leisure life, spiritual and cultural values, and personal satisfaction with life circumstances. Through the PFSH, nurses come to know more about patients as individuals. They gain further knowledge about patients' overall health and their understanding of the factors that affect it.

The personal, family, and social history presents an opportunity for nurse and patient to identify and discuss possible factors that could lead to future health problems. Table 25–2 contains suggested questions for obtaining personal, family, and social history information relevant to wellness and well-being. The following example illustrates the importance of the PFSH.

> Mr. Dodd is admitted to the hospital with a diagnosis of possible peptic ulcer disease after vomiting blood. The nurse pays special attention to his PFSH because of the link between stress and stomach ulcers. Mr. Dodd reports he was an executive in a major corporation but has been unemployed for the past 5 months. He has been looking for a job, but has found nothing satisfactory. He reports frequent arguments about money with his wife, who recently returned to work as a legal secretary. Mr. Dodd said he had stopped smoking several years ago but started again 2 months ago. To get a clearer picture about Mr. Dodd's coping ability, the nurse asks Mr. Dodd about his understanding of the effects of stress on health, whether he exercises regularly, and what he does to relax. This exchange shows Mr. Dodd that the nurse is genuinely concerned, and provides the nurse with a clearer picture of what kind of assistance to offer Mr. Dodd.

Subjective Manifestations

Subjective manifestations (symptoms) can indicate wellness or suggest health problems. Asking questions to cue patients will help them recall symptoms they have experienced recently. Table 25–3 presents sample questions about symptoms according to body system.

WELLNESS AND WELL-BEING EXAMINATION

The wellness examination produces information about the patient's level of fitness, nutrition, stress, and general health. This information is the basis for establishing wellness goals and provides the baseline for evaluating progress once implementation of approaches begins. Normal values and indicators of normal functioning in each body system are presented in Chap. 17. The discussion below highlights changes suggesting altered wellness.

Measurements

Vital Signs. Vital signs including pulse, respiration, and blood pressure are often affected by excessive stress or emotional reactions. Rapid heart rate; shortness of breath with rapid, shallow respirations; and elevated blood pressure may indicate severe anxiety, fear, or pain. Patients exhibiting these signs should be assessed carefully to determine the underlying cause.

Body Weight. Weight is used to assess the nutritional status of a patient. Body weight should be compared to standardized norms and deviations greater than 10 percent should be assessed further with patients.

Objective Manifestations

General Observations. Patients' overall appearance conveys cues about their wellness and well-being. The following elements are especially relevant:

- *Facial expression and speech.* Facial expression reflects feelings such as gladness, excitement, anger, strength, weakness, depression, or powerlessness. Facial expressions can be intentional but often change without a person's awareness in response to emotions. Mode of speech—for example, calm clear, articulate, slow, drawn out, excited, trembling, or garbled—also communicates emotions. Nurses should note facial expressions and verbal statements that do not convey congruent meanings. This observation requires further assessment.
- *Eye movement and gaze.* Assess patients' use of eye contact during interactions. Constant or intense eye contact sometimes indicates anger or lack of trust. Little or no eye contact can indicate anger, withdrawal, hopelessness, or low self-esteem. Because cultural factors influence eye contact, consider a patient's culture of origin when interpreting eye movement and gaze.

(continued on page 632)

TABLE 25-2. WELLNESS AND WELL-BEING HISTORY: PERSONAL, FAMILY, AND SOCIAL HISTORY QUESTIONS

A. Vocational

1. What type of work do you do?
2. Have you changed jobs recently?
3. How do you feel about your work?
4. Are you satisfied with your work?
5. Any problems at work currently? What are you doing to change this?
6. What general stresses are associated with your work? How do you handle them?
7. How do your family members feel about your work?
8. Are you optimistic about your future career prospects?
9. Does your work bring you into contact with pesticides, solvents, x-rays, or other harmful agents?

B. Home and Family

1. What family members live with you? What are their relationships to you?
2. Are there other members of your family who are significant to you? Do you see them often?
3. Are you satisfied with your family life?
4. Have there been any changes in your family group recently? Births? Deaths? Have you recently married, separated, or divorced?
5. What family problems most concern you?
6. What is your financial responsibility for family members?
7. Do any of your family members have a chronic illness or serious disability?
8. Who acts as caretaker for him or her?
9. Where do you live? What type of residence is it?
10. How long have you lived at your current address?
11. Do you keep pesticides, solvents, or other potentially harmful substances in your home? How do you store them?
12. What precautions do you take to prevent fire and accidents in your home?
13. Do your family members wear seatbelts when driving?

C. Social, Leisure, Spiritual, and Cultural

1. What do you do to relax?
2. What hobbies do you enjoy?
3. Do you have a circle of good friends?
4. Do you enjoy your neighbors?
5. What community groups are you a member of?
6. Do you enjoy new people and getting to know them?
7. Are you satisfied with your social relationships?
8. Do you enjoy occasional solitude?
9. Do you feel your life has purpose?
10. Are there any routines or practices based on your cultural ethnic origins that are important in your daily life?
11. Do you practice a religion? Which one?
12. Are there any special religious practices that are part of your daily routine?
13. Do you attend religious services? How often? Would you like to attend religious services or see the clergy while you are in the hospital?

D. Sexual

1. Are you satisfied with yourself in your role as a man/woman?
2. Have you had changes in your sex life recently? Have you noticed a change in your desire for sex?
3. Are you satisfied with your sex life?
4. What precautions do you take to prevent unwanted pregnancies? Sexually transmitted diseases?

E. Habits

Exercise

1. Do you engage in regular exercise? What type? How often?
2. Do you engage in recreational sports?
3. Do you do yoga, limbering, or stretching exercises?
4. Do you feel you are fit? Are you satisfied with your fitness program?
5. Have your exercise habits changed recently?

TABLE 25-2. CONTINUED

Sleep

1. How much sleep do you average a day?
2. Do you wake up feeling fresh and relaxed?
3. Do you fall asleep easily at night?
4. Are you satisfied with the amount of rest you get?
5. Have your sleep habits changed recently?

Diet

1. What is your concept of the foods to include in a healthful diet?
2. What guidelines do you follow for planning meals?
3. Do you pay attention to the ingredients in the food you eat? Vitamins and minerals? Roughage and fiber? Saturated fats, cholesterol, salt, or processed sugar?
4. Do you read the labels for nutrients in packaged foods?
5. Do you avoid any foods for health reasons? What foods? Are you aware of foods suspected to increase the risk of cancer and heart disease?
6. Do you sometimes skip meals? Eat more than you should? Eat between-meal snacks?
7. Are you satisfied with your diet? With your weight? With your nutritional state?
8. Have you changed your diet habits recently? For what reason?
9. What problems do you encounter in providing a healthful diet for yourself and your family?

Beverages

1. Do you drink coffee, tea, water, or cola? How much do you drink per day?
2. Do you drink beer, wine, or other alcoholic beverages? How much do you drink a day?
3. Do you drive after drinking alcoholic beverages?

Tobacco Use

1. Do you use tobacco? How long have you smoked? How many cigarettes/cigars/pipes per day? [or] Did you smoke in the past? How long? How much?
2. What do you know about the effects of tobacco on health?

Other Substances

1. Do you use drugs to feel good? Get high? Relax? Sleep? Reduce pain? What drugs do you use?
2. How often do you use drugs? How many each time?
3. Are there products that you avoid for health reasons? Which ones?
4. Have your substance use habits changed recently?

Hygiene

1. What are your regular personal hygiene habits?
2. Do you brush your teeth and floss regularly?
3. Have you changed your habits recently?
4. What do you do in your home to prevent the spread of illness in your family?

Health Assessment

1. Do you pay attention to the way your body looks and feels?
2. Do you know the seven early danger signs of cancer?
3. (If male) Do you know how to do a testicular self-examination? Do you do testicular self-examinations regularly?
4. (If female) Do you have a Pap smear regularly? Do you know how to do a breast self-examination? Do you do breast self-examinations regularly?
5. Do you take your own pulse or blood pressure? What is your usual pulse? What is your usual blood pressure? Do you know what they should be?

F. Psychological

Stressors

1. Are you aware of any stress factors in your life? What are they?
2. What is your understanding of the effects of stress on health?
3. Do you feel happy, relaxed most of the time? If no: How would you describe your usual mood?
4. Have you had any big changes in your life recently? What were the effects on you, overall?
5. Are you accident prone?

Continued

TABLE 25-2. CONTINUED

Coping

1. What helps you most when you feel stressed?
2. Do you meditate or use any relaxation methods regularly?
3. Have you attended classes to learn relaxation skills?
4. Do you ever pamper yourself?
5. What outlets do you have for your emotions?
6. Are there people close to you with whom you can share problems?
7. Do you consider it acceptable to cry, feel sad, angry, or afraid?
8. Are you able to forget your problems when solutions are not possible?
9. Do you find each day interesting and challenging?
10. Do you look forward to the future?
11. Do you try to keep yourself open to new experiences?
12. Are you able to laugh at yourself or laugh with others over something funny?
13. Do you tend to be shy or sensitive?

Sick Role/Health Beliefs

1. Do you believe that there are things you can do to make yourself well?
2. Do you feel that your health depends on how well you take care of yourself?
3. Do you read articles or books about promoting health?
4. Have you ever attended classes on personal health?
5. Do you feel that you are to blame when you get sick?
6. Does it seem to you that your health is affected by accidental happenings or luck?
7. Whom do you consult when you do not feel well?
8. Do you feel that it is important to consult health care professionals to maintain your health?
9. Do you have regular contact with your physician and dentist?
10. Do you ever question your health care professional or seek a second opinion when you do not agree with the recommended care or treatment?
11. Do your financial resources enable you to maintain routine, preventive health care?

- *Motor behavior.* The manner in which individuals carry themselves implies how they feel about themselves. An erect standing and sitting posture reflects self-confidence and wellness, whereas slouched posture and slumped positioning in a chair may reflect physical illness or emotional distress. Body movements and gestures also reveal feelings. Anxiety can be indicated by many behaviors such as toe tapping, constant, nonpurposeful hand movements, nail or lip biting, picking on hair, or trembling. In contrast, wellness is indicated by relaxed purposeful movements.
- *Grooming and dress.* Evidence of attention to grooming, dress, and cleanliness of the skin, hair, nails, and teeth implies self-esteem. Cleanliness promotes wellness by supporting the body's natural defenses and thereby reducing risk of infection. Poor hygiene can be related to low socioeconomic status or may be a sign of depression or hopelessness. Poor hygiene increases patients' exposure to potential infectious organisms.
- *Mood.* Mood, or affect, reflects the inner experience of an individual. Although mood is a subjective emotional state, observers form impressions of another person's mood by interpreting behavior. Assess affect in the context of the other general observations discussed above. Does the patient suggest an anxious mood by displaying irritability, laughing nervously, or displaying general nervousness? Does the patient demonstrate a flat affect or withdraw from social contact, implying depression or hopelessness? Negative mood states that persist in spite of changes in circumstances suggest altered wellness.

Integument. Healthy skin is dry, warm, and neither pale nor flushed. Physical and emotional stress increases body metabolism and raises body temperature. Vasodilation and increased sweat production promote heat loss by evaporation. Sweat glands on the palms of the hands are activated in response to emotional stressors; therefore, sweaty palms are considered an indication of stress. Severe stress or panic causes a dramatic sympathetic nervous system response characterized by vasoconstriction, causing pallor and coolness of the skin.

HEENT (Head, Eyes, Ears, Nose, and Throat). Clear, alert eyes suggest wellness. Conversely, the eyes also reflect fatigue, sleep deprivation, apprehension, or fear. In a stress state, the sympathetic nervous system stimulates contraction of the radial muscle of the iris, producing pupil dilation. Mucous membranes of the eyes (conjunctiva) and mouth are pink and moist in wellness. Dry, reddened eyes and mouth imply stress, dehydration, or possible disease.

Chest. Even, unlabored respirations indicate a relaxed state, suggesting wellness. Anxiety, fear, pain, or stress cause tachypnea: rapid respirations. Consciously slowing one's breathing can have a calming emotional effect. Lung pathology and other diseases alter

TABLE 25-3. SUBJECTIVE MANIFESTATIONS QUESTIONS RELATED TO WELLNESS AND WELL-BEING

A. General
1. Do you generally feel healthy and energetic? Lethargic? Lacking energy?
2. Do you have any aches, pains, or other symptoms that bother you?
3. Do you ever become angry or agitated over little things?
4. Are you frequently nervous?

B. Integumentary
1. Do you sunburn easily or often? What do you do to protect your skin from the sun?
2. Do you sweat profusely when it is not hot?
3. Do you ever experience rashes or other skin problems?

C. HEENT (head, eyes, ears, nose, and throat)
1. Are you bothered by frequent colds? Allergies?
2. Does your mouth ever feel dry when you are not thirsty?
3. Do you have trouble with your eyesight? Hearing?

D. Chest, cardiovascular
1. Do you ever have difficulty breathing?
2. Do you have a cough even when you don't have a cold? Dry cough or producing mucus?
3. Does your heart ever seem to pound?

E. Gastrointestinal
1. Do you have difficulty digesting your food?
2. Are you bothered by an upset or acid stomach? Gas?
3. Do you have a soft, formed bowel movement regularly without discomfort?

F. Musculoskeletal
1. Do your joints hurt when you move?
2. Do you have neck or back stiffness? Other muscle tension?
3. Do you suffer from muscle twitches?

G. Neurologic
1. Do you have difficulty with balance? Coordination?
2. Do you ever stutter or stammer when you speak?
3. Are you bothered by headaches?
4. Do you ever feel light-headed or faint?

breathing patterns and chest movement and breath sounds (see Chap. 30).

Cardiovascular. Optimum fitness promotes effective cardiovascular functioning, which is reflected in low heart rate and blood pressure and well-perfused tissues throughout the body. Normal values for heart rate and blood pressure vary with age and sex. Heart disease alters the strength, rate, and rhythm of cardiac contractions, often compromising circulation. Other signs and systems of altered heart function are discussed in Chap. 30.

Cardiovascular changes also occur in response to stress-induced sympathetic stimulus. Vasoconstriction raises blood pressure. Increased pulse rate and cardiac contractility increase cardiac output. Anxiety and stress can increase the heart rate to over 100 beats per minute, called sinus tachycardia. Increased sympathetic tone can also trigger a cardiac arrhythmia such as premature heart contractions. Patients may be unaware of stress-related changes in heart rate and rhythm or may notice an irregular heart rhythm which, if sustained may need further evaluation (see Chap. 30). Collaboration in stress management (discussed later in this chapter) is an important nursing intervention for patients who have stress-related cardiovascular signs and symptoms.

Abdomen. Loss of appetite, indigestion, nausea and/or vomiting, abdominal cramping or pain, diarrhea, constipation, bloating, or flatus may be stress related. Gastric motility, blood supply, and acid secretion are increased by anxiety and decreased by depression. The sympathetic nervous system triggers constriction of duodenal blood vessels, making its mucosa vulnerable to trauma from gastric acid. Ulcers in the duodenum are a common result of chronic stress. Chronic stress may also produce parasympathetic dominance causing irritable bowel syndrome with alternating diarrhea and constipation. Chapter 29 addresses gastrointestinal assessment in greater detail.

Musculoskeletal. Anxiety-induced sympathetic stimulation produces increased muscle tension to bolster motor activity in the "fight-or-flight" response. Excessive tension can lead to muscle twitching, stiffness, fatigue, and general body aches and pains, especially in the chest, back, and neck.

Neurologic. Sympathetic nervous stimulation increases mental alertness and mental activity. Sustained stimulation produces symptoms of anxiety but eventually causes lethargy, fatigue, lack of initiative, inactivity, and withdrawal due to exhaustion and parasympathetic dominance. Signs of altered mental status such as confusion, memory loss, and unusual emotional responses may be the result of disease processes, medication side effects, sensory overload or deprivation, depression, or hopelessness. These changes in mental status can be related to chronic stress, illness, or hospitalization. Elderly patients are especially susceptible to confusion as a result of a sudden change in their environment such as a move to an extended care facility or hospital. A new, strange environment may accentuate sensory deficits.

NURSING DIAGNOSIS OF WELLNESS AND WELL-BEING STATUS

Formulating nursing diagnoses requires analyzing and interpreting assessment data that have been collected and validated. Accurate identification of nursing diagnoses is an important, difficult step in the nursing process. It requires an ability to integrate data, using critical thinking skills and sound clinical judgment (Chap. 18). For the diagnostic statement to be useful, it must label the problem, contain a description of the etiology or probable cause of the problem, and list the defining characteristics (subjective and objective data) noted during data gathering. Table 25–4 presents selected examples from these nursing diagnoses with specific etiologies and defining characteristics.

Because of the holistic nature of well-being and wellness, most nursing diagnoses reflect an alteration in well-being and

TABLE 25-4. SAMPLE NURSING DIAGNOSES: WELLNESS AND WELL-BEING

Nursing Diagnosis	Defining Characteristics/Manifestations: Subjective Data	Defining Characteristics/Manifestations: Objective Data	Etiology
Health-seeking behaviors: participates in weight-loss program *5.4*	Asks questions regarding healthy weight-loss methods. Verbalizes concern about weight. Verbalizes concern regarding family health history/personal risk for developing disease due to excess weight. States desire to alter dietary habits.	Actively participates in prescribed dietary/activity program. Joins support group to reinforce lifestyle change.	*Cognitive:* Exposure to information regarding health risks associated with obesity.
Altered health maintenance: substance abuse *6.4.2*	Reports frequently feeling overwhelmed. States worry about using "too much booze and pills." Verbalizes difficulty managing stressors without drugs/alcohol.	Smell of alcohol detected during visit. Displays flat affect (eg, does not participate in care, initiate interaction). Speaks in monotone. Limited eye contact with nurse.	*Emotional:* Ineffective individual coping.
Anxiety *9.3.1*	"I feel so wound up." "My stomach feels like it's tied in knots." "I am so afraid of what they might find."	Heart rate 80. Trembling. Restlessness. Unable to remember instructions given to prepare for diagnostic test. Poor eye contact when speaking. Awake most of previous night.	*Physical:* Threat to health status: uncertainty about result of diagnostic tests.
Diversional activity deficit *6.3.1.1*	Verbalizes "this place is boring." States "the only thing you can do here is read and I hate it."	Wearing T-shirt that says "I'd rather be fishing." Spends 5 hours 3 times/week in the outpatient renal dialysis center.	*Environmental:* Frequent, lengthy treatment: hemodialysis.
Fear of pain *9.3.2*	Reports of distress. States feelings of apprehension: "I'm afraid of severe pain. I can't handle it." Reports of insomnia, nausea, palpitations. "I've never had surgery but I'm sure it is painful."	Pulse increased above baseline. Respiratory rate increased above baseline. Drawn expression when discussing surgery. Refuses meals.	*Cognitive:* Knowledge Deficit: postoperative pain management options.
Powerlessness *7.3.2*	"It doesn't matter what I want—I can't do it anyway." "There's nothing I can do—they make the rules." "What do I know about any of this?"	Lack of participation in treatments or daily regimen. Refuses to participate in decision making (eg, when to bathe). Sleeps more than 12 hours/day.	*Environmental:* Illness-related regimen.
Hopelessness *7.3.1*	Verbal expressions of profound despair: "I'm never going to get better." "Don't waste your time on me." "I don't want to live like this." "Nothing I do will help."	Withdraws from social contact. Passively allows care. Refuses to participate in self-care. Eating less than 50% of diet. Decreased verbalization.	*Physical:* Deteriorating physical condition: AIDS.
Spiritual distress *4.1.1*	"I need my priest to give me communion." "God seems so far away since I can't go to mass." "Why did God let this happen to me?"	Personal clergy unable to visit due to distance.	*Self-Conceptual:* Separation from religious ties.

Nursing Diagnosis	Risk Factors
Risk for infection *1.2.1.1*	*Physical:* Decreased WBCs Receiving chemotherapy Invasive procedures: Foley catheter; peripheral IV fluids while npo; central line for parenteral nutrition

Source: The nursing diagnoses and etiologies on this table and the definitions of nursing diagnoses in the body of the text not credited to other sources are from Nursing Diagnosis: Definitions and Classification, 1997–1998. *Philadelphia: North American Nursing Diagnosis Association; 1996. Manifestation categories for etiologies and specifications of general etiologies on these tables are authors' original work.*

wellness in one form or another. A discussion of some of the most significant diagnoses related to well-being and wellness and their etiologies is presented in the following sections.

HEALTH-SEEKING BEHAVIORS

Health-seeking behavior is a state in which a patient in stable health actively seeks ways to change lifestyle, health habits, and/or the environment to achieve a higher level of well-being and wellness. Unlike the majority of nursing diagnoses, this diagnostic statement reflects a positive condition in which an individual is striving for high-level wellness. The key defining characteristic is a patient's desire to achieve a higher level of wellness.

Specific etiologic factors have not been identified for this diagnosis. It can be appropriately applied, however, to patients who are actively seeking knowledge about health and how to improve it, who are expressing an interest in eliminating personal behaviors that threaten wellness, or who are expressing concerns regarding the impact of environmental factors on their health status.

ALTERED HEALTH MAINTENANCE

Altered health maintenance is the inability to identify or manage resources to maintain wellness. Evidence of unhealthy lifestyle behaviors is a major defining characteristic of this nursing diagnosis.

- *Etiology: lack of or impaired communication skills.* Impaired verbal skills or inability to communicate in the language of the dominant culture prevents a patient from expressing health needs or perceiving information from health care professionals. A patient's inability to describe symptoms accurately can result in erroneous or ineffective treatment. Language differences also impair effective health education and discharge teaching.
- *Etiology: perceptual-cognitive impairments.* Perceptual-cognitive function is the ability to gather information through the senses and process it through intellectual skills such as thinking and reasoning. Impairments include limitation of senses such as blindness or deafness and brain dysfunction such as memory loss or confusion. These impairments interfere with self-care, prevent gaining knowledge about a health condition or prescribed treatment, and can delay seeking professional assistance.
- *Etiology: ineffective individual or family coping.* Coping mechanisms are strategies that enable a person to deal with life difficulties. Ineffective coping implies a response that does not solve the problem or resolve the associated stress. Some types of ineffective coping, such as smoking, alcohol or drug abuse, and eating disorders, have a direct negative impact on health. Prolonged preoccupation with personal or family problems interferes with usual self-care and health maintainance.
- *Etiology: unachieved developmental tasks.* Developmental tasks are projected accomplishments for stages, or age periods, in people's lives. Developmental theorists suggest that each task must be successfully completed before a person can move on to tasks in successive stages. Failure to master developmental tasks can result from intellectual, physical, or emotional deficits or from developmental or situational crises (Chaps. 8 and 11). Not meeting developmental norms may interfere with ability or motivation to take personal responsibility for one's health.
- *Etiology: lack of material resources.* Lack of material resources implies insufficient assets to support a health-promoting lifestyle or access health care. This is a major barrier to health maintenance. Inadequate shelter, poor nutritional intake, and stress associated with limited finances compromise health. The cost of health care services prohibits many individuals from seeking preventive or routine care.

DIVERSIONAL ACTIVITY DEFICIT

Diversional activity deficit describes a state in which patients experience reduced stimulation from or interest in recreational activities. Without pleasurable diversions in life, well-being—the perception of feeling good—and wellness—the full expression of one's potential—are blocked. The major defining characteristic of diversional activity deficit is observed or stated boredom.

- *Etiology: lack of diversional activity in the environment; prolonged hospitalization.* Most individuals seek diversionary stimuli from their environment. The environment in acute or long-term care facilities is bland and sterile. The space allowed there for patients and their personal effects is very small, and opportunities to move about are limited. Restricted visiting hours often reduce contact with friends and family. If a prolonged stay is required, the few diversions available—television, radio, or reading—become monotonous. This situation compounds the threat to wellness that created the need for inpatient care.
- *Etiology: frequent or lengthy treatments.* Patients needing recurring and time-consuming treatments such as renal dialysis, intravenous chemotherapy, or radiation therapy spend many of their waking hours confined to a bed in a clinical environment. As in the above situation, boredom and apathy often develop.

ANXIETY

Anxiety is defined as a vague feeling of uneasiness or apprehension that one cannot relate to an identifiable source or threat. Anxiety is associated with future, anticipated events. Any change or threat of change in an individual's life situation can create anxiety. A degree of anxiety is healthy because it motivates growth. Severe anxiety interferes with normal activity and is detrimental to wellness and well-being.

- *Etiology: threat to or change in health status.* Illness and treatment of illness frequently require individuals to change routines and habits. For many, this loss of control produces anxiety. Changes in health status may also cause changes in body structure and function, which threaten identity and well-being. Anxiety regarding change or threat to health status sometimes serves as the motivation for developing new wellness behaviors but often interferes with coping and problem solving.
- *Etiology: threat to or change in environment.* The environment a person chooses as part of life structure serves as a basis for a sense of security. A change in environment results in loss of familiar landmarks, conveniences, and support systems. It may disrupt usual routines. If the change is involuntary, anxiety may be intense.

FEAR

Fear is defined as a feeling of apprehension that one can validate and relate to an identifiable source. Health problems and their treatment often generate fear. The sensations associated with fear characterize the absence of well-being. Because the source of fear can be identified, the actual threat should be named in the diagnostic statement (eg, fear of pain, fear of mutilation, or fear of death).

- *Etiology: environmental stimuli.* Patients are often threatened by environmental stimuli such as loud noises, darkness, and strangers. Health care environments include many unfamiliar sounds, smells, and images that can be very frightening, especially to children. Children may also fear needles and other equipment used in diagnostic or therapeutic procedures. Adults often fear the discomfort that equipment such as needles or procedures can cause. Nurses can decrease this stress and fear by empathic listening and support.
- *Etiology: knowledge deficit.* Misinformation or lack of information generates fear that may be groundless. Imagined consequences or outcomes typically are more serious than reality. Accurate information about health-related tests or procedures can eliminate unnecessary stress.
- *Etiology: separation from support systems.* Fear is exacerbated during potentially threatening situations by separation from support systems. It is a universal experience, most pronounced in children separated from parents. Patients faced with threatening situations such as hospitalization need the support and comfort of their significant others. Having to face frightening situations alone may be overwhelming.

POWERLESSNESS

Powerlessness is perceived lack of control over a current situation or future outcome. In powerlessness, individuals expect that outcomes are not determined by what they do (internal control) but rather by the influence of outside forces (external control). This is in conflict with well-being, which requires a perception of control over life events and a sense of satisfaction with life circumstances.

- *Etiology: health care environment.* Lack of privacy, altered personal territory, and the forced dependence often found in acute care settings dramatically alter an individual's sense of control. Generally, patients with an internal control orientation experience greater distress than those with an external control orientation because the former are more self-directed.
- *Etiology: illness-related regimen.* Medical care can create a sense of powerlessness, especially when all treatment choices seem as undesirable as no treatment at all. Nurses can promote patients' feelings of control and power with empathic listening and by helping patients define what power they have within the prescribed treatment options. Nurses can then support patients in seizing that power.
- *Etiology: interpersonal interaction.* Insufficient information from caregivers or their failure to involve patients in health care decisions increases patients' sense of powerlessness. Collaborative care is characterized by avoiding paternalism, a philosophy that health care professionals "know best." Even debilitated patients can make some decisions and choices. Retaining a sense of power and control enhances patients' self-esteem and gives meaning to life. Prolonged powerlessness leads to hopelessness.

HOPELESSNESS

Hopelessness is a state in which one feels that positive alternatives are limited or nonexistent. It is the absence of optimism that is such an important part of well-being. Like powerlessness, hopelessness represents personal loss of control, which interferes with self-care and decision making. The major defining characteristic of hopelessness is passivity, which is manifested by decreased verbalization and/or decreased affect.

- *Etiology: prolonged activity restrictions.* Mobility confers independence. Prolonged activity restrictions create feelings of isolation and helplessness. This can have a devastating effect on self-esteem and sense of purpose.
- *Etiology: deteriorating physiologic condition.* Generalized deterioration signifies impending cessation of function, dependence, and eventually death. Heart disease, kidney disorders, cancer, and AIDS are examples of progressive conditions in which patients experience increasing pain and weakness. Prolonged treatments with no positive results or the development of new or unexpected symptoms may leave individuals feeling that no solution is possible.
- *Etiology: long-term stress.* Unremitting stress has many causes. The cumulative effect of daily pressures, environmental stressors, or normal developmental life changes may deplete energy reserves and coping resources. Stress associated with failure to achieve valued life goals may leave individuals feeling exhausted and without options. Extended caretaking responsibilities for a disabled or ill family member saps strength and may eventually overwhelm the caretaker. If an unexpected stressor such as hospitalization or illness occurs, vulnerable individuals may feel completely overwhelmed.
- *Etiology: loss of spiritual beliefs or belief in transcendent values.* Hope is often closely linked with spiritual well-being. Crisis events such as loss of someone or something valued (spouse, child, job) can leave individuals feeling there is no purpose in life. Religious individuals may feel that God has deserted them and may question their most fundamental values. Such profound spiritual distress makes individuals more susceptible to physical and mental deterioration. See also the following nursing diagnosis, spiritual distress.

SPIRITUAL DISTRESS

Spiritual distress describes a disturbance in one's value and belief system: those principles that integrate and give meaning to existence. Spiritual distress causes people to question the meaning of life, death, and suffering.

- *Etiology: separation from religious or cultural ties.* Beliefs and values based on religion and cultural ties provide some patients with a powerful resource for adapting to stress. Therefore, separation from religious rituals and cultural practices because of illness or hospitalization can significantly threaten patients' well-being.
- *Etiology: challenged belief or value system.* Beliefs and values frequently assume increased importance during a time of stress such as loss, serious illness, or hospitalization. Some situations confront individuals with experiences they never imagined could occur. For example, observing a loved one dependent on life-support equipment may challenge family members' defini-

tions of life and death. When events challenge the care values that formerly guided decision making, the sense of uncertainty and isolation that ensues is often profound.

RISK FOR INFECTION

Infection is the invasion and multiplication of pathogens in body tissue. The state of risk for infection implies that an individual is highly vulnerable to pathogens. As discussed in Section 1, disease and hospitalization create risk for infection because of compromised body defenses and a high concentration of organisms within the physical environment. As discussed in Chap. 18, multiple risk factors must be present for a patient to be considered at higher risk for infection than the general hospital population.

- *Risk factor: inadequate primary or secondary defenses.* Compromised primary and/or secondary defenses is generally considered to be the basis for this nursing diagnosis. Chapter 27 addresses the role of the primary and secondary defenses in promoting healing and protecting against infection.
- *Risk factor: increased environmental exposure.* Repeated or prolonged exposure to environmental reservoirs for infectious agents provides more opportunity for pathogens to enter one's body and produce an infection.
- *Risk factor: tissue destruction/invasive procedures.* Any procedure involving invasion of body boundaries with instruments carries with it the risk of providing a vehicle for organisms to enter the body. If other stressors have weakened secondary defenses, the organisms can reproduce in the body.
- *Risk factor: malnutrition.* Adequate nutrition is needed to maintain tissue integrity and promote wound healing. It is also necessary for production of leukocytes for phagocytosis of invading organisms. Malnutrition compromises normal defense mechanisms, increasing the body's vulnerability to infection.
- *Risk factor: effects of pharmaceutical agents.* Some drugs pose a threat to secondary defenses. Immunosuppressive drugs such as corticosteroids interfere with the body's ability to identify and destroy pathogens. Antibiotics destroy normal flora that are part of the body's natural defense against infection. Chemotherapy destroys rapidly dividing cells, including bone marrow, which decreases the number of leukocytes available to fight infection.

RELOCATION STRESS SYNDROME

Relocation stress syndrome refers to physiologic and/or psychosocial disturbances resulting from transfer from one environment to another. A change of environment can be stressful for anyone. For some persons, moving to a new environment produces persistent symptoms such as confusion, depression, and apprehension. Often prior or concurrent stressors play a role, as noted below.

- *Etiology: past, concurrent and recent losses.* A familiar environment often represents security and comfort. This is especially true when significant losses—a job, a relationship, or a loved one—challenge equilibrium. Being without familiar surroundings eliminates a major coping resource.
- *Etiology: feelings of powerlessness.* Powerlessness associated with a change of environment is most likely when the move is not of one's choosing. Elders having to move from their family home to "senior citizen housing" or an "assisted living center" for financial or health reasons exemplify this situation.
- *Etiology: little or no preparation for moving.* A move forced by sudden changes in life situation, for example, financial or health related, is usually more difficult to cope with. Not only is there greater emotional turmoil, but the physical aspects such as packing and relocating possessions are more demanding under pressure of limited time. Moving under these conditions frequently also precludes personal communication: saying goodbye to friends and loved ones.
- *Etiology: impaired physical, psychosocial health status.* These conditions create significant demands on coping capabilities. The challenge of relocation with these overlying conditions can be overwhelming.

IMPAIRED HOME MAINTENANCE MANAGEMENT

Being unable to independently maintain a safe, growth-producing immediate environment can precipitate or result from altered wellness. One's immediate surroundings or "home" provide shelter and security—important basic needs. When the existence or quality of the home environment is threatened, so are wellness and well-being threatened. With nursing care increasingly being provided in patients' homes, there is more opportunity for nurses to diagnose and treat this threat to wellness.

- *Etiology: disease or injury of family member.* This is a very common reason for disruption in a home environment. The physical and emotional demands of caring for an ill family member interfere with home maintenance tasks and nurturing interpersonal relationships among others in the family. Illness of the family member responsible for maintaining the home or of the primary wage earner is especially challenging. The others in the family may lack the maturity or skills to assume these roles.
- *Etiology: insufficient finances.* Poverty is a major reason that some individuals and families are unable to maintain a safe, secure home. Low-income families must often accept poorly maintained or overcrowded housing. They may be unable to pay for adequate home heating or cooling. Needs for extra funds may force working more than one job, leaving little time to carry out home management tasks and little energy for quality family interaction.
- *Etiology: lack of knowledge, impaired cognitive or emotional functioning.* Failure to recognize hazards to home safety, such as accumulations of dirt and wastes or infestations with vermin, precludes taking action to correct them. This can result from acquired impairments in brain functioning related to disease or aging or may be due to never having learned basic home maintenance skills.

INEFFECTIVE MANAGEMENT OF THERAPEUTIC REGIMEN

This diagnosis applies to a person who chooses a treatment program that is not effective for achieving personal health goals to manage a disease or its sequelae or who is unable to follow a treatment regimen recommended by a health care provider.

- *Etiology: knowledge deficit.* Failure to completely understand the correct execution of a treatment plan or the use of necessary equipment or medications is a common reason for failing to effectively manage the plan. Having taught a patient the skills and information needed is no guarantee that learning occurred. Evaluation of the teaching is a critical step to promote effective patient management of the treatment regimen.

- *Etiology: complexity of therapeutic regimen.* Some diseases are best treated by a combination of lifestyle modifications and medications or other therapies. Some therapies require complex pretreatment activities. Intricate adjustments of dosages or schedules may be necessary to attain therapeutic effects of a medication, but avoid negative or toxic effects. Food and drug interactions can present challenges. If persons lack the motivation, ability, or social support to organize their lives to meet all of these demands, the treatment is likely to be ineffective.
- *Etiology: mistrust of regimen and/or health care personnel.* Many variables can generate patient distrust of a particular treatment plan or of those recommending it. Unless providers recognize and correct these problems, there is a high likelihood that a patient will not make a commitment to participating in the plan.
- *Etiology: perceived seriousness, perceived susceptibility, perceived barriers, perceived benefits.* As discussed in Chap. 13, these factors interact to influence individuals' motivation to seek health care and participate in a treatment regimen. A patient who believes a health problem is serious or that personal susceptibility to complications is high will likely work hard to maintain recommended therapy, even though there are barriers such as cost or inconvenience. However, if that patient fails to experience expected benefits, the perceived barriers may then outweigh concerns about seriousness and result in abandonment of the program. Providers who are not sensitive to these patient perceptions miss opportunities to facilitate effective collaborative management of a therapeutic regimen.

STATING THE WELLNESS AND WELL-BEING DIAGNOSIS

A clearly stated nursing diagnosis is the basis for mutual planning. The general etiologies of nursing diagnoses related to altered wellness and well-being discussed above can be made more specific to individual patients. Specificity is important because patient care is often based on the etiology of a problem.

The taxonomy also lists many signs and symptoms, called defining characteristics, that are associated with each nursing diagnosis. No individual patient experiences all of the signs and symptoms listed for a diagnosis. Some of these signs and symptoms are specific, others general. Clearly describing the signs and symptoms a patient exhibits in the diagnostic statement facilitates development and evaluation of desired outcomes.

The following are examples of clearly stated wellness and well-being nursing diagnoses that are an effective basis for planning:

- Relocation stress syndrome R/T an involuntary move to a board and care facility after convalescence from a hip fracture, AEB "I'm scared someone will take my things," "I can't sleep unless I'm in my own bed," "Who are these people that come into my room?", refusal to participate in group social activities, and sad facial expression.
- Risk for infection. Risk factors: 75 years old, 8 days postoperative after colon resection, chronic lung disease, central venous catheter and indwelling Foley catheter in place, eats less than 50 percent of full liquid diet each meal.

Clearly stated nursing diagnoses are the basis for a comprehensive individualized care plan or can be part of a critical pathway.

SECTION 3

NURSE–PATIENT MANAGEMENT OF WELLNESS AND WELL-BEING

Management of wellness and well-being encompasses planning, implementing, and evaluating patient care to promote, maintain, or improve wellness and well-being. Individuals' abilities to meet their own health needs determines the nature and extent of nursing implementation. A primary goal of nursing management is to maintain, restore, or increase individuals' capacity for self-care.

Much of the content in this section deals with clinical procedures and approaches aimed at promoting well-being and preserving or improving patients' current level of wellness even though disease is present. This reflects the philosophy of the authors that wellness-oriented behaviors are as important in the face of disease as they are in a state of health.

PLANNING FOR OPTIMAL WELLNESS AND WELL-BEING

PATIENT CARE PLANS

In a collaborative approach, planning for optimal wellness begins with sharing and validating nursing diagnoses with patients to establish priorities for care. Nurses also address problems that patients and/or families feel are most important. For example, a young woman admitted for treatment of injuries sustained in a motor vehicle accident may have many obvious nursing problems including severe pain, impaired mobility, and risk for infection. However, this patient's greatest concern may be an unfinished project at work. Facilitating communication with one of her co-workers to make arrangements for completing the project during the patient's hospitalization will allay much distress and enable her to focus energy and attention on recovering from her injuries.

The individualized nursing diagnoses and mutually determined priorities are the basis for selecting desired patient outcomes and nursing implementation. The outcomes should reflect the highest level of wellness and independent functioning possible. The level of nursing implementation needed to achieve the desired outcomes depends on the current level of wellness. Four levels of nursing implementation are discussed in later sections.

The patient care plan is not complete until evaluation criteria are drafted. Evaluation criteria are derived from desired outcomes. They specify the patient behavior or status that indicates outcome attainment. Nurses and patients use them to monitor progress toward outcomes during the course of care and outcome achievement on specified target dates.

Table 25–5 presents sample outcomes, nursing implementation, and evaluation criteria for nurse–patient management of some nursing diagnoses related to wellness and well-being. These samples can guide development of individualized care plans based on patient's needs and situations.

CRITICAL PATHWAYS

Critical pathways are another way to organize and evaluate patient care. They are collaboratively developed, standardized

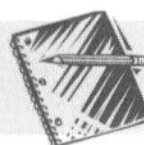

TABLE 25-5. NURSE-PATIENT MANAGEMENT OF WELLNESS AND WELL-BEING

Nursing Diagnosis	Desired Outcome	Implementation	Evaluation Criteria
Health-seeking behavior: participation in weight-loss program R/T exposure to information regarding health risks associated with obesity *5.4*	1. Verbalizes understanding of factors that contribute to current physical condition.	1a. Assess current nutritional patterns (see Chap. 28). 1b. Assess factors that influence eating patterns (stress, boredom, cultural practices/beliefs). 1c. Assess activity patterns (see Chap. 33). 1d. Assess patient's knowledge of basic nutrition/caloric value of favorite foods. 1e. Review diet diary (see Chap. 28) with patient to identify factors that contribute to increased intake.	1a. Patient identifies personal eating patterns that contribute to weight gain. 1b. Patient accurately describes role of exercise in weight control.
	2. Adopts lifestyle changes necessary for attainment of weight-loss goals.	2a. Collaborate with patient to plan a balanced, acceptable diet that considers cultural and personal preferences. 2b. Assist patient in setting realistic weight-loss goals. 2c. Discuss ways to manage stress and emotions instead of eating. 2d. Involve significant others in treatment plan. 2e. Explore alternative exercise programs with patient. 2f. Support selection of exercise program that fits patient's preferences and daily routines. 2g. Provide positive reinforcement for verbal and behavioral indicators of healthy changes in eating and exercise.	2a. Patient reports ability to successfully follow prescribed dietary plan. 2b. Patient reports/describes participation in exercise regimen. 2c. Patient demonstrates weight loss of 1–2 lb/wk.
Altered health maintenance: substance abuse R/T ineffective individual coping *6.4.2*	1. Cessation of excessive use of alcohol and other drugs. 2. Effective stress management.	1a. Assess patient's history of abuse and possible past attempts at reducing substance use. 1b. Discuss effects of drugs and alcohol on health. 2a. Assess patient's other coping skills. 2b. Assist patient in identifying other methods for coping with stress (eg, exercise or relaxation technique). 2c. Be supportive of functional coping behaviors such as use of progressive relaxation. 2d. Assist patient to identify personal strengths and set realistic goals for change. 2e. Explore available resources and support systems with patient. 2f. Refer to a community support group for individuals who are recovering from substance abuse.	1. Patient reports cessation of alcohol and drug use. 2a. Patient reports use of exercise and meditation to manage stress. 2b. Patient participates regularly in a community support group.
Anxiety R/T threat to health status: uncertainty about results of diagnostic tests *9.3.1*	1. Decreased anxiety.	1a. Encourage patient to discuss feelings. 1b. Engage in active listening at least twice a shift. 1c. Encourage patient to explore possible factors contributing to anxious feelings. 1d. Provide clear, concise information about all patient care activities. 1e. Reduce as many stressful environmental stimuli as possible. 1f. Remain with patient during severe anxiety. 1g. Provide opportunities to discuss test results when available.	1a. Patient identifies factors that trigger anxiety. 1b. Decreased anxiety AEB: decreased trembling and restlessness ("I feel calmer now, my stomach isn't so upset"); improved eye contact when speaking; sleeps throughout night.
Diversional activity deficit R/T frequent, lengthy treatment: hemodialysis *6.3.1.1*	1. Patient reports reduced feelings of boredom. 2. Participates in chosen activity.	1a. Encourage patient to discuss feelings. 1b. Discuss patient's favorite topics during treatments. 1c. Make TV and/or radio available during treatments. 2a. Assess patient's hobbies, interests, favorite music, TV, and radio programs. 2b. Explore alternate methods available for getting involved in desired activity. 2c. Plan treatments at time that enables patient to engage in desired activity.	1a. Patient reports satisfaction with use of time during treatment. 2a. Patient reports involvement in chosen activity. 2b. Patient discusses recent activity with caregiver during treatment.
	3. Uses relaxation techniques as needed.	3a. Assess patient's knowledge and experience with relaxation techniques. 3b. Teach relaxation method, eg, guided imagery or meditation.	3. Performs progressive relaxation technique several times a day.

Continued

TABLE 25-5. CONTINUED

Nursing Diagnosis	Desired Outcome	Implementation	Evaluation Criteria
Fear of pain R/T knowledge deficit: postoperative pain management options *9.3.2*	1. Reduction in fear.	1a. Encourage patient to discuss feelings. 1b. Engage in active listening at least twice a shift. 1c. Assess patient's knowledge and experience with relaxation techniques. 1d. Teach a relaxation technique such as guided imagery or meditation.	1. Reduced fear AEB: "I can see now that there's not so much to be afraid of," relaxed expression, pulse and respiratory rate at patient's usual baseline.
	2. Verbalizes accurate knowledge of procedures and methods to control pain.	2a. Provide information regarding techniques to control pain. 2b. Encourage questions. 2c. Discuss procedures within patient's level of understanding.	2a. Patient verbalizes understanding of techniques to control pain. 2b. Patient describes expected sensations and what can be done to minimize unpleasant sensations.
Powerlessness R/T illness-related regimen *7.3.2*	1. Reduction in feelings of powerlessness and recognition of aspects of situation patient can control.	1a. Facilitate verbalization through active listening. 1b. Discuss aspects of treatment regimen that are most difficult for patient; explore possibilities for changes with other health care team members. 1c. Facilitate patient's identifying factors under own control. 1d. Ask patient how he or she prefers to participate in care. 1e. Discuss all treatments and procedures with patient. 1f. Acknowledge the importance of patient's space. 1g. Keep personal effects within reach.	1. Reduced sense of powerlessness AEB: describes changes in environment that give feelings of control, participates in decisions related to care, participates in self-care activities.
Hopelessness R/T deteriorating physical condition (AIDS) *7.3.1*	1. Reduction in feelings of hopelessness.	1a. Facilitate expression of feelings through active listening, open-ended questions, nonverbal acceptance. 1b. Encourage patient to explore and verbalize feelings related to physical condition. 1c. Acknowledge reality of situation; recognize both abilities and deficits. 1d. Assist patient to set realistic goals for progress/future. 1e. Accept negative emotions and avoid false reassurances.	1. Reduced feelings of hopelessness AEB: participation in self-care initiation of interactions with others, reduction in negative remarks about self and situation.
	2. Identifies personal/social resources to facilitate coping with changes in function.	2a. Assist patient in identifying activities that can be performed independently. 2b. Help patient identify personal strengths and sources of support. 2c. Collaborate with patient in planning schedule of daily activities; respect patient preferences as much as possible. 2d. Provide opportunities for social interaction/diversional activities. 2e. Encourage visits by significant others. 2f. Provide positive reinforcement for behaviors that show initiative (eg, self-care, increased appetite, increased interaction). 2g. Inform patient of available agency and community resources. 2h. Introduce patient to other individuals who have coped successfully with a similar situation.	2a. Verbalizes feelings of confidence and self-worth. 2b. Lists agencies to contact for assistance prior to discharge.
	3. Participates in decision making for the future.	3. Facilitate patient's identifying factors under own control.	3. Identifies realistic alternatives for future.
Spiritual distress R/T separation from religious ties *4.1.1*	1. Feelings of spiritual comfort.	1a. Acknowledge patient's spiritual concerns. 1b. Encourage patient to express thoughts and feelings. 1c. Offer to arrange visits by clergy; provide privacy during visit. 1d. Provide patient privacy for religious practices during hospitalization. 1e. Arrange to have objects that provide spiritual comfort at bedside.	1a. Specifies what spiritual assistance is needed. 1b. Verbalizes has achieved restored closeness to God, sense of peace during prayers and after receiving communion from local priest.

TABLE 25-5. CONTINUED

Nursing Diagnosis	Desired Outcome	Implementation	Evaluation Criteria
Risk for infection, RF: invasive procedures, decreased WBCs, receiving chemotherapy *1.2.1.1*	1. Patient remains free of infection throughout treatment regimen.	1a. Monitor vital signs every 4 hours. 1b. Monitor urine for altered color and odor. 1c. Wash hands before patient contact. 1d. Encourage or assist with daily hygiene. 1e. Discontinue invasive procedures as soon as possible. 1f. Adhere to strict aseptic technique for all invasive procedures and IV site care. 1g. Prevent patient exposure to infective visitors. 1h. Teach patient and family techniques to prevent infection.	1a. Patient remains afebrile. 1b. IV sites are free of signs of infection: redness, swelling, heat, purulent drainage. 1c. Urine remains free of bacteria. 1d. Patient verbalizes knowledge of techniques to prevent infection.

Source: See Table 25–4.

multidisciplinary guidelines for care related to a particular medical diagnosis or surgical procedure. Table 25–6, Partial Critical Pathway for Total Hip Replacement: Wellness and Well-being, illustrates portions of a critical pathway that addresses altered wellness associated with a common surgical procedure—total hip replacement. Table 25–7, Partial Critical Pathway for Congestive Heart Failure: Wellness and Well-Being, addresses altered wellness associated with a common medical diagnosis—congestive heart failure.

NURSING IMPLEMENTATION TO PROMOTE WELLNESS AND WELL-BEING

PREVENTIVE CARE

The goal of preventive care is to assist patients attain or maintain a high level of wellness through health protection and disease prevention.

Preventive patient care is provided in a variety of settings including physicians' offices, nurse practitioner clinics, industrial health clinics, schools, homes, and community care facilities. In all of these patient care settings, patients are active participants in health care decision making. Nurses are facilitators and educators. First-level nursing practice focuses on promoting self-care through education, motivation, and development of lifestyle and behaviors conducive to health.

Health Education

Health education is a major focus of preventive patient care. The goal of health education is to foster health-promoting and health protective behaviors. Health education empowers individuals to make responsible, informed lifestyle choices.

Nurses educate patients about elements of a wellness lifestyle, discussed in the first section of the chapter: eating well, being fit, feeling good, caring for self and others, fitting in, and being responsible.[7] Having knowledge of the principles of nutrition, fitness, and stress reduction assists patients to develop a program of high-level wellness (Fig. 25–1). Patient education about the negative effects on wellness and well-being of such habits as smoking, consuming excessive alcohol and drugs, irresponsible sexual activity, unbalanced nutrition, lack of exercise, and prolonged stress enables patients to recognize and eliminate detrimental habits. Teaching patients about the importance of immunizations, basic health maintenance, and principles of safety, sanitation, and hygiene is also part of health protection.

Vehicles for Health Education. Printed material is an important vehicle for education. Many health care professionals use pamphlets and checklists that address specific topics for health education. Patients at risk for a particular problem find these brief resources a useful reference to reinforce teaching by a health care provider. Some managed-care groups emphasize self-responsibility through printed resources. For example, the *Kaiser Permanente Healthwise Handbook*[60] is a 300-page book that advises members about health

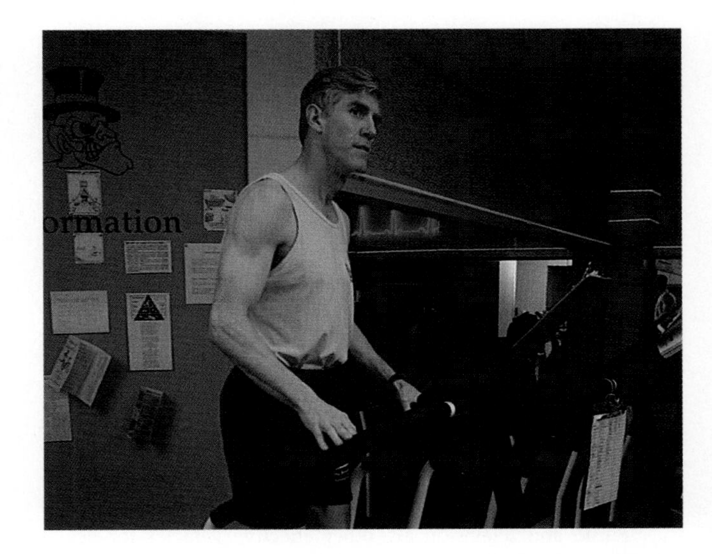

Figure 25–1. Teaching people about the elements of a wellness lifestyle encourages them to take advantage of workplace fitness centers and employee wellness programs.

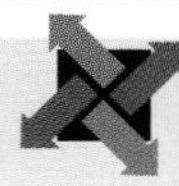

TABLE 25-6. PARTIAL CRITICAL PATHWAY FOR TOTAL HIP REPLACEMENT: WELLNESS AND WELL-BEING

Nursing Dx/Problem	Outcome DOS/Day 1	Outcome Days 2–3	Outcome SNF Days 4–6	Outcome Home Care 3 Weeks (6 Visits)
Fear of pain after surgery R/T knowledge deficit R/T pain relief options	Relaxed body posture Facial expressions relaxed Requests additional meds c̄ pain rated above 3 (1–5 scale)	Verbalizes reduction of fear Self-regulating pain med to below 3 on pain scale	Verbalizes comfort with pain control measures & regimen in SNF	Gives accurate feedback of pain control measures
Implementation	**DOS/Day 1**	**Days 2–3**	**SNF Days 4–6**	**Home Care 3 Weeks**
Assessment	Observe for S/Sx of fear q shift: rapid pulse, sweating, tense facial expression, muscle tightness, verbalizations	Same Knowledge & use of relaxation techniques	Same Same	Same Same
Tests/Consults				
Medications/Treatments	Pain control meds (PCA, epidural, or intravenous analgesia) & comfort measures	Same Assist to use relaxation techniques	Same Encourage to use relaxation techniques	Same Same
Psychosocial	Active listening to elicit current concerns Give clear information about options		Provide information about resources	Arrange for community services
Teaching	Relaxation & guided imagery techniques	Reinforce relaxation and guided imagery techniques	Same	Same
Activity/Safety/Self-care				
Nutrition				
Transfer/Discharge Coordinator/ Case Manager		Communicate outcomes achieved, problems/ interventions to SNF	Communicate outcomes achieved, problems/ interventions to Home Health	Communicate outcomes achieved, problems/ interventions to MD & prepare for discharge

See inside back cover for abbreviations.

promotion, provides information about basic self-care, and explains when to call a provider for over 180 health care problems. Kaiser supplies the book to members. Consumer interest in health information has generated a market for magazines and articles that target health-seeking individuals of all ages and lifestyles. Nurses can use consumer health articles as a basis for patient education, after evaluating them for accuracy. Misinformation can be clarified for patients while accurate information can be reinforced.

Radio and television are other effective vehicles for health education. They are especially useful for patients who are unable to read. The media get health promotion information to individuals with limited access to health care services. Videotape, cable, and closed-circuit systems enable use of television for small group and individual health education in homes and health care facilities.

Computers are also used in patient education. Computer-assisted instruction (CAI) programs are available on many health-related topics. Interactive programs that provide positive reinforcement and feedback are most effective. The Internet is a newer form of computer-based health information. The World Wide Web provides a wealth of information. Its resources are expanding rapidly. Examples of search engines that are useful in accessing health information are Yahoo! (http://wwwyahoo.com), Alta Vista (http://www.altavista.digital.com), or Achoo (http: //www.achoo.com).[61] A computer-literate patient can browse the Internet and

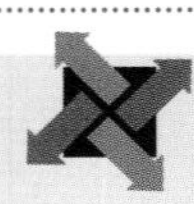

TABLE 25-7. CRITICAL PATHWAY FOR CONGESTIVE HEART FAILURE: WELLNESS AND WELL-BEING

Nursing Dx/ Problem	Outcome Primary Care Visit	Outcome Home Care Week 1 (3 Visits)	Outcome Home Care Week 2 (3 Visits)	Outcome Home Care Weeks 3–4 (3 Visits)
Anxiety R/T situational crisis: exacerbation of chronic illness	Verbalizes decreased anxiety p̄ plan of care outlined	Verbalizes less anxious p̄ included in discussion of plan of care	Reports anxiety resolving	Reports anxiety resolved
Implementation	**Primary Care Visit**	**Home Care Visit Week 1**	**Home Care Visit Week 2**	**Home Care Visit Weeks 3–4**
Assessment	Physical, emotional, cognitive symptoms of anxiety Level of knowledge & experience c̄ relaxation techniques Use of relaxation techniques	Same Same	Same Same	Same
Tests/Consults	Refer to Home Health			
Medications/ Treatments	Reflective listening Explain plan of care Request feedback of understanding	Assist with relaxation techniques Same Same	Same Reinforce as needed	Same
Psychosocial	Reflective listening	Explore adjustment to health status	Same	
Teaching	S/Sx to report to MD, RN, 911 Introduce relaxation techniques Importance of rest	Disease process plan of care, chest pain scale Reinforce as necessary	Review, reinforce as needed Same	Effect of exercise on sleep
Activity/Safety/ Self-care	Bedrest, HOB @ 30–45 degrees c̄ BSC or BRP	Regular rest periods	Progressive ambulation/ activity Regular rest periods	Same Same
Nutrition				
Transfer/Discharge Coordinator/ Case Manager		Communicate outcomes achieved to MD	Same	Same Prepare for discharge

See inside back cover for abbreviations.

obtain information on almost any topic. Nurses can use Internet information in patient health education, but like other forms of consumer-based health information, it needs to be evaluated for accuracy. See Chap. 22 for more information on computers as an aid to collaboration in health education. Radio, video, print, and computer-based information must be available in varied languages and reading levels to be most effective.

Health education can begin in health care facility waiting rooms, where educational materials and video presentations about wellness and health maintenance can be accessible (Fig. 25–2, page 646). Nurses who solicit patients' questions about information presented in the waiting area while assisting them to prepare for the health examination enhance the effectiveness of the educational materials and reinforce their use.

Screening

Screening procedures identify people at risk or in the early stages of disease. Early diagnosis and prompt treatment can often arrest

TABLE 25-8. HEALTH-PROTECTIVE BEHAVIORS THROUGHOUT THE LIFE SPAN

Developmental Level	Immunizations/Prophylaxis	Screening Procedures	Health Education
Infants (0–1 year)	DPT, oral polio, *Haemophilus influenza* B (Hib-conjugate) at 2, 4, and 6 months of age. Hepatitis B at birth, 2, and 6 months of age. Prophylactic erythromycin ointment in eyes, injection of 1 mg vitamin K.	At birth: Inborn errors of metabolism, developmental assessment.	Parent education: normal growth and development, breastfeeding, nutrition practices, safety measures, management of common childhood illnesses, importance of regular health supervision (well baby checks).
Toddlers and preschool children (1–5 years)	Hib-conjugate at 12–15 months of age. MMR at 15 months of age. DPT and oral polio at 18 months of age.	Complete physical examination every 2–3 months. Complete physical examination every 3 months to age 2; every 6 months to age 3; and annually to age 5. Vision and hearing screening. Developmental assessment. TB testing at age 4–6 years.	Parent education: dental health measures, discipline measures, accident prevention, nutritional practices, normal growth and development. Child education: dental self-care, basic hygiene practices.
School-age children (5–12 years)	DPT and oral polio boosters at age 5 or 6. Tetanus booster at age 10. Girls should receive rubella vaccine before puberty if not previously immunized. MMR booster at 12 years. Var. if no history of chickenpox.	Complete physical examination annually. TB test every 3 years. Vision and hearing screening. Dental checkups every 6 months.	Healthy diet habits. Accident prevention and safety measures. Preparation for physical changes of puberty. Substance abuse education. Basic sex education.
Adolescents (12–18 years)	Oral polio at 12–14 years. Tetanus booster, if needed.	Complete physical examination at puberty, including blood pressure, cholesterol, CBC, UA. BSE (female). TSE (male). Pap smear and pelvic examination for females, if sexually active. TB test at 12 years. Dental checkups every 6 months.	Healthful lifestyle practices. Sex education/methods of birth control/sexually transmitted diseases. Safe driving skills. Substance abuse education. Safety practices. Basic stress management. Methods for monthly BSE or TSE.

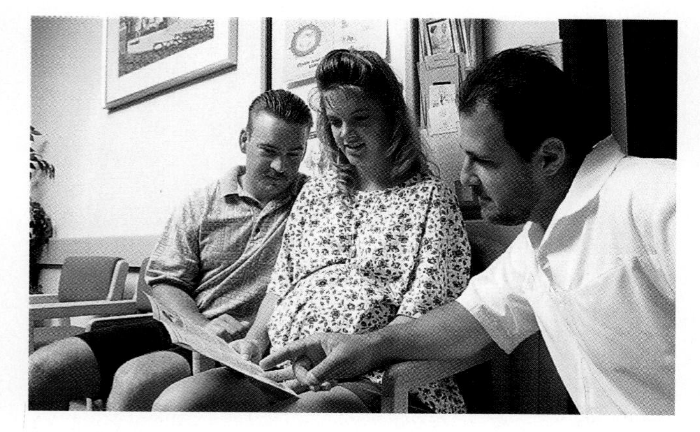

Figure 25–2. A waiting room with educational materials makes good use of time patients spend waiting to see a health care provider.

diseases and prevent disability. Self-responsibility plays a central role in effective screening. Breast or testicular self-examination, checking for occult blood in stools, and monitoring weight are examples of self-screening techniques that many health-conscious adults regularly perform. Individuals should also frequently assess for the seven warning signs of cancer:

- Change in bowel or bladder habits
- A sore that does not heal
- Unusual bleeding or discharge
- Thickening or lump in breast or elsewhere
- Indigestion or difficulty swallowing
- Obvious change in wart or mole
- Nagging cough or hoarseness

Some screening, such as blood pressure checks, are easier if done with the assistance of a family member or significant other. Screen-

TABLE 25-8. CONTINUED

Developmental Level	Immunizations/Prophylaxis	Screening Procedures	Health Education
Young adults (18–30 years)	Tetanus at age 20 and every 10 years. Hepatitis B for high-risk populations/occupations if not immunized as a child. Rubella for females if serum test negative.	Complete physical examination at age 20 and every 5 years. Monthly BSE (female). Monthly TSE (male). Pap smear and pelvic examination every 2 years for healthy females; every year for high-risk groups. Blood pressure screening. VDRL or RPR. Regular dental checkups.	Sexual counseling on birth control, sexually transmitted disease. Lifestyle counseling: stress management, nutrition, physical fitness, parenting skills, environmental health.
Middle-age adults (30–65 years)	Tetanus booster every 10 years. Influenza for high-risk individuals annually.	Complete physical examination every 5 years. Monthly BSE (female). Monthly TSE (male). Pap smear and pelvic examination every 2 years; annually after age 40. Baseline mammogram at age 35; annually after age 40. Stool for occult blood at age 50 and annually after. Sigmoidoscopy at age 50. Glaucoma testing routinely after age 40. Blood pressure screening.	Warning signs of serious illness. Cancer detection. Continuation of lifestyle counseling. Anticipatory guidance for retirement/"empty nest."
Older adults (65+ years)	Annual influenza. Tetanus booster every 10 years. One-time pneumococcal.	Complete physical examination every 2 years. Blood pressure annually. Monthly BSE (female). Monthly TSE (male). Annual mammogram (female). Annual stool for occult blood. Glaucoma screening every 3–5 years. Pap smear and pelvic examination annually. Regular vision and hearing screening.	Home safety/fall prevention. Lifestyle counseling: nutritional changes, retirement/relocation, adjustment to changes related to aging, cancer detection.

DPT = diphtheria, pertussis, tetanus; MMR = measles, mumps, rubella; TB = tuberculosis; Var. = varicella; CBC = complete blood count; UA = urinalysis; BSE = breast self-examination; TSE = testicular self-examination; VDRL = Venereal Disease Research Laboratory (test for syphilis); RPR-rapid plasma reagin (test for syphilis).

ing programs such as annual Pap smear, mammogram, and testing for diabetes, elevated cholesterol, and glaucoma require the services of a health care professional.

Health education is a requisite for effective screening. Individuals need to know about the importance of scheduling screening procedures and they need information about procedures requiring professional assessment that they can perform independently. Knowledge enables patients to exercise self-responsibility. Refer to Table 25–8 for screening procedures that are recommended for each developmental stage.

Preventing Infection

Microorganisms are naturally present everywhere in the environment. Many are harmless, some are beneficial, others, called *pathogens,* are capable of producing infection. Sometimes microorganisms that are typically harmless can cause disease in susceptible individuals. Individual's exposure to disease-producing microorganisms is largely determined by the type of environment in which they live or work. Those having frequent close contact with large numbers of people, for example, are at increased risk for contagious diseases. This includes people living in crowded conditions, such as often exist in shelters for the homeless and in some low-income housing or in school environments. Health care facilities such as hospitals generally have a larger population of microorganisms than other environments. For this reason rigorous infection-control measures are used in health care settings. Many variables determine whether exposure to a pathogen will result in an infection. See Chap. 9 and the discussion in Section 2 of this chapter on the nursing diagnosis, risk for infection.

Infection-control measures control or eliminate the source, transmission, and multiplication of potentially infectious agents. Some of these measures, such as handwashing and use of gloves, are important at all levels of nursing care—preventive, supportive, restorative, and rehabilitative—and in all settings in which care is given. Others apply more readily to a particular level of care. Supporting and facilitating individual efforts to maintain optimum wellness (see Section 1) is the most basic infection-control strategy in preventive nursing care. Then, the natural defense mechanisms that protect people against invading organisms function most effectively. These defenses are discussed in Chap. 27.

CRITICAL QUERY

Research indicates that artificial fingernails and chipped nail polish harbor potentially harmful bacteria.[63] What is your responsibility as a professional when you observe a peer wearing artificial nails when she is on duty?

Handwashing. Handwashing is the single most important means of preventing the spread of infection. The purpose of handwashing is to remove microorganisms that might be transmitted to a new susceptible host. Everyone in the health care community, including patients, visitors, and health care providers, should consistently perform good handwashing. Recent studies have indicated that fewer than half of all patient contacts by health care personnel were preceded or followed by handwashing, even when the patients were known to have infectious diseases.[62] This is a serious concern. Related research indicates that artificial fingernails and old chipped nail polish harbor greater numbers of potentially harmful bacteria than natural, unpolished nails. The organisms are not effectively removed by routine handwashing.[63] The Association for Professionals in Infection Control and Epidemiology (APIC), the Centers for Disease Control and Prevention (CDC), and the Hospital Infection Control Practices Advisory Committee (HICPAC) recommend washing hands thoroughly and promptly between patient contacts and after contact with body substances (blood, body fluids, secretions, excretions) or articles contaminated by body substances.[62,64] APIC further recommends that health care workers who provide direct patient care not wear artificial nails and keep natural nails short with fresh nail polish or none at all.[62]

Various products are available for handwashing. Plain soap is adequate for routine handwashing. Plain soap, however, only removes organisms—it does not kill them. Therefore, in dealing with high-risk patients or in areas where exposure to many virulent pathogens is likely, washing with a product that contains an antimicrobial ingredient is recommended.[62,64] Correct handwashing technique is presented in Procedure 25–1.

Use of Gloves. Gloves provide a protective barrier that reduces the risk of transmitting potentially infectious organisms from patients to health care workers, from health care workers to patients, and from one patient to another via the hands of health care workers. Some procedures require sterile gloves. Their use is discussed in a later section: Surgical Asepsis. The new HICPAC/CDC guidelines for hospital infection control indicate the following recommendations for the use of clean (unsterile) gloves[64]:

- Wear clean gloves when there is the risk of contact with mucous membranes, nonintact skin, and any body substances.
- Put on the gloves just before the expected contact.
- Change gloves between tasks and procedures on the same patient and after contact with material that may contain a high concentration of microorganisms.
- Remove gloves and discard in trash can promptly after use, before touching uncontaminated items and environmental surfaces, and before going to another patient.
- Wash hands immediately after removing gloves.

No special technique is required to put on clean, unsterile gloves. They are designed to fit either hand. A supply of gloves in several sizes should be available in all rooms in which direct care is given (Fig. 25–3). Removing the gloves as one does sterile gloves, described later in Procedure 25–3, step 9, prevents hand contact with soiled gloves. Some facilities may supply special waste containers for gloves and other disposables that are soiled with a large amount of potentially contaminated body substances. The facility then collects and stores this hazardous waste in a central location for collection and appropriate disposal (Fig. 25–4, page 649). Refer to Table 25–9, later in the chapter, for more information about the use of gloves to reduce the risk of transmitting organisms.

(continued on page 649)

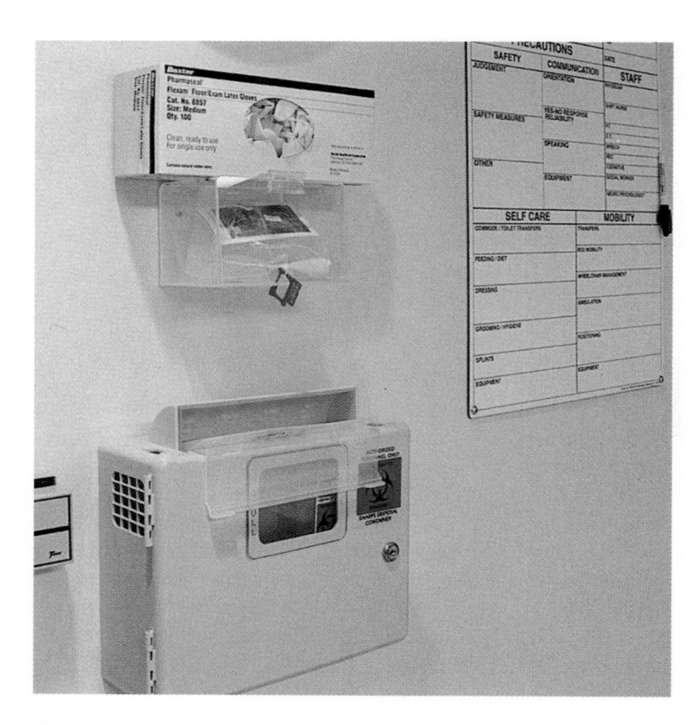

Figure 25–3. A dispenser for clean disposable gloves and a container for disposal of used syringes in each patient's room facilitates carrying out Standard Precautions. *(From Smith S, Duell D.* Clinical Nursing Skills: Nursing Process Model; Basic to Advanced Skills. *4th ed. Norwalk, CT: Appleton & Lange; 1996.)*

PROCEDURE 25–1. HANDWASHING

PURPOSE: To prevent transmission of pathogens from one patient to another by removing soil and transient organisms from the hands.
EQUIPMENT: Liquid or bar soap, warm running water, and paper towels.

ACTION 1. Remove and store all jewelry except watch and plain band-type rings. Push watch and long sleeves above the wrists.

RATIONALE. Jewelry harbors microorganisms that are difficult to remove with normal handwashing technique. These organisms may be transferred to the patient.

ACTION 2. Adjust water flow so no splashing occurs; adjust water temperature to lukewarm. Avoid contacting sink with hands or uniform as you wash.

RATIONALE. The sink is a reservoir of microorganisms. Contact and/or splashed water will transfer organisms to you, which could then be transmitted to patients. Hot water depletes protective skin oils, increasing risk of chapping and breaks in the skin. Chapped or broken skin provides a portal of entry for organisms, increasing infection risk to nurses.

ACTION 3. Wet hands and wrists, keeping hands lower than elbows.

RATIONALE. The hands have a greater microbial population than forearms. Gravity causes water and suspended microorganisms to flow downward and off the hands. If hands are higher than elbows, wrists and forearms will be contaminated by microbes from hands.

ACTION 4. Apply soap and rub hands and wrists to create a generous amount of lather.

RATIONALE. Lather suspends transient microorganisms so they can be flushed from the hands.

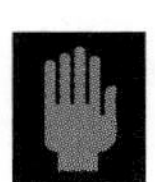

Bar soaps harbor microbes. If used, rinse bar thoroughly to remove them.

ACTION 5. Wash for 10 to 30 seconds, cleaning all surfaces of hands and fingers, with firm, brisk rubbing motions.

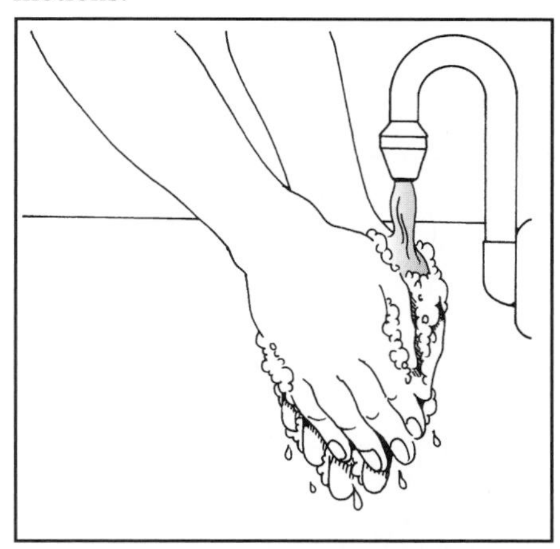

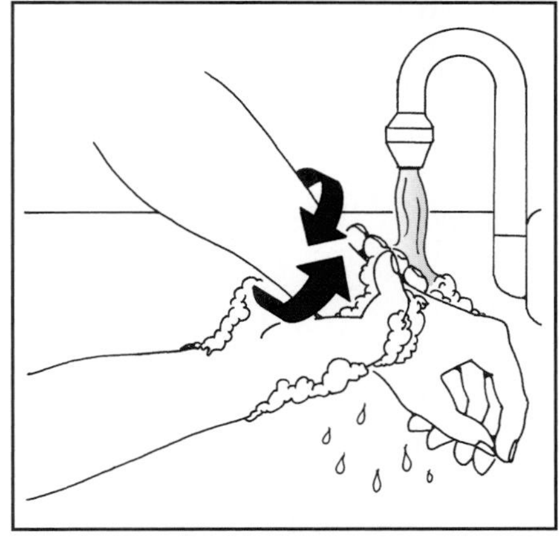

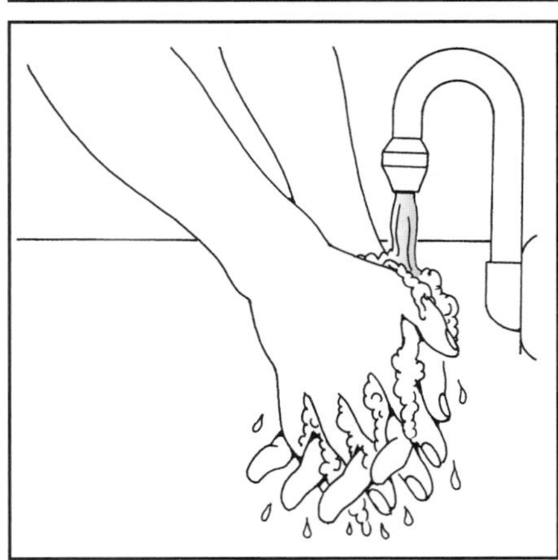

RATIONALE. Firm rubbing creates friction, which dislodges transient microbes.

Continued

ACTION 6. Clean under nails and around nailbeds with fingertips and nails from opposite hand.

RATIONALE. Microbes lodge under and around nails. Transient microbes may become resident flora and colonize if not removed. Short nails are less likely to harbor microbes.

ACTION 7. Thoroughly rinse each hand, holding fingertips downward.

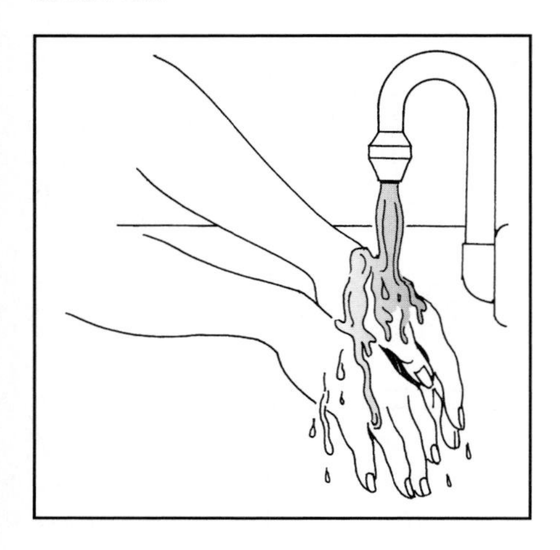

RATIONALE. Rinsing removes lather with suspended microbes. See also Action 3.

ACTION 8. Repeat Actions 4 to 7, if hands were grossly contaminated.

RATIONALE. No studies support a specific length of time for effective washing; however, it is generally accepted that length of washing should correspond to degree of contamination.

ACTION 9. Dry hands thoroughly with paper towels.

RATIONALE. Drying well prevents chapping (which would create a portal of entry for organisms).

ACTION 10. If faucet is hand regulated, protect your hand with a paper towel when turning off the water.

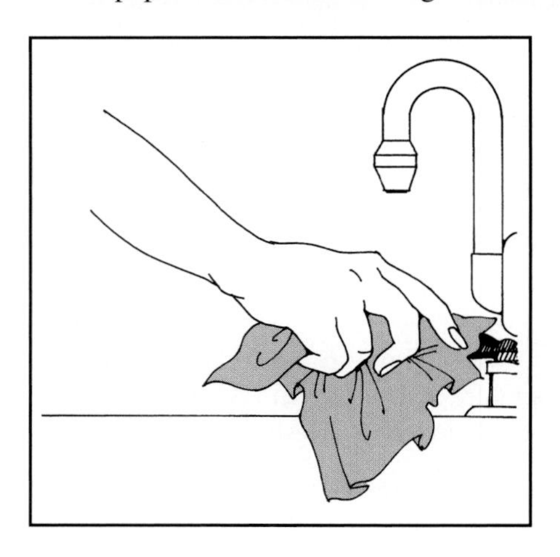

RATIONALE. The faucet handle is contaminated. The paper towel creates a barrier, preventing transfer of microbes to your hands.

ACTION 11. Apply lotion to hands if desired.

RATIONALE. Hand lotions contain emollients, which replace skin moisture lost during handwashing. This prevents cracking and chapping.

Recording:
No recording is necessary.

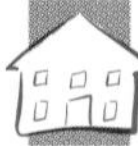

HOME HEALTH ADAPTATION: Carry your own container of liquid soap and paper towels for use in homes lacking these items. If suitable handwashing facilities are not available, thoroughly cleanse hands with an isopropyl-alcohol–based disinfectant rinse. Instruct family members in correct handwashing technique. Emphasize the importance of washing hands before and after providing care.

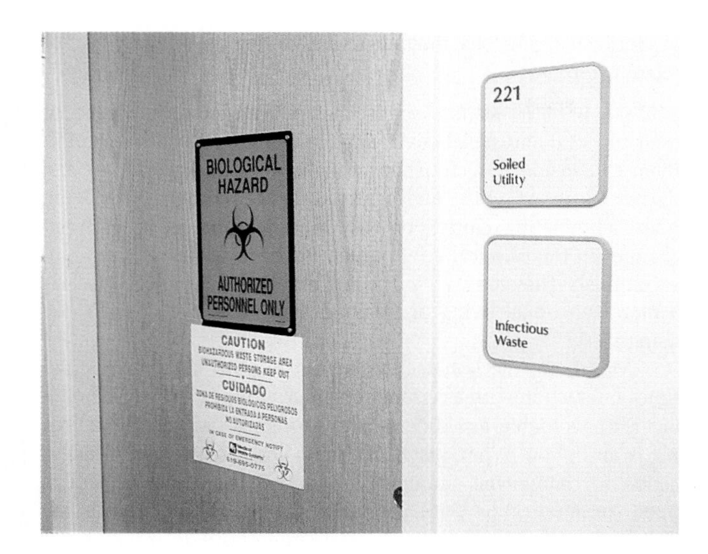

Figure 25–4. **Hazardous waste disposal.**

Most gloves are made of latex with a cornstarch powder applied to glove surfaces to reduce stickiness. Latex hypersensitivity among health care workers and patients has made it necessary to make gloves made from synthetic materials or powderless gloves available as well.[65–67] Refer to Clinical Guideline 25–1 for more information.

Immunization. Routine immunization programs also help to prevent infectious diseases. Although most immunizations are given to children, some are recommended throughout the life span. For example, the tetanus toxoid booster is required every 10 years throughout life, and older adults should receive an annual flu shot to prevent influenza.

Nurses have several responsibilities when administering immunizations. First, informed consent is important. Individuals need to know about the risks and benefits. Some individuals fear immunizations because of concern about possible adverse reactions. In most cases, the consequences of acquiring a disease are more serious than complications from immunizations. Obtaining a thorough history (including allergies) before administering a vaccine and carefully observing patients for immediate adverse reactions after receiving an immunization are also important nursing responsibilities. Finally, it is necessary to maintain an accurate record of immunizations. Usually, health care providers record immunizations in patients' health records, but giving patients a record to keep for personal reference promotes self-responsibility. Table 25–8 lists the immunizations that are recommended at each developmental stage.

Other precautions to reduce the risks of transmitting infections are addressed in the sections on supportive and restorative care.

Managing Stress

Effective stress management promotes the sense of "feeling good," which is essential to well-being. The nurse's role in stress management extends beyond controlling sources of biologic and environmental stressors in health care settings. It also includes

CLINICAL GUIDELINE 25–1

RECOGNIZING AND REDUCING RISKS OF LATEX HYPERSENSITIVITY

TYPES OF REACTIONS	SIGNS AND SYMPTOMS	APPROPRIATE ACTION
Irritant dermatitis: Not a latex sensitivity. Caused by powder.	Localized redness and itching during or immediately after use of gloves.	Try powder-free latex gloves or change glove brands.
Type IV Reaction: Delayed hypersensitivity reaction. Triggered by chemicals used in manufacture of gloves.	Localized redness, itching, urticaria, edema. Flushing, rhinitis, coughing, conjunctivitis. First reactions delayed up to 72 hours; with continued exposure reaction within 30 minutes. Symptoms may resolve within 1 to 2 days without exposure, return or worsen with subsequent contact. May progress to Type I allergy.	Use nonlatex glove until open lesions resolve, then change glove brands. If symptoms persist, be evaluated for latex allergy. Removing latex powdered gloves from work area may be necessary.
Type I Reaction: Latex allergy. IgE-mediated response that can be life-threatening.	Vary with degree of exposure and individual sensitivity; may progressively worsen. Localized or systemic response. Local: urticaria, edema. Systemic: flushing, conjunctivitis, pharyngeal edema, dyspnea, bronchospasm, cardiac arrhythmias, diarrhea, anaphylaxis. Some develop chronic asthma.	Immediate: Vary with severity: antihistamines, epinephrine, corticosteroids, IV fluids, oxygen, intubation. Long term: Use latex-free gloves. Avoid all latex products. Some persons may need all powdered latex gloves removed from working area. May be unable to continue to work in health care.

General: Use gloves only when necessary according to HICPAC/CDC guidelines. Avoid touching face and eyes when wearing latex gloves. Change gloves whenever your hands feel moist. Wash hands well after removing gloves to remove all traces of powder; dry hands thoroughly. Dispose of gloves properly: do not leave them on counters, beds, or other work areas.

Source: *Gritter M. Latex hypersensitivity: what are your risks?* NURSEWEEK. 1997;10:10–11.

assisting patients to assess their current stress levels, evaluate the adequacy of their coping mechanisms, and develop competence in using stress management techniques. The discussion of stress and coping in Chap. 8 provides the information needed to teach patients about stress assessment and coping. The discussion below provides information to facilitate effective stress management.

Minimizing Exposure to Stressful Situations. Attempting to eliminate all stressors is unrealistic and undesirable; however, managing time, avoiding unnecessary change, and modifying one's environment are effective means of preventing overload from excessive stress.[2,68]

MANAGING TIME. Feeling stressed about "not enough time" is a common complaint. The real problem in most cases is poor use of available time. Effective time management strategies enable people to reduce the stress associated with time pressures. Time management involves the following steps:

- *Clarify personal goals.* People sometimes lose sight of their goals and values as they become involved in carrying out routine daily activities. Suggesting that patients take time to review their aspirations and priorities will bring goals and values back into focus.
- *Assess time use.* This activity follows from the clarification of values and personal goals. It involves several steps:
  - List typical daily or weekly activities and estimate time allotted to each.
  - Analyze time allocations in light of personal goals and priorities.
  - Take note of time spent on activities unrelated to goals.
  - Consider whether time is overcommitted.
- *Restructure time use.* Assist patients to plan preferred use of time to achieve personal goals with the least stress, while still allowing time for relaxing and restorative pursuits. Emphasize that executing the plan involves:
  - "Saying no" to activities that are low on the priority list
  - Delegating responsibility to others
  - Seeking assistance when necessary
  - Breaking tasks down into smaller elements
  - Recognizing the value in the accomplishment of each element
  - Recognizing and avoiding procrastination
- *Monitor progress.* Encourage patients to include in their plan a block of time to analyze and reflect on their progress toward improving time management and achieving personal goals.

AVOIDING UNNECESSARY CHANGE. Change is stressful for most people. Encourage patients who are experiencing stress to avoid any unnecessary changes, such as taking on extra responsibilities at home or work, changing jobs, moving, or embarking on a new project or relationship.

MODIFYING THE ENVIRONMENT. Suggest that patients identify aspects of their physical and social environments that are stressful. Then ask them to consider which aspects they can avoid, which they can decrease contact with, and which they can change. Reducing noise, eliminating clutter, or relocating seldom used items are changes in the physical environment that are relatively simple to accomplish. They are well worth the time they take if the result is a more functional living or working space and less stress when using it.

Modifying the social environment is more complex. Sometimes interaction with a certain person or group is stressful. If contact is unavoidable, avoiding sensitive topics when with these people is an option. When neither of these choices is feasible, taking action to change the situation is another alternative. Generally, open communication with the person or people involved is the first step in changing stressful social situations. For example, if a patient is bothered by a co-worker's irritating behavior, encourage asking the co-worker in a tactful manner to change the behavior. Emphasize that using an "I message" (one that expresses a personal desire or need) rather than a "you message" (one that labels another's actions) is more likely to have positive results. For example, "It's hard for me to accomplish what I need to when I'm interrupted. Would you be willing to set a daily meeting time to talk instead of dropping in several times a day? Perhaps you could make a list of things you want to discuss as you think of them" is an "I message." "You're always interrupting me when I'm working and I can't get anything done" is a "you message." Role-playing

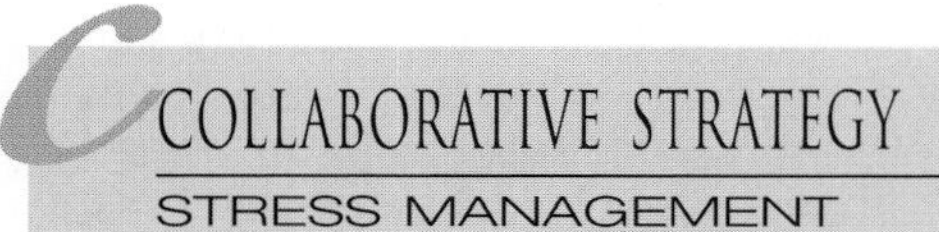

COLLABORATIVE STRATEGY

STRESS MANAGEMENT

Interaction between nurse and patient that accomplishes a reduction in patient stress is an example of successful collaboration. Not only must a nurse understand the sources of patients' stress and the appropriate management techniques, but also patients must trust nurses' understanding and actively participate.

INSIGHTS FROM NURSING LITERATURE

FACTORS IN MAKING HEALTH PROMOTION A HABIT

Bottorf JL, Johnson JL, Ratner PA, Hayduk LA. The effects of cognitive-perceptual factors on health promotion behavior maintenance. Nurs Res. *1996;45:30–36.*

Relatively little research, the investigators noted, exists on the persistence of health-promoting behavior over time, particularly in relation to exercise, weight control, and stress management behavior. Using survey data from the National Center for Health Statistics, they designed a study to illuminate the role of cognitive-perceptual factors in solidifying such behavior. Questions on the survey queried respondents about the degree of control over their own health they perceived themselves to have, how well they felt they were taking care of their own health, and how they rated their health in relation to others their own age. The data, analyzed statistically, showed cognitive-perceptual factors only weakly connected to the stability of health-promoting behaviors. The researchers suggested that motivation or the effect of a person's "self-schema"—organization of knowledge, feelings, and thoughts about oneself in relation to health promotion—could also be at play.

using "I messages" with patients is a useful technique to increase their confidence about asking others to change.

Another way to change some stressful situations is to share personal feelings. For example, sharing with a friend that a certain topic is painful for you to talk about or telling a co-worker that performing a particular task makes you nervous may result in a response that is mutually beneficial.

Sometimes these types of environmental modifications are insufficient to eliminate or reduce the stress. Then a more extreme change (for example, a new job, a new roommate) is another alternative to consider. Often, however, changing oneself as discussed in the next section is a more effective long-term alternative.

Altering Responses to Stressful Situations. As discussed in Section 1, individuals' lifestyle practices and general physical condition greatly influence their perceptions and reactions to stressful events. The importance of good nutrition, rest, and regular exercise in preventing stress-related disorders and promoting physical and mental well-being is well documented. Nutrition, rest, and exercise are discussed in other chapters in this unit.

People can also moderate their physiologic response to stressors. As discussed in Chap. 8, there are a variety of techniques that can interrupt the emotional and physiologic responses to stress that usually are automatic. One method, cognitive reappraisal, is presented in Chap. 8. Two others, the relaxation response and biofeedback, are detailed below. These stress management techniques have been shown to be extremely useful in managing the pain of childbirth, controlling hypertension, and alleviating anxiety-related symptoms such as tension headaches, insomnia, and chronic muscle tension.[11] When used routinely, relaxation and biofeedback techniques can significantly reduce the taxing effect of the "daily hassles" that aggravate almost everyone.

RELAXATION RESPONSE. The **relaxation response,** first described by Dr. Herbert Benson, is a physiologic response that is the opposite of the fight-or-flight response.[69] It is a state of heightened endorphin secretion and parasympathetic nervous system stimulation leading to feelings of well-being and decreased anxiety, tension, and pain. There is a corresponding reduction in sympathetic stimulation, so metabolism slows and heart rate blood and pressure decrease. The relaxation response is not the same as sleeping. To use relaxation effectively requires making the techniques part of one's daily routine. The only necessary components for eliciting a relaxation response are (1) a quiet environment that is free of external distractions; (2) a comfortable position (usually sitting or reclining) that one can maintain for at least 20 minutes; (3) a passive attitude that is gained by emptying all thoughts and distractions from the mind; and (4) an object, phrase, sound, or image to dwell upon.[69] No physician's order is required to teach and use relaxation.

Before learning to relax, individuals first must become aware of the tension in their bodies. Common areas of tension are jaw, neck, shoulder, and back muscles. Encourage patients to "scan" their bodies for these signs periodically throughout the day. The following techniques can be used to evoke the relaxation response.

- *Controlled breathing.* Individuals are usually not conscious of breathing because it is automatically controlled by the respiratory center in the brain. During controlled breathing exercises, individuals concentrate on taking slow, deep breaths that fully expand the lungs. Conscious slowing of breathing counteracts the effects of sympathetic stimulation. Because of this effect, briefly using controlled breathing is also an effective means of responding to acute stress events.
- *Progressive relaxation.* Progressive relaxation works by tensing and relaxing major muscle groups in systematic fashion until all muscles are fully relaxed. With practice, deeper and deeper levels of relaxation are possible.[2,11] By focusing on the feelings associated with relaxation such as heaviness and warmth, individuals can eventually achieve full relaxation nearly instantaneously without the systematic progression through muscle groups.
- *Guided imagery.* This technique quiets the sympathetic nervous system through focus on a mental image that is pleasing and comforting. The emphasis is on the feelings that accompany the image rather than the clarity of the image.
- *Meditation.* Meditation interrupts the stress response through concentration on one thing and blocking out other thoughts. Music, breathing, or a mantra may be used to aid concentration.

Clinical Guideline 25–2 summarizes instructions for eliciting the relaxation response.

BIOFEEDBACK. *Biofeedback* is a technique to develop conscious control of autonomic nervous system functions, such as muscle tension, skin temperature, brain waves, blood pressure, or heart rate. Information about internal body functioning is "fed back" to individuals via machines that detect and signal changes in one or more target function. This feedback enables them to detect negative and desirable internal changes. They can then learn to reproduce the state that resulted in desired changes. The goal of biofeedback is achieving generalized relaxation without feedback devices. Biofeedback training is a long-term process. It is currently used to treat stress-linked conditions such as tension or migraine headaches, hypertension, muscle spasms, insomnia, and asthma.

Self-management

Self-management is a method of achieving personal change that draws principles from several learning theories (see Chap. 21). Self-management theory stresses that knowing and believing in oneself, understanding environmental events that reinforce behavior, and systematic planning are important to success in changing oneself. Motivation and will power alone are usually insufficient to bring about change. Change also requires a plan.

Self-management is a classic model that is useful in health care today because it provides techniques that nurses and other health care professionals can teach to patients who desire to make changes in their lives. A summary of Williams and Long's[70] self-management philosophy and techniques is included under preventive care because self-management is effective for developing new, health-enhancing habits. Adding an exercise program to one's daily activities, for example, is a common new pattern that can be achieved through self-management. It can also be used as a way to change long-established, health-endangering habits such as smoking or overeating. The method can be used just as effectively to achieve supportive and rehabilitative health goals once a health problem has developed. Nurses can make significant contributions to patients' well-being by teaching self-management techniques. By using these techniques themselves, nurses can enhance their own health and well-being.

The Process of Self-management. Applying self-management theory entails three systematic steps: (1) self-assessment and selecting

CLINICAL GUIDELINE 25–2

ELICITING THE RELAXATION RESPONSE

Have patients select the method they feel will work best for them. Begin with the patient in a comfortable sitting or lying position. Reduce environmental stimulation, including lights, noise, and tactile irritants. Practice the selected method with the patient at least once, slowly verbalizing instructions in a soothing tone of voice. Supply the following written or taped instructions for patient's subsequent use.

DEEP RELAXATION BREATHING

- To learn this technique, place your left hand on your chest, your right on your abdomen. If you become dizzy or light-headed during practice, go back to your normal breathing for a short time, then try deep breathing again. Sometimes it takes a little while to adjust to deep breathing. Repeat the exercise for several minutes daily. Use it whenever your feel stressed or nervous.
- Exhale completely through your nose, then inhale slowly and deeply, filling your abdomen with air. Your right hand should rise.
- Continue to inhale, filling your chest with air. As your left hand rises, continue to inhale until your collarbone rises as well.
- Hold your breath for several seconds—as long as is comfortable.
- Exhale slowly, releasing air first from your lungs, then your chest, finally from your abdomen. Contract abdominal muscles briefly to expel all air. Think: "I feel relaxed."
- As you become used to deep breathing, gradually increase the length of time you hold your breath and exhale. The recommended ratio of inhale to hold to exhale is 1:4:2 (eg, 4 counts inhale, 16 counts hold, 8 counts exhale).

PROGRESSIVE RELAXATION

- Begin deep, slow breathing. Then, contract (tighten) your muscles as you inhale for a count of 4 to 6 and relax them as you exhale for a count of 15. You will relax and contract each muscle group until you have progressed through all of the muscles.
- Tense your facial and neck muscles. Relax.
- Tense your left shoulder, arm, and hand. Relax.
- Tense your right shoulder, arm, and hand. Relax.
- Tense your left buttock, leg, and foot. Relax. Notice your body feeling heavy.
- Tense your right buttock, leg, and foot. Relax.
- Tense your chest, abdomen, and buttocks. Relax. Notice you feel heavier.
- Tense your entire body for a count of 15.
- Release your entire body saying "aahh." Notice that your body is completely relaxed. Think: "I feel relaxed."

GUIDED IMAGERY

- Begin deep, slow breathing. Close your eyes. Feel tensions leave your body as you exhale. Repeat 4 to 12 times. Notice your body is feeling heavy and warm.
- "Paint a picture" in your mind. Imagine you are at the top of a staircase with steps numbered 1 to 10.
- Descend the staircase. With each step you will feel more deeply relaxed. 9, more relaxed . . . 8 . . . 7 much deeper . . . 6 . . . 5 more relaxed . . . 4 . . . 3 more deeply relaxed . . . 2 . . . (Narrator: allow 15 to 60 seconds for each number.)
- 1. Look around you. You are in a beautiful safe place. Perhaps it's a place you have been before . . . or it may exist only in your imagination.
- As you look, notice what is there . . . colors? . . . water? . . . trees? . . . Put anything or anyone you wish in your place.
- What smells do you notice?
- Do you feel textures? Sand? . . . grass? . . . a pillow? . . .
- Notice how peaceful and safe you feel in this place. Relax and stay here for a few moments . . . . (Narrator: pause for 1 to 3 minutes.)
- Now, a soft light begins to fill your place.
- It gets gradually brighter, but lovely to look at . . . . The light is healing energy.
- It moves within you now. It is warm and comforting.
- Now it is within and around you. . . . Feel its warmth. . . . Feel your wholeness.
- Bask in the light. . . . Enjoy it. . . . Know you can take this feeling with you. (Pause 1 to 3 minutes.)
- Now the light is dimming, but you still feel its warmth. . . . It's yours to keep.
- Enjoy your place for a few minutes more. . . . (Pause 1 to 3 minutes.)
- Now get ready to leave, knowing you can come back whenever you want . . . Look around. . . . Say good-bye.
- Now you are at the foot of the stairs. Climb up slowly, feeling more refreshed and alert with each step.
- 1 . . . 2 begin to notice your breathing . . . 3 notice your arms and legs . . . 4 . . . 5 . . . 6 feel your body . . . 7 . . . 8 begin to be aware of the room . . . 9 hear the sounds around you . . . move around a little. . . . (Allow 15 to 60 seconds per number.)
- 10. When you are ready, open your eyes. Stretch. Feel refreshed, yet peaceful.

MANTRA MEDITATION

- A mantra is a word or phrase that is repeated to elicit a meditative state. Select a personal word or phrase that makes you feel peaceful ("om," a Sanskrit word, is a common choice; its vibratory sound aids deepening meditation). Some people find classical music, tapes of nature sounds, or tapes designed to enhance meditation help to deepen the meditation. Breathing with inhale, hold, exhale ratio of 1:4:2 also enhances meditation.
- Begin deep, slow breathing.
- As you exhale, repeat your word aloud or silently.
- If distracting thoughts come into your head, "watch" them go by. Then refocus on your word. These intrusions will lessen with practice.
- Maintain meditation for about 20 minutes.

Techniques adapted from Carpenito, LJ. Nursing Diagnosis: Application to Clinical Practice. *Philadelphia: Lippincott; 1995; Kahn S, Saulo M.* Healing Yourself. *Albany, NY: Delmar Pub; 1994; Healing meditation for nurses.* Calif Nurs Rev. *1989;Jan–Feb.*

? CRITICAL QUERY

Self-management[70] is an effective process for making personal changes that nurses can teach to patients. You are a nurse attempting to teach this process to a patient who desires to quit smoking. If you are a smoker, can you effectively assist your patient?

goals, (2) developing an action plan, and (3) measuring progress and maintaining improvement.

SELF-ASSESSMENT AND GOAL SELECTION

- *Assessing outlook.* The process of self-management begins with identifying personal locus of control. Nurses can assist patients to assess their own locus of control using the scale in Fig. 25–5. The scale score indicates one's inclination toward an internal or an external locus of control. Patients who believe in an internal locus of control generally have greater success in personal change. Self-management theorists state that by employing self-management techniques, people can shift locus of control from external to internal. However, patients who are initially externally oriented may require more self-management trials to achieve ultimate success.
- *Assessing behavior.* The next step is selecting behavior to be changed. Williams and Long have devised a self-assessment inventory of behavior patterns (see Fig. 25–6) to target potential changes. They categorize behaviors in four self-management areas—work, social, health, leisure. Positive scores and balance among the scores in each area is desirable. Minimal or negative scores indicate areas for potential change.
- *Setting priorities.* Priority setting is ranking the list of behaviors targeted for change in order of their importance. The object is to decide which changes have the greatest personal importance. A priority list is used to guide goal setting. For example, a personal list might look like this:
  - breaking the habit of interrupting during conversations
  - becoming more self-directive
  - making new friends
- *Assessing personal resources.* Focusing on personal abilities or reviewing personal successes is one way to recognize one's inner

Using the scale −3, −2, −1, +1, +2, +3, indicate the extent to which you agree or disagree with each of the following items. Let −3 represent complete disagreement and +3 complete agreement. Put the number representing the degree of your agreement or disagreement by each item. Directions for scoring your responses are given at the conclusion of the inventory.

1. Whether or not I get to be a leader depends mostly on my ability.
2. To a great extent my life is controlled by accidental happenings.
3. I feel like what happens in my life is mostly determined by powerful people.
4. Whether or not I get into a car accident depends mostly on how good a driver I am.
5. When I make plans, I am almost certain to make them work.
6. Often there is no chance of protecting my personal interest from bad-luck happenings.
7. When I get what I want, it's usually because I'm lucky.
8. Although I might have good ability, I will not be given leadership responsibility without appealing to those in positions of power.
9. How many friends I have depends on how nice a person I am.
10. I have often found that what is going to happen will happen.
11. My life is chiefly controlled by powerful others.
12. Whether or not I get into a car accident is mostly a matter of luck.
13. People like myself have very little chance of protecting our personal interests when they conflict with those of strong pressure groups.
14. It's not always wise for me to plan too far ahead because many things turn out to be a matter of good or bad fortune.
15. Getting what I want requires pleasing those people above me.
16. Whether or not I get to be a leader depends on whether I'm lucky enough to be in the right place at the right time.
17. If important people were to decide they didn't like me, I probably wouldn't make many friends.
18. I can pretty much determine what will happen in my life.
19. I am usually able to protect my personal interests.
20. Whether or not I get into a car accident depends mostly on the other driver.
21. When I get what I want, it's usually because I worked hard for it.
22. In order to have my plans work, I make sure that they fit in with the desires of people who have power over me.
23. My life is determined by my own actions.
24. It's usually a matter of fate whether or not I have a few friends or many friends.

Scoring procedures for the I, P, and C scales

There are three separate scales used to measure one's locus of control: Internal scale, Powerful Others scale, and Chance scale. There are eight items on each of the three scales. To score each scale add up your answers to the items appropriate for that scale. (These items are listed below.) Add to this sum +24. (This removes the possibility of negative scores.) The possible range on each scale is from 0 to 48. Theoretically, a person could score high or low on all three dimensions. The higher the score on a scale, the more inclined the individual is to believe in that particular form of control.

Scale	Items
Internal scale	(1, 4, 5, 9, 18, 19, 21, 23)
Powerful Others scale	(3, 8, 11, 13, 15, 17, 20, 22)
Chance scale	(2, 6, 7, 10, 12, 14, 16, 24)

Figure 25–5. Levenson locus of control scale. *(From Levenson H. Activism and powerful others: distinction within the concept of internal–external control.* J Personality Assess. *1974;38:381–382.)*

Your life is probably characterized by many different behaviors. To learn how you spend your time, indicate how frequently you engage in each of the behaviors listed in the inventory, using the following time distinctions:

Never: Under no circumstances do you ever engage in the behavior.
Rarely: You engage in the behavior a few times a year.
Periodically: You engage in the behavior a few times a month.
Regularly: You engage in the behavior several times a week.
Always: You engage in the behavior every time an opportunity presents itself.

Rate your response in the right column with the answer that *best* corresponds to your level of participation in each behavior by using the following points: 0 = never; 1 = rarely; 2 = periodically; 3 = regularly; and 4 = always.

Behavior	Rate
1. Filing work materials	______
2. Rambling in conversation	______
3. Flossing my teeth	______
4. Creating art objects	______
5. Overextending myself in work commitments	______
6. Keeping my word	______
7. Using hard drugs	______
8. Attending art and cultural exhibits	______
9. Attaining work goals	______
10. Criticizing others behind their backs	______
11. Getting adequate rest at night	______
12. Playing a musical instrument	______
13. Jumping from one task to another	______
14. Initiating conversation	______
15. Eating excessively	______
16. Attending concerts	______
17. Completing work assignments on time	______
18. Interrupting others during conversation	______
19. Participating in vigorous physical activity	______
20 Writing creatively (e.g., poetry, short stories)	______
21. Putting off unpleasant, but necessary, tasks	______

Behavior	Rate
22. Listening closely to others' comments	______
23. Smoking cigarettes	______
24. Reading leisurely (e.g., poetry, fiction, magazines)	______
25. Setting working goals	______
26. Dominating conversation	______
27. Drinking water	______
28. Gardening/working in the yard	______
29. Losing work-related materials	______
30. Encouraging others	______
31. Eating junk food	______
32. Engaging in outdoor nature activities	______
33. Reading course/ professionally related materials	______
34. Reprimanding others	______
35. Doing stretching exercises	______
36. Engaging in a hobby not otherwise listed in questionnaire	______
37. Failing to meet deadlines	______
38. Showing affection towards others	______
39. Gulping meals	______
40. Dancing	______

Scoring Instructions: Give yourself 0 to 4 points credit for never-to-always responses to the positive items, and subtract 0 to 4 points for the never-to-always reponses to the negative items. Total your scores within each of the four areas outlined below. If you gave very few never or always responses, don't be alarmed. We consider the other catagories more realistic alternatives for most individuals.

Work

+ Items	*Positive credit*	*− Items*	*Subtraction points*
1	______	5	______
9	______	13	______
17	______	21	______
25	______	29	______
33	______	37	______
Total A	______	Total B	______

Subtract B from A to get your work self-management score.

Social

+ Items	*Positive credit*	*− Items*	*Subtraction points*
8	______	2	______
14	______	10	______
22	______	18	______
30	______	26	______
38	______	34	______
Total A	______	Total B	______

Subtract B from A to get your social self-management score.

Health

+ Items	*Positive credit*	*− Items*	*Subtraction points*
3	______	7	______
11	______	15	______
19	______	23	______
27	______	31	______
35	______	39	______
Total A	______	Total B	______

Subtract B from A to get your health self-management score.

Leisure activities

All + Items			
4	______	24	______
8	______	28	______
12	______	32	______
16	______	36	______
20	______	40	______
Total A	______	Total B	______

Subtract B from A to get your leisure activity score. Because this subscale contains only positive items, one can score twice as high in this area. For comparison with other subscales, we suggest that you divide by 2 your leisure activities' total.

Figure 25–6. Self-description form. *(From Williams RL, Long JD.* Toward a Self-management Life Style. *3rd ed. Boston: Houghton Mifflin; 1983. Adapted from a presentation by Sandra Thomas, Damaris Olsen, and Robert Williams on "The Development of a Naturalistic Self-management Inventory" at the American Education Research Association, New York, 1982.)*

strengths. Another way is to review situations or actions that generally elicit others' compliments. Compliments from others serve to highlight personal resources that an individual may have come to take for granted.[70] Realizing personal resources is a way to maintain confidence during the process of personal change.

Assessing the influence of the environment is part of resource assessment. Environmental events strongly affect behavior. Identifying setting events, that is, events that set the stage for a particular response, is helpful. For example, a person might notice that he eats more when eating alone than when eating with friends. Eating with friends and eating alone are different setting events for eating behavior. Awareness of setting events and response patterns is helpful in devising an action plan.

- *Establishing baselines.* To judge progress in behavior change, it is necessary to quantify the targeted behaviors, setting events, and consequences of the behaviors over a period of time. This appraisal acts as the baseline for future analysis. For several days or a week, one counts and records how many times or how long the target behavior is repeated in the course of a day. By recording what happens immediately before or after a target behavior occurs, one also can establish the setting events and consequences of that behavior. For example, an individual who is trying to quit smoking would count the number of cigarettes smoked over a period of several days, and also would note the conditions surrounding smoking. Was he or she conversing with others, drinking coffee, or working at the computer while smoking? Did reward or reinforcement accompany any of these activities and, by association, reward smoking? Recording for a week allows an individual to see cycles in personal behavior. The frequencies and patterns are useful to set realistic goals for change.
- *Writing goals.* Self-management experts advocate writing goal lists. Successful people have been found to be more likely to use "to-do" lists than unsuccessful people. Williams and Long recommend breaking down overall priorities into manageable, measurable, daily and weekly objectives. For example, if physical fitness is a long-term priority, the daily objective list would specify a particular physical activity and note the expected duration.

Some goals can be difficult to quantify, for example, reducing anxiety. To quantify such a goal, a person might consider the ways he or she expresses anxiety or what things anxiety prevents them from doing. If anxiety prevents a person from speaking up in a group, a corresponding daily objective could be to make one comment per day in a group setting.

Effective goals are achievable, but they should also provide a challenge. When goals are set too high, they are likely to be dropped; when they are set too low, they provide no stimulation.[70] What represents a challenge varies from individual to individual. Williams and Long suggest that when an individual consistently meets a goal, the level of expectation can be increased.

DEVELOPING AN ACTION PLAN

- *Task analysis.* After establishing goals, an appraisal of strategies or activities to attain them is necessary to create a workable action plan. This process is called task analysis. For example, to accomplish the task of speaking up in a group setting, one needs to consider how to prepare for speaking up. It may be easier to speak at the beginning of a group session than later. Or a person may decide to make a list of appropriate comments to make in the group.

For some goals, activities must also be scheduled. Activities can be grouped and sequenced in such a way as to make them easier to accomplish. Factors to consider are the number of activities and personal energy level.

- *Arranging environmental support.* One object of self-management is to make social influences and external physical events work with one's inner resources rather than in opposition to them.[70] One can reduce the inhibiting impact of some environmental setting events on goal attainment by arranging for social support—asking a friend to provide a cue to help you stay "on track." Avoiding or altering a particular physical environment to minimize the likelihood that it will stimulate an undesirable target behavior is also effective. The internal environment—one's personal thoughts—can contribute to meeting goals for change or can interfere. Many people engage in negative internal dialogue that inhibits success. Consciously changing this internal script to positive, self-encouraging messages is a useful strategy.
- *Arranging helpful consequences.* An important step in self-management is arranging for immediate consequences that reinforce good habits. First, examine target behaviors for intrinsic reinforcers, that is, the natural reinforcement they offer. When these are insufficient, external reinforcers can be added. Pairing enjoyable activities with a desired target behavior, for example, increases the likelihood of repeating the behavior.[70] Joggers wear headsets so that they can listen to music, which makes the activity of jogging more enjoyable, for example.

EVALUATING PROGRESS AND MAINTAINING IMPROVEMENTS

- *Record keeping.* Keeping accurate records of target behaviors while implementing the action plan is important because it lets individuals see what they have accomplished each day and what remains to be accomplished. For most behavior changes, frequency counting is effective. This involves counting a target behavior or some element within it and totaling the number of these events for a day. For example, a jogger might count the number of blocks or miles completed each day. Plotting each day's total on a graph provides a visual display. If the graph shows improvement, it is a form of reinforcement. If not, analyzing the graph can generate possibilities for revising goals or strategies.

Another record-keeping method is product assessment. If the target behavior involves producing a product of some sort, a person who wishes to improve job performance can keep track of tasks, jobs, or projects completed each day to evaluate output increases. Product output can also be graphed cumulatively to show an individual that he or she is accomplishing change goals.

For records to be useful, they must be accurate. Records that are made several hours after a behavior are likely to be inaccurate. On the other hand, some behaviors do not lend themselves to on-the-spot recording. If having a paper and pencil ready is impossible, a wrist counter can be an alternative.

- *Creating internal rewards.* Williams and Long emphasize that long-term success of any self-management program requires that one learn to shift from artificial support to natural support.[70] This needs to be done gradually. The first task is to analyze whether any of the strategies of the action plan should become a permanent part of one's daily routine. For an individual with a tendency to overeat, it may be important to eliminate the cookie jar indefinitely. Another strategy is to find substitutions for artificial rewards. Self-approval statements can be substituted for frequency counts and graph recording. Once self-management has been applied successfully in one life area, most people are able to apply the method to other areas of their lives as they decide to make changes.

Home Health Care

Preventive care in the home encompasses all of the above implementations. Nurses have unique opportunities when providing home care to observe elements of patients' social and physical environments. This information makes possible more personalized education about stress management and self-management. Also, interacting with patients in their homes enables nurses to make informed inferences about patients' environment and lifestyle habits that enhance optimal well-being or place them or their families at risk. While reinforcing and supporting healthful choices, nurses can participate with patients and families in collaborative planning to reduce risks.

SUPPORTIVE CARE

Supportive care focuses on patients who are exhibiting early changes in health status. Physiologic alterations (eg, diminishing eyesight due to a cataract) and psychological alterations (such as fear of blindness) are present; however, patients are coping with the changes and continue to function in a fairly independent manner. These patients often receive care at home or in an outpatient setting. They are sometimes admitted to a hospital for diagnostic testing such as tumor biopsy or minor surgery such as a cataract extraction. A new trend called telehealth is an innovation that permits nurses or other care providers to monitor and advise patients remotely.[71] Telehealth uses computer-based telecommunications equipment. Currently basic assessments such as weight and blood pressure checks can easily be accomplished through telehealth. As technology develops, more complex assessments will become possible.[71]

The goals of supportive care are to correct or improve current problems and prevent more serious disruptions in patients' health. Minor health alterations often motivate patients to develop lifestyle and behaviors more conducive to health. The major categories of supportive care are promoting patient self-responsibility, empowering patients during health care experiences, maintaining comfort and safety, and managing fever.

Promoting Self-responsibility

Entering the health care system, whether as an outpatient or inpatient, may elicit a passive, dependent attitude. Also, although many patients are able to function independently, their daily routines are frequently dictated by physicians' orders or organizational policy. Patients who are used to caring for themselves often find accepting assistance difficult. To promote patient well-being, nurses support self-responsibility by promoting patients' abilities to maintain, restore, or increase involvement in self-care.

This focus requires nurses to examine care routines in light of patient needs and abilities, especially in inpatient settings. For example, nurses generally administer all medications to patients according to an institutional schedule. This schedule does not usually take into consideration the medication schedule patients used at home, nor the fact that many are capable of continuing to manage their medications without nursing assistance. To promote self-responsibility, a nurse could explore self-medication regimens for appropriate patients. Nurses can also involve patients in other aspects of care. Teaching patients how to do procedures such as simple dressing changes, certain irrigations, and mobility exercises are examples. Enhancing patient understanding of their condition and prescribed treatments can decrease anxiety and fear and promote self-confidence and feelings of self-efficacy.

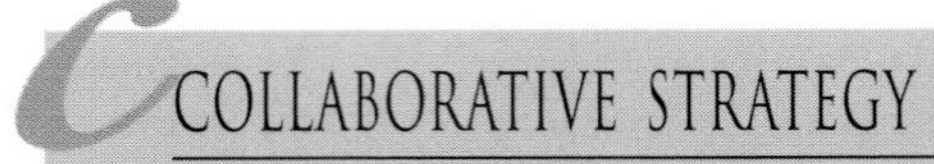

COLLABORATIVE STRATEGY

SELF-CARE

The collaborative philosophy centers on self-responsibility. It acknowledges patients' capacity for self-care and endorses active patient participation in preventive and therapeutic measures.

Promoting self-care should also include family members. Family participation in patient care, not only aids patients' recovery, but also helps family members to feel they are making a positive contribution to their loved one's well-being. Increasing family understanding and involvement also fosters the development of a supportive home environment that enhances patient wellness and participation in prescribed treatments after discharge.

Promoting self-responsibility sometimes requires taking on the role of "patient advocate." Institutional rules and routines are often intimidating. Not all patients who would benefit from taking more responsibility for their care and desire to maintain maximal independence can accomplish this on their own. Interceding on behalf of patients whose needs conflict with established routines demands courage and commitment, but can make a significant impact on recovery from disease and overall well-being.

Informed Consent. **Informed consent** is voluntary, educated participation in a therapeutic regimen. It is central to self-responsibility. Patients have the right to refuse or consent to proposed diagnostic or therapeutic measures based on clear information from health care providers. The information should include a description of the treatment, the expected benefits, possible risks, and any alternative treatments or procedures that might be available. In most states, the law requires that written consent to procedures considered to be invasive be obtained and placed in patients' charts.

For patients' consent to be valid, three conditions must be met: (1) patients must be capable of giving consent; (2) patients must have received sufficient information necessary to make an intelligent decision; and (3) the consent must be voluntarily given—not coerced.

Primary responsibility for informing patients and obtaining consent for treatment rests with the prescriber, usually a physician. However, nurses often play an important supportive role in educating patients and clarifying information. Frequently, nurses are asked to witnesses a patient's signature. In both situations, nurses should assess patients' capability, understanding, and willingness to proceed with the planned procedure. If patients express doubts or hesitation, even after signing a consent form, notify the physician so he or she can verify that the consent is still valid. Legal and ethical considerations related to informed consent are discussed further in Chaps. 2 and 6.

Advance Directives. Nurses can also promote self-responsibility by initiating discussion with patients about advance directives. **Advance directives** communicate a person's preferences about specific health care treatments and designate a person to make health care decisions on their behalf, should they become unable to do so. They are legally binding documents, which usually include a Durable Power of Attorney for Health Care (see also Chap. 2). Health care providers use advance directives in lieu of informed consent when a person's condition makes informed consent impossible to obtain. Although no one is required to prepare an advance directive, some states mandate that health care givers inform patients about their right to have one. This is often done by clerical personnel at the time of admission to a health care facility. For many patients this may be the first time they have heard of such a document. They may need clarification of its significance and an opportunity to explore their feelings about its meaning with a person who is not so emotionally involved in the decisions as a family member might be. Nurses' knowledge and communication skills make them an ideal resource to facilitate patient self-responsibility in this important decision.

Empowering Patients During Health Care Experiences

Anxiety and fear are common reactions when anticipating health care experiences. Admission to a health care facility, diagnostic tests, and surgical procedures are stressful events for many patients and their families. Empathy and respect from caregivers and sufficient information to facilitate knowledgeable participation and decision making enables patients to cope effectively and attain maximum benefit from health care experiences.

Admission to a Health Care Facility. Being admitted to an inpatient facility for diagnosis or treatment of a health problem is often a significant event. There are many unknowns and many potentially negative outcomes. Caregivers' demeanor during admission procedures influences patients' perceptions of the entire care experience.

Generally, unless it is an emergency admission, preliminary information including personal data (name, address, date of birth, next of kin, religion), the reason for admission, physician's name, and expected form of payment is gathered by the admitting office prior to the admission to the nursing unit. Patients are also asked to sign a general consent to treatment form, which permits the health care facility to provide routine care.

Nursing assistants are usually responsible for preparing patient rooms and assisting patients to bed. Prior to a patient's arrival, a bath basin, water pitcher, bedpan or urinal, emesis basin, towels, and hospital gown are placed in the room. Supplies for oxygen administration, suctioning, or other special needs are arranged for immediate use when specified by admission orders. The bed controls, lighting, call bell, oxygen, and suctioning apparatus are checked to ensure that they function properly. The bed should be adjusted to its lowest position unless a patient is arriving by stretcher. Then, high position is best. The bedspread, blanket, and top sheet are folded to the foot of the bed.

Nurses' first opportunity to interact with patients is usually the admission assessment. It is important to remember that for many patients, a hospital has many negative connotations. It is unfamiliar and associated with illness. A friendly, supportive attitude that conveys interest and consideration for patients' needs helps to allay anxiety. Soliciting immediate concerns and promptly attending to them facilitates a sense of security and initiates a trusting nurse–patient relationship. Guidelines for admitting patients to a health care facility can be found in Clinical Guideline 25–3.

Preparing Patients for Diagnostic Tests. Diagnostic tests are frightening experiences for many people. They may fear the pain or discomfort associated with the test, or experience anxiety about what the results may show. An accurate explanation of the procedure eases patients' concerns. Sensory information—how something looks, feels, sounds, and so on—is most useful. When discussing diagnostic tests, consider patients' current level of understanding and how much they need or want to know. Use the following guidelines:

- Give objective information such as where the test will take place, who will do it, how long it will last, and when the results will be available.
- Describe physical sensations, but do not evaluate them. For example, tell patients that they will feel a burning or stinging sensation, but not that it will be "intense" or "unbearable."
- Explain the causes of the sensations.
- Prepare patients only for those aspects of the experience that are noted by most patients. Overpreparation increases fear and anxiety.

Knowing what to expect helps patients mentally prepare for the experience and diminishes misinterpretation or fears that something has gone wrong.

CLINICAL GUIDELINE 25–3

ADMITTING PATIENTS TO A HEALTH CARE FACILITY

1. Introduce yourself to the patient and significant others who are present. Briefly discuss what the admission procedure involves. Introduce the patient to other patients in the room and any other staff members present. No one should be in the patient's immediate environment without introducing themselves and explaining their purpose for being there.
2. Explain and demonstrate the use of the equipment in the patient's area: nurse call system, overhead lighting, bed controls, overbed table, telephone system, and television controls. Show location of bathroom and showers, and available closet or storage space.
3. Place an identification bracelet on the patient's wrist and explain its purpose.
4. Provide information about normal daily routines: mealtimes, visiting hours and restrictions, and smoking regulations. Describe other areas of the facility that the patient or family members may use, such as the cafeteria, lounges, chapel, or gift shops.
5. Inform the patient of agency policies regarding valuables and personal articles. Treat personal articles with respect and store valuables such as money, jewelry, and keys in a secure manner following agency procedures.
6. Obtain and record a nursing and health history. Augment standard admission history/examination forms as needed according to patient condition. Post allergy alerts in appropriate places if needed.
7. Encourage the patient and family members to ask questions and clarify needed information.
8. Begin implementing physician's admitting orders.

The extent of physical preparation depends on the diagnostic test ordered. Some tests, such as a chest x-ray, require only a simple explanation. However, other studies require more extensive preparation measures such as dietary restrictions, bowel preparation, or sedation. Many diagnostic procedures are performed on an outpatient basis. This means that patients are responsible for some aspects of the preparation. Verify that they are adequately informed of the purpose and rationale of the ordered preparation. Written instructions are beneficial and help to avoid misunderstandings. To avoid invalid or inaccurate results, determine whether patients have followed preparation instructions properly before the test is begun.

Preparing Patients for Surgery. Preparing patients for surgery has many similarities to preparing patients for diagnostic procedures. Preoperative patient education, emotional support, and exact physical preparation measures significantly decrease the time of recovery from surgery and the incidence of postoperative complications. Physical preparation varies with the type of procedure. It is specified in detail in admitting orders. Some elements may be completed prior to admission.

Information about preoperative sedation, usual duration of surgery, and the sensations to expect during recovery assists most patients to prepare emotionally for pending surgery. In addition, preoperative education should emphasize pain management options and the postoperative activities necessary to decrease postoperative complications. Repeatedly encouraging patients to voice concerns throughout teaching is a way of normalizing fears that most people have about surgery, but that they may feel are inappropriate for adults to express. Preoperative teaching enables patients to become active participants in postoperative care and enhances individual well-being by fostering personal control. A detailed discussion of perioperative patient care appears later in this chapter in the section Restorative Care.

Home Health Care

Emphasis on self-responsibility is central to supportive care in a home setting. Supporting well-being for those with early or transient changes in health status focuses on promoting comfort and safety and managing fevers.

Promoting Comfort. Many patients needing supportive care experience mild to moderate pain related to their health problem(s). Effective pain control contributes significantly to physical and emotional well-being. Mild pain, although not debilitating or overwhelming, can limit activities, interfere with rest and sleep, and make individuals feel irritable and unpleasant. The main objective in management of mild pain is to assist patients to reduce their own pain. Nurses support self-responsibility in management of mild pain by educating patients regarding nonpharmacologic measures they can use independently to promote comfort. The relaxation and guided imagery techniques discussed earlier are effective pain control techniques. Relaxation not only reduces muscle tension and anxiety but also draws the individual's attention from the pain and provides a sense of personal control.

Positioning and movement are effective comfort measures. Patients often believe that movement will enhance pain. They are surprised that a change of position or mild exercise, such as walking in pleasant surroundings, promotes comfort instead. When counseling patients about position changes, emphasize the importance of maintaining correct anatomic alignment and providing extra pillows to support joints and extremities. More specific information about exercise and positioning is found in Chap. 33.

Hygiene measures also greatly contribute to physical comfort. Besides their cleansing effect, bathing, shampooing hair, shaving, and oral care enhance self-esteem, stimulate circulation, and promote feeling refreshed and relaxed. Applying heat or cold, distraction, and cutaneous stimulation also are effective in managing mild pain. Use of these measures and a detailed discussion of managing moderate and severe pain can be found in Chap. 32.

Enhancing Safety. Patient safety is influenced by personal safety awareness. Individuals receiving supportive care at home may need education regarding potential home and treatment-related safety hazards, particularly if there has been a recent change in health status. Patients can self-manage treatments such as application or heat or cold, for example, but the treatments pose hazards that nurses should call to patients' attention. Some patients have special safety needs. Patients with visual or auditory impairments may be unable to perceive a potential danger. Patients with impaired mobility are at risk because they often need assistive devices or support from another person. They may be unable to maintain basic personal and household cleanliness, creating increased risk for disease. See also Clinical Guideline 33–2 for a mobility-related safety assessment. Those needing oxygen therapy in the home need to be especially aware of fire safety precautions. If electrical devices are needed as part of a home treatment regimen, the wiring may need upgrading to prevent electrical overload and risk of fire. Smoke detectors throughout the home are especially important in these situations. Clinical Guideline 25–4 summarizes a home safety check nurses and patients can perform.

Managing Fever. Fever is an elevation in body temperature caused by disease. Temperature elevation usually produces a sensation of chilliness with shivering due to vasoconstriction. Fever also stimulates sweating to transfer heat from the body via evaporation. With fever, the body's metabolic rate and rate of oxygen consumption increase. Pulse and respiratory rates increase. Energy reserves are depleted, causing lethargy.

Fever is one of the body's defense mechanisms. Fever between 37 and 38C (98.6 and 100.4F) helps to activate the body's immune system by stimulating antibody production. Antibodies work best at temperatures higher than normal, and microorganism growth is inhibited. For these reasons, low-grade fevers are not always treated. However, if body temperature elevates to 41C (105F), the rate of cellular metabolism increases so much that the body's regulatory mechanisms can no longer overcome the rate of heat production. High fever can have serious complications, including brain damage. These fevers require medical treatment.

Therapy for low-grade and high fevers is similar. It consists of fluids, antipyretics, and comfort measures. When a specific organism can be identified as the cause, antibiotics are used as well. With low-grade fevers, these therapies are managed at home by patients. Nurses can facilitate self-management of fevers by reviewing with patients the points in Clinical Guideline 25–5.

RESTORATIVE CARE

Patients requiring restorative care are experiencing significant threats to well-being. The care setting is usually an inpatient health care facility, or in some situations, patients' homes. Nursing care involves measures to support or restore functioning altered by dis-

CLINICAL GUIDELINE 25–4

HOME SAFETY CHECK

FIRE SAFETY

- Is there at least one smoke detector on each floor? Does family test each monthly?
- Does the family have a plan for escape in case of fire?
- Does the family have fire extinguishers suitable for all types of fires available in risk areas such as kitchen and garage? Are extinguishers checked and recharged regularly?
- Are all flammable liquids stored in safe containers (UL or FM certified) away from sources of heat or flame?
- Do family members know how to safely light pilot lights on all gas appliances?
- Do all fireplaces have screens?
- Are areas in which candles are used free from drafts? Away from curtains or other highly flammable items?
- Do family members avoid using aerosols near open flames?
- Are all portable heaters designed to resist tipping and equipped with automatic shut-off switches that activate if the heater is not upright?
- Are cooking areas (range, exhaust hoods, ducts) free of grease? Are grease containers stored away from the stove?
- Are kitchen towel racks positioned so towels are not near burners?
- Is there sufficient space for air circulation around major appliances (eg, TV, refrigerator, microwave)?
- Are electrical cords and plugs in good repair? Located away from traffic patterns?
- Do all extension cords have proper capacity for the tools/appliances used with them?
- Are outlets free from "octopus" cords/connections?
- Do family members know how to replace fuses or reactivate a circuit breaker if a circuit overload occurs?
- If family members smoke, are there adequate ashtrays? Are they emptied frequently? Do smokers refrain from smoking in bed?

EARTHQUAKE SAFETY

- Is there a 3- to 5-day supply of water (1 gal/person/day) in unbreakable containers stored on low shelves in a cool, dark area? Is the supply replaced every 6 months?
- Is there a source of extra water for cooking, hygiene, pets?
- Is there a 3- to 5-day supply of canned foods? A manual can opener?
- Is there a flashlight in every bedroom as well as extra lights and batteries?
- Do all family members have hard-soled shoes stored near their bed to prevent injuries from broken glass?
- Does the family have a battery-operated radio and ample batteries?
- Are crescent and pipe wrenches available to turn off gas and/or water lines? Do family members know how to do this?
- Is tall, heavy furniture secured to walls? Do cabinets have positive catching latches?
- Is water heater strapped? Other heavy appliances (especially gas powered) secured to walls?
- Are pictures hung with closed hooks attached to wooden studs?
- Is there a well-equipped first-aid kit in a secure location? An extra supply of critical medicines?
- Do family members know safe spots in each room to go to during a quake? Dangerous spots to avoid? Do they have earthquake drills?

HOME SECURITY

- Do exterior doors have deadbolts?
- Is there a through-door viewer to scrutinize visitors before opening the door?
- Are window locks secure?
- Do sliding doors have supplementary locking devices (such as a "pin" connecting the two doors or an aluminum bar in the track) and devices to prevent their being lifted off their tracks?
- Is there at least a 60-watt bulb lighting every exterior door? Floodlights with motion detectors on opposite corners of the house and over the garage are even better.
- Are there timers for lights, radios, TV so these can be irregularly turned on when family is away?
- Does family stop delivery of newspapers and mail or have a neighbor collect them when away?
- Do all family members lock all doors upon leaving or when working in the yard?

FALL PREVENTION

- See Clinical Guideline 33–2: Home Assessment for Barriers to Mobility.

ease and to assist with activities of daily living that patients are unable to perform independently. Although nurses assume more responsibility for patient's needs than in preventive or supportive care, promoting patient involvement through education, mutual goal setting, and cooperative planning of care is important to well-being. Nursing interventions that promote patients' beliefs in their own capability to deal with a current health problem facilitate shared responsibility for achieving the highest level of wellness possible. Five broad categories of restorative care are presented here: maintaining a safe physical environment, infection control, perioperative nursing care, administering medications, and restorative care in a home setting.

CLINICAL GUIDELINE 25–5

HOME MANAGEMENT OF FEVER

MONITOR TEMPERATURE REGULARLY

- Check temperature at least every 4 hours while awake, more frequently if temperature is over 103F (39.5C) or continues to rise with each check.
- If antipyretics such as aspirin or acetaminophen (Tylenol) are prescribed, check temperature again within 1 hour after taking the medication.
- Consult your health care provider:
  - If the fever does not respond to antipyretic
  - If the fever rises to 105F (41C)

PROMOTE HEAT LOSS

- During chills, which may precede onset of fever, an extra blanket helps maintain comfort.
- Remove blankets and outer clothing when feeling warm.
- Reduce room temperature with cool circulating air.
- Apply a cool washcloth to the forehead.
- If fever is high:
  - Give a sponge bath with tepid (21.1 to 29.1C or 70 to 85F) water to reduce the body's surface temperature. Do not bathe for more than 30 minutes.
  - Keep the bathed body part exposed to cool air circulating in the room.
  - Apply an icebag to the head during the bath to relieve headache.
  - Apply cold wet compresses on the neck, groin, and axilla to promote cooling of large superficial blood vessels.

LIMIT ACTIVITY

INCREASE INTAKE OF FLUIDS AND FOOD

- Drink at least 3 quarts of fluids a day to replace fluids lost due to increased metabolism.
- If dry mouth persists, brush teeth or rinse with mouthwash.
- Eat light, but balanced meals to provide needed calories to compensate for increased metabolism during fever.

Maintaining a Safe Physical Environment

Safety for acutely ill or debilitated patients is an important nursing responsibility. When patients feel physically safe, they are able to relax and rest while focusing energy on getting well. Safety risks of concern to nurses include fires, falls, and electrical shock.

Fire. The hospital and home environments are always at risk for fires. The most common cause of institutional fires is faulty electrical equipment. All electrical equipment used in health care facilities must be properly grounded, with cords and plugs in good condition. Extension cords are unacceptable. Special fire safety precautions are needed when oxygen therapy is used in patient care. Chapter 30 provides more information on oxygen safety measures.

In the past, smoking was a contributing cause of hospital fires. Now, smoking is not permitted in most health care facilities. Some permit smoking in a few designated areas. All regulations should be clearly explained to all hospitalized patients and family members and should be strictly enforced. Providing adequate ashtrays in smoking areas and the proper disposal of ashes and used matches can help to prevent trash-can fires.

In the event of an institutional fire, nurses have three priorities: (1) to notify authorities of the existence and location of the fire, (2) to protect patients from injury, and (3) to attempt to contain the fire if it poses no immediate threat to patients or self. Health care agencies must have fire extinguishers prominently displayed throughout the facility and established procedures to be followed in emergency situations. Nurses should become familiar with the fire and evacuation policies of their employing institutions and participate in agency fire drills.

Falls. Seriously ill patients are at risk for falls because of altered body function and some aspects of their treatment regimen. The unfamiliar environment of an acute care setting enhances the risk of falls among all hospitalized patients, but falls are the greatest threat for elderly or debilitated patients. Broken bones due to falls are more common in older patients, whose bones have lost density.

Prevention of falls begins with identifying patients at risk for falling. Research indicates the following risk factors[72–74]:

- Altered mental status (confusion, disorientation, uncontrolled restlessness, sedation)
- Cognitive impairment
- Limited hearing or vision, change in vision
- Cervical disc disease, peripheral nerve problems
- Poor balance, poor muscle strength, gait abnormalities, foot disorders
- Physical inactivity, prolonged bed rest, restraints
- More than one disease, use of many medications (polypharmacy)
- Orthostatic hypotension, antihypertensive medications
- Elimination problems: incontinence, urgency, indwelling catheter
- History of falls
- Ill-fitting footwear

Patients who have just had surgery or who are in severe pain for any other reason need close observation or assistance with mobility. Nursing measures to prevent falls are outlined in Clinical Guideline 25–6.

Electrical Shock. The body's natural defense against electrical shock is dry, intact skin. All electrical equipment emits a low-level leakage current, which normally is undetectable by individuals in contact with the equipment. However, in the presence of moisture, including sweat, urine, or wet dressings or when the skin surface is broken, the skin is a less effective barrier. Under these conditions even minor leakage current can produce substantial electrical injury. The following safety measures reduce electrical hazards:

- Keep patients and bed linens dry.
- Use only grounded electrical devices.
- Check cords for fraying or other signs of damage before using. Do not use if damage is evident.
- Do not use extension cords.
- Always pull a plug from the wall outlet by firmly grasping the plug and pulling straight out. Never remove a plug from an outlet by pulling on the cord.
- Avoid overloading outlets.
- Do not touch the bed, patient, or any device attached to the patient when plugging in electrical equipment.
- Report loose or broken electrical receptacles to the engineering department.
- Report any shocks experienced while using equipment. Send equipment to engineering department for assessment and repair.
- Check all patients' personal electrical appliances through engineering department for safe functioning.

Infection Control

In the past, infection control focused on preventing the spread of microorganisms from individuals who were exhibiting manifestations of infection. The term *medical asepsis* was used to describe measures that limit the growth and/or spread of microorganisms. Objects were identified as clean or dirty. *Clean* objects were considered to harbor microorganisms, but not pathogens. *Dirty* or *contaminated* objects were considered to carry microorganisms capable of causing disease. Various isolation protocols were used to protect patients and caregivers from infectious patients or contact with dirty items.

More recently, it has become apparent that pathogens are transmitted, not only from symptomatic individuals, but also from asymptomatic individuals whose body substances (blood, wound drainage, feces, urine, airway secretions) contain infectious agents. As a result, in the 1980s several new infection control recommendations were released. The most commonly used were *Universal Precautions* (UP) developed by the CDC and *Body Substance Isolation* (BSI), developed by infection control experts in two West Coast hospitals.

Infection Precautions. As of 1996, still newer guidelines have been released by HICPAC in collaboration with the CDC.[64] These guidelines supercede all prior guidelines, but may take some time to be fully implemented. Although the guidelines specify hospitals as the location in which they are to be used, many infection control experts suggest that they are applicable to other types of settings.[75–77] The new guidelines contain two levels of precautions. The first, **Standard Precautions** are to be used in care of all patients. They are a blending of the former UP and BSI. The second level, called **Transmission Based Precautions,** are to be used in addition to standard precautions for patients documented or suspected to be infected with highly transmissible pathogens. The usual mode of transmission of the suspected organism(s) is the basis for transmission-based precautions.[64] (See Clinical Guideline 25–7, Significant Routes of Microorganism Transmission, and Table 25–9, Infection Control Measures). Figure 25–7 shows supplies for transmission-based precautions.

CLINICAL GUIDELINE 25–6

NURSING MEASURES TO PREVENT FALLS

- Assign high-risk patients to rooms near the nursing station for close observation.
- Alert all health care providers to patient's "at risk" status (eg, Kardex and chart notations; signs over bed, outside patients' room, or near intercom console at nurses' station).
- Keep beds in low position except while giving care.
- Emphasize to patient and family members the importance of seeking assistance for ambulation or transfers.
- Make sure call light or bell is within easy reach and remind patient where it is before leaving the room.
- Answer all calls promptly and courteously.
- Place all personal items, TV controls, etc, within easy reach.
- Observe patients frequently.
- Provide well-fitting nonskid footwear.
- Schedule frequent toileting or provide a bedside commode.
- Arrange furniture and equipment to allow clear walkways free of obstacles to the bathroom and door.
- Instruct patients in the correct use of ambulatory aids such as canes, crutches, or walkers.
- Provide frequent comfort measures (position changes, pain relief).
- Provide psychosocial stimulation (companionship, recreational activities).

CLINICAL GUIDELINE 25–7

SIGNIFICANT ROUTES OF MICROORGANISM TRANSMISSION IN NOSOCOMIAL INFECTIONS

CONTACT TRANSMISSION

The most frequent mode of transmission. It has two subgroups:

- **Direct Contact:** Direct body surface to body surface contact that permits physical transfer of microorganisms between a susceptible host and an infected or colonized person.
- **Indirect Contact:** Physical contact of a susceptible host with an intermediate object, such as instruments, gloves, or unwashed hands that have been contaminated by contact with an infected or colonized person.

DROPLET TRANSMISSION

- Droplets containing microorganisms are generated by an infectious person, propelled a short distance through the air (eg, by a cough, sneeze, talking, or during suctioning), and deposited on a host's conjunctiva, nasal mucosa, or mouth. Droplets are not suspended in the air, which distinguishes droplet from airborne transmission.

AIRBORNE TRANSMISSION

- Dissemination by air currents of droplet nuclei (small particles of 5 microns or less), evaporated droplets, or dust particles containing microorganisms that are inhaled by susceptible hosts. The microorganism containing particles remain suspended in the air for long periods of time and can be disseminated widely.

Adapted from Garner JS, the Hospital Infection Control Practices Advisory Committee. Guideline for isolation precautions in hospitals. *Infect Control Hosp Epidemiol.* 1996;17: 53–80.

TABLE 25-9. INFECTION CONTROL MEASURES

		Transmission-based Precautions		
	Standard Precautions	*Airborne Precautions*	*Droplet Precautions*	*Contact Precautions*
Purpose	Prevent transmission of microorganisms from all sources of infection.	Prevent transmission of infectious agents contained in small droplet particles or dust.	Prevent transmission of infectious agents contained in large droplets.	Prevent transmission of infectious agents by direct or indirect contact.
Room	Private room is indicated if patient hygiene is poor.	Private room with special ventilation. Door should be kept closed. In general, persons infected with the same organism can share a room. There are additional special precautions for preventing transmission of tuberculosis.	Private room is indicated. In general, persons with the same organism can share a room. Maintain 3-foot separation between infected person and other persons.	Same as Droplet Precautions.
Gowns	Indicated to protect skin and prevent soiling of clothing by splashes or sprays of blood, body fluids, secretions, or excretions.	Same as Standard Precautions.	Same as Standard Precautions.	Indicated for all persons entering the room.
Masks and eye protection	Indicated for activities that are likely to generate splashes or sprays by blood, body fluids, secretions, or excretions.	Indicated for all persons entering room of patient with tuberculosis.	Indicated when working within 3 feet of the patient.	Same as Standard Precautions.
Gloves	Indicated when touching blood, body fluids, secretions or excretions, and contaminated items. Also, when touching mucous membranes and nonintact skin. Apply immediately before contact. Remove promptly.	Same as Standard Precautions.	Same as Standard Precautions.	Indicated for all persons entering the room.
Handwashing	Wash hands after touching blood, body fluids, secretions or excretions, and contaminated items; also after removing gloves and between patient contact.	Same as Standard Precautions.	Same as Standard Precautions.	Same as Standard Precautions.
Patient care equipment	Contaminated articles should not contact skin, mucous membranes, or clothing, or be transferred to the environment. Place contaminated linen and other reusable supplies in a single, sturdy, moisture-proof bag for transport to appropriate departments for cleaning and disinfecting. Place used sharps in sealable puncture-resistant containers. Use care to avoid contacting the outside of bags and containers with the soiled item when depositing items. Facility policies may indicate more specific procedures. No special precautions are needed for dishes and other eating utensils.			Avoid sharing of common equipment.
Patient transport		If transport is necessary, place surgical mask on patient.	Same as Airborne Precautions.	If transport is necessary, take precautions to prevent contamination of environmental surfaces.

Adapted from Garner JS, the Hospital Infection Control Practices Advisory Committee. Guidelines for isolation precautions in hospitals. Infect Control Hosp Epidemiol. *1996;17:53–80.*

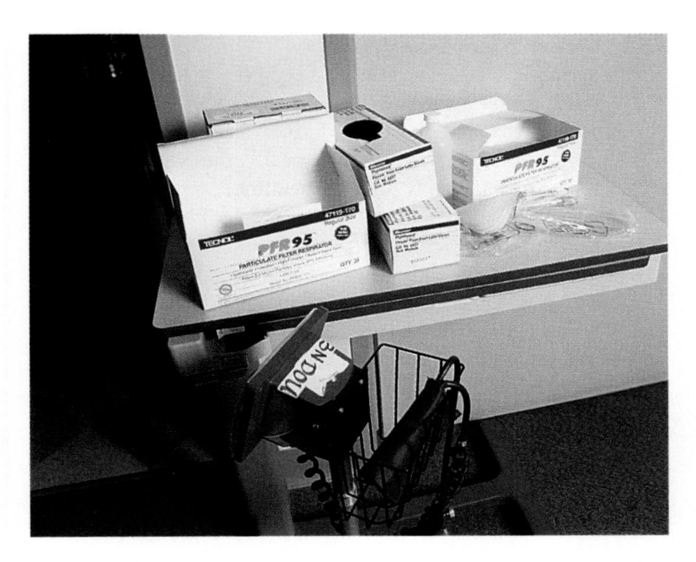

Figure 25–7. Supplies for transmission-based precautions outside a patient's room: gloves, eye protection, and masks.

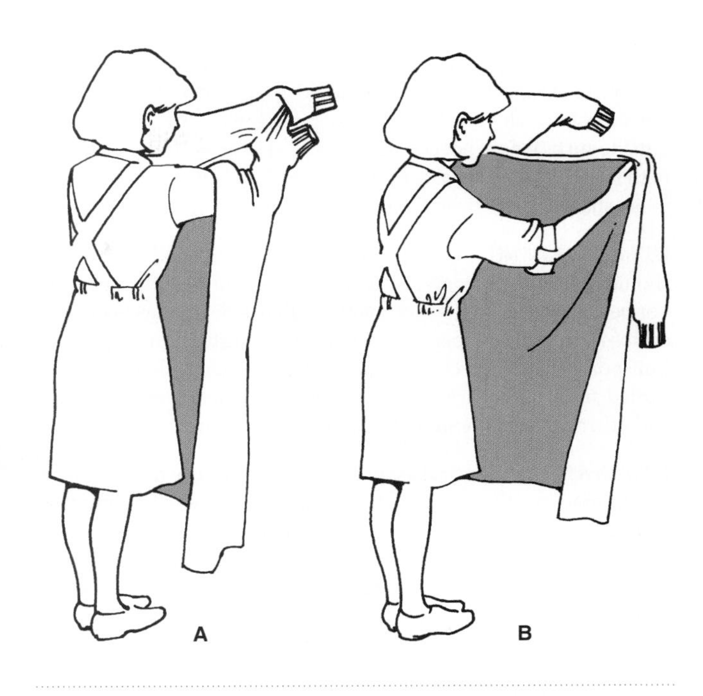

Figure 25–8. A nurse protects herself from contact with organisms when removing an isolation gown by (**A**) slipping her hands out of the sleeves without touching the outside of the gown; and (**B**) pulling the gown off her shoulders and folding it inside out for disposal.

Two elements of Standard Precautions, handwashing and the use of clean gloves, were discussed above in the section on preventive care. Other elements of Standard Precautions are presented below.

GOWNS. Wear a clean nonsterile gown to protect skin and clothing during patient care activities in which splashes or sprays of body substances (blood, body fluids) are likely. Cloth gowns are not impervious to moisture, so a plastic apron over the gown is appropriate when significant contact with fluids is expected. Disposable paper gowns with moisture-resistant backing are another alternative. Gowns are long with long sleeves and tight cuffs to provide maximum protection.

There is no special technique for putting on a clean gown. The opening should be in back with edges overlapping to ensure coverage of clothing. Tie the gown securely at the waist and the neck. After use, remove the gown without contacting the outside. First loosen the ties, then slip your hands inside the gown sleeves (Fig. 25–8A). Then pull the gown off your arms and shoulders, keeping the sleeves right side out. Hold the gown at the inside of its shoulders and fold the outside surfaces together (Figure 25–8B). Discard the gown into a receptacle for soiled linen or trash and wash your hands. If wearing a both mask and gown, remove the mask first.

MASKS. Wear a mask and protective eyewear (goggles, glasses, or face shield) when patient care measures create a risk for patient body substances splattering your eyes, nose, or mouth. Masks also protect against airborne and droplet transmission, so they are indicated as part of these transmission-based precautions (see Table 25–9).

To apply a mask, position the mask over the bridge of your nose, bring the ties above your ears, and tie the upper strings high on the back of your head. If you wear glasses, the top edge of the mask should fit under your glasses to reduce fogging of the glasses as you exhale. Pull the lower edge of the mask so that it fits under your chin. Tie the lower strings at the nape of the neck. Some prefer to tie the lower strings high on the head, above the first ties (Fig. 25–9). Squeeze the flexible metal strip to secure the mask on the bridge of your nose. A properly applied mask should fit snugly over the nose and mouth.

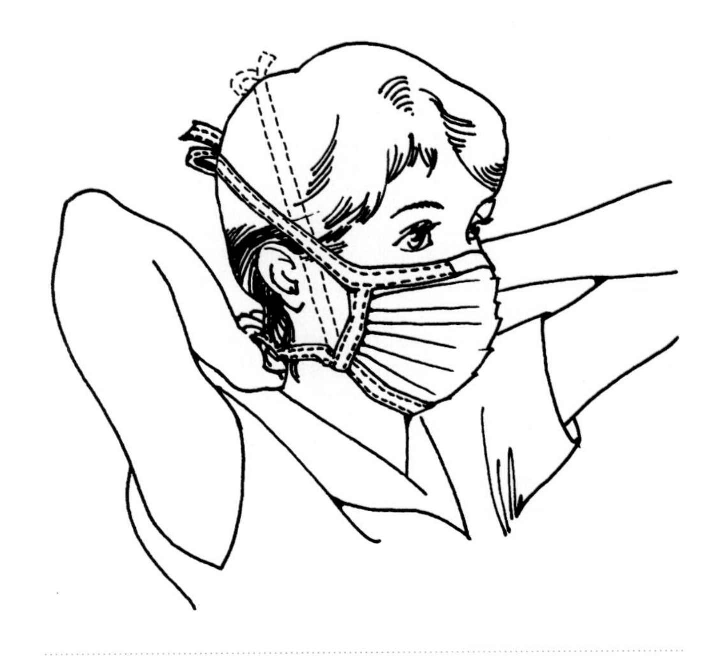

Figure 25–9. Apply a disposable mask so that the top ties go over your ears and tie high on the back of your head and the lower ties tie at the base of the neck or near the top of your head. Adjust the mask to fit over your nose by bending the metal strip at the top of the mask.

Keep talking to a minimum when wearing a mask. Masks that become moist are ineffective and should be discarded. Before removing a mask, wash your hands. Loosen the lower strings first so the outside surface does not contact exposed skin on your neck. Dispose of the used mask in a waste receptacle marked "infectious waste." A mask should never be left tied around the neck and reused.

PATIENT CARE EQUIPMENT. Used equipment soiled with body substances should not contact caregivers' skin, mucous membranes, or clothing nor be transferred to the environment. Reusable articles need to be enclosed in a bag impervious to air and moisture and sealed for transport to a disinfection area. Disposable items should be discarded in designated receptacles. Disposal containers for needles and other sharp items should be puncture resistant and sealable.

Surgical Asepsis. **Surgical asepsis,** also called **sterile technique,** refers to practices that keep areas and/or objects free of all microorganisms. The practice of surgical asepsis requires extreme conscientiousness and strict attention to detail. Surgical asepsis is routinely practiced in operating rooms, labor and delivery suites, and special diagnostic areas. Also, there are many procedures performed in general care areas that require sterile technique. Examples include injections, intravenous therapy, bladder catheterization, tracheobronchial suctioning, and wound care.

Sterile technique demands application of the basic principles listed in Clinical Guideline 25–8: General Principles of Surgical Asepsis. To apply these principles, the following points are important:

- Sterile technique is necessary for any procedure that involves contact with a sterile body cavity or that results in breaking of the skin or mucous membranes.
- A sterile field is a work area for assembling and handling sterile supplies. Only sterile items are placed on a sterile field.

CLINICAL GUIDELINE 25–8

GENERAL PRINCIPLES OF SURGICAL ASEPSIS

- A sterile object is free of all microorganisms.
- Microorganisms are present on the skin, in body cavities with an opening to the exterior of the body, in many body fluids, and on all objects in the environment not subjected to sterilization procedures.
- Intact skin prevents microorganisms from entering the body; mucous membranes and broken skin provide a portal of entry.
- The skin cannot be sterilized; however, rigorous cleaning can remove transient microorganisms and some resident flora.
- A wet, dark environment damages skin and promotes growth of many microorganisms.
- Microorganisms require a mode of transmission to move from one place to another. See Clinical Guideline 25–7.
- Microorganisms cannot penetrate dry cotton fabric, nonwoven paper, or plastic wrappers.
- Sterile items that are not kept within one's visual field are considered contaminated.
- If there is any doubt about the sterility of an item, it is considered contaminated.

- Identify sterile supplies as follows:
  - The outside of commercially packaged sterile items is marked "sterile." Materials sterilized by a health care facility's central supply department may use indicators such as heat-sensitive marker tapes on which a dark stripe becomes visible after exposure to sufficiently high temperature.
  - Check all packages marked "sterile" for sterility expiration dates.
  - Check sterilization indicators inside large packages to ensure that all contents have been exposed to the sterilization process.
  - Any package that appears torn, open, punctured, or wet should be considered contaminated and discarded.
- The outer 2.5 cm (1 in.) margin around the edges of a sterile field is considered contaminated because of its proximity to an unsterile surface. Place all items inside these margins when preparing the sterile field. Any item that contacts the margin is considered contaminated.
- If an item in use during a sterile procedure contacts any unsterile item, it is considered contaminated. The procedure must be started again with new sterile equipment.
- Sterile items (including your sterile gloved hands) that are out of the field of vision or held below waist level are considered contaminated because undetected contact with unsterile items is possible.
- Avoid activities that create air currents when working with sterile equipment. Close doors and keep traffic to a minimum.
- Talking, laughing, sneezing, or coughing over a sterile field can contaminate it with microorganisms from the oral cavity and respiratory tract via droplet transmission.
- Moisture facilitates contact transfer of microorganisms via *gravity* or *capillary action* (movement of fluid against gravity in a tube or fiber). To prevent this,
  - Use moisture-proof barriers for sterile fields whenever possible.
  - Exercise care to avoid splashing or spilling liquids near a sterile field (such as a cotton towel or drape) that is not impervious to moisture.
  - When using sterile forceps or swabs to apply liquids in a sterile procedure, keep the tips of the forceps below the level of the handles throughout the procedure. This will prevent the sterile fluid from flowing from the tips to your hands and becoming contaminated. The contaminated fluid would then flow downward and contaminate the forceps tips as you continue with the procedure.
- Before starting a sterile procedure, assist patients to a comfortable position and enlist their cooperation to prevent inadvertent contamination of sterile items. Ask patients to avoid any sudden movements, refrain from touching any supplies, and avoid talking, sneezing, or coughing over sterile areas.

The following activities are basic to using surgical asepsis:

- *Preparing and maintaining a sterile field.* This is outlined and illustrated in Procedure 25–2.
- *Putting on and removing sterile gloves.* Sterile gloves are sized to promote finger dexterity. They should be snug, but not tight. Procedure 25–3 outlines the steps for gloving.
- *Opening sterile packages.* Most commercially prepared sterilized items are packaged in "peel packs" or peel-back containers. Agency-sterilized items and large commercially prepared procedure kits are typically wrapped in cotton or paper in

(continued on page 669)

PROCEDURE 25–2. PREPARING AND MAINTAINING A STERILE FIELD

PURPOSE: To provide a work area for placement of sterile supplies needed to perform a sterile procedure.
EQUIPMENT: Package containing sterile drape (may be called "barrier towel"), and additional supplies as dictated by specific care to be given.

ACTION 1. Wash your hands.

RATIONALE. Removes transient microbes, thereby reducing possibility of contamination.

ACTION 2. Assemble all necessary supplies. Inspect all packages for dryness, intactness, indication of sterility, and expiration date. Discard any packages marked sterile that appear damp or whose wrappers are damaged.

RATIONALE. A sterile field may not be left unattended to retrieve extra supplies. Because sterility cannot be assured, an unattended sterile field is considered contaminated unless covered by a sterile drape. A torn or wet wrapper permits entry of microbes.

ACTION 3. Select a clean, dry work surface that is at a comfortable working height.

RATIONALE. A wet surface beneath a sterile field permits transmission of microbes through the drape by capillary action, unless the drape is impervious to moisture.

ACTION 4. Open the package containing the drape according to Clinical Guideline 25–9.

RATIONALE. These techniques prevent patient infection by maintaining sterility of supplies.

ACTION 5. Without touching the drape, inspect it to locate the corner that has been diagonally folded. Then grasp the corner with your thumb and forefinger.

RATIONALE. The corner is folded to facilitate holding it. The outer 2.5 cm (1 in.) of a sterile field may be touched during its preparation. The entire border of the field is therefore considered contaminated.

ACTION 6. Lift the drape from its wrapper, allowing it to unfold. Prevent contact with unsterile items by stepping away from the work surface as you lift the drape and by holding your arm well away from your body.

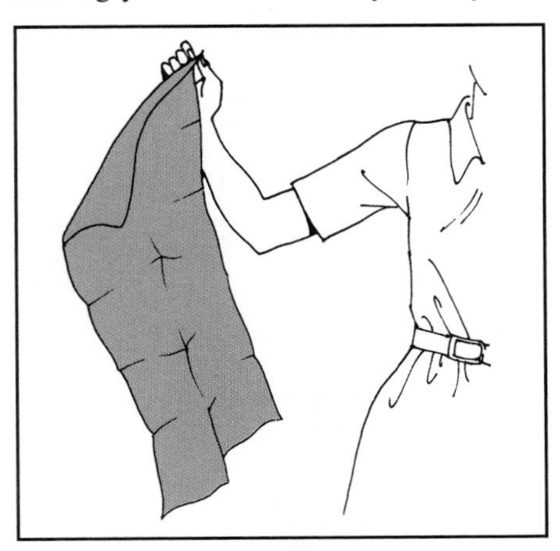

RATIONALE. Microorganisms are transmitted by direct contact with an unsterile object.

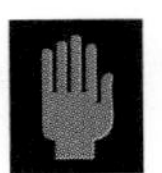

Disposable drapes may not unfold readily. Gently shaking the drape may help, but avoid vigorous movement.

ACTION 7. Grasp the adjacent corner of the drape with your other hand. Place the drape on the work surface. Either side of the drape may be placed facing up. Do not lean or reach over the drape while positioning it or while placing sterile items on it.

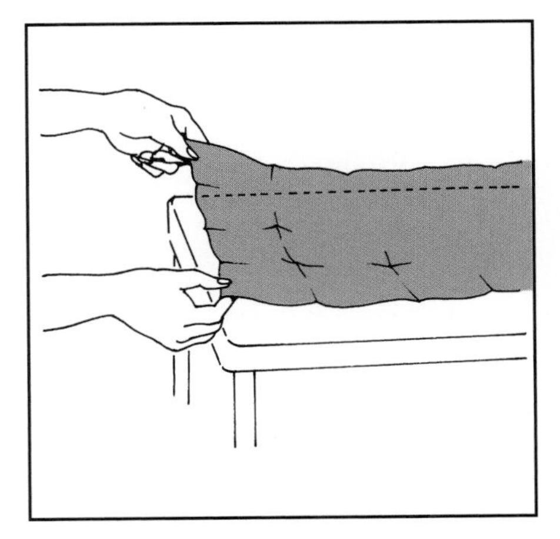

RATIONALE. Leaning or reaching over the drape as it is placed on the table may contaminate it by direct contact.

Continued

ACTION 8. Open sterile supplies needed for the procedure as described in Clinical Guideline 25–9.

RATIONALE. These techniques prevent patient infection by maintaining sterility of supplies.

ACTION 9. Place sterile supplies on the sterile field as follows:

a. Drop small lightweight items near the center of the field from a height of about 15 cm (6 in.).

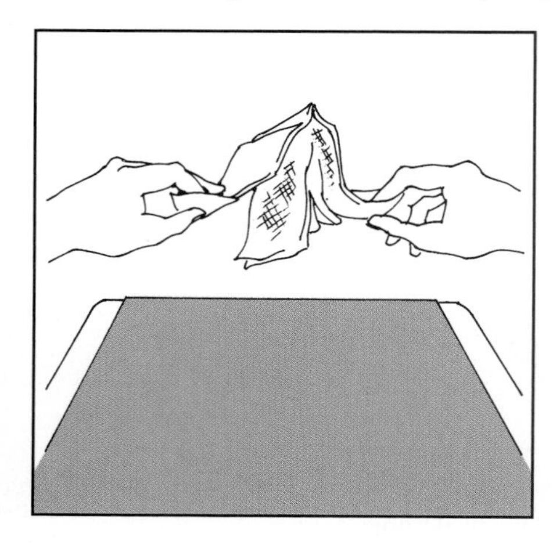

RATIONALE. This distance is small enough to prevent items from contacting the unsterile border of the field.

b. Do not use supplies that touch the 2.5-cm (1-in.) border of the sterile field.

RATIONALE. See Action 5. These supplies are potentially contaminated by direct contact with the unsterile border.

c. Place bulky items such as sterile basins near the margin (see Action 5) of the sterile field, holding one edge of the item in its sterile wrapper as shown.

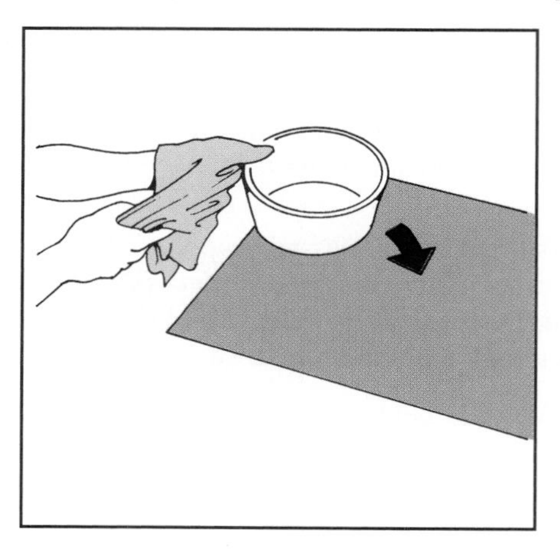

RATIONALE. Dropping bulky items could cause them to bounce or slip off the sterile field. The wrapper provides a barrier between your hand and the sterile item. See Action 6, above.

ACTION 10. If sterile solution is to be used, pour according to Clinical Guideline 25–10.

RATIONALE. These techniques will maintain sterility of field and solution.

ACTION 11. After putting on sterile gloves, rearrange sterile items on field if necessary. See Procedure 25–3.

RATIONALE. See Action 6, above.

ACTION 12. Maintain sterile field during its use by allowing only sterile items to contact the field or items on it. If the field becomes contaminated, it must be discarded and new sterile equipment obtained.

Recording:
Document procedure performed according to guidelines for that procedure. Preparation of a sterile field need not be documented separately.

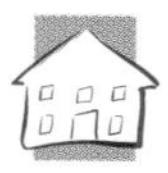

HOME HEALTH ADAPTATION: This procedure adapts well to the home situation.

PROCEDURE 25–3. PUTTING ON AND REMOVING STERILE GLOVES: OPEN GLOVING

PURPOSE: To prevent transmission of microorganisms from caregiver to patient and from one patient to another.
EQUIPMENT: Undamaged package of sterile gloves in caregiver's size. Additional supplies dictated by specific care to be given.

ACTION 1. Wash your hands. Remove rings with stones.

RATIONALE. Handwashing removes transient microbes, thereby reducing possibility of contamination. Rings increase risk of tearing gloves.

ACTION 2. Assemble all necessary supplies. Inspect all packages for dryness, intactness, indication of sterility, and expiration date. Do not use any packages that appear damp or whose wrappers are damaged.

RATIONALE. A sterile field may not be left unattended to retrieve extra supplies. Because sterility cannot be assured, an unattended sterile field is considered contaminated unless covered by a sterile drape. A torn or wet wrapper permits entry of microbes, so contents are contaminated.

ACTION 3. Open the outer wrapper according to Clinical Guideline 25–9. Discard wrap. Place the inner package on a clean, dry work surface that is at a comfortable working height and provides enough space to unfold the glove wrapper without contacting sterile supplies already prepared. Do not place glove wrapper on sterile field.

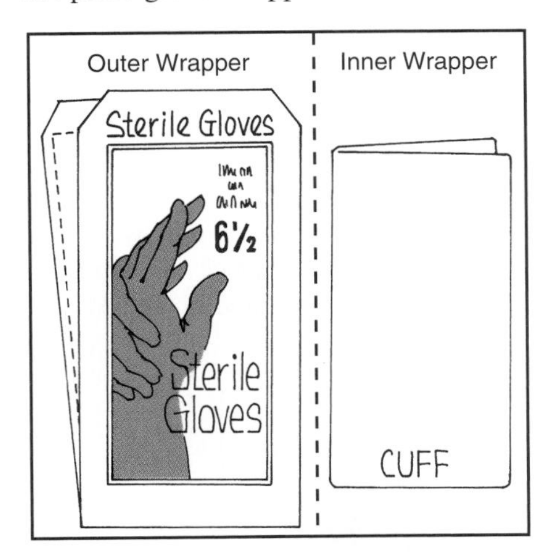

RATIONALE. A wet surface beneath the package would permit transmission of microbes through the wrapper to the gloves by capillary action. Contact between the glove wrapper and the sterile field would transmit microbes to the sterile field, because the outside of the wrapper is not sterile once placed on work area.

ACTION 4. Open inner wrapper according to directions printed on package. Illustration below is typical. Pull wrapper firmly to keep it flat, touching only exposed "cuffs" of wrapper. Gloves will be positioned next to each other, palm up, with thumbs to the outside, bottom cuffed.

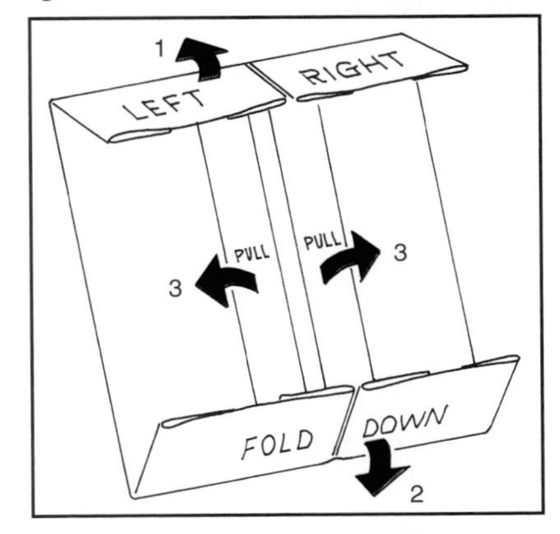

RATIONALE. Correctly opening the inner wrapper creates a sterile field for the gloves. If wrapper returns to folded position after you have touched it, gloves may be contaminated by contact with wrapper.

ACTION 5. Grasp the folded edge of the cuff of one glove. Lift it above the work area and away from your body. Insert your other hand into the glove and pull it on. Do not adjust the cuff or placement of fingers inside the glove. If the outside of the glove touches any unsterile object, the glove must be discarded.

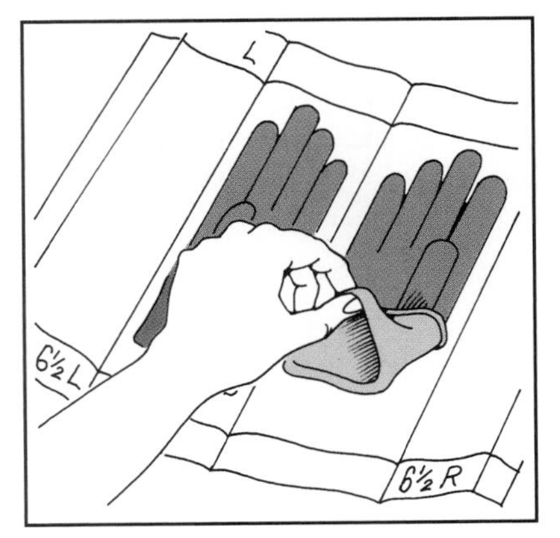

RATIONALE. These actions prevent the outside of the glove from contacting unsterile objects such as your hand, uniform, or the work surface, which would allow transmission of microbes to the glove. Incorrect finger placement can be adjusted when both gloves are on.

Continued

ACTION 6. Slip your gloved hand *under* the cuff of the remaining glove, lift it up as above, and pull it on. Do not flex the wrist of the gloved hand while lifting or putting on the second glove. Hold the gloved thumb away from the opposite hand and arm.

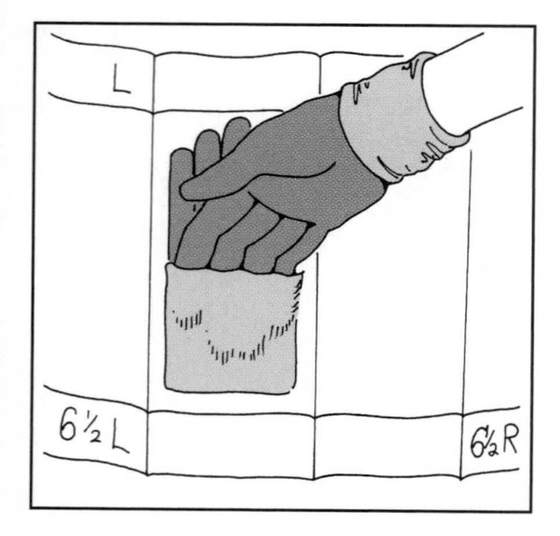

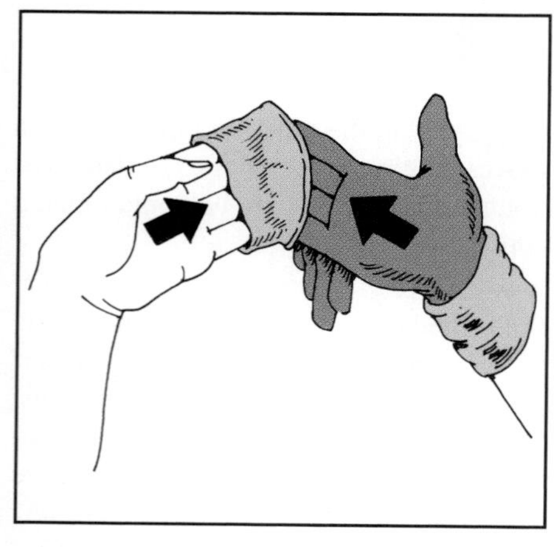

RATIONALE. This technique prevents contact between the sterile surfaces of the gloves and exposed skin, thereby keeping both gloves sterile.

ACTION 7. Touching only the outside of the gloves, adjust gloves so they fit smoothly. Slide fingers under cuffs to shorten them if cuffs extend over palms of gloves.

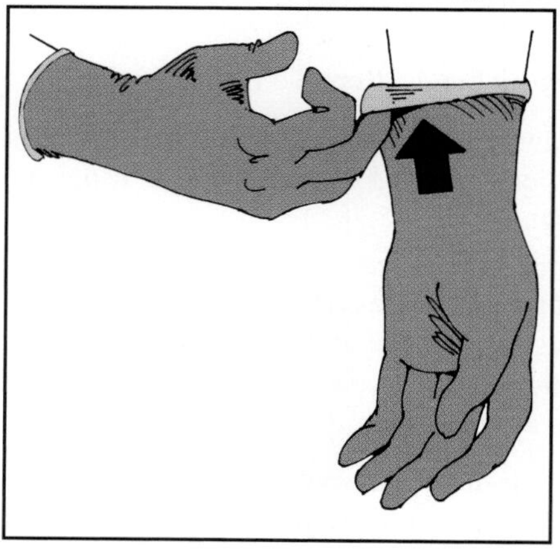

RATIONALE. Contact with the unsterile inside of the gloves would transfer organisms to the outside of the gloves. Smooth fit improves dexterity during procedure.

ACTION 8. Carry out sterile procedure without extraneous movement. Gloved hands must remain in sight above waist level at all times.

RATIONALE. Excessive movement increases risk of contacting unsterile objects and creates air currents that could transmit organisms to patient or sterile field. Keeping gloves in sight assures awareness of accidental glove contamination.

ACTION 9. To remove gloves:

a. Grasp outside of one glove near the wrist and remove it by turning it inside out. Once removed, the glove may be held in the opposite hand or placed with used equipment from procedure.

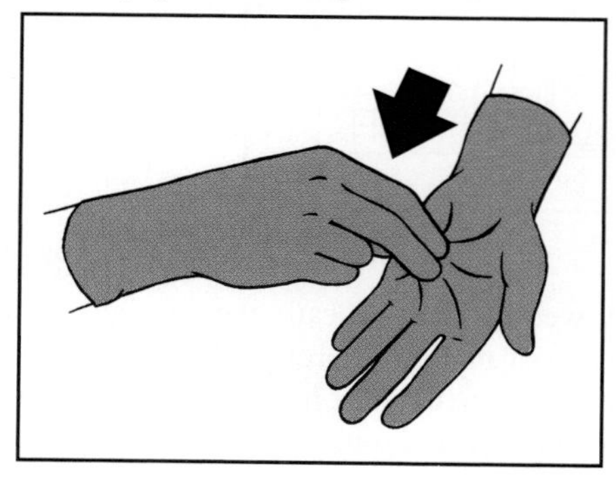

RATIONALE. During the procedure, gloves have contacted organisms from the patient's skin. Touching the outside of the glove and inverting it when removing glove prevents transmitting these organisms to the nurse's hands.

Procedure 25–3. (continued)

b. Slip ungloved thumb or fingers inside remaining glove and remove it by turning it inside out. Do not touch outside of glove.

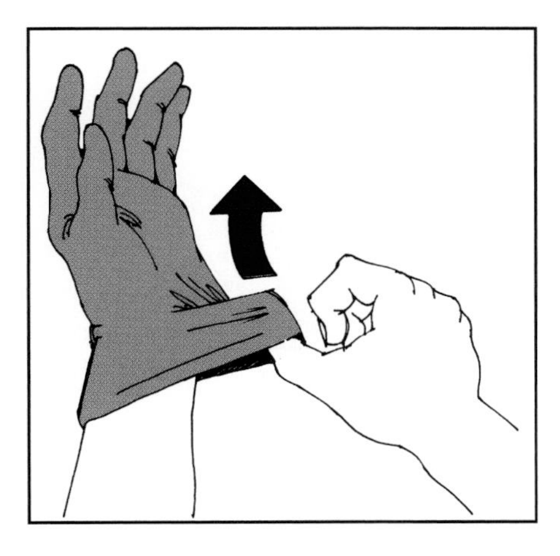

RATIONALE. This prevents contamination of nurse's hand with organisms from outside of glove. If first glove was held, it will be contained inside second glove.

ACTION 10. Discard gloves and other used equipment according to agency policy.

RATIONALE. Equipment contacting certain body secretions requires special handling according to HICPAC/CDC Infection Control.

ACTION 11. Wash your hands. See Procedure 25–1.

RATIONALE. Microorganisms flourish in moist warm environment inside gloves. Thorough washing removes most transient organisms. See Procedure 25–1.

Recording:
Specific reference to use of sterile gloves is not usually required. Documentation of specific procedure should indicate sterile technique was used.

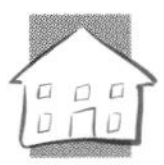

HOME HEALTH ADAPTATION: This procedure is applicable in any setting.

an "envelope style." Clinical Guideline 25–9 illustrates these packages and describes opening them without contamination.

- *Pouring sterile liquids.* See Clinical Guideline 25–10 (page 672).
- *Using sterile forceps.* A forceps is a two-bladed instrument used for grasping or manipulating equipment or body tissue. There are several types. Thumb forceps look like tweezers; ring forceps (sometimes called transfer forceps) have handles like scissors. The blades or tips of forceps are varied according to their intended uses. In some procedures, sterile forceps are used in lieu of sterile gloves. In situations in which the handles of sterile forceps are contaminated (having contacted your hand), but the tips are sterile, they may by placed on the edge of a sterile field with the tips within the sterile area and the handles outside the field.

Perioperative Nursing Care

Surgery is often a component of restorative care. Perioperative nursing refers to surgery-related patient care. Nurses play an important role in enhancing patient well-being in all aspects of the care of surgical patients, from the time surgery is presented to patients as a possible therapy through their recovery and resumption of normal activities.

Preoperative Care. Preoperative care is given before surgery. The preoperative period begins at the time the decision is made that surgery is necessary and extends until a patient is safely transferred to the operating room. Nurses' primary function during the preoperative phase is to prepare patients for the surgical experience.

PSYCHOLOGICAL AND EDUCATIONAL PREPARATION. Surgery represents a significant threat to well-being. Anticipating surgery is often a very frightening and stressful experience for patients and family members. Several approaches help reduce the threat to well-being:

- *Facilitate communicating concerns.* Worries about surgery are difficult for some patients to acknowledge and even more difficult to express. Expressing feelings is the first step in resolving them; resolution alleviates stress. Nurses working with patients at the time they are first told of their need for surgery, those assisting with patients' admission to a surgical unit, and those giving immediate presurgery care need to actively facilitate patient communication of feelings and concerns. One way to do this is by telling patients that fear and anxiety are nearly universal responses to impending surgery. Then, invite them to share their thoughts about their upcoming surgery. Normalizing fears in this way helps patients overcome hesitancy to reveal their personal concerns.
- *Give information about surgery experience.* Accurate information about the purpose of the surgery and what to expect throughout the perioperative experience also alleviates anxiety and fear. Facts are a basis for effective coping; anticipating "the unknown"

CLINICAL GUIDELINE 25–9

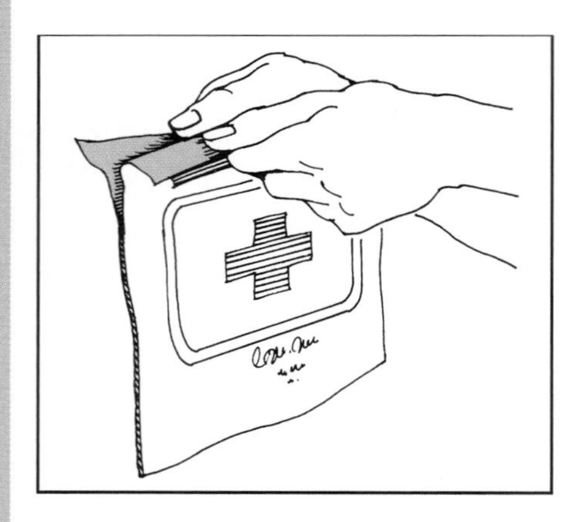

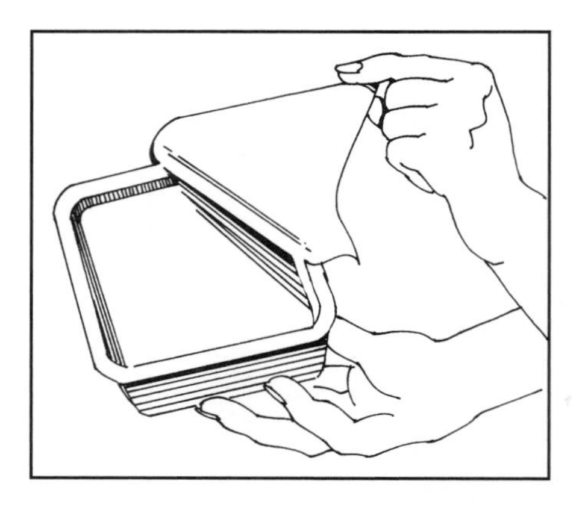

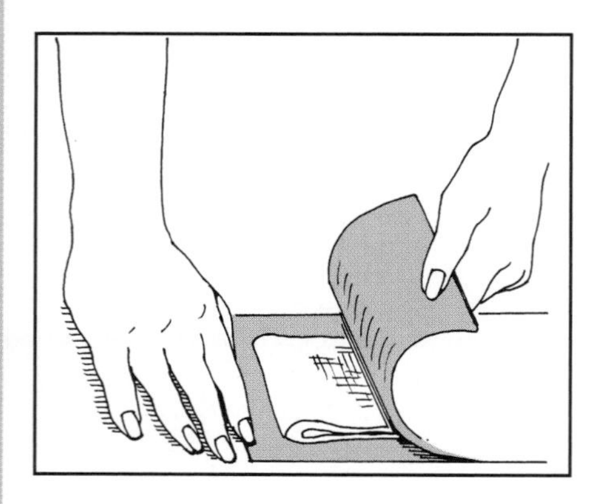

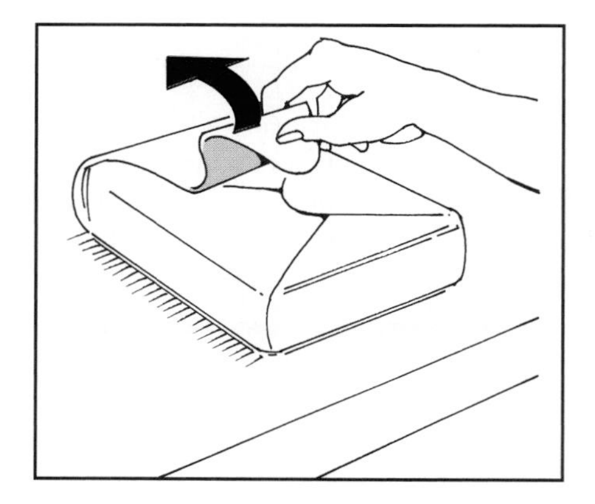

OPENING STERILE PACKAGES

Inspect all packages for dryness, intactness, indication of sterility, and expiration date. Do not use any packages that appear damp or whose wrappers are damaged.

PEELPACKS

1. Grasp the tabs above the sealed edge as shown.
2. Peel edges apart to break seal.
3. Package may be placed on a flat surface and top wrapper carefully removed to completely expose contents as shown, creating a small sterile field for contents of package. Do not allow contents to slip near or over the edge of the wrapper as you open it. This contaminates contents.
4. Or contents may be placed on another sterile field. (See Procedure 25–2.)

PEELBACK CONTAINERS

1. Hold the bottom of the container with one hand.
2. Grasp corner tab of peelback top; pull to remove top.
3. Container may be used as self-contained sterile field and sterile solution added if needed. Or dry contents but not container may be placed on another sterile field and container used to hold sterile solution if needed. Refer to Clinical Guideline 25–10.

ENVELOPE-WRAPPED PACKAGE ON A SURFACE

1. Center the package on the work area so the outer flap of the wrapper faces away from you.

is not. Information enhances individual well-being. It promotes personal control, a sense of accomplishment, and active patient participation throughout the perioperative experience.

A step-by-step overview that addresses procedures, settings, equipment, and sensations to expect during the preparation, the surgery, and the recovery is effective. (Recall the previous discussion, *Preparing Patients for Diagnostic Tests.*) This approach is appropriate when obtaining written consent for surgery or to reinforce the information the patient received at the time consent forms were signed. Informed consent was addressed in the prior section on supportive care. In some facilities, regularly scheduled group classes are used to present information about surgery, including pain management and postoperative activities to prevent complications.

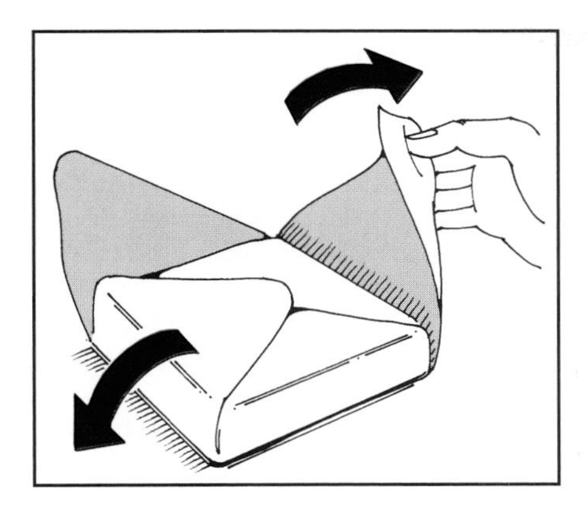

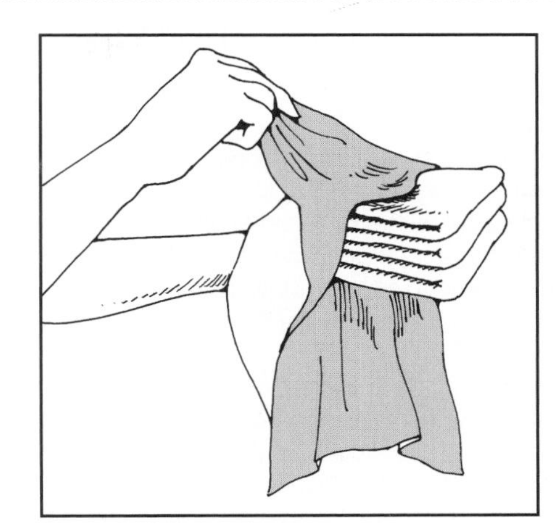

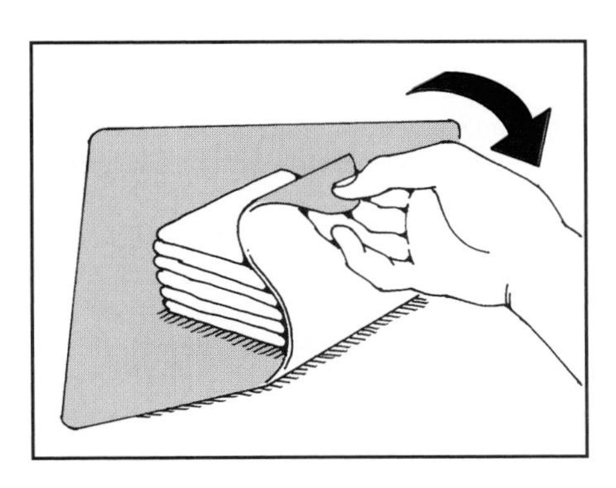

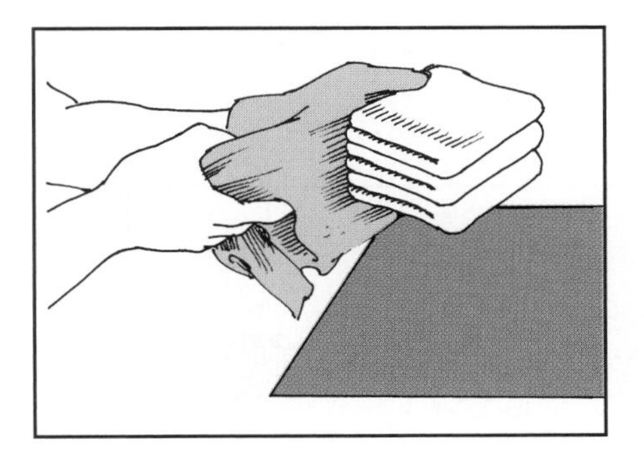

2. Reach around, not over, the package and open the flap, pulling it away from you. Touch only the outside of the wrap.
3. Open side flaps in sequence, using right hand for right flap and left hand for left flap. Touch outside surface only, as shown. Avoid reaching over package.
4. Open inner flap by pulling turned down corner toward you. If flap is large, step away from the table so wrapper does not contact your uniform. If inner corner is not turned down, touch outside of wrap only, as in step 3.
5. Wrapper may be used for sterile field. Additional items may be added as necessary. See Procedure 25–2.

ENVELOPE-WRAPPED PACKAGE HELD IN HAND

1. Hold the package in one hand so the outer flap of the wrapper faces away from you.
2. Open the package as in steps 2 to 4 above, pulling the flaps back toward you as you open each one.
3. Gather the opened flaps with your free hand and hold them against the opposite arm, as shown. The sterile item can now be placed on a sterile field without risk of contacting the field with the parts of the wrapper that you have touched.

- *Pain management.* Patients need to know that effective management of postoperative pain is a reasonable expectation. This implies a tolerable level of pain, but not necessarily freedom from pain. Postoperative pain is most responsive to narcotic medications. They can be given according to several protocols. Traditionally, *intravenous* or *intramuscular* administration *prn* (as needed), with interval restrictions of 2 to 4 hours to prevent oversedation, has been the protocol of choice. It is still used in many health care facilities. Narcotic analgesics can also be administered by the *epidural route,* formerly used only for anesthetics. This provides pain relief for 8 to 12 hours and doses can be repeated if the epidural catheter is left in place.

Patient-controlled analgesia (PCA) is another option. It is a drug delivery system that enables patients to obtain pain

CLINICAL GUIDELINE 25–10

POURING STERILE SOLUTIONS

1. Check order to verify name and strength of solution ordered for procedure.
2. Obtain correct solution. Do not use solution from previously opened bottle unless time and date of first use are written on the label. Most agencies allow solution from an opened bottle to be used for a 24-hour period before discarding remaining contents. Some solutions may have a specific expiration date or time indicated on the label. If solution has been refrigerated, place in a basin of hot water to warm it to room temperature.
3. If using solution from an unopened bottle, write current time and date on the label where it can be readily seen.
4. Prepare sterile field and sterile container for solution as needed. See Procedure 25–2 and Clinical Guideline 25–9.
5. Remove the lid and place it on a nonsterile surface so the inside of the lid is facing up, to prevent contamination of inside surface of lid.
6. Grasp solution bottle with its label facing the palm of your hand to prevent solution, which may drip or run down the side of the bottle, from obliterating the label.

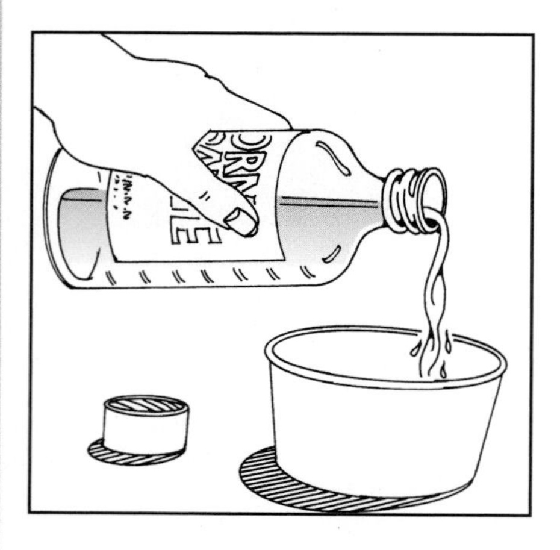

7. Hold the solution bottle about 10 cm (4 in.) above the receiving container and pour slowly to avoid splashing. Do not allow the lip of the bottle to contact the receiving container.
8. Replace lid on the bottle securely. Store according to agency policy.
9. Record specific care given, identifying type and strength of solution used.

medication as they need it. An intravenous infusion pump that administers a small preprogrammed dose of narcotic analgesic when the patient pushes a button is attached to the primary intravenous line. To prevent overmedication, the pump has a "lockout" mechanism that limits the amount of medication delivered in a given time frame. PCA has the advantage of giving patients control over their pain management. Being in charge of their own medication administration reduces patients' anxiety and feelings of powerlessness. This enhances pain relief. Although patients are not always able to choose which of these protocols will be used for their pain management, addressing the options so they can discuss questions and preferences with their surgeon fosters self-responsibility.

McCaffery and Beebe[56] have identified four other important points about postoperative pain management that should be included in preoperative patient teaching:

- Pain medications are most effective if administered at regular intervals around the clock. If pain medications are ordered on a prn (as needed) basis, instruct patients to ask for medication before the pain becomes severe and unbearable. Emphasize that they should not assume that nurses will automatically bring the pain medication, or that nurses will know when they are in pain.
- Encourage patients to notify a nurse if the medication being used is not effective. If the prescribed pain medication is not adequately controlling pain, different medications or dosages can be ordered.
- There is very little danger of addiction to medications when used in the management of postoperative pain. Patients should not "suffer in silence" or delay asking for medication in the first few days after surgery because of fear of addiction.
- Effective pain management facilitates patient participation in the activities and exercises necessary for recovery and prevention of complications.

Teaching should also address how to use relaxation techniques such as deep breathing or guided imagery with analgesics to facilitate pain management during postoperative recovery. See Clinical Guideline 25–1. Additional information related to pain control can be found in Chap. 32.

- *Activities to prevent postoperative complications.* Preoperative teaching that includes a demonstration of the activity, a discussion of the reason it is important, observation of practice, and positive reinforcement or corrective feedback is most effective.
  - *Deep-breathing exercises.* Deep-breathing exercises are done postoperatively to expand the lungs and facilitate oxygenation of tissues, thus preventing many of the respiratory complications of surgery.
  - *Coughing exercises.* Coughing facilitates the removal of mucous that sometimes accumulates in the respiratory tract postoperatively.
  - *Leg exercises.* Pooling of venous blood (venous stasis) due to sluggish blood flow in the legs is common after surgery. Venous stasis increases the risk for deep vein thrombosis (DVT): clot formation in deep veins. Leg exercises stimulate blood flow and reduce DVT risk. Chapter 30 details procedures for effective breathing, coughing, and leg exercises.
  - *Mobilization techniques.* Turning in bed at least every 2 hours and early postoperative ambulation promote circulation and effective lung expansion. Informing patients before surgery that mobilization techniques will be initiated even as they are recovering from the effects of anesthesia will enhance participation. Techniques to assist patients with turning and ambulation are presented in Chap. 33.

PHYSICAL PREPARATION. Some aspects of the physical preparation for surgery are unique to the type of surgery, the surgeon's preferences, and the special needs of individual patients. The nursing care highlighted below is appropriate for all surgical patients.

- *Nutrition and hydration.* Because of the potential danger of patients vomiting and aspirating while under general anesthesia, they are generally required to fast at least 6 to 8 hours prior to surgery. Patients and family members must be informed of the importance of taking nothing by mouth (npo). Patients may rinse their mouths with water or mouthwash and brush their teeth, as long as they do not swallow any fluids. If patients eat or drink during the fasting period, the surgeon must be notified. The administration of intravenous fluids via a large gauge cannula is generally initiated preoperatively. This supports maintaining hydration and provides venous access for medications or blood transfusions, if needed, during and after surgery.
- *Hygiene and skin preparation.* Hygiene and skin preparation prior to surgery removes microorganisms from the skin and reduces the incidence of postoperative infection. The skin is cleansed by scrubbing the operative site one or more times with an antimicrobial soap or solution. Often this can be done by patients in the shower. Removal of hair at the surgical site is no longer a standard practice. Current CDC guidelines recommend that unless the hair around the surgical site is so thick that it interferes with the surgical procedure, it should not be removed. If hair removal is necessary, clipping or a depilatory cream is preferred to shaving.

  Lips, skin, and at least one fingernail bed must be visible during surgery for circulatory assessment. For this reason, lipstick, makeup, and nail polish are removed as part of preoperative hygiene.
- *Elimination.* A Foley catheter is often inserted prior to surgery to prevent bladder distension and accidental bladder injury during surgery. If a catheter is not ordered, patients should void just prior to the administration of preoperative medications.

  Routine enemas prior to surgery are no longer prescribed. However, because anesthetics slow bowel activity, patients who have not had a bowel movement for several days prior to surgery may need an enema or suppository to prevent postoperative constipation.

  Patients undergoing abdominal surgery always require bowel preparation, which usually consists of cathartics and/or a series of cleansing enemas to empty the gastrointestinal tract. Without this preparation, these patients would be at high risk for postoperative abdominal distension, because peristalsis is delayed for 24 to 48 hours after the bowel is handled. An empty bowel also reduces the risk of injury to the intestines during surgery and prevents contamination of the surgical wound if the bowel is opened.
- *Special orders.* Preoperative medications from one or more of the following categories may be ordered for the night before surgery and/or on the day of surgery. Some may be *"on call" medications.* These are medications to be given 45 minutes to 1 hour prior to surgery. They are given when the operating room notifies the nurse giving preoperative care that surgery is imminent.
  - *Sedatives* decrease anxiety and promote sleep. Some also induce amnesia (suppress memories of the surgical experience).
  - *Anticholinergics* reduce oral and respiratory secretions to decrease the risk of aspiration during surgery.
  - *Analgesics* decrease discomfort during preoperative procedures.
  - *H_2-receptor antagonists* increase gastric pH and suppress production of gastric secretions to prevent postoperative nausea and vomiting.
  - *Nonparticulate antacids* reduce gastric pH.
  - *Antibiotics* provide prophylaxis against postoperative infections in certain risk conditions.

For some surgeries, preoperative antiembolism stockings (see Chap. 30) or placement of a nasogastric (NG) tube (a tube inserted into the stomach via the nose—see Chap. 28) is ordered. The stockings promote venous return to the heart by counteracting the venous pooling associated with positioning during surgery and physiologic responses to the stress of surgery. NG tubes remove gastric contents through direct suction to prevent gastric distension, nausea, and vomiting from stasis of gastrointestinal secretions due to absent or diminished peristalsis (see Proc. 25–4).

CARE OF VALUABLES AND PROSTHESES. All prostheses (eyeglasses, contact lenses, removable bridgework, artificial limbs, etc) must be removed prior to surgery, labeled, and stored for safekeeping. It is preferred that valuables such as money and jewelry be given to family members for safe-keeping during surgery. If this is not possible they should be labeled and locked in a secure place such as the hospital safe. Many patients are reluctant to remove their wedding band or religious ornaments. If so, tape the ring or ornament in place to prevent accidental loss during transfers and positioning.

PREOPERATIVE CHECKLIST. In most health care facilities, a preoperative checklist is used to validate that all procedures required for surgery have been completed. Checklists are reminders to verify completion of the preparation measures discussed above, validate the accuracy of information such as the data on the patient's identification bracelet, and record data such as the patient's allergies, height and weight, preoperative lab work results, and latest vital signs on the appropriate forms. The preoperative checklist, patient chart, and operative permit accompany patients to the operating room.

Intraoperative Care. Intraoperative care begins when the patient enters the operating room (OR) and ends with admission to the recovery room. Operating room personnel function as a team to assist one another and meet the needs of patients undergoing surgery (Fig. 25–10, page 678). A discussion of specific nursing tasks in an OR is beyond the scope of this text. Primary patient-focused functions include providing emotional support and maintaining patient safety.

- *Emotional support.* Whether patients are groggy and sedated or awake and alert when they arrive in the OR, the circulating nurse uses touch and soothing verbal communication to show caring in what is often a threatening environment. Instructions and explanations, when appropriate, convey a message of focus on the person rather than the procedure.
- *Safety.* The scrub nurse or technician and the circulating nurse share responsibility for careful patient transfer and positioning, meticulous attention to sterile technique, accurate sponge and instrument counts, and precise documentation of intraoperative procedures.

(continued on page 678)

PROCEDURE 25–4. MANAGING NASOGASTRIC SUCTION

PURPOSE: To maintain patency of nasogastric tube so decompression of stomach is maintained, preventing abdominal distension, nausea, and vomiting. To promote patient comfort and tissue integrity while NG tube is in place.

EQUIPMENT: Regulator and gauge for wall suction or portable suction machine, connecting tubing and collection container, syringe with tip that fits tightly into lumen of NG tube (usually 50-mL size), water-soluble lubricant, cotton-tipped applicators, lemon glycerine swabs or mouthwash, 1-in. hypoallergenic adhesive tape, adhesive remover, and catheter plug for ambulatory patients.

ACTION 1. Check physician's order for type, amount, and duration of suction to be maintained.

RATIONALE. Maintainance of gastric decompression is not an independent nursing function. Suction orders may be for high (80 to 100 mm Hg) or low (30 to 40 mm Hg); intermittent or continuous suction. A specific schedule for suction may also be ordered.

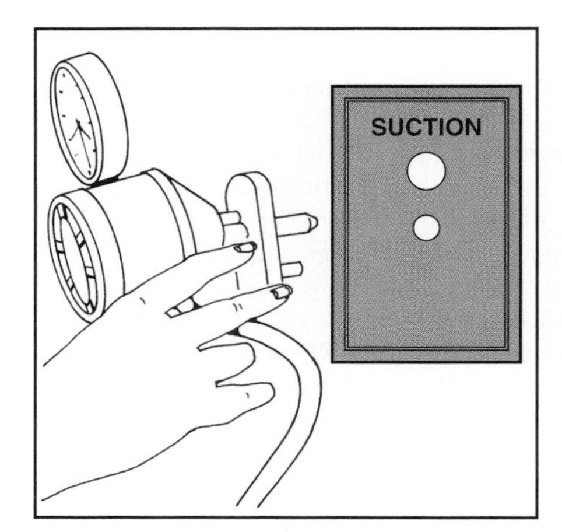

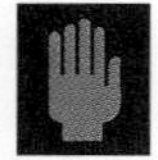

High suction will damage gastric mucosa unless the tube has a double lumen with an air vent such as a Salem sump tube. Also, single-lumen tubes require intermittent suction while double-lumen tubes function best with continuous suction.

ACTION 2. Discuss the purpose of the suction and associated assessments and trouble-shooting, usual sensations, desired patient participation, and expected benefits with the patient.

RATIONALE. Patient will be less anxious and more willing to participate if reasons and expected benefits of procedure are clear.

ACTION 3. Attach NG tube to connecting tubing, and then attach tubing to suction container and suction source, making sure that all connections are tight. Turn on suction as ordered. A five-way adapter may be needed to join NG tube to connecting tubing.

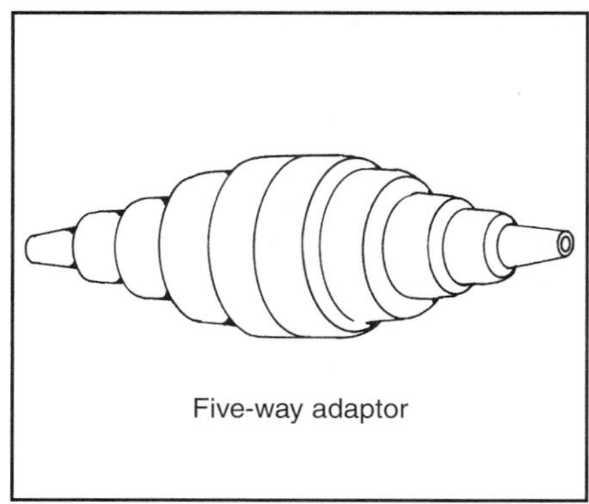

Five-way adaptor

RATIONALE. Connecting tubing allows patient to move freely in bed without pulling on the NG tube. Tight connections prevent pressure leaks, which decrease the effectiveness of the suction apparatus.

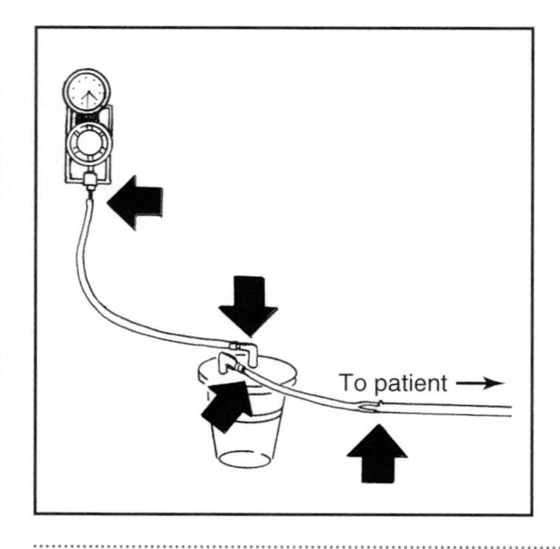

ACTION 4. When system is on, assess for proper functioning at least q2h:

RATIONALE. Patient is receiving no benefit if system is not functioning.

a. Any fluid in the connecting tubing should be moving toward the suction source.

RATIONALE. Lack of fluid movement suggests tube is blocked or placed incorrectly. Check for kinks in tube. See also Action 5.

b. There should be no leaking of fluid at connection points or from the air vent ("pigtail") of a Salem sump tube (See illustration for Action 5c).

RATIONALE. Leaks suggest a block and ineffective connections. Reflux from pigtail has several causes; see Action 6

c. There should be no sounds of air movement, except with Salem sump, which should produce a hissing sound at the pigtail opening.

RATIONALE. Air intake sounds at sites other than the pigtail decrease effectiveness of suction in the stomach. Recheck all connections.

d. If intermittent suction is ordered, suction pump should turn on and off in a cyclic fashion; cycles last several seconds.

RATIONALE. Lack of cycling indicates no suction is occurring. Patient will become distended and nauseous and may vomit. Obtain new suction equipment.

ACTION 5. To troubleshoot a blocked tube:

a. Check suction equipment. Disconnect from NG tube. If liquid in tubing then moves toward collection container, suction is working. (End of tubing may be placed in a glass of water to test if no drainage is present in the tubing.) If water does not move, tighten all connections and recheck.

RATIONALE. Mechanical malfunction is relatively easy to rule out with minimal trauma to patient, so it should be done first. If all connections are tight and liquid does not move when tubing is separated from the smaller lumen of the NG tube, obtain a new suction unit.

b. If collection container is full of drainage or plastic liner is bulging with air, turn off suction and empty container. (Drainage should be measured before discarding in toilet.)

RATIONALE. Overfilled collection container may decrease suction efficiency and may trigger shut off valve.

c. Check placement of the tube by aspirating contents of the lumen of the tube and checking the pH. The mean pH of gastric secretions is 3.02. A pH between 6 and 7 implies the tube is not in the stomach. Alternate method: with suction off, place stethoscope just below the xyphoid process, then inject 15 mL of air via pigtail (separate NG from connecting tube to inject if single-lumen tube). A whooshing or popping sound indicates tube is in the stomach. Clearing the pigtail may also restore suction.

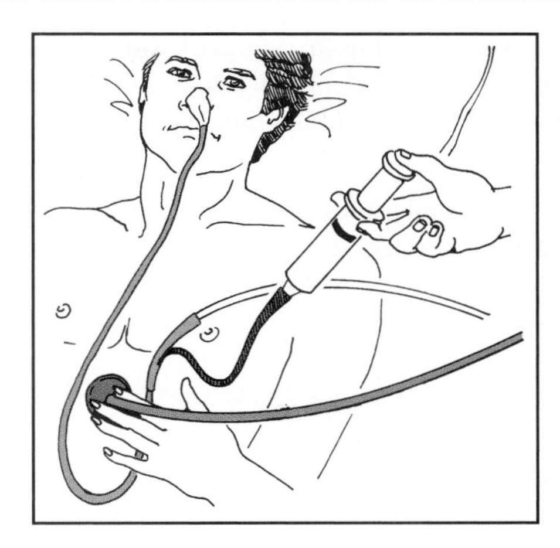

RATIONALE. Suction noise interferes with placement check. Pigtail prevents tube from adhering to mucous membrane because air intake via vent reduces negative pressure at inlet ports of tube. If vent is blocked, adherence to mucosa may occur, interfering with suction. Air movement from the tube into the stomach can be heard with this stethoscope placement. If no sound is heard, tube is not in the stomach. Advance tube 1 to 2 inches and recheck. Do not advance tube if patient has gastric surgery

d. Reposition patient to the opposite side and turn on suction. Reposition tube so pigtail is above level of stomach after position change (see Action 6).

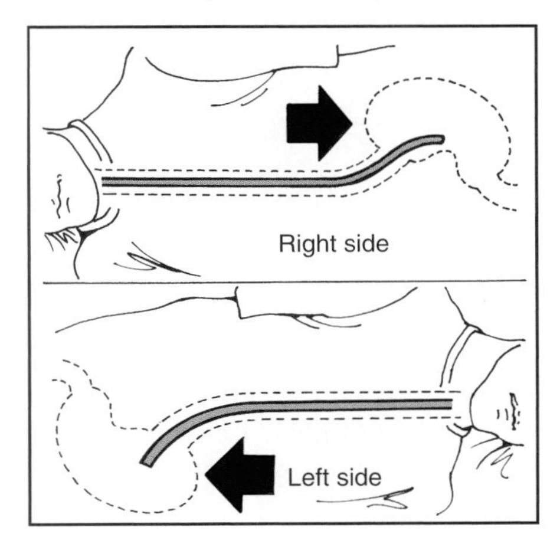

RATIONALE. Position change alters the angle/placement of tube in stomach. It may move tube away from mucosa. This is not effective if suction is on, as tube will adhere to mucosa.

Continued

e. If patient has not had gastric surgery, tube may also be rotated and/or advanced or retracted 1 to 2 inches before suction is turned on. (Tape must be removed and reapplied.)

RATIONALE. These measures also change the angle or position of the tube in the stomach. Movement of tube may disrupt gastric sutures; consult with surgeon before changing position of the tube.

f. Irrigate NG (see Procedure 25–5).

ACTION 6. Correct reflux of gastric contents via the pigtail which may occur because of pressure gradients created by changes in the relative heights of the stomach and the collection container:

a. Pin the NG tube to the patient's gown so that the air vent is above the level of the stomach—if patient is side-lying, NG tube should be pinned to the higher, not the dependent, shoulder. (Pin NG tube to the opposite shoulder when patient turns to other side.)

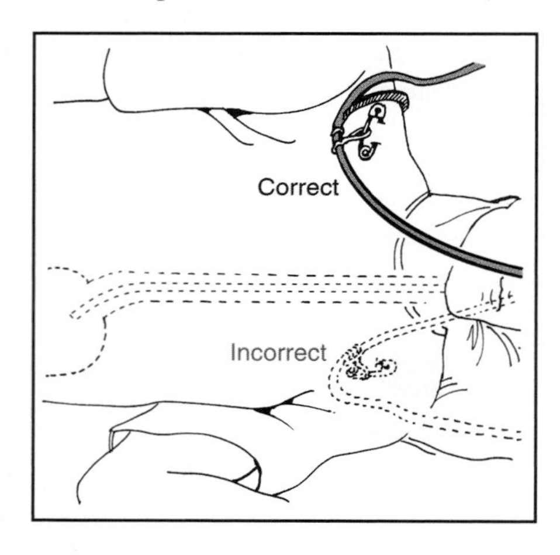

RATIONALE. Gravity prevents fluid in stomach from flowing out of vent. If vent is lower than stomach, syphon effect (movement of fluids from higher to lower level without external suction) will cause reflux out of vent.

b. Keep the collection container below the level of the stomach. It may be necessary to obtain an extension for tubing connecting drainage container to wall suction.

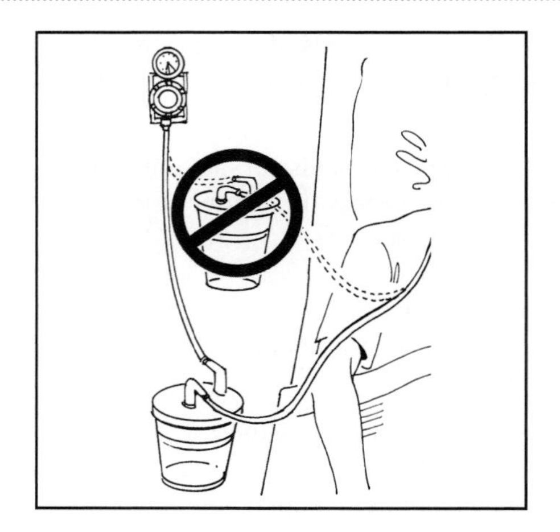

RATIONALE. Fluid levels in two connected containers tend to equalize. If the collection container is higher, fluid will rise in the air vent to seek the level of the container.

c. Maintain patency of both lumina: irrigate drainage lumen (see Procedure 25–5); inject air into air vent. See illustration, Action 5C. Never occlude the air vent to stop reflux.

RATIONALE. Blocked suction lumen will prevent air flow via vent and cause liquid to rise in vent to the level of the block. Positive pressure of air injection clears fluid from vent. If vent is occluded, mucosal damage is likely.

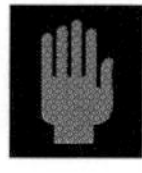

An antireflux valve may be used to prevent spills, if available in your agency (see also Fig. 25–13).

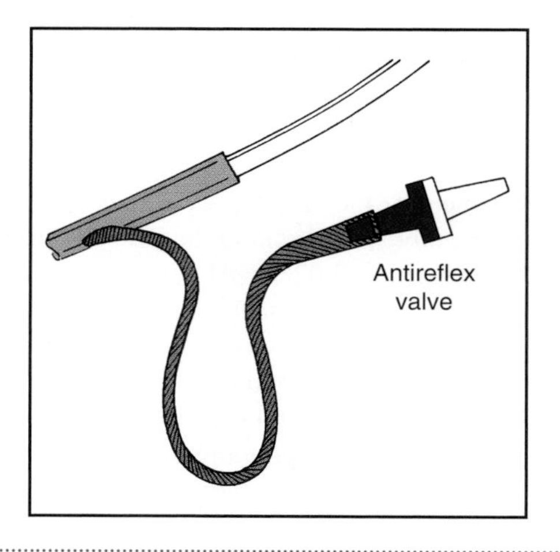

ACTION 7. Supply patients with materials of preference for lubricating mouth: toothbrush/toothpaste, lemon glycerine swabs, NaCl gargle, iced one-half-strength mouthwash, ice chips, chewing gum, lozenges, or hard candy. Offer emollient for lips. Provide mouth care for weak or unconscious patients at least q2h (see Procedure 27–6). Check with physician to verify whether any of the lubrication techniques are contraindicated.

RATIONALE. Patients with NG tubes with suction are NPO; therefore, secretion of saliva is decreased, causing discomfort and cracking of lips. Tube may also irritate throat mucosa. Mouth care increases saliva production and provides supplemental lubrication to mouth, throat, and lips.

ACTION 8. Assist patient to clean nares with moist cotton-tipped applicators prn. Provide water-soluble lubricant for nares.

RATIONALE. Mucus production in the nose is increased because the tube is an irritant. Mucosa may also be eroded because of friction caused by movement of the tube. Dried mucus around the tube increases irritation. Lubricant decreases friction. Water-soluble lubricant is preferred for the nose because it will not cause irritation if accidentlly aspirated into the lungs.

ACTION 9. Retape tube to nose prn (see Procedure 28–2, Action 5C). Remove adhesive residue, if any, with adhesive remover. Recheck tube placement.

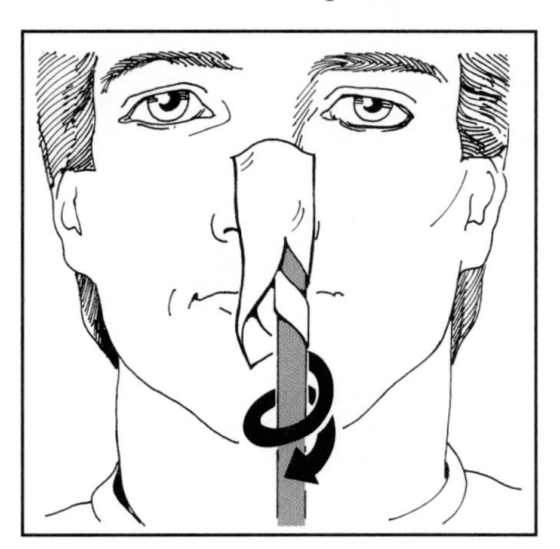

RATIONALE. Skin oils decrease effectiveness of adhesives and may produce a gummy residue, which is not water soluble. Cleaning and retaping promotes comfort and maintains tube placement. Manipulation of tube during care may displace tube, so placement should be rechecked.

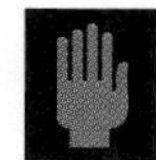

Slight repositioning of tube in nares before retaping will change its point of contact with the nares and the throat, decreasing irritation.

ACTION 10. If patient is ambulatory, suction may be discontinued during ambulation. Disconnect NG from connecting tubing; plug NG tube with catheter plug or the white tip anti–reflux valve. Turn off suction. Be sure pigtail remains above stomach level during ambulation. Resume suction as ordered when ambulation is completed.

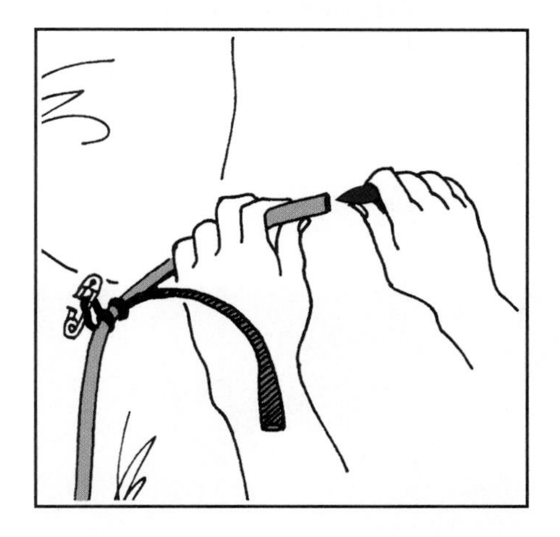

RATIONALE. Short periods without decompression will not cause distension, but secretions will move from stomach out of tube via suction lumen and/or pigtail if end of tube is below level of stomach. (See Action 6.)

ACTION 11. At least q8h, assess:

a. Abdomen for distension and bowel sounds. (Turn off suction to assess for bowel sounds.)

RATIONALE. Abdominal distension indicates buildup of gastrointestinal secretions. Suction is used to prevent this, so suction apparatus should be checked if distension occurs. Presence of bowel sounds in a postoperative patient indicates NG tube is no longer needed, as secretions will be moved via peristalsis.

Continued

Procedure 25–4. Managing Nasogastric Suction (continued)

b. Signs and symptoms of hydrogen, chloride, and potassium depletion (see Chap. 34).

RATIONALE. Gastric secretions are rich in hydrogen, chloride, and potassium, which are removed by suction. Inadequate IV replacement of these electrolytes may result in deficits.

c. Measure and assess color and consistency of drainage. Normal gastric drainage is of slightly mucoid consistency and yellow- or dark-green in color.

RATIONALE. Changes in drainage may indicate complications or improvement in patient's condition. Amount of secretions is expected to decrease as GI function returns.

d. pH and/or hematest if ordered.

RATIONALE. pH is an indicator of tube placement. Occult blood may indicate damage to gastric mucosa. Some blood is expected if gastric surgery was performed.

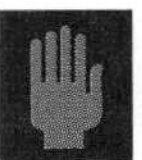

Report presence of drainage that is frankly bloody or with coffee-ground color.

Recording:

Document that suction was maintained as ordered. Describe any problems encountered and action taken to correct them. Record all assessment findings and action taken, if any. Drainage is considered output and is recorded on I&O records.

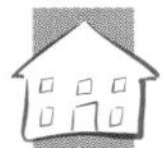

HOME HEALTH ADAPTATION: Initiate a log for family members to record amount and characteristics of gastric contents. Instruct them in reportable signs and symptoms, safety measures and patient comfort measures. This is not a common home health procedure.

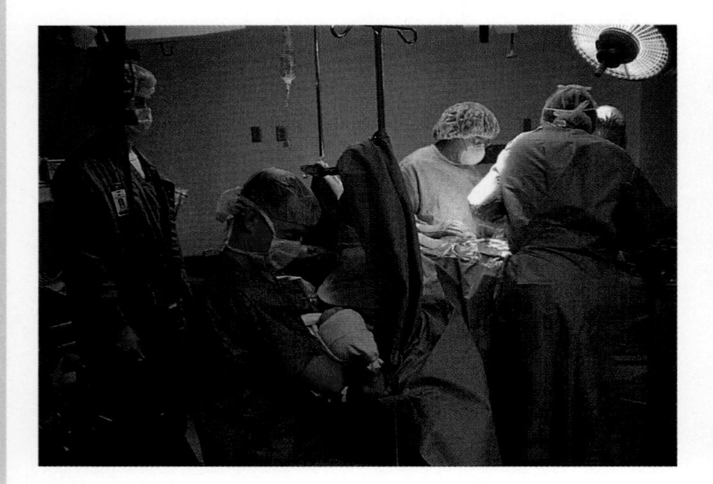

Figure 25–10. The interdisciplinary OR team completes a cesarean section as the father holds his newborn.

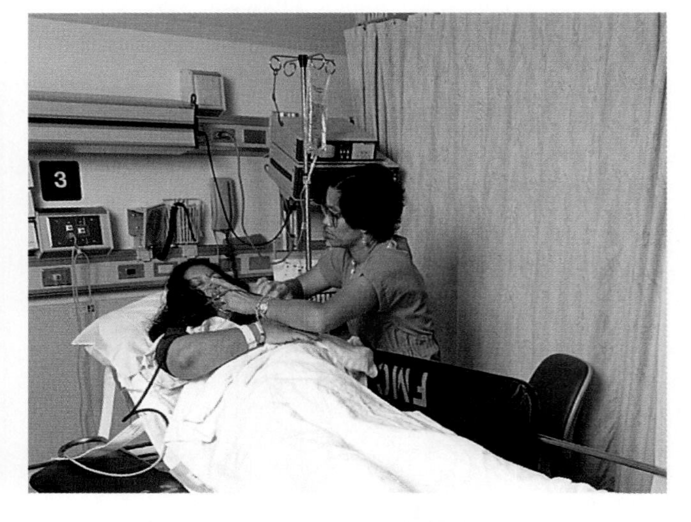

Figure 25–11. Recovery room nurse provides constant assessment and care for patients recovering from the effects of anesthesia.

Postoperative Care

RECOVERY ROOM. The *recovery room* (RR), also called the *postanesthesia room* (PAR) or the *postanesthesia care unit* (PACU), is a special unit for nursing care immediately after surgery is concluded (Fig. 25–11). Patients are carefully monitored using electronic monitoring equipment and direct observation until their physiologic status is stabilized and all effects related to the anesthesia have disappeared. The following are critical postanesthesia assessments:

- Airway and respiratory status: RR, depth, rhythm, breath sounds
- Cardiovascular status: HR, rhythm, BP, color, pulse oximetry, peripheral pulses
- Neurologic status: level of consciousness, return of reflexes, voluntary activity, sensation, pain
- Fluid balance: intake and output (including amount and character of drainage and patency of tubes/drains)
- Wound: condition of dressing, color, consistency of drainage

Nursing measures to promote safety during recovery include positioning to prevent aspiration, suctioning of excessive lower respiratory secretions, administration of oxygen, and initiating deep-breathing exercises when patients are responsive.

Promoting physical and emotional comfort is also important. Most patients need pain relief as the effects of anesthesia wear off. Some may also need antiemetics to counteract nausea and vomiting common during recovery. Many patients complain of feeling cold and may experience shaking and chills. Providing warmed blankets provides welcome relief. The clinical "high-tech" surroundings and absence of loved ones in the recovery room may generate anxiety and rekindle concerns about the findings during surgery. Consistently explaining procedures even when patients seem unresponsive and promptly attending to requests for assistance is reassuring and communicates caring and respect.

CONTINUING POSTOPERATIVE CARE. Postoperative nursing measures after transfer from the recovery room to the general surgical unit support return to normal physiologic functioning and prevent common postoperative complications. These measures include

- *Maintaining respiratory function.* Preventing respiratory complications requires frequent turning, full lung expansion, and aggressive pulmonary hygiene measures. Remind or assist patients to turn to side, back, side and to do deep-breathing exercises every 1 to 2 hours while awake. Incentive spirometers are a practical alternative (see Chap. 30). If secretions accumulate, coughing (see Chap. 30) is added to the breathing routine. As discussed previously, preoperative teaching facilitates effective postoperative execution. Pain relief measures also enhance participation. Suctioning may be necessary for patients who are unable to mobilize and expectorate secretions (see Chap. 30).
- *Preventing circulatory stasis and pathologic clotting.* Frequent position changes, leg exercises, and early ambulation facilitate circulation and prevent pooling of blood in the legs. Many surgeons also order antiembolic stockings or sequential compression devices (SCDs) to enhance venous return. Their application is discussed in Chap. 30.
- *Maintaining fluid balance.* Postoperative patients receive continuous IV fluids until they can take in sufficient fluids by mouth to meet daily fluid requirements. When bowel sounds are noted, oral intake is initiated in small amounts, beginning with clear liquids.
- *Promoting normal urinary elimination.* Urinary function is often suppressed during the immediate postoperative period. Surgery stimulates aldosterone production, so the kidneys conserve fluid. Some anesthetics and narcotics reduce sensation of bladder fullness and temporarily diminish bladder tone. Usually postoperative patients have a Foley catheter in place for the first 24 to 48 hours after surgery. This prevents urinary retention and facilitates monitoring output. About 60 mL of urine per hour is expected; notify the physician if less output is noted. Patients who do not have an indwelling catheter are expected to void within 6 to 8 hours after surgery. If they do not void within that time frame, assess for bladder distension. Techniques to facilitate urinary elimination are discussed in Chap. 29. The same assessment is appropriate after the catheter is discontinued. Accurate intake and output records should be maintained on all surgical patients for at least 48 hours or until a patient demonstrates a normal voiding pattern.
- *Promoting normal bowel elimination.* Typically, bowel function is slowed in the immediate postoperative period as well. Sometimes, the sluggish function is prolonged, a complication called postoperative ileus. It is characterized by nausea, vomiting, absent or diminished bowel sounds, and abdominal distension from accumulated gas and gastrointestinal secretions in the lumen of the bowel. Ileus causes considerable discomfort, particularly in patients with abdominal incisions. Gastric decompression (emptying stomach contents) via a nasogastric tube or a gastrostomy (a surgically created opening through the abdominal wall into the stomach) tube, connected to a source of negative pressure prevents the discomfort associated with sluggish bowel function (Fig. 25–12). The Salem sump tube is a double-lumen tube that is most commonly used to maintain gastric decompression. The Levin tube (a single-lumen tube) is used in some facilities (Fig. 25–13). Procedure 25–4 describes the

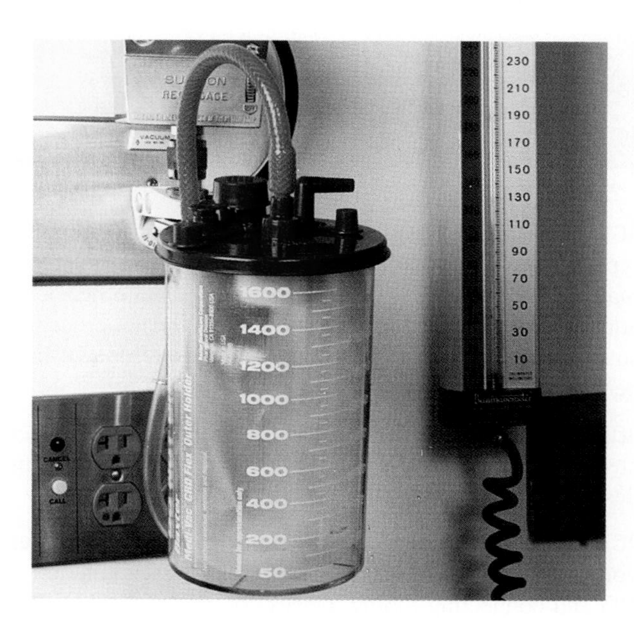

Figure 25–12. Wall suction unit for generating negative pressure for nasogastric decompression. Optimum placement is below the level of the patient's stomach. *(From Smith S, Duell D.* Clinical Nursing Skills: Nursing Process Model; Basic to Advanced Skills. *4th ed. Norwalk, CT: Appleton & Lange; 1996.)*

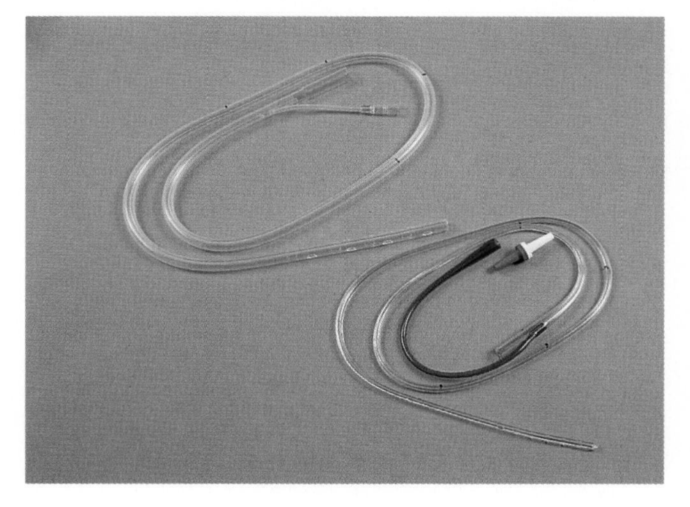

Figure 25–13. Nasogastric tubes used for gastric decompression. **Top left**: Levin (single lumen) tube. **Lower right**: Salem sump (double lumen) tube with anti-reflux value.

PROCEDURE 25–5. IRRIGATING A NASOGASTRIC TUBE

PURPOSE: To clear nasogastric tube of obstruction, so decompression of stomach is maintained, preventing abdominal distension, nausea, and vomitting.

EQUIPMENT: Irrigation set, normal saline or tap water, and disposable waterproof underpad.

ACTION 1. Check physician's order or agency policy for type and amount of solution to be used for irrigation. Normal saline or tap water may be specified. Obtain necessary equipment. NG irrigation is a clean, not a sterile, procedure so equipment may be kept in room and reused for a 24-hour period.

ACTION 2. Discuss the purpose of the irrigation, associated assessments and trouble shooting, usual sensations, desired patient participation, and expected benefits.

ACTION 3. Pour solution (or obtain from tap) into reservoir. Place waterproof underpad on bed under junction of NG and connecting tubing. Check for placement (see Procedure 25–4). If tube is in stomach proceed to Action 4. If not, advance tube 1 to 2 inches and check again. (Tape must be removed and reapplied.)

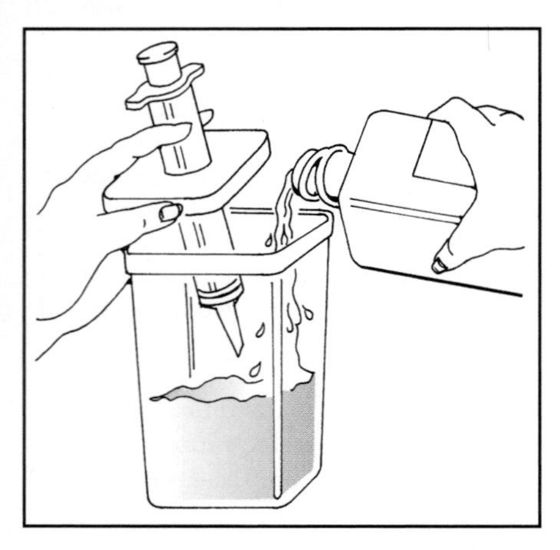

ACTION 4. Draw up 30 to 50 mL in syringe and inject all of liquid into tube. If NG tube is a Salem sump tube, keep pigtail above level of stomach during irrigation to prevent reflux.

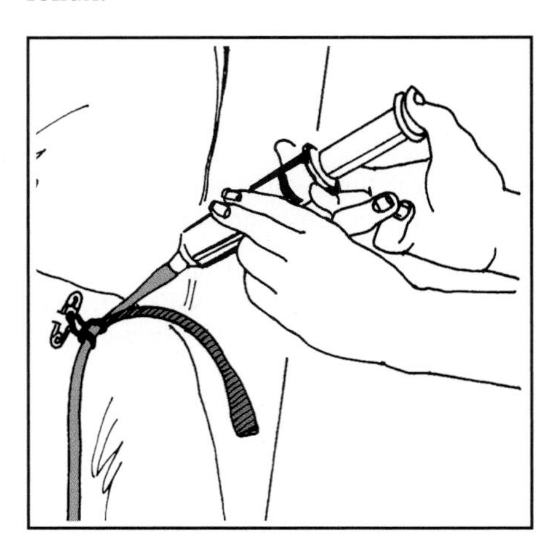

ACTION 5. Reattach NG tube to connecting tubing. If drainage now moves toward drainage collector, check pigtail for hissing sound. Inject 10 mL of air to clear tube if no air movement can be heard.

ACTION 6. Assist patient to comfortable position. Store equipment at bedside for next irrigation.

ACTION 7. If no return of irrigant is obtained, repeat Actions 4 and 5, above. Repeat instillation a third time if second attempt is not successful. If no return is obtained after third instillation of fluid, reposition patient to change angle of tubing in stomach. Tubing may be advanced 1 to 2 inches more to reach pool of liquid in stomach, if fluid still does not return.

ACTION 8. If none of the above measures result in return of fluid, repeat trouble-shooting measures described in Procedure 25–4. If unable to determine cause of problem, do not irrigate again, as fluid in stomach stimulates production of secretions, so is contraindicated if suction is not functioning correctly. Report status of patient and equipment to charge nurse or physician.

Recording:
Document procedure, patient's response, problems, and action taken. Record total amount of fluid instilled as intake.

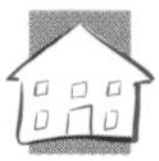

HOME HEALTH ADAPTATION: This procedure requires no adaptations for the home setting, but is not common in home health care.

management of nasogastric suction. To maintain effective decompression, the nasogastric tube must remain patent. Procedure 25–5 describes the technique for irrigating a nasogastric tube to maintain patency. Nasogastric tubes remain in place until peristalsis resumes. Presence of bowel sounds and passage of flatus indicate the return of peristalsis. This means the tube can be discontinued and oral intake resumed. For most patients bowel activity resumes in 1 to 3 days after surgery. Problems with nausea and distension can be minimized in patients who do not have NG tubes by limiting oral intake to small sips of fluids initially and slowly progressing to regular dietary intake. Normal bowel movements are not expected until oral intake is resumed. Early ambulation facilitates return of bowel functioning.

- *Supporting nutrition.* Dietary intake following surgery is dependent upon the extent of the surgery and the organs involved. It is dependent on the return of normal bowel function, as discussed above. When the surgery presents no interference with bowel function, patients can begin oral intake as soon as they are fully recovered from the effects of anesthesia, progressing from clear liquids to a regular diet. Postoperative patients benefit from liberal fluid and protein intake when normal gastrointestinal function returns. Healing is also enhanced by vitamins A and C and zinc. See also Chaps. 27 and 28. Patients who must remain NPO for longer than 3 to 5 days are candidates for total parenteral nutrition (see Chap. 28).
- *Promoting comfort and rest.* Incisional pain, tension and irritation from tubes, tight dressings, muscular aches from positioning in the operating room, and abdominal distension make comfort and rest elusive for many postoperative patients. Relief measures such as relaxation, imagery, diversion, and administration of medications were discussed earlier in this chapter. Other interventions for relief of severe pain can be found in Chap. 32. Effective pain management and adequate rest are vital to healing and uncomplicated recovery.
- *Preventing infection.* As discussed earlier in this chapter, surgical patients are at risk for infection. The bladder, lungs, and the surgical wound are the most common sites of postoperative infection. Many of the nursing measures discussed above protect patients against infection.
  - Postoperative bladder infections are most often traced to poor technique when inserting a urinary catheter or failing to follow established protocols when moving, positioning, and giving catheter care to patients with indwelling catheters (see Chap. 29). Maintaining hydration and promoting urinary elimination also reduce the risk of bladder infections.
  - Aggressive pulmonary hygiene, including hourly deep-breathing exercises, incentive spirometry, and early ambulation promote pulmonary expansion, remove pooled secretions, and prevent the development of postoperative pneumonia.
  - Most surgical wounds are covered with a sterile dressing to prevent contamination and to collect drainage. Enhancing healing by supporting the body's natural defenses, using aseptic technique during dressing changes, maintaining patency of surgical drains, and applying the standard precautions for infection control discussed earlier in the chapter are nursing responsibilities. Wounds, healing, wound infections are discussed in greater detail in Chap. 27.
- *Meeting the psychological needs of postsurgical patients.* The multiple stressors that accompany surgery tax the coping skills of most people. Refer to Table 25–10, Impact of Surgery on Well-being. The primary postoperative psychological issues—altered body image, self-concept, and role performance—may not be prominent during the acute phase of recovery. Although most postoperative patients find their incision and the associated bulky dressings, multiple tubes, and visible drainage containers somewhat distressing, not all express concerns directly. Irritability, frequent demands for assistance, tearfulness, withdrawal, and sleep disturbances are indicators that stressors are stretching coping resources.

Recognizing that patients need control as well as nurturing is the key to effective emotional support. Discussing the rationale for prescribed activities, providing consistent pain relief, offering empathic listening, and promoting rest and relaxation are nurturing. Soliciting patient input in scheduling routine care and inviting and normalizing expressions of anger or other negative emotions are ways of respecting patients' needs for control. Motivating but not coercing patients to participate in treatment measures that will expedite their recovery despite being uncomfortable or tiring requires sensitivity and skilled communication. It does much to support self-worth and self-respect as patients adapt to the challenges in the postoperative period.

As recovery progresses at home, there will be new challenges and adjustments. Anticipatory guidance for patients and their families enables effective coping responses. Asking them to share their expectations about their first several weeks at home is one way to identify misconceptions and teaching needs and to validate and support realistic plans and perceptions. Information for patients and families that will facilitate healthy adaptation after major surgery includes

- Gains in energy, strength, and overall well-being will be gradual. You may even feel that you are regressing or "losing ground" on some days. This is normal. Remember that you

INSIGHTS FROM NURSING LITERATURE

NURSES' ASEPTIC TECHNIQUE IN DRESSING WOUNDS

Bree-Williams FJ, Waterman H. An examination of nurses' practices when performing aseptic technique for wound dressings. J Adv Nurs. *1996;23:48–54.*

Questioning the ritualistic nature of some aseptic practices in light of recent efforts to streamline sterile wound dressing procedure, the researchers designed a study to determine if nurses' practices were simple, were based on up-to-date knowledge, and did not incur an unnecessary waste of resources. They studied 21 nurses on a surgical ward as they performed aseptic dressing changes. The findings showed subjects lacked up-to-date knowledge on aseptic wound care practices. Indeed, most subjects were unaware of the scientific rationale for the new streamlined procedures and used old variations that were complicated and inefficient. The researchers cautioned, however, that their findings, gathered on subjects in one hospital, are not generalizable to other settings.

TABLE 25-10. IMPACT OF SURGERY ON WELL-BEING

Alteration	Associated Stressors
Disruption of skin integrity	Potential infection of surgical incision Potential wound dehiscence or evisceration Change in body image/self-esteem
Disruption of circulatory system	Possible postoperative hemorrhage Excessive fluid losses Problems related to venous stasis (thrombus, thrombophlebitis) Potential infection/inflammation at IV site
Altered respiratory function	Pooling of respiratory secretions in lungs/alveoli Decreased lung expansion related to immobility and pain Potential trauma to larnyx during intubation/extubation
Altered nutrition	Potential negative nitrogen balance Problems with nausea and vomiting
Activation of the stress response	Increased fluid retention/potential fluid overload
Altered elimination	Decreased peristalsis Potential problems with postoperative ileus Abdominal distension Constipation Postoperative urinary retention Potential urinary tract infection related to catheterization
Decreased physical mobility	Increased risk of venous stasis Pooling of respiratory secretions Potential problems with skin breakdown Decreased muscle strength/joint mobility
Altered body temperature	Increased vasodilation from anesthetic agents Exposure of internal organs to cold operating room (OR) environment Infusion of cool IV fluids Fever related to infectious process
Sleep pattern disturbance	Altered normal biorhythms Use of narcotics/anesthetics Round-the-clock monitoring/assessment Postoperative pain
Pain	Incisional pain Irritation from tubes/drains Muscular soreness related to OR positioning
Fluid and electrolyte imbalance	Excessive fluid losses Restricted oral intake Potential fluid overload from IV fluid administration Increased aldosterone and antidiuretic hormone secretion
Altered sensory perception	Loss of consciousness Decreased sensation/orientation related to use of narcotics Sensory overload or deprivation
Altered body image	Loss of body part or function Permanent incisional scar Invasion of body by tubes, equipment Possible alteration in sexual expression
Altered role performance	Changes in family relationships Possible financial difficulties Permanent lifestyle alterations

TABLE 25-10. CONTINUED

Alteration	Associated Stressors
Self-care deficit	Forced to assume dependent role Change in normal hygiene routines Sense of powerlessness Invasion of privacy Loss of self-esteem
Fear/anxiety	Decreased attention span Disturbance of sleep/rest Increased conflict in interpersonal relationships

will need rest periods every day for optimal healing. Let willing family and friends help at first. This will hasten your return to independence.
- Your incision should appear completely healed within a week or two. Itching and soreness are normal during healing. The scar will change gradually for up to 6 months. It will shrink and the redness will fade, but it will not disappear altogether.
- Don't be alarmed if you feel emotional. Irritability, crying, sadness, even mild depression are normal reactions to the changes in your body, not signs of weakness. Talking about your feelings is a good way to help yourself feel better. Usually these feelings begin to resolve as you regain strength and independence. If you feel listless and blue for several weeks, it's a good idea to call your primary care provider.
- Family members can help by providing assistance at first, then encouraging increasing independence. Avoid a "take charge" approach. Be accepting of mood swings, listen without offering advice, and share your own concerns in a nonthreatening way.

For some postsurgical patients, home health care is appropriate. Nursing implementation for restorative care in the home setting is addressed in a later section.

Administering Medications

A **medication** or **drug** is a chemical substance used for therapeutic purposes: diagnosis, treatment, cure, or prevention of disease. Drugs are a component of many patients' medical treatment. Nurses often administer the medications to patients needing restorative care.

Administering medications responsibly requires that nurses (1) understand general basic concepts relating to drugs; (2) understand how the body responds to drugs; and (3) safely and skillfully perform the mechanics of administering medications by all routes.

Collaborative effort contributes to the safe and effective use of medications. Physician, pharmacist, nurse, and patient have important responsibilities in obtaining maximum patient benefit from medications.

General Concepts. Legal responsibilities of nurses, systems of measurement and dosage calculation, drug names and related terminology, and responsibilities to patients are presented in this section.

LEGAL RESPONSIBILITIES. Drug production, distribution, prescription, and administration in the United States and Canada are governed by federal, state, and provincial laws. The Canadian Food and Drug Act was passed in 1953 with many subsequent amendments. The major U.S. federal laws controlling drugs are the Food, Drug, and Cosmetic Act (1938) and its amendments, which require proof of the safety and efficacy of a drug before it can be sold; and the Controlled Substances Act (1970), which sets strict controls on the manufacture and distribution of narcotics and other controlled substances. Nurses have legal responsibilities for administering medications safely and for maintaining the security of controlled substances. All controlled substances are kept in double-locked cabinets. Access to keys is limited to licensed nurses and possession of keys is documented. Nurses keep a precise inventory of all controlled substances received from the facility's central pharmacy and dispensed to patients or wasted (because of contamination or administering only a partial dose) on their unit. Two nurses verify the accuracy of the inventory at the beginning and end of every shift.

Recent federal legislation has extended rights to prescribe medications to nurse practitioners in certain rural areas. Some states have expanded the prescription rights of nurse practitioners to include other settings. State nurse practice acts govern most aspects of medication administration by registered nurses. The following discussion provides a general overview of the important legal responsibilities included in most practice acts.

No medication can be legally administered without a valid, signed order from a qualified health care provider. Verbal or telephone orders are acceptable, but must be received and transcribed on a patient's chart by a licensed caregiver (usually a registered nurse or pharmacist) and must be signed by the prescriber within the time frame specified by institutional policy. A valid medication order contains the following essential components:

- The patient's full name.
- Date (including the day, month, and year) and time the order was written.
- Drug name, clearly written and correctly spelled.
- Dosage: strength, amount, and/or number of tablets.
- Route of administration. Route refers to the way a drug enters the body: eg, by mouth or by injection. A nurse who believes a patient's condition makes the ordered route inappropriate (for example, a patient who is nauseated and vomiting with orders for oral medications) must contact the prescriber before changing the route. However, it is appropriate for a nurse to administer another form of the drug by the ordered route. For example, a nurse can substitute the liquid form of an oral medication for a tablet if a patient is having difficulty swallowing the tablet, so long as the ordered dosage is given. Table 25–11 lists common forms in which drugs are manufactured.
- Frequency. The time of day is also specified for some drugs. A medication order for regular ongoing administration of a drug is called a **routine order.** An order stating a drug is to be given only once is called a **one-time order.** Some one-time orders indicate that a mediation is to be given immediately. This is called a **stat order.** If a drug is ordered to be given as needed by the patient, the order is a **prn order.** Valid prn orders specify the condition of need, for example, "pain" or "fever above 102°F."

Medication orders often contain *abbreviations*. The abbreviations may be used to indicate dosage, routes of administration, and special information for nurses to follow when dispensing the drug. Table 25–12 lists abbreviations commonly used in medication orders.

Nurses are responsible for *questioning* any order that is unclear or incomplete or that seems unreasonable or inappropriate for the patient. Refuse to administer the medication until the order is clarified or corrected. Orders of these kinds not only raise the possibility of harm to patients, they also put nurses at risk for a lawsuit. A nurse who administers a drug according to an incorrect medication order will be held responsible for the error. "Because it was ordered" offers no legal or ethical protection. To evaluate the appropriateness of a medication order for a particular patent, nurses need to know the expected therapeutic benefit for that patient (some drugs have more than one therapeutic effect), the usual dosage, major side effects, and contraindications.

Medication orders are *transcribed* to a form, often called a **medication administration record (MAR),** which is used as a guide for scheduling drug administration and to document drugs given or withheld. Increasingly, hospitals are using computer-generated MARs, which reduce the incidence of errors. The transcription of orders is often a clerk's responsibility. However, a registered nurse must verify all transcribed orders, that is, compare the transcription to the written order in a patient's chart, to ensure accuracy and thoroughness of transcription.

Once a medication has been given, nurses must *document* the time and route of administration and monitor the patient for intended or undesired effects. Document any unexpected responses and notify the prescriber.

SYSTEMS OF MEASUREMENT AND CALCULATING ACCURATE DOSAGES. Three systems of measurement are used in North America for drug therapy: metric, apothecary, and household. Nurses must be familiar with these systems and be able to convert from one system to another.

TABLE 25-11. COMMON FORMS OF MEDICATIONS

Form	Description
Capsule	Powder, liquid, or oil form of medication enclosed in a gelatin shell.
Elixir	Medication in a clear liquid containing alcohol, water, sweeteners, and flavoring. Designed for oral use.
Liniment	Medication mixed with alcohol, oil, or soapy emollient, which is applied to the skin.
Lotion	Drug in liquid suspension designed for topical use.
Lozenge	Flat round preparation containing drug in a flavored or sweetened base that dissolves in the mouth to release the medication. Also known as a *troche*.
Ointment	Semisolid preparation of one or more drugs applied to the skin.
Paste	Semisolid preparation, thicker and stiffer than ointment; absorbed more slowly than ointment through the skin.
Pill	Mixture of powdered drug with cohesive material in round, oval, or oblong shape.
Powder	A drug ground into fine particles from a solid for inhalation or application to the skin.
Solution	A drug dissolved in another liquid substance. May be used orally, parenterally, or externally.
Suppository	One or more drugs mixed into a firm base, such as gelatin, designed for insertion into a body cavity. The preparation melts at body temperature, thus releasing the medication for absorption.
Suspension	Fine drug particles dispersed in a liquid medium. Must be shaken before use.
Syrup	Medication dissolved in a concentrated sugar solution to mask unpleasant taste.
Tablet	A powdered form of medication compressed into a hard small disk or cylinder. May be a variety of colors or sizes. Enteric-coated tablets are covered with a substance that is insoluble in gastric acids, thus reducing possible gastric irritation.
Transdermal patch	A self-adhesive patch containing medication that is absorbed continuously via the skin and acts systemically.

TABLE 25-12. ABBREVIATIONS COMMONLY USED IN MEDICATION ORDERS

Abbreviation	Meaning
ac	Before meals
ad lib	Freely; as desired
bid	Twice a day
c̄	With
cap	Capsule
D/C	Discontinue
elix	Elixir
hs	At bedtime; hour of sleep
IM	Intramuscular
IV	Intravenous
IVPB	IV piggyback
OD	Right eye
OS	Left eye
OU	Both eyes
pc	After meals
po	By mouth
prn	As needed; when necessary
q	Every
qd	Every day
qh	Every hour
qid	Four times a day
qod	Every other day
qs	Sufficient quantity
s̄	Without
SC or SQ	Subcutaneous
$\overline{ss}$	One-half
stat	Immediately
supp	Suppository
tid	Three times a day

- *Metric system.* The metric system is used most frequently. It is a logically organized system with one basic unit for each type of measurement. Larger secondary units are derived by multiplying by 10 (100, 1000) and are designated by Greek prefixes: deka- (10), hecto- (100), kilo- (1000). Smaller secondary units are derived by dividing by 10 (0.1, 0.01) and are designated by Latin prefixes: deci- (0.1), centi- (0.01), milli- (0.001). The measurements relevant to drug administration are volume and weight. The basic units for these measures are the *liter* (volume) and the *gram* (weight). Fractions of units are written in decimal form: for example, one-half of a gram is written 0.5 g. A zero is placed in front of the decimal point to prevent errors in interpretation. Table 25–13 shows the relationships between metric system units for volume and weight that are commonly used in drug therapy.
- *Apothecary system.* The apothecary system was brought to the United States and Canada from England during Colonial days. Although physicians and pharmacists formerly used the apothecary system extensively, it has been replaced by the metric system in most health care facilities. Some of the units of measurement of the apothecary system are familiar because we use them in daily life. We measure fluids in pints and quarts, weight in pounds, and length in feet and inches. However, the basic units and those most often used to order and prepare medications are smaller units. The basic unit of weight is the *grain* (equal to the weight of a grain of wheat in Colonial days), and the basic unit of volume is the *minim* (a volume of water equal to the same grain of wheat). The units of weight in ascending order are the grain, dram, ounce, and pound. The units of volume in ascending order are the minim, fluid dram, fluid ounce, pint, quart, and gallon. When the apothecary system is used for ordering medications, quantities are designated by lowercase Roman numerals. The Roman numeral follows rather than precedes the unit of measure. For example, 3 grains (gr.) would be written as gr. iii.
- *Household measurements.* Household measurements are also familiar to most people: drops, teaspoons, tablespoons, cups, and glasses. However, household measurements are used less frequently for medications because household utensils are not

TABLE 25-13. METRIC SYSTEM: RELATIONSHIPS OF UNITS FOR VOLUME AND WEIGHT

Units	1	0.1	0.01	0.001	0.000001
Prefixes	Gram (g)	Deci-	Centi-	Milli-	Micro-
Weight		Decigram (convert to grams)	Centigram (cg)	Milligram (mg)	Microgram (μg)
Equivalents	1 g	(10 decigrams)	100 cg	1000 mg	1×10^6 (μg)
	0.1 g		1 cg	100 mg	
	0.01 g			10 mg	
	0.001 g			1 mg	1000 (μg)
				0.001 mg	1 (μg)
Volume	Liter (L)	Deciliter (dL)		Milliliter (mL)	
Equivalents	1 L			1000 mL	
	0.1 L	1 dL		100 mL	
	0.001 L			1 mL	

TABLE 25–14. EQUIVALENTS OF MEASUREMENT

Apothecary	Metric	Household
15 or 16 minims	= 1 milliliter (mL)	= 15 drops (gtts)
1 dram (ʒ)	= 4 or 5 mL	= 1 teaspoon (tsp)
4 ʒ	= 15 mL	= 1 tablespoon (tbsp) (3 tsp)
1 fluid ounce (℥)	= 30 mL	= 2 tbsp
1 grain (gr)	= 60 (64) milligrams (mg)	
7½ gr	= 500 mg	
15 gr	= 1 gram (g)	
1 pound (lb)	= 454 g	
2.2 lb	= 1 kilogram (kg)	

manufactured to a uniform standard. When accuracy is not critical, it is safe to use household measures, such as with many over-the-counter drugs (antacids, cough syrups, etc).

Table 25–14 illustrates the most frequently used **equivalents** between the three systems of measurement. Conversions involving household measures and grains and minims are approximate, not exact.

Medications are usually supplied in the dosages most commonly used. If an order specifies a dose other than what is supplied, a *mathematical calculation* is necessary to determine the exact amount of a drug to give. All problems relating to drug dosages can be solved by using a proportion. The dosage on hand is indicated on medication container or package. Write it on the left side of the proportion, the unknown in the right. Figure 25–14 contains a sample dosage calculation.

Sometimes a medication order specifies a dosage in units of one system of measurement (eg, grains) and the drug is supplied in units of another (eg, milligrams). In these instances, you must *convert the dosage* specified in the order to its equivalent in the units supplied (eg, convert grains to milligrams) to determine the quantity of medicine to give. Use the equivalents in Table 25–14 to set up a proportion. Accurately solving a proportion for converting dosages from one measurement system to another requires that only two different units of measure be used in the proportion. For example, do not use grains, milligrams, and milliliters as units in one proportion. In this case, use two separate calculations: grains to milligrams using equivalents in a conversion table, then milligrams to milliliters according to the concentration (milligrams per milliliter) specified on the medication container. Figure 25–15 shows a sample conversion between systems.

Verifying the accuracy of dosages ordered for children requires caution. Because of their small size and relatively immature organ systems, the margin for error is smaller and the response to drugs less predictable. References that designate *pediatric dosages* for specific drugs in milligrams per kilogram of body weight are the most useful resource for validating the appropriateness of pediatric medication orders. Using the dosage parameters specified for a particular drug, rather than a standard formula, is considered the safest method for calculating pediatric drug dosages. If no such reference is available for a given drug, a formula based on **body surface area (BSA)**—a calculation of the quantity in square meters of the surface of a person's body—is recommended.

BSA is determined by using a **standard nomogram** (Fig. 25–16). Plot the child's height and weight on the designated axes and connect the two points with a straight line. The point at which the line crosses the surface area axis (center) is the child's estimated body surface area. For example, a child who is 4 feet, 2 inches (50 inches) tall and weighs 75 pounds has a body surface area of 1.08 m^2. The *BSA-based formula* for calculating a child's dose of medication is:

$$\text{Child's dose} = \frac{\text{Surface area of child}}{1.7\ \text{m}^2} \times \text{Normal adult dose}$$

DRUG NAMES AND CLASSIFICATIONS. Most drugs have three different names. The **chemical name** provides an exact description of the chemical composition of the drug. It is rarely used by health care providers. The **generic name** is a shorter name, often derived from the chemical name. This is the name by which each drug is listed in official pharmacologic publications, such as *The United States Pharmacopeia (USP)* or *The British Pharmacopoeia (BP)*. These references are official listings of drugs used in the United States and Canada, respectively. They describe drugs in detail according to several categories such as source, chemical formulas, physical properties, and usual dosages. The **trade or proprietary name** is the name under which a manufacturer markets a drug. Some drugs are manufactured by many different companies; therefore, a drug may have many trade names. For example, acetaminophen (generic name) is known by the trade names of Anacin-3, Datril, Panadol, Tempra, and Tylenol.

Physician's medication order: Aspirin 650 mg q4h po prn for pain.
Drug available: Aspirin 325 mg tablets.

	Known equivalent		Unknown equivalent
1. Set up proportion: write units of measure in the same position on both sides of proportion.	325 mg / 1 tab	=	650 mg / X tab
2. Cross-multiply.		=	650 x 1 325X
3. Solve for X.	325X / 325 (cancelled)	=	650 / 325 = 2 tabs

Figure 25–14. Sample drug dosage calculation.

Physician's medication order: Phenobarbital gr ¾ po bid. Drug available: Phenobarbital elixir 20 mg per 5 mL.

Step 1: Convert measurements to same system.

	Known equivalent		Unknown equivalent
Set up proportion: Write units in the same position on both sides of proportion (gr in top position on both right and left side of proportion).	$\frac{1\ gr}{60\ mg}$	=	$\frac{3/4\ gr}{X\ mg}$
Cross-multiply.	1X	=	60 x ¾
Solve for X.	X	=	45 mg

Step 2: Calculate amount of drug to be given.

	Known equivalent		Unknown equivalent
Set up proportion: Write units of measure in the same position on both sides of proportion.	$\frac{20\ mg}{5\ mL}$	=	$\frac{45\ mg}{X\ mL}$
Reduce to lowest common denominator.	$\frac{4\ \not{20}\ mg}{1\ \not{5}\ mL}$	=	$\frac{45\ mg}{X\ mL}$
Cross-multiply.	4X	=	1 x 45
Solve for X.	$\frac{\not{4}X}{\not{4}}$	=	$\frac{45}{4}$ = 11.25 mL

Answer: Give 11.25 mL of available phenobarbital elixir.

Figure 25–15. Drug dosage calculation with conversion between systems.

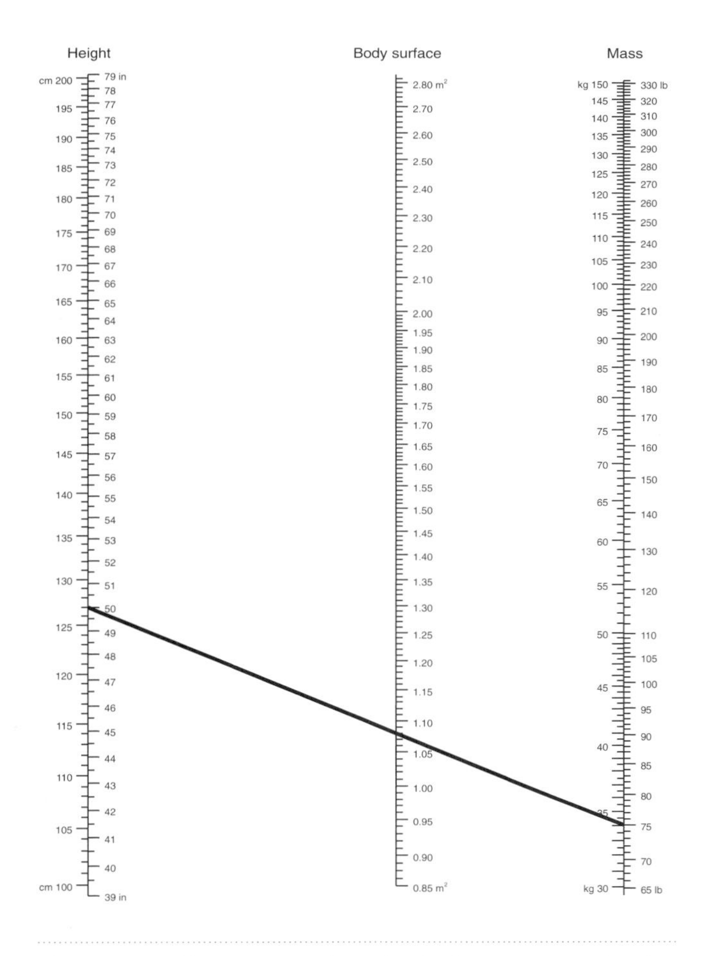

Figure 25–16. Nomogram to determine body surface area by plotting height and weight on the parallel axes.

Drug *classification systems* are designed to organize the vast body of information related to medications. Three systems are in common use: body system (eg, cardiac drugs); clinical indication (eg, antihypertensives, laxatives); and chemical attributes (eg, barbiturates, calcium channel blockers).

RESPONSIBILITY TO PATIENTS. Responsibility to patients, the final general drug-related concept, involves assessment, teaching, and patient advocacy. *Patient assessment* is an essential nursing responsibility associated with administering medications. A **medication history** includes a review of drugs (prescription drugs, over-the-counter medications, and recreational drugs such as alcohol, marijuana, etc) that a patient is taking currently or has taken in the past. Documentation of known or suspected drug allergies or adverse reactions is also part of this history. Prior to the giving a medication, nurses assess the *physiologic* or *psychological* functions the drug is expected to affect, either as a therapeutic or as a side effect. For example, assess blood pressure prior to giving an antihypertensive, pain before giving an analgesic, respiratory rate before giving a narcotic that depresses respirations. This assessment provides information on which to base a decision to give or withhold a drug and a baseline to use in evaluating patients' responses to the medications.

Although health care providers typically refer to medication orders as "prescriptions," nurses must not expect patients to unquestioningly accept every medication they offer. For patients to give *informed consent to medications,* they must be aware of the anticipated therapeutic effects, major adverse side effects, and other available treatment options. Once a patient agrees to take medications, nurses provide information about how to maximize the therapeutic effect and minimize adverse side effects. When patients are taking multiple medications, nurses should collaborate with prescribers and pharmacists to identify undesirable drug interactions and find ways to eliminate or mitigate these effects.

Nurses and patients need to discuss the names and dosages of medications that will be continued after discharge from a health care facility and develop a daily schedule that is compatible with a patient's home routine without compromising the drug's effectiveness. Inquire about over-the-counter drugs and home remedies (herbals, other special preparations) patients use regularly, so their possible interaction with the current drug therapy can be explored. Most patients need teaching and opportunities to *practice administration techniques* for routes other than oral. They should also be made aware of signs and symptoms related to their medications that warrant contact with their primary health care provider. Whenever possible include family members in teaching–learning exchanges.

Be alert for verbal and nonverbal indicators that either patients or family members have personal concerns about maintaining the drug therapy at home. Issues such as cost, inconvenience, anticipated discomfort, and negative feelings about taking drugs are common barriers to effective home management of drug therapy. Frank discussion and exploration of these concerns can result in a decision to make a commitment to carry out the recommended regimen or to seek other options with the help of health care providers.

Drugs and the Body. Once administered, all drugs go through four stages: absorption, distribution, biotransformation or metabolism, and excretion. *Pharmacokinetics* is the study of these four drug processes. Each drug has its own unique pharmacokinetic properties.

ABSORPTION. **Absorption** is the process by which a drug is transferred from its site of entry into the body or **route** to the circulatory system. This process occurs in the gastrointestinal tract, subcutaneous tissue, muscles, skin, and mucous membranes. Several factors influence the rate of absorption.

Drugs given by any route must be in liquid form to be absorbed. Oral drugs administered in a solid form that dissolve easily are absorbed readily. Drug preparations with poorly soluble components delay drug absorption. Sometimes delayed release is desired. For example, oral drugs that are highly irritating to gastric mucosa or that would be inactivated in an acid medium are coated with a substance that is resistant to dissolution in the stomach called **enteric coating.**

Gastrointestinal motility greatly influences absorption of oral drugs as well. If motility is sluggish because of constipation, the time a drug remains in the GI tract is extended. This permits greater absorption, perhaps even in toxic amounts. With diarrhea, the rapid movement of intestinal contents may limit or preclude absorption. The presence or absence of food in the gastrointestinal tract can enhance or hinder the rate of absorption, depending on the drug.

Route determines the nature of the tissue a drug initially contacts. Tissue type influences absorption. Drugs that are injected directly into the bloodstream are immediately absorbed. Drugs are more rapidly absorbed from muscle, because it is more vascular, than from subcutaneous tissue; absorption via both of these routes is faster than via oral administration.

High concentrations of a medication are absorbed more quickly than low doses. Because of this, higher initial doses called **loading doses** are sometimes given to rapidly achieve therapeutic levels. Then smaller **maintenance doses** can be given on a regular schedule.

DISTRIBUTION. **Distribution** is the process by which a drug is transported in body fluids to the site of action. Organs having the most extensive blood supply such as the heart, brain, liver, and kidneys receive drugs the most rapidly. The rate and extent of distribution depend on the physical and chemical properties of the medication and the physiology of the person taking the drug.

Distribution may be general or selective. Some drugs have an affinity for specific tissue. Drugs that are fat-soluble tend to accumulate in adipose tissue. Water-soluble drugs cannot pass through the blood–brain barrier and therefore are relatively ineffective on the central nervous system. The placenta is a less specific barrier, but it blocks the distribution of some drugs to fetal circulation. A drug's *binding to albumin* and other plasma proteins also affects the drug's distribution. When bound to albumin, drugs cannot exert their therapeutic effect. Plasma protein binding acts as a kind of reservoir, because the temporary "storage" in the drug–protein complex allows the drug to remain in the body for a longer period of time, and then exert its therapeutic effect as it is slowly released. Many factors effect the amount of protein binding. Refer to a pharmacology text for a detailed discussion.

BIOTRANSFORMATION. **Biotransformation,** or **metabolism,** is the process that changes a drug into an inactive form and prepares it for excretion. Most of this process takes place in the liver, where a variety of enzymes alter a drug's active chemicals. For this reason, individuals with impaired liver function are at greater risk for drug toxicity. If the liver cannot effectively metabolize a drug, it will remain in the active form for unusually long time periods. Cumulative drug effects result as subsequent doses increase the concentration of active drug.

EXCRETION. **Excretion** is the process by which drugs and their metabolites (breakdown products) are eliminated from the body. The kidneys are the primary organs of excretion, although some drugs are excreted through the intestines, respiratory tract, and sweat, salivary, and mammary glands. Compromised kidney function delays excretion. Changes in urine pH enhance or inhibit excretion of drugs, depending on its pH.

DRUG EFFECTS. Drugs do not introduce new responses in the body, but rather act to alter existing physiologic activity. Drugs interact with the body in several different ways—by interacting with enzymes, by affecting cell membranes or cellular processes, and most commonly by binding or interacting with chemical receptor sites at the cellular level. All medications produce multiple physiologic responses or effects in the body—some desirable and some undesirable. Nurses need to understand the terms used to describe these effects to correctly interpret information about specific drugs and to accurately communicate with others about drug effects that they observe in patients. The **therapeutic effect** is the effect for which the drug was prescribed. To achieve this effect, the **therapeutic level,** the concentration of a drug in the bloodstream needed to produce the therapeutic effect without toxicity, must be reached. The terms *plasma level* and *serum level* are used to refer to measurement of drug concentration in the bloodstream. Therapeutic level is expressed as a range rather than a precise amount. There is variation among individuals in the serum level needed to produce the desired effect of a given drug. For some intravenous medications, plasma levels are drawn just after a dose is given, the point of its **peak concentration,** and again just before the subsequent dose is due. At this time, the plasma concentration is expected to be at its lowest level (**trough concentration**). Sometimes this combination is called simply "peak and trough."

Drugs may also act unpredictably, be harmful, or have unpleasant effects. **Side effects** are unintended effects. They may be undesirable (often called adverse effects), neutral, or even beneficial. Side effects are often tolerated in order to achieve the drug's therapeutic effect. **Idiosyncratic responses** are unusual and unpredictable reactions such as extreme sensitivity to low doses of a drug, resistance (no evidence of effect) to a drug, or abnormally prolonged drug effects. These reactions usually relate to altered drug metabolism; often they are of genetic origin. **Toxic effects** are serious adverse reactions that result from plasma concentrations that are too high. Toxic effects can occur because of a drug overdose or from abnormal accumulation of the drug in the body. They may be localized or systemic, reversible or cause permanent damage.

A **drug allergy** is an immune system reaction to a drug as a result of a previous sensitizing event. Any substance that the body perceives as a foreign substance (called an antigen) triggers an allergic response. Allergies are highly individualized. Allergic reactions may be mild or severe, and may occur immediately after exposure to the antigen or be delayed for hours or days. Urticaria (hives), pruritus (intense itching), wheezing, nausea, vomiting, and diarrhea are examples of signs and symptoms of a drug allergy. **Anaphylaxis,** a severe, life-threatening allergic reaction, results in severe respiratory distress, and may be fatal.

Drug tolerance exists when an individual needs increasing dosages of a particular medication in order to maintain a given therapeutic effect. Opiates, alcohol, and barbiturates are examples of drugs that are known to cause drug tolerance.

Drug interactions occur when one drug modifies the action of another drug. When a drug interferes with the action of another, the interaction is called **antagonism.** Drug interactions can also be additive. When two drugs used together produce an effect equal to the sum of the anticipated effects of each acting independently, it is called **summation. Synergism** refers to an additive effect that is greater than summation; the joint effect is more than the sum of the anticipated effects of each drug used independently. This is sometimes explained as "1 + 1 = 3." When one drug enhances the effect of another, but its own effectiveness is not altered, this interaction is called **potentiation.** Synergism and potentiation permit using a low dose of a drug that produces many side effects at therapeutic doses, in combination with a second drug to achieve a greater benefit than the first drug given by itself.

Response to drugs varies among individuals. Some variations are predictable and are therefore of concern to nurses as they administer drugs and monitor their effects.

Age is a prominent concern. Generally, the very young and the elderly exhibit increased responsiveness to drugs. Infants' immature hepatic and renal systems may promote delayed metabolism and excretion of drugs. Their volume of total body water is high; therefore, water-soluble drugs are distributed widely and plasma levels are rapidly depleted. Because of relatively small fat stores, lipid-soluble drugs remain in circulation and achieve higher plasma concentrations for a given dose. The elderly absorb, metabolize, and eliminate drugs more slowly than younger adults, because of decreased gastric motility, lower levels of circulating serum albumin, and decreased kidney and liver function associated with aging. Drug effects may be delayed due to slower absorption and there is greater risk of cumulative drug effects.

Body weight significantly affects drug action. The greater the body weight, the higher the dosage of drug required to effect the same response. However, individuals with large amounts of body fat tend to store lipid-soluble drugs for longer than the expected duration of action of the drug. Subsequent doses can then produce a cumulative effect.

Time of administration can influence the response to drugs. Giving oral medications at mealtime usually slows absorption of a drug, but may reduce gastric irritation. Recent research suggests that biorhythms can also influence the incidence of adverse or toxic reactions to drugs because of differences in absorption, metabolism, excretion, and drug receptor sensitivity at different phases of biologic cycles.

Psychological factors such as the meaning or significance of taking drugs and the patient's belief in the medication's effectiveness can also affect responses to drugs. This is one of the reasons why nurses tell patients to expect pain relief within in a certain time when administering pain medications. The *placebo effect* (see Chap. 32), in which an inactive substance produces effective pain relief, is a classic example of the impact of patient expectations on drug effect.

The Mechanics of Medication Administration. Administering medications requires efficiency, mental concentration, and skillful technique to achieve patient safety and comfort and maximum drug effectiveness.

For beginning nursing students, the first step toward efficiency is understanding the facility's system of organizing the medication supply. The two methods in common use are individual patient supply and stock supply. The *individual patient supply system* typically employs a mobile cart with small numbered drawers or containers, corresponding to the room numbers of the patient rooms on the nursing unit. The drawers are also labeled with the name of the patient currently in that room. Each drawer contains all the medications, other than controlled drugs, ordered for that patient for a particular time frame (usually 24 hours). The drugs are individually packaged and labeled with drug name, dose, and expiration date. This type of packaging is called a **unit dose system.** The unit dose packaging and the limited supply of any given medication reduces errors in the preparation process. However, a central, double-locked stock supply is necessary for storing controlled drugs, even in facilities that use an individual patient supply system.

In the *stock supply system,* the medications most frequently used on a particular unit are kept in labeled bulk containers in a central location or a mobile cart. The containers are usually organized alphabetically by drug name. Nurses dispense drugs as needed from the bulk containers. Although in the past, only the containers were labeled in a stock supply system—the medications had no individual wrapping or labels—in current practice unit dose packaging is most often used.

Some units use a combination of the unit dose and stock supply systems. *Computerized access systems* (Fig. 25–17) are a variation of the stock supply system that provides simultaneous medication security, inventory, and documentation of withdrawals from the stock supply.

Nurses should administer only medications that they have personally prepared. To minimize errors, avoid interruptions and conversation while preparing medications so your concentration is focused on obtaining the correct drugs. The standard called *"the*

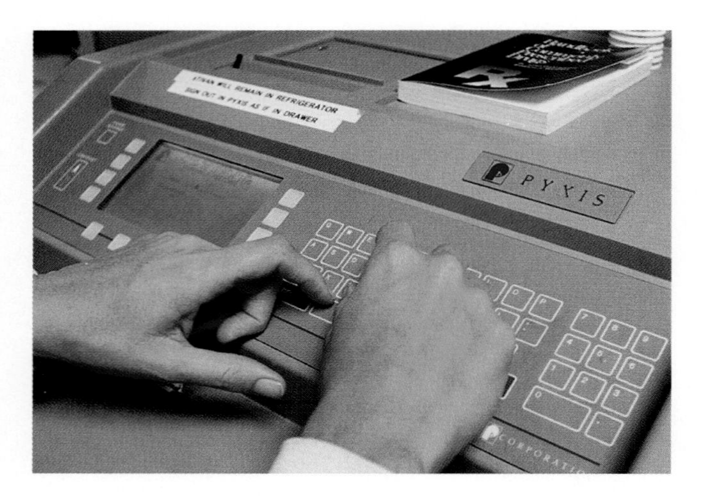

Figure 25–17. Computerized drug access system. *(From Smith S, Duell D.* Clinical Nursing Skills: Nursing Process Model; Basic to Advanced Skills. *4th ed. Norwalk, CT: Appleton & Lange; 1996.)*

five rights" has long been used as a formula for preparing drugs safely. This standard mandates that the right *medication* in the right *dosage* be administered by the right *route* to the right *patient* at the right *time.*

In practice, the application of this standard begins with the *right time.* Most health care facilities have an established time schedule for routine medications ordered at regular intervals (such as bid, tid), but not at specific times. A standard schedule facilitates efficiently organizing the care of several patients. This schedule is used unless the drug order, an individual patient's needs, or a drug's effectiveness would be compromised by using the standard schedule. Nurses have discretion in scheduling routine medications to accommodate patient preferences or to maximize drug effectiveness. When the best time of administration is identified, it is recorded on the MAR. Medications given within 30 minutes of the prescribed time are generally considered to meet the right time standard. For some drugs, such as insulin given prior to a meal, giving the drug at the actual time specified is a high priority.

Next, a nurse must identify all of the drugs to be given at a particular time. To identify the *right drug,* the *right dose,* and the *right route,* first check that the list of medications on the medication administration record (MAR) has been verified for accuracy by an RN, as discussed above in the section on legal responsibilities. Some nurses prefer to validate the accuracy all of their assigned patients' MARs at the beginning of their shift rather than at the time each drug is due to be given. Then, check three times that the name and dosage on the label of the drug container matches that on the MAR and note whether the form of the drug in the supply is appropriate for the route specified in the order. Associate each check with a specific activity to make it purposeful rather than cursory.

Do the *first check* as you locate the drug in the storage area.

Do the *second check* by placing the labeled container next to its name on the MAR. If a calculation is required to deliver the correct dose, double-check it for accuracy. Give special scrutiny if your calculation implies that multiple pills/tablets or the splitting of a tablet is required to deliver the ordered dose. Use careful attention to detail when pouring liquid medications or filling syringes.

Do the *third check* before leaving the drug cart or storage area. Some nurses prefer to take the MAR to the bedside and complete the third check just before administering the drug. Never use drugs from an unlabeled or illegibly labeled container. If a patient questions a medication, withhold the medication until you have rechecked the medication orders. Many patients are aware of the number and appearance of medications prescribed for them, so take their comments seriously.

Administering medications to the *right patient* is vital. Nurses are often responsible for administering medications to several patients within a short time frame. Patients often have similar names, and it may be difficult to associate names and faces accurately. Make it a consistent habit to verify a patient's identity just before giving any medication. Bring the MAR or other written reference such as your organizational plan for the day to the patient's room with the medication. Read the patient's identification bracelet or ask the patient to state his or her name and ascertain that it matches the name on your written reference. Asking "Are you Jennifer Brown?" is not a reliable method for identifying a patient. Some hospitalized patients are confused or scared and may answer "yes" to the wrong name.

Clinical Guideline 25–11 outlines safe medication administration. Consistently apply these guidelines to protect patient safety and well-being. The following sections address the specific techniques for administering medications by all routes.

ADMINISTERING ORAL MEDICATIONS. Oral preparations are the most commonly prescribed forms of medication. Unless a patient has impaired gastrointestinal functioning or is unable to swallow, the oral route is the safest, cheapest, and easiest way to give medications. Some oral drugs have disadvantages such as unpleasant taste, harmful gastric side effects, and delayed absorption associated with food in the stomach at the time of administration. Often these can be mitigated by the timing or technique of administration.

Some patients have *difficulty swallowing* pills, tablets, or capsules. To assist them, suggest they sit upright or stand. Explain that taking a sip of fluid to lubricate the mouth and throat, then placing the medication under or near the back of their tongue and drinking 60 to 100 mL (2 to 3 ounces) of fluid without focusing on the

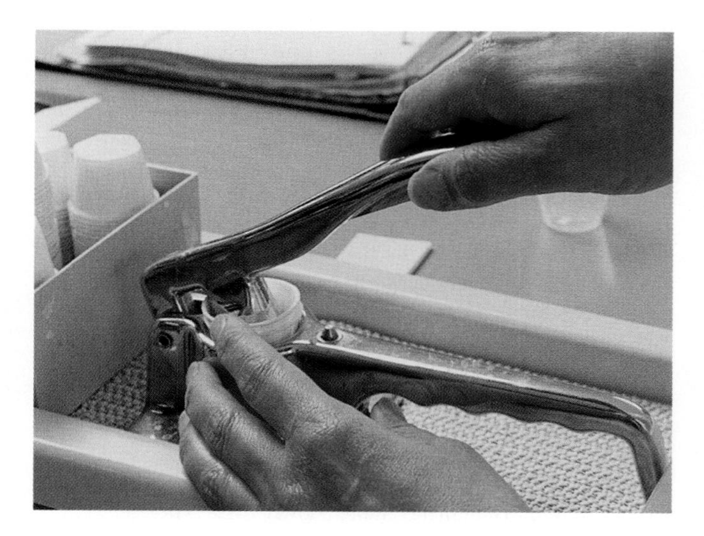

Figure 25–18. Pill crusher. Pill or tablet is placed in a paper medication cup. A second cup is placed on top. Squeezing the handles together crushes the medication. *(From Smith S, Duell D.* Clinical Nursing Skills: Nursing Process Model; Basic to Advanced Skills. *4th ed. Norwalk, CT: Appleton & Lange; 1996.)*

CLINICAL GUIDELINE 25–11

MEDICATION SAFETY

ACTION	RATIONALE
1. Verify prescriber's order prior to administering drugs.	1. Promotes safety and accuracy.
2. Before administering any medication, know patient's diagnosis, purpose of the medication, its therapeutic effects, major side effects, and any pertinent nursing implications.	2. Enables nurses to make informed professional decisions regarding appropriateness of medication order and to teach patients about their medications.
3. Check patient's allergy list before administering a medication.	3. Prevents administration of medications with potentially harmful effects.
4. Wash your hands prior to preparing all medications. Use surgical asepsis for preparing and administering parenteral medications.	4. Protects patients from injury.
5. Check the name, dosage, route, and expiration date of every medication three times.	5. Promotes safety and accuracy. Outdated medications may have reduced potency or be chemically altered from original condition.
6. Do not leave medications unattended. If you must interrupt medication preparation for more urgent tasks, return the medications to their storage area. Repeat safety checks when resuming medication preparation.	6. Unattended medications may be removed by unauthorized individuals. Interruptions cause loss of concentration and possible errors. Repeating safety checks prevents errors.
7. Do not return an unused unlabeled medication to a container or transfer medications from one container to another. An unopened unit dose package may be returned to a patient's medication drawer in the unit dose cart so patient can be credited for unused drug.	7. Prevents inadvertent mixture of medications or placing of medication in incorrect container.
8. Identify patients prior to administering medication by checking their identiband or asking their name.	8. Prevents administering the drug to the wrong patient.
9. Discuss the purpose and side effects of drugs with patients.	9. Promotes self-responsibility.
10. Observe that patients take their medications. Do not leave medications at the bedside, assuming a patient will take them.	10. Ensures correct administration of prescribed drug to the correct patient.
11. Special precautions are required for certain drugs. Most agencies require that two registered nurses double-check the dosages of anticoagulants, insulin, and certain intravenous medications. Check institutional policies.	11. Prevents accidental errors in dosage with potentially lethal drugs.
12. Chart a medication immediately after administering it. It is also acceptable to initial the medication administration record before taking the medication to a patient's room. If the medication is not taken, this is indicated when the drug is returned to the cart or discarded.	12. Prevents potential overdose. Failing to chart promptly may cause another nurse to repeat the dose thinking it has not been given. Initialing when leaving the cart verifies intent to administer medications and prevents repeated doses and omitted charting because of interruptions that interfere with returning to the cart to chart immediately after administering medication.

medication will help the medication slide down the throat. Also, tipping the head forward slightly rather than back facilitates swallowing. If there is no fluid restriction, suggest drinking at least one full glass of water after the drug is swallowed. If swallowing difficulties are due to hemiplegia (paralysis of one side of the body, usually associated with a stroke), place the tablet on the unaffected side of the tongue to facilitate swallowing without choking. If a patient with swallowing problems must remain flat or is on a strict fluid restriction, obtain a liquid form of the medication, if available. Crushing the medication and mixing it with a small amount of liquid or soft food is another option, so long as this does not alter its therapeutic properties. Most nursing units have a pill crusher (Fig. 25–18). Enteric-coated and sustained-release medications may not be crushed.

Crushing can also be used to mask the *unpleasant taste* of medications. Fruit juices, ice cream, crushed ice, or cold carbonated beverages work well for this. Placing medications on the back of the tongue where there are fewer taste buds may help as well. If medications cannot be crushed or diluted, have juices or other beverages on hand to offer immediately after administration. Procedure 25–6 details the steps for administering oral medications.

Patients with nasogastric (NG) feeding tubes can receive oral preparations through the feeding tube. In most instances, liquid preparations are preferred. See Clinical Guideline 25–12.

ADMINISTERING SUBLINGUAL AND BUCCAL MEDICATIONS. The sublingual (placed under the tongue) or buccal (placed in the pocket between cheek and gums) routes are infrequently used. However, drugs given by these routes are rapidly absorbed because of the many capillaries and thin epithelium in the mouth. No liquid is given with these medications and they must be held in the mouth until they are completely dissolved for maximal effect. Explain to patients that these drugs should not be chewed and swallowed. If a small amount of the drug is accidentally swallowed, drug effects may be slightly diminished and delayed.

(continued on page 694)

PROCEDURE 25–6. ADMINISTERING ORAL MEDICATIONS

PURPOSE: To provide medication for a specific therapeutic effect, when rapid absorption is not a major consideration.
EQUIPMENT: Medication supply, disposable medication cups, patient's medication administration record (MAR), drinking water or juice, and straws.

ACTION 1. Follow Clinical Guideline 25–11.

RATIONALE. These guidelines facilitate safe, error-free preparation of medication.

ACTION 2. Before preparing oral medications, verify that no tests or procedures are scheduled requiring the patient to be npo.

RATIONALE. Most oral medications may be safely deferred until test/procedure has been concluded. If in doubt about significance of delayed administration, consult physician.

ACTION 3. Check the patient MAR to determine the medication(s) to be given.

RATIONALE. All routine medications are usually given according to a standardized schedule. Frequently a patient will have several medications ordered for each administration time.

ACTION 4. To prepare tablets or capsules, compare the dosage ordered with the dosage available to determine how many tablets/capsules should be given.

RATIONALE. Many medications are dispensed in several strengths corresponding to the commonly prescribed dosages, but individual patient needs may require that less than 1 or more than 1 tablet be given at each administration time. This comparison of the order and drug label represents the **first** safety check.

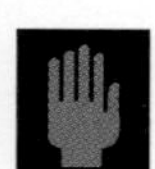

Some tablets are scored to facilitate administration of ½ or ¼ tablet. Do not break capsules or unscored tablets. Consult with physician or pharmacist.

ACTION 5. Remove the correct number of tablets/capsules from the supply. Compare the drug name and strength on the label with the order on the MAR. Do not remove the wrapper of unit dose medications. Place packet into a medication cup.

RATIONALE. This is the **second** safety check. Intact wrapper provides positive identification of the drug at the bedside, providing opportunity for third safety check and ready identification of any drugs refused or held because of assessment data obtained at the time of administration. Unused medications can be returned safely to the supply.

Some nurses prefer to place each wrapped drug on the MAR next to the order. A third check that all medications ordered for the current time have been correctly prepared can then be done prior to placing all drugs into a medication cup.

ACTION 6. If dispensing tablets/capsules from a stock supply, pour the required number into the bottle cap, then into the medication cup. Compare the label to the order a **third** time before returning the bottle to the shelf. Avoid touching medications with your fingers, if possible.

RATIONALE. Extra tablets poured inadvertently can be readily returned to the stock container from the cap before being mixed with other drugs in the medication cup. Third safety check at the bedside is impossible because drugs cannot be positively identified.

ACTION 7. Repeat the above sequence of actions for all medications to be given at this time. Compare the number of drugs ordered for current time to the number of drugs in the cup(s) prior to leaving the preparation area.

RATIONALE. Following a specific routine for each drug reduces medication errors. Comparing the number of drugs ordered with the number prepared prevents omissions.

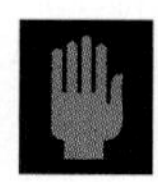

Many nurses place drug(s) requiring specific assessment (eg, pulse, BP) prior to administration in separate cups as a reminder to carry out the assessment prior to giving the medication.

Procedure 25–6. (continued)

ACTION 8. Follow the same safety checks for preparing liquid medications. If available in unit dose form, do not open lid until at the bedside. If pouring from a stock bottle, calculate the correct volume required for ordered dosage prior to pouring liquid.

RATIONALE. See Action 5. Prior calculation reduces likelihood of pouring incorrect amount.

ACTION 9. To pour the correct volume, hold bottle with your palm on the label and pour liquid into a graduated medicine cup held at eye level. If cup is not marked in sufficiently small increments to measure the required amount, use a syringe to obtain the correct dose.

RATIONALE. Palming the label prevents liquid that drips during pouring from obliterating the label. Using appropriately graduated container to measure dosages prevents errors related to incorrect estimation. If a meniscus is not read at eye level, parallax (the apparent displacement of objects caused by a change in the observer's position) will distort perception and result in inaccurate dosage.

ACTION 10. Take medications to patient's room. If supplies (such as juice, foods to mix with crushed medications) are needed, take these in with the medications.

RATIONALE. Taking all necessary supplies to complete the procedure saves nurse time and energy.

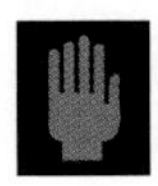

Some nurses also take the MAR into the patient's room to match with ID bracelet and to perform third safety check. Others chart on MAR prior to leaving medication preparation area.

ACTION 11. Identify patient by reading patient's ID bracelet. You may also ask patients to state their name.

RATIONALE Positive identification prevents giving medications to the wrong patient.

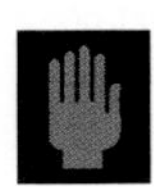

Complete special assessments before giving medications.

ACTION 12. Match drug labels with MAR if third safety check was not previously completed. Discuss drug effects/precautions with patient.

RATIONALE. Informed patients are able to take greater responsibility for decisions regarding health care.

ACTION 13. Remove drug wrappers. Offer medications according to patient's preference for order of drugs, number taken at once, liquid/food of choice, etc. Encourage intake of additional 60 to 100 mL of fluid after medications have been swallowed.

RATIONALE. Respecting patient's preferences promotes trust. Extra fluid facilitates drug moving to stomach rather than remaining in the esophagus.

Placing the medications under the tongue or on the back of tongue facilitates swallowing them. Mix crushed tablets or contents of capsules with food for patients who have difficulty swallowing pills. Do not crush enteric-coated tablets or granules from time-release medications.

ACTION 14. Remain with patient until all medications have been swallowed.

RATIONALE. Verification of actual ingestion of medication is necessary for documentation of administration.

Recording:

Note name, strength, route, and time of administration according to agency policy. The MAR is the usual location for this information. Specific assessment data (P, BP) may also recorded on the MAR in some agencies. Additional information regarding patient response to the medication may be placed in the nurse's notes, but generally only untoward effects are documented for routine medications.

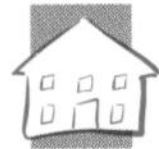

HOME HEALTH ADAPTATION: The role of the home care nurse can include administration of oral medication, but more often it involves teaching the patient and/or family member self-administration. This includes instructing them in frequency, dose, purpose and action, side effects, and contraindications of their medications. This information is prioritized and presented in small increments to avoid mental fatigue and promote retention. To assess the level of understanding of your instructions, request that patient and/or family members restate important points. Preparing a weekly medicine cassette is necessary for some patients to reduce under- and overmedication.

CLINICAL GUIDELINE 25–12

ADMINISTERING MEDICATIONS THROUGH A NASOGASTRIC TUBE

1. Consult with pharmacy to have all drugs that are available in liquid form dispensed as liquids. Liquid forms of medication are most easily administered via NG tube.
2. Crush and mix simple compressed tablets with liquid. Use a glass mortar and pestle, pill crusher (Fig. 25–18), or crush tablets inside the unit dose package.
3. Dissolve a soft gelatin capsule in 20 to 30 mL of warm water rather than sticking a needle into the capsule and squeezing out the contents.
4. Separate capsules containing powders and mix the contents with liquid.
5. Do not crush enteric-coated tablets or sustained-release preparations. These are intended to dissolve in the intestines, not the stomach. Consult with the physician or pharmacist for alternative forms of the drug.
6. Administer buccal or sublingual tablets as intended, if possible.
7. Consult with the physician to arrange intermittent rather than continuous feedings, if an empty stomach is critical to a drug's absorption. Patients receiving continuous tube feedings generally have residual feeding solution in the stomach, so medications that are inactivated by milk (such as tetracycline) are unlikely to be effective. Absorption of most drugs will be slowed by the presence of the tube feeding formula in the stomach.
8. Verify the placement of the NG tube before administering medications. (See Procedure 25–4, step 5.)
9. Use a large syringe to administer medications. Remove the plunger, insert the tip into the NG tube, and pour the medications into the barrel. Reinsert the plunger, creating positive pressure to instill the medications, rather than gravity. Most crushed tablets and viscous liquid medications will not move through small-lumen tubes via gravity.
10. Flush the tubing with 30 to 50 mL of water to clear the tubing after administering medications to prevent their plugging the tube. (See Procedure 25–5.)
11. Record the total volume of liquid (medications and water) instilled on the intake and output (I&O) record.

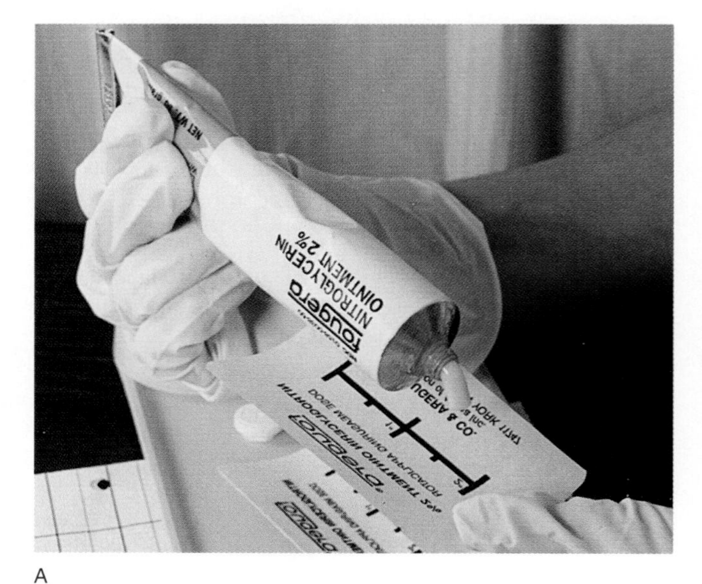

A

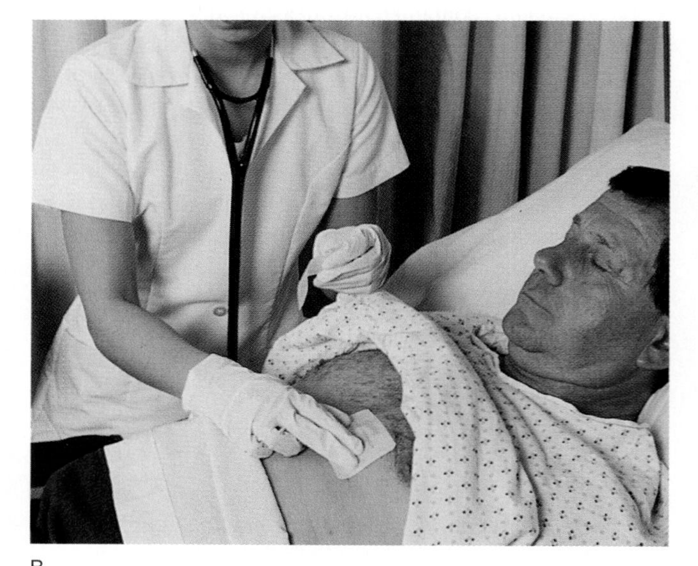
B

Figure 25–19. Application of topical medication. **A.** This topical medication is applied using special papers to measure the dosage. **B.** The paper is applied to the skin and remains in place until the next dose is given. *(From Smith S, Duell D.* Clinical Nursing Skills: Nursing Process Model; Basic to Advanced Skills. *4th ed. Norwalk, CT: Appleton & Lange; 1996.)*

ADMINISTERING TOPICAL MEDICATIONS. Topical medications are applied to the skin or mucous membranes. Thorough cleansing of the skin with soap and water prior to application of topical medications improves their absorption. Most topical medications are used for local effects on the immediate area of application. However, a new modality, the *transdermal patch,* is effective for drugs intended to exert a systemic effect. It is applied to the skin much like an adhesive bandage to supply a low dose of continuously absorbed medication over a period of several days.

Most topical medications are manufactured as creams, lotions, and ointments. They are most often supplied in multiple-use containers such as tubes and jars. A tongue blade, cotton balls, or cotton-tipped applicators are effective tools to apply ointments or topical liquids. Wear gloves when working with systemically acting medications (Fig. 25–19) or when there is a risk of infection transmission.

EYE AND EAR INSTILLATIONS. All procedures involving the eye require the use of sterile technique. The cornea of the eye is extremely sensitive; therefore, preparations intended for use in the eye must be instilled in the lower conjunctival sac to avoid direct contact with the cornea. Typical eye preparations include artificial tears/lubricants, antibiotic drops or ointments, and medications for the treatment of glaucoma. Procedure 25–7 describes installation of medications into the eye.

Medications are placed in the ear for local effect. They may be in the form of drops or medication-impregnated cotton plugs. The technique for instilling ear drops appears in Procedure 25–8. Information about eye and ear irrigations can be found in Chap. 27.

PROCEDURE 25–7. INSTILLING MEDICATIONS INTO THE EYE

PURPOSE: To deliver locally acting medication to the cornea and conjunctiva.
EQUIPMENT: Eyedrops, tissues, cotton balls or washcloth, and patient's medication administration record (MAR).

ACTION 1. Follow Clinical Guideline 25–11.

ACTION 2. Be sure the patient is aware of the purpose, expected benefits, and usual sensations associated with the medication, as well as desired patient participation to facilitate instillation.

ACTION 3. If encrusted secretions are present, cleanse the eyelid and lashes with soft cloth or cotton ball moistened in warm water. Wipe from inner to outer canthus. To avoid possible cross-contamination, use a separate cotton ball or a different portion of the cloth for each eye.

ACTION 4. Ask or assist the patient to assume a supine or a sitting position with head tilted back.

ACTION 5. Rest the heel or the side of your dominant hand lightly on the patient's forehead while holding the dropper or tube vertically between thumb and index finger. Gently pull downward on the lower lid with the other hand, exposing the conjunctival sac. Ask patient to look upward.

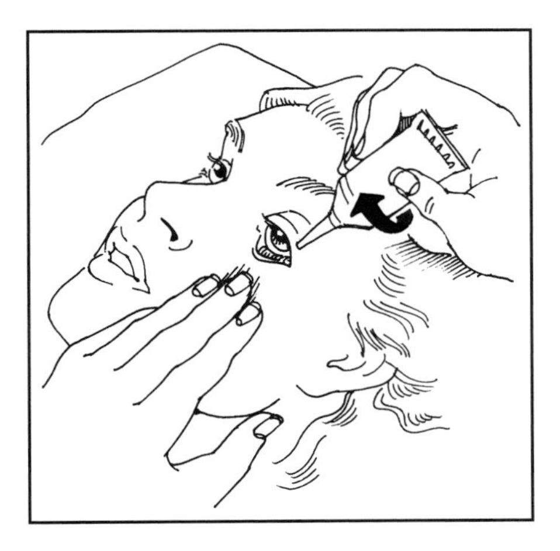

ACTION 6. Squeeze gently to dispense the required number of drops into the conjunctival sac, not on the cornea. If medication is in ointment form, squeeze a ribbon of ointment from inner to outer canthus, rotating your hand toward the forehead to disconnect the ointment strip as you near the outer canthus. Do not touch the eye or surrounding tissue with the dropper or the tip of the tube. If accidental contact occurs, the dropper or tube must be discarded.

ACTION 7. Ask patient to close eye gently and keep closed for 2 to 3 minutes to spread the medication over the surface of the cornea, but not to squeeze the eye tightly closed, as this will force medication out of the eye. If drops were instilled, apply gentle pressure on the lacrimal duct for 1 to 2 minutes to delay medication overflow into the duct. This action will increase local effectiveness of the medication and decrease systemic absorption. Some eye medications cause systemic side effects if drained undiluted into lacrimal ducts. Some patients may prefer to apply duct pressure themselves.

ACTION 8. Repeat for other eye, if ordered.

ACTION 9. Excess medication may be wiped from eyelids from inner to outer canthus, using a tissue or cotton ball.

Recording:
Record medication administration, appearance of eye and/or drainage, and any unexpected reactions to the medication according to agency policy.

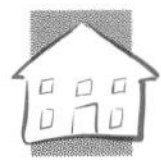

HOME HEALTH ADAPTATION: The procedure for instilling eye medication is the same regardless of the setting. Some patients may be capable of self-administration; teach correct technique to family members also.

NASAL INSTILLATIONS. Nasal medications may be used for systemic or local effects. They may be sprays, drops, or medication-impregnated plugs. To administer nose drops:

- Request patient assume a sitting or recumbent position with the head tilted back.
- Lightly rest the heel of your hand against the patient's chin and place the medication-filled dropper just inside the nostril. Administer the required number of drops. Repeat for the other nostril.
- Instruct patient to keep the head tilted back for several minutes so drops drain into the sinuses rather than out of the nose.

Nasal sprays are administered in the same way. Tell the patient to inhale as the container is squeezed to deliver the medication. Many patients prefer to self-administer nasal medications.

VAGINAL INSTILLATIONS. Vaginal medications are applied as creams, foam, jellies, suppositories, or irrigations (douches). An applicator that facilitates placement of the medication high into the vaginal cavity is provided with many vaginal preparations. Nursing students often feel uncomfortable about administering vaginal medications; many patients have similar feelings. A respectful but matter-of-fact approach eases concerns of nurse and patient. Privacy during the procedure is important. Close the door, draw the

PROCEDURE 25–8. INSTILLING MEDICATIONS INTO THE EAR

PURPOSE: To deliver locally acting medication into the auditory canal.
EQUIPMENT: Medication, cotton balls, washcloth or tissue, and patient's medication administration record (MAR).

ACTION 1. Follow Clinical Guideline 25–11

ACTION 2. Be sure the patient is aware of the purpose, expected benefits, and usual sensations associated with the medication, as well as desired patient participation to facilitate instillation.

ACTION 3. Use medical asepsis for ear instillations unless tympanic membrane is ruptured. Then sterile technique is required.

ACTION 4. The ear is sensitive to cold. Warming medication to body temperature will diminish discomfort, although this may be contraindicated for some medications. Carrying the container in your uniform pocket for 15 minutes or immersing the container in a cup filled with warm water for several minutes will warm contents.

ACTION 5. Ask or assist the patient to assume a side-lying position with the affected ear facing upward. Clean discharge from external ear with a soft cloth, cotton ball, or cotton-tipped applicator. Do not attempt to clean inside auditory canal.

ACTION 6. Gently straighten the auditory canal to facilitate entry of medication: Pull the pinna slightly upward and backward for adults; for a child under 3, pull downward and backward. This may cause slight discomfort if the patient has an ear infection. Rest the heel of your hand lightly on the patient's head near the ear as you introduce the medication to prevent injury to the ear should the patient move unexpectedly.

ACTION 7. Direct the flow of drops against the side of the canal, as direct application on the tympanic membrane is uncomfortable. Administer the prescribed amount of medication. Gently massage the tragus (area directly anterior to the ear) to facilitate dispersing medication into the canal.

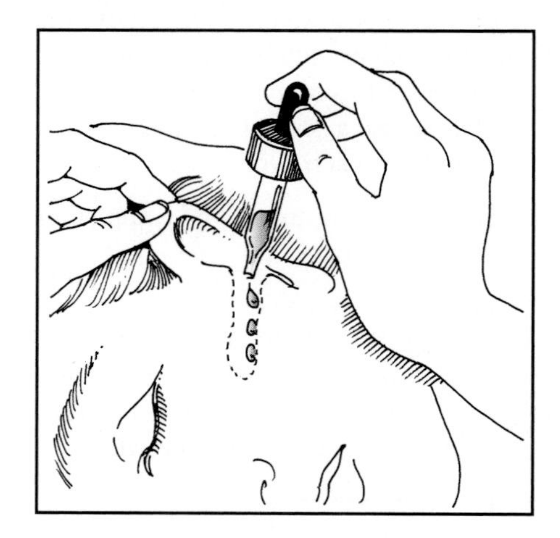

ACTION 8. Inform the patient of the importance of remaining on the side for 5 minutes to prevent immediate drainage of the medication out of the ear. A cotton ball may also be placed loosely in the ear to absorb drainage after the patient sits up.

ACTION 9. Repeat for other ear, if ordered.

Recording:
Record medication administration, appearance of the ear and/or description of drainage, and any unexpected reactions to the medication according to agency policy.

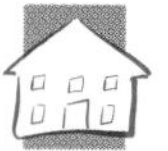

HOME HEALTH ADAPTATION: The procedure for instilling medications into the ear is the same regardless of the setting. Some patients may be capable of self-administration; teach family members also.

curtains around the bed, and offer draping to minimize exposure. Many women prefer to self-administer vaginal medications. In this case, review the correct technique and assist with at least one application to ascertain that she is able to correctly insert the medication. To administer vaginal medications:

- Instruct the woman to lie on her back with her knees bent and legs rotated outward at the hip. Drape as for insertion of a Foley catheter (Procedure 29–9).
- Wearing clean gloves, spread the labia major and minora with one hand, gently insert the filled applicator or suppository approximately 5 cm (2 in.) into the vagina, and push the plunger until the applicator is empty.
- Instruct the woman to remain in a supine position for at least 10 minutes to facilitate absorption of the medication. A sanitary napkin may be needed to absorb excess drainage.

INSERTING RECTAL SUPPOSITORIES. Usually rectal suppositories are given to stimulate evacuation of the bowel; however, the rectal route is useful to deliver systemic medications to patients unable to tolerate medications by mouth. Absorption of rectal medications is somewhat unpredictable. When a systemic effect is desired, absorption is improved if an enema is given prior to inserting the suppository. Procedure 25–9 describes the technique for administration of a rectal suppository.

ADMINISTERING MEDICATIONS BY INHALATION. Medications such as bronchodilators and decongestants are often administered by inhalation. A hand-held metered dose inhaler is used to dispense medication in the form of a fine mist (Procedure 25–10). Inhalation medications via metered dose inhaler are most effective when self-administered by patients, as the ejection of the mist must coincide with deep inhalation. Aerosol therapy can also be delivered with specialized respiratory equipment such as a nebulizer.

ADMINISTERING INJECTIONS. An injection is considered parenteral medication. **Parenteral** means administration by any route other than oral. In common usage the term refers to medications given via a needle, therefore including injections and intravenous medications. Injections are used when medications by mouth are contraindicated, for medications (such as insulin) that cannot be given orally, and when relatively rapid absorption is desired. Therapeutic and toxic effects develop rapidly, so close monitoring is important.

Receiving medications by injection is a source of anxiety and discomfort for most patients. Nurses can reduce physical discomfort through careful choice of site, proper patient positioning, and skillful injection technique. Encourage apprehensive or fearful patients to express their concerns. Explain the techniques you will use to minimize their discomfort. Clinical Guideline 25–13 outlines measures to minimize patient discomfort associated with injections.

To prepare injections correctly and efficiently requires familiarity with injection equipment: needles, syringes, and the containers in which injectable medications are supplied. Figure 25–20 illustrates the parts of a syringe and needle.

Needles are sized according to gauge and length. **Gauge** refers to the diameter of the needle shaft. The *smaller* the gauge number, the *larger* the needle diameter (eg, an 18-gauge needle has a *larger diameter* than a 25-gauge needle). Needle lengths vary from ⅜ in. to 2 in. Clinical Guideline 25–14 outlines criteria for selecting appropriate needles and syringes. Needles have a slanted or beveled tip (Fig. 25–20). The bevel is designed to make a narrow slit-type opening in the skin that seals easily when the needle is removed to minimize seepage of blood or medications. When attaching a needle to a syringe, you may touch the hub of the needle and twist to ensure a tight connection; however, the shaft and the tip must remain sterile.

Syringes vary in capacity from 1 to 50 mL. One- to 5-mL sizes are most commonly used for injections. The three types of syringes used most commonly for injections are illustrated in Fig. 25–21A. Figure 25–21B shows a safety syringe, designed to protect care givers from postinjection needle sticks. Larger syringes are used

(continued on page 700)

CLINICAL GUIDELINE 25–13

NURSING MEASURES TO REDUCE INJECTION DISCOMFORT

1. Select the smallest gauge needle appropriate for the site and solution to be administered.
2. Do not administer more fluid in one injection than is recommended for the selected site or route; divide large doses and give two injections. Recommended volumes:
   Intradermal: 0.1 to 0.5 mL
   Subcutaneous: 1.5 mL maximum
   Small muscle: 2 mL maximum
   Large muscle: 5 mL maximum
3. Make sure the outside of the needle is free of medication that may be irritating to the subcutaneous tissues.
4. Respect patient preferences for injection site when feasible. Carefully locate site using anatomic landmarks. Do not give an injection where skin is irritated or damaged.
5. Rotate injection sites to avoid repeated trauma to tissues.
6. Applying ice to the insertion site prior to administration to numb pain receptors is an option. Some patients find the ice more painful than the injection.
7. Position the patient comfortably. Ask patient to assume a position that will relax the muscle at the selected site:
   Deltoid: hand open, arm hanging down
   Dorsogluteal: side-lying with knee flexed or prone with internal hip rotation
   Ventrogluteal: sitting or side-lying
8. Divert the patient's attention from the injection through conversation or relaxation techniques.
9. Stabilize skin at the site by stretching or pinching. Use a quick dartlike motion to insert needle.
10. Hold the syringe steady while aspirating and injecting the medication.
11. Inject the medication slowly.
12. Stabilize skin as in item 9 before removing needle from muscle.
13. Massage the area of injection after administration with a dry gauze square unless contraindicated.

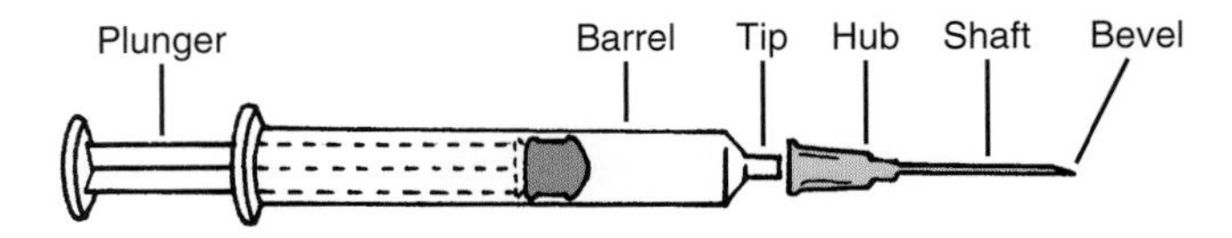

Figure 25–20. Parts of a syringe and needle.

PROCEDURE 25–9. INSERTING A RECTAL SUPPOSITORY

PURPOSE: To provide local effect on gastrointestinal tract or systemic effect when oral route is impossible or contraindicated.

EQUIPMENT: Clean gloves, water-soluble lubricant, disposable waterproof underpad, suppository, and patient's medication administration record (MAR). If laxative suppository: bedpan, commode, and toilet tissue.

ACTION 1. Follow Clinical Guideline 25–11

ACTION 2. Be sure the patient is aware of purpose, expected benefits, and usual sensations associated with the medication, as well as desired patient participation to facilitate administration.

ACTION 3. Provide privacy. Ask or assist patient to assume a side-lying position. Raise bed to comfortable working height. Arrange bed covers so buttocks are exposed, but patient is otherwise covered. Place underpad under buttocks.

ACTION 4. Unwrap suppository. Don clean glove. Lubricate tapered end of suppository and your index finger.

ACTION 5. Raise patient's buttock to expose anus. Ask patient to take a deep breath to facilitate relaxation. Touch anal sphincter lightly with suppository, then wait several seconds. Sphincter will contract, then relax as a reflex response to being touched.

ACTION 6. Gently insert suppository. Use your index finger to direct the suppository 3 to 4 inches (2 inches for children) along the rectal wall, toward the umbilicus. It must be inserted beyond the internal sphincter to prevent expulsion. Do not insert it into a fecal mass. The suppository must contact the rectal mucosa to be absorbed.

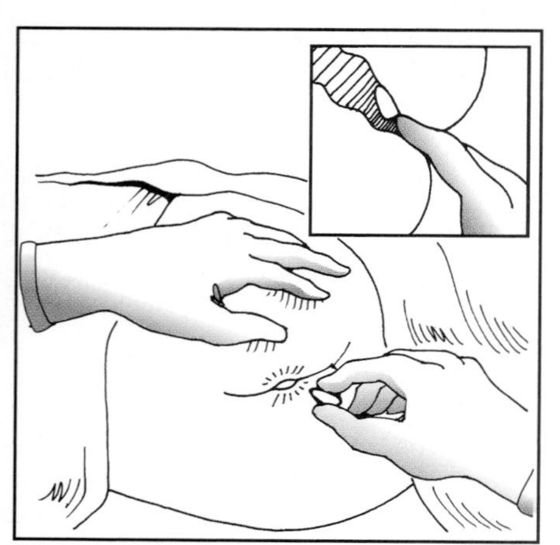

ACTION 7. Withdraw your finger. Applying slight pressure over the anus with tissue or holding the buttocks together briefly will assist the patient to overcome the reflex urge to defecate.

ACTION 8. Turn glove inside out to remove it, and discard. Cover patient. Wash hands. Inform patient that remaining in side-lying position for up to 30 minutes will enhance absorption of systemic medication. If suppository is a laxative, urge to defecate may be strong within 5 to 10 minutes. Leave call bell in reach. Some patients may prefer a bedpan and toilet tissue be left in the bed to prevent soiling.

Recording:
Record medication administration and any unexpected reactions to the medication according to agency policy.

HOME HEALTH ADAPTATION: The procedure for inserting a suppository is the same regardless of the setting. Some patients may be capable of self-administration; teach family members also.

PROCEDURE 25–10. ADMINISTERING MEDICATIONS VIA A HAND-HELD INHALER

PURPOSE: To deliver medication to the respiratory tree, usually for local effect.
EQUIPMENT: Medication cannister, metered dose inhaler (some patients may also use aerochamber), and patient's medication administration record (MAR).

ACTION 1. Follow Clinical Guideline 25–11

ACTION 2. Be sure the patient is aware of purpose, expected benefits, and usual sensations associated with the medication, as well as desired patient participation to facilitate instillation.

ACTION 3. If patient is unfamiliar with the inhaler, provide opportunity for the patient to manipulate the equipment and ask questions as you explain. Use a placebo as you explain.

ACTION 4. Discuss the critical elements for correct use of the inhaler. If no method is specified by the prescriber, teach the open-mouth method.

OPEN-MOUTH TECHNIQUE

a. Shake cannister/inhaler unit; remove mouthpiece cover.

b. Invert inhaler. Hold it with index and middle fingers on cannister, thumb supporting mouthpiece.

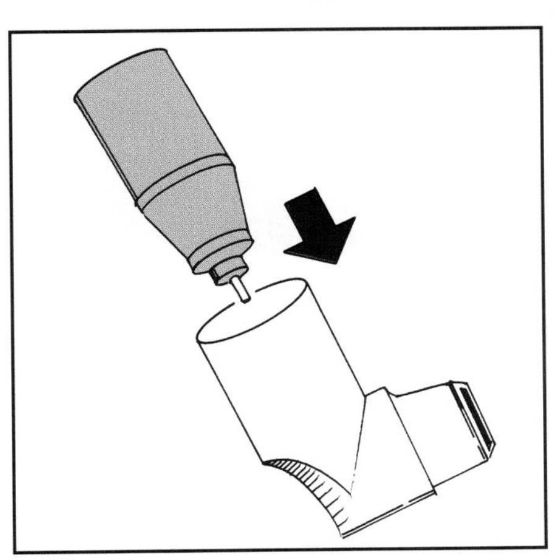

c. Hold the inhaler about 1½ inches in front of widely opened mouth.

d. Exhale, then inhale slowly through your mouth as you press down firmly on the cannister.

e. Hold breath for 10 seconds to allow medication to reach deeper airways.

f. Exhale normally.

g. If more than one dose at each use is ordered, wait 30 seconds to 1 minute before inhaling second dose.

h. Caution patient about the risks of overuse: development of drug tolerance and possible increased side effects.

i. Inhaler should be rinsed with warm water and dried after use or at least once per day.

CLOSED-MOUTH TECHNIQUE

a,b. See open-mouth technique.

c. Place mouthpiece into open mouth, and then place teeth and lips firmly around mouthpiece.

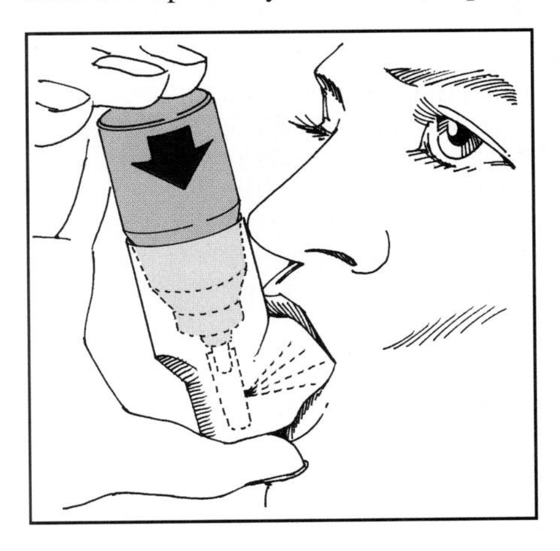

d. Exhale; then *while inhaling* slowly and deeply through the nose, press down on cannister to deliver measured dose of medication into airways.

e–i. See open-mouth technique.

ACTION 5. Request that patient verbalize steps for using inhaler to assess level of understanding. Clarify misunderstandings, if any.

ACTION 6. Ask patient to self-administer medication with inhaler while you observe. (Nurse must observe each use if medication administration is to be charted on MAR.)

Recording:
Record medication administration, level of patient participation, and any unexpected reactions to the medication according to agency policy.

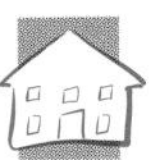

HOME HEALTH ADAPTATION: The patient may need assistance to establish and maintain a routine at home to avoid over- or underuse. As a reminder, connect and cue use of the inhaler to patient's daily schedule.

CLINICAL GUIDELINE 25–14

CRITERIA FOR SELECTING NEEDLES AND SYRINGES

NEEDLES

1. *Route of administration.* Select a needle that will deposit the medication accurately into the specified tissue.
   - Intradermal: 25 to 26 gauge; $\frac{3}{8}$ to $\frac{5}{8}$ in.
   - Subcutaneous: 25 to 27 gauge; $\frac{1}{2}$ to 1 in.
   - IM: 21 to 23 gauge; 1 to $1\frac{1}{2}$ in.
2. *Patient's size.* Patients with large amounts of subcutaneous fat require longer needles to reach muscle tissue. If the needle is too short and medication is injected into the subcutaneous tissue, absorption will be slower and drug effect delayed.
3. *Viscosity of medication solution.* Viscous fluids require a larger-gauge needle.
4. *Patient comfort.* To avoid unnecessary discomfort, select the smallest-gauge needle that is appropriate for site and medication.

SYRINGES

1. *Amount of medication.* Check that the syringe is marked in increments that allow for accurate measurement of the required dose (eg, accurate delivery of 0.25 cc of medication requires a syringe marked in increments of one-hundredths of a cc). Select a syringe slightly larger that the volume of medication (eg, 5-cc syringe used for 3 cc of medication). Syringes filled to capacity are difficult to manipulate.
2. *Type of medication.* Insulin syringes must be used when administering insulin injections.

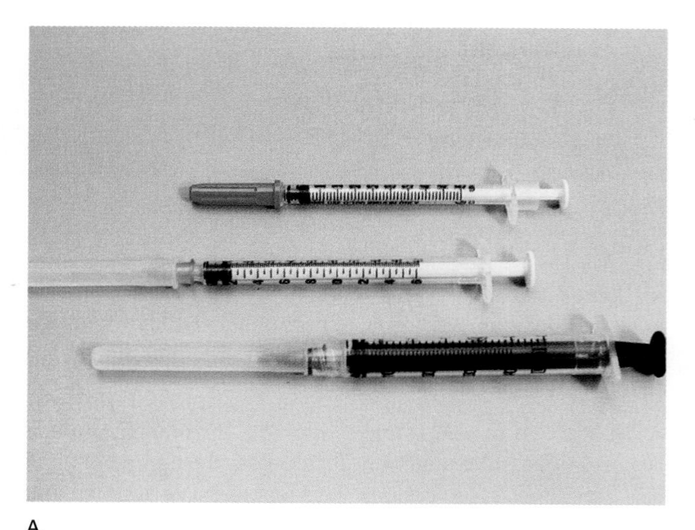

A

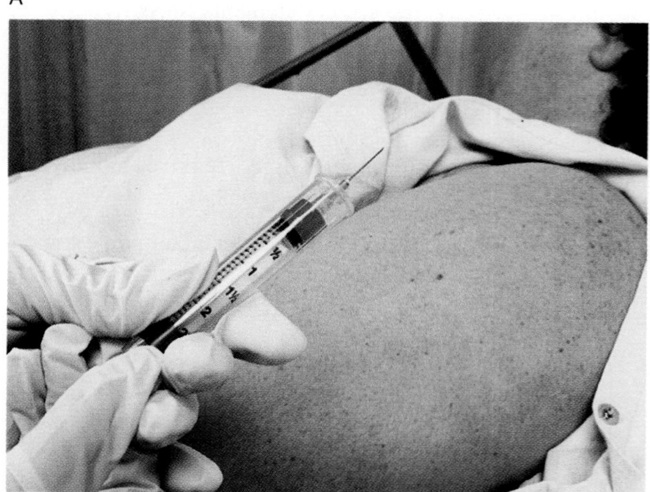

B

Figure 25–21. **A.** Three types of syringes: (from top): insulin, tuberculin, and 3 mL. **B.** Safety syringe to prevent postinjection needle sticks. *(From Smith S, Duell D.* Clinical Nursing Skills: Nursing Process Model; Basic to Advanced Skills. *4th ed. Norwalk, CT: Appleton & Lange; 1996.)*

for adding medications to IV fluid or for irrigations. Most syringes are made of plastic and are disposable. They are individually packaged with and without an attached needle, in a sterile wrapper or rigid plastic container.

Parenteral medications are supplied in ampules, vials, and prefilled syringes or cartridges. An **ampule** is a one-piece glass container with a constricted neck that holds a single dose of medication. Procedure 25–11 illustrates how to remove medication from an ampule.

A **vial** is a plastic or glass container with a self-sealing rubber top. Procedure 25–12 describes removing medication from a vial. Vials may be single-dose or multiple-dose containers. Some drugs deteriorate when stored as liquids. They are supplied in powdered form in single-dose vials. Reconstitute these medications with a sterile diluent or solvent (generally sterile water or sterile normal saline) according to the directions printed on the label. It is important to use the type and amount of diluent specified for optimum drug effect. Rotate rather than shake the vial to thoroughly dissolve the medication. The reconstituted solution should be clear and free of particles prior to administration.

Prefilled single-dose cartridges or syringes save time and reduce errors. The cartridges have attached needles, but must be loaded into a reusable cartridge holder to administer the medication (Fig. 25–22). Many narcotics and emergency medications are available in this form.

Sometimes two parenteral medications are ordered to be given at the same time to achieve optimal drug effectiveness. If the two drugs are compatible and the resulting volume is not greater than 2 mL, it is advisable to mix them in the same syringe and administer as a single injection. Drug compatibility charts are usually available in medication preparation areas. If you have any question about the compatibility of two medications, consult a pharmacist or drug reference book. When mixing drugs supplied in multiple-dose vials, it is important that neither vial be contaminated with medication from the other vial (Procedure 25–13). If only one of the drugs is supplied in a multiple-dose vial, withdraw the correct dose of that medication first.

All syringes, glass vials, and ampules must be discarded in specially marked containers, called *sharps disposal containers* located in the medication preparation area (Fig. 25–23, page 706) and in all patients' rooms (Fig. 25–3). These containers also prevent needle stick injuries to personnel handling trash because they are impervious to penetration by needles. When full they are

(continued on page 703)

PROCEDURE 25–11. REMOVING MEDICATION FROM AN AMPULE

PURPOSE: To withdraw medication contained in an ampule in preparation for parenteral administration.
EQUIPMENT: Ampule containing ordered medication, sterile syringe and needle, filter needle, alcohol swabs, and patient's medication administration record (MAR).

ACTION 1. Follow Clinical Guideline 25–11

RATIONALE. These guidelines facilitate safe, error-free preparation of medications.

ACTION 2. Remove medication trapped in the neck of the ampule by holding it upright and rotating your wrist several times, by moving the ampule downward as if to trace a large circle, or by flicking the stem with your finger.

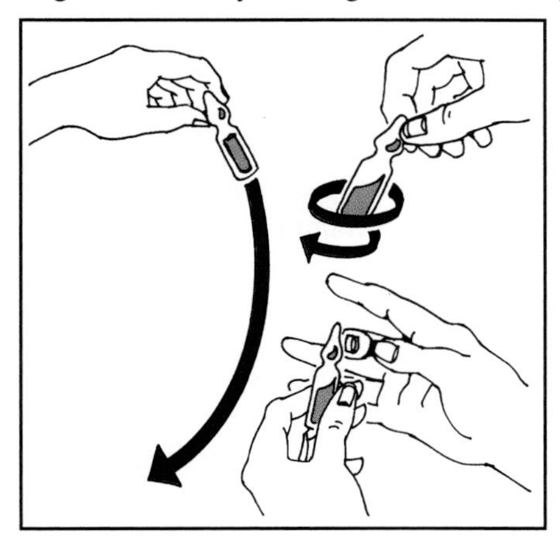

RATIONALE. Circular or rotational movement creates centrifugal force; flicking creates turbulence. Both will overcome the surface tension holding the liquid in the neck and move the medication into the lower portion of the ampule.

ACTION 3. Place an alcohol swab around the neck of the ampule. Keeping your fingers away from the neck, break off the top of the ampule.

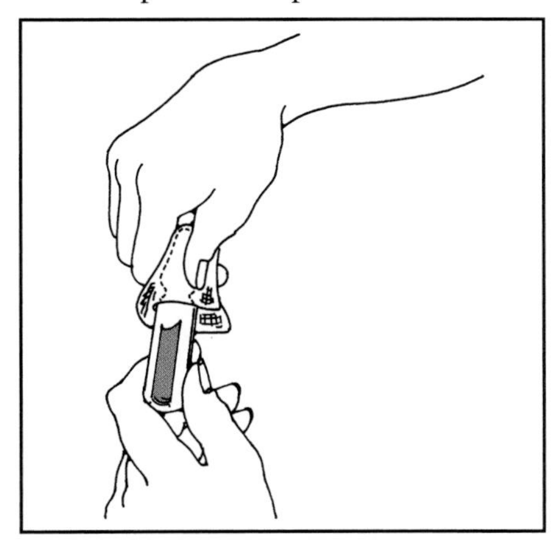

RATIONALE. The alcohol swab protects the nurse's fingers from the sharp edges of the ampule as well as from glass fragments.

ACTION 4. If filter needles are available in your agency, place one on the syringe without touching the needle shaft or the tip of the syringe. Use a firm twisting motion to secure needle.

RATIONALE. Filter needles prevent tiny glass shards, deposited in the medication when the ampule is broken, from entering the syringe with the medication. Although patient injury related to these glass shards has not been documented, experts recommend use of a filter needle as a precaution. Contact with the syringe tip or needle would transfer organisms to the syringe, to the medication, and subsequently to the patient. Medications injected through the skin must be sterile.

ACTION 5. If the syringe has a preattached needle, the needle may be reserved and reattached to give the medication. Remove the needle in its protective cap using a twisting motion and place it on a clean dry surface.

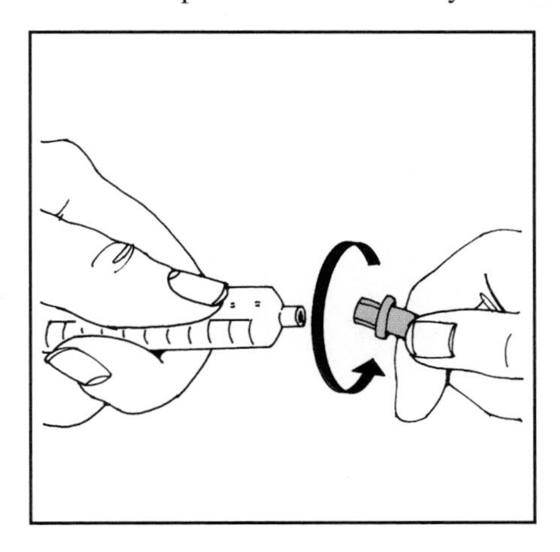

RATIONALE. Filter needles may not be used to administer medications. Pulling on the needle rather than twisting will remove the needle cap rather than the needle. The reserved needle and cap will remain sterile because the flange on the needle cap prevents contact between the inside of the needle hub and the surface of the work area.

ACTION 6. Pull firmly to remove filter needle cap. Insert the needle into the ampule without its touching the rim of the ampule.

RATIONALE. See Action 5, above. The rim of the ampule is considered contaminated. Contact would contaminate the needle and therefore, the medication, creating potential for patient infection.

Continued

Procedure 25–11. Removing Medication from an Ampule (continued)

ACTION 7. Keeping the tip of the needle below the level of fluid, pull on the plunger to withdraw the ordered amount of medication. The ampule may stand upright on a flat surface or be inverted. If inverted, the ampule and syringe should be held in the nondominant hand, as shown, and must not be tipped at an angle. You might need to pick up and tip an upright ampule slightly to withdraw the last part of the fluid if needle is short.

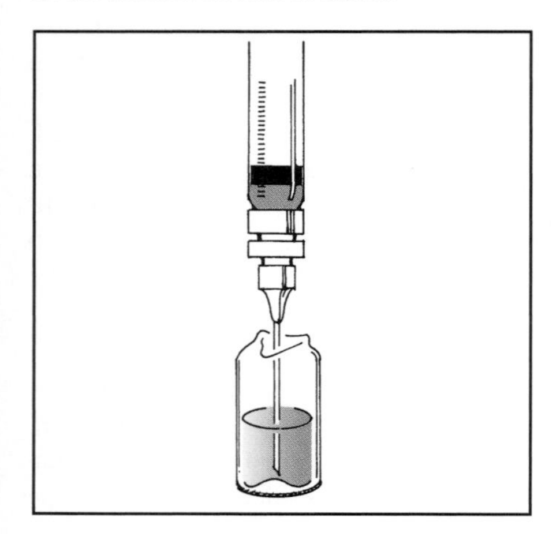

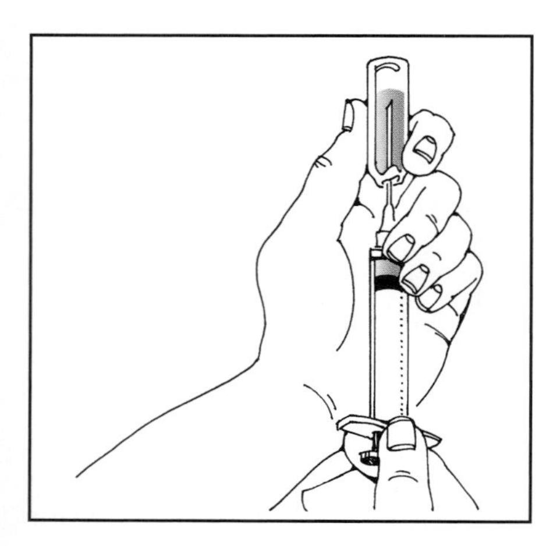

RATIONALE. Pulling on the plunger creates negative pressure within the syringe, causing fluid to move from the ampule into the barrel of the syringe. Air will also move into the syringe if the needle tip is not below the surface of the fluid. Surface tension will prevent the fluid in the ampule from running out when it is inverted, but unless the opening is very small, holding the inverted ampule at an angle will break the surface tension and allow the fluid to run down the needle.

ACTION 8. Remove filter needle; discard in sharps disposal containers. Replace it with reserved needle or another sterile needle of appropriate length and gauge for medication administration. Do not touch the syringe tip, needle shaft, or inside of needle hub when changing needles. Use a firm twisting motion to attach the new needle.

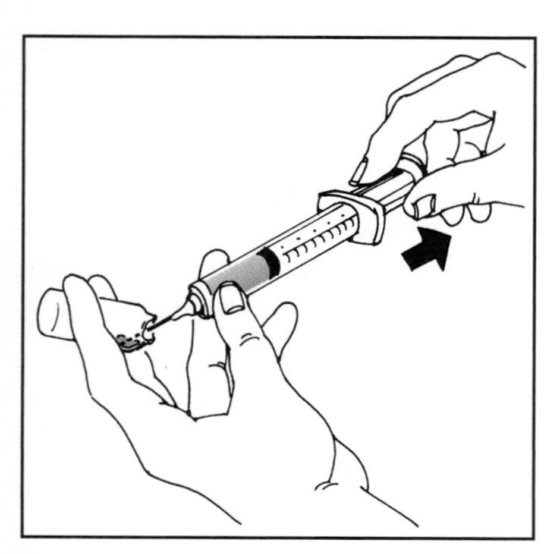

RATIONALE. Filter needle must be removed prior to expelling fluid because particles trapped in the filter needle would be expelled with the medication as fluid flows through it in the opposite direction. See also Action 4. A twisting motion will secure needle.

ACTION 9. Remove needle cap; place it on work surface. Hold syringe vertically, needle up. Tap sharply on syringe barrel to release air bubbles trapped in the liquid. Pull back slightly on plunger, then push it upward to expel air that has moved to the top of syringe.

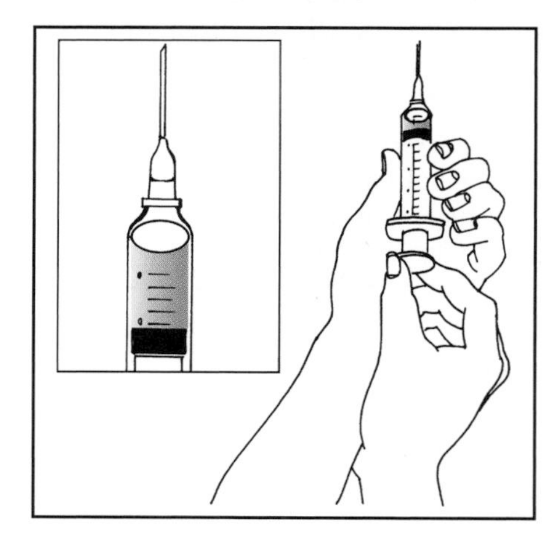

RATIONALE. Cap may trap air or fluid. Air must be expelled to assess accuracy of medication dosage. Syringe position described facilitates removal because air bubbles suspended in a liquid rise. Tapping on the barrel of the syringe releases surface tension, freeing trapped bubbles. Pulling back on plunger before expelling air moves any medication still in needle into the syringe, so it is not expelled with the air.

Procedure 25–11. (continued)

ACTION 10. Recheck the amount of medication to assure accurate dosage. If there is excess, hold the syringe vertically, needle down over a trash container or sink and push downward on plunger until excess is expelled. Do not allow needle to contact sink or trash container.

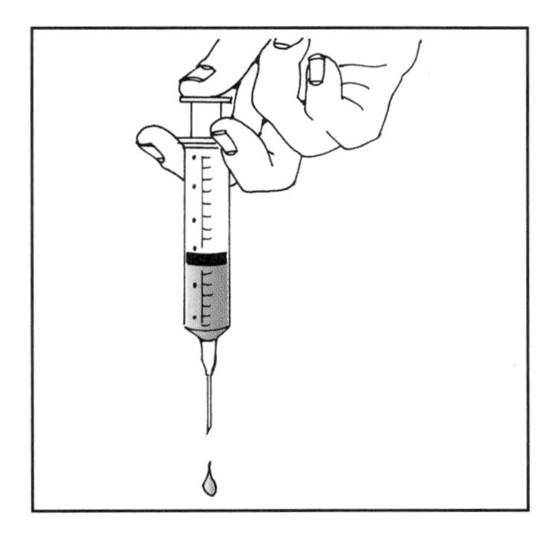

RATIONALE. Accurate dosage is necessary for therapeutic effect and prevention of patient injury. Excess is discarded by inverting syringe to avoid medication running down needle and syringe. Medication on outside of needle can cause tissue irritation. Vertical position allows accurate reading of amount.

ACTION 11. Carefully recap needle, using care not to touch needle with outside of cap or your hand. Do not recap if medication is to be added to another container at the same work area.

RATIONALE. Recapping the needle creates potential needle stick injury to the nurse, so is *not* done except to maintain the sterility of the needle during transport to another area.

ACTION 12. Discard ampule in sharps disposal container. Leave work area clean and dry.

RATIONALE. Glass may cause injury when trash is removed, so glass items are separated from other trash.

Recording:
Record administration of medication according to agency policy.

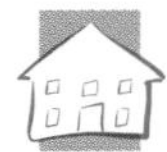

HOME HEALTH ADAPTATION: If medication is supplied in this form in the home and the patient and/or family are involved in the administration, teach them the technique to safely open and withdraw from an ampule as outlined above. Assist and supervise practice until they have successfully mastered the technique.

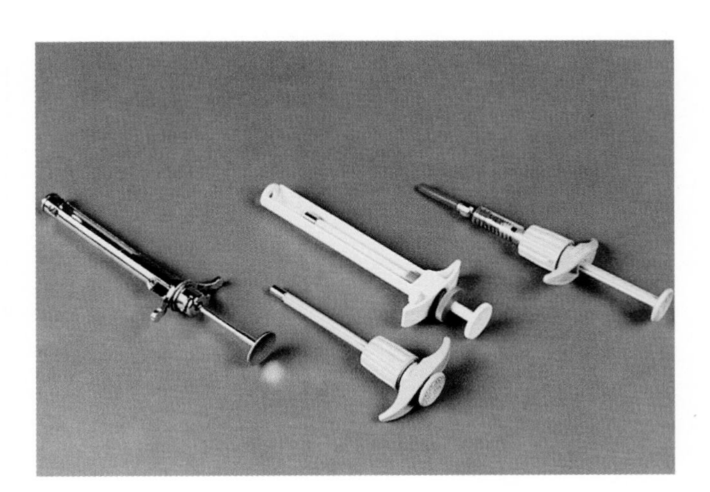

Figure 25–22. Samples of prefilled cartridge-type syringes and holders. From left: 2 types of Tubex® cartridge holders, Carpuject® cartridge holder, and Tubex® holder with cartridge in place *(From Smith S, Duell D.* Clinical Nursing Skills: Nursing Process Model; Basic to Advanced Skills. *4th ed. Norwalk, CT: Appleton & Lange; 1996.)*

destroyed with infectious wastes, not emptied. *Never recap the needle on a used syringe before discarding it.* Recapping used needles is the most common cause of needle stick injuries.

Injections can be given into any of three tissue layers: **intradermal** (into the dermal layer of the skin), **subcutaneous** (into the subcutaneous tissue), and **intramuscular** (into muscle tissue). Figure 25–24 (page 706) illustrates these layers of tissue. Each of these routes has a different purpose and requires a different injection method. All injections require aseptic technique.

The intradermal route is commonly used for diagnostic purposes—primarily allergy and skin testing. It has the slowest absorption rate of any of the parenteral routes. Only very small volumes (eg, 0.1 mL) can be given intradermally. These injections are typically administered in readily observable locations such as the inner forearm, upper chest, and upper back. To avoid inaccurate test interpretation, do not use irritated, discolored, heavily pigmented, or extremely hairy areas. Careful documentation of the injection site is also important for determining results. Most skin tests are evaluated within 48 to 72 hours. Procedure 25–14 outlines steps involved in an intradermal injection.

(continued on page 706)

PROCEDURE 25–12. REMOVING MEDICATION FROM A VIAL

PURPOSE: To withdraw medication contained in a vial in preparation for parenteral administration.
EQUIPMENT: Vial containing ordered medication, sterile syringe and needle of length and gauge appropriate for mode of administration and size of patient, alcohol swabs, and patient's medication administration record (MAR).

ACTION 1. Follow Clinical Guideline 25–11.

RATIONALE. These guidelines facilitate safe, error-free preparation of medication.

ACTION 2. Remove the metal or plastic cap on the top of the vial. If vial is multidose, label with current date and time. A previously used multiple-dose vial will have no cap.

RATIONALE. Protective cap covers rubber seal, maintaining its sterility. Most open multidose vials may be used for 24 hours before discarding contents.

ACTION 3. Cleanse rubber seal of previously used vial with alcohol swab, using firm circular motion. An unused vial need not be cleansed unless seal was touched during cap removal.

RATIONALE. Friction removes bacteria from surface. Although alcohol is an antiseptic, its effectiveness varies. It is not effective unless allowed to dry.

ACTION 4. Obtain syringe. Pull firmly on needle cap to remove it. Pull down on plunger to draw a volume of air into syringe equal to the volume of medication to be given.

RATIONALE. The vial is a closed container, so fluid withdrawn must be replaced with air to keep the pressure inside the vial equalized. If air is not injected, negative pressure is created by withdrawal of fluid, making withdrawal of correct volume difficult.

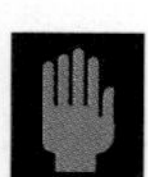

Injecting too much air will create positive pressure inside the vial. The compressed air will displace the plunger and may eject it from the barrel of the syringe.

ACTION 5. Insert the needle through the stopper and inject the air into the air space in the vial to avoid creating bubbles.

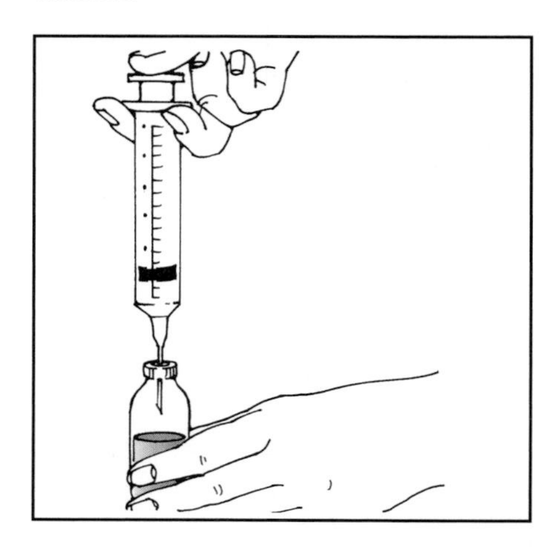

RATIONALE. See Action 4. Air bubbles are to be avoided because they make withdrawing the correct amount of medication more difficult.

ACTION 6. Invert the vial and syringe unit. Stabilize both syringe and needle in the nondominant hand, using one of the grips illustrated.

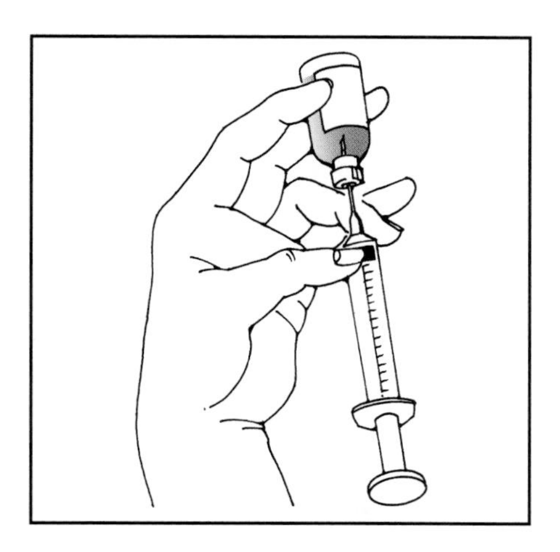

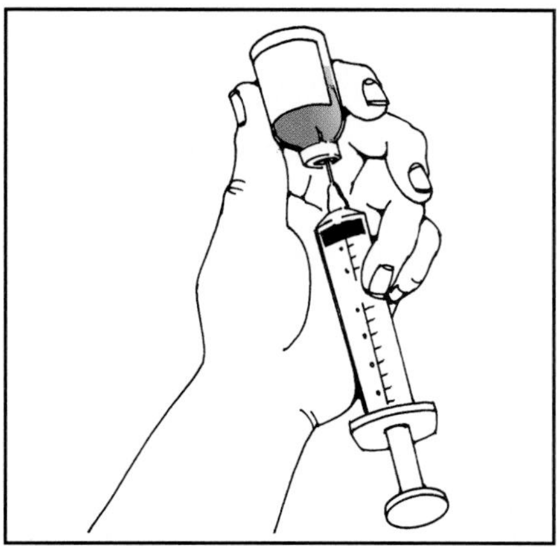

RATIONALE. Either method leaves the dominant hand free to manipulate the plunger with minimal risk of inadvertently withdrawing needle from vial and contaminating it.

ACTION 7. Holding syringe at eye level, with the needle below the fluid–air interface, pull down on plunger slowly to withdraw the required amount of medication.

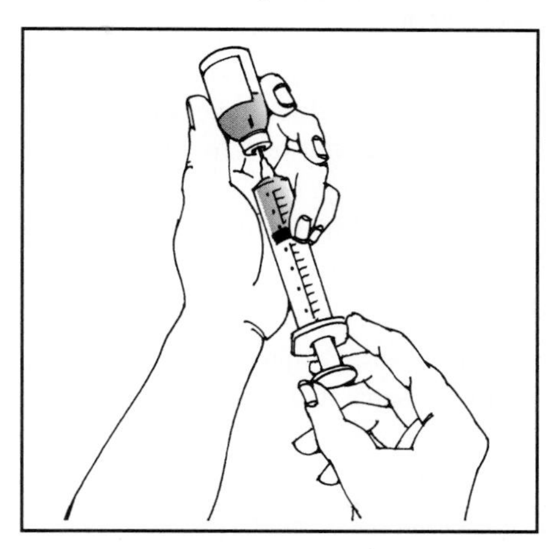

RATIONALE. When a meniscus is not viewed at eye level, parallax (the apparent displacement of objects caused by a change in observer's position) will distort the nurse's perception and result in an inaccurate dosage. If the needle is in the air space, air will be drawn into the syringe. Rapidly withdrawing the medication creates turbulence with resulting air bubbles.

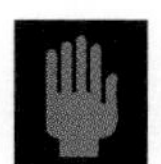

Some experts advise withdrawing enough medication to wet the inside of the syringe, replacing it into the vial, and then removing measured amount. Wetting the syringe decreases air bubbles.

ACTION 8. Check for air bubbles before removing needle from vial. Tap syringe barrel sharply to move air to the top of the syringe, then eject air into vial. Recheck medication volume; return excess or obtain more as needed. Remove needle from vial.

RATIONALE. Tapping on the barrel of the syringe releases surface tension, freeing trapped bubbles so they can rise. Assuring accuracy of dosage before removing needle eliminates need to recleanse and repuncture stopper to obtain additional medication, thereby saving time.

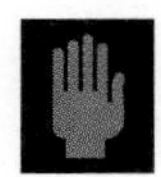

Air bubbles that lodge in the shoulder of the syringe may be difficult to remove. Withdrawing a bolus of air from the vial will often trap the bubble so it can be expelled.

Continued

Procedure 25–12. Removing Medication from a Vial (continued)

ACTION 9. Carefully recap needle, using care not to touch needle with outside of cap or your hand. Do not recap if contents are to be added to another container (eg, IV container) at the same work area.

RATIONALE. Recapping the needle creates potential needle stick injury to the nurse, so is *not* done except to maintain the sterility of the needle during transport to another area.

ACTION 10. Discard empty vial in sharps container. Store vial containing medication according to agency policy. Leave work area clean and dry.

RATIONALE. Glass may cause injury when trash is removed, so glass items are separated from other trash.

Recording:

Record administration of medication according to agency policy.

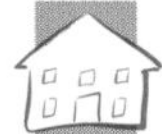

HOME HEALTH ADAPTATION: Teach patients or family members how to withdraw medication from a vial. Assist and supervise their practice until they have successfully mastered the technique.

Subcutaneous (SQ) injections are given into the loose tissue between the skin and muscle. Because there is subcutaneous tissue all over the body, many sites are acceptable. The most commonly used sites are illustrated in Fig. 25–25. Ordinarily no more than 1 mL of solution is administered subcutaneously. Absorption is slower than with intramuscular or intravenous routes; however, the entire dose is absorbed if the patient's circulatory status is adequate. Insulin and heparin are examples of drugs given SQ. Patients who require repeated subcutaneous injections (eg, diabetics) must rotate injection sites in an orderly fashion to minimize tissue damage, avoid patient discomfort, and facilitate absorption. Procedure 25–15 describes the steps for administering a subcutaneous injection.

Intramuscular (IM) injections are used for medications that are irritating to subcutaneous tissue or that need to be absorbed more rapidly. Procedure 25–16 outlines the technique for adminis-

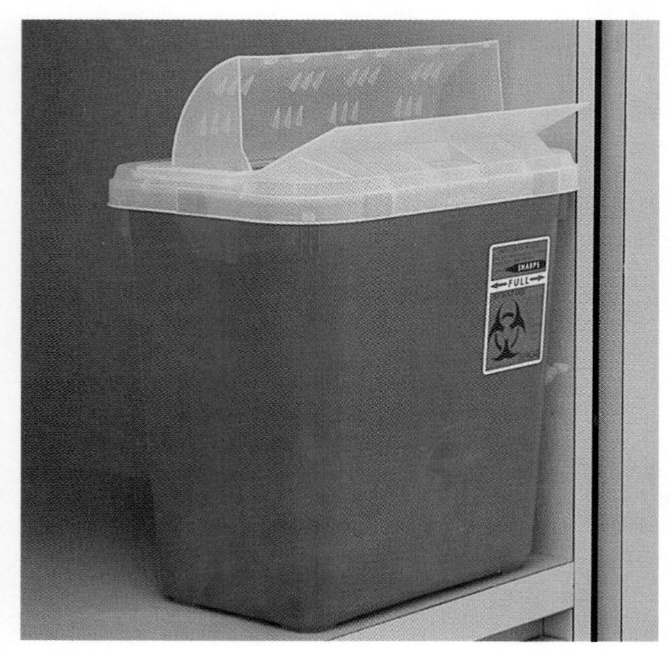

Figure 25–23. Puncture-resistant sharps container for disposal of used syringes and needles in medication preparation area. *(From Smith S, Duell D.* Clinical Nursing Skills: Nursing Process Model; Basic to Advanced Skills. *4th ed. Norwalk, CT: Appleton & Lange; 1996.)*

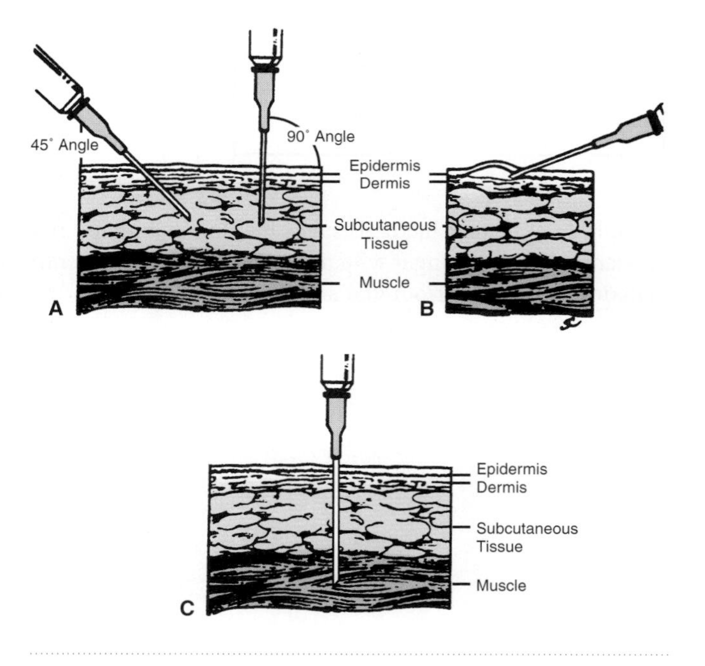

Figure 25–24. Schematic drawings of tissue layers, illustrating locations for parenteral medications. **A.** Subcutaneous. **B.** Intradermal. **C.** Intramuscular. *(From Smith S, Duell D.* Clinical Nursing Skills: Nursing Process Model; Basic to Advanced Skills. *4th ed. Norwalk, CT: Appleton & Lange; 1996: 379.)*

PROCEDURE 25–13. MIXING TWO MEDICATIONS IN ONE SYRINGE

PURPOSE: To simultaneously administer two compatible drugs via subcutaneous or intramuscular routes, thus sparing patient the discomfort of two injections.

EQUIPMENT: Vials and/or ampules containing ordered medications, sterile syringe and needle of appropriate length and gauge based on mode of administration and size of patient, alcohol swabs, and patient's medication administration record (MAR).

ACTION 1. Follow Clinical Guideline 25–11 and the techniques for preparing medications from vials and ampules (Procedures 25–11 and 25–12) to maintain accuracy and asepsis in preparation of medications.

ACTION 2. Determine which drug should be withdrawn from its container first. To minimize the possibility of contaminating a multiple-dose vial and most easily obtain the correct amounts of both drugs, follow these guidelines:

a. If one container is a single-dose vial and the other is a multiple-dose vial, withdraw from the multiple-dose vial first.

b. If one container is a vial and the other is an ampule, withdraw from the vial first.

c. If mixing two forms of insulin, withdraw regular insulin first.

ACTION 3. If both medications are in vials, inject air into both before withdrawing either medication. This will decrease the likelihood of mixing medications when adding air. The vial containing the medication to be withdrawn first ("vial 1"), should be injected with air last.

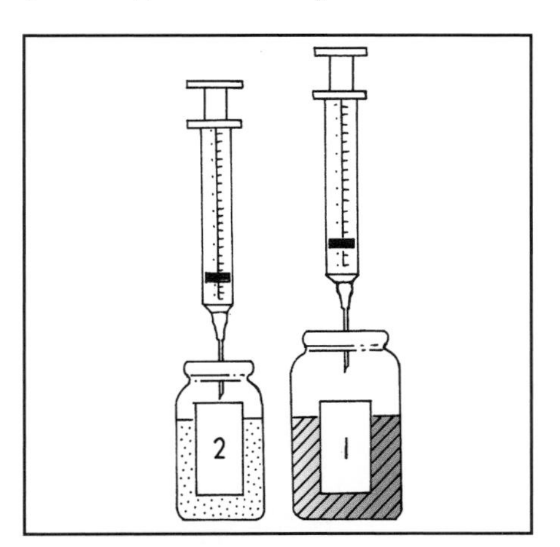

ACTION 4. Withdraw medication from vial 1.

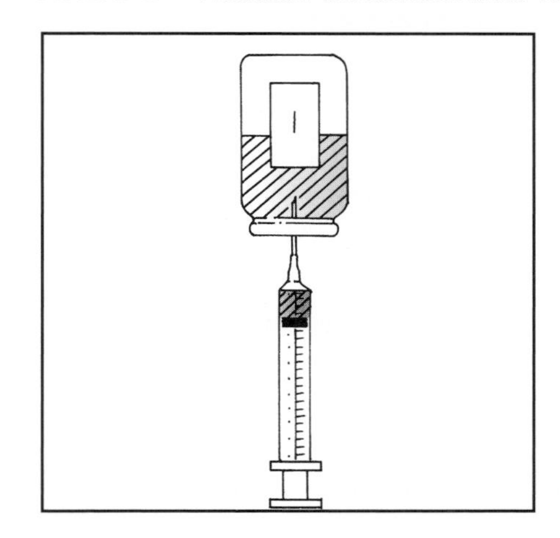

ACTION 5. Withdraw medication from vial 2. Use extreme caution to withdraw only the ordered amount of medication and to avoid creating air bubbles. Excess medication cannot be returned to vial 2, because syringe now contains a mixture of two medications. If air bubbles enter the syringe, they must be expelled into the air, not into vial 2 because some fluid is likely to be expelled with the air. Some experts recommend changing needles prior to withdrawing medication from vial 2. This cannot be done when mixing insulin, as the needles on insulin syringes are not removable. The needle will not carry medication into the second vial, as withdrawing it through the rubber stopper of vial 1 will remove residual medication from the outside of the needle.

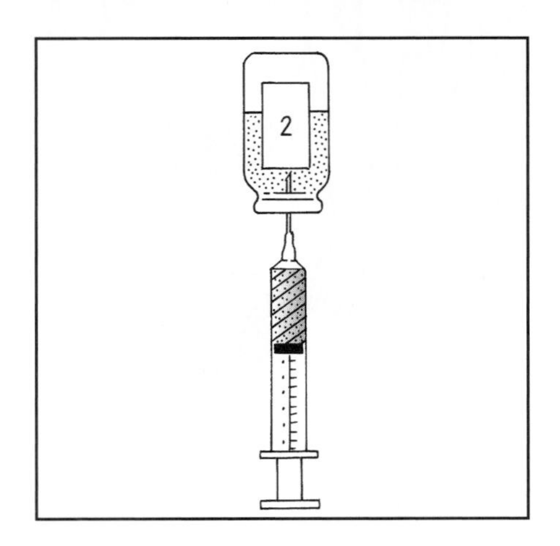

Continued

ACTION 6. Medications are now ready for administration as ordered.

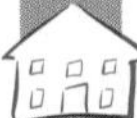

HOME HEALTH ADAPTATION: Teach patients or family members how to correctly withdraw two medications in one syringe. Label the vials "1" and "2" to help them identify which drug to withdraw first and second. Assist and supervise their practice until they have successfully mastered it.

Recording:
Record administration of medication according to agency policy.

tering intramuscular injections. Two variations, the air-lock technique and Z-track technique, minimize drug leakage via the needle track. This techniques are recommended by drug manufacturers to prevent skin staining or abscess formation when administering iron dextran (Imferon) and the diphtheria and tetanus toxoids prepared with aluminum adjuvant. They minimize injection irritation by any IM medication.

For the *air-lock technique,* aspirate a small amount of air (0.2 mL) into the syringe after the desired amount of medication has been prepared. Invert the syringe to move the air toward the plunger. When the injection is administered, the air clears the needle of medication and prevents leakage of medication through the subcutaneous tissue as the needle is withdrawn.

For the *Z-track method,* displace the skin and subcutaneous tissue overlying the injection site laterally, prior to insertion of the needle and hold in this position (Fig. 25–26). Insert the needle and administer the medication. Wait 10 seconds for the medication to disperse, then simultaneously remove the needle and release the skin. This technique forms a zigzag needle path through the patient's tissue and seals the medication into the muscle.

Four sites are appropriate for IM injections: ventrogluteal, dorsogluteal, vastus lateralis, and deltoid. Carefully locate all intramuscular sites using specific anatomic landmarks to avoid damage to major nerves. When selecting a site, consider the condition of the tissue and suitability of the site for the type and volume of medication to be administered.

(continued on page 713)

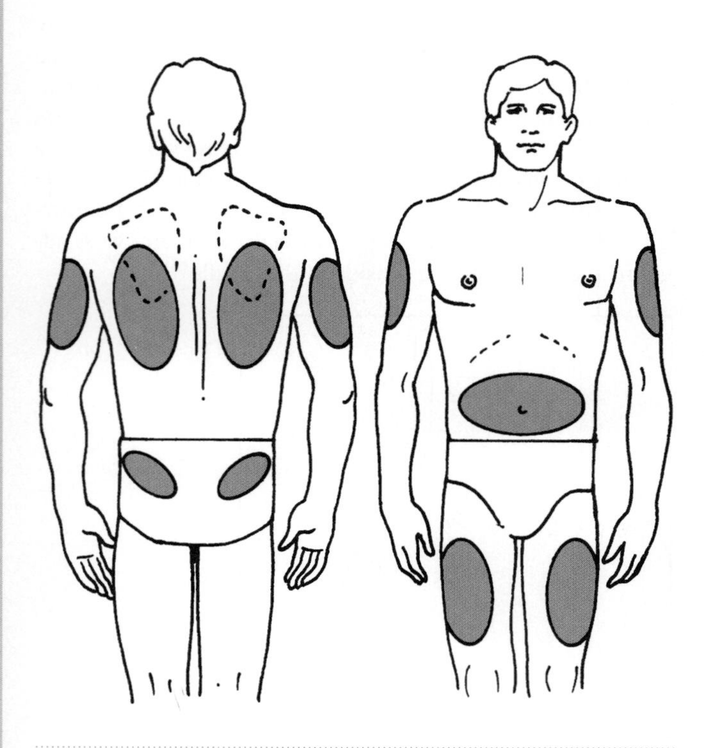

Figure 25–25. Sites for subcutaneous injections. Site rotation is important to prevent tissue damage.

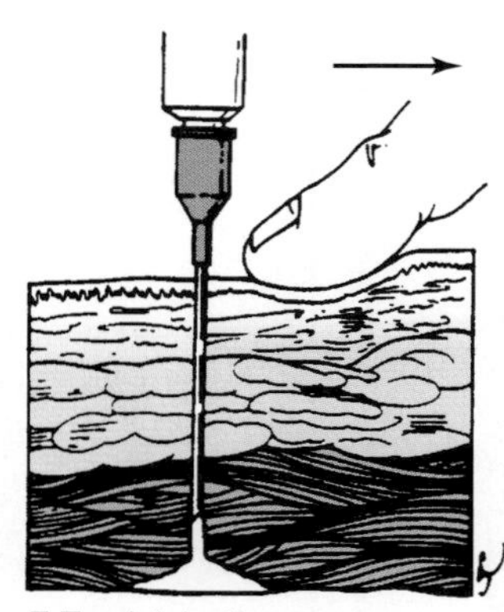

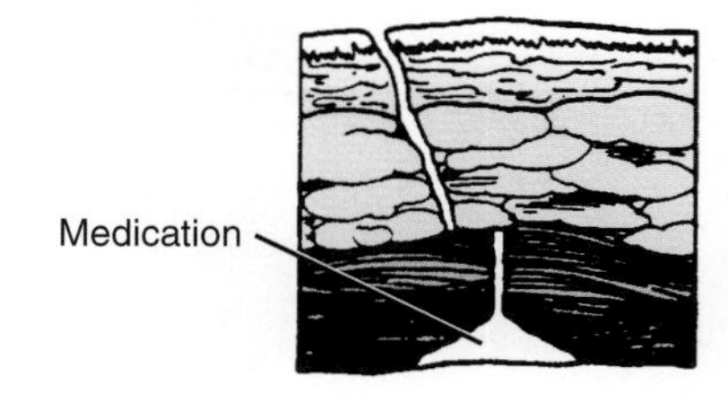

Figure 25–26. Z-track technique for intramuscular injections prevents tracking of medications to the skin. *(From Smith S, Duell D.* Clinical Nursing Skills: Nursing Process Model; Basic to Advanced Skills. *4th ed. Norwalk, CT: Appleton & Lange; 1996.)*

PROCEDURE 25–14. ADMINISTERING AN INTRADERMAL INJECTION

PURPOSE: To inject medication into the dermal skin layer. Generally used for sensitivity testing (allergies, presence of antibodies).

EQUIPMENT: Sterile tuberculin syringe, ⅜- to ⅝-inch 26- or 27-gauge needle, alcohol swabs, medication/allergen to be administered, patient's outpatient record or medication administration record (MAR), and one clean glove.

ACTION 1. Follow Clinical Guideline 25–11 for administration of medications.

RATIONALE. These guidelines facilitate safe, error-free preparation of medication.

ACTION 2. Prepare correct drug dosage from vial or ampule (see Procedures 25–11 and 25–12).

RATIONALE. This method results in aseptic administration of required amount of drug.

ACTION 3. Discuss reason for the procedure, usual sensations, desired patient participation, and expected benefits.

RATIONALE. Patient will be more willing to participate if reasons and benefits are clear. Because many patients are apprehensive about procedures involving needles, extra efforts to inform and relax patient are warranted.

ACTION 4. Discuss possible injection sites with patient. Determine patient's site preference. Screen patient if patient desires.

RATIONALE. Respecting patient's rights of choice regarding their bodies promotes trust in the nurse and diminishes patient's feelings of powerlessness.

ACTION 5. Cleanse the skin at the site using a firm circular motion from center outward, not a back-and-forth motion. Alcohol and/or acetone swabs may be used depending on agency policy. Remove needle cap from syringe.

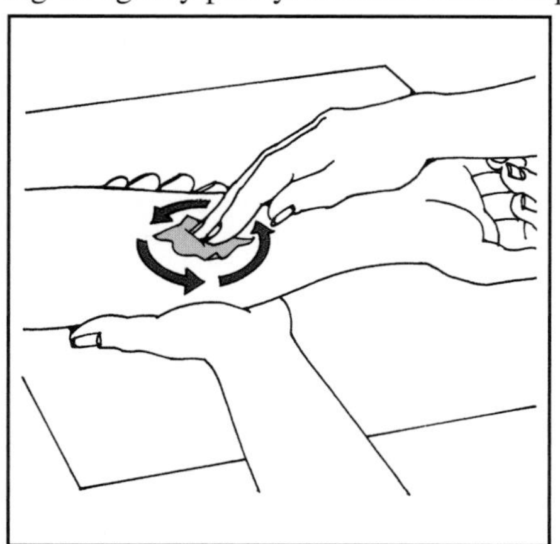

RATIONALE. Alcohol and friction remove surface organisms, preventing their being transmitted through the skin via the needle. A back-and-forth motion is less effective because it moves skin flora from surrounding skin to site. Acetone removes skin oils, which may affect test results in some cases.

ACTION 6. Pull skin taut over injection site by spreading skin between thumb and index finger on nondominant hand. If forearm is used, skin may be stretched by grasping arm from below while it is resting on a table.

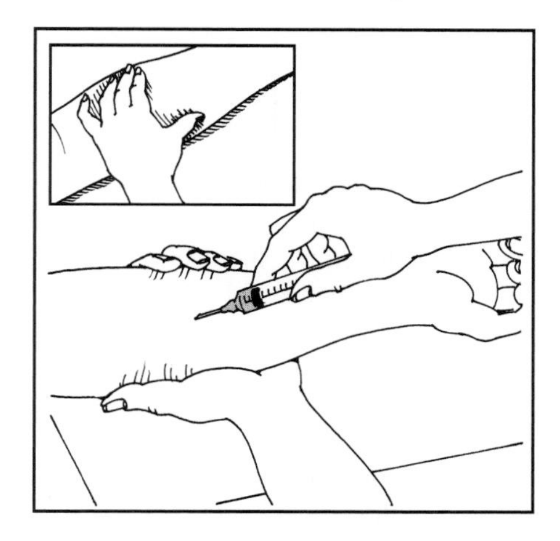

RATIONALE. Taut skin is easier to pierce with needle, so patient discomfort is lessened.

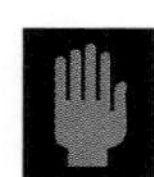

Some nurses prefer to wear a clean glove on the nondominant hand to prevent blood, however, bleeding is *not* usual with intradermal injections.

Continued

Procedure 25–14. Administering an Intradermal Injection (continued)

ACTION 7. Hold syringe as shown, parallel to skin with needle bevel up. Resting your fingers on patient's skin helps to stabilize the syringe during insertion. Insert needle at a 15-degree angle or less. Advance needle far enough to place bevel just under the surface of epidermis. Outline of the bevel will be clearly visible under skin surface.

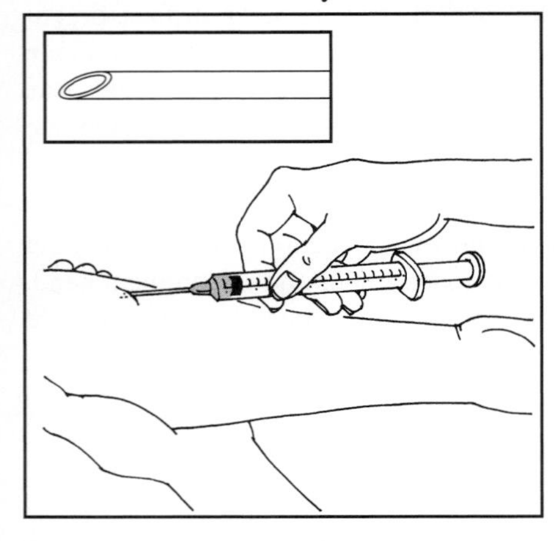

RATIONALE. Insertion of the needle at a greater angle will cause needle to enter subcutaneous tissues, not dermis. When entire bevel is under skin surface, medication will be deposited between dermal layers, as desired.

ACTION 8. Holding syringe steady with dominant hand, slowly push plunger with nondominant hand to inject medication. You should feel slight resistance as medication is injected. A wheal (small raised area like a blister) should be produced on skin surface, as fluid is injected, but no fluid should leak from wheal.

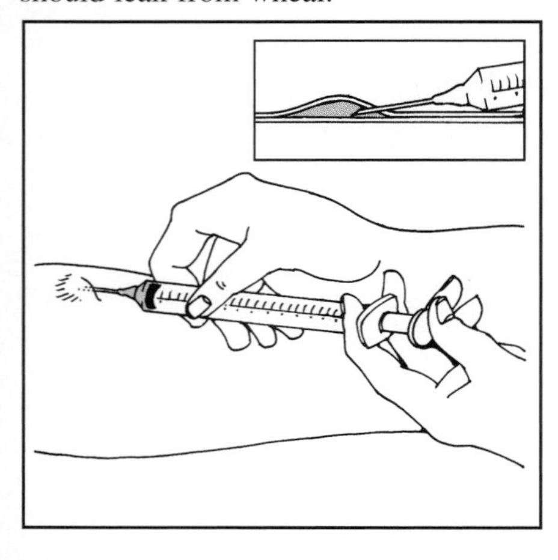

RATIONALE. Syringe movement and tissue distension are sources of injection pain. Slow injection causes gradual distension and less pain. Resistance is created by skin layers. Fluid pushes a small area of epidermis upward, creating a wheal. If no wheal develops, needle insertion was too deep. Leaking indicates needle insertion was too shallow.

ACTION 9. Withdraw needle at same angle it was inserted, without massaging site.

RATIONALE. This method minimizes discomfort. Massage may disperse medication, preventing observation of local reaction.

ACTION 10. Place syringe and needle in puncture-proof container, labeled for used needle disposal. Do not recap needle. Dispose of glove, if used, in a trash receptacle.

RATIONALE. Recapping used needles creates a risk of needle stick injuries and subsequent infection. Labeled puncture-proof container protects other personnel from injuries.

ACTION 11. Wash your hands.

RATIONALE. Washing removes transient organisms, preventing transmission to other patients or personnel.

ACTION 12. Observe site for unusual itching or redness. Provide patient information about site care and reassessment for reaction. Site may be marked to aid later assessment.

RATIONALE. The most common reason for intradermal injections is allergy or antibody testing. Reactions take several days to appear.

Recording:
Note time, date, and location of injection. State name and strength of medication. Describe any immediate local or systemic patient reactions.

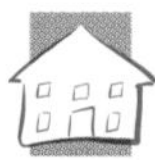

HOME HEALTH ADAPTATION: The procedure for giving an intradermal injection is the same regardless of the setting. This route is not a common one for routine medications.

PROCEDURE 25–15. ADMINISTERING A SUBCUTANEOUS INJECTION

PURPOSE: To inject medication into subcutaneous tissue. This route is preferred for nonirritating medications when sustained effect is desired.

EQUIPMENT: Sterile syringe (insulin or 2- to 3-mL size), ⅝-inch 25-gauge needle, alcohol swabs, medication to be given, patient's medication administration record (MAR), and one clean glove.

ACTION 1. Complete Actions 1 through 4 of Procedure 25–14.

ACTION 2. Choose an area of the selected site that is free of lesions, tenderness, or inflammation.

RATIONALE Medication is more readily absorbed from healthy tissue.

ACTION 3. Cleanse the skin at the site with an alcohol swab, using a firm circular motion from center outward, not a back-and-forth motion. Allow alcohol to dry before penetrating skin with needle.

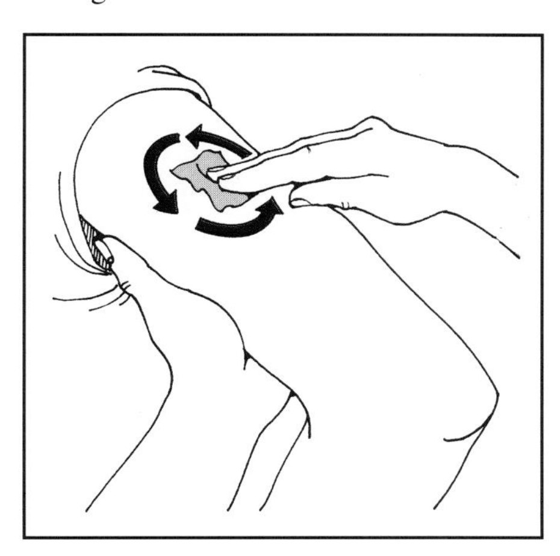

RATIONALE. Alcohol (if allowed to dry on the skin) and friction remove surface organisms, preventing their being transmitted through the skin via the needle. A back-and-forth motion is less effective because it moves skin flora from surrounding skin to site.

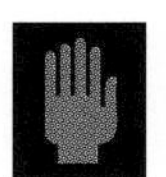

Wearing a clean glove on the nondominant hand while injecting medication is recommended because needle penetration of a capillary may cause a small amount of bleeding from the injection site.

ACTION 4. Remove needle cap from syringe. Stabilize the skin by pinching a fold of skin between thumb and index finger (A) or spreading skin with thumb and index finger of nondominant hand (B).

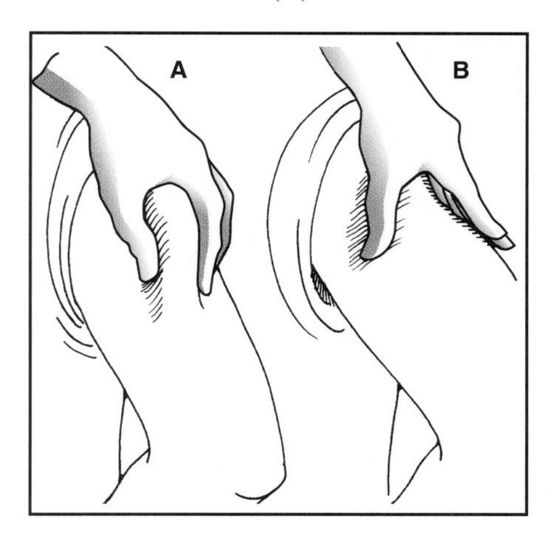

RATIONALE. Spreading skin facilitates piercing of skin by needle, decreasing pain. Some experts recommend pinching a fold of skin when patient is very thin to prevent injecting medication into muscle.

Continued

ACTION 5. Grasp syringe with thumb and four fingers (A) or with thumb and index finger (B, C). Hand or wrist can be stabilized several different ways on the patient's skin, as shown.

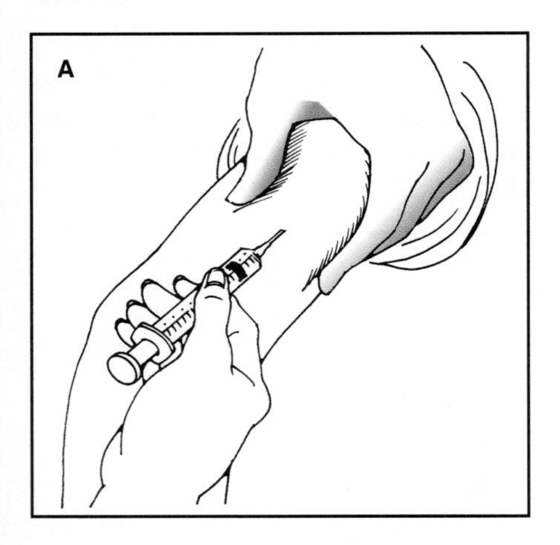

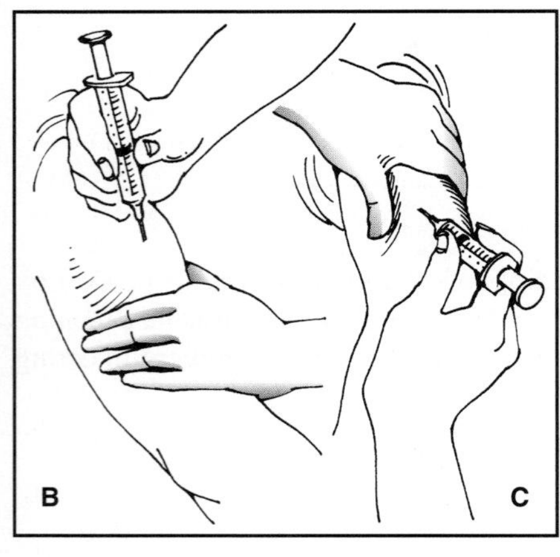

RATIONALE. Either grip facilitates needle entry. Stabilizing hand helps to control the force and distance of needle insertion.

ACTION 6. Quickly insert needle at a 45- to 90-degree angle, depending on the amount of subcutaneous tissue.

RATIONALE. Quick needle insertion reduces stimulation of cutaneous nerves, reducing discomfort. For patients with minimal subcutaneous tissue, inserting needle at a 45-degree angle prevents injection into muscle, which may result in medication being absorbed too rapidly with decreased duration of action.

ACTION 7. Release skin and pull back on plunger with nondominant hand while stabilizing syringe with dominant hand.

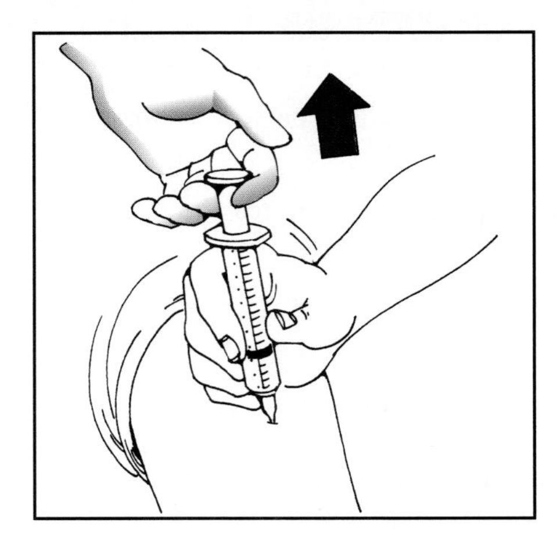

RATIONALE. Stabilizing the syringe with the same hand that was used to insert needle (rather than changing hands so dominant hand aspirates) prevents syringe and needle movement, which would stimulate nerve endings, producing pain.

ACTION 8. If blood enters syringe, withdraw needle and obtain new medication. If aspiration produces no blood, push slowly on plunger with nondominant hand to inject medication into subcutaneous tissue.

RATIONALE. Blood indicates needle is in a blood vessel, so needle is withdrawn to prevent intravenous injection of medication, which could cause patient harm. Medication is injected slowly to prevent rapid tissue distension, which would increase nerve stimulation and increase discomfort.

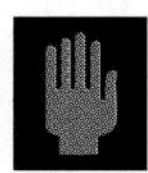

When administering heparin, an anticoagulant, do not pinch the site or aspirate for blood.

ACTION 9. Spread skin around needle, then quickly withdraw needle.

RATIONALE. Taut skin and rapid withdrawal minimize nerve stimulation, reducing pain.

ACTION 10. Massage injection site with gloved hand unless contraindicated for specific medication.

RATIONALE. Massage stimulates circulation, enhancing absorption of medication.

Procedure 25–15. (continued)

ACTION 11. Discard glove in trash receptacle and place needle and syringe, without recapping needle, in specially marked puncture-proof container.

RATIONALE. Recapping used needles creates a risk of needle stick injuries and subsequent infection. Labeled puncture-proof container protects other personnel from injuries.

ACTION 12. Assist patient, if needed, to a comfortable position; replace covers.

RATIONALE Comfort promotes well-being.

ACTION 13. Wash your hands.

RATIONALE. Washing removes transient organisms, preventing transmission to other patients or personnel.

Recording:

Note time, date, and location of injection. State name and strength of medication. If the patient is an inpatient, this recording is usually done on the MAR. Additional recording regarding patient's response to the medication, including desirable and/or undesirable effects, may also be necessary. This is done on the nurse's notes.

HOME HEALTH ADAPTATION: The procedure for giving a subcutaneous injection is the same regardless of the setting. Teach patients or family caregivers how to administer a subcutaneous injection if repeated injections are necessary. Allow ample opportunity for them to practice the technique until they demonstrate proficiency and verbalize confidence. Provide them with a diagram of sites appropriate for subcutaneous injections.

- *Ventrogluteal site* (Fig. 25–27). Landmarks: greater trochanter, *anterior superior iliac spine.* Use your right hand to identify landmarks on the patient's left hip, your left hand for the right hip. With your index finger on the anterior superior iliac spine, extend your middle finger back toward the buttock until it points toward the iliac crest. Your palm should be over the patient's greater trochanter. Give the injection in the lower portion of the "V" formed by your index and middle fingers.

  This site is an excellent choice for both children and adults. It is situated away from major blood vessels or nerves, and generally has a thinner layer of subcutaneous tissue than the dorsogluteal site. It can be used for deep IM, Z-track, and large-volume injections and is accessible with the patient in a sitting, supine, prone, or side-lying position.
- *Dorsogluteal site* (Fig. 25–28). Landmarks: *greater trochanter, posterior iliac spine.* Palpate the posterior iliac spine and the greater trochanter. Draw an imaginary line between them. Acceptable injection sites are above and lateral to the imaginary line.

  The dorsogluteal site can be used in adults and older children; however, it is generally not appropriate for children under the age of 3 years because the muscle is not well developed until a child has been walking for several years. Although many nurses select this site, it provides the slowest absorption rate and the greatest risk for injury to nerves and major blood vessels of all the intramuscular sites. Excessive fat accumulation in this area may result in a subcutaneous rather than intramuscular injection and make visualization of anatomic landmarks difficult. The site is acceptable for large-volume injections. It is accessible with the patient in a prone or side-lying position.
- *Vastus lateralis site* (Fig. 25–29). Landmarks: *greater trochanter, top of patella.* Use the anterolateral aspect of the middle third of the muscle: one hand-breadth below the greater trochanter and one hand-breadth above the patella define the upper and lower borders of the site. Then place one hand perpendicular to the middle of the thigh anteriorly, the other perpendicular to the middle of the thigh laterally to define the lateral borders. Avoid the midanterior portion of the thigh (rectus femoris muscle). Injections in this muscle are uncomfortable for many patients. The vastus lateralis muscle is the site of choice for infants and small children because it is usually well developed and is located away from major nerves and blood vessels.

(continued on page 716)

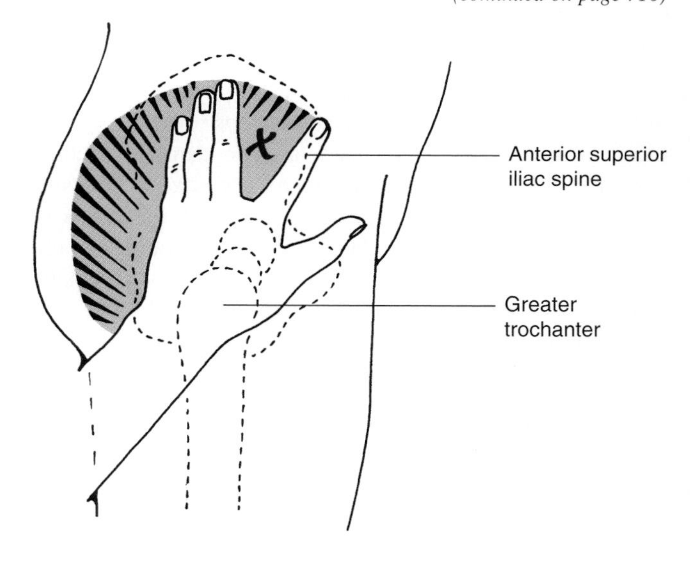

Figure 25–27. Anatomic landmarks for locating **ventrogluteal site** for intramuscular injections. Give injection at the bottom of the V formed by the fingers. (Hand need not remain in place while injection is given.)

PROCEDURE 25–16. ADMINISTERING AN INTRAMUSCULAR INJECTION

PURPOSE: To inject medication into a muscle. Provides more rapid absorption, but shorter duration of effect than subcutaneous injection.

EQUIPMENT: Sterile syringe (3-mL size), 1- to 1½-inch, 22- or 23-gauge needle, alcohol swabs, medication to be given, patient's medication administration record (MAR), and one clean glove. Note: A longer needle is required for obese patients.

ACTION 1. Complete Actions 1 through 4 of Procedure 25–14.

ACTION 2. Determine if needle is of sufficient length to penetrate muscle at site selected by assessing the amount of subcutaneous tissue, as follows: Gently squeeze tissue over muscle with your thumb and index finger. Lift pinched tissue slightly. Estimate the distance between your thumb and finger. One half of this distance is the length of needle needed to reach, but not penetrate, the muscle. Add an additional ½ inch to assure muscle penetration. Obtain new needle of appropriate length, if necessary.

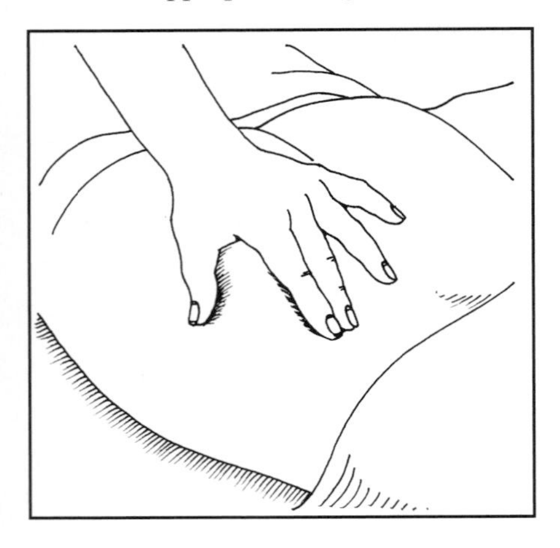

RATIONALE. Subcutaneous tissue is loose and easily isolated from muscle, which has greater density. Method described raises two thicknesses of subcutaneous tissue, hence ½ the thickness represents depth of tissue above muscle. Medications given IM are usually irritating to subcutaneous tissue and if injected they may cause severe pain, sterile abscesses, or tissue necrosis, so the additional ½ inch is important to prevent inadvertent subcutaneous injection. While a 1- or 1½-inch needle is sufficient for most sites in average-sized patients, obese patients may require a 3- to 6-inch needle.

ACTION 3. If necessary, assist the patient to assume a position that provides easy access to the selected site. Adjust covers and gown so sites can be visualized with minimal exposure of patient. Use bony landmarks (Figs. 25–27 to 25–30) to precisely locate correct location for injection. Site should be free of lesions, tenderness, hardness, or inflammation.

RATIONALE. Good access to site allows use of optimum body mechanics and correct injection technique. Minimizing patient exposure prevents chilling and demonstrates respect for patient's privacy. Use of landmarks identifies muscle region without major arteries or nerves. Avoid sites with lesions, tenderness, or inflammation, because medication is more readily absorbed from healthy tissue.

ACTION 4. Cleanse the skin at the site with an alcohol swab, using a firm circular motion from center outward, not a back-and-forth motion. Allow alcohol to dry before penetrating skin with needle.

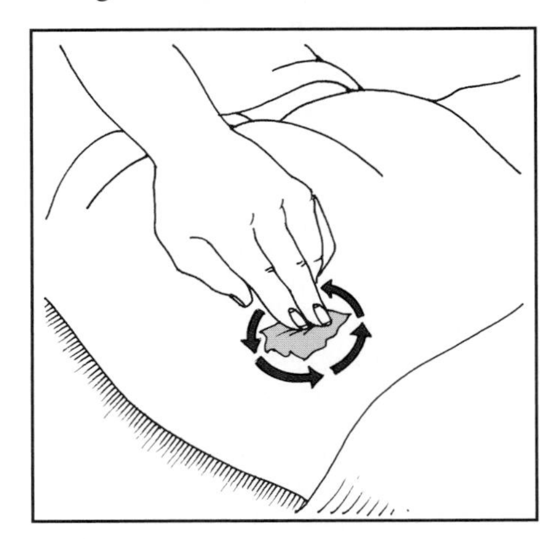

RATIONALE. Alcohol (if allowed to dry on the skin) and friction remove surface organisms, preventing their being transmitted through the skin via the needle. A back-and-forth motion is less effective because it moves skin flora from surrounding skin to site.

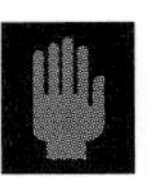

Wearing a clean glove on the nondominant hand while injecting medication is recommended because needle penetration of a capillary may cause a small amount of bleeding from the injection site.

ACTION 5. Remove needle cap from syringe. Stabilize the skin by spreading skin with thumb and index finger of nondominant hand.

RATIONALE Spreading skin facilitates piercing of skin by needle, so fewer nerve endings are stimulated and pain is minimized.

ACTION 6. Grasp syringe with thumb and index finger. Stabilize your hand or wrist on the patient's skin, as shown.

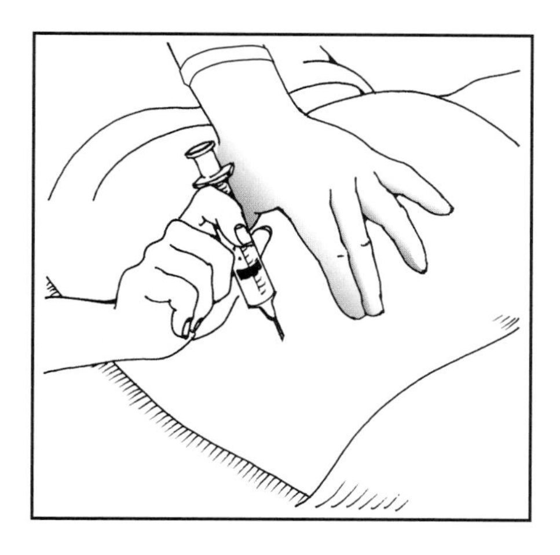

RATIONALE. This grip facilitates needle entry. Stabilizing hand helps to control the force and distance of needle insertion.

ACTION 7. Quickly insert needle to the hub at a 90-degree angle.

RATIONALE. Quick needle insertion reduces stimulation of cutaneous nerves, reducing discomfort. Inserting entire length of needle at 90-degree angle deposits medication well into muscle.

ACTION 8. Release skin and pull back on plunger with nondominant hand while stabilizing syringe with dominant hand. Do not allow partial withdrawal of needle while aspirating.

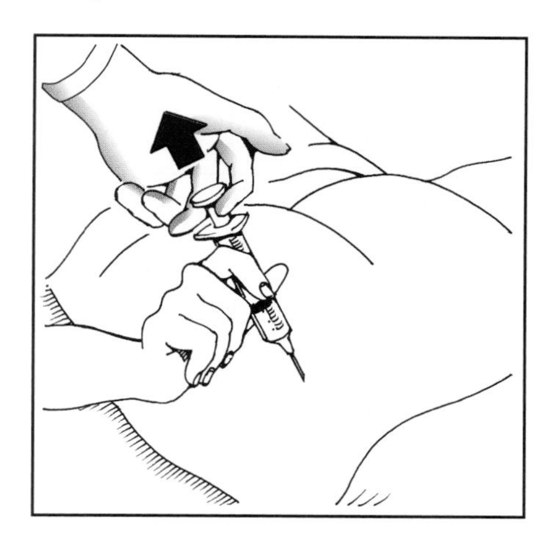

RATIONALE. Stabilizing the syringe with the same hand that was used to insert needle (rather than changing hands so dominant hand aspirates) prevents syringe and needle movement, which would stimulate nerve endings, producing pain. Partial withdrawal of needle could result in subcutaneous injection.

ACTION 9. Follow Procedure 25–15, Actions 8 to 13.

ACTION 10. If drug was a prn pain medication, return in 30 to 40 minutes to observe whether desired effects were obtained.

RATIONALE. Observation is necessary to make a decision regarding subsequent administration of this drug to the patient and the need for additional relief measures.

Recording:
Note time, date, and location of injection. State name and strength of medication. If the patient's is an inpatient, this recording is usually done on the MAR. Additional recording regarding patient's response to the medication, including desirable and/or undesirable effects, may also be necessary. This is done on the nurse's notes.

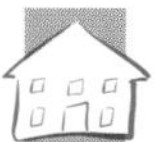

HOME HEALTH ADAPTATION: The procedure for giving an intramuscular injection is the same regardless of the setting. Teach patients or family caregivers how to administer intramuscular injections if repeated injections are necessary. Allow ample opportunity for them to practice the technique until they demonstrate proficiency and verbalize confidence. Provide them with a diagram of sites appropriate for intramuscular injections.

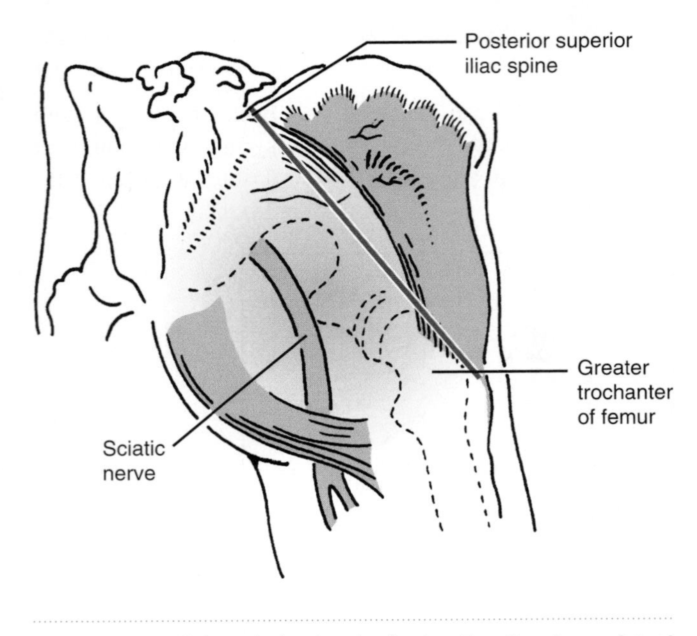

Figure 25–28. Anatomic landmarks for locating the **dorsogluteal site** for intramuscular injections. Place the injection above the diagonal line.

- *Deltoid site* (Fig. 25–30). Landmarks: *acromion process, axilla.* Locate the upper border of the site by measuring three finger-breadths below the acromion process. The top of the axilla marks the lower border. Visualize the middle third of the arm front to back to define the lateral borders. The major advantages of the deltoid site are its easy accessibility and rapid absorption. The deltoid is used primarily in adults for small-volume (1 mL) injections.

ADMINISTERING INTRAVENOUS MEDICATIONS. The **intravenous** (IV) route is chosen when an immediate effect is desired. It is also appropriate for medications not readily absorbed by other routes. None of the interfering factors that delay or limit drug absorption apply to medications given IV. However, the immediacy of transport to the target organ confers risk as well as benefit. The effects of IV medication errors are extremely difficult to counteract; therefore, nurses must always use utmost caution when administering IV drugs. Monitor patient response frequently throughout the infusion. Use meticulous aseptic technique when preparing and administering IV medications.

Many intravenous medications are extremely irritating to tissues. Assess the IV site for irritation and displacement of the cannula (IV needle) before all infusions to prevent injury to subcutaneous tissue. Appropriate dilution of medications protects the vascular system. Infuse extremely irritating medications such as potassium

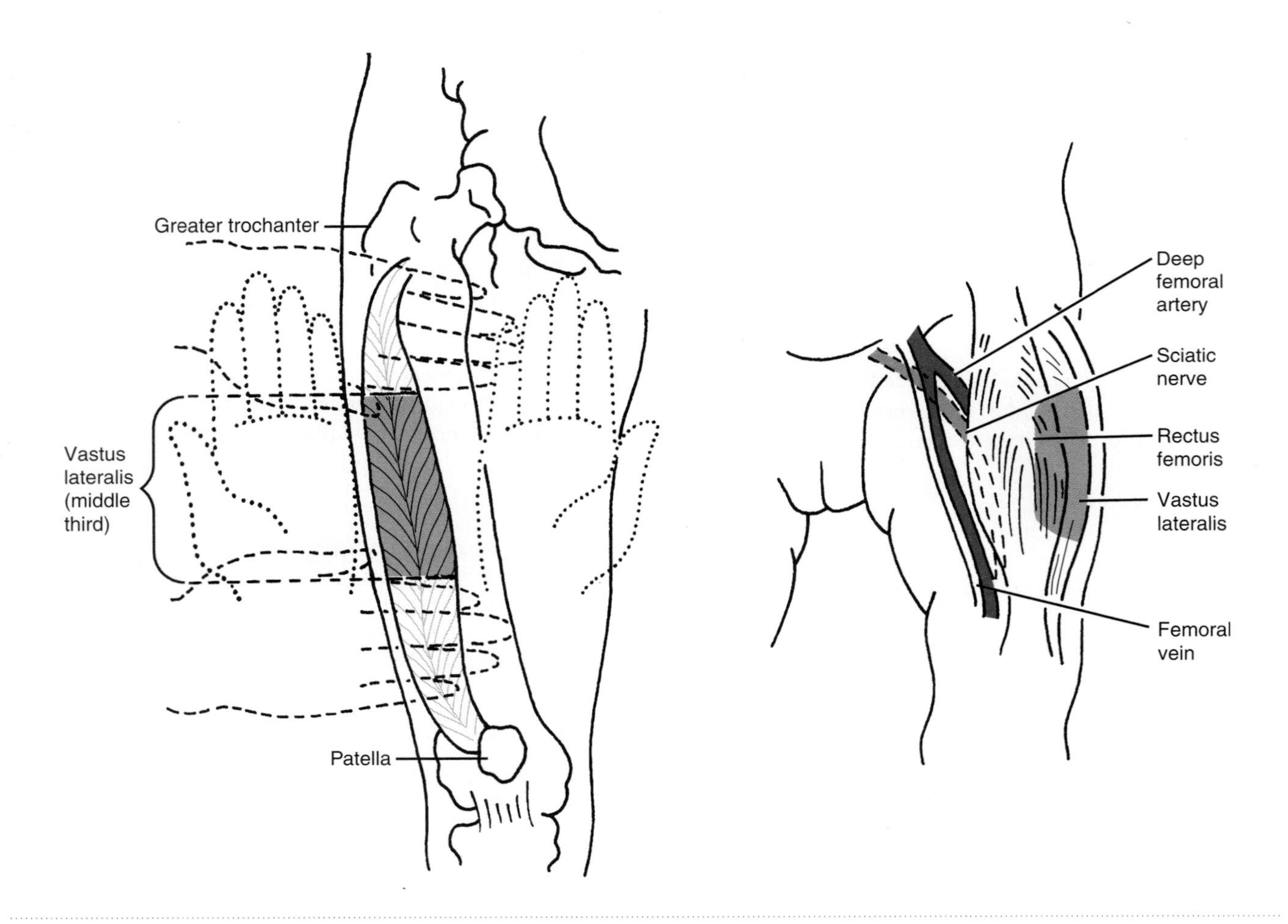

Figure 25–29. Anatomic landmarks for locating the **vastus lateralis site** for intramuscular injections: left, adult; right, infant or small child. Give injection in the middle one-third of the muscle (rectangular space formed by hand placement).

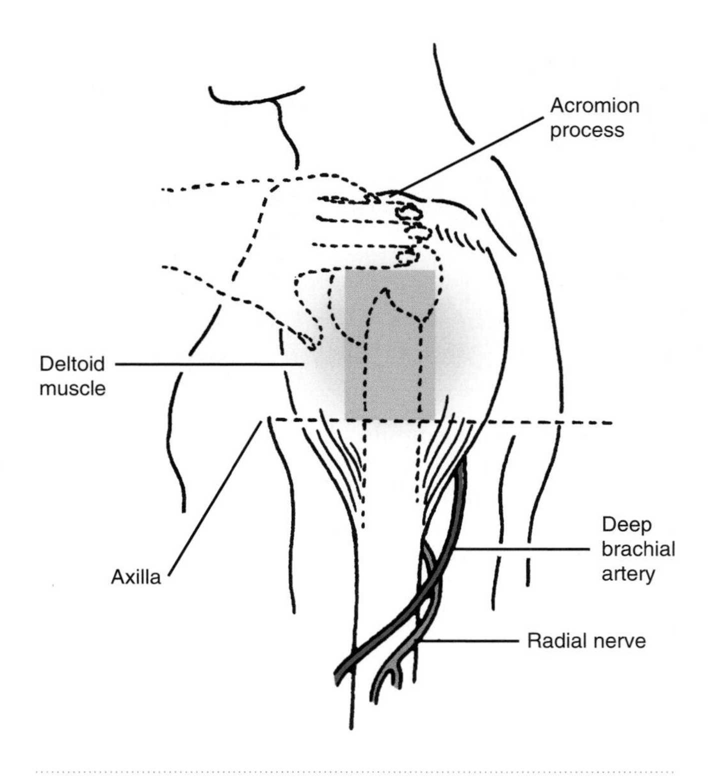

Figure 25–30. Anatomic landmarks for locating the **deltoid site** for intramuscular injections. Give injection in the rectangle formed by the planes of the landmarks.

preparations at a slow rate. Warm refrigerated medications to room temperature prior to administration to reduce venous spasm.

Many of the patient concerns about needles and injections discussed above also apply to intravenous medications. Patients are usually protective of the venipuncture site, fearing that their own movement or tension on the tubing will dislodge the cannula. Nurses' manipulation of the IV equipment, particularly near the cannula insertion site, generates apprehension. The need to "restart" the IV because of *phlebitis* (inflammation of the vein wall) or *infiltration* (infusion of IV solution into the tissue surrounding the blood vessel) is received with dismay. Remember to show empathy for these feelings. Reassure patients that precautions to protect the IV site and minimize discomfort are your priority as well as theirs. A detailed discussion of basic IV procedures can be found in Chap. 34.

There are three methods for administering an IV medication: IV push, as an intermittent small-volume dose using piggyback or volume-controlled devices, and as an additive to a large-volume container of IV fluids.

An *IV push* (bolus) is a concentrated dose of medication injected directly into the systemic circulation via the Y-port on an existing IV line, an intermittent infusion device, or direct venipuncture. This method is used in emergency situations or when a very rapid response to the drug is desired. IV push is the most dangerous method for administering drugs as the entire dose is administered within 1 to 7 minutes. Administration of IV push medications is an advanced procedure. Health care institutions have detailed protocols that identify specific medications and conditions under which nurses can administer IV push medications.

Intravenous medications are most often administered intermittently through the use of small-volume infusions, called *piggybacks* (Procedure 25–17). Drugs to be given as piggybacks are mixed with a compatible solution, usually saline or dextrose, in a 50- to 100-mL IV container. These small-volume containers are called *partial-fill* or *additive sets*. Some piggybacks are prepared in the pharmacy, others by nurses. The solution containing the medication is connected to the uppermost injection site of the primary intravenous line via short IV tubing called *secondary tubing*. The piggyback is regulated to infuse over a 30- to 90-minute interval. IV antibiotics and postoperative pain medications are frequently administered by the piggyback method. Intravenous drip medications are also used when a patient is not receiving intravenous fluid therapy and therefore has no primary IV line. An intermittent infusion device is connected to the IV cannula for venous access (see Chap. 34). Procedure 25–18 outlines the technique for administering an IV drip medication via an intermittent infusion device.

IV drip medications also are administered through the use of volume control sets (eg, Soluset, Buretrol, Pediatrol) or mini-infuser pumps. *Volume-control sets* are small-volume containers (100 to 150 mL) that are attached directly below the primary IV container (Fig. 34–11). The volume-control set is filled with a prescribed amount of fluid from the primary IV and medication is added to it through an injection port. The infusion procedure varies according to manufacturer's design (see Chap. 34). *Mini-infuser pumps* are battery-operated devices that control the infusion of small amounts (5 to 60 mL) of medication in a syringe connected in tandem to a primary IV line (Fig. 25–31).

Medication *additives to large-volume containers* (usually the primary IV solution) are administered continuously over several hours. Potassium chloride and multivitamin solutions are examples of two drugs commonly administered in this way. Often IV solutions with additives are prepared in the pharmacy. The steps for adding medications to intravenous containers are outlined in Procedure 25–19.

(continued on page 727)

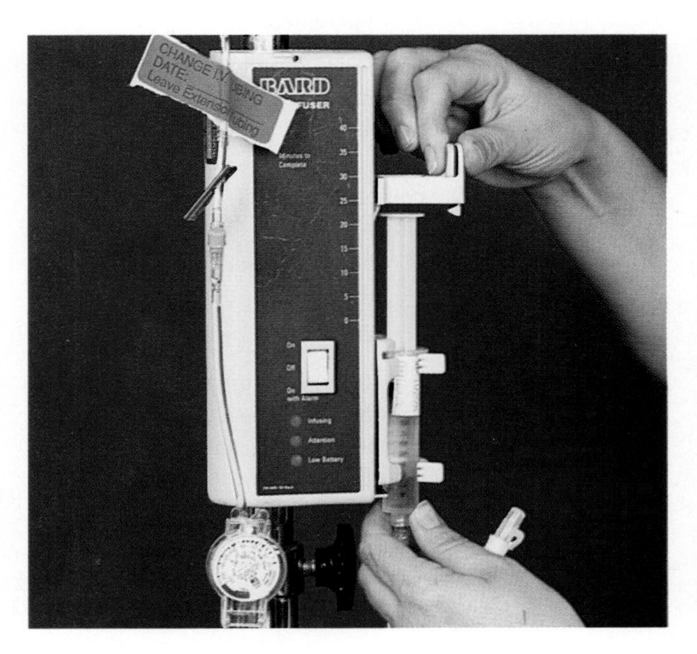

Figure 25–31. Mini-infuser or syringe pump for administration of IV medications. *(From Smith S, Duell D.* Clinical Nursing Skills: Nursing Process Model; Basic to Advanced Skills. *4th ed. Norwalk, CT: Appleton & Lange; 1996.)*

PROCEDURE 25–17. ADMINISTERING IV DRIP MEDICATIONS VIA PIGGYBACK (ADDITIVE SET)

PURPOSE: To deliver medications by intravenous drip.

EQUIPMENT: Ordered medication in a 50- to 250-mL infusion bag, alcohol swabs, sterile 18- to 19-gauge 1-inch needle or needleless adapter, patient's medication administration record (MAR), and IV secondary administration set if tubing change is needed, based on agency policy.
If medication has not been prepared by pharmacy: Vial/ampule of ordered medication, sterile syringe and needle, and 50- to 100-mL infusion bag of D_5W or 0.9% NaCl (often called "partial-fill" or "addit"). *If medication is not compatible with patient's IV solution:* Also obtain a 250-mL container of 0.9% NaCl or D_5W and a standard IV administration set with additive ports, and an additional 18- to 19-gauge needle.

ACTION 1. Follow Clinical Guideline 25–11. If medication has not been prepared by pharmacy, follow techniques for preparing medications from vial or ampule (see Procedures 25–11 and 25–12).

RATIONALE. These guidelines facilitate safe and error-free preparation and administration of medications.

ACTION 2. If ordered medication has not been prepared for IV infusion by pharmacy, inject medication into infusion bag of NaCl or D_5W, using technique for new container described in Procedure 25–19. Affix medication label.

RATIONALE. This will result in aseptic preparation of correct medication for infusion readily identifiable by all personnel during infusion.

ACTION 3. If pharmacy-prepared medication has been refrigerated, remove 30 minutes prior to administration to warm container to room temperature.

RATIONALE. Administration of cold medication is uncomfortable; may chill some patients. Flush line prevents mixing of incompatible solutions.

ACTION 4. Check compatibility of medication and patient's IV solution. If incompatible, prepare 250 mL NaCl or D_5W to use as a flush line. See Procedure 34–3.

ACTION 5. Assess IV site for redness, swelling, warmth, and tenderness. If none are present, proceed with next step.

RATIONALE. These are indicators of inflammation due to vein irritation by solutions. Medications are often more irritating than standard IV solutions, so it may be advisable to consider a new venipuncture if vein is already irritated.

ACTION 6. If the medication is compatible with the primary IV solution, remove and discard empty medication container from prior infusion and spike the new medication container with secondary tubing still connected to port on primary line (clamp should be closed).

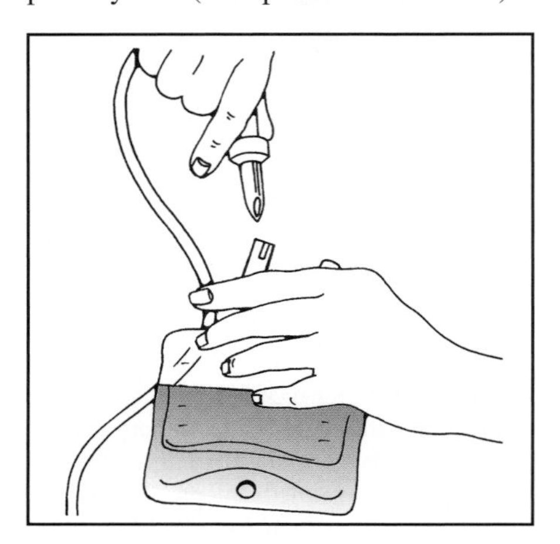

If using new tubing, close the roller, clamp, spike the medication container, and attach the needle or needleless adaptor. Then cleanse the highest port on the primary line with an anchol swab and insert the needle/needless adaptor into the port.

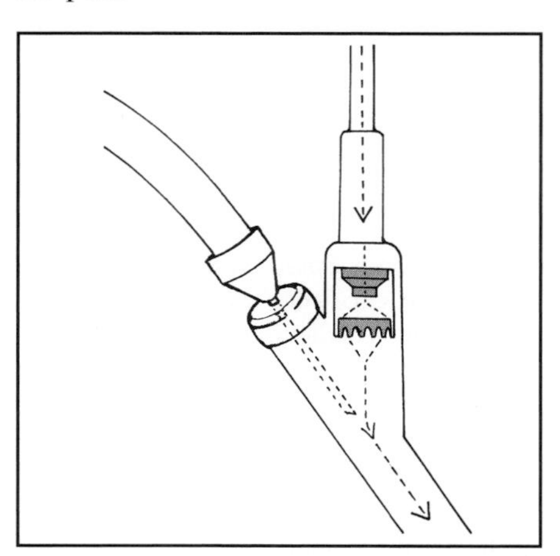

Procedure 25–17. (continued)

Backfill secondary tubing by opening clamp and holding the container lower than the port. When drip chamber on secondary line is half full, hang container, leaving clamp open. If medication is not compatible with IV solution, or if several medications not compatible with each other are ordered, see Actions 12–14.

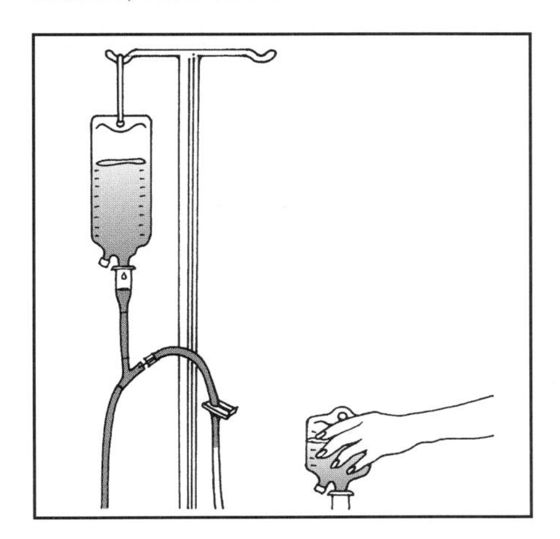

RATIONALE. Setup from previous medication is usually left connected to the primary line after the medication has infused to minimize disruption of closed system (which creates possibility of contamination). Backfilling rather than priming the tubing also introduces air into the medication container. When the container is a plastic bag, adding air is necessary to prevent creation of a vacuum as medication infuses (bag will collapse). A vacuum in the bag prevents all of the medication from infusing. Backfilling is preferred, but not necessary for other types of containers or if vented secondary tubing is used.

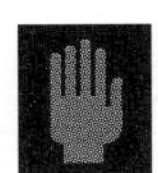

The highest port has a check valve that temporarily stops the flow of the primary infusion while the secondary infusion is running. If other ports are used, the primary infusion will continue to flow while medication is infusing because these ports have no check valves.

ACTION 7. Hang the primary container so it is lower than the secondary (medication) container. If multilevel overhead IV hanger is not available, use extension hook contained in secondary administration set to lower the primary bottle. Use the clamp on the primary line to regulate flow of medication at the ordered or recommended rate. Medications may be infused over 15 to 90 minutes; 30 minutes is most common.

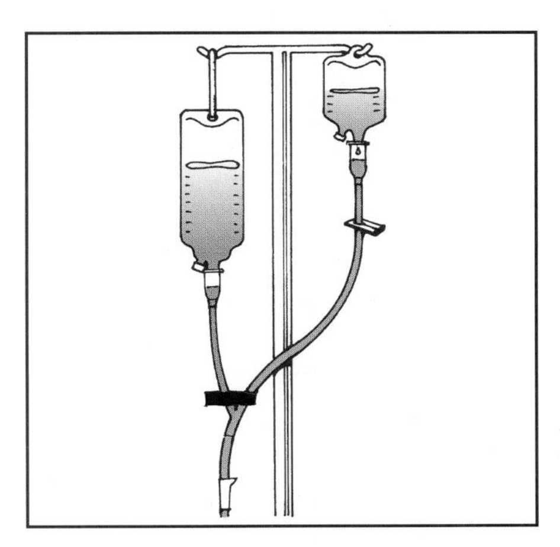

RATIONALE. The greater the height of a column of liquid, the faster the flow. The faster flow from the higher secondary container will close the check valve so medication will infuse according to the setting on the primary tubing. When the level of fluid in the secondary tubing is even with the drip chamber of the primary line, the primary line will have the greater height so the check valve will open and the primary line will resume infusing.

Continued

ACTION 8. If using new tubing, secure secondary line with tape or needle-lock device so it cannot accidently pull out of the port. Tubing used for previous piggyback should already be taped in place.

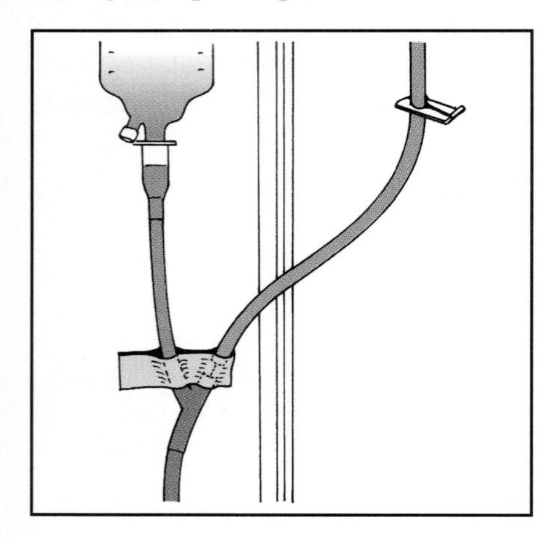

RATIONALE. Accidental separation of secondary line is one cause of needle-stick injuries to health care personnel and would cause loss of medication to floor or patient's bed.

ACTION 9. Assess the infusion, the site, and the patient periodically during the infusion. Reregulate drip if necessary, or reposition limb to improve flow. If severe pain or swelling occurs at site, or other untoward effects occur, discontinue infusion and consult physician.

RATIONALE. These actions promote early detection and correction of problems related to infusion mechanics and/or undesirable reactions to the medication.

ACTION 10. When infusion is complete, close clamp on secondary line, reassess and/or reregulate primary infusion at ordered rate.

RATIONALE. Promotes fluid and electrolyte balance.

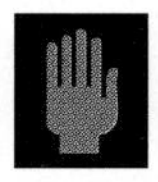

Some agency IV policies recommend pinching off primary line just above the port so medication remaining in secondary tubing will run in, then closing secondary clamp.

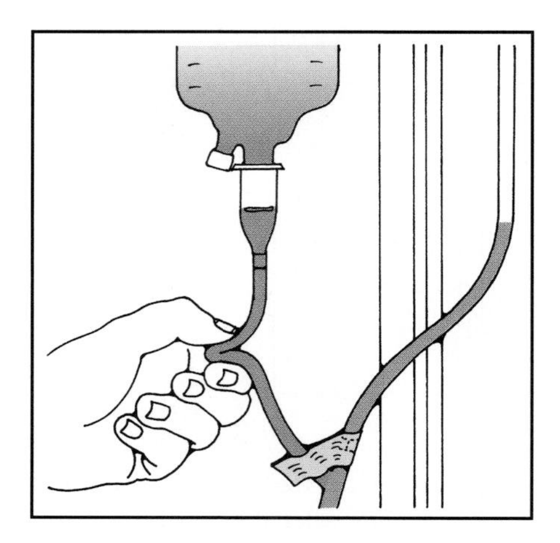

ACTION 11. If medication previously infused is not the same as current medication, but is compatible, above procedure can be followed. If medications are not compatible, use separate secondary tubing for each medication. It is permissible to leave the secondary tubing still attached to the previous medication container hanging on IV stand for use at the next administration time, but needle guard should be securely in place and a new needle or needleless adaptor used for next infusion. Connect and backfill as for new tubing (see Action 6).

RATIONALE. Medications that are not compatible may precipitate, clogging venipuncture device, or may inactivate one another.

ACTION 12. If primary solution and the medication are incompatible, obtain 0.9% NaCl or D_5W to prevent mixing of primary solution and medication (called a "flush line"). Set up the flush line as you would a primary IV (see Procedure 34–3), but attach a needleless adaptor or an 18- to 19-gauge, 1-inch needle to the needle adaptor at the end of the tubing and secure the needleless adaptor or needle on primed flush line into one of the lower ports on the primary tubing; secure as above. Close the clamp on the primary line and open the clamp on the flush line to keep vein open (KVO) rate.

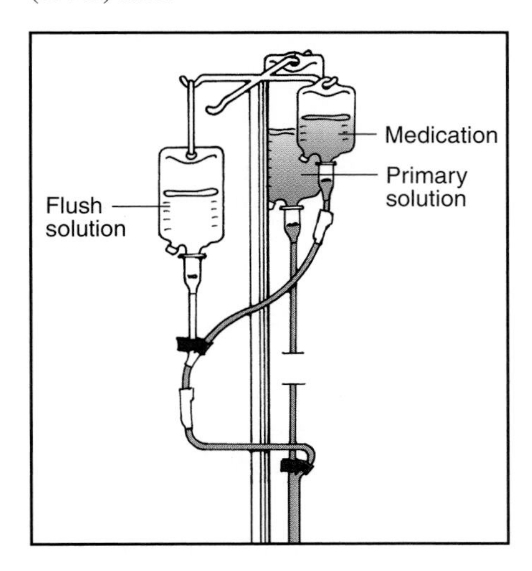

RATIONALE. Solution in flush line acts as a buffer, preventing mixing of medication and primary IV solution.

ACTION 13. Connect medication to container and tubing flush line and administer medication as described in Actions 6–9. When medication container is empty, allow flush solution to flow for 5 minutes, and then separate flush line from primary line, recap or replace needle or needleless adaptor, and leave in room for future use. Readjust flowrate of primary solution to ordered rate.

RATIONALE. When medication has infused, the solution in flush line will flush medication into patient's vein (see rationale for Action 7). This prevents mixing of primary solution and medication.

Recording:
Record administration of IV medications and solutions according to agency policy. Usually recording will be necessary on both the MAR and the I&O record. Narrative recording on nurse's notes may also be expected for some medications or if unexpected reaction to medication occurs.

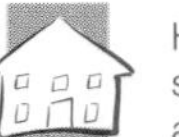

HOME HEALTH ADAPTATIONS: This procedure is the same regardless of the setting. Family caregivers who are conscientious and capable of safely giving medications via piggyback can be taught the procedure. Be cognizant of their anxieties and allow them ample opportunity to practice until they demonstrate proficiency and verbalize confidence. Instruct them in signs and symptoms of an adverse reaction and the immediate action necessary. Many family caregivers will not want to accept responsibility for this level of care.

PROCEDURE 25–18. ADMINISTERING IV DRIP MEDICATIONS VIA AN INTERMITTENT INFUSION PORT (SALINE LOCK)

PURPOSE: To deliver medications by intravenous drip to a patient not receiving continuous IV fluids.

EQUIPMENT: Ordered medication in a 50- to 100-mL infusion container (or vial/ampule of medication, sterile syringe, and 50- to 100-mL infusion container of NaCl or D_5W); IV administration set with sterile 18–19 gauge 1-inch needle or needleless adaptor; sterile syringe/needle (22 gauge, 1 inch) filled with 1- to 2-mL of sterile normal saline (or heparin flush solution in some agencies); alcohol swabs, tape and patient's medication administration record (MAR). If agency policy specifies that medications be infused as a piggyback to a "flush solution setup," rather than directly into the intermittent infusion port, a secondary administration set is required.

ACTION 1. Follow Clinical Guideline 25–11 and techniques for preparing medications from vial or ampule (Procedures 25–11 and 25–12) to prepare syringes of sterile saline and ordered medication (if it is not preprepared in IV solution by pharmacy).

RATIONALE. These guidelines facilitate safe and error-free preparation and administration of medications.

Check agency policy. Although saline is the currently preferred solution, some agencies may specify that a heparin flush solution be used instead to flush and maintain patency of an intermittent infusion port between uses. Also, flushing with a saline-filled syringe before and after infusing medication is unnecessary if a flush IV setup is used; see Actions 10 and 13.

ACTION 2. If ordered medication has not been prepared for IV infusion by pharmacy, inject medication into infusion bag of NaCl or D_5W, using technique for new container described in Procedure 25–19. Affix medication label.

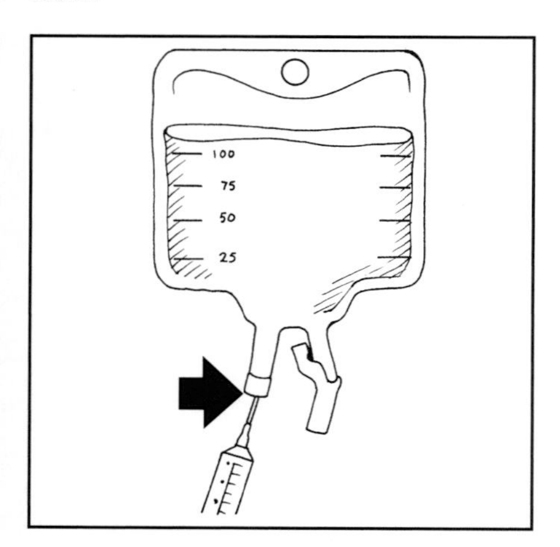

RATIONALE. This will result in aseptic preparation of correct medication for infusion readily identifiable by all personnel during infusion.

ACTION 3. Attach 18-gauge, 1-inch needle or needleless adaptor to apppropriate IV tubing and prime tubing with medication solution. Leave protective caps on. Label all tubing with date and time.

RATIONALE. Secondary tubing is of appropriate length for piggyback administration, but too short to allow patient movement if medication is to be infused directly into intermittent infusion port.

IV tubing used for prior infusion of the same drug may be reused for a 48- to 72-hour period. Check agency policy.

ACTION 4. Discuss the reason for the procedure, expected patient participation, usual sensations, and expected benefits with the patient.

RATIONALE. Patient will be more willing to participate and less anxious if there is an opportunity to clarify concerns and the reasons and benefits for the procedure are clear.

ACTION 5. Assess IV site for redness, swelling, warmth, and tenderness. If none is present, proceed with next step.

RATIONALE. These are indicators of inflammation. IV flow may be sluggish, even if intermittent infusion port is patent. Insertion of a new port at another site may be necessary.

ACTION 6. Hold intermittent infusion port with one hand to stabilize it. Cleanse port with alcohol swab, using firm rotational motion. Let dry.

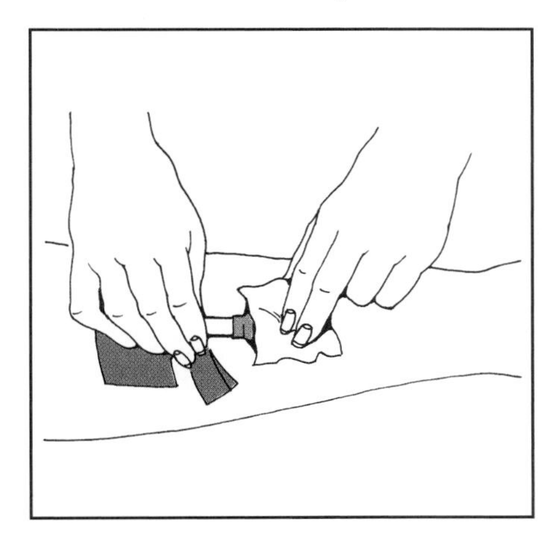

RATIONALE. Stabilizing intermittent infusion port prevents its moving, which causes discomfort and may dislodge cannula. Alcohol (if allowed to dry) and friction remove microbes, preventing their being introduced into the patient's circulatory system when the needleless cannula or needle is introduced.

ACTION 7. To infuse medication directly into the intermittent infusion port, first insert needle or needleless cannula of syringe with sterile saline. Aspirate for blood return. If there is blood return, gently flush IV cannula with saline and continue with next step unless patient complains of pain or burning.

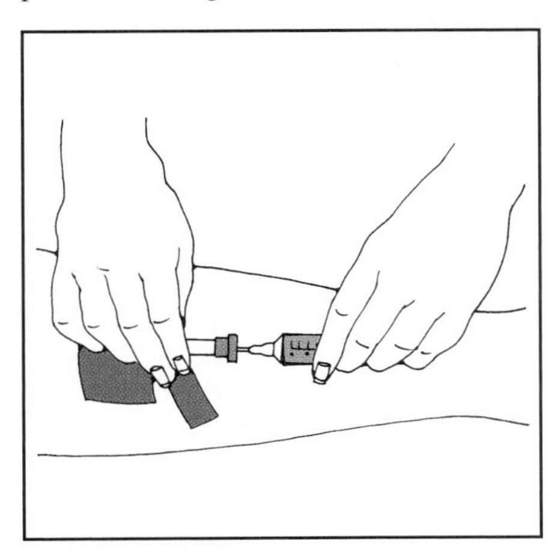

RATIONALE Aspiration is a means of assessing patency of cannula. Lack of blood return suggests cannula has been dislodged from vein or is clotted. Patient discomfort suggests vessel is inflamed. New site may be required. Do not flush forcefully to dislodge clot. You may try to aspirate clot.

ACTION 8. Cleanse port as in Action 6. Insert needle or needleless adaptor attached to IV tubing/bag containing medication. Regulate drip rate according to medical order, your drug research, or agency policy.

RATIONALE. See rationale for Action 6. Optimum infusion rate is determined by type of medication, its stability, and how irritating it is to vein.

ACTION 9. Secure needle/tubing to skin adjacent to port with tape (see Procedure 34–6). Needleless adaptor is secured with threaded guard, but tubing should be taped.

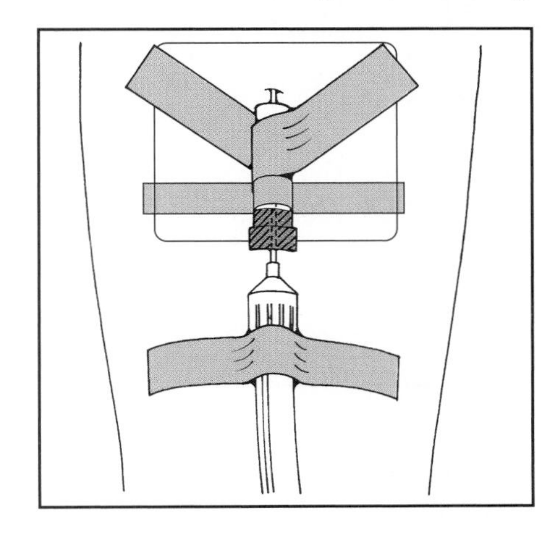

RATIONALE. Threaded guard or tape prevents accidental separation of tubing from intermittent infusion port during infusion.

Continued

ACTION 10. If a flush setup will be used, insert and secure its needle or needleless adaptor into intermittent infusion port. Partially open the roller clamp on the flush line to infuse IV solution. If solution flows readily, insert needle or needleless adaptor on secondary line into highest injection port on flush line and backfill secondary tubing (see Procedure 25–17). Close roller clamp on secondary line. Secure secondary tubing with tape if needle-lock device not available.

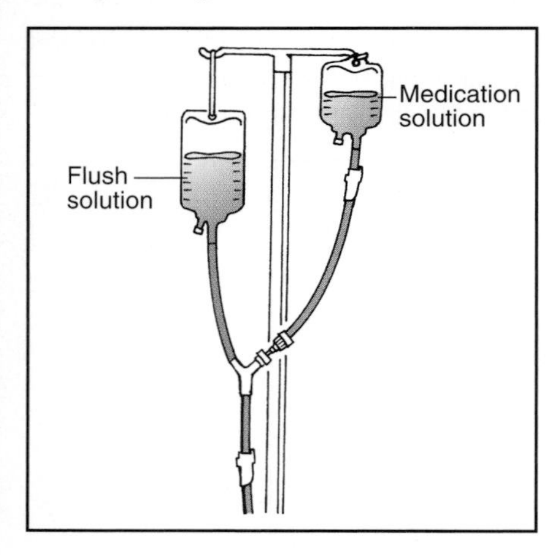

RATIONALE. If solution in "flush" setup infuses readily, intermittent infusion device is patent and drug can be infused.

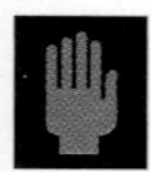

If solution does not flow, disconnect flush line. Obtain syringe with sterile saline and aspirate intermittent infusion device to remove clots. If site is infiltrated, new venipuncture is needed.

ACTION 11. After infusing several mL of "flush" solution, open roller clamp on secondary line. Regulate infusion with clamp on primary line (see Procedure 25–17).

RATIONALE. See rationale for Actions 8–10.

ACTION 12. Assess the infusion, the site, and the patient periodically during the infusion. Reregulate drip if necessary, or reposition limb to improve flow. If severe pain or swelling occurs at site, or other untoward effects occur, discontinue infusion and consult physician.

RATIONALE. These actions promote early detection and correction of problems related to infusion mechanics and/or undesirable reactions to the medication.

ACTION 13. When medication infusion is complete, allow several mL of "flush" solution to infuse. Then close roller clamp and withdraw needle/tubing. Remove and discard used needle or needleless adaptor in specially labeled container. Replace with sterile, capped 18-gauge, 1-inch needle, or needleless adaptor. The empty medication container and secondary tubing may remain connected to flush setup.

RATIONALE. Flush solution clears medication from IV cannula and leaves it filled with saline solution. Needle is discarded rather than recapped to prevent needle-stick injury to nurse. New needle maintains sterility of tubing and solution.

ACTION 14. If medication was infusing directly into intermittent infusion port, via primary tubing, remove needle/-tubing from the port and replace needle or needleless adaptor as in Action 13. Then cleanse port as in Action 6, and flush intermittent infusion port using syringe of sterile saline.

RATIONALE. See rationale for Action 13.

ACTION 15. If intermittent infusion device is not used regularly for medications, normal saline flush solution should be reinjected regularly according to agency policy.

RATIONALE. See rationale for Action 13, above.

Recording:

Record administration of IV medications and solutions according to agency policy. Usually recording will be necessary on both the MAR and the I&O record. The heparin flush solution is also considered a medication and is recorded on the MAR. Narrative recording on nurse's notes may also be expected for some medications or if unexpected reaction to medication occurs.

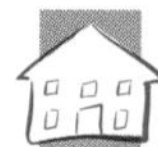

HOME HEALTH ADAPTATION: This procedure is the same regardless of the setting. Family caregivers who are conscientious and capable of safely administering IV drip medications via an intermittent infusion device can be taught the procedure. Be cognizant of their anxieties and allow them ample opportunity to practice until they demonstrate proficiency and verbalize confidence. Instruct them in signs and symptoms of an adverse reaction and the immediate action necessary. Many family caregivers will not want to accept responsibility for this level of care.

PROCEDURE 25–19. ADDING MEDICATIONS TO AN IV SOLUTION CONTAINER

PURPOSE: To deliver intravenous medication continuously over several hours.
EQUIPMENT: IV fluid container containing ordered solution, ampule or vial containing ordered medication, sterile 5- to 20-mL syringe and 19- to 20-gauge needle, alcohol swabs, medication label, and medication administration record (MAR).

ACTION 1. Follow Clinical Guideline 25–11 and technique for preparing medication from an ampule or vial (Procedures 25–11 and 25–12).

RATIONALE. These guidelines facilitate safe, error-free preparation of medication.

FOR NEW IV CONTAINER

ACTION 2. Remove protective cover from injection port:
Glass bottles: metal ring, disc (leave latex disc in place).
Plastic bottles: screw-cap.
Plastic bags: plastic pop-off or pull-off cap. Do not touch tip of port or top of bottle. If accidental contact occurs, cleanse with friction and alcohol swab. Let dry.

RATIONALE. Cover prevents transfer of microbes from environment to port and fluid by direct contact. If contact of opened port occurs, friction and antiseptic action of alcohol will remove or kill microbes. (Alcohol must dry for antiseptic effect.)

Vacuum in glass bottles causes depressions in latex disc over openings in stopper, so their location can be determined without breaking seal.

ACTION 3. Insert the needle of the syringe containing medication into medication port (pierce latex seal on glass bottle) and inject medication. Do not inject medication into air vent port on glass bottle or port for tubing insertion on plastic bag. With glass bottle, medication may be injected into triangular or larger round opening. Vacuum will draw medication into bottle.

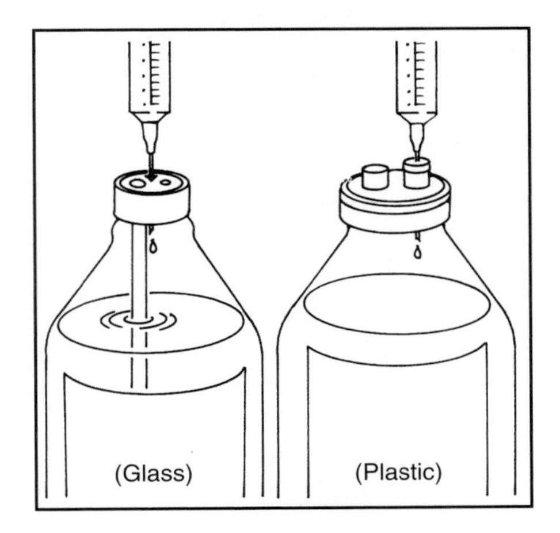

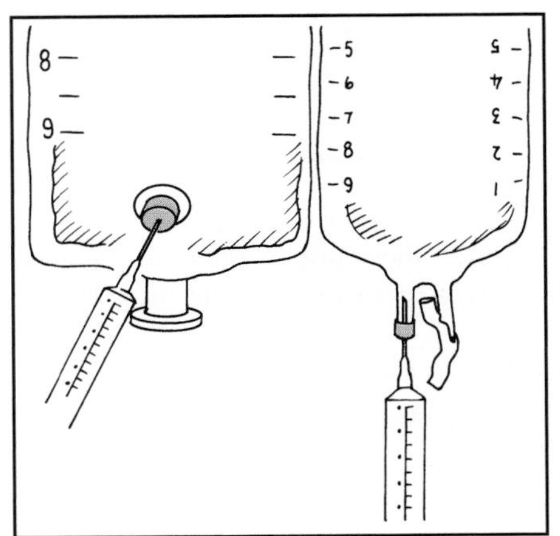

RATIONALE. Port is provided for easy addition of medications. It is self-sealing to prevent leaking. Tubing port is not self-sealing. Injection of liquid into air vent may result in spilling.

Continued

ACTION 4. Remove and discard syringe without recapping in specially marked puncture-proof container.

RATIONALE. Recapping needles creates risk for needle-stick injuries. Container prevents injury to other personnel.

ACTION 5. Gently agitate container.

RATIONALE. Movement increases rate of diffusion of medication throughout container. Complete mixing of medication in IV solution assures uniform rate of administration of drug to patient.

ACTION 6. Fill out and affix medication label to IV container. Spike container with IV tubing (see Procedure 34–3). Set is now ready for administration (see Procedure 34–6). If patient has existing IV, new tubing may be necessary (see Chap. 34).

MEDICATION ADDED

PATIENT *Mendell* RM *207-A*
DRUG *K-Cl*
AMOUNT *40 mEq*
ADDED BY *N.W. Peters, RN*
DATE *12/5/92* TIME *0900*
START TIME *0900* DATE *12/5/92* FLOW RATE *40*
EXP. DATE —

THIS LABEL MUST BE AFFIXED TO ALL INFUSION FLUIDS CONTAINING ADDITIONAL MEDICATION

RATIONALE. Label alerts other staff to presence of medication so precautions related to the specific drug can be observed.

ACTION 7. Take IV container to patient's room, identify patient (see Action 9), and infuse as ordered (see Procedure 34–16).

RATIONALE. See rationale for Action 9 and Procedure 34–16.

FOR CURRENTLY INFUSING IV

ACTION 8. Determine whether the amount of solution remaining in container is sufficient to adequately dilute drug to be added.

RATIONALE. IV drugs have immediate effect. Insufficient dilution may irritate vein as well as intensify drug effect, causing potential harm to the patient.

ACTION 9. Identify patient and discuss purpose of additive as outlined in Clinical Guideline 25–11.

RATIONALE. Promotes self-responsibility and prevents medicating the wrong patient.

ACTION 10. Slow IV to keep vein open (KVO) rate (see Chap. 34).

RATIONALE. Medication port is near tubing insertion site. At a normal infusion rate, concentrated drug may enter tubing before adequate mixing can occur.

ACTION 11. Cleanse medication port with alcohol swab, using firm rotational motion. Insert needle, and inject medication.

RATIONALE. See rationales for Actions 2 and 3.

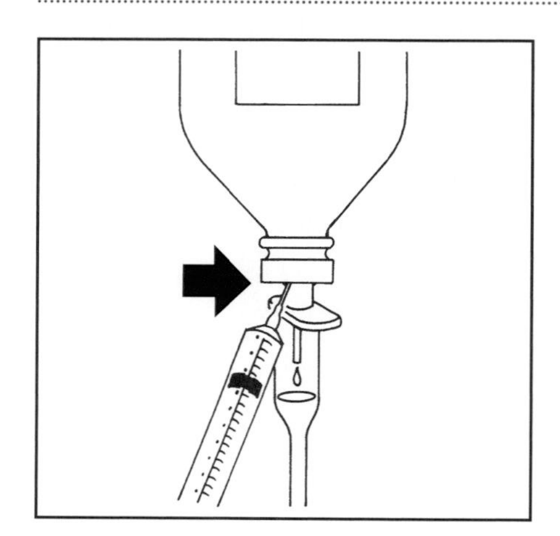

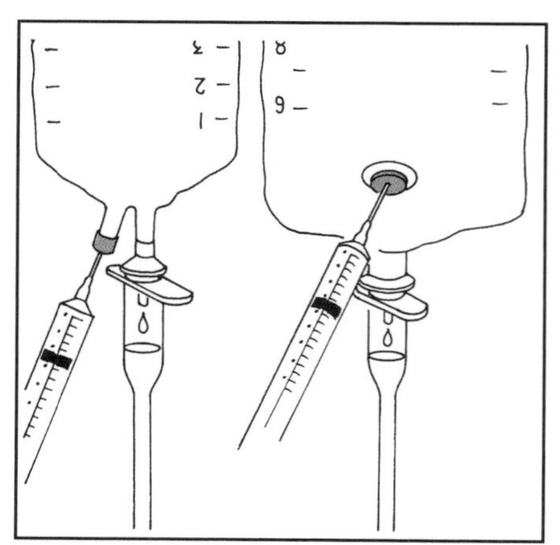

Procedure 25–19. (continued)

ACTION 12. Remove syringe, agitate container, discard syringe as above.

RATIONALE. See rationales for Actions 4 and 5.

ACTION 13. Readjust IV flowrate to ordered infusion rate. Affix completed medication label as above.

RATIONALE. See rationale for Action 6.

ACTION 14. Assess the infusion, the site, and the patient periodically during the infusion. Reregulate drip if necessary, or reposition limb to improve flow. If severe pain or swelling occurs at site, or other untoward effects occur, discontinue infusion and consult physician.

RATIONALE. These actions promote early detection and correction of problems related to infusion mechanics and/or undesirable reactions to the medication.

Recording:
Record IV solution and medication according to agency policy. Some agencies require entry on MAR and I&O/IV record; others indicate medication as IV additive on IV record without MAR recording.

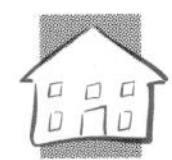

HOME HEALTH ADAPTATION: This procedure is the same regardless of the setting, but is unusual for a home setting. Family members who are conscientious and capable of safely adding medications to IV solutions can be taught this procedure. Be cognizant of their anxieties and allow them ample opportunity to practice until they demonstrate proficiency and verbalize confidence. Instruct them in signs and symptoms of an adverse reaction and the immediate action necessary. Many family caregivers will not want to accept responsibility for this level of care.

Home Health Care

With the trend toward downsizing of acute care facilities, the care given by nurses and family caregivers in home settings has become increasingly more acute.[78] Patients are discharged very soon after surgery, for example, while still needing wound care and IV medications. Many patients with infections receive care at home. Some basics of wound care and infection control do not change in a home setting, but modifications are necessary in most cases. Family members need to learn many skills to manage care for a recuperating loved one in the context of ongoing family life. Home care that is specific to particular functional dimensions is presented in other chapters in this unit. Facilitating recovery after surgery, home infection control, and managing medications are discussed below.

Facilitating Recovery After Surgery. Providing wound care is often the primary reason home care is ordered postoperatively. When a nurse provides wound care at a patient's home, sterile technique is expected to prevent wound infection. Sometimes the goal is for the patient's family to learn to care for the wound. Some experts suggest that wound care and many other procedures for which nurses use sterile technique can be taught to patients and families as clean procedures.[78] The home environment does generally not harbor the types of organisms that are common in inpatient care facilities.

Assessing the progress of wound healing and teaching patients activities to promote healing such as increasing intake of foods high in vitamins A and C, protein, and zinc; planning regular and progressive activity to stimulate circulation; and scheduling activities to allow time for extra rest and sleep are associated nursing activities (see also Chap. 27). Body image and role performance may be issues for some patients. Empathic listening and reinforcing the concepts listed in the discussion of postoperative recovery will facilitate healthy adaptation (see also Chap. 26).

Home Infection Control. Just as is true in health care settings, home infection control begins with basic handwashing and environmental cleanliness. Stress the importance of washing hands before and after caring for the ill family member. Bar soap is often a reservoir for microorganisms; therefore, liquid soap in a pump-type dispenser is recommended. Daily cleaning of the "patient's" room is also important. Caring for equipment and supplies used in home care presents a challenge for families. Clinical Guideline 25–15 summarizes important family education points for home infection control.

Managing Medications at Home. The topics that are important to address in patient and family teaching about medications were addressed previously in the section on administering medications. Maintaining consistent time schedules for taking medications is important to maintaining a constant, therapeutic concentration of medication in the bloodstream. A review of daily activities is important in planning a medication schedule. Nurses can use this review to help patients incorporate medication times into daily routines. For example, a drug ordered four times a day may have been given at 9 AM, 1 PM, 5 PM, and 9 PM in the hospital, but may be easier for the patient to remember if taken with meals (at 8 AM, 12 noon, and 5 PM) and at bedtime (11 PM). A schedule appropriate for the prescribed medication worked out with a patient is usually more acceptable.

Most medications that patients take at home are oral medications. However, some patients learn to self-administer injections such as insulin at home. Home health nurses doing follow-up care for newly diagnosed patients should observe patients' injection techniques. This is a good opportunity to review and reinforce correct technique and correct errors. Intravenous medications are also given at patients' homes. Often venous access devices (VADs) are used for home IV medication (see Chap. 34). In some situations,

CLINICAL GUIDELINE 25–15

FAMILY EDUCATION FOR HOME INFECTION CONTROL

Give the following instructions to family caregivers:

PATIENT CARE

- Always wash your hands before and after providing care to the ill family member.
- Wear disposable gloves when touching blood or other body substances if you have been told that these substances are infectious.
- Wash your hands immediately after removing disposable gloves.
- If you have been told that your family member's infection can be spread through the air, make a "Stop" sign and put it up outside her/his room to remind everyone who goes into the room to wear a mask. Use each mask only once.
- Put trash and disposables used in patient care in leak-proof bags and seal. Keep separate from family trash.
- Soiled dressings and other disposables that have contacted infectious body fluids should be disinfected with 10% bleach solution before discarding. Use double bags for extra strength, if necessary.
- If linen is contaminated, bag and launder it separately from household laundry. Use very hot water, laundry detergent, and 1 cup of bleach per load. Clean the washer by running it (empty) through a full hot water cycle with 1 cup of bleach added.

GENERAL CLEANING

- A 10% bleach solution (1 part bleach to 10 parts water) is an effective home disinfectant. Make fresh bleach solution daily.
- Wear "rubber" utility gloves for all cleaning. Wash gloves with soap and water after use, then disinfect with 10% bleach solution. Throw away gloves with cracks or tears.
- Soap and water is appropriate for cleaning items such as books, toys, furniture; a commercial disinfectant is recommended for trash containers and floors.
- The 10% bleach solution is effective for cleaning up spills of blood, urine, or feces.
- Use 10% bleach solution to clean bathrooms, bedpans, and bedside commodes.
- Usually the regular trash disposal system can be used for all trash, but it is advisable to check with the local public health department.

Adapted from Rice R. *Home Health Nursing Practice: Concepts and Application.* St. Louis: Mosby–Year Book; 1996.

nurses administer the medications, remaining in the home to observe the patient's response, but some IV medications can be managed by patients or family members. Home infusion pumps (Fig. 25–32) are a relatively recent innovation that permits self-medication of certain IV medications.

REHABILITATIVE CARE

Rehabilitative care focuses on long-term management of health problems. As stressed earlier in the chapter, wellness and well-being do not exist only in individuals free of health problems. Those recovering from acute health problems or coping with chronic disease/disability are candidates for rehabilitative care. The goal of rehabilitative care is restoring individuals to the maximum level of wellness and well-being that is possible for them. Nurses in the role of case manager (see Chap. 20) have a pivotal role in facilitating that goal. Identifying the ideal setting for care and the relevant community services for rehabilitative care is the basis for promoting lifestyle change and supporting optimum adaptation.

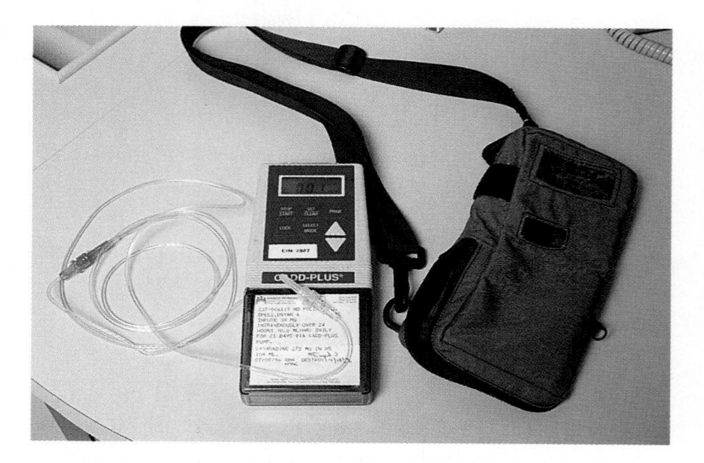

Figure 25–32. **Mini-infuser pump used with VADs makes self-management of IV therapy at home possible for many patients.**

Choosing the Optimal Setting

Many different settings, such as rehabilitation centers, adult day-care centers, patient's homes, long-term care facilities, and hospice are appropriate for rehabilitative care. *Rehabilitation centers* facilitate lifestyle changes needed because of loss of a body part, such as amputation, or loss of physical function, such as occurs with a stroke. Their aim is to assist individuals experiencing changes of this magnitude to return to their optimal level of physical and emotional functioning. Rehabilitation is an educational process that promotes self-responsibility. Patients must participate actively for the process to be effective.

Adult day care provides an alternative to inpatient care for patients who need limited amounts of assistance in daily activities. Day care centers provide services for patients able to remain at home at night. Families caring for patients at home while continuing their employment or other routine activities find adult day care centers a crucial support. It is an ideal setting for health education to promote wellness lifestyle behaviors in older adults.

Respite care is intermittent short-term assistance for a dependent family member who is routinely cared for in the home by family. It enables permanent caregivers to have a rest from the daily responsibilities of caring for a dependent family member. This is frequently a much needed support. It enables a dependent family member to remain in the home, while permitting others in the family to experience an opportunity for a vacation, professional enrichment, or other activities that would ordinarily be impossible with full-time caregiving responsibilities.

Home health care and *homemaker services* are another support for recovering independence and well-being. Home health aides and other nonprofessional workers provide homemaker services for patients who need assistance with self-care, activities of daily living, and managing household tasks.

Nurses giving rehabilitative home care assess patient and family adaptation to long-term illness and provide guidance to facilitate adaptation when needed. They teach self-care and collaborate with patients and families in planning and administering direct care. All of the home care measures discussed under preventive, supportive, and restorative care are appropriate for patients receiving rehabilitative care. Two concerns more specific to rehabilitative care are managing multiple medications, **polypharmacy,** and detecting and treating elder abuse or neglect.

Chronically ill adults, in particular elders, are likely to be taking many medications, often prescribed by several different providers. This puts them at risk for adverse reactions. If the medication regimen is poorly managed, the risk is compounded. If the household consists of an elderly couple, both taking multiple medications, the potential for problems is even greater. To assess for medication-related risks, home health nurses caring for chronically ill elders should ask to see all of the medications, including over-the-counter preparations, that are in the home.[78] Query them about the purpose and schedule for each, how long they have been taking each medication, and how they deal with a forgotten medication. This approach will reveal how they store medications and whether outdated medications are part of the "supply" and will suggest potential adverse drug interactions. Clinical Guideline 25–16 highlights strategies to help patients prevent problems related to polypharmacy.

Elder abuse and neglect is challenging to identify. Often, elders do not report incidents that constitute abuse or neglect, as it is difficult for them to admit.[78] Abusers include spouses, other family members, and caregivers not related to the victim. Nurses providing home care must be alert to potential indicators of abuse or neglect, but must keep in mind that even conscientious caregivers may find meeting impaired elders' care needs a significant challenge. Abuse may be physical or behavioral. Abrasions, bruises, burns, fractures, and drug toxicity may indicate physical abuse. They should be objectively and thoroughly documented in nursing care records and follow-up assessments conducted.[79] Behavioral abuse is more subtle and therefore more difficult to detect. Signs of abuse include passivity, indifference withdrawal and a fearful or guarded manner.[79] Neglected patients may appear dirty and poorly groomed and may develop pressure ulcers, weight loss, and dehydration. A nurse's initial response to any of these symptoms should be to provide nursing care to correct the presenting problem and teaching and support services for the caregiver to prevent its recurrence. If symptoms persist or recur, notifying the adult protective services branch of the local public health department is warranted.

Living in a *long-term care facility* may be necessary for some adults with declining health and increasing dependence. These facilities provide extended care, including personal and psychosocial services. Several levels of service are available, including independent living, intermediate care, and personal care for patients who are no longer able to care for themselves without skilled assistance. Whatever the level of care, these institutions become "home." Patients and family need support and information as they consider institutional care.

Nurses can assist patients and families to choose a long-term care facility by helping them define their options, and then supporting a choice of facilities that matches patients' psychosocial and physical needs. As noted in the earlier discussion on the nursing diagnosis relocation stress syndrome, a life change as significant as moving to a care facility is stressful for patients and families. Institutional care brings changes in interpersonal relationships. An important intervention during this transition is fostering patients' and families' personal support systems. Counsel patients and family regarding the normalcy of the feelings of anger and guilt that accompany the transition to long-term care. These emotions underlie many family interactions, but frequently are not directly expressed. Facilitate communication through active listening and paraphrasing family statements. This helps family members clarify their thoughts and feelings, enabling resolution of conflicts.

Promote quality of life for patients living in extended care facilities by helping them to find ways to maintain their preferred lifestyle. Personal freedom is important. Also, personal possessions such as pictures, photographs, and other items of special significance create homelike surroundings.

Hospice care is a resource for terminally ill individuals. Its focus is meeting the physical, psychosocial, and spiritual needs of dying patients and their families. The goal of hospice care is

CLINICAL GUIDELINE 25–16

STRATEGIES TO PREVENT PROBLEMS RELATED TO POLYPHARMACY

Share the following ideas with elders taking many medications:

1. If medication labels are difficult to read, place the prescription bottle in a large envelope. Write the name of the medication and the time it is due on the outside of the envelope in large black letters.
2. Keep a magnifying glass in the medication storage area.
3. Color-code the tops of medication bottles using a different color for different medications. Post a "key" to the code in your medication storage area.
4. Use a separate labeled plastic storage container for bottles of medications due in the morning, noon, evening, and bedtime. If a medication is taken several times a day, place the bottle in the container for the next time it is due immediately after taking it.
5. Use a "cross off the pill chart" with a square for each time a medication is due. Mark the square with an "X" when you take each medication.
6. Use a plastic organizer marked with days of the week or time of day for each medication.
7. Use a talking medication dispenser (purchased).
8. Check the labels of all of your medications for expiration date every 3 months. Throw outdated medications into the toilet and flush.
9. Make a list of all of your medications (or ask your nurse or pharmacist to help). Take it with you to all of your doctor appointments. Show it to each doctor and ask her or him to add names of newly prescribed drugs.

CRITICAL QUERY

Signs and symptoms of elder abuse are subtle and its victims often do not report it.[79] You are a home health nurse. You observe signs and symptoms suggestive of abuse in a patient in your care. How would you approach discussing your concerns with the patient? The family?

improving or maintaining the quality of life prior to death. Communication, comfort, and pain relief are common needs of terminally ill patients. Coming to terms with dying is a major life task. Achieving resolution and acceptance is truly rehabilitative. It permits living the remainder of one's time to the fullest.

Facilitating Lifestyle Changes

Successful rehabilitation usually demands lifestyle change. Patients confronted with this reality feel confused, overwhelmed, and, often, angry. Change is challenging, no matter what the potential rewards or the consequences of failure. When the consequences of failure to adapt seem extreme, the challenge is magnified. Nurses who desire to effectively facilitate lifestyle change must recognize its impact. Convey your awareness and acceptance of the feelings of anger and powerlessness in all of your discussions with patients about altering their habits.

The self-management process presented in the section on preventive care is equally applicable to rehabilitative care. When assisting patients to use self-management, emphasize that attempting to bring about too much change at one time is an invitation to frustration. Setting short-term goals and building in rewards for progress contributes to feelings of achievement. The positive feelings encourage continued efforts to attain the long-term behavior change.

Promoting Adaptation to Chronic Disease or Disability

Patients with chronic disease or disability comprise the major group needing rehabilitative wellness and well-being care. Chronic disease or disability is a threat to self-esteem. There are permanent changes in body appearance or functioning and interference with role performance that alter feelings of competence, ability to carry out satisfying work, opportunities for enjoyment, and meaning in life. Feelings of inferiority interfere with social interactions and commitment to self-care. Maintaining self-worth in the face of these changes requires examining one's life patterns and clarifying values. Self-efficacy and coping styles are important variables in determining the degree of personal threat, the nature of the response, and need for assistance. Successful adaptation requires determination, a strong social support network, and effective use of other resources.

Nurses can promote healthy adaptation by working with patients to evaluate resources and options. Start by helping patients reexamine personal strengths based on abilities that remain, rather than limitations. This is a good basis for setting achievable rehabilitation goals. Most patients require ongoing medical therapy and monitoring. Control over the treatment regimen facilitates adaptation. Patients who feel intimidated by the demands of a treatment program or dependent on others to provide it have more difficulty. Nurses play a pivotal role in empowering patients to learn to manage their treatment program independently.

Encourage exploring alternatives for work and recreation if patients cannot return to their previous activities. Facilitate contact with others who have similar problems. Reinforce renewing contact with church, friends, or hobbies. Stress that well-being involves a balance between meaningful endeavors and play. Point out achievements and progress toward goals.

Referral to Support Groups and Community Resources

Support groups and community resources are an important component of a comprehensive rehabilitative care plan. Support or "self-help" groups are organized to bring together people with similar chronic health problems. Examples include the American Cancer Society's Reach for Recovery program for recent mastectomy patients, Weight Watchers, the United Ostomy Association, and Alcoholics Anonymous. There are local chapters of major groups in many communities. Groups influence how their members think, feel, and act. They are sources of peer support and personal experience. Participation in support groups enhances self-esteem and encourages commitment to goal attainment. They are a valuable resource for assisting patients to adapt to change. Many groups also include significant others in their programs or meetings.

The availability of other community resources such as visiting nurses, Meals-on-Wheels, or organized transportation assistance is often a critical factor in determining whether a patient can independently function in the community setting during rehabilitation. Nurse case managers are instrumental in locating community resources and obtaining their services for patients that need them. Payment for these resources is often an issue. Ongoing changes in the health insurance industry and in Medicare and Medicaid make funding a challenge.

EVALUATION

Evaluation is the final step in the nursing process. Evaluation of nursing implementation to promote wellness and well-being is based on the outcomes on critical pathways or on desired outcomes and evaluation criteria that nurse and patient developed for each wellness-related nursing diagnosis in the patient care plan. Refer to the samples in Tables 25–4 through 25–7.

Evaluation of patient well-being is an ongoing process that is part of all levels of care: preventive, supportive, restorative, and rehabilitative. Nurses monitor progress toward outcomes as they provide care. On the specified target dates, nurse and patient collaboratively evaluate patient status. If the patient does not exhibit the conditions specified in the evaluation criteria, the outcomes have not been achieved. Nursing implementation is continued, or new strategies considered to meet the outcomes. Sometimes a nurse and patient may decide that the desired outcome was unrealistic. They may agree to choose a new goal and plan new approaches to attain it. If the behavior or status specified in the evaluation criteria has been achieved, the desired outcomes are considered to be met. The related nursing care can be terminated or continued to maintain the current level of wellness. If a still higher level of wellness is possible, patient and nurse can formulate new outcomes and evaluation criteria to reflect the improvement they desire.

SUMMARY

Wellness and well-being are broad, interrelated concepts. Wellness encompasses dimensions that relate to all aspects of individuals' lives, including eating well, being fit, feeling good, caring for self and others, self-responsibility, and fitting in with the environment. Wellness and well-being are manifested through individuals' optimism, self-confidence, energy, sense of purpose, inner peace, and overall satisfaction with their lives.

Many variables influence wellness. Values, lifestyle, culture and socioeconomic status, self-concept, self-efficacy, locus of control, age, and personality traits such as hardiness and resilience affect behavior and choices, and in turn, wellness. Wellness is altered by life experiences such as life change, crisis, and disease. Health care experiences also alter wellness. Becoming a patient and, in particular, being hospitalized can threaten wellness and well-being in a profound way. People manifest altered wellness in many different ways. Fear, anxiety, pain, stress, fatigue, depression, loneliness, powerlessness, confusion, and dissatisfaction with life circumstances are examples.

Because wellness and well-being encompass all aspects of the individual—physical, psychosocial, and spiritual—nurses consider all aspects of a patient's lifestyle when they assess and manage wellness. Nursing diagnoses related to altered wellness and well-being are based on a wide variety of patient problems, including those that are cognitive, physical, emotional, social, and environmental. An effective collaborative relationship requires mutual participation between patients and nurses during the entire process of wellness assessment and management. Threats to well-being and wellness cannot be corrected without the patient's active participation, which is facilitated in a collaborative nurse–patient relationship.

Nursing implementation to promote patient wellness and well-being involves all four levels of patient care. Wellness and well-being care includes screening, counseling, teaching, and/or direct physical care. Patient education is important in promoting a wellness lifestyle, in facilitating self-responsibility, and in empowering patients for health care experiences. Wellness and well-being care also includes infection control and prevention measures, protecting patient safety, perioperative care, and administering medications.

Wellness and well-being are highly individualized. Nurses support wellness and well-being in all their patients, even those experiencing significant alterations in health, by demonstrating respect and caring and promoting patient involvement and self-responsibility through collaboration.

LEARNING OUTCOMES

Upon completing this chapter, the student should be able to

1. Discuss the relationship between an individual's health and lifestyle practices.
2. Describe the basic elements of a wellness lifestyle.
3. Describe the objective and subjective manifestations of wellness and altered wellness.
4. Identify factors that enhance or alter wellness.
5. Identify wellness tasks for major developmental stages.
6. Describe the impact of disease.
7. Discuss health care experiences that can influence an individual's level of wellness.
8. Outline the elements of the health history that are pertinent to assessing wellness and well-being.
9. Discuss the implications of selected objective manifestations for assessing wellness and well-being.
10. List the nursing diagnoses that are most commonly associated with altered wellness and well-being.
11. Describe preventive care measures to promote wellness and well-being.
12. Discuss the nurse's role in assisting patients with stress and describe several stress management techniques.
13. Discuss the relevance of self-management techniques for making lifestyle changes.
14. Describe measures to prevent and control infections in health care facilities and when providing home care.
15. Discuss ways nurses can promote patient self-responsibility.
16. Describe supportive, restorative, and rehabilitative care measures to assist patients.
17. List caregivers' responsibilities when admitting a patient to a health care facility.
18. Discuss the nurse's role in maintaining a safe environment and preventing accidents.
19. Discuss basic principles of surgical asepsis and their application in patient care.
20. Outline the key aspects of patient care prior to, during, and after surgery.
21. Outline the principles of safe medication administration.
22. Describe three systems of measurement in current use for prescribing drugs.
23. Describe the procedures for giving medication by the oral, topical, inhalation, subcutaneous, intramuscular, intravenous, rectal, and vaginal routes.
24. Describe the procedure for eye and ear instillations.
25. Discuss the nurse's role in assisting patients and families to manage multiple medications.
26. Identify indicators of elder abuse and appropriate nursing implementation.

REVIEW OF KEY TERMS

absorption
advance directives
ampule
anaphylaxis
antagonism
biotransformation
body surface area (BSA)
chemical name
distribution
drug
drug allergy
drug interactions
drug tolerance
enteric coating
equivalents
excretion
fitness
gauge
generic name
hardiness
idiosyncratic responses
informed consent
intradermal
intramuscular
intravenous
loading doses
locus of control
maintenance doses
medication
medication administration record (MAR)
medication history
metabolism
nosocomial infection
one-time order
parenteral
patient-controlled analgesia (PCA)
peak concentration
polypharmacy
potentiation
prn order
relaxation response
resilience
route
routine order
self-efficacy
side effects
standard nomogram
Standard Precautions
stat order
sterile technique
subcutaneous
summation
surgical asepsis
synergism
therapeutic effect
therapeutic level
toxic effects
trade (proprietary) name
Transmission Based Precautions
trough concentration
unit dose system
vial

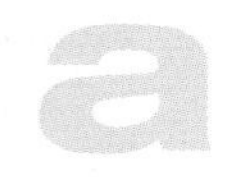

Having Read the Chapter, consider again the opening scenario, page 615, and the following responses to the questions concerning Barbara McMaster's level of wellness and well-being.

Because Barbara's wound has not altered her daily functioning, she has maintained a sense of wellness. Her statement that she does not know "what to think" about the wound not healing indicates that it is threatening her sense of wellness. She might change to an illness orientation if involvement in her social activities were altered. A complete wellness and well-being assessment will provide her nurse with an understanding of how Barbara's current health problem may have occurred and how it can be resolved.

As Barbara had not seen a health care professional in some time, her nurse can use the current threat to wellness as an opportunity to enhance Barbara's overall health and wellness. Her nurse will assess Barbara's level of wellness by reviewing her current health-promoting practices including eating habits, physical fitness, stress level, what she does to care for herself and others at the retirement community, and how she feels about her current living arrangements. A social support system is important in health promotion. Friends from her social activities at the retirement community are an important resource to be considered in her plan of care.

Barbara has demonstrated self-responsibility by seeking the advice of a health care professional regarding the wound that is not healing. Her nurse should assess her sense of self-responsibility further by inquiring about such practices as smoking and drug or alcohol use. Her sense of self-responsibility will be enhanced as the nurse promotes Barbara's sense of wellness by collaborating on a plan of care to promote healing of her wound. Barbara's health care practices reflect a possible internal locus of control with strong self-efficacy. Her nurse will want to validate these assessments as she interacts with Barbara because the findings will have impact on her implementing the plan of care.

Given Barbara's age, her nurse will want to focus her health promotion on teaching regarding a well-balanced diet, safety measures, and exercise. Proper nutrition and exercise will promote wound healing as well as overall wellness and well-being. Her nurse can support Barbara's involvement in social activities and could also encourage social activities that include increased physical activity, such as an exercise group to promote physical fitness.

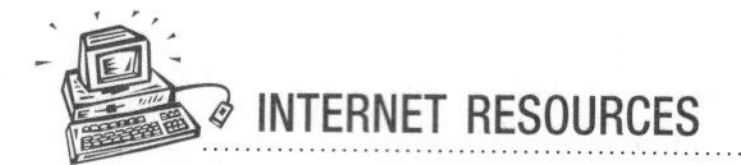

INTERNET RESOURCES

Web Sites and URLs

Drug formulary (enter brand name, obtain generic name):
http://www.intmed.mcw.edu/drug.html

PPS On-line (tm) System—pharmacy resources:
http://www. pps.ca/pps.htm

RxList (searchable drug index):
http://www.rxlist.com

PharminfoNet (online formulary):
http://pharminfo.com

Laboratory values (online book):
http://www.ghso.nwu.edu./ Norm.html

Centers for Disease Control (*Emerging Infectious Diseases* online):
http://www.cdc.gov

Put Prevention into Practice (PPIP)—Office of Disease Prevention and Health Promotion, US Public Health Service:
http://www.os.dhhs.gov:81/PPIP

Jacobs Institute of Women's Health:
http://members.aol/jacobsinst/welcome.html

REFERENCES

1. (National Center for Health Statistics NCHS). *Health in the United States, 1995.* Hyattsville, MD: US Dept of Health & Human Services, Public Health Service, CDC; 1996.
2. Pender NJ. *Health Promotion in Nursing Practice.* Norwalk, CT: Appleton & Lange; 1996.
3. Hafen BQ, Hoeger WK. *Wellness: Guidelines for a Healthy Lifestyle.* Englewood, CO: Morton Publishing Co; 1994.
4. Terborg JR et al. Behavior change at the worksite: does social support make a difference? *Am J Health Promot.* 1995;10: 125–131.
5. Sisney KF. The relationship between social support and depression in recovering chemically dependent nurses. *Image.* 1996;25:107–112
6. Cookman CA. Older people and attachment to things, pets, places, and ideas. *Image.* 1996;28:227–232.
7. Clark CC. *Enhancing Wellness: A Guide for Self-care.* New York: Springer; 1981.
8. Wardlaw GM, Insel PM. *Perspectives in Nutrition.* St. Louis: Mosby; 1996.
9. Floyd PA, Mimms SE, Yelding-Howard C. *Personal Health: A Multicultural Approach.* Englewood, CO: Morton Publishing Co; 1995.
10. Carson VB, Arnold N. *Mental Health Nursing: The Nurse–Patient Journey.* Philadelphia: Saunders; 1996.
11. Kolkmeier LG. Relaxation: opening the door to change. In: Dossey BM, Keegen L, Guzzetta CE, Kolkmeier LG. *Holistic Nursing: A Handbook for Practice.* Norwalk, CT: Appleton & Lange; 1993.
12. Pender NJ, Barkausas VH, Hayman L, Rice VH, Anderson ET. Health promotion and disease prevention: toward excellence

in nursing practice and education. *Nurs Outlook.* 1992;40: 106–112.
13. Schwinam PM et al. Health behavior, life orientation, and health decline among older adults. *J Ment Health Aging.* 1995;10:111–125.
14. Schwart RM. Health locus of control and health promotion behaviors for southern West Virginians and eastern Kentuckians. *KY Nurse.* 1994;42:23.
15. Jenkins RA. Health locus of control, chemotherapy related distress and response to behavioral interventions in cancer patients. *Psychol Health.* 1995;10:463–475.
16. Levinson H. Activism and powerful others: distinction within the concept of internal–external control. *J Personality Assess.* 1974;38:381–382.
17. Wallston B, Wallston K, Kaplan G, Maides S. Development and validation of the health locus of control (HCL) scale. *J Consult Clin Psychol.* 1976;44:580–585.
18. Jenkins LS. Self-efficacy theory: overview and measurement of key components. *Cardiovasc Nurs.* 1988;24:36.
19. Bandura A. Human agency in cognitive theory. *Am Psychol.* 1989;44:1175–1184.
20. Kobasa S, Maddi S, Courtington S. Personality and constitution as mediators in the stress–illness relationship. *J Health Soc Behav.* 1981;22:368–378.
21. Laferriere RH, Hamel-Bissel BP. Successful aging of oldest old women in the Northeast Kingdom of Vermont. *Image.* 1994; 26:319–323.
22. Brooks E, Wilkenson JM, Popkess-Vaughter S. Promoting situational support for nurses in practice. *Image.* 1994;26: 305–308.
23. Tartasky DS. Hardiness: Conceptual and methodological issues. *Image.* 1993;25:225–229.
24. Spector RE. *Cultural Diversity in Health and Illness.* Stamford, CT: Appleton & Lange; 1996.
25. Stanhope M, Lancaster J. *Community Health Nursing: Process and Practice of Promoting Health.* St. Louis: Mosby; 1995.
26. Friedman MM. *Family Nursing: Theory and Practice.* Stamford, CT: Appleton & Lange; 1997.
27. Szafran K. Family health protective behaviors. In: Bomar PJ, ed. *Nursing and Family Health Promotion: Concepts, Assessment and Interventions.* Philadelphia: Saunders; 1992.
28. Harvard University School of Public Health. As reported by *Morning Edition,* National Public Radio, Nov 19, 1996.
29. Eschleman MM. *Introductory Nutrition and Diet Therapy.* Philadelphia: Lippincott; 1996.
30. NCHS (National Center for Health Statistics). *National Health and Nutrition Examination Survey: 1991–1994.* Hyattsville, MD: US Dept of Health & Human Services, Public Health Service, CDC; 1996.
31. Mortality patterns—United States, 1993. *MMWR.* 1996; 45:161–163.
32. Young A, Dinan S. Fitness for older people. *Br Med J.* 1994; 309;331–333.
33. COC Director stresses changing ideas about physical activity. *In Touch.* Jacobs Institute of Women's Health; 1996;4:1, 4.
34. Health objectives for the nation: adults taking action to control their blood pressure—United States, 1990. *MMWR.* 1994; 43:509–510, 517.
35. Friedman M, Rosenmann RH. *Type A Behavior and Your Heart.* New York: Knopf; 1974.
36. State specific prevalence of cigarette smoking—United States, 1995. *MMWR.* 1996;45:962–966.
37. McGinnis JM, Foege WH. Actual causes of death in the United States. *JAMA.* 1993;270:2207–2212.
38. US Department of Health, Education and Welfare/Public Health Service. *Health People 2000: Midcourse Review and 1995 Revisions.* DHEW (PHS) 71-50212. Washington, DC; 1995.
39. Projected smoking-related deaths among youth—United States. *MMWR.* 1996;45:971–974.
40. Update: mortality attributable to HIV infection among persons aged 25 to 44 years—United States, 1994. *MMWR.* 1996; 45:121–125.
41. US Bureau of the Census. *Statistical Abstract of the United States: 1995.* 115th ed. Washington, DC: US Bureau of the Census; 1995.
42. US Dept of Justice, Bureau of Statistics. *Selected findings, domestic violence: violence between intimates.* 2–3. Washington, DC: US Dept of Justice; Nov 1994.
43. EDK Associates. *Men Beating Women: Ending Domestic Violence—A Qualitative and Quantitative Study of Public Attitudes on Violence Against Women.* New York: EDK Associates; 1993.
44. Bachman R. *Violence against women: A National Crime Victimization Survey Report.* Washington, DC: Bureau of Justice Statistics, 1994 Jan. Report No.:NCJ-145325.
45. Pogebrin LC. Pistols for the women of America. *The Nation.* 1989; 666.
46. Sugarmann J, Rand K. *Cease-fire: A Comprehensive Strategy to Reduce Firearms Violence.* Washington, DC: Violence Policy Center; 1994:19.
47. Bonderman J. Armed by fear: self defense, handguns, and women's health. *Women's Health Issues.* 1995;5:3–7.
48. Kellerman AL, Rivara FP, Rushforth NB, et al. Gun ownership as a risk factor for homicide in the home. *N Engl J Med.* 1993;329:1084–1091.
49. US Bureau of the Census. *Statistical Abstracts of the United States: 1992.* 112th ed. Washington, DC; 1992.
50. Betz CL, Hunsberger M, Wright S. *Family Centered Nursing Care of Children.* Philadelphia: Saunders; 1994.
51. Famularo R, Kinscherff R, Fenton T. Parental substance abuse and the nature of child maltreatment. *Child Abuse Neglect.* 1992;16:475–483.
52. Costa AJ. Elder abuse. *Primary Care.* 1993;20:375–389.
53. Commentary. Firearm violence and public health. *JAMA.* 1994; 271:1281–1283.
54. Contraceptive method and condom use among women at risk for HIV infection and other sexually transmitted diseases—selected US sites, 1993–1994. *MMWR.* 1996;45:820–823.
55. Holmes TH, Rahe RE. Short-term intrusion in the life style routine. *J Psychosomat Res.* 1976;14:121–123.
56. McCaffery M, Beebe A. *Pain: Clinical Manual for Nursing Practice.* St. Louis: Mosby; 1989.
57. Martone WJ, Jarvis WR, Culver DH, Haley RW. Incidence and nature of endemic and epidemic nosocomial infections. In: Bennet JV, Brachman PS. *Hospital Infections.* Boston: Little, Brown; 1992.
58. Barry PD. *Psychosocial Nursing Assessment and Intervention: Care of the Physically Ill Person.* Philadelphia: Lippincott; 1996.
59. Beare PG, Myers JL. *Principles and Practice of Adult Health Nursing.* St. Louis: Mosby; 1996.
60. Kemper DW, Healthwise Staff, Physicians and Staff of Kaiser Permanente. *Kaiser Permanente Healthwise Handbook: A Self-care*

Guide for You and Your Family. Boise, ID: Healthwise Publications; 1995.
61. Newbold SK. Making the World Wide Web work for you. *Nursing.* 1996;26:24f–24h.
62. Larson EL. Association for Professionals in Infection Control and Epidemiology Guidelines Committee. APIC guidelines for handwashing and hand antiseptics in health care setting. *Am J Infect Control.* 1995;23:251–269.
63. Jacobson AE. Fancy fingernails may promote infection. *Am J Nurs.* 1997;97:24.
64. Garner JS. The Hospital Infection Control Practices Advisory Committee. Guidelines for isolation precautions in hospitals. *Infect Control Hosp Epidemiol.* 1996;17:53–80.
65. Kelly K, Sussman G, Fink J. Stop the sensitization. *J Allergy Clin Immunol.* 1996;98:857–858.
66. Korniewicz DM, Garzon LS. How to choose and use gloves. *Nursing.* 1994;24:18.
67. Tomazic V. Cornstarch powder on latex products is an allergen carrier. *J Allergy Clin Immunol.* 1994;93:751–758.
68. Dossey BM, Keegan L, Guzzetta CE, Kolkmeier LG. *Holistic Nursing: A Handbook of Practice.* Rockville, MD: Aspen; 1995.
69. Benson H, Klipper M. *The Relaxation Response.* New York: Random House Value; 1992.
70. Williams RL, Long JD. *Towards a Self-management Life Style.* 3rd ed. Boston: Houghton Mifflin; 1983.
71. Canavan K. New technologies propel nursing profession forward. *Am Nurse.* 1996;28:1–3.
72. Galindo-Ciocon DJ, Ciocon JO, Galinda DJ. Gait training and falls in the elderly. *J Gerontol Nurs.* 1995;21:10–17.
73. Wagner EH et al. Preventing disability and falls in older adults: a population-based ramdomized trial. *Am J Public Health.* 1994;84:1800–1806.
74. Brungardt GS. Patient restraints: new guidelines for a less restrictive approach. *Geriatrics.* 1994;49:43–50.
75. Cahill CK, Rosenberg J. Guideline for prevention and control of antibiotic-resistant microorganisms in California long term care facilities. *J Gerontol Nurs.* 1996;22:40–46.
76. Jackson MM. "Isolation" in the nursing home setting. *J Gerontol Nurs.* 1996;22:8–9.
77. Preston GA. HICPAC guideline for isolation precautions in hospitals: community hospital perspective. *Am J Infect Control.* 1996;24:207–208.
78. Rice R. *Home Health Nursing Practice: Concepts and Application.* St. Louis: Mosby–Year Book; 1996.
79. Lynch SH. Elder abuse: what to look for, how to intervene. *Am J Nurs.* 1997;97:27–32.

26

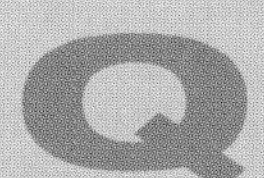

Monica Brown, a 35-year-old high school teacher, wife, and mother, has entered the hospital for surgery to remove an ovarian tumor, which she fears is malignant. Similar cancers caused the deaths of her mother and an aunt. Monica has a 6-year-old daughter, who is being temporarily cared for by her grandmother, Monica's mother-in-law. Monica's husband, an attorney, is struggling to manage at home and support Monica during her treatment and convalescence. Monica, who has taken a leave of absence from her job, has confided in Judy Simon, a staff nurse, that she feels a heaviness in her chest and becomes fatigued easily. Judy notices that Monica does not get up or attempt to make conversation with her husband when he visits.

What are some of the concerns that Monica might have related to her illness and her life situation?

What are the considerations Judy Simon should make in caring for Monica?

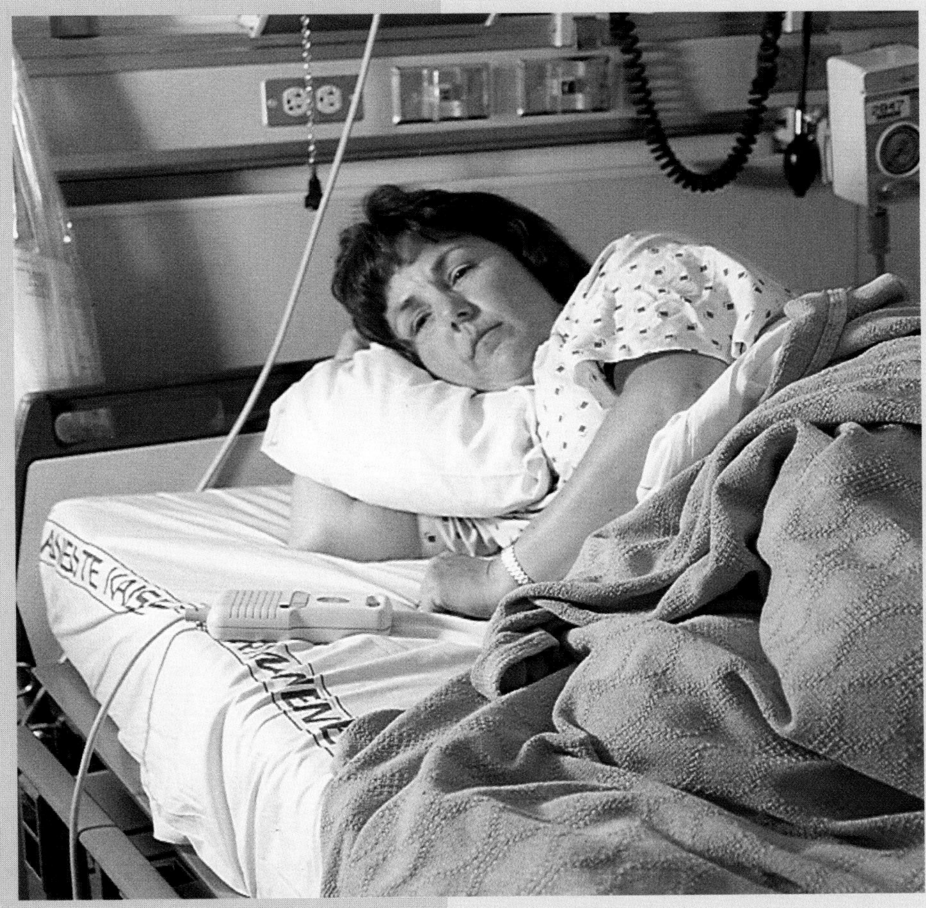

Self-expression

CHAPTER OUTLINE

The expressive character of human behavior is among those features that distinguish humans from other beings. Indeed, humans are unique in their capacity to transcend physical and biologic limits and even the social order of their existence and express themselves in creative, personally satisfying ways.[1]

People express themselves in almost every aspect of living. Virtually any sphere of activity—physical, intellectual, cultural, or social—provides outlets for self-expression. For most people, however, the opportunities for self-expression are discovered in a social context, where they are in some relationship to other human beings.[1] Such opportunities occur in vocational and leisure activities, as well as within individuals' family and spiritual lives.[2,3] People express themselves through their roles as working person, parent, spouse, lover, friend, group member, churchgoer, artist, athlete, citizen, enthusiast, and opinion holder. All of these roles enable individuals to structure an identity and live it out in the world.

Opportunities for self-expression also present themselves in the important transitions of life, such as adolescence and marriage. By participating in the rituals and traditions that surround developmental events, people express the meaning they find in life changes. Even birth and death are occasions for self-expression.[1] As Banerjee points out, the cries of a newborn and the last gasps of a dying man are highly expressive, representing that most basic motive—the desire to live. Symbolically, they too provide evidence of the human urge for self-expression.

Self-expression embodies personal values and aspirations that give meaning to life. Indeed, acts of self-expression affirm and convey the meaning that people attach to their lives.[1,4] Illness, on the other hand, may change an individual's capacity for self-expression, temporarily or permanently. When a catastrophic illness strikes, the person may be forced to seek new meanings in life.

Collaboration between nurse and patient entails a give-and-take characterized by an exchange of personal feeling within the context of a helping relationship.[5–14] Indeed, collaboration involves mutual self-expression between patient and nurse. Empathy, warmth, genuineness, immediacy, and self-disclosure, described in Chap. 15, are aspects of the interaction that are forms of self-expression found in successful therapeutic interactions.[15]

In collaborating with the patient, the nurse facilitates the patient's self-expression and fosters healing.[16] Facilitating self-expression has restorative value for the patient and may be a primary aspect of the patient's care in certain situations. This chapter builds on the concepts presented in Chaps. 11 through 15, relating them to a practical understanding of how nurses support and facilitate patient self-expression.

SECTION 1

UNDERSTANDING SELF-EXPRESSION

OPTIMUM SELF-EXPRESSION

DEFINITION OF SELF-EXPRESSION

For much of the 20th century, researchers in psychology and the social sciences have focused on investigating the expressive nature of human behavior. The result is a substantial body of research on human self-expression. Studies have been undertaken on the universality of self-expression,[17,18] the cultural rules for self-expression,[19,20] the role self-expression plays in determining experience,[21–26] individual differences in expression,[27] and the use of expressive behavior in a social context.[28–31] Nevertheless, the concept of self-expression has for the most part eluded definition.

A Dictionary Definition

The term *expression,* as defined by *Webster's New Collegiate Dictionary,* refers to an action, a gesture, or an utterance by which individuals make their opinions or feelings known to others. *Webster's* emphasizes that expressions give a true or vivid, accurate impression of a person's emotions, moods, or sentiments as aroused by objects or events in the environment, but also refers to expression as related to a person's artistic and creative abilities and impulses.

A Scholarly Concept

Although dictionary definitions are helpful, scholarly ideas add depth and precision. Zajonc[24] notes that expression is an "efferent process." The term *efferent* means to carry or conduct outward. In the strict neurologic sense, it refers to the motor contraction of any tissue or organ in response to impulses from the central nervous system. Thus, certain types of involuntary behavior, such as sweating or blushing, can be classified as expressive.[32–34] However, the term also refers to facial or postural displays, gestures, vocalizations, laughter, crying, or other behavior that corresponds to a person's immediate feelings.[35–37]

Expression implies an internal state composed of thoughts and feelings that forces itself to the surface.[24] Traditionally, experts have viewed this internal state as the "cause" of expression; however, a growing number of experts now agree that expression also plays a role in creating or changing a person's experience.[23–26] Nevertheless, expression as the externalization of thoughts and feelings remains the prevailing view.

This concept of expression is important to nurses because it highlights the assumption on which much of nursing assessment is based—that nurses gain important clues about patients' immediate experience from their involuntary and communicative behavior.

The concept of self-expression, however, involves more than an individual's passing thoughts or momentary moods. Indeed, self-expression presupposes a self.

Chapter 11 describes the self as a dynamic, unified integration of consciousness and identity that is connected to the environment in a self-consistent way. The private self (the subjective self) is the self that is not necessarily apparent to others, comprised of the ideas, attitudes, and feelings a person holds subjectively about who she or he *really* is. The public (external or objective) self is apparent to others in one's manner, behavior, appearance, and surroundings.

> **COLLABORATIVE STRATEGY**
> **MUTUAL SELF-EXPRESSION IN CAREGIVING**
>
> Self-expression by the patient helps the nurse to understand the patient's needs. Sharing of self by the nurse helps communicate empathy and caring. To facilitate the patient's sharing, the nurse can invite the patient to relate his or her "story."

As conceived in this text, the self incorporates private attitudes and public identities and roles that people value and live out in every day life. Integration of the private and public selves into a consistent whole connected in meaningful ways to the world is of central importance to the individual. That unity, as this chapter suggests, is achieved through **self-expression,** the act of sharing one's inner world with others. In other words, self-expression is the process by which the private self becomes public and available for others to know.

ASPECTS OF SELF-EXPRESSION

Aspects of the private self that an individual might elect to share with others include a person's wishes, values and ideals, modes of feeling, thought, and action. Conflicts, fears, and anxieties and ways of resolving and controlling them may also be shared. Other aspects of the private self that people often choose to express are family, ethnic, religious, social class, political, peer group, and sexual identifications.[2,38]

The aspects of self shared with others vary in the importance that individuals attach to them and in the modes by which they are conveyed. In everyday communication, persons' attention is frequently on their own passing feelings, moods, thoughts, and desires that are elicited in social interchanges.[31] Important social identities are conveyed through appearance, dress, and manner.[28] The deepest personal values are revealed in a person's commitments and pattern of life.[2] Intimate feelings are usually expressed through touch and closeness. Such expressions are reserved for the closest relationships.[31]

Expressive behavior may be divided into two fundamental categories, "expressions given," which refers to the traditional use of words and gestures in communication, and "expressions given off."[28] Expressions given off are the messages about self that are conveyed through one's setting (place, situation) and its characteristics (decor, size, physical layout) and through one's appearance as represented in dress and personal adornment, especially the insignia of role, office, or rank.[28] For example, the practice many hospital health providers have of wearing a stethoscope draped around the neck might be looked upon as a symbol of role or status identity.

Longer term aspects of expression deal with the life patterns that endure over time. Levinson and colleagues,[2] for example, argued that life-structure, as the basic design of a person's life, is expressive in the sense that its various components represent an individual's personal choices for life and living. Thus, vocation, avocation, relationships, and social and institutional identifications are an important part of self-expression. Moreover, life structure is expressive in that it provides a framework for establishing social relationships and for building and enacting the self-concept.

Banerjee, an authority on human expression, lists many different types of expressive activities that link individuals with society. Among others, he mentions an effort to improve human relations through acts of personal diplomacy or a study of history to gain a better understanding of others. Banerjee also points to the activities that people undertake to control or satisfy basic needs—technological or medical discovery—as well as the creation of new ideas in, for example, art, music, dance, literature, and poetry.[1]

The Importance of Choice

Choice making lies at the heart of self-expression. Choices reflect personal preference. Preferences, in turn, are an integral aspect of one's inner life and result from the interaction between the environment and the internal state of the individual.[39] Because preferences are so strongly associated with emotion, people may not always be conscious of the inner needs or urges on which their choices are based.

Because choice making is central to expression, freedom of choice is a necessary condition for self-expression. Indeed, without freedom of choice, an individual's actions cannot be considered expressive.[1] According to Banerjee, any behavior that is heavily influenced, manipulated, or forced by others reflects little about that individual's self. Thus, the music played by a child forced to practice would not be classified as expressive, but the child's reluctance to practice, as an exercise of free choice, might. Nevertheless, choice making is almost always constrained to some degree by society, usually on an ethical, legal, or economic basis. An individual's choices are thus as much determined by the resources, opportunities, and limitations of the environment as by personal preference.[2] As a consequence, some aspects of self may never be expressed.

The Importance of Self-reflection

Self-reflection, the process by which people accumulate self-knowledge and develop an awareness of themselves as a unique and separate identity, becomes increasingly evident as individuals mature to adulthood. During self-reflection, people ponder cues from the environment and consider what those cues mean about their own personal qualities. People reflect, for example, on how they behave in particular situations, how others react to them, or what experiences give them pleasure or pain. Such thoughts help people come to know their own attitudes and preferences, and thus confer on them a sense of individual identity. As they mature, self-reflection helps people form judgments about whether or not they are achieving their self-ideals. Self-reflection is particularly evident as people undergo important life transitions (eg, graduation, marriage, divorce, or serious illness). It is also the process by which people become aware of the changes in personal attitudes and preferences that accompany an identity-altering experience.

Styles of Expression

Self-expression occurs on a continuum. At one end is behavior that ties people to others and the world. At the other is behavior that reflects withdrawal from the social world.[1] Both are self-expressive. Indeed, self-expression, although frequently social is not always a social process. Although social withdrawal is sometimes an unhealthy sign, it is also an aspect of yoga and other forms of meditation, and it is a way some people cope with stress. For some individuals, the most self-expressive times are those spent alone.

Functions of Self-expression

Self-expression has several functions, which, as the previous discussion makes clear, are:

- self-identification
- social relationship construction and maintenance
- need satisfaction
- stress reduction and coping

Certainly a major function of self-expression is to communicate "who I am" in the world. Schlenker[40] argues that **self-identification,** the consolidation of identity psychologically and socially, is accomplished through self-reflection and self-disclosure. Because the self evolves and develops over time and with experience, self-identification is a lifelong process. Identity is thus always a "becoming" in the sense that an individual's potentialities are developed and actualized during the entire course of life.[2,41,42] The image of self conveyed at any particular time represents how individuals perceive themselves and how they desire others to perceive them.[40]

Other functions of self-expression are the establishment of interpersonal relationships, and need satisfaction. Relationships, particularly intimate ones, offer a sense of closeness and relief from the isolation inherent in our individual separateness. The sharing of self that occurs with self-expression is thus essential to bridging the gulf between individuals. Further, because social relationships constitute an important part of an individual's experience, self-expression can be viewed as essential to meeting the basic human needs for love, belonging, and esteem.[42]

Another function of self-expression is coping, behavior by which individuals attempt to change their situation for the better. Frank[14] documented the powerful effect of self-expression as a means of coping with the dire circumstances imposed by extreme threat. *Hardiness,* a characteristic that makes a person resistant to stress, reflects an individual's capacity to interpret stressful situations as challenges rather than threats (see Chaps. 8 and 25).

SELF-EXPRESSION AS A CLINICAL CONCEPT

The concept of self-expression is fundamental to the clinical practice of nursing. Indeed, many nursing authorities believe that health is achieved or restored in the context of a caring relationship.[43–45] Caring is an aspect of expression in which there is a social give and take between nurse and patient, which Marck[9] labels "therapeutic reciprocity." Clinical examples include inviting the patient's participation in decisions about care, sharing control of the professional relationship with the patient, mutual self-disclosure and exchanges of humor, and respect for the other's personal space. Through a genuine exchange of feelings, thoughts, and experiences relevant to the patient's care, reciprocity reduces the emotional distance between nurse and patient.[9]

The words nurses use, their facial expressions, the tasks they perform, and how they perform them reflect the nurse's caring. How willing patients are to share may depend to an important extent on the meanings conveyed by the nurse's appearance and behavior. Behavior that contradicts the nurse's words can negate the communication of caring. For example, the patient's trust is at risk when a nurse asks, "How can I help you?" and then fails to promptly answer the patient's call light.

DIMENSIONS OF SELF-EXPRESSION

Self-expression, based on the process of self-reflection, has two behavioral dimensions: self-presentation and self-disclosure (Fig. 26–1).

Self-presentation

Self-presentation, one important dimension of self-expression, refers to the attempts that individuals make to control the images they convey to others through their appearance and behavior.[46] "Control" implies that people try to give a particular type of impression.[46]

Behavior associated with self-presentation falls into four basic categories: verbal, nonverbal, appearance, and situational context. Almost any verbal statement can be construed as an act of self-presentation. Even a simple, "Hello, how are you?" suggests that the speaker has knowledge of standards of politeness. Verbal behavior as self-presentation often takes the form of a self-report—statements individuals make about themselves. Individuals often make statements to convey virtues such as honesty or competence. Their statements may or may not be judged as accurate by others, but are important for what they reveal about how the individual wants to be perceived.[47]

Nonverbal self-presentation includes behaviors such as smiles frowns, yawns, eye contact, brow knitting, head nodding, stooping, or slumping.[47] People who want social approval, for example,

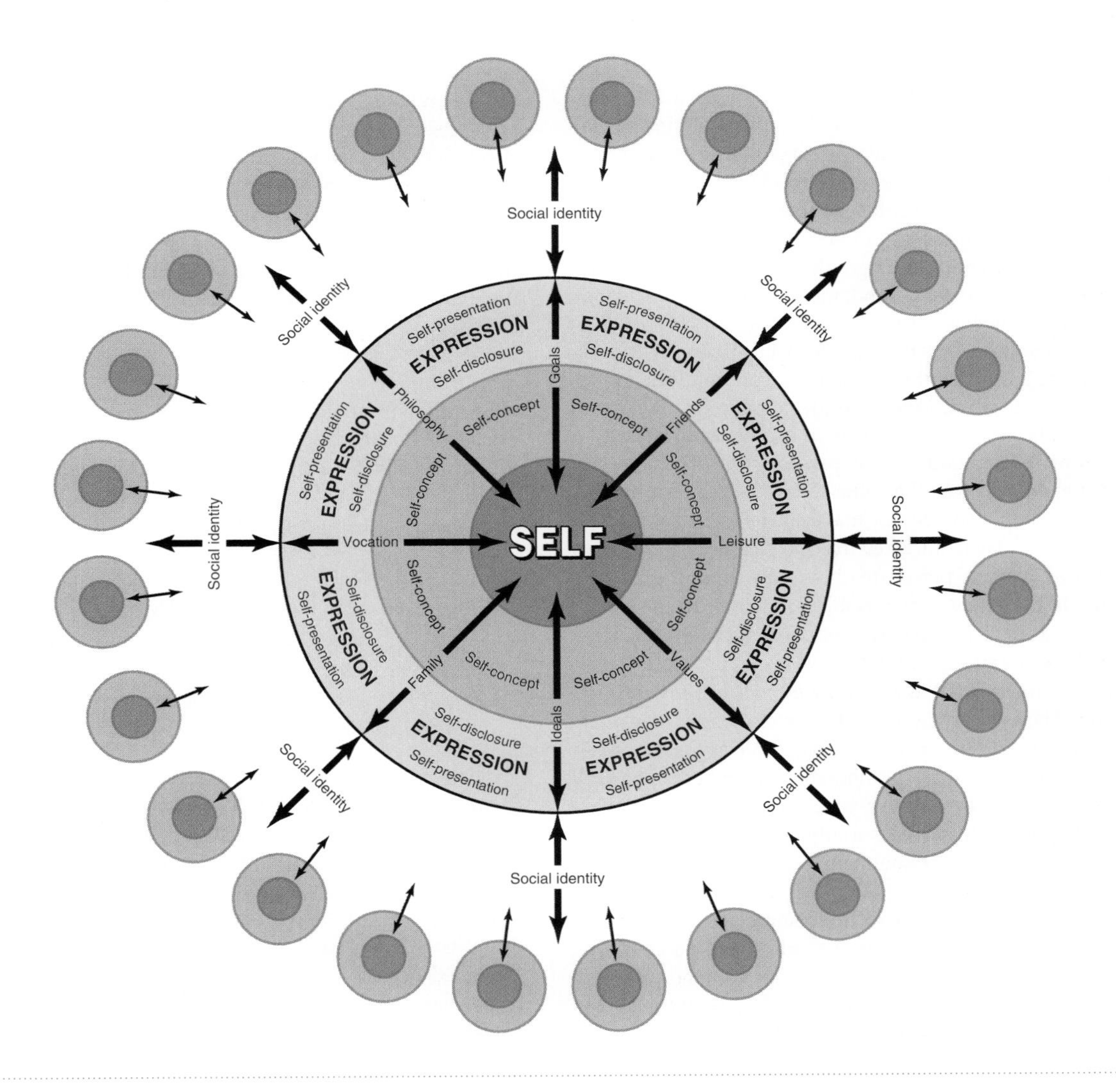

Figure 26–1. Self-expression has two behavioral components—self-presentation and self-disclosure—which are the means by which individuals communicate their self-concept to others and reinforce their self-concept. The spokes (life structures) that extend from the self out into the environment represent the social framework for building and enacting the self-concept. Individuals relate with others by presenting and disclosing themselves. The arrows depict the mutual influence between the self and social environment.

may nod their head frequently to affirm the opinions and ideas of others. Nonverbal behaviors convey a personal style. They create impressions—warmth, intensity, sincerity, modesty, shyness, or aggressiveness. A simple "hello," when accompanied by a smile, eye contact, and a friendly handshake, communicates warmth, and gives an impression about the kind of person the individual is striving to be.

Physical appearance also gives impressions, as do situational contexts such as one's neighborhood or the places a person goes. They convey messages about the type of person an individual is or wishes to be. Similarly, activities—particular long-term pursuits that reflect an enduring commitment—create an impression on others. A display of athletic skill attained through years of training, for example, reveals qualities about the athlete, such as self-discipline.

There are many motives for self-presentation, such as to construct a social role, maintain self-esteem, consolidate power and social influence, and gain social approval and avoid disapproval.[48] Most authorities agree, however, that the common underlying motive is the universal desire for social approval.[49] Social approval is a prime source of self-esteem. Successful self-presentation elicits social approval from others.[50] When others confirm the impressions a person is trying to make, self-esteem is enhanced—the real self becomes closer to the ideal self.[51] People also engage in self-presentation to define themselves in social interaction. Because people convey their identity through their manner, dress, and behavior, self-presentation is a fundamental process for fixing identity in social situations.

Control is important because people want others to regard them in a way that is consistent with their self-concept. When self-presentations are successful, others assign positive qualities and behave in ways that reinforce the positive aspects of an individual's self-concept.[48] The success of a person's self-presentations varies depending on how well the values projected match with the group's values.[40] People sometimes make mistakes in conveying their social identity.[48] Their mistakes may be harmless and easily corrected, such as when a person inadvertently fails to greet an acquaintance. Or they may carry social consequences and elicit negative labels that depict a negative social identity. Serious mistakes, such as those exemplified by types of social deviance (public drunkenness, violence), are associated with varying amounts of social rejection. These carry the risk of a severe loss of personal reputation, and may lead to social ostracism.[52] When their reputation is damaged severely, some individuals construct an entirely new identity. Most, however, strive to avoid self-presentational predicaments, preferring to project socially acceptable identities.[46] Over time, patterns of self-presentation become automatic and unconscious.

Self-presentation is important to understand because all people have identities to affirm and protect—nurses and patients are no exceptions. Human relationships are enhanced when people understand the significance of another's self-presentations. As Chap. 13 establishes, patients who take on the sick role assume a new identity, at least for a period. Such transitions are stressful, and nurses who are able to ease them contribute to the patient's health. Successful nurses get to know their patients as individuals by conversing with patients about their lives, by assisting patients with their personal identity rituals (makeup, grooming, hair arrangement), by listening to patients' self-reports, and by protecting patients' privacy when appropriate. Such actions ease identity transitions between wellness and illness and illness and wellness.

Failure to support a patient's presentation of self, on the other hand, may unnecessarily complicate the patient's transition to the sick role. Nurses generally accept responsibility for developing a positive relationship but may vary the character of their responses with the impressions they gain from the way patients present themselves. It is well documented, for example, that nurses too often differentiate between patients who are "good" and patients who are "bad."[53–56] Good patients, as described in the literature, are cheerful, control their feelings, and appreciate what nurses do for them. Bad patients, on the other hand, are those nurses view as highly anxious, depressed, hostile, challenging, overly dependent or independent, aggressive, impatient, unappreciative, or nonconforming, or whose care necessitates greater energy and effort on the part of the nursing staff.

Although some "bad" patients may be manifesting long-established personality traits, others are simply reacting to the identity transition that frequently accompanies the sick role.[55]

COLLABORATIVE STRATEGY

SELF-PRESENTATION, SELF-IDEAL, LOSS, AND ILLNESS

Self-presentation is the process by which individuals attempt to control the impressions they make on others. It communicates individuals' understanding of how they are and how they would like to be. Illness, however, often interferes with an individual's capacity to fulfill a self-ideal. Effective nurse–patient collaboration provides opportunities for the patient to address issues related to changes in one's self-ideal.

INSIGHTS FROM NURSING LITERATURE

LABELING PATIENTS AS DEVIANT

Carveth JA. Perceived patient deviance and avoidance by nurses. Nurs Res. *1995;44:173–178.*

The researcher studied the effect of labeling patients as related to the amount and quality of care given to patients by nurses. Carveth's focus was the well-documented tendency of nurses to avoid patients labeled as deviant. She chose a convenience sample of 52 staff nurses educated in all types of nursing programs and had them classify patients as "ideal," "difficult," or "neutral" using a controlled card-sorting procedure and then employed a standardized scale to rate the nurses' performances as they gave care to the patients classified. The author found, consistent with the findings of previous research, that the characteristics assigned to patients classified as difficult were negative, but that nurses interacted more rather than less frequently with patients so classified. She further found that such patients received care rated less supportive than that given patients classified as nondeviant.

? CRITICAL QUERY

Carveth[56], in a study of patient deviance, found that nurses interacted more frequently and spent more time during each contact with patients labeled "difficult." She interpreted this as a possible indication the nurses were attempting to change the deviant behavior. If correct, what implications would Carveth's finding have for patients' opportunities for self-expression in a clinical setting?

However, their behavior may cause the nurse to feel ineffective and to react defensively.[54] Too often, nurses label patients "difficult" or "demanding" when they impede the nurse's work with complaints or a failure to cooperate. Such labels signal the nurse's disapproval and perception that the patient's behavior is deviant. Unfortunately, labels serve to fix the identity of the patient in the nurse's eyes. This can have a negative effect on caregiving.[57,58] As Jankin points out, once nurses label patients, they no longer see the total person or process patient data effectively.[59] There is evidence, moreover, that nurses who express personal frustration and anger may avoid or ignore those patients labeled as difficult.[56,59–61]

Self-disclosure

As defined by Jourard, **self-disclosure** is the process of telling another person about oneself and of sharing one's inner thoughts and feelings with another person.[62] Self-disclosures are distinguished from acts of self-presentation in that they are uncontrived, spontaneous, and, thus, more truly expressive of an individual's self-understanding. The goal of image control typical of self-presentation is absent or generally less important in self-disclosure. What truly distinguishes self-disclosure from self-presentation, however, is the level of self-understanding conveyed. Self-disclosures involve more than simple self-reports; they are the communication of one's most closely guarded self-understandings.

Because self-disclosure involves highly personal information, it is often a feature of close, even intimate, relationships.[31] Indeed, the intimacy of a relationship can be defined in terms of the amount of self-disclosure that takes place.[31]

Acts of self-disclosure require decisions about what, how much, when, and where a person reveals his or her private thoughts. As a feature of a relationship in which people feel free to express themselves, self-disclosure can be viewed as a correlate of interpersonal trust.[63]

There are two types of self-disclosure: cognitive and affective.[64] *Cognitive self-disclosure* involves the communication of personal thoughts and beliefs about oneself. It is often conveyed by verbal statements that begin with the words "I think that I . . ." or "I believe that I . . . ." This type of self-disclosure characterizes the early phases of a relationship and helps people develop mutual understanding. The information conveyed generally includes peoples' ideas about their own appearance, behavior, or personality. As the relationship develops, the range of information increases, and the focus often shifts to affective self-disclosure.

During *affective self-disclosure,* people share their feelings. They focus on how they feel about themselves, each other, and the relationship. Partners generally negotiate a relationship in which both are comfortable with the intensity of the emotion exchanged. Even in close relationships, norms, such as those pertaining to sex-role behavior, regulate how, when, and to what extent a person expresses feeling. Some people, for example, have difficulty expressing personal fears or weaknesses, or negative attitudes toward others. Others, anticipating tension or conflict, try to match the intimacy of their own disclosures to those made by other people in an effort to maintain a balanced social exchange.[65]

Self-disclosure, like self-presentation, has many motives; for example, to establish, maintain, and enhance relationships; achieve closeness; or reduce anxiety.[66] Individuals present their thoughts to others and thereby clarify and obtain social validation for what they believe. In addition, individuals identify their similarities and their shared beliefs and expectations, which contributes to a process of mutual accommodation and negotiation of complementary roles. This interdependence provides individuals with the help they need to cope with the challenges of living. Among the benefits of self-disclosure is reduced anxiety. Trust and a sense of confidence in each other's integrity, truthfulness, and commitment frequently follow.

Self-disclosure, like self-presentation, is not without risks. Revealing personal information of a deep, sometimes secret nature makes an individual vulnerable to hurt. A hallmark of self-disclosure is that it places an individual in a vulnerable position, which may explain the pressure for reciprocation that partners frequently experience as relationships develop. Risks stemming from self-disclosure include rejection, embarrassment, and exploitation by others. Individuals may counter the fear of being rejected or exploited by refraining from disclosure. The alternative, however, is social isolation and loneliness.[67]

Nurse–patient interaction, although professional in nature, shares many of the features of other types of close relationships. In health assessment, for example, nurses ask patients to disclose a significant amount of extremely personal information. Patients are responsive because implicit in the interaction is a mutual understanding that it is unethical for the nurse to violate the patient's trust.

Patients, however, often bring their anxiety and fears into the interview situation. As they respond to questions, they may observe the nurse for subtle indicators of the nurse's personal attitudes and worry that the nurse will reject them for their answers. Further, effective caregiving involves counseling the patient about health-related problems. Nurses, educated to understand the psychological impact of illness, can use this special opportunity to get to know the patient to build a therapeutic relationship.

Nurses are uniquely well prepared to aid patients with the distress that commonly accompanies illness. **Distress** is the state of mental anguish that patients often experience during the course of an illness. Distress may be relieved by disclosing intense feelings to others, a process sometimes referred to as **distress disclosure** but more commonly as **catharsis.**[68] There is evidence, for example, that relieving distress benefits a person's physical and mental health. Thus, nurses, understanding that the first impressions they make may enhance or hinder the development of trust are justifiably concerned with the way they present themselves in the health interview. Chapters 15 and 17 discuss interview approaches for enhancing the impressions nurses make as caring professionals.

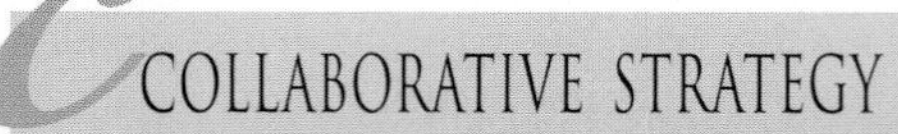

COLLABORATIVE STRATEGY
SELF-DISCLOSURE, DISTRESS, AND LOSS

Distress is the emotional experience of stress; it often accompanies the experience of loss. Illness may initiate changes in self-concept, role performance, sexual behavior, or future plans, changes often experienced as loss. Opportunities for distress disclosure in the context of a caring relationship may help the patient cope with loss.

FACTORS AFFECTING SELF-EXPRESSION

AGE

Age is an important determinant of an individual's pattern of self-expression. (Chapter 11 presents various theories of development and age-related identity changes.) An individual's self-expression develops over time, beginning with the neonate's reflex behaviors and vocalizations to secure food and warmth. Patterns of self-expression are tied to the phases of life and development, with age and self-expression patterns generally corresponding to one another. Development is never complete, however, and even in adulthood, people make significant changes in their lives with the objective of finding satisfying, personally fulfilling self-expression patterns.

PERSONALITY

Personality encompasses the whole of an individual's behavioral and emotional tendencies (see Chap. 11). Personality influences how a person thinks, feels, and acts in any given situation. One of the most important aspects of the personality is the self-concept, the images of the self formed and stabilized over years of personality development. The images most central to an individual form the core self-concept. Self-concept is a fundamental determinant of self-expression.

Most individuals perceive a gap between their self-concept (how they see themselves) and self-ideal (how they would like to be). A wide gap may be accompanied by low self-esteem, whereas a narrow gap may correspond to high self-esteem. Usually people hold self-ideals that are realizable and seek to balance the ideal with the possible.[69] Balance is revealed by an individual's self-confident pursuit of personal goals. An imbalance may be revealed in expressions suggesting emotional insecurity or negative self-concept. Such persons may tend to think or talk about their shortcomings or even withdraw from social interaction. When self-concepts are impossible to realize, as sometimes happens when people become seriously ill, a negative change in self-concept may occur.

Patients whose self-concepts are threatened by illness can learn new patterns with the help of others. Mastery over the most difficult circumstances can be achieved when others engage in teaching strategies to empower the individual to achieve the necessary changes.[70]

INSIGHTS FROM NURSING LITERATURE
CATHARSIS

Kettles AM. Catharsis: an investigation of its meaning and nature. J Adv Nurs. *1994;20:368–376.*

The author emphasizes that catharsis, defined as the process by which a person becomes purged of an overload of distress, is a means of helping patients. Using questionnaires, she studied 142 nursing instructors and students. Her results showed her subjects understood catharsis as a process related to emotion. Half (50 percent) defined it as a "release of emotion," while 27 percent defined it as an "expression of emotion." Although they recognized catharsis as having psychotherapeutic value, the author's subjects also believed that emotional expression was more acceptable for women than men, and did not endorse catharsis as a central therapeutic goal. The author recommends more research to identify the contexts in which catharsis has positive outcomes and therapeutic value.

NEUROSENSORY VARIABLES

Self-expression is also a product of the neurosensory mechanisms for communication. Although factors outside the individual influence self-expression, expression is modified by neurosensory information processing (Chap. 32).

The two hemispheres of the brain, for example, play distinctly different roles in self-expression. Researchers have established the relative superiority of the left cerebral hemisphere for speech and language-related activities.[71] For most right-handed people and the majority of left-handed people, disease or injury of the left hemisphere will result in language disorders. Such individuals may be unable to comprehend oral communications, or speak and write clearly. Right-hemisphere disorders disturb the affective aspect of speech, altering both the comprehension of emotion in others' speech and the expression of emotion in one's own.[71]

Major sense organs play an especially important role in self-expression. Sensory input from vision and hearing is extremely important to communication. The loss of eyesight or hearing raises significant barriers to communication and an individual's capacity for social interaction or other expressive activities that rely on vision or hearing.

SOCIOCULTURAL AND ECONOMIC VARIABLES

In pluralistic, culturally diverse societies such as the United States and Canada, social groups often vary considerably in character. Their rules for regulating social situations may coincide with the rules of the dominant, or majority, culture or with the society's minority cultures—ethnic, religious, or class. Individuals learn the rules of the groups they are a part of, and those rules influence their choices for self-expression.

The groups with which an individual identifies are **reference groups.** Reference groups influence individuals' patterns for speech and dress, their habits and rituals, their goals and attitudes, their personal philosophies, and their choices for work, family, and leisure. Reference groups also provide the standards for the social comparisons that people make when interacting with others. Those standards are the yardsticks people use to evaluate themselves in relation to others.[72]

People tend to look at themselves as better or worse off than others and to adjust their self-appraisals accordingly.[73] Patients also rely on social comparisons when evaluating the advantages and disadvantages of their personal situation. When seeing others with similar health problems in a hospital or clinic situation, patients may feel threatened or fortunate, depending on how well off they see themselves in relation to others they encounter.[74]

PERSONAL VALUES AND PHILOSOPHY

Personal values and philosophy influence self-expression. Personal values derive from an individual's personal beliefs, as modified by social and moral learning. These beliefs often reflect a spiritual identification with a particular religion or ethical code. People may identify with a particular spiritual framework and yet retain a unique perspective that allows them to adhere selectively to its teachings. One can never assume that individuals' affiliations wholly determine their behavior.

HEALTH AND ILLNESS

General health is another important factor. Nutrition and fitness, psychological well-being, and social satisfaction are all important for a vibrant pattern of self-expression. Illness often acts to alter self-expression by its effect on physical, psychological, and social processes. When severe, illness can have a profound effect on the way people communicate as well as on the content of their communication and their opportunities for social interaction.

STRESS

Health, stress, and illness (Chaps. 7 and 8) affect self-expression. Stress disturbs the body's physiologic and psychological regulatory mechanisms. When unchecked, stress can overtax a person's homeostatic capacity and contribute to the development of illness.

To the extent that it interferes seriously with health, stress may lead to distress and altered self-expression. Stressful events commonly generate in an individual a sense of "bottled-up" pressure derived from such emotions as anger, fear, remorse, and despair.[75] That pressure, as indicated above, may be relieved by telling others about one's feelings.

Indeed, people who are distressed often have a need to disclose their discomfort to others. Powerful emotion motivates catharsis—the process for purging or getting rid of emotion. Once catharsis is achieved, the need to disclose is inhibited.[75] Some authorities view the need for catharsis as analogous to a fever, which is both a sign of disturbance and part of the restorative process.

Distress disclosure has decided benefits and often facilitates self-reflection. **Insight,** the mental ability to see into a situation and perceive its meanings, may often result from self-reflection and lead to psychological growth. Further, people may be less likely feel depressed when they confide their feelings to others and, as a result, may have fewer stress-related physical symptoms.[76] Indeed, authorities have suggested that catharsis improves the survival of people who have certain types of serious illness. Derogatis and associates, for example, found that patients with metastatic breast cancer (breast cancer spread to other organs) who expressed their anger and depression survived longer than those who kept their troubles to themselves.[77]

Distress is generally disclosed in such statements as "I've been very lonely lately," or "I'm afraid that I may have cancer." Although the benefits of disclosure are considerable, people who talk openly about their distress risk social rejection. Chronically ill persons, for example, frequently have a persistent need to talk about their feelings, but may find that people close to them tire of hearing about their suffering and problems. Nurses therefore have an important role in providing such patients with opportunities for catharsis.

MEDICATION AND SUBSTANCE USE

Medications and drugs also influence self-expression. Some drugs alter mental functions, acting to change a person's mood (narcotics, alcohol, antidepressants), allay anxiety (antianxiety agents, tranquilizers), stimulate or depress the mind (amphetamines, barbiturates), or alter thought processes (antipsychotic agents, hallucinogens). Such agents, while they may improve an individual's overall social functioning, may also create psychological dependence and physical addiction that results in mental, physical, and social deterioration.

Other drugs may influence self-expression, not by modifying mental processes, but by changing an individual's bodily sensations. Drugs that relieve pain (analgesics), stomach acidity (antacids), vomiting (antiemetics), coughing (antitussives), constipation (laxatives) or that reduce fever (antipyretics) or edema (diuretics) indirectly improve a person's mental outlook by relieving discomfort so that the person is able to refocus on the external world. Still other drugs support self-expression by correcting the causes of distressing symptoms. Drugs that cure infection (antibiotics), improve cardiac function (cardiac glycosides, antiarrhythmics), aid metabolism (insulin), reduce inflammation (corticosteroids), or destroy tumors (antineoplastic agents) may act to improve overall health, and thereby enhance an individual's outlook and opportunities for self-expression.

SEX AND SEXUALITY

Sex (or gender) refers to an individual's anatomic differentiation as male or female. **Sexuality,** on the other hand, is a characteristic of personality reflected in the totality of a person's feelings, attitudes, beliefs, and behavior related to being male or female. Sexuality refers broadly to the human desire for love, warmth, sharing, and physical intimacy that is present throughout the life span (Fig. 26–2). **Gender identity,** a person's psychological identification with a particular sex as reflected in his or her masculine or feminine behavior traits, is also an important aspect of sexuality.

Psychological and social identity are heavily influenced by biologic heritage. The capacity to engage in sexual acts is a vital factor in the consolidation of male and female identity and is an extremely important aspect of self-expression. Indeed, the ability

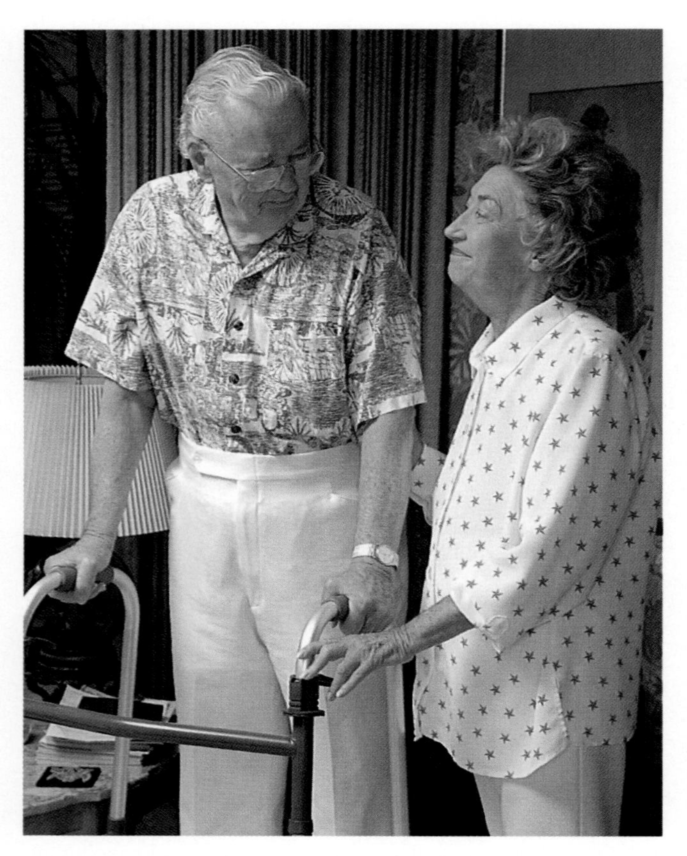

Figure 26–2. Sexuality, including the need for love and sharing, is present throughout the life span.

to have an intimate relationship with a sexual partner is central to the self-esteem of most individuals. Conversely, *sexual incapacity*, the inability to engage in sexual acts, is often accompanied by a loss of self-esteem and confidence in one's masculine or feminine appeal. Such feelings often carry over to relationships where sexual activity may not be involved, but where sexuality is a factor in interpersonal attraction. Self-esteem lost to sexual incapacity, for example, may interfere with an individual's general confidence, reducing a person's influence over others, and leading, in severe cases, to social isolation and loneliness.

Public awareness of sex and sexuality has increased in recent years, and more opportunities for sex education are available.

COLLABORATIVE STRATEGY

SEXUALITY

Sexuality constitutes a central aspect of self-concept. Many illnesses alter the ability to engage in sexual activity or experience sexual feelings. The experience of altered sexuality can be extremely distressing. Individuals who have such experiences may desperately need to examine the nature of their problem. Nurses who are comfortable talking about sex and sexuality make a significant contribution to the patient's well-being.

Nevertheless, myths about sex persist. Some are listed below. All are untrue.

- Elderly people do not want or need sexual intimacy.
- A large penis is of great importance to a woman's sexual gratification.
- Menopause or hysterectomy terminates a woman's sex life.
- Contraception reduces sexual pleasure.
- Condoms eliminate the risk of sexually transmitted disease.
- Sexual intercourse should be avoided during pregnancy.
- Women cannot get pregnant while they are lactating.
- Alcohol is a sexual stimulant.
- Masturbation causes mental illness.
- A couple must have simultaneous orgasms to achieve sexual satisfaction or for conception to occur.
- There is an absolutely "safe" period in a woman's sexual cycle in which coitus cannot cause impregnation.
- Male impotency is incurable.
- AIDS is spread by kissing.
- Contraception eliminates the risk of pregnancy.
- AIDS is a disease of homosexuals only.
- Sex is not important when you are sick.

To more fully understand sex and sexuality, the reader is referred to any of the numerous textbooks on these subjects, which provide a detailed discussion of biosexual development, the consolidation of gender identity, sexual orientation, and modes of sexual expression, all of which are important to the student of nursing but beyond the scope of this discussion. Tables 26–1 and 26–2 summarize the physical aspects of the sexual response.

CHARACTERISTICS OF HEALTHY SELF-EXPRESSION

Healthy self-expression generally reflects a healthy self. Over the years experts have identified numerous characteristics of the healthy personality. Primary among them are that healthy people

- show self-awareness
- have self-esteem
- are self-actualizing
- respect others
- have a personal philosophy and ethical code
- are autonomous
- display resilience

Healthy individuals are able to accurately depict their own abilities and limitations and have realistic self-expectations. They can be open about their desires, intentions, and strong feelings. They are neither self-conscious nor uncomfortable with themselves. They do not mistake how they would like to be with how they are.[78]

Healthy people have self-esteem. They present themselves in keeping with their self-understanding and communicate believable identities to others. They are unburdened by feelings of unreality, self-diffusion, and depersonalization characteristic of people undergoing profound developmental and situational changes.[78]

Healthy people are self-actualizing. They are motivated toward personal development and making an investment in living. Self-actualizing individuals have goals, but their needs for love,

TABLE 26-1. PHYSIOLOGIC SEXUAL RESPONSE: WOMEN

Phase	Site	Response
Excitement	Vagina	Vaginal lubrication occurs
		Inner two thirds of vagina lengthens and distends; color changes to dark purple
		Over one third of vagina fills with blood
	Labia	Labia minora enlarge, become more deeply colored
		Labia majora flatten and thin, move away from midline
	Uterus	Uterus elevates, pulling on vagina and making a tent or open area at inner one third of vagina
	Breasts	Breasts increase in size
		Nipples become erect
	Cardiovascular/respiratory	Heart rate slows early, then increases in rate
		Breathing may increase in rate
		Blood pressure increases as phase progresses
	Skin	Sex flush, measleslike rash occurs on chest or upper abdomen
Plateau	Vagina	Vaginal opening decreases in size by one third
	Labia	Sex skin reaction: labia minora change from pink to bright red in nulliparous women and from red to deep wine in multiparous women
	Clitoris	Clitoris retracts from unstimulated position to inaccessible place under clitoral hood
	Skin	Sex flush spreads to all areas of breast, chest, and abdomen
Orgasmic	Vagina	Contractions begin in outer one third of vagina; at 0.8-second intervals and recur from 3 to 15 times; time between contractions becomes longer and strength of contractions decreases
	Uterus	Uterus contracts as in labor
	Rectum	Rectal contractions are linked in time with vaginal contractions
	Muscular	Muscular spasm is released; some loss of voluntary control occurs, with spasms and contractions of many muscle groups
	Cardiovascular	Heart rate is twice normal
		Blood pressure increases by one third
	Respiratory	Breathing rate is three times normal
Resolution	Breasts	Nipple erection decreases; slower loss of breast volume
		Sex flush and swelling around nipples disappear
	Skin	Perspiration covers body
	Vagina	Within 5–10 seconds clitoris returns to normal position; loss of vasocongestion is slower
		Congestion in outer one third of vagina disappears
		Congestion in vaginal walls disappears in 15 minutes or more
	Labia	Labia majora return to unstimulated size
		Labia minora: prestimulation color returns in 15 seconds; size returns more slowly
		Cervix descends to unstimulated position
	Respiratory/cardiovascular	Breathing, heart rate, and blood pressure return to prestimulation condition
	Urinary	Urge to urinate is felt, particularly in nulliparous women

belonging, and esteem are basically met, thus allowing them to concentrate their energy on their goals and pursuits and to focus on problems outside of themselves.[78]

They are able to express concern for others and balance their own needs with meeting those of others. They generally evoke a compassionate, warm response from others.[79] People who express themselves in healthy ways generally have the ability to love, are competent in interpersonal relations, have the capacity to adapt and adjust, and are able to be assertive without alienating people with their aggressiveness. They respect the personhood of others and refrain from expressing themselves in ways that would impose on the rights of others.[80]

Healthy people display a unified outlook on life which they may not articulate, but that gives them a sense of private, inner harmony and a feeling of purpose and meaning in life.[78] Their philosophy unifies their behavior and sustains them as they move toward long-range goals. Further, healthy people regulate their behavior from within, in accordance with internalized standards.

Healthy people are able to balance a need for the approval of others with their own sense of self-approval.[78] They consider others' opinions but are not unduly dependent on them for their sense of self-esteem.[78] They are able to conform but remain free to choose whether or not to conform. Their capacity for autonomy stems

TABLE 26-2. PHYSIOLOGIC SEXUAL RESPONSE: MEN

Phase	System	Response
Excitement	Penis	Penile erection caused by blood engorgement; penile size increases
	Scrotum/testes	Skin of scrotum tenses, becomes congested and thick
		Testes rise higher in scrotum, increase in size as much as 50%
	Breast	Nipples become erect and swell
	Muscular	Increasing spasm of long muscles of legs and arms and abdominal muscles occurs
	Rectum	Some voluntary contractions occur late in phase
	Respiratory	Breathing may increase late in phase
	Cardiovascular	Heart rate slows initially, then quickens
Plateau	Skin	Sex flush occurs (not as frequent as in women) over chest, neck, and face
	Muscular	Muscular tension of face, neck, abdomen, and limbs increases
	Penis	Penile glans enlarges
	Testes	Testicular size increases from 50 to 100%
		Elevation of testes is fully accomplished
	Blood pressure	Blood pressure increases as phase progresses
Orgasmic	Respiratory/cardiovascular	Breathing, heart rate, and blood pressure increase—generally higher than in women
	Testes	Testes, prostate gland, and seminal vesicles contract as they collect sperm and seminal fluid and expel them into the entrance of the urethra
	Muscular	Muscular spasm is released, some loss of voluntary control occurs, with spasms and contractions of many muscle groups
	Penis	Penile muscle contraction and urethral contractions result in actual ejaculation of seminal fluid out of the penis
	Rectum	Contractions are linked to genital contractions
Resolution	Penis	After ejaculation one half of erection is lost quickly; second stage is slower
	Testes/scrotum	Scrotal wall reverts to uncongested state
		Testes descend rapidly in most men; swelling decreases
	Skin	Skin flush disappears
		Perspiration is usually confined to palms and soles of feet, but sometimes is widespread
	Nipple	Nipple erection lost
	Muscular	Loss of muscle tension over a 5-minute period
	Cardiovascular/respiratory	Heart rate, breathing, and blood pressure return to prestimulation state

from a deep private sense, derived from early childhood relationships, that they have a right to express themselves and that their fundamental personal worth makes their expressions valuable to others around them.[80]

People who express themselves in healthy ways generally show a resilience in adverse situations. They adapt with new patterns when old patterns of self-expression are no longer possible. They are able to laugh at themselves and discharge tension through humor.

ALTERED SELF-EXPRESSION

Alterations in self-expression occur naturally over the life span. Changes are generally manifested in the way people present themselves and in their disclosures to others. Nurses encounter individuals undergoing developmental change, but more commonly encounter people undergoing alterations related to illness. The relationship between self-expression and illness is complex. Illness may cause changes in self-expression, but illness may also be caused by the very choices that individuals make in the course of expressing themselves.

Illness impinges on self-expression in several ways. First, the pain and other serious physical symptoms that accompany illness are a recognized source of psychological stress. As already mentioned, breathing difficulty, nausea, vomiting, fatigue, or any of a number of other symptoms may interfere with a person's ability to communicate with others and meet basic needs for love, belonging, esteem, and intimacy. Illness may place at risk a person's social roles, job, goals, and even the possessions and economic assets important to one's personal and social identity.

Ill persons communicate in various ways the threat that occurs with illness. Often there are changes, sometimes subtle, in an individual's pattern of self-presentation. Ill persons, for example, may suddenly or gradually show less concern for the impressions they make on others, or they may show increased concern, even avoiding those people from whom they fear rejection. Alterations in self-expression are also manifested by changes in an individual's pattern of self-disclosure. Ill persons commonly experience an urgent need to disclose their distress.

ILLNESS, SELF-CONCEPT, AND SELF-EXPRESSION

Whatever the nature of an illness, its underlying threat is to the self-concept. People cherish and protect their wholeness but derive their self-ideals from values in the environment. Media images corresponding to a culture's values of health and beauty focus attention on those people who satisfy the cultural standards, not on those who have deformities or other problems associated with misfortune. Such images serve as a constant reminder to the healthy and ill alike that illness is a deviation from the ideal human state. When an individual can no longer conform but continues to aspire to the ideal, a conflict often results, contributing to the difficulty many people experience in adapting to body changes that are permanent in nature.

ALTERED BODY IMAGE

Body image, the ideas people hold about their bodies that comprise a part of their self-concept, can be profoundly affected by illness.[81,82] Illness and its treatment may change the body structurally and functionally and lead to changes in the mental images a person holds about his or her body and its functions. Body image in turn is tied to self-esteem, in illness as well as in health. As the body image changes, one's self-esteem may also suffer from the changes of illness.[83] Self-esteem, learned early in life, has both stable and evolving aspects. Luckily, diminished self-esteem, when it accompanies illness, need not be permanent.

The impact of an altered body image on the self-esteem derives from the interaction of several factors: (1) the individual's body ideal (the mental measuring stick against which an individual judges the actual body); (2) the sociocultural significance of the altered body part or process; (3) an individual's concept of the importance of the body part altered; (4) a person's age, gender, and marital status. Body changes associated with the breasts and reproductive organs, organs strongly associated with interpersonal attractiveness, are extremely powerful in their potential to effect a negative change in body image.[81] However, the impact of such changes often varies with an individual's circumstances. The loss of a breast may have a different meaning for a young, unmarried, sexually active woman than for an elderly widow, for example.

Virtually any illness can alter a person's body image. For some people, merely being ill is an affront to their concept of themselves as independent persons. However, illnesses that involve physical deformity, mutilation, or loss of a body part or that change the way people communicate, eat, eliminate body wastes or their capacity to move from place to place are particularly likely to alter body image and diminish self-esteem, at least temporarily. Further, illnesses, injuries, or surgeries that significantly alter the face, which is central to a person's identity, are likely to result in a negative change. Even cosmetic surgery can negatively affect an individual's body image when the changes are unanticipated or considered undesirable by the individual.

Treatments that cure or alleviate illness, on the other hand, may reverse the negative effects in some cases.[82] It is also important to keep in mind that the effects of illness on body image are highly individualistic. Attempts to predict who will and who will not face a significant adjustment require an understanding of the meaning that the specific illness has for the individual.

ALTERED SEXUALITY

The relationship between illness and altered sexual functioning is widely recognized.[84] Illness may alter an individual's ability to function sexually and consequently change a person's sense of self as a man or woman. Some chronic diseases are known for their ability to interfere with the sexual function. Diabetes, for example, causes impotence in some males and renders women who have the disease vulnerable to vaginal infection.[85] Likewise, spinal cord injury may interfere with a male patient's ability to function sexually and result in severely diminished self-esteem for those afflicted.[86,87] Acute illness, on the other hand, may cause a person to temporarily lose interest in sex. Individuals may fear that sexual activity will aggravate their illness. Aspects of the sick role may also serve to threaten a person's sexual identity. Admission to the hospital, given the numerous psychological threats associated with it, may serve to dampen sexual feelings and reduce a person's desire for intimacy. Some individuals, however, react with an apparent increase in sexual interest manifested by a use of overt sexual behavior to express a variety of needs. When nurses are confronted by or inadvertently witness patients' sexual activity, their ability to respond in a nonjudgmental manner is crucial.

ALTERED ROLE PERFORMANCE

Role performance is another important aspect of self-concept. Each role individuals perform carries a corresponding definition of self that becomes a part of self-concept. Roles also compose an important aspect of social identity. Roles involve activities that enable an individual to demonstrate personal skill and competence to others. Role behavior thus may be considered self-expressive. Further, people reinforce one another for competence in their respective roles. For that reason, roles are frequently tied to a person's self-esteem.

Not infrequently, illness interferes with an individual's physical capacity for role activity. Indeed, certain roles may become

> **INSIGHTS FROM NURSING LITERATURE**
> **SELF-EXPRESSION AND SUPPORT**
>
> *Bowers JE, Clark-Mahoney JP, Forshee T, Reiner K, Shilling JE, Snyder BS. Analysis of a support group for young spinal cord–injured males.* Rehab Nurs. *1987;12:313–322.*
>
> The authors used Goffman's concept of spoiled identity and Erikson's model of development to study a support group for young males who had sustained a spinal cord injury and permanent paralysis. They noted that the group process was most beneficial when it focused on developing greater independence, communication, and self-expression among members, and when the leaders put a major emphasis on creating an environment in which patients could deal with their feelings about being injured and dependent on others and about public attitudes toward the handicapped. As a result of participating, group members derived support from one another, coped better, and engaged less in dysfunctional behavior.

impossible, and role relationships become difficult to sustain. When that happens, the individual may suffer a loss of self-esteem. Consider a family man who sustains temporary, and possibly permanent, leg paralysis in a work-related accident. Not only will he be unable to work, but his paralysis will also make it difficult to continue the activities associated with being a husband and father. Even with years of treatment, he may be unable to resume some of the activities from which he derived his self-esteem, making it necessary for him to learn new patterns and roles. How these changes influence his self-esteem will depend on his success in finding new sources of reward.

ADAPTATION TO ILLNESSES THAT THREATEN SELF-CONCEPT

Adaptation is a complex process involving the nature of the threat, its perceived outcomes and consequences, and the person's resources for coping.[88] Adaptation generally occurs in four phases: impact, retreat, acknowledgment, and reconstruction.[89]

Impact

When a person becomes seriously ill or injured, there is often an initial period of shock during which the person moves from little awareness of the change that has occurred to at least partial awareness of what has happened. When the crisis involves a permanent change of the appearance of the body, such as the loss of a limb, it quickly becomes apparent to everyone that a return to previous routines is impossible and adjustment is necessary. When the crisis does not involve such changes, however, recognition of an altered state may depend on more subtle cues. Because the altered state is not readily apparent, realization of altered circumstances may take time for the individual and family to integrate, and caregivers may need to intervene to establish the significance of what has happened.

Once an awareness begins to develop, depending on the severity of the problem and its perceived consequences, the individual may express strong emotions, including despair, discouragement, hostility, and anger. The despair expressed may be for others as well as themselves, as those afflicted realize that others' lives are also affected. Anger and hostility may also be expressed. Further, the anger that individuals may feel toward themselves for becoming ill may be projected onto others.

Retreat

In the retreat phase, the individual steps back from the problem to gather energy and mourn the loss of the old self, to reflect on the meaning of his or her situation, and marshal the resources and strength necessary to confront the patterns that must be changed.

During retreat, individuals may try to reduce the threat they feel by denying that an illness exists. Subtle behaviors, such as refusing to take medication, inattention to symptoms, or even a cheerful presentation of self may constitute a denial of illness.

Denial is a largely unconscious mechanism, that is, it is not a deliberate attempt to mislead oneself or others. In addition, there are differences in the degree to which reality is denied. At the extreme, there is verbal denial of what is plainly apparent; for example, a person who has lost a limb may insist that the limb is still there. This *complete denial* suggests the existence of a serious psychological problem. A more common form of denial is ignoring or disowning limited aspects of the problem. An individual having lost a limb may acknowledge its absence but deny any consequences from the loss. Even more common is the tendency of some people to minimize aspects of the problem rather than denying the problem outright. "It's not so bad!" is a statement frequently made by those who wish to deflate the importance of what has happened to them. *Partial denial* is common in everyday life. When it aids individuals without interfering with their long-term adaptation, it is not considered unhealthy. With appropriate support, denial generally gives way to growing awareness.

Acknowledgment

During the acknowledgment phase, people begin to deal openly with threat and make necessary changes. At this point, they have a substantial awareness that change is unavoidable and understand that life roles cannot be resumed without significant modifications to their patterns of coping.

Individuals often experience strong challenges to their personal identity during the phase of acknowledgment. They may question who they are and who they are becoming. This is a highly stressful state in which the bodily symptoms of stress in combination with unusual disturbing feelings of detachment, loss of contact, *self-diffusion*, and *depersonalization* are not uncommon. Persons may feel as if they were observing what is happening to them rather than actually experiencing it. Further, they may have a strong need to talk about their feelings and to share the meaning of their experience with others.

Reconstruction

During the reconstruction phase, the individual repairs old concepts of self or builds what amounts to a new self-concept. Individuals slowly begin to involve themselves in activities and engage in social interaction. This phase is fraught with risk and ambivalence. Individuals still mourn the past, fearing not only that its satisfactions are out of reach but also that their new circumstances will fail to hold comparable satisfactions. Often they experience conflicting emotions and display opposing attitudes about their situation, an emotional state known as **ambivalence.** For example, a paralyzed accident victim may return to sports activities as a wheelchair athlete. Although gratified by new accomplishments, the person may nevertheless mourn the loss, view the emerging self as somehow unwhole, feel anger for whatever personal responsibility he or she may have had for the accident, and therefore experience pride, anger, and remorse all at the same time.

These emotional polarities consume energy and need to be resolved as completely as possible.[90] Part of the process of working through conflicting feelings involves disclosing them to others and examining their implications for health. Individuals experiencing conflicting feelings need the opportunity to express their feelings in the context of a relationship that minimizes the risks of disclosure.[91] Certain conditions are generally required for a person to disclose strong, confusing emotions. These include a high level of interpersonal trust, communication of empathy and caring from the helper, and the opportunity to safely put aside concerns about the impressions one is conveying to others.[91] Humor is particularly important in resolving ambivalence. Humor allows a socially acceptable expression of aggressive feelings, while laughter enables people to discharge the tension associated with difficult situations.[92]

INSIGHTS FROM NURSING LITERATURE

HUMOR

Ruxton JP. Humor intervention deserves our attention. Holistic Nurs Prac. *1988;2:54–62.*

The author reviews the various reasons that humor has been ignored historically as a mode of intervention with patients.

In the author's opinion, humor has an important therapeutic role. Humor is important in establishing a comfortable atmosphere and neutralizes emotionally charged events. Humor in the form of the "jocular gripe" turns individual experiences into a collective experience and can strengthen the social structure of the health care setting. Humor also enhances persons' ability to look at situations from a new perspective, which, in turn, helps them generate new alternatives for themselves. Physically, humor provides benefits similar to those of exercise in the form of stimulation and relaxation. There also may be chemical–neurologic connections involving the endorphins, the natural opiates found in the brain, which have implications for the use of humor for patients with stress-related conditions.

The success of the reconstruction phase depends greatly on the quality of support found in the environment, particularly from significant others. *Feedback* during this phase is critical. The supportive behavior and reactions of others help the person learn that satisfying social relationships are still possible, that a rewarding social identity can be reestablished, and that self-esteem can again develop. Individuals look for indications of their worth in others' acceptance and are sensitive to nuances in the behavior of family and friends.

Conversely, a lack of support may have serious consequences. Reconstruction is a period of profound tension during which the self-concept and self-ideal must undergo substantial revision for adaptation to occur. During this period, the person may experience feelings of *shame*, a feeling of consciousness of guilt derived from the reality that an unalterable change has occurred that may have rendered one undesirable to loved ones. Shame is a highly stressful experience. It may be communicated by a complete or partial withdrawal from others as manifested in avoiding eye contact, bowing of the head, or turning of the back. Other indicators include autonomic skin reactions such as blushing and blanching, nervous gestures such as playing with hair or clothes, twisting fingers, hand tremors, facial tics, and showing a hesitating manner.[93] Individuals who experience shame can be helped to cope when those around them show respect for their manner of self-presentation and their personal and physical privacy and help to discharge tension with humor. Feelings of worth are also reinforced and restored when the individual receives encouragement and positive feedback from others, is given opportunities for realistic problem solving, and experiences the caring interest of those in the environment.

GRIEVING, DYING, AND SELF-EXPRESSION

Perhaps the greatest threat posed by illness is that of death. The fear of death is pervasive among humans. Indeed, humans may be unique among the species for having the capacity to contemplate their own final eventuality.

Death is a biologic process, yet one of the most human experiences an individual can have. At a symbolic level, the process of dying is a process of losing relationships—relationships to others, to valued objects such as one's home and possessions, to important roles and activities, and to one's future and personal goals.[94] Thus, the meaning of death is one of profound loss. **Loss** can be defined as the state of being without something one has had.[94] It is an integral part of the human experience and has far-reaching implications over the entire course of individual development and is a part of the threat to self-concept that accompanies illness, discussed above. Most people have many experiences with loss during their lifetimes.

Paradoxically, the experience of loss may be necessary for the growth of one's sense of mastery over life. Loss can be a real event or a perception of loss derived from an individual's interpretation of events. The more individuals have invested emotionally in a person, object, or even an aspect of self, the more likely they are to feel threatened when what they value is taken away. Generally, it is the loss of a significant other, a person idealized and loved, however, that is likely to be accompanied by grief.

Grief and Grieving

Grieving is a normal process not unlike the adaptation to illness (the loss of health) discussed above, necessary to persons anticipating loss or who have sustained a loss critical to their sense of well-being.[95] **Grief** is a profound state that often affects how a person thinks, eats, sleeps, or copes with the events of the day. Grief involves the strong emotions such as rage, despair, and fear that are common to the stage of acknowledgment of illness described above. Grieving people often show many of the signs of acute stress, among them, a feeling of choking or shortness of breath, a need for sighing, and an empty feeling in the abdomen; they may suffer from insomnia and have mental symptoms such as absentmindedness, confusion, and difficulty concentrating.

Loss, which can be a feature of the experience of any serious illness, is a critical feature of the experience of a terminal illness.[96] **Loss** is a sense of being deprived of something valued. Accompanied by grief, loss is experienced by those who are being left behind and by the dying individuals themselves. Grief experienced before death occurs is known as **anticipatory grief.**

Bereavement is a term associated with grief. **Bereavement** is the role transition that survivors undergo on the death of someone close.[95] The child becomes an orphan, the spouse a widow or widower. Bereavement may or may not be accompanied by grief, depending on the closeness of the relationship, the circumstances of the death, and how disruptive the changes prove to be for the bereaved.

Mourning, related to both grief and bereavement, is a bereaved person's expression of grief. Individuals convey their grief to others through culturally sanctioned attitudes and customs. Because of the cultural plurality in North America, many patterns of mourning are found among the subgroups in the United States and Canada.

INSIGHTS FROM NURSING LITERATURE

DEALING WITH LOSS

Carmack BJ. Balancing engagement/detachment in AIDS-related multiple losses. Image. *1992;24:9–14.*

The author used an interview process to study how persons manage multiple losses and deal with cumulative grief. She noted that when individuals are confronted by losses occurring in rapid succession, they may suffer "bereavement overload," a form of overwhelming grief precipitated when the time available to grieve any one loss is insufficient. Such circumstances, common to war survivors, the elderly, and AIDS patients, cause grief to "accumulate." The author found that her subjects, a sample of 19 people living in the same gay community, coped by varying their involvement in the life of the community to maintain a personally acceptable balance between engagement and detachment. Subjects who remained involved protected themselves from excessive emotional pain by periodically detaching themselves from some aspects of their lives. Getting away on the weekends, for example, served to lessen pain and prevent burnout.

The Experience of Grief

Because nurses encounter, not only people who are dying, but also the people who are grieving for them, it is important that they understand the nature of grief and how it is experienced. Carter asked 30 bereaved individuals about their experience with grieving and found five core themes that convey what it means to grieve[96]:

- *Being stopped,* a theme referring to how death interrupts life's usual flow, is experienced as a state of "falling apart" or being unable to hold oneself together. Although some of Carter's subjects characterized the interruption as a pause in their activities, most experienced it as a more profound change and had difficulty dealing with the associated feelings of being overpowered and helpless.
- *Hurting* is characterized by a cluster of intensely painful emotions that tax the grieving person's coping capacities. As one subject commented on his experience, "I can't stand it." Feelings of sorrow and sadness, often accompanied by crying, were so strong that subjects described them as painful. Some described the experience as similar to being hit, wounded, stabbed, shattered, or crushed, or as an immense heaviness or weight. Painful guilt, burning anger, and sorrowful wishing were also reported. The pain was unrelieved by anything.
- *Missing* is the acute awareness of what has been lost. It includes yearning for the loved one's presence. The loss of the loved one was perceived by Carter's subjects as a kind of emptiness or void that left the bereaved with a sense of desolation, deprivation, abandonment, and even loneliness. Expressions of missing the loved one were simple and direct, as for example, "I miss him so much."
- *Holding* is the desire of the bereaved to preserve the loved one's lost existence. Ways of holding in Carter's sample included "honoring the deceased's wishes" and "carrying on the deceased's legacy." Talking about the life of the deceased in great detail was also important to the bereaved. Holding was a sorting process by which the subject's separated out the good memories and recalled them, while pushing back the painful memories.
- *Seeking* is a search for help, which takes the form of a search for comfort and meaning. Comfort, in Carter's sample, was sought in rituals, prayer, staying busy, writing and reading about bereavement, and seeking out others who "really understood." The search for meaning was represented in frequent questioning "why?" or in a determination to use the experience to help others.

From this picture it is clear that grief is an experience for which there may be no comparison. Cody, another researcher, also documented the pain of grief. In a study of four bereaved individuals, he found there were negative and positive aspects to grieving.[97] Losing someone close gave rise to immobilizing agony, yet a profound change in self also occurred, one that allowed subjects to move forward with a new perspective. One subject viewed his grieving as a rite of passage through which he became more mature.

Understanding the experience of bereavement, nurses are prepared to assist in the resolution of grief. Carter's subjects sought help and gained a sense of comfort by communicating with those they perceived as understanding their feelings, especially those perceived to have been in the same situation.[96] That suggests a sharing of the grief experience is both possible and helpful.

The Process of Grieving

Many authorities have described models of grieving. Generally their models depict the grieving process as occurring in predictable stages and unfolding within certain time parameters. Lindemann,[98] Engle,[99] Kübler-Ross,[100] and Bowlby[101] all described patterns of grieving in a typical sequence. Their models, which are similar to each other, depict stages of response not unlike the stages outlined previously—impact, retreat, acknowledgment, and reconstruction—which can be viewed as a classical model of grieving.

Newer models, however, challenge the assumption that grieving is time limited and proceeds in a static manner.[102] The manifestations of grief are in fact highly variable, and people often progress and regress in unpredictable ways in their journey toward integrating loss. Despite these variations, it is possible to outline clusters of experience that typify the grief reaction:

- *Shock and disbelief.* The immediate response following a death—whether or not the loss is anticipated—often involves shock, numbness, and disbelief. The feeling of numbness gradually gives way to a profound sense of pain and loss, often associated with physical symptoms such as muscular weakness and feelings of exhaustion. Grieving individuals may exhibit extremes of behavior and mood and may have dreams in which the deceased is alive.[103]
- *Yearning and protest.* Strong feelings frequently well up as numbness wears away and grieving individuals begin to adapt to the loss. Such feelings may last weeks or months and include anger toward the deceased for dying and leaving them, anger toward God or caregivers for allowing the death to happen, and even feelings of jealousy and resentment toward others who still have their loved ones. The strength of feeling may cause grief-stricken individuals to question their own mental stability, and

INSIGHTS FROM NURSING LITERATURE

GRIEVING

Cody WK. The meaning of grieving for families living with AIDS. Nurs Sci Q. *1995;8:104–114.*

The author studied several families living with AIDS using a qualitative methodology. Family members were asked to describe their experiences of grieving. The author used their descriptions to compile narratives, and from those identified several concepts of grieving. He concluded that (1) grieving is a transition in which families adapt constantly to welcome and unwelcome changes; (2) grief is a common experience in which family members are related but alone with their feelings—that is, they are co-participants in a kind of existential loneliness; (3) grieving is a time when family members confirm what really matters to them—whom they love and what they love; (4) grieving is a process in which family members are mutually involved in change and choice making and identify new meaning in their lives.

they may therefore hesitate to disclose their feelings, fearing they will be judged to be mentally ill.[103]

- *Anguish, disorganization, and identification.* As anger is exhausted and the reality and permanence of the situation are recognized, many grieving individuals experience confusion, aimlessness, loss of motivation, and a general immobility akin to the sense of being "stopped," described previously. At this point, the grieving often suffer depression and loss of meaning in their lives, and may be overcome by feelings of loneliness. Memory lapses, difficulty concentrating, and frequent loss of emotional control are common. They may display a strong need to cry and will often seek out opportunities to reminisce on idealized memories of the deceased. Grieving individuals may also adopt the behavior, admired qualities, and mannerisms of the loved one.[103]
- *Reorganization.* The process of reorganization often begins months after the death and may last a few years. Data from clinical studies fail to support the idea that grief resolves itself in one year and, in fact, indicates a variable time schedule.[104] During reorganization, periods of depression may be interspersed with periods of well-being. As time passes and opportunities for sharing feelings accumulate, sadness decreases and aspects of ordinary life are resumed.[103]

Elements of Griefwork

The desired outcome of grieving is a resolution of emotional pain so that the grieving are able to remember their loved one and yet preserve the capacity to love and reinvest in living.[105] The process of emotional resolution is stressful and has come to be associated with work, hence the term *griefwork.*

Four elements of griefwork outlined in the classical models include:

- severing the strong emotional bonds to the deceased
- adjusting to an environment without the loved one
- developing a new social pattern
- learning to live with memories of the deceased[103]

Newer models dispute the idea that the grieving should totally detach themselves from emotional ties to the deceased.[102] However, adaptation requires that those who grieve work through the disturbances created by their loved one's death. The bereaved individual must establish a new identity or revise a former identity and fill the roles formerly assumed by the deceased. That means finding new ways to spend time formerly spent together and becoming comfortable with the symbols of the deceased that remain in the bereaved's daily life. Developing new relationships requires the bereaved to reenter social life; it also requires that the loss be integrated into the bereaved person's belief system, so that the individual is able to deal realistically with the loss, remembering the pleasures without forgetting the disappointments of the relationship.[103]

When griefwork is incomplete or unsuccessful, prolonged grief occurs, making reorganization impossible for the survivor. The hallmark of prolonged grief is a sustained sense of personal hopelessness and lack of involvement in the future.[103] Delayed grief, another outcome of incomplete griefwork, is associated with situations in which people have been unwilling to grieve, preferring to keep busy and to appear to cope well while making no reference to the loss. Symptoms and responses resembling the grieving process finally emerge after a long period of absent grief.[103]

Dying

Because of the advances in medical technology, some diseases that routinely caused death in the past are now curable, or their progression can be substantially forestalled. Terminal diagnoses no longer mean that an individual will die now or even in the next month or year. Further, more people are treated for chronic illnesses over far longer periods than was formerly the case.

Technological advances are prolonging life, yet in a sense they are also prolonging death. Today, people with serious illnesses often must cope with living and dying simultaneously. Periods of relative health and energy are often interspersed between periods of deterioration. Terminal illnesses may inexplicably remit, compounding the uncertainty. Because the best possible result, no further deterioration, may be impossible for health professionals to guarantee, the specter of death remains.

Faced with this situation, individuals are forced to deal mentally with their own mortality while continuing an investment in life and living. For some people, a satisfactory adaptation may be possible. They may view their ambiguous situation as an opportunity rather than a danger.[106] For others, the ambiguity and uncertainty may be more difficult than dying itself. Both possibilities have profound implications for an individual's self-expression.

The Meaning of a Potentially Fatal Diagnosis

From the moment they receive a diagnosis of potentially fatal illness, individuals experience many losses over which they may grieve:

- Loss of being a healthy person functioning in society
- Loss of the ability to live without the interruption of hospitalization, clinic appointments, and painful treatments
- Loss of the ability to plan for the long-term future
- Eventual or sudden loss of job role

- Loss of present or future ability to care for home and family
- Loss of present or future ability to perform sexually
- Loss of present or future ability to care for one's own bodily needs and functions[107]

For some individuals, the grieving may begin immediately; for others, it may be substantially delayed. A person's reaction to his or her diagnosis affects significant others with varying degrees of intensity, and the reactions of significant others, in turn, affect the individual. Mutually, they define the situation in a way that makes it possible for them to cope.

One possibility is that they will choose not to acknowledge the possibility of death, at least at first. So long as the person's physical status remains uncertain, inattention to the likelihood of death may actually enhance coping by influencing ill individuals to adhere to their treatment programs.[108] However, as the physical condition deteriorates, new definitions become necessary for adaptation. People who fail to acknowledge the possibility of death as the terminal phase develops may have a need to conceal their feelings from one another, which may affect their ability to grieve.[107] If they and their families persist in ignoring death as an outcome, not only will they become isolated from one another, but the long-term adjustment of the survivors may be placed at risk as well.[106]

The reactions of caregivers from prediagnosis to death and bereavement can facilitate or hinder the emotional response of the patient and family as illness progresses. Caregivers who cope by avoidance may deny the patient and family an important means of support in dealing with their impending losses.[107]

The Experience of Dying

Grieving is an element of dying, just as it is an element of bereavement. Kübler-Ross,[100] in her classic work on death and dying, was one of the first to investigate the experience of dying. She outlined the stages of grieving through which the dying individual passed. They included denial (of the seriousness of the condition), anger ("why me?" with rage directed at anybody and everybody), bargaining (making an arrangement with God or fate), depression (sense of loss and inevitable finality), and acceptance (an acknowledgment that the struggle is over).

Kübler-Ross awakened a generation of people to the needs of the dying person, and her work has been extremely influential; however, critiques of her work have emphasized that the concept of stages ignores the complexity and depth of the dying person's experience and encourages those who use the theory to dismiss the dying person's reactions as a matter of developmental course, rather than to deal existentially with the content and intensity of the dying person's expressions.[109]

Kastenbaum and Costa,[109] in contrast to Kübler-Ross, emphasized that grieving as a part of dying is individualistic. The clusters of grieving, described earlier, can be viewed as having relevance to the experience of the dying, but should not be taken as prescriptive.

The experience of dying often includes loneliness, discomfort, anxiety and fear, and depression. Certainly, an important part of the experience of dying derives from the social context of death. Dying may involve prolonged hospitalization, although the length of hospitalization, even for treatments such as cancer chemotherapy, has been shortened by technology that allows home and even self-administration. During hospitalization, however, the dying person is separated from loved ones. In the course of this separation, the dying person may experience profound *loneliness*, mitigated to a greater or lesser extent by the perception that the separation is temporary.[110] However, loneliness is a distressing experience that, if intense enough, can heighten the ill individual's physical symptoms.

Sometimes, the separation is emotional or social in nature, rather than physical, and this, too, can cause loneliness. Dying persons may find themselves isolated, as others seek to maintain their own composure and coping ability by ignoring the reality of the situation. Dying persons may even find themselves confronted with the necessity to comfort others who are unable to handle the intensity of their own emotions. Even health care professionals, who are vulnerable to becoming emotionally overwhelmed by the frequency of their encounters with death, are sometimes prone to defensive behavior.[111]

All of these situations reinforce the loneliness of dying. The extent and duration of communication changes may be mediated by factors such as pre-illness family function and communication patterns. Generally, stable relationships are less disrupted than unstable relationships by the diagnosis and treatment of terminal illness.[81]

Another aspect of the experience of dying involves *physical suffering*. Pain, anorexia, nausea, vomiting, fatigue, elimination difficulty, sexual dysfunction, and breathlessness are a few of the physical problems that may accompany dying.[112] These changes, in turn, compound the emotional experience, including anxiety, and fear. Terminal illness does not uniformly involve pain, but when it does, the pain is often a prominent feature of the individual's experience. The pain of terminal illness is often of a chronic and progressive nature. Although it may vary in intensity, it frequently requires aggressive pharmaceutical and nonpharmaceutical interventions for control. Narcotics are often used on a regularly scheduled rather than an intermittent basis in the treatment of cancer pain.[112] Pain control is one of the most important contributions that nurses make to care of the dying.

Another important feature of the experience of dying is the emotions associated with dying itself. *Fear of the unknown* is a prominent feature of the distress of many dying individuals. This fear may be so strong as to consume the limited time and energy available. Fears and anxieties may be made more tolerable when the individual has the opportunity to disclose them to caring others. An individual's spiritual beliefs may be comforting. Personal beliefs and philosophy relevant to the dying experience may be shared through self-disclosure and can be reinforced by caregivers as a way of expressing caring and providing comfort.

Depression, another feature of the experience of dying, is often related to the fact of dying, but may also be related to the dying person's physical symptoms. Thus, relief from physical suffering may also be instrumental in bringing relief from depression.[112]

Adaptational Tasks of the Dying Person

Griefwork encompasses coping with the dying experience and, by completing a series of adaptational tasks, moving toward acceptance. The relative importance of each task varies with the characteristics and needs of the dying person. Humphrey[107] identifies several adaptational tasks that the dying person may undertake, the importance of which varies with the individual's needs.

- *Getting affairs in order while coping with loss.* This task involves attention to the arrangements for survivors that a person may wish to make. This task may be delayed because the individual lacks the physical or mental capacity to participate. Indeed, the dying person may be overwhelmed by loss, as he or she begins to contemplate that life will go on without him or her. As Humphrey points out, this issue is especially poignant for the dying person.[107]

- *Considering future health care needs.* Careful planning for the physical care of the dying person should be addressed in advance of the terminal phase and is important not only to the dying person but also to the survivors. The options for care have increased with the development of the hospice movement over the course of the last decade. **Hospices** are homelike institutions specializing in the care of the dying in the terminal phase of illness.
- *Planning for the time remaining.* With an awareness that limited time remains, an individual's choices for the use of time become especially important. Dying persons may contemplate how to use the time available to maximize their opportunities for self-expression.
- *Anticipating pain and other physical problems contributing to a loss of identity.* The issue of pain may have to be addressed and solutions anticipated. Further, changes in physical appearance and body functions may interfere with self-presentation and often are extremely threatening. Loss of hair, for example, a common side effect of cancer chemotherapy, is a source of social embarrassment for many individuals. It is also a constant reminder to the individual of altered identity and approaching death.
- *Considering being a nonperson.* Considering one's own transition to death is like looking at the sun; it cannot be done for long without looking away. Life review may be helpful as the individual undertakes this task and may provide a sense of fulfillment and satisfaction that will aid the dying in letting go. Religious and philosophical discussions may also be helpful.
- *Deciding to speed up or slow down the dying process.* In losing life, one loses ultimate control. Nevertheless, individuals may retain some control over the timing of death. At an emotional level, individuals may decide to fight or give up. Once a person lets go, death often quickly follows. Individuals have the right to refuse life-prolonging treatment, which also gives them some control over the temporal aspect of death. More controversial is whether they have the right to be assisted in their own death.

Hope

Hope is a confident, yet uncertain, expectation of future good, which to the hoping person seems realistically possible and personally significant.[113] Hope is generally regarded as a future-oriented state.

Instilling hope, as part of the care of the dying is controversial.[114] One viewpoint holds that hope is appropriate only if realistic. The other holds that hope is an emotion the purpose of which is to maintain emotional well-being in the face of both everyday and unusual circumstances, and thus is always valuable.[115] The latter view comes from the work of Erick Fromm,[116] who proposed that hope is a shared human experience essential to life.

Hall[114] stresses that hope is integral to humanness, and that loss of hope can be equated with loss of life itself. In a study of 11 individuals who tested positive for the human immunodeficiency virus (HIV), Hall found that all of her subjects had mechanisms for maintaining a positive outlook and that those mechanisms were essential to their sense of well-being. One individual, for example, declined to join an AIDS support group because the members' constant talk of death scared him. Others looked at their survival predictions as a challenge, Hall believed, to maintain hope. Hall emphasized that nurses have an important role to play in helping terminal patients maintain hope, and that trust between nurses and patients is enhanced when nurses relate to the terminally ill in the same future-oriented way they relate to anyone else. Although nurses may provide opportunities for the dying to talk about the meaning and quality of their lives, whether or not to talk about death must be the dying individual's choice.

> **COLLABORATIVE STRATEGY**
> **UNCERTAINTY AND HOPE**
>
> The outcome of illness is often uncertain. Many illnesses are said to be terminal in nature; that is, they rapidly accelerate the process of dying. Nevertheless, individual variability makes it impossible to predict with certainty what the timetable will be. Hope enables people to cope with difficult situations, illness included, in our future-oriented society. Nurses assist ill individuals to preserve their dignity by supporting hope.

Other Spiritual Needs

The dying often have an urgent need to consider the meaning of their lives and to search for forgiveness and love.[117] The consideration of meaning represents a need to make death significant, less fearful, and more tolerable; to deal with the frustration that dying causes; and to affirm the value of one's life. Some individuals find answers in their religious beliefs; others have the ability to articulate their own meaning of death.

The dying may seek relief from feelings of guilt as they review their lives and consider the unfulfilled expectations they had for themselves.[117] Forgiveness from God or particular people may become extremely important. Many find comfort in spiritual counseling from their clergy as they experience these feelings, or they may have a need to express their feelings to others as they strive to identify and deal with the source of their discomfort.

Family and friends, important sources of love, may themselves need assistance from others as they struggle to deal with their own needs and those of their loved one. Professional caregivers are an important source of support, especially when family and friends are unavailable or nonexistent.

Interdisciplinary collaboration to meet the needs of the dying is important. People vary in their ability to balance involvement and objectivity in the care of the dying, and members of the health care team can assist each other to both help the dying and maintain their own ability to carry on.

Definition of Death

Although the definition of death might appear to be self-evident, it is a subject of substantial scientific, social, and public policy controversy. Indeed, the technology of organ donorship and transplant has brought the issue to the forefront of bioethical and medical concern. Nurses who work in hospitals, particularly in critical care settings, are frequently confronted by the human problems that surround the definition of death—the social, ethical, and legal issues that may not soon be resolved, but which are of vital interest to all who work in health care.

In the past, a person was considered dead when the vital functions—heartbeat and respirations—ceased, and when the individual was unarousable, with no nervous reflexes, speech, or movement. Today, technology has rendered traditional approaches to the diagnosis of death inadequate. Is a person dead when the heart, mechanically supported, still beats, when the chest rises and falls, the lungs exchange gases, and the nervous reflexes are intact, even though he or she shows no signs of cognitive functioning?

Kastenbaum[95] has identified several ways of being dead, all of which occur in health care settings:

- The person is dead. The vital processes, although temporarily ceased, potentially may be revived. However, the individual fails to respond and is unable to express thoughts or feelings by any means.
- The person is dead, however, the vital processes function with the use of an elaborate life-support system.
- The person is dead, however, the vital processes continue to function without an elaborate life-support system.
- The body is dead. All vital functions have permanently ceased.

A question that arises, one subject to ethical and legal debate, is how important is the distinction between death of the person and death of the body. Another important question is, what difference, if any, is there between a body that continues to function on a vegetative (involuntary) level with a life-support system and a body that functions on the same level without a life-support system? Still another issue to be resolved is, how long are people obliged to continue elaborate life-support measures for those who are in a vegetative state, and what criteria are applicable to the cessation of life support? These questions are all of practical and ethical significance to health professionals.

Medical Definition. For the past 40 years, the health care and legal communities have attempted to answer these difficult questions as well as the more basic question of what death is. In the late 1960s, a committee of faculty at the Harvard Medical School formulated the Harvard Criteria for determining a permanently nonfunctioning brain.[118] The criteria include the following. The person

- *Is unreceptive and unresponsive.* There is no awareness of external stimuli (including stimuli that ordinarily would be extremely painful) or inner need.
- *Shows no movements and no breathing.* There is a complete absence of spontaneous respirations and all other spontaneous muscular movement.
- *Has no reflexes.* The reflexes elicited in a neurologic examination, including pupillary constriction to light, are absent.
- *Displays a flat electroencephalogram for 24 hours.* Scalp electrodes fail to elicit a printout of electrical activity from the brain, and the stylus records an essentially flat line, indicating a lack of electrophysiologic activity.
- *Has no circulation to or within the brain for 24 hours.* Procedures such as the use of Doppler ultrasound fail to detect the flow of blood in the brain, the loss of which is accompanied by death of the brain cells.

The Harvard guidelines have received widespread application. Generally, the first three criteria are enough to establish a diagnosis of death, and the others are reserved for situations in which traditional criteria are inadequate.

Nevertheless, controversy remains over the extent of loss of brain activity that constitutes brain death. The argument continues over whether the whole brain, the cortex and the brainstem, must cease to function, or whether the cessation of cortical function alone is sufficient for death. The current medical and legal standard requires that all brain functions cease, including the activity of the brainstem and higher structures.[119]

Legal Dilemmas. Despite widespread medical use of these criteria, legal dilemmas exist for those who find themselves confronted with social questions surrounding the definition of death. Right-to-die cases have raised questions about the rights of individuals who find themselves coping with problems stemming from the failure of social policy to keep pace with technology. These cases are gradually providing answers to questions about the withdrawal of support from those who meet the medical criteria of death. The 1976 case of Karen Ann Quinlan, a young woman in a persistent vegetative state, established that surrogate decision makers could speak for individuals who could not speak for themselves and exercise their right to decline extraordinary medical treatment in certain situations.[120] Further, the 1990 case of Nancy Cruzan, another young woman in a persistent vegetative state who required only tube feeding to continue to survive, established that states could restrict the right of surrogate decision makers to act on behalf of previously competent individuals by requiring clear and convincing evidence of the person's expressed decision while competent.[120]

Undoubtedly more issues will find legal resolution as the state courts take positions on similar and different cases. Still under debate, for example, is the proper standard of evidence to apply in hopeless cases involving the withdrawal of nutrition and hydration supplied by artificial means.[121,122] At issue is what standard of proof of a patient's prior intent the courts should require in cases where no advanced directive exists.

The legal requirements for acknowledging death in cases where technology prolongs life artificially will continue to be refined. In deciding cases, the courts are currently turning to guidelines issued by The Hastings Center (a center for legal scholarship) stipulating that such decisions should first of all be based on knowledge of the patient's preferences and values.[121] Thus, even in death, a person's self-expression continues to have a powerful influence over his or her personal fate and the behavior of others.

SECTION 2

ASSESSMENT OF SELF-EXPRESSION

Nursing assessment focuses on both the content and the process of self-expression. The content of self-expression refers to a patient's verbalized feelings and thoughts as well as observable actions and behaviors, particularly those reflecting personal attitudes, values, and priorities. The process refers to the meaning that patients place on their own expression and behavior. Nurses

TABLE 26-3. COMPONENTS OF SELF-EXPRESSION ASSESSMENT

Components	Aspects of Self-expression Evaluated
History	Perception of illness, life structure, self-presentation styles, self-concept, problems, goals, preferences
Primary concern/current understanding	Self-disclosure related to immediate concern, perception of illness
Past health problems/experiences	Health practices, lifestyle choices, body image, interaction patterns
Personal, family, social history	Sexuality, self-concept, vocational choices, life structure, activity patterns, values, social distance/closeness, beliefs, public and private self, interpersonal relationships, role performance, sense of meaning, self-esteem, reference group, life satisfaction
Subjective manifestations	Self-presentation and self-disclosure related to self-concept, body image
Examination	Body image, self-concept, self-esteem
Measurements	Body image
Objective manifestations	Self-presentation, posture, facial expression, speech, dress, manner, grooming

attempt to understand the meaning of the patient's behavior—what significance the experience has for the patient from the patient's point of view.

Assessment provides data about the patient's overall state of wellness, goals, expectations for recovery, care, and future well-being. Important aspects of self-expression—self-concept, body image, role performance, life structure—revealed through a patient's self-presentation and self-disclosures, provide a holistic view of the patient and a basis for effective planning and management of care. Table 26–3 provides an overview of the components of assessment and the aspects of self-expression that are evaluated for each component.

▲ SELF-EXPRESSION DATA COLLECTION

SELF-EXPRESSION HISTORY

History taking is especially important to assessing self-expression. During history taking, nurses try to discern the themes and patterns of the patient's life. A history of the patient's life course, including present and past health problems, assists the nurse to make formulations about the patient's coping ability and capacity to adapt to current and future stressors, including the challenges of illness.

The nurse's approach is extremely important. By asking questions about the patient's life, the nurse communicates interest in the patient as a person. These expressions let the patient know that caregiving is a process of sharing.

In taking a history, the nurse need not strictly follow an interview outline. Generally people do not talk about themselves in an orderly sequence. Indeed the patient's spontaneity is often promoted by avoiding a set format and by inviting patients to tell their own story as they know it, without interruption. Newman,[123] a nursing theorist, notes that by avoiding requests for bits and pieces of information, she is able to glimpse her patients' situations at a more holistic level. It is not common for people to discuss their intimate relations, thoughts, and feelings openly with strangers. Asking patients to tell their own story gives them the ability to control the situation and may help them feel more comfortable with the process of history taking.

In addition to identifying the potential problems in self-expression brought on by illness, history taking helps nurses identify patient strengths and resources. Effective coping is an important strength. Information about how patients are currently coping and how they have coped with similar problems in the past assists nurses in planning care. Further information about the patient's interpersonal network, creative outlets, leisure pursuits, and other activities that serve to enhance self-esteem also helps nurses to select implementations relevant to the patient's situation.

After the patient has completed telling his or her story, the nurse is free to ask questions to clarify points or fill in aspects of the health history the patient has not addressed. Ideally, all or most of the relevant aspects will be touched on spontaneously and those requiring the nurse's prompting will be few. The information provided by the patient is then sorted into the standard history format, primary concern, current understanding, past health care experiences, and so on.

Primary Concern

This portion of the history focuses on the current health problems most bothersome to the patient. When these involve the dimension of self-expression, the potential for impact on the patient's self-concept exists. For example, the patient facing body-altering surgery may fear a loss of identity, an impact on role performance, or an altered ability to have intimate relationships. The following case example illustrates a common health care situation and depicts the patient's primary concern, which is in italics.

> Mr. Foster is a 62-year-old clerical worker, hospitalized for abdominal pain of 2 weeks' duration. He recently lost his wife of 30 years to an unexpected cardiac illness. *Mr. Foster, who has been treated with medication and is now comfort-*

able, *states that he is worried about returning to work, and adds that he hopes his hospital stay will be short.*

Table 26–4 presents other examples of primary concern statements and identifies their potential meaning for the patient's self-expression.

Current Understanding

The nurse in the situation above, aware that Mr. Foster's physician suspects he is suffering from an obstruction of the intestines and may require surgery, recognizes the need to clarify Mr. Foster's understanding of his current health problem. The nurse focuses on Mr. Foster's previous experiences with surgery, his understanding of his current condition, and the treatment and care he anticipates. Further, Mr. Foster's recent bereavement cues the nurse to observe for indicators of Mr. Foster's mental and emotional state and, assess his understanding of its relevance to his current condition.

In assessing current understanding, areas to focus on are the impact of the patient's health problem on his or her self-concept/ body image, self-esteem, role performance, and life satisfaction. The nurse notes factors contributing to the present crisis and those that may facilitate or interfere with the patient's adjustment. To identify the impact of illness on the patient's self-concept, it is helpful to evaluate the patient's highest level of functioning before the illness occurred. The nurse elicits this information by asking several questions: "At what point in your life did you feel the best about yourself?" "What were you doing at the time?" "How did you see yourself functioning during that period?"

Reviewing patients' expectations about how illness will affect their life pattern is also essential. Patients' accounts should include statements about the impact of illness on their mood, interest in activities, involvement with others, and future choices. Understanding how the patient's day-to-day life is affected by illness helps the nurse determine plans for implementation. Patients' attitudes toward their illness and their expectations for care are important data. Some patients may feel helpless in coping with the illness, which may affect their ability to engage in problem solving and to participate with the nurse in identifying the concerns to be addressed and goals to be attained. Further, the patient may describe (or the nurse may observe) modifications of dress, grooming, or personal habits brought on by illness, which provide clues to the patient's inner emotional state. Patients may report mood changes that leave them less interested in how they present themselves to the world, an indication that illness is taking a toll on their emotional well-being. Or they may report an alteration in their energy level that prevents them from paying attention to grooming and hygiene.

Further, patients coping with loss of a loved one from death or divorce may report distress manifesting in weight changes, headaches, pain, or other symptoms. A careful description of the social circumstances in which the symptoms evolved should be obtained. Exploring whether the patient has experienced deaths, separation, or losses of significant others is particularly pertinent to assessing the potential for problems related to self-expression.

Past Health Problems/Experiences

It is important to review the patient's feelings about previous illnesses or injury and its effects on body image, self-concept, and self-esteem. The nurse should also ask about chronic physical conditions to which the patient has had to adapt. For instance, a patient who has undergone drug treatment for cancer and who

TABLE 26–4. EXAMPLES OF PRIMARY CONCERN STATEMENTS

Primary Concern as Expressed by Patient	Aspect of Self-expression Potentially Affected
"I can't manage at home anymore."	Self-esteem, leisure pursuits, social relationships, sexuality, life satisfaction
"My test results show I'm going to need a mastectomy."	Body image, sexuality, self-presentation, self-esteem, self-concept, self-disclosure
"I haven't been able to walk as well as I should."	Self-presentation, self-esteem, vocation, leisure pursuits, social relationships, life satisfaction
"I'm having problems taking care of my baby."	Role performance, self-esteem, psychosocial development, life satisfaction, self-awareness
"My breathing has been getting worse." (words barely audible)	Body image, self-concept, vocation, leisure pursuits, self-disclosure, social relationships
"My heart condition is worse and my doctor thinks I can't work anymore."	Vocation, role performance, body image, self-presentation, life satisfaction
"My wife passed away and I haven't been able to eat very much since."	Self-esteem, self-concept, self-disclosure, role performance, self-presentation, grieving and loss

experienced subsequent hair loss may be angry or depressed, may experience lowered self-esteem related to body-image changes, or may withdraw socially because of concerns about changes in self-presentation. Patients' descriptions of past recoveries, including descriptions of their coping mechanisms, provide information for assessing the potential for problems in self-expression. Support systems and interpersonal contacts the patient has used to aid recovery in the past may suggest resources as well as a direction for current management.

Particularly important is the patient's response to prior episodes of the current illness. The nurse should explore the meaning of the patient's experience by asking the patient questions such as "Did you feel differently about yourself after your surgery last year?" "Did you view your body differently or think of yourself differently after you received the diagnosis of . . . ?" "Did you ever have negative feelings about yourself during the last episode of . . . ?" "Do you think others look at you differently since . . . ?" The following example illustrates the importance of such data.

> Mr. Morton, a 64-year-old patient hospitalized for cardiac surgery, suffered a stroke 1 year ago that left him with a mild paralysis of the left side of his face, as well as sensory loss, numbness, and weakness of the left leg, which has limited his mobility. Mr. Morton is quite anxious about facing major surgery, but is more concerned about the chronic sensory loss in his legs, which restricts his ability to dance and interferes with his relationship with a female companion.

This past history cues the nurse to explore the possibility that Mr. Morton sustained a negative body-image change, a sense of diminished role performance, and general loss of life satisfaction.

Personal, Family, and Social History

Through the personal, family, and social history, nurses discover many dimensions of the patient's self-expression. As described in Chap. 11, the self has many aspects. One important aspect is the social self. It is this aspect of the self that is best revealed in the personal, family, and social history. Another aspect is the individual's sense of personal uniqueness, or identity. The feeling of individuality or distinctness is communicated through one's choices and experiences in personal, family, and social arenas and helps the person answer questions such as "How am I special?" "How am I different than others?" "What makes me unique?"

Vocation/Occupation. The vocation/occupation component of the personal, family, and social history provides information about the patient's vocational or occupational pursuits as well as data about formal and informal education. A job history can provide information about the patient's functional level, goals, personal values, life satisfaction, and self-esteem. Choice of vocation demonstrates how one expresses oneself through work (Fig. 26–3). Work roles usually provide a sense of importance, productivity, mastery, and usefulness, and often determine one's perceptions of self. Work relationships often have a powerful influence, positive or negative, on self-esteem. Exploring the meaning the patient finds in work is helpful to understanding his or her self-concept. Is work the central focus of the patient's life, or does it merely provide a livelihood? Is work activity balanced with other areas of activity such as family or leisure pursuits? These are some of the questions that nurses ask as part of the vocational/occupational history.

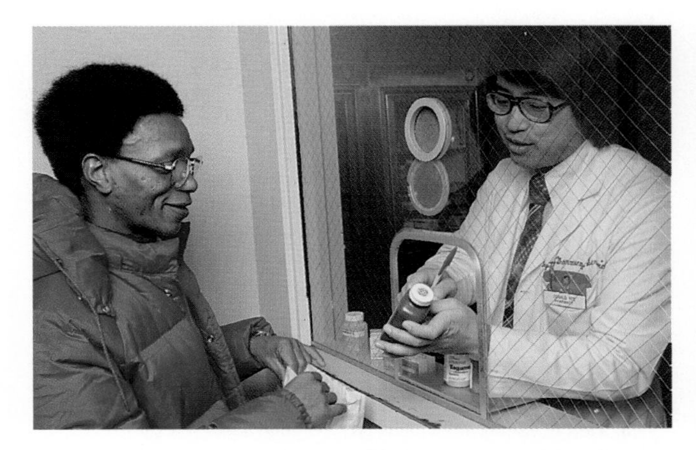

Figure 26–3. Career is an important aspect of self-expression for many people.

Social and Leisure Activities. A review of social and leisure activities gives clues about what provides the patient with a sense of meaning and life satisfaction. An absence of leisure pursuits may demonstrate a lack of stress-reducing mechanisms. Leisure activities contribute to positive feelings about the self, as well as a sense of uniqueness and mastery. They often provide an expressive outlet for patients. Thus, a disruption in leisure activities may result in further crisis for the patient. For example, an illness that leaves a patient unable to exercise may deprive the patient of his or her usual outlet for coping with day-to-day stress, if working out has served as a primary stress reducer.

Sexual History. The sexual history provides important information about the patient's sexual patterns and orientation, sexual satisfaction, and problems with sexual dysfunction. Sexual patterns, as indicated above, are a significant form of self-expression. They affect and are affected by one's body image, self-concept and self-esteem, life satisfaction, and close interpersonal relationships. A review of each of these areas may help to identify significant problems in self-expression. Aspects of the sexual history can also be woven into a discussion related to the patient's significant relationships or health problems. For instance, in discussing the patient's significant others, the nurse might ask "How do you and your partner get along?" "Are there problems in your relationship?" "Do you feel you can talk about most things with your partner?" "Are there areas you would like to see changed in your relationship?" "Do you think your physical condition has affected other areas of your life?" "How so?" For a complete sexual history, however, direct questions may also be required.

Psychological State. The patient's mood and affect are important indicators of psychological state, which in turn affects and is affected by one's self-expression. How patients describe themselves and their strengths and achievements can reflect self-esteem,

TABLE 26–5. SELF-EXPRESSION HISTORY: PERSONAL, FAMILY, AND SOCIAL HISTORY QUESTIONS

A. Vocational
1. What kind of work do you do?
2. What kind of training/schooling did that require?
3. How long have you been doing this kind of work?
4. Have you changed jobs recently? What made you change?
5. What kind of experience did you have in the military? (Include combat experience.)
6. Does your work provide satisfaction?
7. What are your career goals?
8. How close do you feel toward your career ideals?
9. How does your work make you feel good about yourself?
10. How has your work affected your health?

B. Home and Family
1. Do you live alone or with someone?
2. Tell me about your family/spouse. (Include ages, children, duration of marriage.)
3. How is your family or spouse reacting to your illness?
4. What is a typical day like in your home?
5. What roles and responsibilities do you have in your family?
6. Does your family do things together?
7. Have you lost any family members recently?
8. Are you currently having family or marriage problems?
9. How does your family or spouse solve problems with you?
10. Would you describe your family as close?
11. How has your health problem affected your family relationships?

C. Social, Leisure, Spiritual, and Cultural
1. What do you do to relax, have fun?
2. Are you involved in activities outside work or your home?
3. Are you involved in church/synagogue/community activities?
4. What helps you feel good about yourself besides work and family?
5. Are you involved in sports or exercise on a regular basis?
6. Do you have friends you see on a regular basis?
7. Are there things you feel strongly about or are active in?
8. How do you feel around other people?
9. Are there groups you belong to or are active with?
10. How has your health affected your involvement with friends or activities?

D. Sexual
1. Are you single? Married? Divorced? Seeing someone?
2. Do you have a sexual preference (eg, heterosexual, homosexual)?
3. Are you concerned about sexually transmitted diseases?
4. Are you worried about sex?
5. Are there areas about sex that you would like more information about (eg, effects of medication on impotence)?
6. Are you satisfied with your current sexual relationship?
7. Has your health affected your sex life?
8. Are there emotional concerns/issues that have affected your sex life?

E. Habits

Exercise
1. Do you get regular exercise?
2. What type of exercise do you do? How often? For how long?

Diet
1. Are you on a special diet?
2. What do you pay most attention to in the foods you eat (eg, fat content, salt, calories)?
3. Has your health affected your interest in or intake of food?

Sleep
1. Do you have problems sleeping, falling asleep, or staying asleep?
2. Has your health affected your sleep patterns?

Substance Use
1. Do you smoke? How much? How long have you smoked? Are you concerned about its effects on your health?
2. Do you drink alcoholic beverages? How much and how often?
3. Do you use drugs? What kind and how often? How long have you used them?

F. Psychological
1. How would you describe yourself?
2. What do you like best about yourself? Least?
3. What accomplishments are you proud of?
4. Has your appearance changed because of your illness? If so, how has that affected you?
5. What do your friends, family, co-workers say about you?
6. Would you describe yourself as a private person? A loner? Social?
7. Do you think people see the real you?
8. Do you feel depressed or anxious?
9. How do you cope with stress? What helps the most?
10. Are you anxious or self-conscious around people?
11. Do you have certain fears that upset you?
12. Do you ever feel hopeless or that you don't want to go on?
13. Do you feel sad for prolonged periods?
14. Do you feel discouraged? About anything in particular?
15. Have any changes (eg, death or loss) affected your mood?

components of the self-concept, inner emotional state, and capacity for coping. Suggested questions for all areas of the personal, family, and social history appear in Table 26–5.

Subjective Manifestations. A thorough assessment of problems in self-expression should include questions related to each body system. In this aspect of the history, the nurse notes symptoms that imply altered capacity for self-expression, as well as symptoms that suggest emotional distress. Aspects of the neurologic history, for example, may provide information on the former, especially when patients are found to have intellectual, memory, attention, or communication deficits. Patients may report changes in these and other mental functions during the history, cueing the nurse that mental status testing, discussed below, is appropriate. During history taking, the nurse may note that the patient is unable to recall previous experiences, reports difficulty concentrating on even simple tasks, or displays difficulty communicating in words. Any of these findings may represent significant changes in an individual's capacity for self-expression.

SELF-EXPRESSION EXAMINATION

A thorough assessment includes data obtained from the nurse's observations and physical examination of the patient. Observation is especially useful because many important aspects of self-expression are communicated indirectly, subtly, and nonverbally.

Measurements

Measurements of height and weight may suggest a potential for body image problems, particularly when the patient displays an attitude or opinion in relation to the findings. Statements such as "I should lose some weight" or "I have always been too tall and skinny" reflect on the patient's self-concept and may point to a self-esteem problem.

Objective Manifestations

Illnesses that affect body image, such as those associated with the loss of a limb, facial scarring, or other readily apparent body change, have the capacity to negatively affect individuals' self-expression by altering how they feel about their bodies. Further, loss of sensory input or changes in spatial-perceptual abilities may also affect whether patients are able to care for themselves, and thus how they present themselves to others, express themselves through activities, and even adapt to their environment following these changes.

General Observations. The patient's general appearance, gender, age, nutritional status, gait, energy level, speech, color, eye contact, gestures, and motor behavior provide a wealth of information.

GENERAL APPEARANCE. Note characteristics of dress and grooming as well as facial expressions and gestures that are part of an individual's manner of self-presentation (eg, poor eye contact, stooped posture); these provide clues to how a patient views him- or herself. Grooming is an important indicator of patients' ability and/or willingness to care for themselves. Likewise, manner of dress may reveal clues to a patient's group identification, self-concept, or level of self-esteem. Apparent changes in dress or grooming, as well as the patient's behavior, whether agitated, tense, open, or relaxed, can provide helpful clues to a patient's inner emotional state.

POSTURE AND MANNERISMS. Posture and mannerisms reflect self-presentation styles, as does motor activity, which also reflects mood states such as depression, anxiety, agitation, and fear, and thus provides useful data. Note the patient's quality of movement. A patient who has a self-concept or self-esteem problem may express his or her feelings through slumped body posture and timid movements, for example. A patient who is experiencing depression may display a slowness of movement or speech or be withdrawn.

SPEECH. Speech that is pressured or rapid may reflect anxiety. Speech that is slowed or hesitant may reflect an inner state of mistrust, fear, or depression. Note the quality and quantity of speech. Is conversation coherent or disorganized? Is the patient open in describing himself or herself? Guardedness may reflect a reticence for self-disclosure. Conversely, a patient who speaks unusually freely and openly about private matters may have a need to please others, suggesting overcompliance or a loss of personal autonomy.

AFFECT. Affect, the character of a patient's subjective, emotional state, is recognized from general appearance and also from statements reflecting the patient's emotions. Note whether the patient appears happy, calm, and at ease with him- or herself, or instead angry, depressed, anxious, tense, nervous, sad, or irritable. Also note whether the patient's affect is congruent with the content of his or her conversation. An example of incongruent, inappropriate affect would be a patient's smiling when describing the death of a loved one.

THOUGHTS AND PERCEPTIONS. The patient's ability to perceive reality accurately and communicate thoughts in an organized and coherent manner are important to self-expression. Note whether the patient's thoughts are presented in a clear, logical way. The content of thought may provide possible clues to the patient's inner world. What is the patient preoccupied with? Do the thoughts expressed reflect on the patient's ambitions or dreams? Are the thoughts confused? Does the confusion reflect an inner emotional state, a stress response, or possibly even an organic cause (such as a metabolic imbalance)? Can the content of the patient's thoughts be followed? Is the patient oriented to time, place, and situation? Does the patient represent facts accurately? Is the patient's self-perception realistic? Does the patient claim powers or skills he or she clearly does not possess?

SOCIAL INTERACTION PATTERN. The way in which the patient relates to the nurse may reflect the way the patient relates to other strangers and provide clues to the patient's general social patterns and skill. Several observations help the nurse evaluate this aspect. Does the patient seem to boast or brag? Does the patient seem uncomfortable or shy? Does the shyness reflect an inner feeling of low self-esteem or problems in self-concept? Is there a confidence about the patient that communicates a positive self-concept? Does the patient demonstrate eye contact during the interview or seem guarded in the kinds of information she or he shares?

Integument. Disfiguring scars, discolorations, or other anomalies may affect self-concept and body image. Note in particular lesions that readily call the observer's attention because of their size and location.

HEENT. Note losses of function such as blindness, hearing loss, and speech difficulty. Any of these may interfere with the patient's communication and, hence, self-expression.

Breasts. Observe for normal and abnormal characteristics (size, scarring, amputation) that may potentially affect the patient's body image and sexual expression.

Cardiovascular. Rapid heart rate, increased respiratory rate, or elevated blood pressure may accompany an emotional state (fear, anxiety, shock) and a high level of distress.

Genitourinary. Examine for structural abnormalities of the reproductive organs or organs of elimination that may affect the patient's social interaction and sexual functioning and/or satisfaction.

Musculoskeletal. Examine for paralysis, amputation, limited movement or mobility, findings that may potentially affect the patient's body image and self-concept. Loss of a body part such as an arm, leg, or breast, in particular, usually involves a change in body image.

Neurologic. The mental status examination can confirm mental changes noted during history taking. For example, a report of memory changes can be further refined on examination to identify problems with immediate recall, recent memory, or remote memory. Examine the following areas (see Chap. 17 for techniques): immediate recall, recent memory, remote memory, orientation, concentration, knowledge and vocabulary, judgment and abstraction, and behavior/mood/thoughts.

In addition to the mental status component, it is important to assess for coordination, muscle function and movement, and balance, which may affect the patient's mobility and thus capacity for self-expression.

NURSING DIAGNOSIS OF SELF-EXPRESSION STATUS

The final step in assessing self-expression is to analyze the history and examination findings to generate nursing diagnoses. The following section discusses nursing diagnoses related to self-expression approved by the North American Nursing Diagnosis Association (NANDA). Diagnoses are grouped according to four categories: diagnoses related to self-concept/coping, life structure, sexuality, and death and dying. The list covered here is not exhaustive. Diagnoses sometimes contributing to self-expression problems or resulting from altered self-expression are listed in Table 26–6.

DIAGNOSES RELATED TO SELF-CONCEPT/COPING

Nursing diagnoses related to self-concept/coping include self-esteem disturbance, body image disturbance, and personal identity disturbance; anxiety; ineffective individual coping; and impaired adjustment. The etiologies and defining criteria for these diagnoses are discussed below and appear in Table 26–6 under self-concept/coping. To establish a nursing diagnosis related to self-expression, the nurse reviews the data collected in the assessment phase with the patient, and together they consider its implications.

Self-esteem Disturbance

Self-esteem disturbance is a negative self-evaluation about self or self capabilities that may be expressed directly or indirectly. A disturbance in self-esteem can have many sources. The patient may lack a sense of belonging, or competence that results in a deficiency of self-esteem. Defining characteristics include self-negating verbalizations and expressions of shame or guilt. A patient may rationalize or reject positive feedback and/or exaggerate negative feedback about self, or demonstrate a hesitancy to try new experiences or fail to follow through on stated plans. Patients with self-esteem disturbance may project blame or responsibility for their problems onto others, or rationalize personal failures or see themselves as unable to deal with events. Self-destructive behavior, such as substance abuse, may be evident, or the patient may decline to participate in therapy. Patients with a self-esteem disturbance may present themselves in a grandiose (overinflated) way, display a hypersensitivity to criticism, or show poor eye contact or a lack of attention to grooming and dress.

No etiologies are currently specified for self-esteem disturbance. However, illness, surgery, or accidents that significantly change a person's life may decrease feelings of self-worth. Other factors that affect self-esteem include conditions that lead to a loss of independence, situations or stressors that interfere with pursuit of valued life choices, and a loss of significant others or social relationships that provided the nurturing and positive feedback needed for building self-esteem.

Body Image Disturbance

Body image disturbance is a disruption in the way an individual perceives his or her body. Body image disturbances may come from numerous sources, many of which have already been discussed. Defining characteristics include negative verbal statements or gestures or other nonverbal behavior indicating a negative attitude in response to actual or perceived changes in body structure or function.

- *Etiology: biophysical.* Body image, derived from many factors including height, weight, skin color, attractiveness, body build, and physical features, is affected by acute or chronic illness, trauma, surgery, or aging.
- *Etiology: cognitive–perceptual.* Perceived body changes are often the foundation of a body image disturbance. However, the patient's cognitive appraisal may or may not agree with the somatic reality of body dimensions, and distortion can lead to a loss of self-esteem. The patient may state, for example, "I'm too fat" (cognitive appraisal), when the actual somatic dimensions of body weight are within normal limits.
- *Etiology: psychosocial.* Reactions of significant others and society may contribute to body image problems.
- *Etiology: cultural or spiritual.* Society often creates a cultural ideal that is unobtainable or in conflict with the person's own ideal, either of which may lead to a body image disturbance.

Personal Identity Disturbance

Personal identity disturbance refers to a confusion over the distinction between self and nonself manifested by feelings of depersonalization and an inability to separate one's own needs from those of others. No official etiologies have been established for this diagnosis.

Anxiety

Anxiety is defined as a vague, uneasy feeling caused by threat of a nonspecific nature signaling something is not right. Defining characteristics may include apprehension, increased tension, persistent helplessness, uncertainty, fearfulness, feelings of inadequacy, shakiness, fear of unspecific consequences, and expressed concern about change in life events. Objective manifestations often include poor eye contact, trembling hands, extraneous foot or hand movements, facial tension, quivering voice or other signs of increased wariness, and perspiration or sympathetic changes such as pupil dilation, rapid heart rate, rapid breathing, vasoconstriction.

- *Etiology: threat to or change in health status.* Any change or potential change in health may present a threat that causes anxiety, but the level of anxiety present may not be in proportion to the nature of the change. For example, a patient admitted to the hospital for removal of a noncancerous skin lesion may, nevertheless, experience a high degree of anxiety. It is thus important for nurses to identify the significance of the patient's feelings.

- *Etiology: threat to or change in socioeconomic status.* Illness may affect the patient's ability to perform work and alter his or her future work options, which, in addition to other threats, may pose an economic threat leading to significant anxiety.
- *Etiology: threat to self-concept.* Many life and health care experiences, as established above, have potential to threaten individuals' views of themselves as competent, whole, respected by peers, and loved by significant others. Because self-concept is an integral part of the self, a threat to self-concept can produce significant anxiety.
- *Etiology: threat to or change in interaction pattern.* Because of the role of social relationships in affirming self-worth, even a threat of disruption may cause anxiety. Again the threat may be real or perceived; what is important is how the patient views the situation.
- *Etiology: change in role functioning.* Most patients enact multiple roles—worker, mother or father, daughter or son, friend, professional, volunteer—and illness can affect one or more of these roles. Some roles are more critical to a person's self-expression, sense of meaning, and self-concept than others; higher levels of anxiety result when significant roles are threatened.
- *Etiology: threat of death.* A person confronted with death can experience intense anxiety. Threat of loss of one's life is perhaps the ultimate threat. In health care, this threat is most often experienced in the form of a life-threatening illness, such as cancer or AIDS. Those who view death as the cessation of existence may find coping with life-threatening illness particularly difficult.
- *Etiology: maturational crises.* Maturational crises, crises related to aging, create a demand for personal change and often arouse a state of anxiety. Adapting, which requires adjustments in one's thoughts, feelings, and abilities, can also provoke a state of anxiety.
- *Etiology: situational crises.* Situational crises, crises related to an occurrence in the environment, are often unexpected and evoke uncertainty and anxiety. Anxiety will be particularly high if maturational and situational crises occur at the same time, such as when the birth of a new infant coincides with a parent's illness.

Ineffective Individual Coping

Coping includes behavioral and cognitive patterns that are used by individuals in the face of difficult or problematic situations.[124] Illness, as already established, is such a situation, which makes the assessment of coping patterns an important aspect of nursing care.

Ineffective individual coping implies an inability to adapt and problem-solve to meet life's demands and role responsibilities. Defining characteristics include verbalized inability to cope; inability to ask for help, problem-solve, meet role functions, or meet basic needs; altered social participation, including destructive behavior toward self or others and inappropriate use of defense mechanisms; or a change in communication pattern. The first two examples are considered critical defining characteristics; that is, evidence of these behaviors is necessary to validate the presence of the diagnosis.

- *Etiology: personal vulnerability.* A state of personal vulnerability exists when an individual lacks effective adaptive responses. Such a state may occur when persons lack the skills or intellectual capacity for problem-solving or are in an emotional state that interferes with cognitive functioning.

Impaired Adjustment

Impaired adjustment is defined as the state in which an individual is unable to modify his or her lifestyle or behavior appropriate to changes in health status. Processes normally used to maintain a satisfactory equilibrium with the environment are compromised in some way. Defining characteristics are several; a patient may verbalize his or her nonacceptance of the health status change, lack ability to be involved in problem-solving or goal-setting, be immobilized by shock or disbelief, or lack the capacity for future-oriented thinking.

- *Etiology: disability requiring change in lifestyle.* Physical illness often mandates a change in the patient's present style of living. Patients with impaired adjustment are not able to meet the challenge of required changes.
- *Etiology: inadequate support systems.* Crisis theory stresses the importance of a support network to help restore patients' equilibrium following a stressor or crisis.[125] Patients without adequate support are likely to experience compromised adjustment, as well as other problems such as anxiety, loneliness, and depression.
- *Etiology: impaired cognition.* The patient with impaired cognition may well be ill-equipped to problem-solve effectively. Problem-solving is essential in adapting to changes from illness, exploring new options, and managing adjustment.
- *Etiology: assault on self-esteem.* An assault on self-esteem, such as often accompanies the loss of a body part or function or body disfigurement, challenges adaptation. Interpersonal changes such as death, divorce, and altered sexual capacity or role changes such as job loss or change or retirement can also lead to an assault on self-esteem that results in impaired adjustment.

DIAGNOSES RELATED TO LIFE STRUCTURE

Life structure, the philosophical, vocational, and social framework of a person's life, is a way of looking at the choices individuals make throughout life that structure a person's life and participation in the social environment. Addressed in this section are the diagnoses of impaired social interaction and altered role performance. Etiologies and defining characteristics for these diagnoses are presented in Table 26–6 under life structure.

Impaired Social Interaction

Impaired social interaction is defined as the state in which an individual participates in an insufficient or excessive quantity or ineffective quality of social exchange. When a patient is unable or unwilling to maintain relationships with significant others and casual acquaintances, isolation results. This isolation can lead to further problems such as ineffective coping, changes in self-esteem, and depression. Some patients exhibit excessive dependency as a pattern of behavior, burdening their caretakers and family members, who subsequently withdraw resulting in patient isolation. Defining characteristics include verbalized or observed discomfort in social situations; an inability to receive or communi-

TABLE 26-6. SAMPLE NURSING DIAGNOSES: SELF-EXPRESSION PROBLEMS

Nursing Diagnoses	Defining Characteristics/Manifestations: *Subjective Data*	Defining Characteristics/Manifestations: *Objective Data*	Etiology
Self-concept/Coping			
Self-esteem disturbance *7.1.1*	Reports self-deprecating thoughts Makes self-critical remarks "I'm no good any more. I can't do anything since I've been so sick." "Having other people take care of me makes me feel worthless." Rejects positive feedback	Makes poor eye contact Has low voice volume Refuses to try new things/situations	*Social/Life Structural:* Loss of independence secondary to chronic disease
Body image disturbance *7.1.2*	Verbal response to change in structure and/or function: "I can't believe I no longer have part of my bowel and I have to go to the bathroom through this bag." States nonacceptance of body change Verbalizes fears of rejection by others	Bowel elimination via colostomy Surgery 10 days ago Stoma healing well Does not look at stoma Does not participate in colostomy care	*Physical:* Change in body structure and function: colostomy
Impaired adjustment *5.1.1.1.1*	Family members and patient verbalize unrealistic goals Refusal to discuss/acknowledge change in health status: "I'm not really that sick. I don't need to do all that."	Family visits infrequently Spouse repeatedly makes negative comments about patient's prescribed diet restrictions Patient has been admitted to health care facility several times with symptoms suggesting diet restrictions have not been followed	*Social:* Inadequate support systems
Ineffective individual coping *5.1.1.1*	Verbalizes inability to cope: "This is too much for me. I don't know what to do." "I'm supposed to take this medicine, but what difference will it make? I'll just skip it."	Demonstrates difficulty meeting basic needs: awakens frequently during night, eats less than 50% of food at mealtime, refuses to participate in ambulation Shows impaired judgment or problem-solving: unable to make a decision regarding which treatment option to select	*Physical:* Situational crisis: serious illness
Life Structure			
Impaired social interaction *3.1.1*	Verbalizes discomfort in social situations: "It's different being with friends now." Verbalizes inability to participate in satisfying relationships: "I just can't get around to see my friends."	Confined to wheelchair	*Physical:* Change in physical mobility due to illness
Altered role performance *3.2.1*	Verbalizes inability to perform role-related activities	Physical change that interferes with role: no longer able to work Verbalizes conflict in performing roles: "I can't see myself staying at home looking after the house. My work was my whole life."	*Physical:* Loss of function secondary to cardiac illness resulting in premature retirement
Sexuality			
Sexual dysfunction *3.2.1.2.1*	Verbalizes problem: conflict involving values: "My priest taught us that sex was for reproduction. Now that I've had my uterus removed I don't know what to do." Alteration in achieving perceived sex role: "I don't feel as feminine as I used to since the hysterectomy."	Recent hysterectomy	*Physical:* Altered reproductive system in structure or function: hysterectomy

TABLE 26-6. CONTINUED

Nursing Diagnoses	Defining Characteristics/Manifestations: Subjective Data	Defining Characteristics/Manifestations: Objective Data	Etiology
	Alteration in relationship with significant other. "I seem to withdraw from my husband sexually even though I know he's interested." Seeking confirmation of desirability: "I'm constantly asking my husband how I look since the surgery."		
Altered sexuality patterns *3.3*	Reports difficulties: "Ever since my abortion I'm not that interested in sex." Verbalizes change in sexual behavior or attitudes	Actual limitations: "I don't know what to do since I can't afford birth control pills."	*Cognitive:* Knowledge deficit: contraception alternatives
Death and Dying Anticipatory grieving *9.2.1.2*	Reports change in sleep pattern and eating patterns States feels depressed mood Reports changes in activity patterns: "I don't go to church or the club any more." Expresses guilt, anger, sorrow Reports change in libido Reports change in communication pattern	Displays sad expression Experiences mood swings: sometimes angry responses to nurses Withdraws and is not interactive	*Emotional:* Significant other diagnosed with terminal illness
Dysfunctional grieving *9.2.1.1*	Reports verbal expression of distress: "I still miss her very much." "Every day I look for her at breakfast—wait for her to come home from school." Reports alteration in eating habits Reports alteration in sleeping habits Expresses guilt: "I should never have let her go out that night." "If only I'd made her stay home."	Cries frequently Demonstrates poor problem solving Has minimal social interaction Unable to maintain focus on conversation	*Cognitive:* Perceived significant loss: daughter killed in accident 3 years ago

OTHER NURSING DIAGNOSES RELATED TO SELF-EXPRESSION

PHYSICAL
Fatigue
Impaired physical mobility
Impaired verbal communication
Sensory perceptual alterations
Pain
Altered nutrition, less than body requirements
Altered nutrition, more than body requirements

COGNITIVE
Altered thought processes
Impaired verbal communication

EMOTIONAL
Powerlessness
Fear
Hopelessness
Altered health maintenance
High risk for violence
Spiritual distress
Noncompliance
Self-care deficits: bathing, hygiene, grooming, dress

SELF-CONCEPTUAL
Chronic low self-esteem
Situational low self-esteem
Decisional conflict
Defensive coping
Ineffective individual coping

SOCIOCULTURAL/LIFE-STRUCTURAL
Impaired home maintenance
Diversional activity deficit
Social isolation
Altered family processes
Altered parenting
Parental role conflict

DEVELOPMENTAL
Altered growth and development
Developmental lag related to illness/hospitalization

SEXUAL
Rape/trauma syndrome

ENVIRONMENTAL
Impaired adjustment
Health-seeking behavior

Source: The nursing diagnoses and etiologies on this table and the definitions of nursing diagnoses in the body of the text not credited to other sources are from *Nursing Diagnosis: Definitions and Classification, 1997–1998.* Philadelphia: North American Nursing Diagnosis Association; 1996. Manifestation categories for etiologies and specifications of general etiologies on these tables are authors' original work.

cate a satisfying sense of belonging, caring, or interest; unsuccessful social interactions with peers, family, and/or others; or a change in any of these areas reported by family.

- *Etiology: knowledge/skill deficit about ways to enhance mutuality.* Mutuality, a two-way process of communicating concern, interest, caring, and involvement with another, is required to develop and maintain satisfactory relationships. If individuals lack the skill necessary to communicate feelings or are unaware of the kinds of exchanges and behaviors that strengthen relationships, their efforts to interact with others may discourage rather than enhance relationships, and their social interactions will remain ineffective and unsatisfying.
- *Etiology: communication barriers.* Several factors create barriers to effective communication that lead to impaired social interaction. Language and speech problems, culturally determined communication barriers, cognitive or emotional problems, or inattention to others' messages all influence the effectiveness of communication and create impairments in social interaction. (See Chap. 15 for a full discussion of effective communication.)
- *Etiology: self-concept disturbance.* How one views oneself influences many aspects of self-expression, including how one engages with others. An individual with a poor self-concept often displays modes of self-presentation and self-disclosure that are not conducive to establishing and maintaining effective social relationships. Others frequently are not attracted to individuals with low self-esteem, and such individuals may lack confidence to initiate interaction.
- *Etiology: absence of available significant others or peers.* Absence of significant others may be a self-imposed condition resulting from an isolated lifestyle, a temporary state resulting from a current stressor or life situation, or loss of a loved one to death. Hospitalization or recovery, if prolonged, can interrupt a patient's social network and lead to impaired social interaction. Mood states such as severe depression or anxiety may also prompt an individual to withdraw socially.
- *Etiology: limited physical mobility.* Limited physical mobility caused by illness or trauma can result in a state of isolation and reduced social interaction. The reduced frequency of contact with close friends may lead to their withdrawal (from perceived neglect of friendship), resulting in insufficient interpersonal contact for the patient.
- *Etiology: sociocultural dissonance.* Lack of familiarity or comfort in certain sociocultural settings may deter social interaction. (See Chap. 10 for more on how sociocultural factors influence health care interactions.)

Altered Role Performance

Altered role performance is defined as a disruption in the way one perceives one's role performance. Defining characteristics include a change in self-perception of adequacy or capacity to perform a role, deal with a conflict between roles, or carry out the responsibilities of a new role. No official etiologies are specified in the taxonomy for this diagnosis; however, several conditions or situations may lead to altered role performance. Such a condition may develop when individuals and their significant others have differing expectations for role performance or when conflicts between roles—the incompatibility of one role with another—exist. Role overload or role strain may result when a person is unable to fulfill the demands of a role.[126]

DIAGNOSES RELATED TO SEXUALITY

Lack of satisfactory sexual relations or lack of ability to express oneself through sexuality, as established above, can contribute to problems in self-expression. Two diagnoses related to sexuality, sexual dysfunction and altered sexuality patterns, are therefore discussed below and presented in Table 26–6, under sexuality.

Sexual Dysfunction

Sexual dysfunction is defined as the state in which an individual experiences a change in sexual function that he or she views as unsatisfactory, unrewarding, or inadequate. Sexual problems may result from physical or emotional illness, but also commonly occur in persons who function well in other areas. Defining characteristics include verbalizations of problems in sexual function such as alterations in achieving perceived sex role, actual or perceived limitation imposed by disease and/or therapy, conflicts involving values, alteration in achieving sexual satisfaction, seeking of confirmation of desirability, alteration in relationship with significant other, and change of interest in self or others.

- *Etiology: biopsychosocial alteration of sexuality related to ineffective or absent role models.* For most children, learning, identification, and cognitive organization all contribute to the development of sex roles, gender identity, and a sense of masculinity or femininity. Restrictive upbringing, on the other hand, may serve as a source of sexual conflict. The lack of effective role models both in childhood and as adults can also affect sexual identity, sexual comfort, and the ability to engage in sexually appropriate behavior.
- *Etiology: misinformation or lack of information.* A person's sexual information may contain fallacies that influence sexuality and sexual functioning. Sexual dysfunction may occur when individuals base their behavior on erroneous assumptions and beliefs. Further, patients may be hesitant to ask for information or clarification and may be reticent to disclose information about their sexuality.
- *Etiology: values conflict.* Because of negative societal influences and values, individuals may experience conflict in trying to reconcile their own sexual behavior with social norms. For example, a patient's belief that sexual pleasure is sinful, derived from religious proscriptions, may interfere with his or her sexual satisfaction or sexual expression. Messages received in childhood about sexual expression may also lead to conflict and guilt in adult relationships.
- *Etiology: lack of privacy.* For most people, privacy is an essential requirement for maintaining comfort in sexual behavior, especially sexual intercourse. Thus, settings that do not allow for adequate privacy may inhibit sexual expression.
- *Etiology: lack of significant other.* Physical and/or psychological separation from one's significant other can interfere with sexual functioning. Loss of a significant other through divorce, illness, hospitalization, or death alters sexual expression.
- *Etiology: altered body structure or function.* A person who feels ill or is in pain may not be interested in pursuing sexual activity. Illnesses such as diabetes or high blood pressure or diseases of the cardiovascular, pulmonary, neurologic, or genitourinary systems may have a direct effect on erectile function or alter one's desire for or interest in sex. Surgery to the reproductive

system or other areas of the body can also affect sexual ability or perceptions of one's capacity for sexual performance. Injury to the pelvic area can temporarily or permanently alter one's interest and ability to engage in sexual activity.

Altered Sexuality Patterns

Altered sexuality patterns is defined as the state in which an individual expresses concern regarding his or her sexuality, which serves as a source of anxiety and conflict. Defining characteristics include reported difficulties or limitations and changes in sexual behavior or attitude.

- *Etiology: knowledge/skill deficit about alternative responses to health-related transitions.* Many patients who lack information about the normal range of human sexuality and behavior, sexual techniques, or necessary adjustments in sexual behavior following an illness feel concerned about themselves as sexual beings or fear they will no longer be desirable to their partners. They may also feel conflict about desires for sexual expression and fears that may be painful or detrimental to their recovery.
- *Etiology: altered body function or structure.* Many illnesses, medications, or treatments such as surgery can interfere with sexual functioning or affect an individual's perceptions of personal attractiveness or desirability.
- *Etiology: conflicts with sexual orientation or variant preference.* Society, subject to social trends, dictates what is considered appropriate sexual behavior, and those dictates extend to sexual orientation—one's preference for partner gender. An individual's personal sexual orientation may be consistent or inconsistent with the dictates of his or her social reference group. When inconsistent, individuals may experience conflict, feelings of guilt, shame, and ambivalence and experience difficulty with sexual expression related to conflicted feelings about sexual orientation.
- *Etiology: fear of acquiring a sexually transmitted disease (or fear of pregnancy).* Problems in sexual satisfaction or sexual functioning can result from fear of rejection or abandonment by one's partner, fear of penetration, fear of punishment, fear of failure, or fear of pregnancy. Today it is common for people to fear sexually transmitted diseases like herpes, gonorrhea, or AIDS. All of these fears can negatively affect sexual expression and may be based on inadequate information or misconceptions about sex. Understanding the specific fear and its origin is important to the planning of appropriate implementations.

DIAGNOSES RELATED TO DEATH AND DYING

The death of a significant other is recognized as one of the most severe psychological stresses a person can experience.[104] An individual's ability to cope with loss is influenced by many factors, including the significance of the person lost, the conditions under which the loss occurred (sudden death or death after a prolonged illness), and the relationship to the person lost. The threat of death to self-concept and self-esteem is often enormous. Two nursing diagnoses, anticipatory grieving and dysfunctional grieving, are relevant to self-expression. Examples of subjective and objective data, defining characteristics, and established or suggested etiologies for these diagnoses are presented in Table 26–6 under death and dying.

Anticipatory Grieving

Anticipatory grieving is defined as the coping, planning, and psychosocial reorganization that occur when a person discovers that he or she is about to lose a loved one.[127] Defining characteristics include the potential loss of the significant other and expression of distress at this loss. Individuals may experience many emotions, including denial, guilt, anger, and sorrow. Behavioral manifestations may include changes in eating habits, altered sleep patterns and activity, and/or altered communication patterns. Sexual energy and interest are often affected. There are no official etiologies for this diagnosis in the approved taxonomy, but any threat of death or separation can lead to anticipatory grieving. Indeed, Rando[127] suggests that the dying person also experiences a kind of anticipatory grief. The chronic nature of many terminal illnesses often includes extended periods of remission and exacerbation, the exacerbation phases of which may evoke the response of anticipatory grieving.

Dysfunctional Grieving

Dysfunctional grieving is defined as grieving that is unusually prolonged or that remains unresolved. Grief can be unanticipated, conflicted, or chronic.[95] Defining characteristics include verbal expressions of distress. Emotional responses, including denial, anger, sadness, guilt, crying, and anxiety, may be present. The individual may idealize the lost person, have difficulty expressing the loss or express unresolved issues related to the loss, and may display sleep, appetite, activity, or sexual pattern changes. Daily functioning and social involvement may be affected. The patient may regress psychologically to an earlier stage of development or demonstrate altered concentration or cognitive functioning.

- *Etiology: actual or perceived object loss (including possessions, job, status, home, ideals, part or processes of the body).* This etiology, which encompasses more than just the loss of an object or significant other, reflects emphasis on the life structure, values, and areas that provide the individual with a sense of meaning in life.

STATING THE SELF-EXPRESSION DIAGNOSIS

The nursing diagnosis is a specific statement about the problems identified during the assessment process. An effective diagnosis includes three components: problem, etiology, and signs and symptoms or defining characteristics. Making the etiology and defining characteristics as specific to the individual patient as possible makes the diagnostic statement more effective as a basis for planning and evaluating patient care. Many of the nursing diagnoses related to self-expression have general etiologies and defining characteristics. While these are sufficient to explain the diagnosis conceptually, they do not provide enough clarity to guide care planning unless made specific to individual patients. For example, several diagnoses have etiologies of situational or maturational crises. To plan effective care, it is necessary to identify the nature of the crisis underlying the diagnosis and the unique way a particular patient is demonstrating the problem. For example, the nursing diagnosis for a new diabetic who reacts to situational crisis of illness with self-destructive behavior and poor problem solving should identify the problematic behaviors so they can be addressed. Ineffective Individual Coping related to newly diagnosed diabetes, as evidenced by eating binges, skipping meals, missing medical appointments, and erratic testing of blood sugar, is a complete diagnostic statement that provides clear guidance for nursing implementation.

SECTION 3

NURSE–PATIENT MANAGEMENT OF SELF-EXPRESSION PROBLEMS

The nurse–patient management of problems related to self-expression addresses current problems, but also focuses on optimizing the patient's potential for handling and preventing future problems. It includes nurse–patient collaboration in planning desired outcomes and nursing implementation, and in evaluating the plan's effectiveness.

PLANNING FOR OPTIMUM SELF-EXPRESSION

Identifying self-expression problems requires that patients disclose aspects of their experience they do not ordinarily share. In planning care it is important that the implementations selected reflect the patient's perceptions as well as the nurse's professional assessment. A collaborative approach that solicits patient input and promotes self-disclosure is needed. Prioritizing nursing diagnoses also requires patient participation, as does identifying available resources. Table 26–7, Nurse–Patient Management of Self-expression Problems, presents sample outcomes, nursing implementations, and evaluation criteria related to self-expression. Table 26–8, Partial Critical Pathway for Total Hip Replacement: Self-expression, and Table 26–9, Partial Critical Pathway for Congestive Heart Failure: Self-expression, show collaborative plans of care that incorporate concepts from this chapter.

NURSING IMPLEMENTATION TO PROMOTE SELF-EXPRESSION

Nursing implementation is a collaborative process through which nurse and patient identify nursing approaches to promote the patient's self-expression. It is important that patients participate in this process. Nurses can promote a climate that encourages patient self-disclosure by communicating empathy, respect, and warmth. Nurses' self-disclosure is helpful in communicating empathy and genuineness to patients.[14] Sharing experiences or feelings relevant to the patients' concerns helps promote self-disclosure by the patient. Specific nursing approaches are described below.

PREVENTIVE CARE

Preventive care is directed toward patients who currently are experiencing no change in self-expression but who may be at risk for developing such a problem. Individuals at risk are identified at this phase with the intention of preventing problems by reducing or eliminating the risk factors.

Conditions That Create Risk

Situational crises such as illness or physical trauma create a need for preventive care. Life changes such as starting a new job, being promoted, forming a new relationship, losing an old relationship, pregnancy and childbirth, or changing one's place of residence all have an impact on coping, adaptation, and self-expression.[128] Thus, any patient who has an important life change or anticipates one should be viewed as being at risk for problems in self-expression. Examples of changes that often result in a situational crisis are presented in Table 26–10, along with nursing approaches to address those crisis situations. Crisis prevention involves working with patients to alter their perception of their situation, provide situational supports, and strengthen their coping mechanisms.[129]

The normal process of growth and development creates changes that may lead to problems in self-expression (see Chap. 11). When these changes are perceived by the patient as crises, intervention is necessary. Examples of maturational crises are presented in Table 26–11, along with nursing approaches for addressing them.

Health Education

Health education is a particularly important preventive approach. It is important to understand a patient as a total person when determining the need for health education. The patient's culture, religion, environment, developmental stage, life structure choices, self-concept, and ability for self-disclosure affect the patient's understanding and the nurse's subsequent teaching.

Appropriate timing and patient receptivity are critical to success in teaching. So are information resources. A vast new resource available to nurses and patients alike is the Internet. Websites and URLs for accessing information on self-expression are listed at the end of this chapter. The focus of health teaching for a patient at risk for problems in self-expression is described in the following sections.

Developmental Milestones. Each stage of development with its associated developmental tasks provides not only an opportunity for potential change or growth but also the potential for maturational crisis. Education provided by nurses about normal stages of development will assist patients to prepare for and cope with these changes. Parents, in particular, need to appreciate the different stages of development to help their children learn to express themselves in satisfying and healthy ways.

Nurses can assist patients by providing education about age-appropriate behaviors and tasks. Chapters 11 and 12 describe these behaviors and tasks in detail. Examples include the following:

- During early infancy, newborns have no separate sense of self apart from the mother, but have the capacity for expression.
- Toddlers begin to learn that their identity is separated from others and to display patterns of individuality in their self-expression.
- Adolescents are challenged by body image changes as they grow and develop. It is important to assist parents to provide appropriate support during this period.
- Adults must deal with building a life structure by making important choices and, when faced with situational challenges, periodically revise those choices.

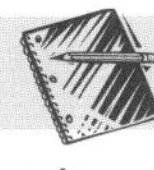

TABLE 26-7. NURSE-PATIENT MANAGEMENT OF SELF-EXPRESSION PROBLEMS

Nursing Diagnosis	Desired Outcomes	Implementation	Evaluation
Self-esteem disturbance R/T loss of independence secondary to chronic disease *7.1.2*	1. Recognition of personal strengths	1a. Accept expressions of negative emotions regarding present condition 1b. Provide opportunities to discuss specific concerns about changes in levels of independence 1c. Encourage patient to identify current aspects of independent functioning	1. Makes realistic positive statements about abilities
	2. Participation in developing plan to maximize abilities and use supportive resources appropriately	2a. Discuss aspects of daily living in which independence is most important; problem-solve strategies to maintain self-responsibility for these areas 2b. Engage patient in discussions of realistic alternatives for coping 2c. Refer to mental health professional	2a. Engages in collaborative problem-solving with nurse 2b. Identifies some daily activities in which independence is possible 2c. Identifies acceptable assistance when independence is not possible
Body image disturbance R/T change in body structure and function: colostomy *7.1.1*	1. Recognition and acceptance of change in body appearance and function	1a. Accept expressions of negative emotions regarding body changes 1b. Provide opportunities to discuss specific concerns about change in appearance and function 1c. Engage-patient in discussions of realistic alternatives for coping 1d. Encourage viewing ostomy, then progressing to participating in care as patient demonstrates readiness 1e. Provide contacts with local self-help group for patients with ostomies 1f. Positively reinforce attempts at self-care, grooming, and other behaviors that suggest progress toward acceptance of body change	1a. Patient statements about colostomy are descriptive and factual rather than negative 1b. Participates in care of colostomy
	2. Recognition of aspects of appearance and physical capacities are intact and positive		2a. Maintains usual grooming and hygiene activities 2b. Positive statements about appearance, abilities to carry on usual daily activities
Impaired adjustment R/T inadequate support system *5.1.1.1.1*	1. Recognition of change in health status	1a. Discuss changes in health status 1b. Facilitate expression of feelings about changes in health status through active listening	1. Acknowledges change in health status
	2. Modification of lifestyle in response to change in health status	2a. Discuss specific problems patient and spouse are having with prescribed diet 2b. Identify options for menus and recipes that meet diet prescriptions 2c. Confer with other members of the health care team about possibility for less restrictive diet 2d. Explore alternate support systems, including other patients with same diagnosis and diet 2e. Refer to appropriate community resources	2a. Verbalizes intent to adhere to modified diet 2b. Indicates that talking to others with same problem is helpful and plans to continue relationship

Continued

TABLE 26-7. CONTINUED

Nursing Diagnosis	Desired Outcomes	Implementation	Evaluation
Ineffective individual coping R/T situational crisis: severe illness *5.1.1.1*	1. Use of problem-solving strategies to deal with current crisis	1a. Accept expressions of negative emotions regarding illness 1b. Provide-opportunities to discuss current situation; focus on identifying specific problems 1c. Discuss past problems and past coping to resolve them 1d. Engage patient in discussions of realistic alternatives for coping with current illness 1e. Involve family in problem-solving discussions 1f. Provide a list of relevant community resources	1a. Identifies problems needing immediate attention 1b. Identifies past successful coping strategies 1c. Participates in planning to cope with current situation
	2. Recognition and effective use of available support	2. Same as 1a–f above	2a. Identifies resources is willing to use 2b. Initiates involvement with resources (family, community)
Impaired social interaction R/T change in physical mobility related to illness *3.1.1*	1. Improvement in quality and quantity of social interactions	1a. Discuss perceived barriers to social interaction 1b. Explore ways patient has altered communication/interaction after change in mobility 1c. Identify communication approaches patient can use to initiate contact with friends 1d. Discuss alternatives available for transportation to meet with friends 1e. Provide a list of community resources for social activities appropriate to health condition	1a. Reports improved social interactions: initiates contact with friends when interaction desired; has joined community group that sponsors social events; uses varied modes of transportation including friends, public transportation
Altered role performance R/T loss of function secondary to cardiac illness resulting in premature retirement *3.2.1*	1. Adaptation to new role/ alternative role definition	1a. Accept expressions of negative emotions regarding present condition 1b. Explore possible positive outcomes of role change 1c. Engage patient in discussions of realistic coping 1d. Involve family in problem-solving discussions 1e. Refer to mental health professional or community resources	1a. Actively participates in exploration of alternative role definition/role activities 1b. Positive statements about changed lifestyle, life activities 1c. Active involvement in new/changed role
Sexual dysfunction R/T altered reproductive system structure and function: hysterectomy *3.2.1.2.1*	1. Satisfying sexual relationship	1a. Provide opportunities to discuss specific concerns about change in appearance and function 1b. Provide opportunities for further discussion about values conflict regarding sexual expression, now that procreation is impossible 1c. Provide factual information about physical sexual functioning after hysterectomy 1d. Involve partner in discussions, if patient and partner are willing 1e. Refer to mental health professional if unable to resolve conflicts	1. Reports able to discuss concerns with her partner; able to enjoy satisfying sexual relationship with partner

TABLE 26-7. CONTINUED

Nursing Diagnosis	Desired Outcomes	Implementation	Evaluation
Altered sexuality patterns R/T knowledge deficit about contraception alternatives *3.3*	1. Concerns regarding sexuality resolved	1a. Explore concerns about loss of interest in sexual expression 1b. Determine what patient knows about contraception 1c. Correct misconceptions, if any, and provide factual information about contraceptive techniques in which patient is interested; include information on correct use, effectiveness, risks, and necessary associated health assessment and care	1a. Reports able to enjoy satisfying sexual relationship 1b. Selects affordable contraception; reports satisfaction with selected method
Anticipatory grieving R/T significant other diagnosed with terminal illness *9.2.1.2*	1. Expression of grief	1a. Provide opportunities to talk about anticipated loss 1b. Encourage grieving person to share feelings with spouse, other family members 1c. Provide anticipatory guidance about grieving: physiologic, emotional responses; typical pattern of progression, regression, resolution 1d. Provide information about community resources, support groups	1. Verbal and emotional expressions of grieving
	2. Recognition of importance of experiencing the present as well as preparing for the future	2a. Encourage collaborative decision making with spouse regarding care, treatment, amount of personal involvement desired 2b. Encourage life review with spouse 2c. Encourage taking time for sharing special experiences as spouse's health allows 2d. Provide opportunities to discuss life after loss	2a. Participates with spouse in day-to-day decisions related to current illness 2b. Describes special time shared with spouse 2c. Makes realistic statements about personal needs after spouse is gone
Dysfunctional grieving R/T loss of daughter in accident 3 years ago *9.2.1.1*	1. Resolution of grief, allowing resumption of productive personal life	1a. Accept, then confront, expressions of loss, grief, guilt 1b. Provide health teaching about healthy grieving process 1c. Encourage identification of realistic choices for personal growth and fulfillment 1d. Encourage removal and appropriate disposition of daughter's personal effects 1e. Refer to mental health professional	1a. Resumes active involvement in career/home responsibilities 1b. Resumes social interaction with peers 1c. Reports return to regular eating and sleeping habits

Source: See Table 26–6.

- Older adults are often faced with role changes, losses, and self-esteem and body image changes related to aging.

Healthy Self-Expression. Most people have a general awareness of what healthy self-expression means. Nevertheless, many lack a clear understanding of the characteristics of the healthy self and the relationship of these characteristics to self-expression. Thus, it is often beneficial for the nurse to review these characteristics, summarized in Section 1, with patients. Sample focuses for teaching include:

- Healthy individuals acknowledge their emotions and have energy available to bring meaning to life. They have a realistic view of others and an ability to relate to them in satisfying ways.
- Healthy individuals cope effectively with the realities and problems of life and demonstrate realistic dimensions of self-concept, among them a positive body image, adequate self-esteem, and competent and satisfying role performance.

Sexual Patterns and Practices. Many patients benefit from information on sexual self-expression. Despite the greater openness of

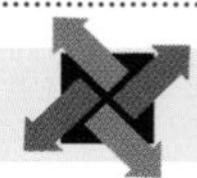

TABLE 26-8. PARTIAL CRITICAL PATHWAY FOR TOTAL HIP REPLACEMENT: SELF-EXPRESSION

Nursing Dx/Problem	Outcome DOS/Day 1	Outcome Days 2–3	Outcome SNF Days 4–6	Outcome Home Care 3 Weeks (6 Visits)
Ineffective individual coping R/T situational crisis: unsatisfactory support system		Initiates contact with 1 support person	Selects 3 community resources	Utilizes 3 community resources appropriately
Implementation	**DOS/Day 1**	**Days 2–3**	**SNF Days 4–6**	**Home Care 3 Weeks**
Assessment	Note visits or contact by family	Patient/family interaction Willingness/ability of family support system	Same Same	Same Same
Tests/Consults		Refer to social worker		
Medications/ Treatments		Reflective listening	Same	Same
Psychosocial		Assist patient to identify potential support systems (Lifeline, Meals-on-Wheels, Medical Transportation Service, Home Health Nursing Services, In-house Social Services)	Provide information about resources	Arrange for community services
Teaching			Problem-solving strategies	Same
Activity/Safety/Self-care				
Nutrition				
Transfer/Discharge Coord./Case Manager		Communicate outcomes achieved, problems/ interventions to SNF	Communicate outcomes achieved, problems/interventions to Home Health	Communicate outcomes achieved, problems/ interventions to MD & prepare for discharge

See inside back cover for abbreviations.

today's society about issues relating to sex and sexuality, many individuals lack information that might enable them to limit the risks encountered in sexual activity. Age-appropriate education by nurses can be instrumental in preventing problems in sexual expression. For example, nurses who care for adolescent patients beginning to develop secondary sex characteristics may allay anxiety or prevent body image disturbances by discussing with the patient the normal physiologic changes of adolescence.

Patients needs for information about sex and sexuality vary. Possible topics include normal anatomy and physiology of sexuality, stages of sexual development, effects of various illnesses on sexuality, preventing sexually transmitted diseases (STDs), and contraception (Fig. 26–4). Patients whose behavior puts them at risk for contracting a sexually transmitted disease benefit greatly from learning about preventive care. Patients may take risks because they lack information about "safe sex" practices. Current, accurate information about STD incidence and transmission helps patients identify behaviors that increase their risk for contracting STDs such as acquired immunodeficiency syndrome (AIDS), syphilis, and gonorrhea. Educating sexually active patients about the importance of limiting the number of sexual partners and using "safe sex" practices, such as wearing latex condoms and

TABLE 26-9. PARTIAL CRITICAL PATHWAY FOR CONGESTIVE HEART FAILURE: SELF-EXPRESSION

Nursing Dx/Problem	Outcome Primary Care Visit	Outcome Home Care Week 1 (3 Visits)	Outcome Home Care Week 2 (3 Visits)	Outcome Home Care Weeks 3–4 (3 Visits)
Altered role performance R/T exacerbation of chronic illness	Accepts family assistance	Accepts outside assistance	Identifies alternative role	Endorses alternative role

Implementation	Primary Care Visit	Home Care Visit Week 1	Home Care Visit Week 2	Home Care Visit Weeks 3–4s
Assessment	Feelings about role	Feelings about role change	Same	Same
Tests/Consults	Refer to Home Health	Refer to social worker		
Medications/ Treatments				
Psychosocial	Reflective listening	Explore feelings about role change	Involve family in problem solving Explore realistic solutions	Reinforce role adaptations
Teaching	S/Sx to report to MD, RN, 911	Disease process care plan	Review, reinforce as needed Review alternative roles	
Activity/Safety/Self-care	Bedrest, HOB, 30–45 degrees c̄ BSC or BRP			
Nutrition				
Transfer/Discharge Coord./Case Manager		Communicate outcomes achieved to MD	Same	Same Prepare for discharge

See inside back cover for abbreviations.

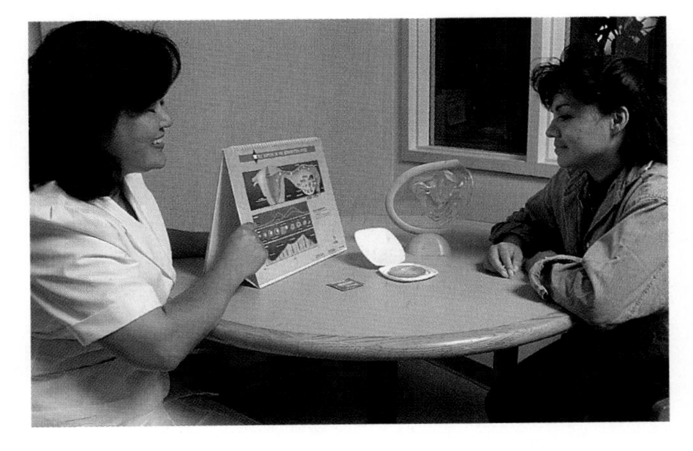

Figure 26–4. Counseling about contraceptive methods is one way that a nurse can address a patient's concerns about sexuality.

avoiding anal intercourse, can help them avoid contracting an STD. Further, providing information about the physical signs of common STDs alerts individuals when to seek care.

Impact of Crisis/Illness. Educating patients about normal responses to illness and other types of stress promotes new coping patterns and averts escalation of stress to crisis. For instance, a patient experiencing a severe emotional loss who is bothered by disruptions in sleep or eating patterns may fail to associate these symptoms with the crisis; not recognizing this connection may amplify the associated anxiety. Educating patients about the feelings they may experience and communicating that such feelings are normal may reduce the inner sense of turmoil and encourage further verbalization and self-disclosure.

Patient Support Organizations. Patients at risk for alterations in self-expression can benefit from information about patient support organizations, agencies or groups such as church groups, secular

TABLE 26-10. SITUATIONAL CRISES AFFECTING SELF-EXPRESSION

Situational Event/Stressor	Crisis	Nursing Approaches
Birth of new infant	1. Low self-esteem in mothering role 2. Inadequate support from family 3. Lack of knowledge about child care	1. Encourage verbalization of inadequate feelings 2. Encourage family intervention to strengthen support base 3. Provide health teaching/parent class to increase knowledge base
Loss of job	1. Self-esteem changes resulting from loss of role 2. Inadequate problem-solving skills	1. Promote self-esteem–building activities 2. Explore resources with patient for job search and/or training, eg, vocational rehabilitation counselor, job retraining seminar
Diagnosis of physical illness	1. Body image changes 2. Temporary loss of leisure pursuits 3. Interruption of interpersonal network	1. Assist patient to work through feelings associated with body image changes 2. Promote realistic adaptation and assist patient in exploring substitute activities 3. Provide support to patient and encourage continued contact with significant others

support groups, or local clubs. These community systems frequently have services that support patients' coping. For example, a patient who is suddenly widowed may find a great deal of support and assistance in a self-help group such as Suddenly Alone—a group that helps people cope with the initial stages of grief and assists them to rebuild their lives and social networks. See Internet Resources at the end of the chapter.

Screening

Screening for risks can be done during group-oriented screening programs targeted to identify the needs of a specific population or in one-to-one encounters with patients. In reviewing patients' personal, family, and social history, nurses can identify areas of potential risk that may require preventive implementation. As discussed earlier, poor eye contact, low voice volume, or an unkempt appearance may indicate an emerging self-esteem or body image problem. Early signs of coping problems include changes in social patterns such as withdrawal from social interaction or meaningful activities, less effective functioning in various roles, and sexual disinterest. Group-oriented screening, such as breast cancer screening programs, and standard wellness inventories for knowledge assessment provide nurses opportunities to interact with patients who are at risk for self-expression problems and to elicit data about risk factors.

TABLE 26-11. MATURATIONAL CRISES AFFECTING SELF-EXPRESSION

Stage of Maturation or Development	Crisis	Nursing Approaches
Adolescence	Development of secondary sex characteristics leading to body image changes	Encourage verbalization of feelings of private self related to body changes Provide education about sexuality, normal secondary sex characteristics, and responsible sexual expression
Adult/middle age	Retirement with loss of role and self-esteem	Discourage withdrawal Explore alternative activities that bring life satisfaction and build self-esteem, eg, volunteer work
Late adulthood	Isolation and loneliness as a result of chronic illness	Explore resources to decrease withdrawal, eg, senior centers, church, volunteer work, support groups Encourage contact with significant others, building new social network

Risk factors include physical, developmental, environmental, age-related, familial, or lifestyle changes, such as hospitalization, the onset of a severe or chronic illness, loss of social contacts, sudden roles changes, and changes in support systems or socioeconomic resources, as well as developmental milestones such as marriage, career choice, childbirth, and retirement. Familial problems manifested in parental overcontrol or inability to set limits may also result in acting out by children.

Age-related Approaches

Preventive measures are appropriate to address possible problems in self-expression throughout the life cycle. Approaches include anticipatory teaching directed at promoting healthy self-expression. Examples of age-appropriate approaches are presented in Table 26–12.

- *Infants and toddlers.* Consistent, sensitive, loving care by the mother or caretaker lays the foundation of trust and is essential to a healthy self-image. Nurses can teach parents about the importance of self-esteem and the conditions that promote healthy self-concept.
- *School-age children.* The child's sense of self continues to develop during preschool and school years. Parents need to understand the importance of creating a stable environment, which is essential to the development of their child's self-esteem and self-concept. A parental dyad that is free of excessive tension, promotes autonomy in the young child, provides adequate attention, affection, and consistent and firm rules, reinforces positive behavior, and gives the young child ample positive appraisals will foster a stable environment for the young child. Providing parents with information about family roles and normal family conflicts (ie, sibling rivalry) promotes improved parenting skills.
- *Adolescents.* The rapid growth during adolescence may cause fluctuations in body image, self-esteem, and self-concept. As adolescents become more independent, they are confronted with life choices involving leisure activities, school curriculum, peers and friends, and sexual choices. The need for individuality is particularly great during this stage. Rejection of parental values and beliefs can lead to role conflicts and family adjustment problems. Anticipatory teaching can help to prevent family crises at this stage.
- *Young and middle-aged adults.* During early adulthood, individuals continue to experience changes in self-concept. Rossan suggests that many changes in identity result from changes in social settings and reflected appraisals from others.[130] The developmental tasks of early adulthood include choosing a career, choosing a partner, starting a family, and building additional meaningful activities; all are areas for potential risk to self-expression. Even the process of decision making in building a life structure may present a risk to some patients. For example, ambivalence about career choice or educational path may threaten self-esteem. Counseling patients who are faced with overwhelming life decisions can help prevent problems in self-expression. Nurses often encounter individuals who are making life choices. The anxiety surrounding decision making sometimes provokes an emotional crisis, which interferes with carrying out the decision. Nurses are in a position to identify such problems, to provide patients with opportunities to disclose and examine confusing feelings, and to refer patients for further counseling.
- *Older adults.* Late adulthood holds potential for change and growth in many areas. Often this stage of development also includes multiple losses. Retirement, the "empty nest" syndrome as children grow up and leave home, death of family

TABLE 26–12. PREVENTIVE NURSING IMPLEMENTATION ACROSS THE LIFE SPAN

Developmental Stage	Nursing Approach
Infant/toddler	Educate parents about needs of infant or toddler: establishing trust and a nurturing environment and promoting normal developmental tasks
Child	Provide health teaching to parents about body image, beginning separation, self-expression needs, socialization needs, and self-concept formation Educate about need for physical mastery and health and safety maintenance
Adolescent	Provide health teaching to adolescents and parents about continued growth of self-concept, identity formation, and body image integration Educate about sex role, sexuality, need for leisure pursuits, and continued development of interpersonal relationships Educate about tobacco, drug, and alcohol use, fertility, and contraception
Young and middle-aged adults	Provide health teaching about role acquisition and changes, normal sexual expression, and intimacy needs, review safe sex measures Educate about life structure, choices, and decisions (eg, work, marriage)
Older adult	Provide health teaching about changing life structure, body image changes, role changes, response to losses, grieving, and self-esteem changes

and friends, and economic changes may occur. During this stage, patients are at risk for problems with social adjustment, loss of self-esteem, loss of roles, loss of meaningful activities, losses related to health changes, and losses of significant others. Indeed, the losses may be so many that they accumulate to cause overwhelming grief.[131] The existential issue of meaninglessness may be particularly salient during this stage.[132] Nurses can assist patients to redefine meaning and restructure significant activities during this period. Approaching older patients with respect communicates that they are viewed as capable adults who can make their own choices and promotes a positive self-concept and sense of individuality. Hospitalized older patients require privacy and should be encouraged to adorn their space with personal, meaningful belongings. The nurse's role also includes assisting older patients to adapt to the changes occurring at this stage of life.

Making Referrals to Community Agencies

Patients identified as being at risk may require special, ongoing assistance. It may be necessary to refer patients to an agency of professionals who deal with their area of difficulty. There are a variety of community agencies that provide support to patients experiencing an alteration in self-expression. Community-based agencies include local home health care services and crisis intervention centers, drug or alcohol centers, family planning agencies, and day-care agencies. Voluntary agencies encompass the American Cancer Society, American Lung Association, Arthritis Foundation, Hospice Association, and local parent teaching classes. Self-help organizations include Alcoholics Anonymous, Cocaine Anonymous, Overeaters Anonymous, Codependents Anonymous, Suddenly Alone, and Parents Without Partners. Governmental agencies that might assist include unemployment agencies, vocational rehabilitation services, Social Security, and the public health service. By collaborating with patients to identify risks, nurses can facilitate the acceptance of and willingness to follow through on the referral.

Home Health Care

Much health care today is performed in the home, and more nurses than ever before work in the home setting. Increasingly, agencies and managed care organizations are integrating mental health services into their home care programs.[133,134] Nurses therefore find themselves screening patients, particularly the elderly and home-bound chronically ill, and their family members for needs such as grief counseling, depression treatment, family dynamics and coping assessment, crisis identification and intervention, motivation to participate in recreational activity, and monitoring patient adherence to medication and treatment plans. As the need for health care economy continues, nurses undoubtedly will find their preventive role in home health care greatly expanded. At present nurses in home health regularly incorporate therapeutic listening and other principles of therapeutic communication, described in Chapter 15, into home health nursing plans to assist patients with the numerous self-expression problems that may accompany illness.

SUPPORTIVE CARE

Supportive care focuses on patients whose situation places them at high risk for developing self-expression problems or who may already have concerns about some aspect of self-expression and whose problems may be alleviated or their impact reduced through early intervention. Patients entering the hospital for an illness, those receiving a diagnosis of a serious disease or who have recently experienced a death (or other significant loss), patients whose chronic illnesses have entered a progressive phase, and patients facing body-altering surgery, trauma, or death are all examples of those requiring supportive care. Supportive nursing implementation focuses on preventing further disruption and minimizing the impact of early changes.

Not all patients who demonstrate problems experience crisis as a result. Indeed, those who receive supportive care usually recover and go on to cope with their situation. For example, a patient who experiences body changes due to illness may already have sought out appropriate resources (such as a support group for diabetics) and applied effective problem-solving skills to overcome a self-expression problem. The nurse need only survey the patient's problems, needs, and risk factors related to self-expression and assess the patient's resources for coping effectively. In some cases, however, the patient may require short-term assistance to overcome a problem.

Caring for Patients with a Self-esteem Problem

The nursing care of patients with a self-esteem problem begins with a nurse–patient relationship that is collaborative, caring, warm, genuine and respectful. Nurses assist by employing implementations directed toward helping the patient achieve a realistic self appraisal and by helping patients acknowledge their own positive attributes. They contribute by honestly pointing out patients' strengths and successes. Nurses can provide a model for patients by accepting compliments and positive appraisals of their own behaviors and actions without minimizing or devaluing them. Nurses can also assist patients to accept tasks or accomplishments that will provide sources of positive feedback.

Body image, a central component of self-concept, can be altered by a variety of physical, psychosocial, and cultural factors. (See the discussion of *Body Image Disturbance* in Section 2.) Patients with physical body changes such as those undergoing surgery and chemotherapy for breast cancer often need assistance to develop a realistic perception of their body image.[135] Nurses help such patients by providing them with understanding and support as they explore their feelings about their newly altered body and by supporting behaviors that suggest a positive adaptation to their body change (eg, interest in self-preservation, interest in interpersonal relationships). Further, patients often benefit from the additional support provided by participating in groups of other individuals who have similar body changes.

Caring for Patients with a Social Interaction Problem

Several etiologies, as previously noted, may contribute to problems in social interaction. A collaborative nurse–patient relationship, one using effective interpersonal communication and conveying genuineness, empathy, and warmth, promotes trust and self-disclosure, and thus is an important component of care for patients displaying a social interaction problem. The nurse's role includes promoting appropriate social contact with others. In a study of the institutionalized elderly, Nelson identified common social support sources, among them spouses, relatives, friends, neighbors, health care providers, counselors, and ministers.[136] These provide a basis for assisting patients to establish or reestablish adequate social interaction and social support. Guidelines for promoting increased social interaction include the following:

- With the patient, plan times during which visiting is convenient.
- Encourage social contact via phone or letter with important persons.
- Help the patient identify barriers to initiating contact with others.
- Assist the patient to initiate new contacts for support when appropriate (eg, contacting clergy).
- Encourage self-disclosure in areas that might interfere with making contact (eg, embarrassment, humiliation, fears of rejection, feelings of being a burden).
- Educate the patient about the need for support systems to assist in coping with crisis and promoting self-esteem.
- Encourage contact with other patients, when appropriate, to reduce isolation or loneliness.

Caring for Patients with Concerns About Sexuality

Because self-esteem and body image are integral aspects of sexuality, patients with illnesses affecting aspects of the body involved with sexual expression often require nursing care to support healthy sexual functioning. Sexuality also is a concern to many patients hospitalized for cancer and other illnesses. Indeed, a recent study of women with breast cancer found that sexual concerns ranked in importance with subjects' concerns about treatment options and likelihood of a cure.[137] Talking with patients who express concerns about sexuality helps the nurse understand the specific causes for these concerns as well as their effect on the patient's sexual behavior patterns and is an important part of care. To help the patient with sexual concerns, it is important that nurses examine their own attitudes and beliefs about sexuality. The following guidelines will assist nurses who care for patients with concerns about sexuality:

- Work toward developing comfort in discussing sexuality with patients.
- Develop a nonjudgmental, caring, and supportive attitude.
- Avoid imposing your own values and beliefs concerning sexuality on patients.
- Develop sufficient knowledge to understand the effects of disease on sexuality and sexual functioning.
- Become familiar with the language used by patients to express sexuality and sexual functioning.
- Acquire experience in interviewing patients regarding sexual matters.
- Provide a private, quiet, and relaxed atmosphere for discussion.
- Include the patient's significant other, whenever possible.
- Prevent premature disclosure; avoid overwhelming or rushing the patient to disclose more than he or she is comfortable disclosing.[138]

The PLISSIT Model

The PLISSIT model, a classical model described by Annon in 1976, provides a useful framework for the care of patients with concerns about sexuality.[139] The model outlines four levels of implementation: permission, limited information, specific suggestions, and intensive therapy. Generally, nursing care addresses only the first three levels of implementation. Nurses must recognize the limits of their own personal comfort, knowledge, and expertise in handling problems related to sexuality and know when to refer the patient to the appropriate professional.

- *Permission.* Patients sometimes fear that feelings, thoughts, or concerns related to sex are inappropriate; providing patients with an opportunity to address their fears and concerns related to sex may help resolve problems with a potential to hinder the patient's recovery.
- *Limited information.* Information about normal anatomy, physiology, and the effects of certain medications or diseases on sexual functioning can assist patients to change behaviors and attitudes about sexuality and accept limitations.
- *Specific suggestions.* Nurses may be able to suggest courses of action to improve a patient's sexual functioning or sexual satisfaction.[140] Referral to a support group may be indicated.
- *Intensive therapy.* Referral to an appropriate professional is indicated when the preceding interventions are not helpful or have not met a patient's goals. Marital therapy, sex therapy, or urologic/gynecologic intervention require expertise outside of the scope of the nurse's role.

Caring for Patients Who Are Having Difficulty Coping

Coping with stressors, illness, or life changes necessitates resourcefulness and an ability to problem-solve. Assessment of patients' responses to stressors helps nurses' determine whether the patient's coping behaviors are effective. Nurses can assist patients by helping them develop alternative coping mechanisms as well as evaluate whether new coping behaviors are effective. For example, a patient coping with work stress by drinking excessively may be encouraged to attend an Alcoholics Anonymous meeting after-which nurse and patient review the patient's response to the meeting and what was learned. Nurses also can teach patients how to recognize signs of stress and how to reduce stress to a manageable level through exercise, meditation, or relaxation techniques.

Caring for Patients with a Role Performance Problem

Patients displaying a serious change in health status usually experience some interruption in role performance. The personal, family, and social history provides the nurse with information about the roles the patient is engaged in, the responsibilities these entail and their centrality to the patient's self-concept and life satisfaction. Role performance problems include *role stress* (role demands exceeding patient skill), *role conflict* (role demands that conflict with one another), *role overload* (roles demands exceeding patient resources), and *role ambiguity* (role demands that are unclear). Nurses can assist by teaching patients how to adapt to and cope with role changes that occur as a result of illness and the concepts of role sharing and role negotiation to reduce the stress.[141] Once the patient's limitations are identified, nurses can assist the patient to define realistic role expectations congruent with the changes caused by illness. At times, referral to a family therapist or other professional may be necessary to assist families in adjusting to a family member's altered role performance.

Caring for Patients Who Are Faced with a Difficult Life Choice

Levinson and colleagues describe the importance of life choices in building an individual's life structure.[2] The process of making major life choices involves change, which is often stressful. Patients undergoing life transitions may experience a state of crisis as they deal with the implications of their situation. Emotions may include ambivalence, uncertainty, fear, sadness, depression, or anger. The act of making a choice may result in a gain, but also frequently a loss. For example, in choosing to leave a job to return to school, the individual gains the means to realize a goal, but also loses the resources provided by the job. Even a desired change, one expected to provide a pathway to fulfillment, may evoke an emotional crisis because it involves giving up something. Ambivalence associated with choice making may itself create problems in coping (eg, sleep disruption, poor concentration, social withdrawal). Nurses assist patients facing a difficult life choice by inviting them to verbalize their conflicting emotions. Such discussions may help patients clarify their feelings as they gain a perspective on what is important to them. The nurse's role is not to suggest a course of action, but to prepare the patient to make his or her own choice. Nurses may also assist patients by raising questions regarding aspects of the decision the patient may have overlooked. For example, a patient who is considering moving to another city to obtain a job may not have considered all of the ramifications of the move. The nurse can ask questions to help the patient examine these factors. For example, the nurse might ask, "How long do you think your finances will last while you're looking for work?" or "What might happen if you don't find work?" Assisting patients to make decisions without making the decision for them is an important nursing skill and one often needed in providing supportive nursing care.

Caring for Newly Hospitalized Patients

Hospitalization has the potential to disrupt many dimensions of the patient's life—physical, social, intellectual, sexual, and psychological. For some patients, the loss of control of their daily routine is the most disruptive aspect of hospitalization. Other patients may perceive the loss of privacy, the loss of contact with significant others, or the loss of valued roles as more disruptive. Nurses must understand the impact of hospitalization on the individual patient and use that understanding to plan approaches that will minimize the negative effects of the experience. Anxiety may be reduced by explaining hospital routines, procedures, and tests and, whenever possible, by inviting patients to participate in the management of their care. The following are guidelines for supporting patients' self-expression during hospitalization:

- Address the patient by name. Ask the patient how he or she prefers to be addressed.
- Express interest in the information the patient reveals during history taking. Take the opportunity to share a few items about yourself that communicate who you are as a person and that might be likely to create a social bridge to the patient.
- Invite the patient to continue wearing his or her own clothing if the patient is not acutely ill and no immediate diagnostic or therapeutic procedures are to be performed.
- Invite the patient to display personal artifacts (photos, greeting cards, small figurines, and so on) at the bedside.
- Ensure that the patient and the patient's significant others understand visiting policies and know about facilities for visitors such as parking, cafeterias, and rooming-in arrangements. Provide space for patient and family interaction.
- Discuss daily schedules with the patient so that he or she will have a mental framework of the day's activities and can make appropriate arrangements for support from significant others as well as prepare himself or herself mentally.
- Make an effort to identify the patient's identity reference groups and express interest in the role identities from which the patient gains self-esteem.
- Protect the patient's physical privacy by closing the door to his or her hospital room and knocking before entering and by providing and using screens or drapes during all diagnostic, therapeutic, or caregiving procedures.
- Protect the patient's psychological privacy by giving the patient time to reveal aspects of self and personal situation at his or her own pace.
- Communicate warmth and empathy while providing the patient with opportunities for self-disclosure.
- Offer to assist (eg, to comb the patient's hair, shave the patient, put on makeup) if the patient has difficulty with self-care activities.
- Inform the patient about in-hospital church services or clergy available for spiritual counseling.
- Use humor when possible to relieve the tension associated with the embarrassments of hospitalization.

Caring for Patients Who Receive a Diagnosis of Serious Illness

Patients who have recently been diagnosed with a serious illness usually experience many threats to their self-expression; among these are shock and anxiety. Shock is the momentary or lasting numbing emotional response that often accompanies traumatic news such as the loss of a loved one or a diagnosis of serious or life-threatening illness. Patients experiencing shock may appear to be in a normal state, but if asked to describe their inner feelings use phrases such as "I'm in a fog," "I can't think clearly," or "I'm numb—I can't feel much of anything." The following guidelines are relevant in caring for patients experiencing shock in response to traumatic news:

- Do not rush the patient through this stage; provide the patient with time to integrate the information.
- Offer the patient support and comfort, both physical and emotional.
- Provide the patient with opportunities to describe what he or she is experiencing.
- Anticipate expressions of emotion and provide the patient with opportunities for catharsis.
- Use nonverbal gestures of support, such as staying with the patient who expresses emotion and providing tissues for the patient who becomes tearful.
- Assist the patient to define areas in which he or she needs assistance (eg, contacting a family member).
- Recognize that the patient may at first deny the diagnosis, but do not attempt to alter the patient's coping pattern; in time the denial will give way to growing awareness.
- Monitor the patient's level of distress by inviting self-disclosure.

Patients who receive a diagnosis of serious illness usually experience a period of anxiety that progresses in intensity. They may deny the threatening information at first or fail to recognize its implications. They may experience fear of dying or worry that they will endure suffering and pain. Because patient responses to the news of illness vary, nurses must explore each individual's responses and the meaning of the diagnosis to that person. That is achieved by promoting patient self-disclosure. Nurses facilitate self-disclosure by the following approaches:

- Provide a private, comfortable, unhurried environment.
- Convey a warm, concerned, interested, and permissive attitude.
- Listen actively to the patient's concerns, beliefs, and attitudes regarding his illness.
- Use open-ended verbal techniques that encourage patients to expand.
- Demonstrate empathy by accurately reflecting back to the patient the feelings he or she expresses.
- Recognize symptoms of anxiety that may interfere with self-disclosure.
- Communicate in an unobtrusive way, and without interrupting the flow of the patient's disclosure, any personal experiences you may have had with the patient's problem. It is not necessary to volunteer the specifics of the experience. Patients who desire to know will respond with their own inquiries.

Mischel suggests that managing the uncertainty associated with an illness and its treatment may be an essential task of adapting to illness. In fact, patients coping with the uncertainty of an illness use various coping mechanisms, among them, information seeking.[106] Information commonly sought by women who receive a diagnosis of breast cancer, for example, incorporates facts on stage of illness, likelihood of a cure, and treatment options.[137] Nurses should make themselves available to assist patients in their efforts to cope. Nursing approaches include the following:

- Encourage patients' self-disclosures regarding their expectations for the outcome of their illness.
- Provide clarification, education, and health teaching as necessary according to collaborative agency protocols about the specifics of the patient's illness.
- Talk to patients about the resources and support networks available.
- Encourage patients to verbalize their feelings in response to the information provided.
- Monitor patients' responses to teaching. Do not provide more information than the patient is ready to receive. Watch for behavior indicating stress; for example, the patient may appear distractable or change the subject.
- Using the guidelines above, support patients' need to experience the normal emotions, such as shock, fear, denial, and sadness, associated with a diagnosis of illness. (These emotions are discussed in more detail later under *Restorative Care*.)
- Explore the patient's need for additional support (eg, from clergy, nurses, support groups, therapist).
- Assist the patient to develop coping patterns for dealing with role changes or other necessary life-structure adaptations.
- Talk to the patient about future needs. This will also aid the problem-solving process in coping with a future crisis.

Caring for Patients Who Anticipate Body-altering Surgery

To anticipate the impact of surgery on a patient, the nurse needs to understand how patients view themselves and their bodies. Nurses may ask patients what they currently think of their body, what they like best about their body, and what aspect of their body makes them feel the best about themselves. They may also ask patients to describe the ways in which they think they will be different after surgery, what abilities related to their body they expect to change, what limitations they imagine living with after surgery, and what kind of scarring or disfigurement they expect.

Patients facing body-altering surgery commonly experience a variety of strong emotions (see *Caring for Patients Who Are Grieving a Loss*.) Assisting patients to verbalize their emotional responses to anticipated changes communicates support and understanding. Folz[142] describes several useful strategies for working with patients at risk for body image changes. One important strategy is patient-to-patient visitation programs. Such programs ensure that a patient undergoing breast or ostomy surgery, for example, is visited preoperatively by someone who has had the same surgery and is coping well. Such visits can be enormously helpful to patients anticipating surgery by assisting them to resolve concerns they may have about the effect of surgery on their self-presentation. An effective postoperative strategy is to employ desensitization techniques. Such techniques help patients gradually adjust to aversive stimuli such as surgical body changes. Patients undergoing desensitization are slowly encouraged to address their body change, at first by providing a mirror to help the patient look at the surgical site, and then by inviting the patient to participate in the care of the wound, little by little increasing his or her role.[142]

Sexual functioning may also be affected by body image changes. Particular sensitivity is required to assist patient's to make disclosures regarding sexuality and sexual functioning. Patients may require referral to other health care professionals or sex therapists, but nurses can be helpful by assisting patients to understand the abilities and disabilities brought on by surgery and helping them adjust accordingly.[143]

Caring for Patients Who Are Chronically Ill

Patients who have illnesses that are generally incurable and last longer than several months are considered chronically ill. Such patients have special needs and are often faced with loss of health, body image, self-esteem, or sense of self-control or mastery over the environment. Commonly, they also face changes in relationships and roles, changes in lifestyle activities and leisure pursuits, and changes in sexual functioning. Chronically ill patients may also face major disruptions in lifestyle that are stressful, time consuming, fatiguing, and frustrating. Such disruptions include frequent clinic or physician visits, regular laboratory or other tests, medication trials and adjustments, and possible rehospitalizations for exacerbations of the illness. Chronically ill patients often suffer from chronic fatigue related to the illness and emotional exhaustion from coping with exacerbations and remissions. All of these variables have the potential to affect self-expression.

Encouraging patients to verbalize their feelings may assist them to deal with these feelings and will help nurses to plan appropriate implementations. Similar to patients who face body-altering surgery, chronically ill patients must cope with a variety of emotional responses. These include feelings of anger, depression, and anxiety, but also, in many cases, hopelessness. Nurses' realistic assessment of patients' health, when communicated to the patient, may help to provide a sense of hope. Patients may come to acknowledge the aspects of self-expression unaffected or minimally impaired by illness (Fig. 26–5). Often patients with chronic illness suffer from loneliness and isolation. Nurses may help by working with these patients to establish a plan to reduce their isolation and increase their social contacts. Nurses may also provide support by facilitating expression of spiritual beliefs through enlisting the help of a pastoral care representative, for example, a priest, rabbi, or minister who might be asked to visit the patient.

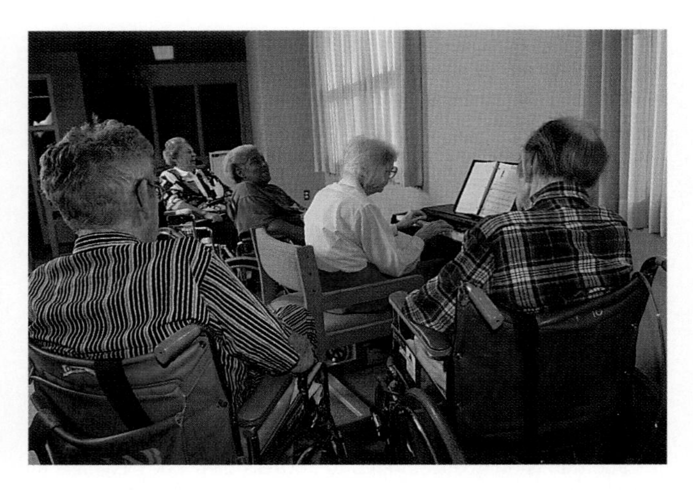

Figure 26–5. Group activities facilitate self-expression in chronically ill individuals.

Patients with chronic illness often have difficulty pacing their activity at a level appropriate to their limitation. Patients who are coping with a chronic illness may withdraw from activities that could provide a sense of meaning in their lives because of embarrassment, lack of energy, or lack of resources. Nurses can assist patients to minimize their withdrawal by emphasizing the importance of such activities to well-being and, as necessary, by helping patients reengage or identify new meaningful activities.

Patients with chronic illness require support during times of exacerbation and remission of the illness. Referrals to support groups can help meet this need. Groups like Better Breather, for patients with chronic lung disease, provide ongoing support for patients suffering the many problems associated with chronic disease.

Caring for Patients Who Receive a Terminal Diagnosis

Perhaps no threat to self-expression is greater than a diagnosis of a terminal illness. Leming and Dickinson emphasize that a patient's whole view of himself and his relationship to the world undergoes an enormous change upon receiving a terminal diagnosis.[144] Such patients experience the range of strong emotions, described under *Caring for Patients Who Are Grieving a Loss*, below, but also one that may be more pronounced in this than in other situations—the experience of shock.

Shock and disbelief are usually the first responses to a terminal diagnosis. Patients numbed by this news may appear dazed, sit motionless, cry, or demonstrate extreme behavior or mood changes. Nurses may provide support by remaining with patients, providing privacy, or assisting patients to contact family members during this emotional phase. The shock phase (impact) usually gradually gives way to acknowledgment when patients are treated with empathy and understanding. Nurses should clarify the reality of the patient's health situation. Some patients, upon hearing they have cancer, assume the illness will quickly lead to death, when in fact treatment options may significantly extend their lives. Helping patients to understand their options is a way to allay anxiety.

Patients who are terminally ill may or may not be anxious themselves but often elicit anxiety in others, including health care providers and family. The nurse's role involves, not only helping patients to identify, express, and cope with the feelings associated with receiving a terminal diagnosis, but assisting family members to do the same. Encouraging family members to visit by giving them extended visiting hours to accommodate their needs or by inviting them to room-in or dine with the patient communicates to family members that their needs and concerns are important.

Caring for Patients Who Are Grieving a Loss

Patients who are grieving a loss, whether of a body part, an aspect of self or personal identity, a treasured object, or a loved one, will generally experience a variety of intense emotions during the course of their adaptation process and often must cope with sadness, depression, anger, guilt and anxiety.[145]

Anger. A natural response whenever a person feels deprived of someone or something valued, anger is a common, normal response during grieving. It signifies an innate predisposition to find and recover what has been lost and derives from failure to recoup the loss, but also an inability to find meaning in the loss, which often results in a profound sense of injustice. A grieving person often asks, "Why me?"

Anger, hostility, and frustration are manifested in negative verbalizations, aggressive behavior, sarcasm, irritability, tension, anxiety, or withdrawal, which may be directed at the object of the loss, at the self, or at other people. Most people, including nurses, do not welcome others' expressions of anger. Grieving people therefore may fear alienating others with expressions of their bitterness and disappointment, and become isolated with their feelings, sometimes directing their anger inward. Internalized anger, in turn, leads to guilt and depression.

Dealing with anger is thus an important part of the care of the grieving. Permission to ventilate anger in the context of interaction provides an important outlet, one which carries no risk to the patient's relationships. Physical outlets, such as exercise, may also help to siphon energy otherwise available to fuel aggressive expressions. Nurses should remember, however, that individuals vary and should avoid communicating preset expectations for patients' feelings or behavior. It is also important to help significant others to understand the patient's anger and the role of anger expression in the adaptation process. Guidelines for caring for patients who expresses anger include the following:

- Help patients "get in touch" with their anger by providing feedback about how they are presenting themselves to others. Point out behaviors such as rising voice volume, furrowed brow, clenched fists, hand waving, rapid breathing, or sarcastic comments.
- Give patients time to verbalize and describe their anger.
- Explore with patients reasons for anger (avoid the use of "why" questions, which may be perceived as a challenge).
- Help patients distinguish appropriate anger expression from aggressive behavior.
- Assist patients to identify alternatives to a direct expression of anger such as exercise or other physical-release activities.
- Do not counter with a response of anger toward patients.

Anger that has been denied or suppressed for a long period is often expressed in the form of hostility. Hostility, which arises from a sense of conflict or frustration, may be expressed openly or may be oblique and subtle. A husband angry at his wife for routinely failing to be on time may express hostility by remarks such as "Can't you get a watch?" A more direct expression of the anger he feels, on the other hand, is, "I'm angry with you for keeping me waiting." Direct expressions may alleviate the pent-up anger that leads to indirect hostile expression. Guidelines for assisting patients who cope with illness by expressing hostility include the following:

- Recognize the patient's hostile response with a statement that conveys concern and willingness to help, such as "I sense that you are feeling troubled about something."
- Encourage the patient to identify and express the underlying anger or conflict.
- Give permission for the expression by acknowledging what you perceive to be the patient's feelings, such as, "You seem upset or angry that I kept you waiting so long."
- Demonstrate empathy with the patient's emotional state by paraphrasing what was said and what emotions are communicated.
- Do not counter with a response of hostility.

Guilt. In adapting to loss, many people experience some amount of guilt, usually in association with other strong feelings. For example, guilt may accompany feelings of anger felt toward the deceased for having died or be experienced in relation to a sense of responsibility for the loss, whatever its nature. Nurses should look for signs that their patients are experiencing guilt, often revealed in self-disparaging statements such as "We should have gone to the doctor sooner," or "If only I had been there when he got sick." The significance of guilt feelings often eludes those who are grieving. Patients may not understand, for example, that dwelling on the negative is a way of severing the ties with the object of the loss, and thus an important part of adaptation. Nurses may help by pointing this out. Moreover, people who experience guilt may be unaware of its relationship to other emotions. Thus, when a patient expresses strong emotions such as anger, it may be helpful to encourage such expressions and reassure the patient that such feelings are a normal part of grieving. Pointing out to the patient the relationship between guilt and anger is often helpful.[146]

Sadness. Feelings of sorrow, sadness, pain, and anguish are commonly associated with the experience of loss. Indeed, feelings of sadness are a hallmark of grieving. Sadness is often expressed through crying, but may be expressed through other behaviors such as a downward cast of the eyes, a blank stare, monotone or low-volume voice, or a slumped posture. Some patients fear being overcome by feelings of sadness. Others overcompensate by becoming aggressive or demanding, behaviors that hide their true vulnerability.[146] Nurses working with patients experiencing the emotion of sadness may find the following approaches helpful:

- Encourage the patient to put the feeling of sadness into words.
- Help patients understand their feelings of sadness and sorrow as part of grieving.
- Assist patients to recognize their own need for emotional release and catharsis as part of the adaptive process.
- Encourage the patient to express sadness through crying, even if the patient's crying makes you uncomfortable. Provide tissue in a nonverbal gesture of support
- Stay with the patient, but be mindful that some patients prefer solitude when crying and be prepared to provide privacy.
- Point out that, with time, the feelings of sorrow and pain will diminish.
- Be mindful of patients' limits for expressing strong emotion. Monitor patients' expressions and assist them to close conversations when it appears they may be overwhelmed by their emotion.

Self-control is an important value for most adults, and patients may need help to express emotions at a pace and with a degree of intensity consistent with their self-esteem. People who fear being overwhelmed by their sadness may distance themselves from others to avoid the embarrassment of losing control and, thus, presenting themselves in a way they will later regret.

Depression. Depression, a state marked by feelings of profound sadness accompanied by functional inactivity, is part of the grieving process, often associated with some degree of behavioral disorganization.[127] Among the symptoms of depression are:

- Weight loss or gain
- Sleep difficulties
- Decreased energy, fatigue
- Loss of interest in sex
- Anorexia
- Social withdrawal
- Dependency on others
- Lack of initiative, motivation
- Restlessness
- Agitation
- Irritability
- Confusion
- Disorganization
- Poor concentration
- Difficulty with decision making
- Tearfulness
- Sense of meaninglessness
- Loneliness
- Sadness
- Anguish
- Despair
- Hopelessness

These symptoms may manifest themselves at any time in the process of grieving. Depression may be short-lived or prolonged; it may remit, only to recur. When it promotes new patterns necessary to meet future problems, depression is adaptive. Guidelines for helping patients who are depressed include the following:

- Monitor the patient for the signs and symptoms of depression.
- Encourage the patient to express feelings—anger, guilt, sadness—associated with the loss.
- Assist the patient to identify and label specific emotions experienced; this promotes the patient's understanding of the grief experience and prevents the accumulation of emotions in an undifferentiated mass of painful stimuli.
- Encourage the patient to talk not only about the tangible aspects of his or her loss, but also the symbolic and psychosocial aspects.

Anxiety and Fear. Anxiety represents a threat to a value essential to an individual's existence and thus is a predictable experience when something is lost. Anxiety has no readily identifiable source and thus often accompanies the uncertainty associated with serious illness. Causes include unexpressed emotions or thoughts that well up during grieving, a sense of vulnerability or helplessness, distressing memories, or anticipation of mental disorganization.[146] Fear differs from anxiety by the fact that fear has an identifiable source. Patients who fear something, for example, pain or disfigurement, are able to identify a cause for their feeling. Guidelines to help the patient experiencing anxiety or fear include the following:

- Explore with the patient his or her perception of the threat.
- Provide time for self-disclosure to allow the patient to verbalize his or her fears.
- Identify aspects of the perceived problem which the patient controls and which can be changed; this process may help to reduce fear.
- Clarify areas of misinformation that may unnecessarily magnify the fears.
- Provide grieving patients with information, which may ease the uncertainty of the unknown.
- Recognize that individuals vary in their capacity to cope with information; some people require smaller amounts given at a slower pace.
- Help patients to identify realistic self-expectations and to make the adjustments appropriate under the circumstances.
- Assist family members to understand the patient's anxiety or fear. Helping significant others to understand increases the likelihood that they will be able to support the patient.[146]

Patients experiencing the stress of illness often cope by expressing strong emotions. Such reactions are sometimes viewed by nurses as "difficult" patient behavior. Such behavior may elicit anger and frustration in the nurse, leading to responses such as criticism or withdrawal from their emotionally distraught patients.[147] Expressing their own angry feelings to the patient is rarely beneficial. Further, nurses who understand the patient's emotional expression as a form of coping behavior are less likely to label patients and more likely to respond in a helpful, caring manner such as by helping the patient to work toward an understanding the reasons for his or her strong emotion. Kettles[148] stresses the value of catharsis for patients experiencing strong emotion. Nurses who withdraw from the patient fail to provide opportunities for catharsis that may benefit the patient's grieving process.

Caring for Patients Who Are Dying

Because dying often arouses a sense of helplessness in caregivers, nurses, first of all, should find outlets for their own feelings, to ensure their own capacity to cope.

Patients who are dying often seek opportunities to review their lives, recall and share important memories, and review decisions and choices they have made during their lives. The therapeutic value of "life review" as a support to the patient's own grieving cannot be underestimated. Dying patients also frequently struggle to put their affairs in order. Nurses may provide support by listening as patients plan for the future and as they talk about the decisions that must be made. A form of practical help, this also serves to alleviate the sense loss of control and loneliness that patients experience.

The patient's family and significant others may experience emotional distress and may require assistance coping as they anticipate the patient's death. They too may need to discuss the dying patient's life, the circumstances of the patient's illness, and what he or she has meant to them.[146] When grief interferes with a family member's everyday functioning, the nurse may wish to refer him or her for professional bereavement counseling.[145]

As discussed previously, patients and their families experience many emotions as they adjust to the reality of the patient's dying. The nursing care of the dying involves providing informational, familial, and social support.[107] Humphrey offers several general guidelines for nurses who care for dying patients:

- Get to know the patient as an individual.
- Facilitate meaningful discussions by assisting the patient to review the values that have meant the most during his or her life.
- Do not take over for the dying person or family, but encourage their participation in care.
- Assist the patient to maintain important relationships by providing practical supports.
- Spend adequate time with the patient.
- Monitor your own feelings to prevent being overwhelmed by accumulated emotion.

In addition, Humphrey suggests the following guidelines for working with family members of dying patients:

- Encourage open communication to the extent the family communication style allows.
- Support family members' unique identities and assist them to differentiate their own needs, legitimately experienced, from those of the dying person, for example, need for a period of solitude away from the patient.
- Assist family members to assume new roles.
- Encourage family members' expression of emotion and support them in sharing their emotions.
- Assist family members to understand pertinent information about the dying person's illness and its treatment so that they may plan for the future.
- Assist family members to recognize signs that the end is near.[107]

Acknowledging Patients' Feelings. Dying patients grieve for their loss of health, plans for the future, ability to care for self, ability to perform roles, and eventual loss of significant others. Emotional responses vary. Patients who face these losses often experience moments of awareness and terror as they engage in the internal processing that is part of grieving.

Nurses who work with dying patients have a unique opportunity to respond empathically to the varied emotions patients share. Nurses can be helpful by displaying a genuine effort to understand the unique meaning of the patient's life experience,

? CRITICAL QUERY

Kettles[148] found that the nurses in her study understood the nature of catharsis, but did not consider it a central therapeutic goal. She further found that her subjects believed displays of emotion were more appropriate for women than men. What are the implications of these findings for the care of patients undergoing body-altering medical treatments or surgery?

past and present, to the dying patient.[149] Nonverbal behaviors are powerful tools for communicating empathy. Concern for the dying patient is conveyed by the nurse's focused attention and interest, expressed through eye contact, body posture, and gesture. For example, sitting down with the patient, facing him or her in a relaxed position, communicates a desire to understand, as may a gentle touch or speaking in a softly modulated voice.

Dying patients forced to face their own mortality often fear pain, the procedures that are carried out in their care, and loss. Nurses who care for them should encourage verbalization of these fears and, when possible, assist coping by providing support and education. Feelings experienced by dying persons in addition to fear and the shock, anger, sadness, and depression already discussed, include loneliness and a desire for hope.

LONELINESS. Dying patients often experience loneliness, both from facing death and from their isolation from significant others. Zack proposes several approaches for working with patients experiencing loneliness:

- Teach significant others about the patient's needs for closeness and belonging.
- Use empathic skills, such as listening attentively and inviting the expression of feeling.
- Employ measures to conserve the patient's energy and relieve symptoms; this enables the patient to meet needs for closeness and social interaction.
- Explore use of nonsocial, creative/solitary pursuits, when indicated.[110]

In addition to the approaches above, nurses may encourage contact with significant others via the telephone and/or face-to-face visits and provide a sense of connection to others through inviting patients to display photographs at the bedside.

HOPE. Much literature on care of the dying patient stresses the importance, in our future-oriented society, of hope as a coping mechanism. Assisting patients to maintain hope in the face of a terminal diagnosis requires sensitivity on the part of the nurse. It is important to understand the patient's emotional state and knowledge of the illness situation. Understanding the patient's need for hope enables the nurse to assist the patient in maintaining hope. For many patients, hope may derive from an assurance that they are cared about, will not be alone, and will be pain free during their final hours.

Promoting Independence. Promoting independence is another aspect of the care of the dying. Encouraging the dying patient to remain independent for as long as possible promotes self-esteem and a sense of dignity. Encouraging patients' participation in decisions about their care also reinforces independence and a sense of control.

Maintaining Physical and Spiritual Comfort. Dying patients have many physical needs. The alleviation of pain is a particularly important physical need, but other important needs include skin care, oxygenation, movement, nutrition, elimination, and personal hygiene. Patients whose mobility is limited are at risk for pressure uclers and compromised respirations, but vigilant nursing care will ensure comfort and optimal physiologic functioning.

Providing spiritual comfort requires that nurses have an understanding of patients' values, belief systems, and religious affiliation (see Chap. 10). Facilitating contact with clergy may assist patients with their spiritual needs. Prayers, Bible readings, meditation, and spiritual counseling are some of the ways patients find spiritual comfort. Further, encouraging self-disclosure about such issues as the meaning of death, belief in afterlife, and feelings associated with dying may also be helpful.

Promoting an Optimal Situation for the Dying—Hospice Care. Hospice care provides a change from hospital-based curative care to palliative/supportive care and helps terminally ill patients continue their lives with minimal disruptions. Hospice care is provided in a home-like setting by a team of health care professionals and support staff specially trained in the care of the dying. Nurses should be informed about local hospice services and the scope of services available. Nurses can be helpful to patients and families by explaining the option of hospice care.

Home Health Care

Supportive home health care for self-expression problems often focuses on the elderly, whose losses are frequently multiple and who are therefore at risk for problems of grieving. The supportive role of the home health nurse is not to assist such patients directly, but to assist their family caregivers—often their spouses—in helping them cope. This role may involve helping caregivers understand their loved one's experience of illness and loss.[150] Not uncommonly, supportive home care is interrupted as a patient's health situation deteriorates, and a move to a long-term care facility becomes unavoidable. Again, the home health nurse has an important role to play during these transitions, as patients and caregivers often experience the additional losses that accompany a change in their relationship.[151] Elderly patients may experience difficulty adjusting to their new surroundings, just as their spouses may experience difficulty redefining their role as caregiver. Such problems may involve a period of grieving. During this period, home health nurses may help by applying the principles of caring for those grieving a loss, discussed previously.

RESTORATIVE CARE

Restorative care focuses on the care of patients who display a severe self-expression problem. Restorative care, like preventive and supportive care, may occur in the home, clinic, or hospital setting. Patients with severe health problems may have many problems with implications for self-expression. The nurse's role includes planning implementations to treat the existing problems as well as to prevent the progression of problems that may be detrimental to the patient.

Caring for Patients Who Grieve Dysfunctionally

Dysfunctional grief is another term for unresolved grief, that is, grief that continues for a prolonged period and interferes with an individual's adaptation to living and coping with loss. Ordinarily grief diminishes with time—although the time taken varies with the individual. While in some cases grief never completely disappears, the feelings do not interfere with an individual's functioning.[102] Dysfunctional or unresolved grief, however, is similar to a wound that fails to heal properly, and in such cases, the feelings continue to overwhelm the individual.

Causes of Unresolved Grief. Unresolved grief results from a variety of social and psychological factors. The causes include the following:[152]

- *Social negation of loss.* Ordinarily members of a person's social network are supportive following losses, such as the loss of a parent or a child. Some losses accompanied by grief, however, may not be recognized by society. These include losses associated with abortion, miscarriage, the death of parent or child surrogates (substitutes), or of one in a relationship not always socially acknowledged, such as that of unmarried lovers (homosexual or heterosexual). Because such losses may not be recognized, other people may not offer the social support to the grieving they otherwise would.
- *Losses deemed inappropriate for social acknowledgment.* Some losses may be acknowledged, but because of their nature, deemed inappropriate to discuss. These include deaths caused by the bereaved either intentionally or accidentally and death by suicide. Such deaths often leave the bereaved feeling embarrassed, ashamed, or humiliated and are commonly avoided as topics of social conversation.
- *Social isolation.* Social isolation, which has many causes, can interfere with an individual's ability to find the social support necessary for griefwork. Many elderly, for example, are confined to nursing homes and lack a social network, thus limiting their social resources in a time of need.
- *Lack of opportunity to grieve.* Under ideal conditions the bereaved are permitted to give up some responsibilities to take time to grieve. However, many situations and make it necessary for some individuals to continue in their usual roles without outside assistance. Forced to carry the burdens of everyday living in addition to dealing with grief, some individuals fail to grieve.
- *Uncertainty over loss.* In some situations, it is unclear whether a person has actually died (kidnapped children, soldiers missing in action, comatose patients on long-term life support), and thus it is difficult for relatives to begin the process of grieving.
- *Guilt.* People who are prone to guilt or who feel intensely ambivalent toward the deceased may have difficulty grieving. They may unconsciously anticipate an experience of enormous guilt should the process of grieving begin. Often individuals who fail to grieve feel a sense of responsibility for the death through something they did or failed to do.[152]
- *Reawakening of an old loss.* Some people are unable to grieve a current loss because they have not dealt with a previous unresolved loss and, at some level of awareness, may fear that acknowledging a current loss will reawaken the pain of the old loss.
- *Multiple losses.* Individuals who experience multiple losses simultaneously or close in time may have difficulty grieving because they are psychologically overwhelmed.
- *Individual resistance to grieving.* Some individuals resist grieving because they view grieving as a sign of weakness, fear a loss of emotional control, or fear their grief will hurt other people.

Identifying Patients with Unresolved Grief

Several characteristics may help nurses recognize persons who experience unresolved grief:[152]

- Manifestations and symptoms of depression.
- Experience of prolonged grief in the past.
- Expressions of guilt, self-reproach; panic attacks; physical symptoms such as choking sensations, or shortness of breath.
- Physical symptoms similar those manifested by the dead person—often those manifested during the terminal illness.
- Searching behavior—looking for something that cannot be found.
- Difficulty remembering dates that are anniversaries in the life of the deceased.
- Statements indicating the death occurred yesterday, even though it may have been years ago.
- Unwillingness to remove the material possessions of the deceased—refusal to give away or pack the deceased's clothes.
- Diminished participation in religious and other ceremonial activities such as visits to the grave, participation in memorial services.
- Inability to discuss the deceased without crying.

Patients who suffer from unresolved grief rarely identify their problem as grief, but instead complain of depression or difficulty with interpersonal relationships. Nurses must be alert to the possibility of unresolved grief and confirm or disconfirm that possibility through the health history.

Implementation for Unresolved Grief

The goal of care is to help patients with unresolved grief accomplish the griefwork they previously had been unable to complete. However, in many clinical settings, nurses may have insufficient time to fully address the problem. Therefore, one of the nurse's most important roles is to encourage the patient to seek support in the form of bereavement counseling.

The process of getting the patient appropriate support may be complicated by the fact that many patients fail to recognize their grief, and thus it may be necessary to help patients identify the nature of the problem before any action can be taken. In settings where there is time to assist patients with griefwork, there are several ways in which the nurse may be helpful. These include the following:

- Encourage the patient to express painful emotions when they surface.
- Encourage the patient to recollect the deceased through inquiring or speaking about the deceased or reviewing photos and other memorabilia. It is acceptable for the nurse to ask questions such as, "What kind of a person was your husband?" "What did he look like?" "How long was he ill?" "When did he die?" Such questions encourage recall so that catharsis can be achieved.
- Support the patient as he or she expresses ambivalent feelings by acknowledging the feelings and putting them into context for the patient. Use soft words. The patient may be unwilling to open up if the nurse makes reference to "anger," "hate," or "hostility," but may be willing to discuss feelings of "disappointment," "irritation," or "annoyance."

Once patients have grieved their losses, they generally experience a change in their feelings.[152] Sadness diminishes; the bereaved are able to discuss the deceased without losing control; holidays and other occasions become enjoyable again; searching behavior ceases; the deceased is remembered more positively.

It is never too late to grieve a loss. Anderson described a case of unresolved grief that was grieved over four decades after the death occurred.[153] Thus, sharing pain long suppressed can have therapeutic effects for the individuals involved.

Helping Patients at High Risk for Unresolved Grief

The AIDS epidemic in the United States and elsewhere is significant, not only for the lives taken each year, but also for the number of bereavements created. Because of the social stigma attached to AIDS, the AIDS bereaved, especially the partners of deceased gay men who never publicly acknowledged their orientation, may find themselves excluded from the social rituals of bereavement.[154] Such individuals are at high risk for unresolved grief. Nurses who care for patients dying of AIDS may be in the best position to offer support to their significant others. Nurses may provide assistance by being available and by helping the dying and their partners to express their grief at their own pace and in their own way.

Caring for Patients Who Deny Illness

Denying illness is not the same as maintaining hope. Denial involves the inability to accurately integrate and use information about one's health status. Denial serves a useful function in the early stages of illness but can be detrimental as illness progresses. Patients who deny illness may not seek treatment that, if provided early, could speed or ensure recovery. After establishing that the patient is in a state of complete or partial denial, nurses should work with such patients to facilitate acceptance. The first step is to encourage self-disclosure so that the nurse may better understand what the illness experience means to the patient. Some patients may need information about the illness to understand the implications of the diagnosis. Others may need help in working through their fears about the illness or its impact on various aspects of their lives.

Caring for Patients Unable to Accept Body Changes

As discussed above, many illnesses and medical treatments cause profound changes in body function and appearance. Cancer, for example, may require medication or surgery that alters a person's appearance. Sometimes the results are unsightly, even though the treatment itself may be life-saving. Such changes represent an assault on a person's body image and self-concept and, in our society, with its emphasis on wholeness, are difficult for many people to accept. Some individuals, however, may be unable to accept the reality of an altered appearance and may present a wide variety of needs—physical, psychological, and social—that, if unmet, increase the risk of adaptation failure.

Care of individuals at risk begins after diagnosis, before any treatments are rendered, as patients are given information about their disease and what to expect from its treatment. It continues during the treatment phase as the patient is assisted physically and psychologically through the ordeal and its aftermath. Even so, patients may have questions about their disease or surgery that go unanswered.[155] Frequently these questions concern issues related to sexuality and how they will function as a social person.[156]

Caregiving during treatment is usually oriented around the patient's immediate physical needs. As the patient's condition improves and the patient becomes aware of the profound changes in his or her body, the staff may have redirected its energies to others more acutely ill, leaving the patient to cope with the shock of the new reality alone. Because patients are often unable to communicate their concerns, busy staff members may assume they are coping well. Such patients often experience a period depression upon discharge. Restorative care should therefore address emotional needs regarding body changes as well as physical care. Assistance to deal with problems of body image and self-concept includes providing information on common physical and psychological symptoms and a time frame for measuring one's progress.

Identifying Patients at Risk. Nurses make an important contribution by identifying individuals at risk for an adaptation problem. Denial is a common response in the phase leading up to treatment and may or may not signify impending adaptation problems. Nevertheless, patients who seem to be unable to absorb information or who seem completely unaware of the reality of their situation should be monitored closely for signs of adaptation problems following treatment.

One of the most important signs of an impending problem is the patient's reaction to the altered body part. Some patients completely ignore the altered area, declining to look at or touch it. They may act as if nothing were different. While such behavior may be adaptive in the acute phase of recovery, persistent inability to acknowledge a change should be regarded as a problem. Patients likely to encounter problems are those who have mutilating changes. Northouse studied women undergoing mastectomy (breast removal) and found that their reactions varied considerably.[157] Nearly one half reported looking at their incision within 1 to 3 days after surgery, while in the hospital. Another one third viewed their incisions within the first 2 weeks after returning home; the remaining women first looked at their incision between 2 and 4 weeks later. All had seen the incision by 1 month after surgery.

Adaptation to body changes takes time. Persistent inability to look at, touch, or care for the affected body part, however, is a sign of an adaptation failure and is an indication that the patient is suffering from an unmet need. With proper care, most patients will adapt within several months of surgery. However, persistent denial or resistance to acknowledging change beyond this period should be regarded as an indicator that the patient needs professional assistance.

Assisting Patients to Accept a Body Change. Readiness is a factor in the progression toward health. Some women in Northouse's sample were reluctant to look at their incisions even though they had the opportunity do so. They described a need to "work up the nerve."[157] One said, "I didn't want to look." Another said, "I was scared and didn't know what to expect." Many were concerned about what their husbands' reactions would be, and husbands in the study reported being unprepared for what to expect.[157]

Readiness can be encouraged by helping patients progress through the grieving process associated with body changes. Encouraging patients to express their feelings before, during, and after treatment can facilitate the grieving process. Often catharsis will help the individual prepare to acknowledge deficits that are real and permanent. Nurses also may be helpful by teaching patients about what they should expect from their altered body part. Such teaching should be paced according to the individual's ability to integrate the information.

- Begin by presenting small pieces of information, and gradually build a foundation. Patients able to handle information at a faster pace will generally respond with questions for clarification or make requests for more information.
- Clarify information that patients have previously received. Sometimes patients have significant misunderstandings that may inhibit readiness to progress.

- Gently encourage patients to consider their affected body part. Patients who are paralyzed, for example, may benefit from information about how their injury or disease is affecting various body functions.
- Gently encourage patients to care for the affected region of the body.
- Develop realistic short-term goals for the patient's participation, beginning with a small, simple activity and gradually progressing to more complex aspects.
- Invite the patient to participate in the decision-making process; this also encourages the patient to become involved in care.
- Make contracts with patients who are reticent to join in caregiving activities.
- Involve family members in decision making and care planning. Information is helpful, not only for patients, but also for family members.
- Encourage family members to express their feelings. Sometimes this may mean interacting privately with spouses and other close relatives to assist them in coming to terms with their own feelings.
- Encourage patients to interact with others who have similar illnesses and have successfully undergone similar treatments. Patients often derive strength from seeing others who have adapted successfully to what they are experiencing and feel less isolated and alone when given a chance to talk to them.
- Be sensitive to patients' sexual concerns by gently acknowledging their importance and by implicitly or explicitly inviting patients to ask questions on these topics and to express their feelings.
- Monitor patients' needs for ongoing counseling.

By having the opportunity to address the issues involved, patients may be helped to adapt to major body changes. Those who have a profound body change may benefit from ongoing group or individual counseling during the course of recovery. Whenever possible, such support should be encouraged and provided.

Caring for Patients With a Sexual Dysfunction

The care of patients with a sexual dysfunction builds on the approaches outlined earlier. The etiology of the sexual dysfunction will determine appropriate nursing approaches. As noted in the earlier discussion of etiologies, childhood development, lack of role modeling, and religious and values conflicts may influence an individual's sexual functioning. If a sexual dysfunction is suspected or identified, a thorough sexual history is warranted to identify a long-term or situational problem. The information gathered through the sexual history enables the nurse to determine whether referral is appropriate, an important step since problem resolution often necessitates referral to other providers, such as sex therapists. General approaches for the patient with a sexual dysfunction problem include the following:

- Identify the obstacles as perceived by the patient to satisfactory sexual functioning—whether illness, psychological conflicts, loss of physiologic function, anxiety, problems in a relationship, partner rejection, or other sexual fears.
- Provide opportunities for the patient to discuss sexual concerns.
- Provide practical information as appropriate to allay the patient's sexual fears.
- Assist patients to resolve their practical concerns related to illness and self-presentation. Such concerns often impinge on sexuality and personal self-esteem. For example, cancer patients may fear a loss sexual attractiveness from the hair loss associated with chemotherapy. Practical solutions, such as fitting the patient with a wig, may alleviate the patient's sexual fear.
- Encourage patients with sexual dysfunction to focus on sensual pleasure and reduce the demands they place on themselves for sexual performance.
- Evaluate the need for referral to a sex therapist or other appropriate provider.

The management of sexual dysfunction is a sensitive and often difficult endeavor, as patients are often embarrassed to engage in discussions of intimate sexual functions. Nurses who demonstrate concern and professionalism help build patients' trust and comfort, thus facilitating communication of their sexual needs and functioning.

Home Health Care

Restorative home health care often focuses on patients recuperating from body-altering illnesses or treatments, many of whom may have related self-concept problems and sexual concerns. The home health nurse's role is to identify patients at risk, monitor their progress, and refer them to groups or providers for long-term counseling should they fail to adapt within a reasonable period of time. Although the approaches described above apply whether the patient is at home or in the hospital, the home health nurse may be constrained by the limited number of home visits allotted such patients by their insurance carriers, and referral for special counseling may be necessary to meet the patient's needs for restorative care.

REHABILITATIVE CARE

Patients who have undergone an acute change in health status may have short-term or long-term needs during the rehabilitative phase. Rehabilitative care, which may go on in the home or an inpatient facility, often focuses on the phase of reconstruction, the last phase in the psychological adaption to illness, and involves tasks sometimes referred to as "identity work,"[158] that is, those involved with the integration of the positive aspects of the changes in self-expression undergone as a result of health problems. This focus includes the patient's efforts to develop new life patterns and build a new self-concept. Patients often need a great deal of support during this period, both from significant others and from health care professionals. Regaining a sense of self-esteem is critical. Nurses may be instrumental by providing feedback and encouragement as patients endeavor to reenter or establish a new niche in the social world.

Patients recovering from an acute health alteration may require support to reestablish their former life structure and role patterns or to initiate changes in previous patterns necessitated by health alterations.

Counseling

Counseling is frequently a component of rehabilitative care for patients with self-expression problems. Patients who undergo an alteration in self-concept, body image, or an aspect of their social identity or role performance that lowers their self-esteem often experience a prolonged period of adjustment and coping. Referral for appropriate counseling is an important component of care. Psychologists, psychiatrists, psychiatric social workers and nurses, sex therapists, and marriage and family counselors are some of the providers who engage in such counseling. The nurses role is to identify the need and refer the patient to find an appropriate provider.

Referral to Support Groups

Many support groups are available to aid patients coping with various health problems, including grief and loss, and may be helpful to patients who are trying to establish a new sense of who they are and how they will relate to the social world. The nurse can help by providing information on such groups and assisting the patient to establish contact. The Internet can hep nurses and patients find support resources.

EVALUATION

The evaluation of care related to self-expression is the final component of nurse–patient management of self-expression. Nurse and patient jointly evaluate progress toward the desired outcomes. Reassessment and replanning are sometimes necessary to achieve outcomes. Progress toward goals is monitored throughout the course of care. As outcomes are met, the results are recorded in the patient's chart. Outcomes not met, along with reassessment plans, are also recorded.

SUMMARY

Self-expression, the process by which individuals share their self-understanding with those around them, is vital in health and illness. It is the process by which people find meaning in their lives, come to know themselves and be known by others, establish and maintain relationships and live out their values. Self-expression has two essential aspects—self-presentation and self-disclosure. Both convey important messages about an individual's self-concept and self-esteem. Through self-presentation, people project a valued image of themselves to those around them, one they hope will strengthen their relationships with others and reinforce their desired social identity. Through self-disclosure, they share the deepest aspects of themselves with trusted others to reduce loneliness and further strengthen the social bonds they value.

Illness interrupts the flow of events in everyday life and often creates conditions that inevitably alter a person's self-perception and identity. This situation often creates a crisis as the individual faces unavoidable and sometimes permanent change. Changes in one's body are accompanied by changes in self and social behavior, which in turn may change social relationships of all kinds, most particularly the close, intimate relationships where the capacity to function in important roles, including sexual roles, may also be affected. Such changes are experienced as a loss and are often accompanied by great distress, initiating a process of grieving, a painful but necessary process for healthy adaptation. Grieving a loss and resolution of grief require repeated opportunities for sharing one's distress.

Death is sometimes the outcome of illness. It is a source of wrenching emotion and also elicits grieving. During the process of dying, the dying and the bereaved alike deal with urgent issues of identity change. Nurses are in an pivotal position to come to the aid of those confronting death, to assist them with the threat they inevitably experience, and to assist them to meet their needs as they adapt to profound change and loss.

LEARNING OUTCOMES

Upon completing this chapter, the student should be able to:

1. Define self-expression.
2. State the importance of self-expression to health and well-being.
3. Discuss three functions of self-expression.
4. Discuss the concept of self-expression in relation to identity, self-concept, life structure, sexuality, and development.
5. Identify common modes of self-expression observed in every-day life.
6. State the importance of self-presentation and self-disclosure to self-expression.
7. State several characteristics of optimal self-expression.
8. Describe the impact of life change, illness, and loss on self-expression and state the implications for nursing practice.
9. Describe the grieving process.
10. Outline components of the patient history and examination pertinent to assessing self-expression.
11. Outline nursing diagnoses related to self-expression, listing etiologies and defining characteristics.
12. Discuss nursing implementation related to self-expression for patients undergoing self-concept or body image changes, patients with concerns about sexuality, grieving patients, and dying patients.
13. Discuss the collaborative role of the nurse in assisting patients with self-expression problems.

REVIEW OF KEY TERMS

ambivalence	insight
anticipatory grief	loss
bereavement	mourning
catharsis	reference groups
distress	self-disclosure
distress disclosure	self-expression
gender identity	self-identification
grief	self-presentation
grieving	self-reflection
hope	sex
hospice	sexuality

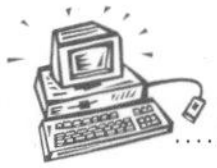

INTERNET RESOURCES

Web Sites and URLs

1-800 Numbers for Patient Support Organizations:
http://infonet.welch.jhu.edu/advocacy.html

Grief/grieving information, transition/loss, self-help resources:
http://fohnix.metronet.com/~tic

Death/dying; home care/hospice information:
http://www.lib.umich.edu/hw/nursing.html

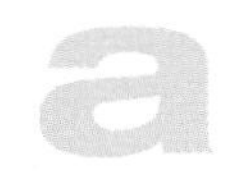

Having Read the Chapter, consider again the opening scenario, page 735, and the following responses to the questions concerning Monica Brown's care following surgery to remove an ovarian tumor.

Monica Brown, who has not yet received a diagnosis, is awaiting treatment for a disease that she worries may be terminal. She may not have identified specific fears related to the effects of surgery and subsequent treatments and may benefit from an opportunity to discuss her situation with the nurse. Given that the diagnosis is uncertain, the nurse, Judy Simon, should provide Monica with information on the procedure she will undergo and encourage Monica's hope for a positive outcome. On the other hand, the nurse should recognize that Monica already shows signs of depression and may require substantial support should her diagnosis be unfavorable. The nurse will want to explore with Monica her thoughts about the impact that illness might have on her roles as teacher, mother, and wife. They should discuss Monica's experience with the illnesses of her mother and aunt and her knowledge about the effect that surgery might have on her body.

REFERENCES

1. Banerjee SP. Dimensions of self-expression: Freedom and constraints. In: Banerjee SP, Moitra S, eds. *Communication, Identity, and Self-Expression.* Delhi: Oxford University Press; 1984.
2. Levinson DJ, Darrow CN, Klein EB, Levinson MH, McKee B. *The Seasons of a Man's Life.* New York: Ballantine Books; 1978.
3. Whitbourne SK. *The Me I Know: A Study of Adult Identity.* New York: Springer-Verlag; 1986.
4. Frankl VE. *Man's Search for Meaning.* Boston: Beacon Press; 1962.
5. Kasch CR. Establishing a collaborative nurse–patient relationship: A distinct focus of nursing action in primary care. *Image.* 1986;18:44–47.
6. Morse J. Reciprocity in care: Gift giving and the patient–nurse relationship. *Can J Nurs Res.* 1989;21:33–45.
7. Cooper MJ. Covenantal relationships: Grounding for the nursing ethic. *Adv Nurs Sci.* 1988;10:48–59.
8. Davies MD. An ode to being human. *Nurs Clin North Am.* 1971;6:695–701.
9. Marck P. Therapeutic reciprocity: A caring phenomenon. *Adv Nurs Sci.* 1990:13:49–59.
10. Paterson JG, Zderad LT. *Humanistic Nursing.* New York: John Wiley & Sons; 1976.
11. Sarvimaki A. Nursing care as a moral, practical, communicative and creative activity. *J Adv Nurs.* 1988;13:462–467.
12. Thorne SE, Robinson CA. Reciprocal trust in health care relationships. *J Adv Nurs.* 1988;13:782–789.
13. Yuen FKH. The nurse–patient relationship: A mutual learning experience. *J Adv Nurs.* 1986;11:529–533.
14. Young JC. Rationale for clinician self-disclosure and research agenda. *Image.* 1988;20:196–199.
15. Gazda GM, Asbury FS, Balzer FJ, Childers WC, Walters RP. *Human Relations Development.* 4th ed. Boston: Allyn & Bacon; 1991.
16. Bowers JE, Clark-Mahoney JP, Forshee T, Reiner KA, Schilling JE, Snyder BS. Analysis of support groups for young spinal cord–injured males. *Rehab Nurs.* 1987;12:313–322.
17. Ekman P, Sorenson ER, Friesen WV. Pancultural elements in facial displays of emotion. *Science.* 1969;164:86–88.
18. Ekman P, Oster H. Facial expressions of emotion. *Annu Rev Psychol.* 1979;30:527–554.
19. Ekman P, Friesen WV. Origins, usage and coding of nonverbal behavior. In: Vernon E, ed. *Communication Theory and Linguistic Models in the Social Sciences.* Buenos Aires: DiTella; 1968.
20. Ekman P. Universal and cultural differences in facial expressions of emotion. In: Cole J, ed. *Nebraska Symposium on Motivation.* Lincoln: University of Nebraska Press; 1972.
21. Cupchik GC, Leventhal H. Consistency between expressive behavior and the evaluation of humorous stimuli. *J Pers Soc Behav.* 1974;30:429–442.
22. Zuckerman M, Klorman R, Larrance DT, Spiegel NH. Facial, autonomic, and subjective components of emotion: The facial feedback hypothesis versus the externalizer–internalizer distinction. *J Pers Soc Behav.* 1981;41:929–944.
23. Riskind JH. They stoop to conquer: guiding and self-regulatory functions of physical posture after success and failure. *J Pers Soc Psychol.* 1984;47:479–493.
24. Zajonc RB. Emotion and facial efference: A theory reclaimed. *Science.* 1985;228:15–21.
25. Winton WM. The role of facial response in self-reports of emotion: a critique of Laird. *J Pers Soc Behav.* 1986;50: 808–812.
26. Izard CE. Facial expressions and the regulation of emotions. *J Pers Soc Behav.* 1990;58:487–498.
27. Rosenthal R. *Skill in Nonverbal Communication: Individual Differences.* Cambridge, MA: Oelgeschlager, Gunn, & Hain; 1979.
28. Goffman E. *The Presentation of Self in Everyday Life.* Garden City, NY: Doubleday Anchor Books; 1959.
29. Schneider DJ, Hastorf AH, Ellsworth PC. *Person Perception.* 2nd ed. Reading, MA: Addison-Wesley; 1979.
30. Tedeschi JT, ed. *Impression Management Theory and Social Psychological Research.* New York: Academic Press; 1981.
31. Derlega VJ. *Communication, Intimacy, and Close Relationships.* Orlando, FL: Academic Press; 1984.
32. Notarius CI, Levenson RW. Expressive tendencies and physiologic responses to stress. *J Personality Social Psychol.* 1979; 37:1204–1210.
33. Ekman P, Levenson RW, Friesen WV. Autonomic nervous system activity distinguishes among emotions. *Science.* 1983; 221:1208–1210.
34. McBride G, King M, James JW. Social proximity effects of galvanic skin responses in adult humans. *J Psychol.* 1965; 61:153–157.
35. James WT. A study of the expression of bodily posture. *J Gen Psychol.* 1932;7:405–437.

36. Ekman P, Friesen WV. The repertoire of nonverbal behavior: categories, origins, usage and codings. *Semiotica.* 1969; 1:49–97.
37. Chelune GJ, ed. *Self-Disclosure: Origins, Patterns and Implications of Openness in Interpersonal Relationships.* San Francisco: Jossey-Bass; 1979.
38. Rose A. *Human Behavior and Social Processes.* Boston: Houghton Mifflin; 1962.
39. Zajonc RB. Feeling and thinking: preferences need no inferences. *Am Psychol.* 1980;35:151–175.
40. Schlenker BR, ed. *The Self and Social Life.* New York: McGraw-Hill; 1985.
41. Bonner H. *On Being Mindful of Man: Essay Toward a Proactive Psychology.* Boston: Houghton Mifflin; 1965.
42. Maslow AH. *Toward a Psychology of Being.* Princeton, NJ: Van Nostrand; 1962.
43. Gadow SA. Nurse and patient: the caring relationship. In: Bishop AH, Scuder JR Jr, eds. *Caring, Curing, Coping: Nurse, Physician, Patient Relationships.* Tuscaloosa, AL: University of Alabama Press; 1985.
44. Benner P, Wrubel J. *The Primacy of Caring: Stress and Coping in Health and Illness.* Toronto: Addison-Wesley; 1988.
45. Watson MJ. New dimensions of human caring theory. *Nurs Sci Q.* 1988;1:175–181.
46. Schlenker BR. Identities, identifications, and relationships. In: Derlega VJ, ed. *Communication, Intimacy and Close Relationships.* Orlando, FL: Academic Press; 1984.
47. Schneider DJ. Tactical self-presentations: toward a broader conception. In: Tedeschi JT, ed. *Impression Management Theory and Social Psychological Research.* New York: Academic Press; 1981.
48. Tedeschi JT, Riess M. Identities, the phenomenal self, and laboratory research. In: Tedeschi JT, ed. *Impression Management Theory and Social Psychological Research.* New York: Academic Press; 1981.
49. Arkin RM. Self-presentational styles. In: Tedeschi JT, ed. *Impression Management Theory and Social Psychological Research.* New York: Academic Press; 1981.
50. Tedeschi JT. Private and public experiences and the self. In: Baumeister RF, ed. *Public Self and Private Self.* New York: Springer-Verlag; 1986.
51. Tedeschi JT, Norman N. Social power, self-presentation, and the self. In: Schlenker BR, ed. *The Self and Social Life.* New York: McGraw-Hill; 1985.
52. Goffman E. *Relations in Public.* New York: Basic Books; 1971.
53. Podrasky DL, Sexton DL. Nurse's reactions to difficult patients. *Image.* 1988;20:16–21.
54. Sarosi GM. A critical theory: the nurse as a fully human person. *Nurs Forum.* 1968;7:349–363.
55. McGregor FC. Uncooperative patients: some cultural interpretations. *Am J Nurs.* 1967;67:88–91.
56. Carveth JA. Perceived patient deviance and avoidance by nurses. *Nurs Res.* 1995;44:173–178.
57. Larson PA. Nurse perceptions of patient characteristics. *Nurs Res.* 1977;26:416–421.
58. Ruiz MJ. Open-closed mindedness, intolerance of ambiguity and nursing faculty attitudes toward culturally different patients. *Nurs Res.* 1981;30:177–181.
59. Jankin JK. The nurse in crisis. *Nurs Clin North Am.* 1974; 9:17–26.
60. Flaskerud JH, Halloran EJ, Janken J, Lund M, Zetterland J. Avoidance and distancing: a descriptive view of nursing. *Nurs Forum.* 1979;18:158–174.
61. Williams F. The crisis of hospitalization. *Nurs Clin North Am.* 1974;9:37–45.
62. Jourard S. *The Transparent Self.* Princeton, NJ: Van Nostrand-Reinhold; 1964.
63. Derlega VJ. Self-disclosure and intimate relationships. In: Derlega VJ, ed. *Communication, Intimacy, and Close Relationships.* Orlando, FL: Academic Press; 1984.
64. Hill CT, Stull DE. Gender and self-disclosure: strategies for exploring the issues. In: Derlega VJ, Berg JH, eds. *Self-Disclosure: Theory, Research, and Therapy.* New York: Plenum Press; 1987.
65. Berg J. Responsiveness and self-disclosure. In: Derlega VJ, Berg JH, eds. *Self-Disclosure: Theory, Research, and Therapy.* New York: Plenum Press; 1987.
66. Carpenter BN. The relationship between psychopathology and self-disclosure. In: Derlega VJ, Berg JH, eds. *Self-Disclosure: Theory, Research, and Therapy.* New York: Plenum Press; 1987.
67. Stokes JP. The relation of loneliness and self-disclosure. In: Derlega VJ, ed. *Self-Disclosure: Theory, Research, and Therapy.* New York: Plenum Press; 1987.
68. Coates D, Winston T. The dilemma of distress disclosure. In: Derlega VJ, Berg JH, eds. *Self-Disclosure: Theory, Research, and Therapy.* New York: Plenum Press; 1987.
69. Schlenker BR. Self-identification: toward an integration of the private and public self. In: Baumeister RF, ed. *Public Self and Private Self.* New York: Springer-Verlag; 1986.
70. Ozer EM, Bandura A. Mechanisms governing empowerment effects: a self-efficacy analysis. *J Pers Soc Psychol.* 1990;58: 472–486.
71. Guyton AC, Hall JE. *The Textbook of Medical Physiology.* 9th ed. Philadelphia: Saunders; 1996.
72. Schachter S. *The Psychology of Affiliation.* Stanford, CA: Stanford University Press; 1959.
73. Buunk BP, Collins RL, Taylor SE, VanYperen NW, Dakof GA. The affective consequences of social comparison: either direction has its ups and downs. *J Pers Soc Psychol.* 1990; 59:1238–1249.
74. Wood JV, Taylor SE, Lichtman RR. Social comparison in adjustment to breast cancer. *J Pers Soc Psychol.* 1985;49: 1169–1183.
75. Stiles WB. "I have to talk to somebody." A fever model of disclosure. In: Derlega VJ, Berg JH, eds. *Self-Disclosure: Theory, Research, and Therapy.* New York: Plenum Press; 1987.
76. Pennebacker JW, O'Heeron RC. Confiding in others and illness rates among spouses of suicide and accidental death. *J Abnorm Psychol.* 1984;93:473–476.
77. Derogatis LR, Abeloff MD, Melisaratos N. Psychological coping mechanisms and survival time in metastatic breast cancer. *JAMA.* 1979;242:1504–1508.
78. Jahoda M. *Current Concepts of Positive Mental Health.* New York: Basic Books; 1958.
79. Jourard SM. *Personal Adjustment.* New York: Macmillan; 1963.
80. Price GM. Empathic relating and the structure of self. In: Honess T, Yardely K, eds. *Self and Identity: Perspectives Across the Lifespan.* London: Routledge & Kegan Paul; 1987.

81. Bello LK, McIntyre S. Body image disturbances in young adults with cancer. *Cancer Nurs.* 1995;18:138–143.
82. Wright JE. Self-perception alterations with coronary artery bypass surgery. *Heart Lung.* 1987;16:483–490.
83. Crouch M, Straub V. Enhancement of self-esteem in adults. *Fam Community Health.* 1983;6:76–78.
84. Katzin L. Chronic illness and sexuality. *Am J Nurs.* 1990; 90:55–59.
85. Isselbacher KJ, Braunwald E, Wilson JD, Martin JB, Fauci AS, Kasper DL. *Harrison's Principles of Internal Medicine.* 13th ed. New York: McGraw-Hill; 1994.
86. Goddard LR. Sexuality and spinal cord injury. *J Neurosci Nurs.* 1988;20:240–244.
87. Chicano LA. Humanistic aspects of sexuality as related to spinal cord injury. *J Neurosci Nurs.* 1989;21:366–369.
88. Archer J. The process of grief: a selective review. *J Adv Health Nurs Care.* 1991;1:9–37.
89. Lee JM. Emotional reaction to trauma. *Nurs Clin North Am.* 1970;5:577–587.
90. Wortman CB, Silver RC. The myths of coping with loss. *J Consult Clin Psychol.* 1989;57:349–357.
91. Young JC. Rationale for clinician self-disclosure and research agenda. *Image.* 1988;20:196–199.
92. Ruxton JP. Humor intervention deserves our attention. *Holistic Nurs Pract.* 1988;293:54–62.
93. Lange S. Shame. In: Carlson C, ed. *Behavioral Concepts & Nursing Intervention.* Philadelphia: Lippincott; 1970.
94. Peretz D. Development, object relationships, and loss. In: Schoenberg B, Carr AC, Peretz D, Kutscher AH, eds. *Loss and Grief: Psychological Management in Medical Practice.* New York: Columbia University Press; 1970.
95. Trunell EP, Caserta MS, White GL. Bereavement: current issues in intervention and prevention. *J Health Educ.* 1992; 23:275–280.
95a. Kastenbaum RJ. *Death, Society, and Human Experience.* 3rd ed. Columbus, OH: Charles E. Merrill; 1986.
96. Carter SL. Themes of grief. *Nurs Res.* 1989;38:354–358.
97. Cody WK. Grieving a personal loss. *Nurs Sci Q.* 1991;4:61–68.
98. Lindemann E. Symptomatology and management of acute grief. *Am J Psychiatry.* 1944;101:141–149.
99. Engle GL. Grief and grieving. *Am J Nurs.* 1964;64:93–98.
100. Kübler-Ross E. *On Death and Dying.* New York: Macmillan; 1969.
101. Bowlby J. *Attachment and Loss: Loss.* New York: Basic Books; 1980.
102. Horecek BJ. A heuristic model of grieving after high-grief deaths. *Death Studies.* 1995;19:21–31.
103. Martocchio BC. Grief through bereavement: healing through hurt. *Nurs Clin North Am.* 1985;20:327–341.
104. Sowell RL, Bramlett MH, Gueldner SH, Gritzmacher D, Martin G. The lived experience of survival and bereavement following the death of a lover from AIDS. *Image.* 1991;23:89–94.
105. Alty A. Adjustment to bereavement and loss in older people. *Nurs Times.* 1995;91:35–36.
106. Mischel MH. Uncertainty in illness. *Image.* 1988;20:225–232.
107. Humphrey MA. Effects of anticipatory grief for the patient, family member, and caregiver. In: Rando TA, ed. *Loss and Anticipatory Grief.* Lexington, MA: Lexington Books; 1986.
108. Capritto K. *The Effect of Perceived Ambiguity on Adherence to the Dietary Regime in Chronic Hemodialysis.* Unpublished master's thesis, California State University, Los Angeles.
109. Kastenbaum R; Costa PT. Psychological perspectives on death. *Annu Rev Psychol.* 1977;28:225–249.
110. Zack MV. Loneliness: A concept relevant to the care of dying persons. *Nurs Clin North Am.* 1985;20:403–413.
111. Glaser BG, Strauss AL. *Awareness of Dying.* Chicago: Aldine; 1965.
112. Moseley JR. Alterations in comfort. *Nurs Clin North Am.* 1985;29:427–438.
113. Dufault K, Martocchio BC. Hope: its spheres and dimensions. *Nurs Clin North Am.* 1985;20:379–391.
114. Hall BA. The struggle of the diagnosed terminally ill person to maintain hope. *Nurs Sci Q.* 1990;3:177–184.
115. Stoner M. Measuring hope. In: Frank-Stromberg M, ed. *Instruments for Clinical Nursing Research.* Norwalk, CT: Appleton & Lange; 1988.
116. Fromm E. *The Revolution of Hope.* New York: Harper & Row; 1968.
117. Conrad NL. Spiritual support for the dying. *Nurs Clin North Am.* 1985;20:415–425.
118. Ad Hoc Committee of the Harvard Medical School to Examine the Definition of Brain Death. A definition of irreversible coma. *JAMA.* 1968;205:337–340.
119. Youngner SJ, Landefeld CS, Coulton CJ, Juknialis BW, Leary M. Brain death and organ retrieval: a cross-sectional survey of knowledge and concepts among health professionals. *JAMA.* 1989;261:2205–2210.
120. Annas GJ. Nancy Cruzan and the right to die. *N Engl J Med.* 1990;323:670–673.
121. Leibson CM. The role of the courts in terminating life-sustaining treatment. *Issues in Law & Medicine.* 1995;10:437–451.
122. Wintersheimer DC. The role of the courts in terminating nutrition and hydration for incompetent patients. *Issues in Law & Medicine.* 1995;10:453–465.
123. Newman MA. Theory for nursing practice. *Nurs Sci Q.* 1994;7:153–157.
124. Rohde P, Tilson M, Lewinsohn P, Seeley J. Dimensionality of coping and its relation to depression. *J Pers Soc Psychol.* 1990;153:499–511.
125. Wooley N. Crisis theory: a paradigm of effective intervention with families of critically ill people. *J Adv Nurs.* 1990; 15:1402–1408.
126. Heiss J. Social roles. In: Rosenberg M, Turner R, eds. *Social Psychology: Sociological Perspectives.* New York: Basic Books; 1981.
127. Rando TA. A comprehensive analysis of anticipatory grief: perspectives, processes, promises, and problems. In: Rando TA, ed. *Loss and Anticipatory Grief.* Lexington, MA: Lexington Books; 1986.
128. Sheehan DV, Hackett TP. Psychosomatic disorders. In: Nicholi AM, Jr. *The Harvard Guide to Modern Psychiatry.* Cambridge, MA/London: Belknap Press of Harvard University Press; 1978:319–353.
129. Aguilera D, Messick J. *Crisis Intervention: Theory and Methodology.* 5th ed. St. Louis: Mosby; 1986.
130. Rossan S. Identity: its development in adulthood. In: Honess T, Yardley K, *Self and Identity: Perspectives Across the Lifespan.* London/New York: Routledge and Kegan Paul; 1987.

131. Carmack BJ. Balancing engagement/detachment in AIDS-related multiple losses. *Image.* 1992;24:9–14.
132. Erikson E. *Childhood and Society.* New York: WW Norton; 1963.
133. Kozlak J, Thobaben M. Psychiatric home health nursing care of the aged: a selected literature review. *Geriatr Nurs.* 1994;15:148–150.
134. Pessin N, Lindy P, Stricoff DJ, et al. Integrating mental health and home care services for AIDS patients. *Caring Mag.* 1993;May:30–34.
135. Trief PM, Donohue-Smith M. Counseling needs of women with breast cancer: what the women tell us. *J Psychosoc Nurs Ment Health Serv.* 1996;34:24–29.
136. Nelson PB. Social support, self-esteem, and depression in the institutionalized elderly. *Issues Ment Health Nurs.* 1989; 10:55–68.
137. Bilodeau BA, Degner LF. Information needs, sources of information, and decisional roles in women with breast cancer. *Oncol Nurs Forum.* 1996;23:691–696.
138. Unsain IC, Goodwin MH, Schuster EA. Diabetes and sexual functioning. *Nurs Clin North Am.* 1982;17:387–393.
139. Annon JS. *The Behavioral Treatment of Sexual Problems: Brief Therapy.* New York: Harper & Row; 1976.
140. Dale KG. Intimacy and rheumatic diseases. *Rehab Nurs.* 1996;21:38–40.
141. Winston K. Family roles. In: Bomar P, ed. *Nurses and Family Health Promotion: Concepts, Assessment and Interventions.* Baltimore: Williams & Wilkins; 1989:55–66.
142. Folz AT. The influence of cancer on self-concept and life quality. *Semin Oncol Nurs.* 1987;3:303–312.
143. Wilson RE. The nurse's role in sexual counseling. *Ostomy Wound Manage.* 1995;41:72–74.
144. Leming MR, Dickinson GE. *Understanding Dying, Death and Bereavement.* New York: Holt, Rinehart and Winston; 1985.
145. Cooley ME. Bereavement care: a role for nurses. *Cancer Nurs.* 1992;15:125–129.
146. Rando TA. Understanding and facilitating anticipatory grief in the loved ones of the dying. In: Rando TA, ed. *Loss and Anticipatory Grief.* Lexington, MA: Lexington Books; 1986.
147. Podrasky D, Sexton DL. Nurses' reactions to difficult patients. *Image.* 1988;20:16–21.
148. Kettles AM. Catharsis: an investigation of its meaning and nature. *J Adv Nurs.* 1994;20:368–376.
149. Tyner R. Elements of empathic care for dying patients and their families. *Nurs Clin North Am.* 1985;20:393–401.
150. O'Neill C, Sorenson ES. Home care of the elderly: a family perspective. *Adv Nurs Sci.* 1991;13:28–37.
151. Ade-Ridder L, Kaplan L. Marriage, spousal caregiving, and a husband's move to a nursing home: a changing role for the wife? *J Gerontol Nurs.* 1993;19:13–23.
152. Lazare A. Unresolved grief. In: Lazare A, ed. *Outpatient Psychiatry.* Baltimore: Williams & Wilkins; 1979.
153. Anderson DB. Never too late: resolving the grief of a suicide. *J Psychosoc Nurs.* 1991;29:29–31.
154. Alonzo AA, Reynolds NR. Stigma, HIV and AIDS: an exploration and elaboration of a stigma trajectory. *Social Sci Med.* 1995;41:303–315.
155. Deeny P, McCrea H. Stoma care: the patient's perspective. *J Adv Nurs.* 1991;16:39–46.
156. Nishimoto PW. Sex and sexuality in the cancer patient. *Nurs Pract Forum.* 1995;6:221–227.
157. Northouse LL. The impact of breast cancer on patients and their husbands. *Cancer Nurs.* 1989;12:276–284.
158. Matheison CM, Stam HJ. Renegotiating identity: cancer narratives. *Sociol Health Care Illness.* 1995;17:283–306.

27

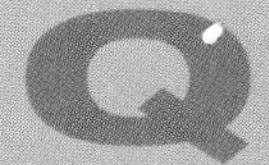

Harry Jones, a 62-year-old man, lives alone in a small house in Florida. His hobby is gardening and his yard is ablaze with the colors of the flowers and vegetables he cultivates. He tells Ms. Evans, the staff nurse, that he grew up on a farm where he worked with his arms, head, and shoulders bare and frequently got sunburned. Lately he has noticed scaling of the skin on his nose.

Ms. Evans observes on the patient's arms obvious signs of sun exposure and, during the assessment, notices that Mr. Jones's facial skin is reddened over the forehead and nose, areas vulnerable to overexposure. His skin has many age spots *(lentigos)*. Ms. Evans discovers an area on the back of his neck (another area vulnerable to overexposure) about 0.75 cm in diameter. The lesion appears smooth-surfaced and well circumscribed, has an indentation in the center, and is just beginning to break down into an ulcer with slight crusting. Ms. Evans, recognizing the possibility that the lesion may be cancerous, makes a mental note to refer Mr. Jones to a physician for further dermatologic assessment.

What should the nurse teach Mr. Jones about his skin care?

What should Mr. Jones know about skin exposure?

What should Mr. Jones know about how to perform skin self-assessment?

What additional information does this patient need to know?

Skin and Tissue Integrity

Janet-Beth McCann Flynn

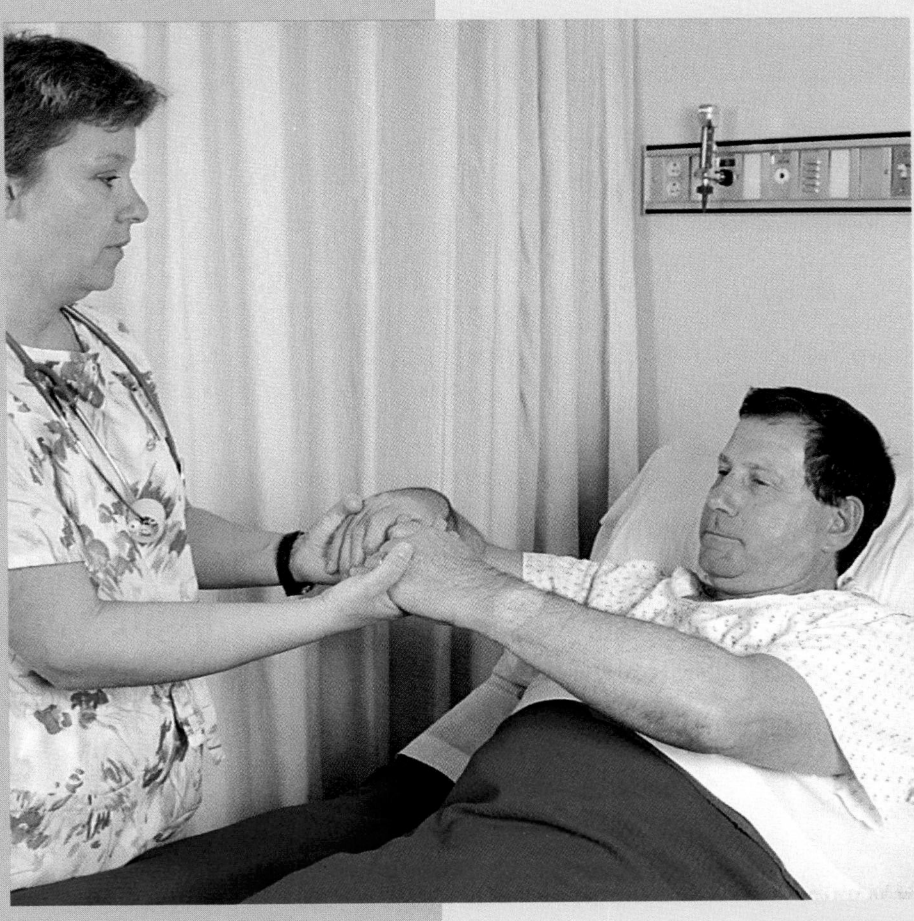

CHAPTER OUTLINE

The integument—including skin, hair, nails, and mucous membranes—comprises the body's largest organ. The skin, a major part of the integument, forms 8 percent of the total body mass.[1] The integument has protective, excretory, secretory, sensory, and metabolic functions.

People often describe skin in terms of its appearance: firm and youthful, smooth and tan, wrinkled and leathery. Individuals' first impressions of others are often based on the appearance of skin, hair, and teeth. The appearance of skin affects the way people feel about themselves. Many individuals moisturize and apply cosmetics to their skin, color their hair, and paint their nails in an effort to improve their appearance. Body odors also affect people's responses to others. The glands of the skin release odors that act to attract people to each other and are part of our sexuality. Various cultures have differing ideas as to which body odors are pleasant and which odors are repulsive.

Many variables affect skin, including age, exposure to sun, nutrition, ethnic background, and occupation. Some of these factors cause disruptions in skin and tissue integrity. Disruptions in skin integrity have been documented for thousands of years. Ancient cliff writings and Egyptian hieroglyphics contain references to syphilitic lesions, leprosy, and wounds. The Bible describes types of lesions and their healing. Early medical texts described the care of wounds.

Because many alterations in health status alter skin, the assessment and care of the skin is a primary nursing concern. This chapter addresses:

- the anatomy and physiology of the various integumentary structures
- common skin disruptions
- assessment for integument problems
- nursing diagnoses related to skin and tissue integrity
- nursing implementation for prevention of integumentary problems

SECTION 1

UNDERSTANDING SKIN AND TISSUE INTEGRITY

OPTIMAL SKIN AND TISSUE INTEGRITY

Intact skin and mucous membranes are part of the body's primary defense against microorganisms. Integrity of skin and mucosa protects tissue integrity throughout the body. Conversely, skin and mucosal changes often reflect changes in internal tissue integrity. Understanding the structure and function of skin and mucous membranes contributes to effective nursing assessment and management of integumentary health and overall health, as well.

ANATOMY OF SKIN AND MUCOSA

Skin

The skin varies in thickness and character according to the area it covers. Indeed, it varies from 0.5 mm over the tympanic membrane to 6.0 mm on the palms of the hands.[2] Some areas are devoid of hair, whereas thick hair grows on the scalp and softer hair on the trunk and limbs.

The skin owes its adaptability to its three anatomic regions: the outer epidermis, the dermis (which is below the epidermis), and the subcutaneous fat. Each region has unique functions and components while sharing specialized cells that give the skin its general properties.

Epidermis. The **epidermis** is the outer surface of the skin. It is composed of four layers. The innermost layer is the layer that produces skin cells. These cells, called basal keratinocyte cells, move up through the other epidermal layers to replenish the skin surface. This process normally takes 30 days, but is shortened in wound healing and in aberrant conditions such as basal cell skin cancer and psoriasis, in which overproliferation of skin cells is the basis of the pathology.

The two middle epidermal layers are very active metabolically and contain a variety of cell types. Melanocytes are found here; they produce melanin, the substance that determines skin pigment and filters ultraviolet radiation from the sun. Other specialized epidermal cells provide cell-to-cell adhesion, participate in the initial identification of antigens, function as touch receptors, and give each epidermal layer its characteristic appearance.

The surface layer of the epidermis is composed of layers of large cornified, flattened, polyhedral cells. The cells overlap at the margins and form interlocking ridges. This layer varies in thickness from 15 cells on the face to 100 cells on the plantar surfaces. This layer possesses properties of physical toughness, strength, flexibility, elastic return, and electrical impedance, and has a dry surface that resists moisture and microorganism growth.

Appendages. Epidermal appendages include hair, the nails, sebaceous glands, eccrine sweat glands, and apocrine sweat glands.

HAIR. Hair develops from follicles that arise from the dermis and is found over the entire body surface except for the soles of the feet, palms of the hands, fingertips, glans penis, and lips. Free nerve endings and arterioles and venules surround each follicle, nourishing and stimulating it. Autonomic nerve action causes hair to "stand on end" due to pilomotor stimulation.

Hair may be straight, spiral, or wavy. Straight hair is due to straight vertical hair follicles and is typical in Asians. Spiral hair, seen in blacks, arises from curved follicles having the lower portion of the follicle horizontal to the skin surface. The white race has a combination of all three types.

Hair has five important functions. It is a sexually attractive body element, acts to filter irritants in the nasal passages, protects the scalp and skin, serves as a shield for the eyes from sun and sweat droplets, and aids in tactile perception.

NAIL UNIT. The nail unit consists of the nail plate and the tissue surrounding it. The nail plate is hard, convex, rectangular, and translucent. Nail growth is continuous. Fingernails grow at a rate of about 1 mm per week; toenails grow more slowly. The fingernails and toenails protect the terminal phalanges, participate in tactile stimulation, scratch, and allow humans to grasp minute objects.

SEBACEOUS GLANDS. The sebaceous glands produce sebum, a lipid substance. They are usually associated with hair follicles. Sebum regulates skin absorption of fluid and chemicals, lubricates the hair and skin surface, carries out antibacterial and antifungal activity, and is a vitamin D precursor.

ECCRINE SWEAT GLANDS. The eccrine sweat glands, the true sweat glands, are present all over the body. Their primary function is to produce sweat during periods of internal or external heat stress to cool the body through evaporation.

Sweating also can occur during periods of emotional stress. The palms, soles, axilla, and forehead have sweat glands that react to emotions. Sweaty palms or beads of perspiration on the brow are often indicators of fear or anxiety.

APOCRINE SWEAT GLANDS. The apocrine sweat glands are distributed primarily in the axillae, anogenital area, abdomen, face, and scalp. Specialized apocrine glands produce cerumen (wax) in the external ear canal. Apocrine secretion occurs in response to both physical and emotional stress. In lower animals, apocrine secretions allow species identification.

Dermis. The **dermis** lies directly below the epidermis and contains the specialized capillaries, nerve ends, and lymph channels of the skin.

The dermis is composed mostly of noncellular connective tissue, including collagen, elastin fibers, and ground substance. It is divided into two layers, a thin zone that interfaces with the epidermis in wavelike projections called papillae, and a thicker layer that contains a variety of specialized cells.

Subcutaneous Fat. A lipid layer lying below the dermis, **subcutaneous fat** contains major vascular networks, the lymphatics, and nerve fibers. Its thickness varies: it is absent in the eyelids, penis, and scrotum, but prominent on hips, thighs, and buttocks. Women generally have more subcutaneous fat than men, but there is considerable variation in amount among individuals of both sexes.

Subcutaneous fat serves several protective functions. It acts as an insulator, preventing loss of body heat in cold environments. The body retains heat because fat is a poor conductor of heat. Fat protects internal organs from impact trauma, acting as a shock absorber. It is also a storage form of energy that can be mobilized when nutritional intake is diminished.

Dermal–Epidermal Junction. This area between the dermis and epidermis, called the basement membrane, appears to play an integral role in the inflammatory process (discussed later in the chapter) and also acts as a filter barrier that regulates the passage of molecules into the dermis.

Musoca and Related Structures

Mucosa, a membrane that secretes mucus, lines many organs.

Oral Cavity. The mouth contains several types of mucosa, as well as the tongue, salivary glands, and the teeth.

ORAL MUCOSA. The oral mucous membranes form a continuous covering extending from the lips through the oral pharynx. The fibrous tissue covering the alveolar surfaces of the jawbone and surrounding the teeth is called the **gingiva,** or gums. The membrane covering the interior surface of the cheeks is called the **buccal mucosa.**

TONGUE. The tongue is a highly specialized organ. Its functions are taste, speech, mastication, and sensation. The tongue has a rough, rosy texture due to the papillae on its dorsal surface. The ventral surface is smooth and delicate.

SALIVARY GLANDS. The salivary glands are located under the tongue, at the base of the jaw, and beneath the ear. *Saliva*—a clear, odorless, tasteless, and somewhat viscid (sticky) liquid—lubricates the oral cavity, facilitating chewing and swallowing of food, and initiates the digestion of starches. Saliva also acts as a solvent for waste excretion and assists in the regulation of water balance. The dry mouth that occurs during stress is due to adrenergic (sympathetic) nervous system suppression of salivation. Saliva becomes ropey and more viscid when a person becomes dehydrated, breathes through the mouth, or ingests drugs like atropine or antihistamines.

TEETH. Children have 20 deciduous teeth that begin to erupt at about 6 months of age and are lost during the early school-age period. Thirty-two permanent teeth gradually replace them. The teeth are living structures with a circulatory and nerve supply that is contained in the inner core of the tooth, called the pulp. Dentin, the primary tissue of the tooth, surrounds the pulp. Enamel, a hard substance, covers the exposed portion of the tooth, called the crown. The primary functions of teeth are to bite and masticate (chew) food.

Eyes. Fibrous membranes called the sclera and the cornea cover the eye. The sclera, white and opaque, extends from the optic nerve to the cornea. The cornea is continuous with the sclera, but is transparent and colorless. The cornea plays a role in refraction. The mucous membrane that lines the eyelids is called the *conjunctiva;* it is attached to the sclera (see Figs. 17–20 and 17–21). Tears, secreted by the lacrimal glands, keep the conjunctiva, sclera, and cornea moist. Tears cleanse the eye and protect it from contamination by pollutants.

Nose and Pharynx. The mucous membranes and accessory structures in the nose filter, warm, and moisturize incoming air. Nasal hairs screen out larger particles, while cilia on the mucosa remove smaller particles. The mucus-producing goblet cells lining the nasal passages moisturize incoming air. The abundant blood vessels in nasal mucosa also warm the air as it passes to the lower respiratory tract.

The *pharyngeal (throat) mucosa* is continuous with nasal mucosa and extends to the base of the larynx. It is similar to the mucosa of the respiratory tract and contains lymphoid tissue, which makes up the tonsils. A dry sensation in the pharyngeal mucosa is part of the mechanism that stimulates thirst.

Genitalia. Glandular vaginal epithelium, which lies in folds called *rugae,* covers the smooth-muscle walls of the vagina. This mucosa produces a continuous flow of fluid that serves to maintain vaginal cleanliness. The vestibule (the area between the labia majora in females) contains the vaginal opening and the urinary meatus. It is covered with very thin, almost mucosal skin. Bartholin's and Skene's glands, both of which produce mucus, especially during sexual excitement, also open into the vestibule.

Mucosal tissue also lines the urethra in the male reproductive tract. The bulbourethral glands open into the urethra and produce a rather viscid secretion that lubricates the urethra.

Anus and Rectum. Mucous membranes line the rectum and anus. The rectal mucosa lies in transverse folds that contain rectal smooth muscle. In the upper third of the anal canal, the mucosa forms vertical folds containing arteries and veins. The mucous membrane merges into skin in the distal third of the anal canal.

FUNCTIONS OF SKIN AND MUCOSA

Protection

The outer layer of the epidermis is a relatively impermeable layer of interlocking cells that provides a mechanical barrier to protect underlying tissue from the environment. The epidermis resists penetration by mechanical forces as well as bacteria and is moisture resistant. It minimizes the loss of body fluids or absorption of liquids on the surface of the skin, which affects the efficacy of topical medicines and the intensity of hypersensitivity allergic responses.

Antimicrobial action is another form of protection afforded by the skin and mucosa. Even when a break occurs in the skin, the basement membrane of the dermal–epidermal junction acts as an effective filter to limit invasion of foreign substances. The cells of the dermis marshal the body's defenses if microbes do gain entrance, initiating the inflammatory response and, in some cases, a specific immunologic response. **Collagen,** a component of the dermis, is essential for wound healing and scar formation; it gives the healing wound tensile strength. Elastin fibers give the skin its ability to return to its original shape after stretching. Ground substance promotes cell migration in wound healing, acts as a glue to hold skin surfaces together while healing occurs, and influences the skin's osmotic properties because of its ability to retain water (up to 1000 times its own weight).

Fibroblasts, macrophages, and mast cells are the primary functioning cells within the dermis. **Fibroblasts** act in the building and rebuilding of connective tissue. They are active in wound healing. **Macrophages** are phagocytes; they are particularly important in the inflammatory process. Mast cells are highly specialized cells that also play a role in inflammation. The skin also hosts a variety of nonpathogenic organisms known as **normal flora.** These organisms provide further protection against invasion by pathogenic bacteria. Normal flora create a biologic niche for themselves, thereby effectively competing with other bacterial strains for nutrients and space.

When intact, mucous membranes are impermeable to bacteria, although viruses are able to penetrate them. The most effective protection afforded by mucosa is related to the secretion of mucus, which traps microbes and other foreign materials so they can be more readily disposed of, for example, by coughing. Mucous secretions also contain antimicrobial enzymes that are lethal to many invading bacteria.

Temperature Regulation

The hypothalamus and receptors in the dermis regulate body temperature. When skin receptors sense a change in environmental temperature, specific responses to conserve heat or to prevent an increase in core temperature occur.

When an individual is exposed to cold, constriction of blood vessels in the skin and subcutaneous tissue minimizes the amount of heat energy carried by the blood from the interior to the surface of the body. **Pilomotor activity,** or "gooseflesh," appears, trapping a layer of warm air next to the surface of the body, which acts as an insulator against heat loss.

An increase in environmental or core body temperature, on the other hand, stimulates vasodilation, facilitating heat transfer from the body to the environment. Sweating occurs, enhancing heat loss by evaporation. More than 80 percent of the body heat loss occurs via the skin by radiation, conduction, convection, and/or evaporation. See the discussion of heat loss in Chap. 17.

Sensation

Skin is an important organ of sensation. A person's ability to discriminate touch, pressure, pain, and temperature is due to a complex network of nerve fibers in the dermis. Specialized receptors as well as free nerve endings transmit the varied impulses that communicate information about the immediate environment as well as initiate important reflexes that are important in adapting to the environment. These receptors react to different thresholds of stimulation and sensation depending on the region of the body in which they occur.

Excretion

Although the skin is not a major excretory organ, excretion of varied amounts of water, salts, and urea occurs via the skin. Under certain abnormal conditions, water loss via the skin can be substantial enough to cause fluid imbalance.

Lubrication

Lubrication is primarily a function of mucosa. When mucosa are irritated by chemical or mechanical stimuli, mucus is produced. The mucus protects the fragile membranes from damage that could result from such stimuli. Mucus also provides needed lubrication for bodily functions such as bowel elimination and sexual activity.

FACTORS AFFECTING SKIN AND TISSUE INTEGRITY

AGE

Infants

At birth, the newborn is covered with a protective substance called *vernix caseosa,* a whitish creamy secretion produced by the sebaceous glands. It is absorbed by the skin or removed during the infant's first bath. *Lanugo,* the precursor to body hair, may be present, particularly over the shoulders and back. Newborns' skin is particularly vulnerable to environmental irritants.

Many newborns develop physiologic jaundice at 24 to 48 hours of age. This is because the number of red blood cells needed for oxygenation in utero is greater than that needed after the transition to extrauterine life, so unneeded red blood cells are destroyed after birth, producing jaundice. **Desquamation** (peeling or sloughing of the outer epidermal layer) is also common during the first several weeks of life.

Common skin variations include *milia* (small white papules caused by plugged sebaceous glands) over the bridge of the nose and forehead; *acrocyanosis* (bluish tinged hands and feet, related to uncoordinated vasomotor responses to temperature changes and oxygen demands); **petechiae** (red pinpoint capillary hemorrhages) over the head and face; and *mongolian spots* (area of darker pigmentation over the lower back and buttocks due to uneven melanocyte distribution in dark-skinned babies). Some newborns have birthmarks such as capillary *hemangiomas,* which usually disappear by the age of 1 year; or permanent birthmarks such as strawberry marks, nevus flammeus, and port wine stains.

Toddlers Through School Age

During this time the skin takes on the appearance and functions of adult skin. Nevertheless, abrasions and lacerations associated with play activities, and allergic or infectious forms of **dermatitis** (inflammation of the skin characterized by redness and itchiness), do occur.

Adolescents

Adolescents experience skin changes associated with physical maturation. The sebaceous glands begin to produce *sebum,* a complex mixture of cholesterol, fatty acids, and waxy alcohols, several years prior to puberty because of stimulation by sex hormones. The larger glands of the face and scalp are particularly sensitive to androgens (male sex hormones produced by testis, adrenal glands, and ovaries), giving rise to acne and other skin eruptions. Apocrine glands become active at the onset of puberty and secrete a substance that exudes odor in the presence of bacteria. Boys and girls develop pubic and axillary hair. Body hair becomes thicker and more noticeable. Boys begin growing facial hair. In girls, there is an increase in subcutaneous fat deposits over the hips, thighs, and breasts.

Middle-aged and Older Adults

There are few age-related skin problems affecting middle-aged adults. The skin of older people gradually loses elasticity, appearing wrinkled, with folds because of collagen changes and loss of subcutaneous fat. This increases vulnerability to epidermal tears, which occur as a result of even minimal friction or shearing.[3] Blood vessels are more fragile and less protected because of collagen tissue changes, and so even minor trauma results in localized hemorrhages into the skin, initially having a red to purplish appearance, and then fading to yellowish-brown before disappearing. This is called *senile purpura.* Skin tears are a frequent complication of purpura.

Pigmentation changes related to altered melanocyte activity—such as mottling, darkened spots ("age spots" or lentigo), particularly on the face and back of hands are common. Sebum production diminishes after menopause in women, and in the late 70s in men; the loss of lubrication causes dry, flaky skin and dry hair. Some hair follicles cease to function, so scalp hair is thinner. Nails become thicker and brittle because of overgrowth of keratin, and may appear yellow due to deposition of calcium. The skin is a less effective barrier against infection, and immune function is somewhat diminished. Vascular insufficiency is more common among older adults; shiny, hairless skin and stasis ulcers are manifestations of this.

EXPOSURE TO SUN

Sun exposure is damaging to skin. Premature development of skin changes associated with aging occurs in individuals who experience frequent and regular exposure to sun without use of protective skin preparations. Sunburn is even more serious. It damages deeper skin layers and its destructive effects are cumulative. For further discussion refer to *Protection from Sun Exposure* later in this chapter.

NUTRITIONAL STATUS

The integument is particularly vulnerable to deficiencies in essential nutrients, because of the rapid turnover of its cells. Protein and vitamin deficiencies in particular result in diminished skin integrity and poor wound healing. Vitamin deficiency diseases typically produce skin manifestations such as **dermatitis** (vitamin B_6, niacin, riboflavin); cracks in the corners of the mouth (vitamin B_6, riboflavin); edema (thiamin); petechiae and bleeding gingivae (vitamin C). Insufficient vitamin A results in epithelial cells becoming plugged with excess keratin, forming unsightly bumps on the skin. Hyperkeratinization interferes with mucus production as well, so mucosa throughout the body becomes dry and hardened.

PERSONAL HYGIENE

Poor hygiene makes the integument vulnerable to insult and can even cause breakdown and deterioration. For example, inadequate oral hygiene promotes dental caries and permits buildup of excessive amounts of dental plaque, which eventually causes severe periodontal disease and loss of teeth.

Infrequent bathing causes skin irritation from accumulated oil, dead skin cells, perspiration, and bacteria. Skin folds are particularly vulnerable; skin in these areas may break down. Genital and anal–rectal mucosa may become excoriated from residue of urine and fecal matter. Conversely, excessive bathing, or bathing with harsh soaps, hinders the protective actions of sebum, producing dryness and compromised antibacterial action.

HEALTH STATUS

The integument reflects overall health state. A healthy person generally has a healthy integument. Ill health may alter the integument.

Acute Conditions

Some acute illnesses cause temporary changes in skin and mucosal status. For example, any condition in which there is abnormal body fluid loss, such as vomiting or diarrhea, will eventually produce dry skin and mucosa, thickened or diminished secretions (mucus, tears, saliva) and loss of skin turgor. The effects of dehydration are discussed in greater detail in Chap. 34.

Many minor infectious diseases have skin rashes as one manifestation. In some of these the skin is the target organ of the infectious agent; in others the skin manifestations are secondary. Dermatitis is a common response to environmental allergens; inflammation of nasal, pharyngeal, and respiratory mucosa also may occur because of allergens. Some acute illnesses such as upper respiratory infections or vaginal infections cause mucosal irritation, resulting in increased mucus production. Continuous drainage of mucosal discharge also may irritate surrounding skin.

Pressure ulcers are another example of skin changes related to health status. **Pressure ulcers** are lesions caused by unrelieved pressure resulting in damage to underlying tissue.[4] They are usually located over bony prominences. Pressure ulcers are discussed in greater detail later in this chapter.

Integument alterations associated with acute conditions are usually self-limiting, that is, they heal spontaneously when the causative agent is no longer present.

Chronic Conditions

Many chronic diseases generate integumentary manifestations. Some of these are diseases in which the primary pathology involves the skin. The specific type of skin change or lesion depends on the specific disease. In other cases, the effects on the skin are secondary to pathology in other organs. For example, skin is particularly vulnerable to circulatory disorders. Interference with circulation causes a wide range of skin changes. Manifestations include thinning of skin layers, decreased sebum production, and loss of hair. More pronounced disruption of circulation produces *stasis ulcers* and tissue death. Diabetes mellitus is one cause of poor peripheral circulation. Some individuals with respiratory conditions suffer similar skin changes because of low oxygen concentration in the blood, even though circulation to the skin is intact.

ALTERED SKIN AND MUCOSAL INTEGRITY

SKIN PIGMENTATION CHANGES

Hyperpigmentation

Some variations in the skin are the result of an increase in pigmentation. Normal color variation between races is a result of the increase in the number and size of melanocytes and the rate at which melanin is produced. An increased production of melanin produces hyperpigmentation. A suntan is one example of hyperpigmentation. Sunlight activates increased production of melanin. The ability to tan varies among individuals. Light-skinned, blue- or green-eyed individuals produce pigment more slowly than those whose skin is normally darker. Sunburn results when sun exposure exceeds an individual's ability to produce melanin. The result is redness and tenderness, often appearing several hours after the sun exposure.

Hyperpigmentation also occurs in freckles, skin changes in pregnancy (chloasma and linea nigra), aging (age spots on upper body and face), and certain drug and allergic reactions (silver nitrate, perfumes, and the antimalarials).

COLLABORATIVE STRATEGY

ASSESSING LIFESTYLE

Lifestyle is a frequent cause of skin problems. Personal choices regarding hygiene, diet, and sun exposure, for example, may cause or contribute to various skin conditions. A collaborative approach to dealing with skin problems involves the nurse's recognition of the importance of a patient's personal preferences. Sensitive information sharing is likely to result in trust and effective problem resolution.

Hypopigmentation

Decreased or absent melanin production is quite rare. It results in a decrease in pigmentation. *Albinism* is a congenital lack of pigmentation that may be total or partial. *Vitiligo,* in which areas of normal coloring surround patchy areas without pigmentation, is an acquired condition that is thought to be due to decreased cholinesterase activity in the skin or to an autoimmune process.

Color Changes

The skin changes in color in response to a variety of internal conditions. A decrease in capillary flow or in blood components is visible on the skin surface, causing **pallor** (pale skin). **Erythema** is a generalized area of redness that blanches when palpated. It is due to dilation of superficial capillaries. **Cyanosis,** a bluish-gray skin color, occurs when oxygen content of the intravascular hemoglobin is diminished or when blood flow rate is slowed, for example, when a person is chilled. Increased serum bilirubin level will cause the skin to have a yellowish cast, called **jaundice.**

SKIN LESIONS

A **lesion** is a circumscribed area of pathologically altered tissue. Skin lesions may be primary or secondary.

Primary Lesions

Primary lesions appear in previously healthy skin. They are classified according to their size, shape, and contents. Primary lesions may be flat or raised, circular or lobulated. They may be filled with clear fluid, pus, or solid matter. There are many causes of primary lesions, including trauma, allergens, infectious agents, and cancer. Advise patients to bring persistent skin lesions to the attention of a health care provider to determine cause and appropriate treatment. The terms used when describing primary lesions, with accompanying illustrations and definitions, appear in Table 17–15.

Secondary Lesions

Secondary lesions are alterations in primary lesions, such as erosion of deeper skin layers or cracking of skin surrounding a primary lesion. They can also be caused by scratching or infection. Scars are also considered secondary lesions because they represent dermal changes following a primary lesion. Table 17–16 provides definitions and descriptions of common secondary lesions.

MUCOSAL DISRUPTIONS

Oral Mucosa

Oral mucosal lesions include mechanical trauma, stomatitis, tooth and gum problems, and malignant changes.

Mechanical Trauma. Mechanical trauma to oral cavity structures is due to accidental occurrences or chronic irritants. The resultant lesion may be erosion of oral mucosa, puncture wounds, lacerations, or burns.

Examples of accidental causes of trauma include overly vigorous tooth brushing, chewing on sharp objects, biting oneself, and ingesting very hot foods or beverages. Chronic irritation develops from orthodontic braces, loose-fitting dentures, and cigarette and pipe smoking. Some treatment modalities such as oral airways and nasotracheal or orogastric tubes may cause irritation to the oral cavity.

Stomatitis. **Stomatitis** is inflammation of the mouth. Causative factors include pathogens (bacteria, fungus, yeast, or viruses); chemical substances (ingredients in mouth-care products, medications, especially cancer chemotherapy); systemic infections (measles, syphilis); and vitamin deficiencies.

Typically, stomatitis presents with numerous small vesicles on the cheeks, palate, gums, or oral pharynx. Sometimes there are also lesions on the tongue. The vesicles soon break and leave shallow ulcers with reddened edges. The lesions are uncomfortable and may make eating difficult. Some causative agents of stomatitis produce agent-specific lesions; for example, thrush produces white plaque-like lesions; measles produce small red spots with blue-white centers.

Tooth and Gum Problems. The most common tooth and gum problems are associated with the accumulation of dental plaque because of ineffective or infrequent oral hygiene. **Plaque** is a mixture of saliva, bacteria, and sloughed epithelial cells. Sugary foods tend to make plaque more adherent to teeth. The presence of plaque on the tooth can cause demineralization of the tooth enamel. As the enamel wears away, bacteria enter the dentin of the tooth and cause **caries** (tooth decay or "cavities"). Bacteria present in the plaque are often odor producing, causing halitosis.

Plaque also irritates the gingiva. When plaque is not removed from the teeth by regular oral hygiene, plaque is transformed into **tartar,** a hard yellowish substance that forms along the gum line. Prolonged contact of the gingiva with tartar causes inflammation and bleeding of the gums, called **gingivitis.** Chronic gingivitis often progresses to periodontal disease, in which the supporting structures of the teeth degenerate, resulting in loosening and loss of teeth.

Other gum problems include hyperplasia (overgrowth of epithelial tissue), most frequently secondary to use of certain anticonvulsant medications, and *sordes,* a crustlike accumulation of dead cells, food debris, and microorganisms.

Malignant Lesions. Malignant lesions in the oral cavity occur on the tongue, gums, and associated bony processes. The original lesions may be whitish-gray plaques, lumps, or small ulcerations. As the disease extends, the ulcerations become more extensive and may cause numbness. Early treatment is often curative, but extensive lesions usually require radical surgical dissection. For this reason, persistent mouth sores or mouth pain should be investigated to determine their origin.

Corneal Mucosa

Disruptions of corneal mucosa result from foreign bodies or chemical injury. Foreign bodies are often small airborne particles such as dust that blow into the eye. They are easily removed and usually do little harm, although they may cause considerable discomfort, as the cornea is very sensitive. When a foreign body penetrates the sclera or cornea, damage to the eye may result. The injury is a medical emergency and must be treated immediately.

Contact lens wearers may experience corneal abrasions because of poorly fitting lenses or foreign bodies trapped under the lens. These problems are more common with hard contact lenses.

Many chemicals are toxic to the conjunctival mucosa, sclera, and cornea. They create a burn or ulcer. Immediately flushing the eye with water for 5 minutes or more may remove the chemical before damage results. If irritation persists after flushing, medical assistance is advisable.

Nasal and Throat Mucosa

Rhinitis (inflammation of nasal mucosa) and **pharyngitis** (inflammation of throat mucosa) are common minor illnesses. The usual cause of acute inflammation is viral or bacterial invasion of the tissues. Mucosa become reddened and painful and mucus production increases. With bacterial infection, discharge is often purulent. Smoking causes a chronically irritated, reddened throat and a characteristic "smoker's cough" from frequent need to clear the airways of accumulated mucus.

Genital Mucosa

Disruptions of genital mucosa include **vaginitis** (inflammation of vaginal mucosa) and **urethritis** (inflammation of the urethra). Infection by bacteria, viruses, protozoa, or yeast is the most common cause of genital mucosal disruptions. The infectious agent may be sexually transmitted or be transmitted from the anal area because of incorrect wiping of the perineum in women. Occasionally, yeast infections result from disruptions in normal vaginal flora after a course of systemic antibiotic therapy. **Neoplasms** (tumors), foreign bodies such as a retained tampon, or chemical irritation from strong douches are other causes of vaginitis.

Symptoms include discharge that is sometimes malodorous, **pruritus** (itching) of the vulva and perineum, and painful urination. The vaginal mucosa appears red and may have superficial ulcerations; the urethra in males is not visualized to diagnose this condition.

Atrophic vaginitis frequently occurs in postmenopausal women, or women experiencing disruption of estrogen production for other reasons. The vaginal mucosa becomes thinner and vaginal mucus secretion declines. Some women experience pruritus with this condition. Painful intercourse is sometimes associated with atrophic vaginitis, because lubrication is diminished.

Anal and Rectal Mucosa

Hemorrhoids (enlarged veins in the mucosa of the anal canal) and anorectal *fissures* (cracklike lesions) are common problems of anal and rectal mucosa. Hemorrhoids have varied causes; frequently straining at stool is a contributing factor (see also Chap. 29). Anal fissures are often trauma related, resulting, for example, from passage of extremely hard stool or anal intercourse. Local pain, particularly upon defecation, and itching are symptoms of both problems.

WOUNDS

A **wound** is an injury to tissue that disrupts normal cellular processes. It may involve a break in the integrity of the skin or mucous membranes and/or damage to deeper tissue. Wounds may result from mechanical, thermal, chemical, or radiation trauma or from invasion by pathogens. Surgical incisions, accidental scrapes and cuts, and pressure ulcers are examples of wounds.

Classifying Wounds

Several overlapping descriptive categories, including severity, cause, and contamination, may be used to classify wounds.

Severity. Severity relates to type and amount of tissue damage. In closed wounds, the skin remains intact, but soft tissue or deeper structures are damaged. Open wounds are those in which skin or mucosa is damaged. Wounds are also described in terms of extent of injury. Superficial or partial-thickness wounds involve only the epidermis and/or part of the dermis. Tissue-loss wounds are deeper, with damage or destruction of subcutaneous fat, muscle, bone, or other structures.

Cause. How a wound is acquired, or its cause, is another way to describe it. In an **abrasion,** all or part of the skin or mucosa is scraped away. Skinned knees and dermabrasions (a cosmetic skin procedure) are examples.

Burns are injuries due to heat, radiation, chemicals, or electricity. Thermal and electrical burns are classified by degrees, depending on the depth of tissue injury. First-degree burns are minor, injuring only the outer epidermis; second-degree burns extend into the dermis, causing blisters; third-degree burns destroy epidermis and dermis and damage underlying tissue as well. Tissue may be charred or coagulated.

A **contusion** is a blow from a blunt object that entails soft tissue damage, but no break in the skin. Often bleeding is associated with contusions. Diffuse bleeding into surrounding tissue is called an **ecchymosis** (bruise); encapsulated bleeding is known as a **hematoma. Lacerations** are tears of tissue having uneven edges and often contaminated with dirt, grass, or other debris. Lacerations can involve skin and muscle layers.

A **puncture wound** is a wound made by a sharp pointed instrument that penetrates the dermal layer. Getting a splinter and stepping on a nail are examples of minor puncture wounds. Puncture wounds are prone to become infected because they bleed little and are difficult to cleanse. A foreign object entering deeper tissue or a body cavity such as the chest or abdomen causes a **penetrating wound.** If the foreign object enters and then exits an internal organ, the wound is called a **perforating wound.** An **incision** is a clean-edged cut made with a sharp instrument. Most incisions are intentional surgical wounds.

A **pressure ulcer** is a wound caused by unrelieved pressure that results in damage of underlying tissue. Pressure ulcers are graded from stage 1 to stage 4, according to the extent of tissue damage.[5] The stages are summarized in Table 27–1 and illustrated in Fig. 27–1.

? CRITICAL QUERY

Bergstrom and others[5] state that 9 percent of all hospitalized patients have serious problems with pressure ulcers. This percentage jumps to 23 percent in nursing home patients. Pressure ulcers add to pain, suffering, and increased hospital stay, and their treatment has always been a problem in health care. What economic and social factors might explain the persistence of pressure ulcers as a health care problem?

TABLE 27-1. STAGES OF PRESSURE ULCERS

Stage	Illustration	Description
Stage 1		Involves epidermis only. Ranges from swollen pinkish-red mottled skin that does not return to normal color after pressure is relieved.
Stage 2		A partial-thickness skin loss involving the epidermis, dermis, or both. The ulcer is superficial and is characterized by abrasions, blisters, or shallow craters.
Stage 3		A full-thickness ulceration involves subcutaneous fat where extensive undermining occurs. Deep fascia limits the depth of penetration of necrosis.
Stage 4		Full-thickness ulcer penetrates deep fascia and muscle and may expose bone and supporting structures. Undermining and sinus tracts may be associated with this stage.

Sources: Adapted from Shea J. Pressure sores: Classification and management. Clin Orthop. *1975;112:89–100. Updated from National Pressure Ulcer Advisory Panel. NPUAP Report.* Adv Wound Care. *1995;8:32–33.*

Wound Contamination. Wounds are classified on the basis of actual or potential contamination. **Contaminants** are agents in the wound that may cause infection, render a surgical site less clean, or interfere with healing. Examples of contaminating agents are bacteria, fecal material, soil, and gravel particles. There are four levels in the classification.[6]

- *Clean wound.* Surgical sites in which no inflammation occurs. The wound makes no contact with body cavities having bacterial populations (normal flora). Occurs in tissue that is not infected. Example: breast surgery.
- *Clean-contaminated wound.* Wound enters an organ that has normal flora or that connects with an organ having normal flora. Example: lung surgery.
- *Contaminated wound.* Open accidental wounds; surgery with a break in sterile technique or in which gastrointestinal drainage or drainage from an infected area contacts the wound. Example: ruptured appendix.
- *Infected wound.* Wound in which microorganisms are multiplying and producing injurious effects. Example: drainage of an abscess.

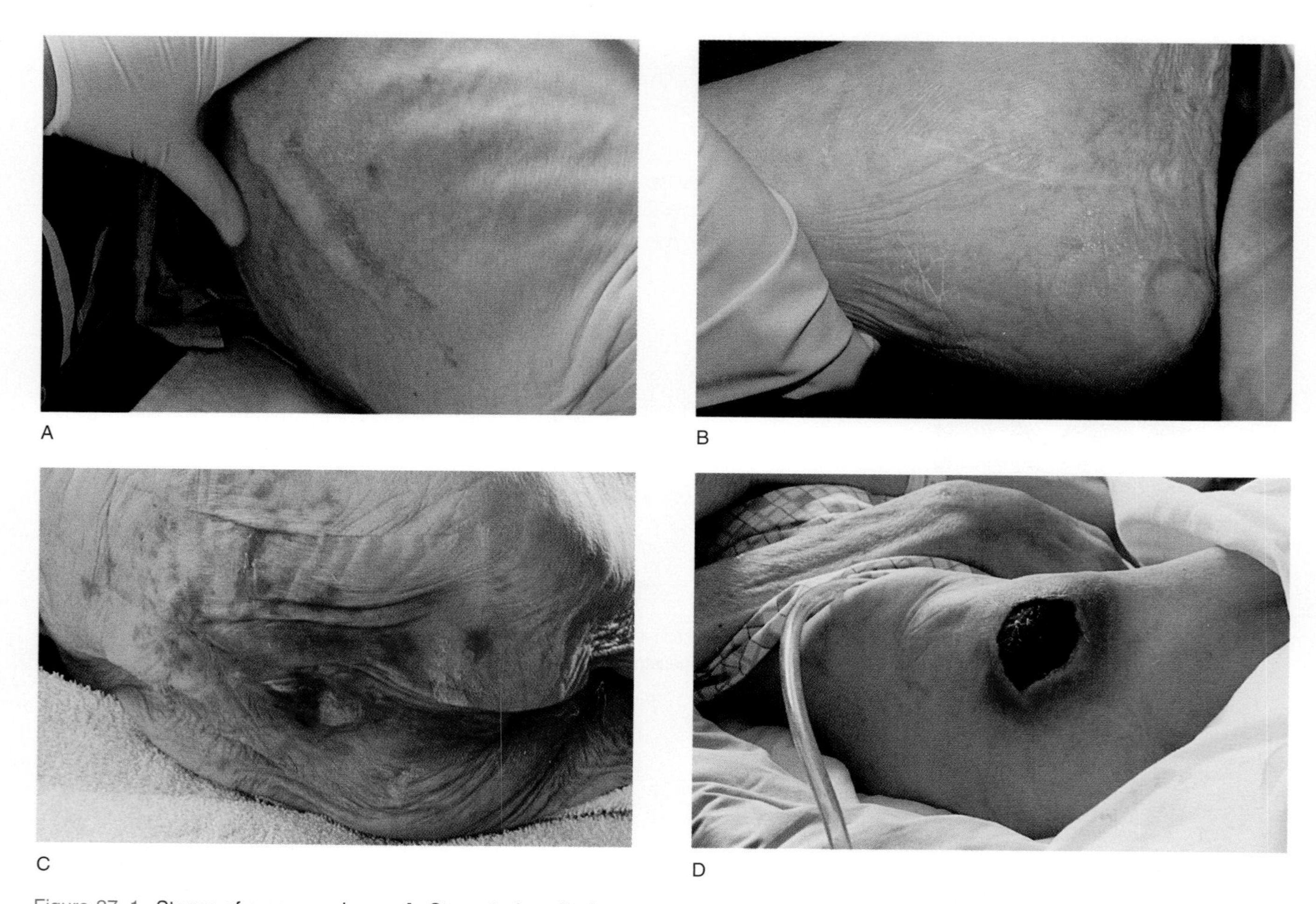

Figure 27–1. Stages of pressure ulcers. **A.** Stage 1 ulcer. **B.** Stage 2 ulcer. **C.** Stage 3 ulcer. **D.** Stage 4 ulcer.
(From Smith S, Duell D. Clinical Nursing Skills: Nursing Process Model; Basic to Advanced Skills. *4th ed. Norwalk, CT: Appleton & Lange; 1996:690.)*

▲ WOUND HEALING

Wound healing is a spontaneous restorative process that is initiated immediately after a wound occurs. The nature of repair and the length of each stage vary with the type of wound as well as with local and systemic host factors. Good health is predictive of good wound healing. Conversely, health-related factors, such as stress and many chronic diseases, are detrimental to healing.

PROCESS OF WOUND HEALING

The healing process consists of three overlapping phases: inflammation, proliferation, and maturation.

The Inflammatory Phase

Inflammation is a nonspecific defensive response to injury, beginning at the instant of injury and lasting 3 to 6 days.[7,8] It is initiated by the release of intracellular chemicals from injured tissues. Inflammation serves to control bleeding, prevent bacterial invasion, remove debris from tissue injury, and prepare for repair.[9]

Mechanisms in Inflammation. Immediate vasoconstriction at the site of an injury and the accumulation of platelets along damaged blood vessel walls accomplish the goal of controlling bleeding. The clotting mechanism, involving a complex series of interactions among coagulation factors, produces a platelet and fibrin plug called a clot or **thrombus** to seal off the site of the injury from further blood loss.

Protection from bacterial invasion results from **phagocytosis** (ingestion and digestion of foreign cells and debris) and **epithelialization** (migration of epithelial cells to close the wound site), which occur simultaneously. Phagocytosis also accomplishes removal of debris and preparation for repair.

PHAGOCYTOSIS. Vascular changes support initiation of phagocytosis. Immediately after the initial vasoconstriction, arterioles, venules, and capillaries dilate. Vasodilation increases vascular permeability, allowing cells, plasma proteins, and fluid to flow into the injured tissues from blood vessels surrounding the injury (Fig. 27–2). These

INSIGHTS FROM NURSING LITERATURE

EVALUATING RISK OF PRESSURE SORES

McCormack HC. A pressure sore risk scale for use with older people. Prof Nurs. *1996;11:673–676.*

Acknowledging the enormous economic cost to society and the physical and emotional cost to the patient of treating pressure sores, the researcher studied pressure sore risk-assessment scales in the interest of promoting prevention. Several existing scales, she found, tended to overpredict the risk of sore formation in the elderly. However, one scale, the Stratheden scale, which uses indicators, such as body build for height and nutritional status, omitted by other scales proved helpful. It includes factors such as skin status, urinary and fecal continence, mobility, and mental awareness all important in evaluating the likelihood of pressure ulcers. Each factor is assigned a number. Fully mobile elderly patients, for example, are allotted zero points (low risk), whereas those with restricted mobility get three points (moderate risk), and chairbound patients get five points (high risk). Overall risk scores can be computed by adding the numbers assigned to each factor.

responses underlie formation of inflammatory exudate and produce some of the signs and symptoms characteristic of inflammation, discussed below.

Leukocytes (white blood cells) are the cells that migrate (through processes known as margination and diapedsis) to the site of injury to carry out phagocytosis. Neutrophils are the primary leukocyte in the initial phase of the inflammation. Macrophages (defined earlier as reticuloendothelial cells whose primary function is phagocytosis) present in loose connective tissue are also active. As neutrophils die, monocytes become the dominant leukocyte. The monocytes are transformed into macrophages to replace those consumed in the process of clearing the wound site of debris that would interfere with the next phase of healing.

EPITHELIALIZATION. Epithelialization begins within a few hours of the creation of a cutaneous wound.[1] The reproduction and migration of cells occurs from the edge of the wound toward its center. New epithelial cells continue to form, until they cover the surface of the injury, and the epidermis is as thick as before. In sutured incised wounds, a layer of epithelial cells usually covers the wound surface within 24 hours (Figs. 27–2 and 27–3).

Inflammatory Exudate. The fluid that accumulates around the site of an injury is called an **exudate.** The characteristics of exudates depend on the type of injured tissue, cause of the injury, and duration of the inflammatory response. Serous exudate, the liquid component of blood, is produced in mild to moderate injuries. The fluid that collects inside a blister is a familiar example. Other types of exudates are:

- *Serous:* Clear exudate that accumulates in interstitial tissue in mild to moderate injuries and is produced with injury to serous membranes such as peritoneum or pleura.
- *Serosanguineous:* Reddish, pink exudate containing red blood cells with serous drainage produced when an injury involves blood vessel damage.
- *Catarrhal:* Exudate produced with mucosal irritation such as in a cold; appears as clear liquid with strands of mucus.
- *Fibrinous:* Sticky exudate produced in severe injury or prolonged inflammation. Increased capillary permeability permits escape of fibrin molecules into interstitial space. This promotes adherence of membranes to one another, causing, for example, intestinal adhesions or pleural friction rubs. May appear as grayish, opaque membrane over tissue-loss wounds.
- *Purulent:* Thick exudate containing dead bacteria and leukocytes produced when an infection is present at the site of an injury. Color varies with causative organism; yellowish, grayish, green are most common. Collection of purulent drainage is called an *abscess.*

Large amounts of exudate significantly delay healing. The circulatory system must reabsorb the exudates before healing can progress.

Signs and Symptoms of Inflammation. The cardinal signs and symptoms of inflammation are redness, heat, swelling, pain, and loss of function (Table 27–2). If inflammation is severe or prolonged, systemic manifestations, such as weakness, malaise, and a low-grade fever, are noticeable as well. White blood cell counts show elevations in neutrophils in the acute phase of inflammation, with increased monocytes in the recovery phase.

Duration of Inflammation. Inflammation overlaps with the next phase of healing, proliferation. Usually, acute inflammation peaks 24 to 48 hours after an injury, and then subsides. Inflammation is prolonged when the response is insufficient to accomplish preparation of the site for healing, as with individuals with compromised nutritional status or other physiologic stressors.

INSIGHTS FROM NURSING LITERATURE

EVALUATING PRESSURE ULCER HEALING

Reprinted from NPUAP Report. NPUAP position on reverse staging of pressure ulcers. Adv Wound Care. *1995;8:32–33.*

Officials of the National Pressure Ulcer Advisory Panel (NPUAP) note that the staging system which describes pressure ulcer severity by the layers of tissue involved is meant to help clinicians define the progression of a wound, but should not be used to assess healing. They stress that full thickness pressure ulcers, according to clinical studies, do not heal by replacing the same tissue layers (muscle, fat, dermis), but fill with granulation tissue composed primarily of endothelial cells, fibroblasts, collagen, and extracellular matrix. Therefore, attempts to describe healing by applying the staging system in reverse produces erroneous results and may lead to inappropriate wound care.

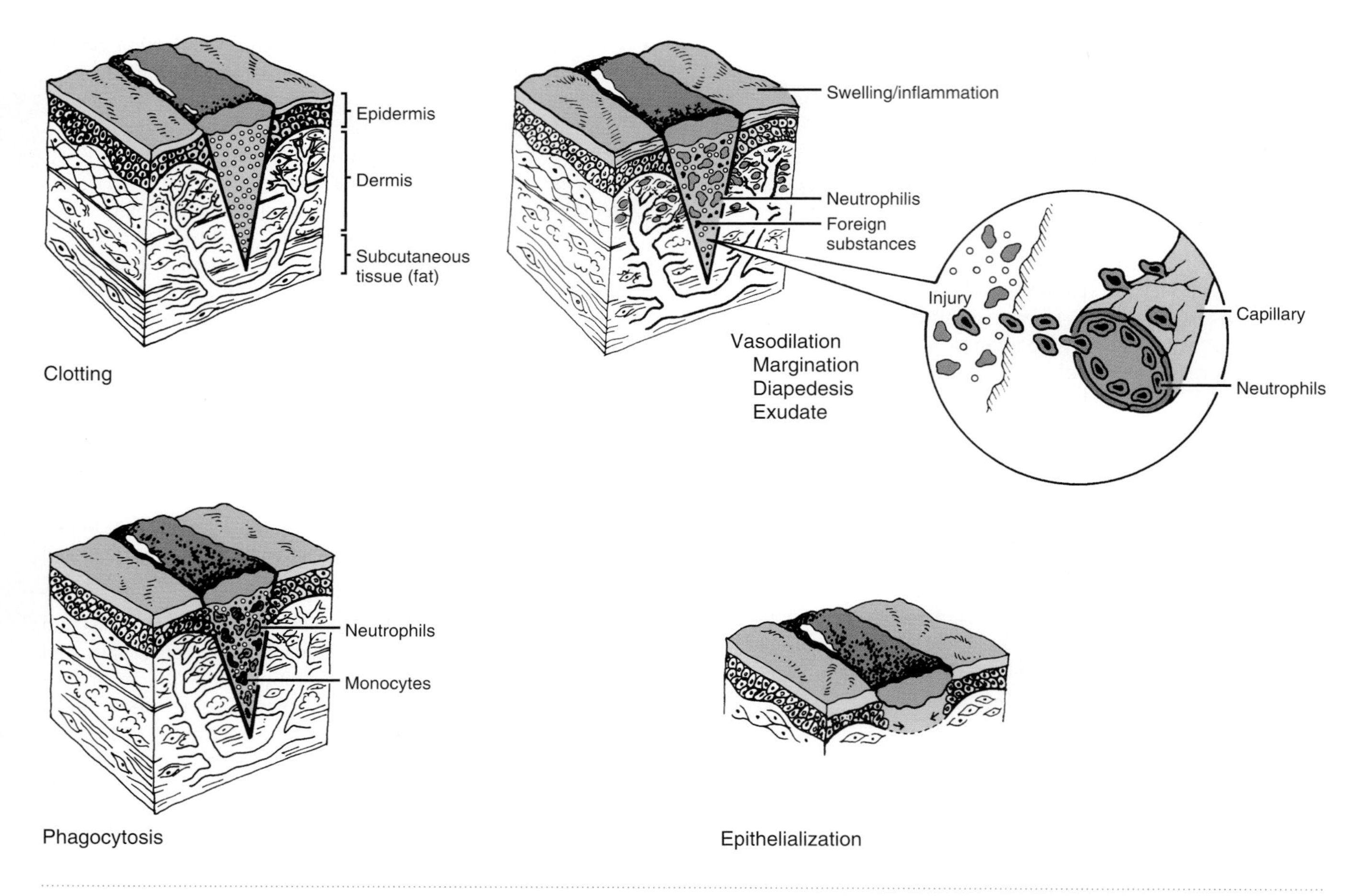

Figure 27–2. Inflammation: the first phase of wound healing.

TABLE 27-2. CARDINAL SIGNS AND SYMPTOMS OF INFLAMMATION

Manifestation	Produced By
Redness	Increased blood flow to site of injury. Capillary dilation produces reddened skin.
Heat	Increased blood flow transfers body heat to site of vasodilation.
Swelling	Exudate distends interstitial tissue.
Pain	Stimulation of nerve endings by tissue distension, and by chemicals released by injured tissues.
Loss of function	Death of cells, limited mobility because of swelling and pain.

The Proliferative Phase

The proliferation of several types of cells that form new tissue and, when possible, restore the function of the injured area initiates tissue reconstruction (Fig. 27–3). The new tissue may be identical to the injured tissue, or be connective (scar) tissue. The amount of connective tissue required for reconstruction varies with the extent and location of the injury. In some tissue, such as muscles and nerves, minimal regeneration is possible, so considerable scarring results if the injury is extensive.

Cellular Migration. Within a few hours of an injury healthy cells at the wound margins migrate toward the center of the wound. Migrating cells include epithelium and parenchymal cells. *Parenchymal cells* are the functional cells of internal organs—that is, those cells that actually carry out the functions of the organ, rather than giving it structure. Cellular migration continues until the cells migrating from all of the wound edges meet one another. In an incised sutured wound, the surgeon approximates all tissue layers, so cellular migration is relatively rapid. In a large tissue-loss wound, granulation tissue replaces both parenchymal cells and

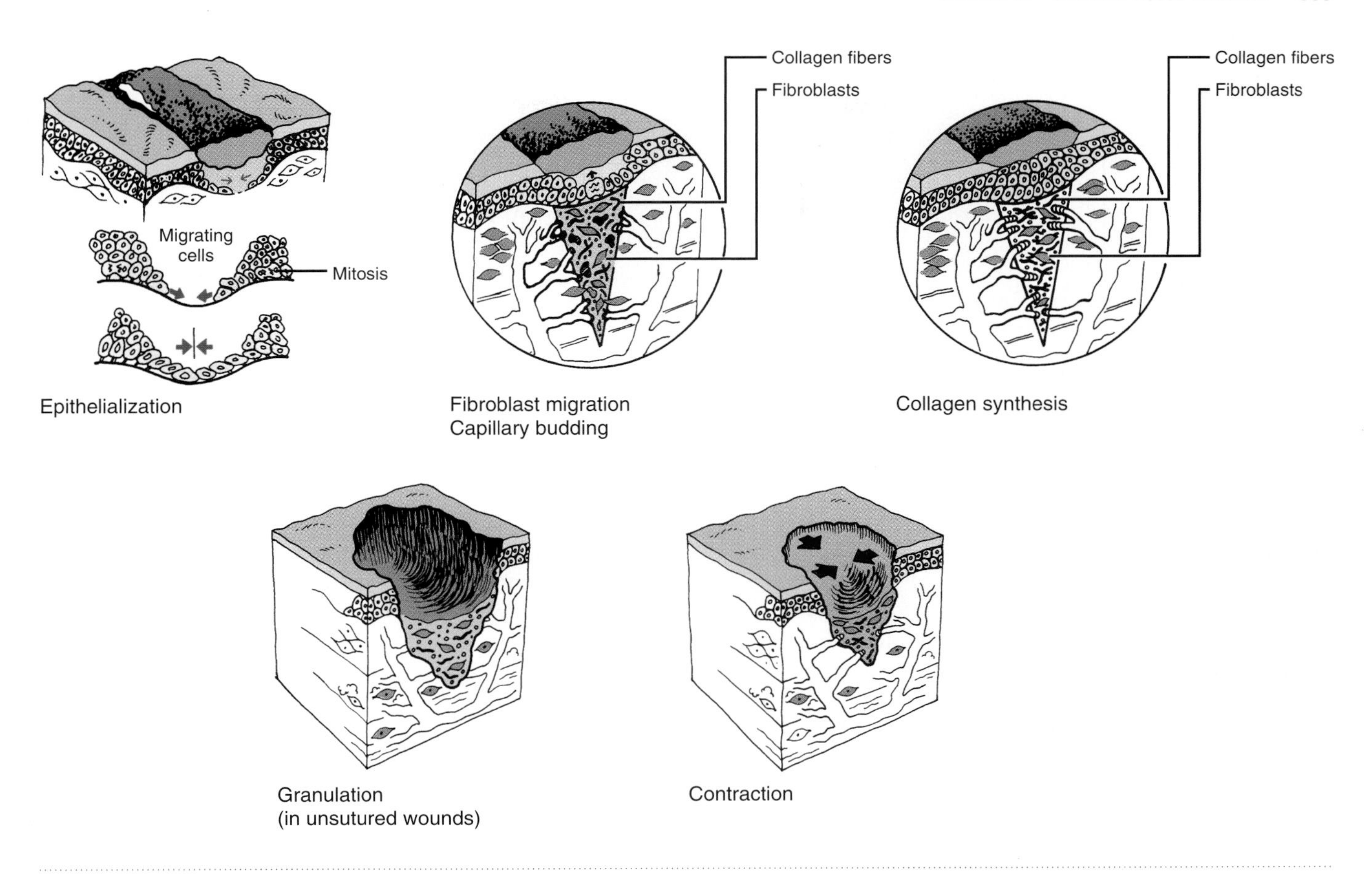

Figure 27–3. Proliferation: the second phase of wound healing.

epithelial cells (see *Capillary Budding*, below). Epithelial cells eventually cover the wound surface. The process of epithelialization is enhanced and more efficient when the wound surfaces are kept moist.[10] To cover a scabbed wound, epithelial cells must migrate under the thick layer of dried protein and dead cells, called **eschar.** A great deal of the metabolic energy of epithelial cells is expended in secreting enzymes to dissolve the eschar, greatly prolonging the process.[10]

Fibroplasia. Connective tissue cells called *fibroblasts* appear at the wound site about 2 days after an injury. These cells are the precursors of collagen, the protein molecule that makes up most connective tissue in the body. Over the course of wound reconstruction, the fibroblasts produce collagen fibers of increasing size that cross-link and overlap. Collagen supports the junction of migrating cells and gives scar tissue tensile strength.

Capillary Budding. At the same time that collagen production is progressing, blood vessels adjacent to the wound site produce capillary buds. These capillary branches eventually create a network that bridges the wound space, providing ample oxygen and nutrients to support the growth of new tissue. The new tissue that fills a large wound space or bridges the small gap between margins of a sutured wound is called **granulation tissue.** It is made up primarily of collagen, new capillaries, macrophages, and fibroblasts. Granulation tissue is pink to red because it is highly vascular. It is quite fragile and bleeds easily if traumatized.

Contraction. Myofibroblasts, cells with contractile properties similar to cardiac muscle, begin to gather around the wound edges in this phase of healing. As these cells contract in unison, they significantly reduce the surface area of the wound in a process called **contraction,** facilitating epithelial coverage.[11]

The proliferative phase lasts for 2 or more weeks after an injury. An extended proliferative phase is necessary to heal large tissue-loss wounds.

The Maturation or Remodeling Phase

Maturation consists of reorganization and remodeling of the scar. It involves continued production and alignment of collagen, balanced by selective collagen reabsorption and continued contraction (Fig. 27–4). Contraction shrinks the scar. Extra blood vessels are reabsorbed and compressed as maturation proceeds, so the scar becomes pale in color like surrounding skin. Eventually, the collagen fibers become interwoven with the fibers of original tissue surrounding the wound and with each other, resulting in a serviceable scar that is nearly as strong as the original tissue. Maturation lasts several months in sutured surgical incisions and takes considerably longer in tissue-loss wounds.

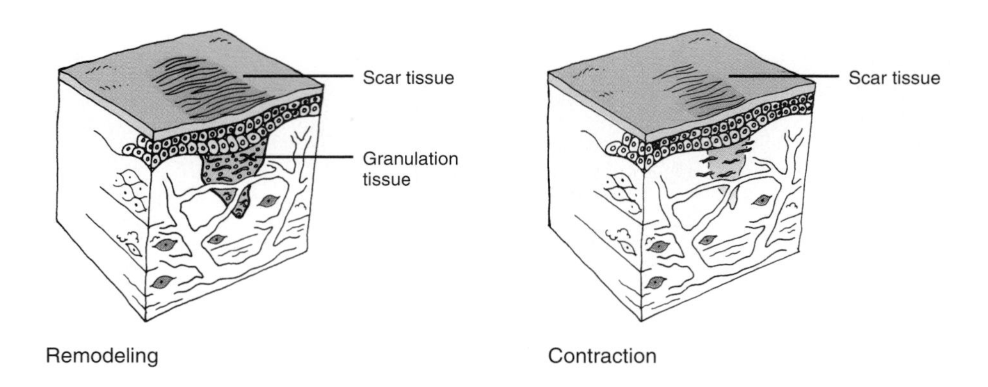

Figure 27–4. Maturation: the third phase of wound healing.

FACTORS AFFECTING WOUND HEALING

Type of Wound

Although healing proceeds through the same phases regardless of the type of wound, the length of healing time and the appearance of the scar differ with the type of wound. These differences are summarized by the terms primary and secondary intention.

Healing by Primary Intention. **Primary intention healing** refers to the healing of a wound in which there is no tissue loss (Fig. 27–5A). An incised surgical wound is an example. The approximation and securing of the corresponding tissue layers enhances cellular migration and facilitates healing. In surgical incisions, this is accomplished when the surgeon sutures the wound edges together.

In primary intention inflammation is minimal, because damage is not extensive. Epithelialization is rapid, usually occurring within 72 hours, so the infection risk is slight. Little or no granulation tissue forms, because migration of matching tissue types from the wound margins facilitates tissue regeneration. A small scar is typical.[12]

Healing by Secondary Intention. **Secondary intention healing** is the process by which tissue-loss wounds heal by granulation (Fig. 27–5B). In secondary intention, all phases or healing are prolonged. Inflammation may be significant. Often there is more debris and necrotic tissue in tissue-loss wounds, extending the period of phagocytosis. Infection risk is greater. These wounds need more fibroblasts to provide a framework for granulation tissue. Considerable granulation tissue is often needed to fill the wound cavity. Often epithelial cells cannot close the tissue defect, and eschar covers the wound surface. Parenchymal migration may be impossible, resulting in more scar tissue. Deformities are common with contraction of the large scar.

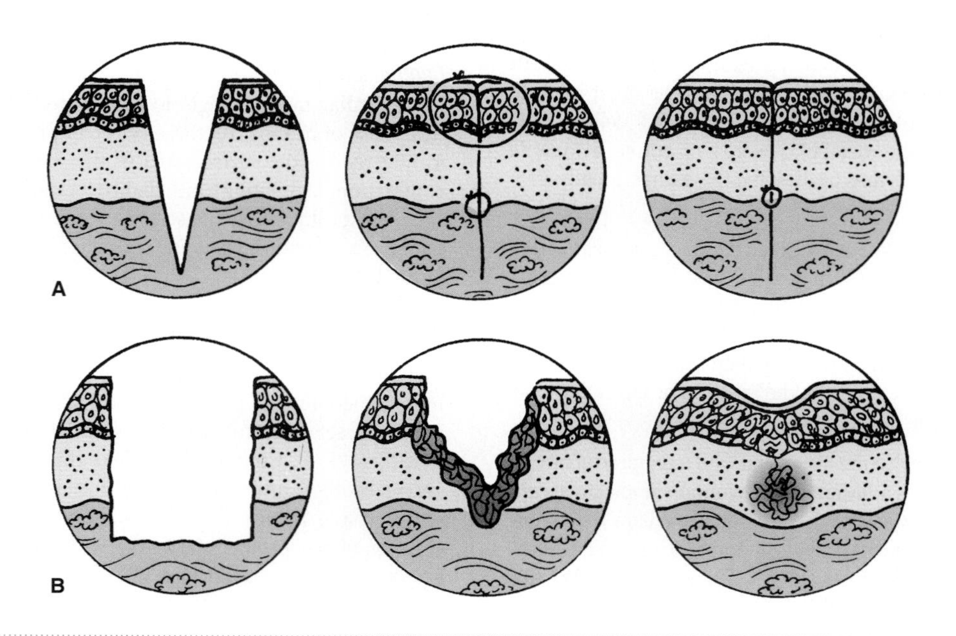

Figure 27–5. Wound healing: **(A)** primary intention and **(B)** secondary intention.

Healing by Tertiary Intention. **Tertiary intention healing** refers to a wound that is not sutured initially because of infection or high risk for infection. More satisfactory healing occurs when this type of wound is left open and the development of granulation tissue is promoted by special wound care and simultaneous treatment of the infection. After a time, the wound can be closed to allow healing to conclude by primary intention.

Age

Generally, extremes of age compromise wound healing. Several physiologic variables affect healing in neonates and premature infants. These include:

- respiratory compromise
- decreased tissue perfusion
- ineffective phagocytosis and cellular immunity

Because of rapid metabolism, growth, and limited nutrient reserves, basal energy needs are high. Wound healing increases energy needs, and it is therefore important to provide sufficient calories for both.

Older adults are also at risk for delayed healing. Age-related changes in immune function and circulatory efficiency delay onset of inflammation and prolong its phases. Cellular migration, replication, and maturation slow with age, extending reconstruction.[13] Moreover, diminished amounts of slow-wave sleep (see Chap. 31) reduce production of growth hormone, contributing to slower anabolic processes.[9] Nutritional deficits are relatively common among elderly individuals, an added risk factor, as discussed in the next section.

Nutritional Status

Healing is a significant energy demand. Rebuilding tissue at the site of injury requires protein, which individuals can synthesize only if they take in sufficient amounts of essential amino acids. Carbohydrate and fat calories are also important. Average-sized individuals must ingest about 4000 kilocalories a day in order to use protein for tissue repair rather than for basal metabolic activity.[14] Vitamin C is required for collagen synthesis, capillary formation, and capillary stability.[12,15,16] Vitamin A enhances epithelialization.[15] Zinc enhances epithelialization and the rate of gain of collagen strength.[17]

Even well-nourished patients who remain on nothing-by-mouth status for several days, and then on a clear liquid diet for more than a day, are at risk for developing deficiency states that can delay healing.[18] Standard dextrose and electrolyte solutions deliver 170 calories per 1000 mL. This marginal calorie intake depletes carbohydrate reserves within 1 to 2 days, making gluconeogenesis (formation of glycogen from noncarbohydrate sources, such as amino acids) necessary and therefore depleting amino acids available for tissue replacement.[19]

State of the Tissue

Variables such as the general condition of the wounded tissue, tissue perfusion, surgical dead space, and microorganism population influence the healing process.

General Condition. Healthy tissue heals best. A surgical wound made in otherwise undamaged tissue is likely to heal rapidly and without complication. On the other hand, a traumatic wound that damages a large area of tissue and disrupts surrounding circulation takes longer to heal. Tissue compromised in other ways, such as by radiation (often part of therapy for cancer), or tissue exposed to extremes of heat or cold, heals slowly. Radiation also threatens the immune system, because of its interference with the production of fibroblasts.[7]

Tissue Perfusion. The vascular system is a primary factor in initiating and maintaining tissue repair. Many of the cells responsible for phagocytosis and the immune response are blood components. Phagocytosis and cell migration, cell replication, and protein and collagen synthesis require a good oxygen supply.[17] Highly vascular tissue, such as in the head and face, heals more rapidly than less vascular tissue. Early mobility after surgery or injury improves overall circulation, and so enhances healing. Any condition that compromises circulation—such as obesity, anemia, vascular occlusion, or smoking—interferes with healing. Obesity increases the amount of adipose tissue, which is not highly vascular. Anemia reduces the amount of oxygen that is transported to healing tissue.[17] Smoking reduces hemoglobin's oxygen-carrying capacity (see Chap. 30). It is the most common cause of wound hypoxia.[10] Wound oxygen tensions have been measured at 0 for 20 minutes after smoking 1 cigarette.[20] Hypoxia and ischemia can also be caused by excessive tension on sutures.[6]

Dead Space. Dead space refers to areas within a sutured wound in which tissue layers on opposite sides of the wound are not aligned and in contact. Dead space is inevitable when surgery involves removal of a large amount of tissue, but dead space disrupts healing because it interferes with cellular migration and tissue perfusion. Exudates that collect in or around a wound increase dead space and distort tissue because of increased tension on the wound.[21] Large amounts of wound fluid decreases oxygen availability in the wound. Therefore, whenever surgeons expect a significant amount of inflammatory exudate to form after surgery, they place a drainage system adjacent to the wound to facilitate fluid removal from the incision site. Recent data show that the sutures themselves may promote infection and the extra stitches themselves that are used to close a layered incision may be the cause of infection.[21] Surgical drainage systems are discussed in Section 3 of this chapter.

Microorganism Population. The presence of microorganisms in a wound site increases the chance of wound infection and delayed healing. Accidental wounds are contaminated wounds and carry a greater risk of infection than wounds that occur under surgically aseptic conditions. Surgical wounds that enter body cavities having a normal bacterial population are more likely to become infected than those in which only sterile organs or cavities are entered. If drainage from a nonsterile body cavity, such as the bowel, contaminates the wound site, the infection rate is greater still.

Type of Wound Care

The materials used to dress and cleanse wounds can support or inhibit healing. If the selection of wound antiseptic is inappropriate, tissue irritation, and even destruction of granulation tissue, is possible.[17] Vigorous cleaning of wounds destroys developing granulation tissue even when using mild solutions. Dry gauze or wet to dry dressings adhere to healing tissue and remove viable tissue when they are removed.[17] Wound care that enhances drying of the wound surface retards epithelial regeneration, as noted previously.

COMPLICATIONS OF WOUND HEALING

Hemorrhage

Hemorrhage is excessive loss of blood. Traumatic wounds hemorrhage if damaged blood vessels are not effectively compressed. Hemorrhage in surgical wounds results when severed blood vessels are not completely sealed by suturing or cautery, or when sutures are disrupted. Unchecked hemorrhage is life threatening. Hemorrhage from closed surgical wounds may be visible as an accumulation of bright red drainage on wound dressings or occult if bleeding is internal. Other symptoms of hemorrhage include rapid, irregular, thready pulse; pallor; and cool, moist skin. Postoperative wound hemorrhage is most common within the first 48 hours after surgery, but late hemorrhage also occurs. Late hemorrhage is often secondary to infection and typically happens on the sixth to the tenth postoperative day.

Wound Infection

Wound infections are the result of microbial contamination at the time a wound occurs, or during the healing process. Microorganisms can enter a wound at any time prior to completion of epithelialization. When microorganisms multiply and cause injurious effects, the wound is considered infected. A well-functioning immune system usually effectively contains and destroys small numbers of microorganisms. With highly virulent organisms or grossly contaminated wounds, however, bacteria multiply faster than the body's defenses can destroy them. Other risk factors, such as malnutrition, poor perfusion, extremes of age, chronic diseases, and a history of steroid therapy, predispose patients to wound infections.[19] Environmental factors such as breaks in asepsis during wound care, a lengthy surgical procedure, or delayed treatment of contaminated wounds also contribute to infection risk.

Signs and symptoms of wound infection include local heat, redness, edema, pain, high-grade fever, elevated white blood count, and purulent wound drainage. Clinical signs of infection become apparent within 2 to 7 days following surgery.

Wound Separation

Several degrees of wound separation may occur in surgical wounds. Superficial separation refers to separation of approximated skin on the wound surface. This usually occurs in small spaces between sutures or skin staples, but may involve larger portions of the incision. Usually, superficial separation is minor and presents no risks other than possible widening of the scar at the point of separation. **Dehiscence** is separation of previously closed wound edges. It may be complete, involving all tissue layers, or partial. It is a serious complication and requires immediate correction. *Evisceration,* that is, the spilling out of the abdominal contents, may accompany dehiscence of abdominal incisions. In some cases, partial dehiscence occurs, involving the muscle and fascia layers only. This often leads to an incisional hernia. Dehiscence is not a common complication of surgery, but is two to three times more frequent in patients over the age of 60 than in younger patients. It is also more common in individuals with diabetes, immunocompromise, cancer, and obesity, and with those receiving steroid therapy.

Keloids

A **keloid** is a raised, firm, thickened scar that results from deposition of abnormal amounts of collagen into the tissue surrounding a wound. The excess collagen is not lysed during the maturation stage of healing, allowing the disproportionate tissue to continue to grow for some time after wound closure. This complication is more common among African-Americans.

Contracture

A **contracture** is the pathologic shrinking of a scar causing loss of mobility. It should not be confused with contraction, which is a normal part of wound healing. Contractures sometimes need surgical correction.

SECTION 2

ASSESSMENT OF SKIN AND TISSUE INTEGRITY

SKIN AND TISSUE DATA COLLECTION

Skin and tissue alterations often affect an individual's appearance and threaten self-concept, so some patients may be sensitive about discussing or exposing skin or tissue lesions. Discomfort related to pain, itching, or irritation may also be a feature of integumentary problems. Keeping these points in mind when gathering data about skin and tissue guides the nurse's approach to data collection. Particular attention is paid to any wounds or lesions.

SKIN AND TISSUE HISTORY

The focus of the history is to obtain patients' perceptions of integumentary problems and the effects these problems have on their daily activity.

Primary Concern

A primary concern related to the integument may relate to the appearance of a lesion, its interference with activities, its cause, or other features, such as whether it is contagious or likely to recur. The nature of the patient's distress guides the data-collection process as well as treatment approaches. A primary concern related to the skin may imply a need for a comprehensive data collection, because the skin and mucosa reflect general health and provide clues to problems in other functional areas. Conversely, a skin and tissue assessment may be appropriate with other kinds of primary concerns, such as dietary or elimination problems. The following example demonstrates a nurse's use of primary concern data.

> Brenda Thomasen seeks help for a recurring rash on her face. Although this is the first time she has sought health care for this problem, she recalls two previous occurrences of this rash in the same location. Her son has a history of herpes skin lesions and she is concerned that her rash may have the same etiology. Although her son has not required treatment, she is worried that she will be unable to work if her lesions are not treated, because she has just started a job in a newborn nursery, and she realizes that newborns are highly susceptible to this infection. The nurse assures her that if the diagnosis is positive for herpes simplex type 1, medication to prevent or limit the duration of future outbreaks is available.

Current Understanding

It is helpful to determine what a patient believes precipitated the problem, what makes it worse or better, and what has been tried as a home remedy. Since skin and tissue alterations can result from injuries, infectious diseases, topical contact with an irritant or toxin, or food ingestion, it is necessary to explore environmental factors with patients. Sometimes the appearance of a lesion implies its cause and helps to focus nurses' assessment questions. Other appropriate inquiries about the current eruption or exacerbation include, for example: When did the eruption appear? Have there been previous episodes? Are there other problems associated with the lesion such as itching, cold-type symptoms, localized swelling, warmth, redness, bleeding or oozing of fluid, or odor? Has the skin around the lesion changed in texture, color, or turgor? Has there been any change due to the treatment? The following is an example of current understanding.

> Anita, age 13 years, reports to a clinic with bilateral redness and swelling of the conjunctiva. She reports she has been bothered by these symptoms for 3 days, but has never had them before. She reports that she has tried rinsing her eyes with warm water, but has gotten no relief. In discussing Anita's usual skin care, the nurse learns that Anita and her friends have been trying out new makeup. The nurse suggests that discontinuing the makeup until the irritation clears and then using hypoallergenic products may solve the problem.

Past Health Problems/Experiences

Many skin conditions are chronic or recurring. Medications or treatments for other medical conditions may underlie skin or mucosal symptoms, or they may be sequelae or complications of other health problems. An example of nurses' use of past health problem data follows.

> Salvador Lopes is admitted to Ward B for treatment of leg ulcers on his lower left leg. He has a history of diabetes mellitus and reports difficulty following his dietary and skin care assessment regimen. Nurse Cataldo notices irregular scars on both legs, and asks about their cause. He states that they were the same kind of sores, but "I just can't seem to keep them from happening." Nurse Cataldo makes a mental note to explore what barriers prevent Mr. Lopes from engaging in preventive practices and seeking early care when symptoms first appear.

Personal, Family, and Social History

Lifestyle influences environmental exposure and ingestion of substances that may cause skin and tissue alterations. For example, hygiene habits affect oral cavity and skin health. Sun exposure for leisure or because of work increases risk for skin cancers. Occupational exposure to chemicals is a frequent cause of mucosal and skin lesions. Stress may precipitate skin rashes. A patient who smokes or who has poor nutrition habits may have difficulties with healing. Smokers are also more susceptible to oral cancers. Skin and integumentary alterations are the primary manifestations of many nutritional deficiencies. Pets in the home may cause allergic lesions.

The following example illustrates a nurse's use of data from a patient's personal, family, and social history. Table 27–3 provides sample questions to elicit relevant information about personal, family, and social influences on integumentary health.

> Sam Carruthers seeks health care for a small red lesion on his forehead that has been present for several weeks. The nurse notices that he also has a sunburn, and so asks about his usual leisure and occupational activities. He indicates that although his office job keeps him indoors most of the time, he participates in sailing and golf every weekend. He relates a family history of skin cancer. He admits "I'm a little lazy about the sunscreen—I don't get all the SPS, SPX stuff and I keep forgetting to take it with me." The nurse realizes that Mr. Carruthers is at risk for skin cancer and resolves to problem-solve with him to help integrate sun protection into his regular habits.

COLLABORATIVE STRATEGY

ASSISTING SKIN AND TISSUE HEALING

Nurse–patient collaboration during the skin and tissue history is an effective means of assuring accurate determination of patient concerns. Skin problems often have broad impact on psychosocial and physical well-being. Nurses who obtain patient participation in the assessment process are able to gain more understanding of patient distress and how a skin problem affects that patient's general functioning.

Subjective Manifestations

The last part of the skin and tissue history is subjective manifestations. As discussed in Chap. 17, this portion of the history is a general overview of common symptoms that serves as a means of assuring that no relevant symptoms go unreported. Chapter 17 provides sample questions relevant to skin and tissue.

SKIN AND TISSUE EXAMINATION

The primary modalities in the skin and tissue examination are inspection and palpation. Measurements are occasionally used.

Measurements

Measurements are relevant when lesions are present. Health care providers measure lesions to diagnose the type and evaluate remission or exerbation.

Assessment of weight and weight changes is important for postsurgical patients and patients with skin and tissue disruptions who do not have good oral intake. Weight loss may be an indicator of risk for nutrition-associated complications of surgery, such as infection and wound dehiscence.

Objective Manifestations

General observations, integument, eye, ear, nose, mouth, throat, breast, cardiovascular, genitourinary, and anal–rectal examinations provide information that contributes to assessment and diagnosis of skin and tissue problems. Chapter 17 summarizes normal findings relevant to skin and tissue integrity. The following discussion addresses alterations.

General Observations. Overall appearance suggests actual or potential problems, as well as healthy functioning. Note whether the skin appearance is congruent with the stated age. Note facial skin color. Changes, such as pallor or jaundice, usually are visible first in the face. This may be difficult to evaluate in a patient with dark skin.

TABLE 27-3. SKIN AND TISSUE HISTORY: PERSONAL, FAMILY, AND SOCIAL HISTORY QUESTIONS

A. Vocational
1. What type of work do you do?
2. How long have you had this job?
3. Where did you work previously?
4. Does your current or prior work involve contact with chemicals, dyes, or fibers?
5. What precautions or safety measures do you take when handling these materials?
6. Have you ever had a rash or sore that seemed related to contact with these materials?
7. Does your job involve frequent or prolonged exposure to the sun?

B. Home and Family
1. What are your usual home activities?
2. Do you live in an urban neighborhood? Rural?
3. Are there many kinds of plants growing around your neighborhood? Do you notice many insects around your home?
4. Does your family have pets? What kind? Who cares for the pets?

C. Social, Leisure, Spiritual, and Cultural
1. What are your favorite leisure activities?
2. Do you spend a lot of time in outdoor recreation?
3. Do you often get sunburned? How often do you use sunscreen?
4. Has your skin problem ever interfered with participation in social or leisure activities?

D. Sexual
1. Are you sexually active?
2. How do you protect yourself against sexually transmitted diseases?
3. Have you ever been treated for a sexually transmitted disease?
4. Has your skin problem ever interfered with sexual expression?

E. Habits

Sleep
1. Have your skin problems ever interfered with getting a good night's sleep?

Nutrition
1. What foods do you eat daily?
2. Are you allergic to any foods? What foods? What symptoms do you experience?
3. What kinds of snack foods do you prefer? Do you eat them often?

Beverages
1. How often do you drink sugared beverages, such as soda, sweetened iced tea, or coffee?
2. How much water do you drink each day?
3. Do you drink alcoholic beverages? How often? How much?

Tobacco Use
1. Do you smoke? Cigarettes, cigar, pipe?
2. How much do you smoke each day?

Other Substances
1. How often do you take nonprescription medications, such as aspirin?
2. Do you take any prescription medications? Any that you apply to your skin?
3. Are you allergic to any medications?

F. Psychological/Coping
1. Do you ever feel nervous or stressed? How often does this happen?
2. Do you notice flare-ups of your skin problem when you feel nervous?
3. Is there anything about your skin problem that worries you?
4. Has having this skin problem changed the way you feel about yourself? Your body?
5. Has your skin problem caused you to miss activities or events that are important to you? Do you ever avoid going out when it flares up?
6. How do you deal with your skin problem?

Body odors, and general cleanliness of the hair, body, and apparel, give clues about hygiene practices. Patients with poor oral or general hygiene habits are likely to have poor skin and mucosal health. Extensive lesions are also noticeable on general inspection, but will need more meticulous examination in the integumentary examination. Guarding or scratching suggest lesions in unexposed areas that should be inspected later in the examination.

Integument. Examination of the integument should address skin (including lesions and wounds), skin appendages, and mucosa over all body areas. For the sake of efficiency and convenience, the integument assessment is not conducted all at once, but is integrated into the head-to-toe observations of other organs and functions. Chapter 17 describes the integument findings expected in healthy individuals. Selected indicators of problems are addressed here.

SKIN LESIONS. Characteristic primary and secondary lesions are described in Tables 17–15 and 17–16. It is useful to compare lesions to intact skin areas. When describing lesions, include distribution, size, shape, color, and configuration.

- *Distribution.* Distribution refers to the location and symmetry of lesion placement. Symmetric distribution means that lesions appear on corresponding body parts on opposite sides of the body. Asymmetric distribution means that only one side of the body is affected. Skin folds are an important area to scrutinize when assessing for the distribution of lesions, as this is a common location for lesions.
- *Size.* Measure lesion size. If many lesions of varying sizes are present, describe the range of sizes found or the size of a typical lesion. It may be useful to compare the size of lesions to familiar objects, such as "dime-sized."
- *Shape.* Lesions may be regular or irregular in shape. In some cases, a characteristic shape may be diagnostic of a specific lesion, for example, ringworm presents in an annular or ringlike formation.
- *Color.* Lesions may be red, purple, yellow, white, or black. Some lesions are of mixed color. Note whether the color is uniform and widely distributed throughout the lesions (diffuse) or limited to the edges (circumscribed).

- *Configuration.* Configuration refers to the general arrangement of lesions. Lesions may be singular or grouped. Grouped lesions may cluster in regular patterns, such as linear or annular, may follow the course of a cutaneous nerve, or may cluster randomly with no particular pattern.

WOUNDS. The wounds that nurses encounter most frequently are traumatic wounds, surgical wounds, and pressure ulcers.

- *Traumatic wounds.* Initial assessment of traumatic wounds includes location, type, size, and the amount of bleeding or other drainage. When patients have experienced trauma, it is important to assess their overall condition, including adequacy of breathing, pulse, and the presence of other injuries. Initially hemostasis of all bleeding wounds and maintenance of cardiorespiratory function are critical. When cardiorespiratory status is stable, examine the wound for the presence of foreign bodies such as particles of dirt, clothing, or glass and note changes in drainage or appearance since the initial assessment. Many traumatic wounds need suturing or surgical repair. After treatment, assessment should be the same as for any other wound. The elements of a routine wound assessment are summarized in Clinical Guideline 27–1.
- *Surgical wounds.* It is common practice to cover surgical wounds with dressings. The type of dressing varies with the kind of procedure, complications (if any), and provider's preference. It is important to assess both the dressing and the wound regularly. If a dressing has fresh bloody drainage, assess for additional drainage in the bed. When a wound is hemorrhaging, blood flow is often too rapid for the dressing to absorb it; instead it flows into the bed under the patient due to gravity. If hemorrhage is suspected, assess vital signs and notify the physician or charge nurse immediately and chart findings.

  Surgeons often place one or more devices to evacuate and contain drainage in surgical wounds. Assess output in these devices for color, odor, consistency, and amount. Sutures or staples used to approximate the wound edges at the surface of the wound may be visible (Fig. 27–6). Staples are removed 48 to 72 hours after surgery; sutures are absorbed.
- *Pressure ulcers.* Pressure ulcers are preventable wounds. Assessment of the bony prominences of all patients and implementation to relieve pressure at the first sign of a stage 1 ulcer (see Chap. 33 and Table 27–1) are vital. Once an ulcer has advanced beyond stage 1, the appearance of the wound guides the selection of treatment. It is important to note the color of the wound and the nature of the drainage. This will help identify healing tissue and necrotic areas and will suggest the presence of infection.

SKIN APPENDAGES. Changes in the nails and hair often accompany skin diseases and nutritional deficiencies. If nails are brittle, dry, and cracked, or hair is dull and brittle, look for other signs of nutritional deficiencies (see Chap. 28).

Alopecia (hair loss) is sometimes a side effect of cancer chemotherapy. Hair that grows after therapy is discontinued, is often sparse and of fine texture. Spotty areas of alopecia may indicate disease, and warrant further investigation. One possible cause is ringworm. If there are scalp lesions, look for lice infestation (pediculosis). When checking for lice, a flashlight is useful. Eggs (nits) on the hair shaft have a pearlized appearance in the light.

CLINICAL GUIDELINE 27–1

ROUTINE WOUND ASSESSMENT

PRIMARY INTENTION

1. *Inspect dressing*
   - Is the dressing secure?
   - Drainage: What is the color, odor, and amount (measure diameter of soiled area on dressing and number of gauze pads soaked)
2. *Inspect incision*
   - Are wound edges approximated or are they separated?
   - Is healing proceeding favorably—is there moderate swelling and redness?
   - Are there signs of infection—red, puffy wound edges surrounded by tautly stretched tissue? Does the drainage appear purulent, with a yellow, green, or gray discoloration?
   - Does the exudate have an odor?
3. *Inspect drainage devices*
   - Are they intact and functioning correctly? Do they need emptying and recompression?
   - Measure liquid drainage.
4. *Palpate incision.* Note tension, heat, and healing.
   - Are incision edges and surrounding tissue taut and moderately swollen? Are they warmer than other parts of the body?
   - Is a healing ridge (1-cm wide) detected around the wound about a week following surgery?
5. *Assess pain.* Note location, intensity, onset, duration, character, and exacerbating factors.
   - Is pain around the incision or elsewhere? Is it deep?
   - How severe is pain, on a scale of 0 (none) to 10 (most severe)? Less severe than before? Building in intensity?
   - Did pain occur suddenly or gradually?
   - Ask patient to describe character of pain. Sharp? Dull? Knifelike? Constant?
   - What brings on pain—a specific event or movement? Movement in general?

SECONDARY INTENTION

1. *Assess dressing, drainage,* and *pain* as described above.
2. *Inspect wound*
   - Do wound color and texture suggest healing (pink, red, velvety)?
   - Does the wound appear to need debriding (color yellow or black; texture dry, rigid, or crusted)?
   - Note size, shape, depth. Is size changing?
3. *Inspect the surrounding tissue*
   - Does it appear healthy? If not, what is the extent of involvement?
   - Are the edges well defined, rolled toward base? Is there evidence of undermining?

TERTIARY INTENTION

1. *Inspect the site of the wound, and note drainage and devices*
   - What is the condition of dressing and the closure material if used?
   - Inspect surrounding skin, as above.
2. Note frequency of irrigations and dressing changes.

MUCOSA. Examine the mucosa of the eye, nose, mouth and throat, and perineal–rectal area for color changes, hydration, discharge, and evidence of disruptions. Common problems specific to each body area are discussed below in the corresponding examination sections. Table 27–4 summarizes causes of mucosal disruptions.

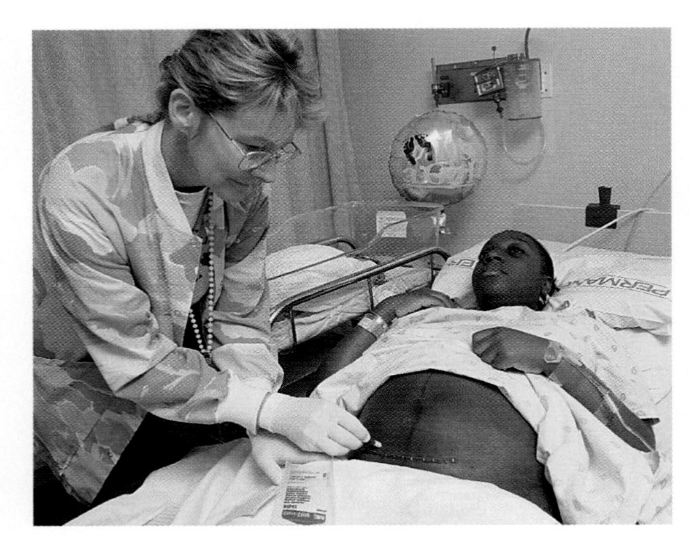

Figure 27–6. Nurse removes staples from a surgical incision that is healing well.

HEENT. The aspect of the head, eyes, ears, nose, and throat (HEENT) assessment that is most germane to skin and tissue assessment is mucosal assessment. See Chap. 17 for a discussion of the examination of these areas. It is important to note that dehydration and mouth breathing are common causes of altered oral and throat membranes. The teeth and tongue may appear coated, and saliva sticky. Without frequent mouth care, open lesions can develop. Oral mucous membranes quickly reflect fluctuations in hydration status and also suggest changes in nutritional health. For this reason assessment of oral mucous membranes should be part of nurses' routine head-to-toe assessment every shift.

Cardiovascular. The elements of the cardiovascular examination that are important to skin and tissue assessment relate to perfusion. Palpate peripheral pulses, particularly in the lower extremities, and note coolness, pallor, and mottling of the skin of the legs, indicative of acute arterial occlusion. Chronic arterial occlusion results in hairlessness, thinning skin, and color changes related to gravity: redness when dependent, pallor when elevated. Ankle edema, with shiny bluish or brownish thin skin, or open ulcers on the lower leg suggest chronic venous insufficiency.

Genitalia, Anus, and Rectum. The mucosa of the genital and anal–rectal region is vulnerable to fissures; infectious lesions, such as jock itch (tinea cruris), herpes, or venereal warts; infestations, such as scabies or lice; and irritation from accumulated secretions or excretions, warts, or hemorrhoids. When patients remain in bed for treatment of illness, nurses need to conduct perineal assessment and provide perineal hygiene several times a day. Increased perspiration, indwelling urinary catheters, and diminished ability for self-care increase patients' vulnerability to skin and mucosal disruptions.

DIAGNOSTIC TESTS

There are few diagnostic tests related to skin and mucosal functioning.

Culture and Sensitivity

Cultures identify causative organisms of infections. Culture samples are obtained from wounds with suspicious drainage and from skin or mucosal lesions of unknown origin. Sensitivity testing is a means of determining the antibiotics to which the causative organism of an infection is sensitive. Specific techniques for this procedure are discussed later in this chapter.

Erythrocyte Sedimentation Rate

The erythrocyte sedimentation rate (ESR) test is a general test for an acute inflammatory process. It is a measure of the rate at which red blood cells settle to the bottom of a test tube of anticoagulated blood in 1 hour. Inflammation tends to increase the protein content of plasma, so the sedimentation rate increases when inflammation is present. The ESR does not identify the location of the inflammation. There are no food or fluid restrictions for this test. The normal range is 0 to 7 or 0 to 10 mm/h for males and 0 to 15 or 0 to 20 mm/h for females, depending on the method used.

C-reactive Protein

C-reactive protein is virtually absent from the blood serum of healthy persons and appears in the blood serum about 6 to 10 hours after an injury and the onset of an acute inflammatory process, peaking in 48 to 72 hours. It is not present in viral infections, but bacterial infections and tissue destruction produce the protein. It is not specific to location, but it is useful in determining if a bacterial infection is the cause of an inflammatory response and is helpful in monitoring the wound-healing process. Patients must remain npo for 8 to 12 hours before the test. Normally the protein is not present (negative); a titer of greater than 1:2 is positive.

Antibody Titers

Antibody titers measure the presence or concentration of antibodies. Some are specific to particular antigens (a foreign substance that initiates formation of antibodies); others detect the presence of a general type of antibody, but do not conclusively identify the antigen. The presence of a high concentration of a particular antibody implies the presence in the body of the organism or substance that it attacks. There is no preparation for antibody titer tests. Diagnostic titers vary with the specific antibody.

Skin Sensitivity Tests

Skin sensitivity tests identify allergens, often the cause of skin and mucosal symptoms. Small amounts of the allergens commonly responsible for the type of symptoms an individual is experiencing are injected into the dermis. The sites of the injections are examined after a period of time (usually 48 to 72 hours). Local inflammation is indicative of sensitivity to the antigen.

Biopsy

Tissue is excized from the most characteristic area of a lesion. Tissue is sent to the laboratory for microanalysis.

▲ NURSING DIAGNOSIS OF SKIN AND TISSUE INTEGRITY

Data analysis and data clustering assist nurses to determine if a patient has any skin and tissue problems that nursing therapies can address. Five nursing diagnoses apply specifically to skin and tissue. Four are discussed here. They are impaired tissue integrity, impaired skin integrity, risk for impaired skin integrity, and altered

TABLE 27-4. CAUSES OF MUCOSAL DISRUPTIONS

Location	Internal/Biologic	External/Mechanical
Eye (conjunctiva)	Infection: bacterial, viral Allergy	Abrasions (eg, from contact lenses) Chemical burns Foreign bodies
Mouth/pharynx	Infection: bacterial, viral, fungal Dehydration Mouth breathing Emesis Plaque Cancer Cancer chemotherapy	Poorly aligned teeth Trauma: braces, toothbrushes, toothpicks, biting self, hot liquids Oral airways Ortracheal tubes
Nose	Upper respiratory infections	Foreign body Manual extraction of secretions Chemicals: cocaine, caustic gas Nasogastric tube Nasotracheal tube
Vaginal/perineal	Infection: bacterial, fungal, viral, protozoal Age-related atrophy Irritation: poor hygiene, obesity	Trauma: sexual abuse Foreign body: retained tampon Foley catheter Chemical irritation: soaps, contraceptive foams, creams, sponges; douches
Penile/perineal	Infection: bacterial, fungal, viral, protozoal Irritation: Poor hygiene, obesity	Foley catheter Condom catheter Sexual abuse
Rectal	Infection: bacterial, viral, parasitic Trauma: hard stools Irritation: diarrhea, medications, poor hygiene, obesity Cancer	Foreign body Sexual abuse

oral mucous membranes. The latter three diagnoses are subcategories of the first. The last, impaired tissue perfusion, is discussed in Chapter 30. Refer also to Table 27–5, Sample Nursing Diagnoses of Skin and Tissue Problems. Examples of diagnoses that may accompany, result from, or produce skin and tissue problems are listed following the table.

IMPAIRED TISSUE INTEGRITY

Impaired tissue integrity is the state in which an individual experiences damage to mucous membrane, corneal, integumentary, or subcutaneous tissue.

- *Etiology: altered circulation.* Interference with circulation to body tissue, **ischemia,** prevents the adequate transport of oxygen, nutrients, and cellular waste products. Ischemia rapidly produces hypoxia, and eventually cellular death or necrosis. Altered circulation can result from diseases such as diabetes, arterial insufficiency, and internal blockage of vessels by plaque or clots, and from external pressure. Immobility is a factor in pathologic clotting as well as a major cause of external pressure. Poor perfusion also delays wound healing. Although nurses cannot independently treat medical diagnoses as etiologies of altered tissue integrity, collaborating with other members on the health care team, teaching and preventive measures to eliminate additional contributing problems, such as pressure, friction, and shearing, are essential.
- *Etiology: nutritional deficit.* Deficiencies in essential nutrients, particularly vitamins, produce lesions in tissues with rapid cell turnover, such as mucosa and skin. Nutrient deficits also impair wound healing, as discussed in Section 1. Ischemia is likely when patients with excessive adipose tissue are immobile, because fatty tissue is not highly vascular and becomes less resilient when it is dense. Conversely, muscle and a moderate amount of subcutaneous fat provide a cushioning effect against pressure that is lacking in underweight patients. Nursing studies identified underweight as the most effective predictor of skin breakdown.[22,23]
- *Etiology: fluid deficit or excess.* Dehydration produces shrinking of cells. To maintain life-sustaining functions, fluid shifts to the intravascular space occur when total body water diminishes. Therefore, skin and mucosal changes are among the first clinical signs of dehydration. Secretions, such as tears and mucus, decrease, with resultant tissue damage due to friction and irritants.

TABLE 27-5. SAMPLE NURSING DIAGNOSES OF SKIN AND TISSUE PROBLEMS

Nursing Diagnosis	Defining Characteristics/Manifestations: *Subjective Data*	Defining Characteristics/Manifestations: *Objective Data*	Etiology
Impaired tissue integrity *1.6.1.2.1*	"It's harder to breathe lying on my side, I need to sit up—but my tailbone hurts too."	1-in, diameter sacral ulceration extending through dermis. Selects semi-Fowler's position unless reminded to change positions. Frequently slips down in bed.	*Physical:* Pressure and shearing from continuous use of semi-Fowler's position.
Altered oral mucous membranes *1.6.2.1.1*	"My mouth feels like cotton." "It's really sore at the edge of my tongue."	Xerostomia. Coated tongue. Reddened area on lateral surface of tongue. Saliva sticky, ropey. Halitosis.	*Physical:* Dehydration.
Impaired skin integrity *1.6.2.1.2.1*	"I feel so weak." "It hurts on my left hip." "I just can't turn myself, it's too hard."	Reddened area over left greater trochanter, does not disappear after 1 hour in supine position.	*Physical:* Generalized muscle weakness and physical immobilization.

Nursing Diagnosis	Risk Factors
Risk for impaired skin integrity *1.6.2.1.2.2*	Altered sensation: "I notice a sore or a bruise, but I never remember getting it, and it doesn't hurt." Does not recoil and is unable to describe sensation when lightly pricked with a sterile needle while eyes are closed.

OTHER NURSING DIAGNOSES RELATED TO SKIN AND TISSUE INTEGRITY

PHYSICAL
Altered nutrition: more than body requirements
Altered nutrition: less than body requirements
Risk for infection
Hypothermia
Hyperthermia
Diarrhea
Bowel incontinence
Urinary incontinence
Fluid volume excess
Fluid volume deficit
Decreased cardiac output
Impaired gas exchange
Risk for disuse syndrome
Altered protection
Impaired physical mobility
Activity intolerance
Fatigue
Sleep pattern disturbance
Impaired swallowing
Unilateral neglect
Pain

COGNITIVE
Sensory–perceptual alterations
Knowledge deficit
Altered thought processes

EMOTIONAL
Hopelessness
Powerlessness
Dysfunctional grieving
Anxiety
Ineffective coping
Impaired adjustment

SELF-CONCEPTUAL
Body image disturbance
Self-esteem disturbance

SOCIOCULTURAL/LIFE STRUCTURAL
Social isolation
Altered role performance
Sexual dysfunction

DEVELOPMENTAL
Feeding self-care deficit
Bathing self-care deficit
Toileting self-care deficit

ENVIRONMENTAL
Risk for injury
Risk for trauma

Source: The nursing diagnoses and etiologies on this table and the definitions of nursing diagnoses in the body of the text not credited to other sources are from Nursing Diagnosis: Definitions and Classification, 1997–1998. *Philadelphia: North American Nursing Diagnosis Association; 1996. Manifestation categories for etiologies and specifications of general etiologies on these tables are authors' original work.*

Localized fluid excess, edema, is an abnormal expansion of the interstitial space. This increases the distance between the cells and the capillaries that deliver oxygen, compromising local cellular profusion.

- *Etiology: knowledge deficit.* Lack of knowledge may result in behaviors that result in skin, mucosal, corneal, or deeper tissue injury. Examples of knowledge deficits that can lead to impaired tissue integrity include nutrition, optimal hygiene, appropriate skin care, effective use of sunscreen, correct contact lens care, and the risks associated with immobility.
- *Etiology: impaired physical mobility.* Individuals with intact musculoskeletal and neurologic function relieve pressure on body parts through spontaneous movement, prompted by discomfort. Compromised sensory perception and capacity for independent movement, altered level of consciousness, and muscle weakness impair mobility. Impaired mobility exposes patients to pressure sore risks from altered circulation and mechanical forces. Other debilitating effects of immobility that may interact to further increase pressure sore risk are discussed in Chap. 33.

- *Etiology: chemical irritants.* Many chemicals destroy superficial skin layers, resulting in an injury that is similar to a burn. Body excretions are a source of irritating chemicals. Urine and feces contain urea and intestinal enzymes that are destructive to skin. Moreover, *Candida albicans*, a component of intestinal flora, often colonizes in fecal matter left on the skin, causing painful excoriation. Body secretions such as blood and mucus also serve as growth media for microorganisms that subsequently cause skin irritation and breakdown.
- *Etiology: thermal (temperature extremes).* Mild burns characterized by local erythema involve only the epidermis and cause minor tissue damage. More serious burns damage dermis or even deeper layers. Hypothermia damages skin by causing cellular dehydration.[23] Ice crystals form between cells, pulling intracellular fluid to them as they grow. Milder forms involve transient blanching and numbness. These injuries can occur through unsafe use of heat or cold as a treatment for other injuries.
- *Etiology: mechanical.* Pressure, friction, and shearing are the mechanical forces responsible for disruptions in tissue integrity. Pressure is created on body tissue when it is compressed between a bony prominence and a firm surface, blocking capillary blood flow. The tissue appears blanched and pale. On release of pressure, reactive hyperemia occurs, giving the skin a flushed appearance.[23] When the redness does not disappear, tissue damage has occurred. This is a stage 1 (or grade 1) pressure ulcer.

  Tissue tolerance for pressure is influenced by intrinsic factors, such as nutritional status, age, and circulatory status; and extrinsic factors, such as moisture, friction, and shearing.[3] The amount of pressure and the length of time the pressure is exerted are also factors. Studies designed to define the lowest amount of pressure needed to cause tissue injury have not produced uniform results. Pressures as low as 35 mm Hg to as high as 350 mm Hg have been reported as the threshold for injury within time periods of 1 to 2 hours.[24]

  Friction is the rubbing together of two surfaces. It weakens epithelium by removing cells from the epidermis, making breakdown more likely. A common source of friction is nurses' pulling patients across bed sheets when moving and repositioning them. Friction on heels, elbows, and sacrum also occurs with self-repositioning, in particular when patients move themselves toward the slightly elevated head of the bed.

  In mechanics, **shearing** is the stress created from the sliding of one load against another. As this concept applies to patients in bed, one load is a patient's weight, and the other is the bed. Shearing occurs most often when a patient in a semi-sitting (semi-Fowler's) position slips toward the foot of the bed. Because of friction, the skin surface in contact with the sheets moves less than the deeper tissues attached to the skeleton, often damaging capillaries and compromising circulation, besides damaging other cells.
- *Etiology: radiation.* Radiation can produce multilayered tissue destruction similar to that caused by burns. The destruction in radiation depends on the level of radiation, length of exposure, and area of the body exposed. Radiation burns occur in people undergoing radiation therapy for malignancies, as well as in those accidentally exposed. Side effects from radiation therapy range from mild erythema and dryness to a severe skin loss that appears raw and moist with clear exudate. Sometimes there is scarring accompanied by loss of hair follicles, sebaceous glands, and sweat glands, and residual hyper- or hypopigmentation.[25] Although nurses do not independently treat lesions caused by radiation, nurses treat responses to the lesions, such as discomfort and body image changes, and take measures to prevent secondary lesions or infection.

IMPAIRED SKIN INTEGRITY

Impaired skin integrity is a state in which an individual's skin is adversely altered, including disruption of the skin surface and/or deeper layers. External (environmental) factors or internal (somatic) factors cause impaired skin integrity. Many of the etiologic factors for this diagnosis are the same as or similar to those discussed above for impaired tissue integrity. Two additional factors are discussed here.

- *Etiology: mechanical factors, restraint.* Caregivers use restraints to restrict the mobility in patients who are at risk for injury or who may harm others. Restraints also are used to prevent patients from dislodging treatment modalities, such as nasogastric tubes or intravenous lines (see Chap. 33). Often patients are restrained because they are confused or are too young to understand the importance of remaining at rest. In both cases, patients pull against restraints in an effort to move or free themselves. Even restraints that are applied correctly can cause skin damage from the pressure and friction this resistance generates. The elderly are particularly vulnerable.
- *Etiology: developmental factors.* Diaper dermatitis is a skin alteration that is common among newborns and infants. The cause is prolonged skin exposure to urine and feces, which contain urea and intestinal organisms. The use of rubber pants, which prevent evaporation of moisture and therefore enhance absorption of the irritants by the skin, aggravates the rash. The perineal skin appears reddened and thickened. In 80 percent of cases lasting more than 4 days, *Candida albicans* can be cultured from the lesions.[26]

  Another example of a developmental skin alteration is epidermal skin tears in older adults, discussed in Section 1.

RISK FOR IMPAIRED SKIN INTEGRITY

Risk for impaired skin integrity refers to a state in which an individual's skin is at risk of being adversely altered. The risk factors for this diagnosis are the same as the etiologies for actual impaired skin integrity. Nurses can spare a patient at risk from actual skin damage by taking appropriate preventive actions.

ALTERED ORAL MUCOUS MEMBRANE

This is the state in which an individual experiences disruptions in the tissue layers of the oral cavity. Etiologies may be chemical or mechanical, or related to hydration or radiation. Mechanical and chemical etiologies of oral mucosa lesions are discussed in Section 1. The section on *Impaired Tissue Integrity* addresses changes related to hydration.

Head and neck exposure to radiation decreases saliva production, with a resulting dry mouth (xerostomia). Erythematous lesions progressing to ulceration can occur. Radiation also may affect mucosal appendages including taste buds and dental structures. As with radiation injuries to the skin, nurses do not independently treat these lesions.

STATING THE SKIN AND TISSUE DIAGNOSIS

Although damaged or destroyed tissue is the only defining characteristic for the diagnosis of impaired tissue integrity, including information about the size, depth, and location of the damaged tissue provides more guidance for developing desired outcomes, evaluation criteria, and nursing implementation. Similarly, definitive statements of etiology help focus implementation effectively.

Patients with skin and tissue disruptions commonly experience more than one of the related factors listed on the taxonomy. For example, a debilitated person who develops a pressure ulcer may have a protein–calorie nutritional deficiency causing weakness and therefore impaired mobility. As a result of this, pressure over a bony prominence alters circulation, which finally results in the ulcer. To guide corrective nursing action effectively, the diagnostic statement should include the related factors most basic to the problem. For example: impaired tissue integrity related to protein–calorie malnutrition, weakness, and physical immobility as evidenced by stage 2 pressure ulcer, ½ inch diameter, on left hip.

The same guidelines apply to the other skin and tissue diagnoses. Make etiologies and defining characteristics as precise as possible.

SECTION 3

NURSE-PATIENT MANAGEMENT OF SKIN AND TISSUE INTEGRITY

PLANNING FOR OPTIMAL SKIN AND TISSUE INTEGRITY

Management of skin and tissue integrity involves collaborative planning, nursing implementation, and evaluation. A care plan for skin and tissue integrity describes:

- expected changes in skin and tissue
- criteria for evaluating the achievement of desired changes
- nursing implementation to bring about the improvements in skin and tissue condition
- statements of desired outcomes (expected changes in skin condition)
- the related evaluation criteria reflecting patient and nurse input

For most skin and tissue problems, the desired outcome is healing of the wound or lesion. Evaluation criteria specify the expected indications of progressive healing for the particular type of wound or lesion a patient is experiencing. Patients may have unrealistic expectations about how the skin will look after a deep lesion heals. A pleasing appearance is important to body image, and scarring may be difficult to accept. While healing of lesions is primary, nurses need to be sensitive to concerns voiced by the patient about disfiguring scars when developing collaborative outcomes and evaluation criteria. Implementation must also be acceptable to patients. Because a variety of etiologies generate skin problems, implementation must incorporate multiple approaches. Refer to Table 27–6, Nurse–Patient Management of Skin and Tissue Problems, for sample standard care plans with desired outcomes, evaluation criteria, and nursing implementation for patients with selected nursing diagnoses related to skin and tissue.

Table 27–7, Partial Critical Pathway for Congestive Heart Failure: Skin and Tissue Function, and Table 27–8, Partial Critical Pathway for Total Hip Replacement: Tissue Integrity Promotion, are examples of collaborative plans that incorporate concepts from this chapter. Collaborative plans are the basis for productive, cost-effective implementation.

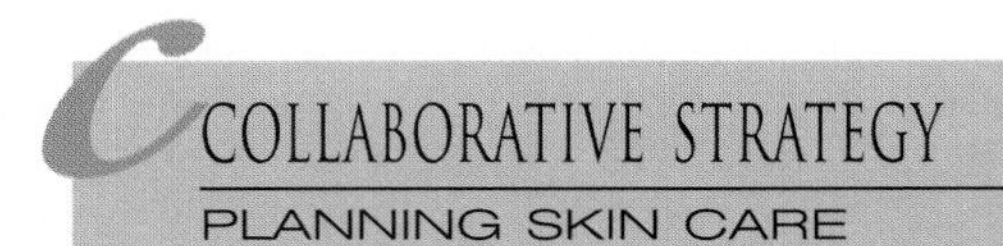

Planning is a collaborative nurse–patient function. Mutual development of outcomes and implementation is appropriate for problems of all types. Skin problems often present a challenge, because the outcome most patients see as ideal—complete healing without scarring—is not always achievable. Accepting patients' feelings while encouraging participation in planning and in care requires empathy and skill.

NURSING IMPLEMENTATION TO PROMOTE OPTIMAL SKIN AND TISSUE INTEGRITY

PREVENTIVE CARE

Preventive care related to skin and tissue integrity includes health teaching about topics such as basic hygiene, prevention and treatment of minor skin injuries, and sun protection; and screening for patients at risk for skin and tissue injury.

Health Education

Nurses provide preventive health education about skin and skin care in locations such as schools, occupational sites, clinics, wellness centers, private practice settings, and as part of home care. Often group presentations are effective, such as teaching oral hygiene to school children or protective measures against common toxic materials encountered in a particular job setting.

Teaching Basic Hygiene. Personal hygiene is influenced by advertising, cultural background, socioeconomic status, and personal preferences. Although most individuals value basic cleanliness, poverty and crowded living conditions may make adhering to hygienic practices difficult. A sensitive and nonjudgmental approach is essential.

School and community health nurses often teach hygiene practices, such as washing hands before eating and after toileting, brushing teeth after meals, and the importance of regular bathing and hair washing. Changes in hygiene needs corresponding to growth and development, such as use of deodorants, menstrual hygiene, and the need for more frequent facial cleansing, bathing, and shampooing during puberty are other topics that school, public health, and clinic nurses address. Teaching new mothers about

(continued on page 817)

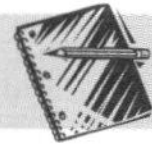

TABLE 27-6. NURSE-PATIENT MANAGEMENT OF SKIN AND TISSUE PROBLEMS

Nursing Diagnosis	Desired Outcomes	Implementation	Evaluation Criteria
Impaired tissue integrity R/T pressure and shearing from continuous use of semi-Fowler's position *1.6.2.1*	1. Intact skin over sacrum.	1a. Establish a turning schedule that is acceptable to patient and that avoids pressure on sacrum. 1b. Collaborate with physician to obtain pressure relief bed, mattress, or overlay. 1c. Maintain clean, dry, and wrinkle-free bed linen. 1d. Discuss the value of leg exercises and other movements in promoting circulation and therefore healing. Encourage use of exercises with each position change. 1e. Apply hydrocolloid dressings over ulcer. Assess dressing q shift, change according to manufacturer's directions. 1f. Clean or irrigate wound with isotonic solution such as normal saline or Ringer's lactate.	1. Progressive healing of sacral ulcer AEB: • Decreased depth and diameter. • Pale pink wound margins. • Presence of pink granulation tissue at base of wound, gradually filling in cavity.
	2. Avoidance of semi-Fowler's position until ulcer is healed.	2a. Discuss with patient how shearing and pressure caused sacral ulcer. 2b. Obtain foam or other supports to assist patient to maintain correct alignment in a side-lying position with HOB sufficiently elevated to facilitate breathing without difficulty. 2c. Obtain footboard if needed to prevent shearing in above position.	2. Patient maintains turning schedule, is observed to avoid semi-Fowler's position.
Altered oral mucous membranes R/T dehydration *1.6.2.1.1*	1. Intact oral mucosa.	1a. Assist as needed with mouth care after meals and prn. Use foam toothettes instead of toothbrush if gums inflamed. 1b. Provide emollient for lips prn. 1c. If npo, assist to rinse mouth q1–2 hours. Use ¼ strength H_2O_2, normal saline, or ½ strength low-alcohol mouthwash. Discuss irritating effect of alcohol, tobacco, acidic foods.	1. Tongue and oral mucosa uniformly pink.
	2. Healthy fluid balance.	2a. Provide oral fluids, if allowed, to compensate for losses and meet basal requirements (see Chap. 34). 2b. Maintain intravenous fluids as ordered.	Oral mucosa pink, shiny. Saliva of watery consistency. Breath fresh smelling.
Impaired skin integrity R/T generalized muscle weakness and immobilization *1.6.2.1.2.1*	1. Intact skin over left greater trochanter. 2. Increased muscle strength appropriate to patients age, sex, and health status.	1a. See *1.6.2.1,* 1a–1d, except avoid trochanter pressure in turning schedule. 2. Provide progressive strengthening exercises to patient's tolerance twice daily.	1. Skin over trochanter without redness or ulceration. 2. Serial testing of muscle strength shows progressive improvement.
	3. Improved mobility, appropriate to age and health status.	3a. Discuss relationship between mobility and healing and mobility and prevention of pressure ulcers. 3b. Collaboratively develop and use progressive ambulation regimen to patient's ability.	3. Progressive increase in mobility without fatigue.
Risk for impaired skin integrity *1.6.2.1.2.2*	Skin will remain free of lesions or wounds.	Establish preventive measures in keeping with patient's mobility status. Eg, if mobile reduce or eliminate environmental hazards; if bedridden, establish and maintain a regular turning schedule and exercises to stimulate circulation.	

Source: See Table 27–5.

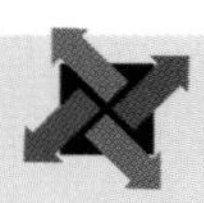

TABLE 27-7. PARTIAL CRITICAL PATHWAY FOR CONGESTIVE HEART FAILURE: SKIN AND TISSUE FUNCTION

Nursing Dx/ Problem	Outcome Primary Care Visit	Outcome Home Care Week 1 (3 Visits)	Outcome Home Care Week 2 (3 Visits)	Outcome Home Care Weeks 3–4 (3 Visits)
Risk for impaired tissue integrity, RF chronic ankle edma	Verbalizes need to keep legs elevated	Applies elastic stockings when up Extremities' skin intact	Same Ankle edema <2+ Same	 Ankle edema <1+ Same
Implementation	**Primary Care Visit**	**Home Care Visit Week 1**	**Home Care Visit Week 2**	**Home Care Visit Weeks 3–4**
Assessment	Degree of edema Skin integrity Capillary filling Measure ankle circumference	Same Same Same Same	Same Same Same Same	Same Same Same Same
Tests/Consults	Refer to Home Health			
Medications/Treatments	Diuretics, K supplements Digoxin Measure for & obtain antithromboembolism stockings	Same	Same Same	Same Same
Psychosocial	Reflective listening			
Teaching	 S/Sx to report to RN, MD, 911 Protect feet & legs Antithromboembolism stocking application Medications: correct use, SE, precautions Elevate legs when up	Plan of care, disease process Reinforce as needed Reinforce as needed Skin care Reinforce as needed Reinforce as needed Reinforce as needed Food & fluid restriction	Reinforce as needed Reinforce as needed Reinforce as needed	Reinforce
Activity/Safety/Self-care	Bedrest, HOB 30–45 degrees c̄ BSC or BRP	Chair c̄ legs elevated tid Remove obstacles to ambulation Bedside commode	Regular rest periods Progressive ambulation/ activity	Same
Nutrition	Fluid restrict 1 L/d 2 g Na diet	Same Same	Same Same	Fluid 1.5 L/d Same
Transfer/Discharge Coord./ Case Manager		Communicate outcomes achieved to MD	Same	Prepare for discharge

See inside back cover for abbreviations.

TABLE 27–8. PARTIAL CRITICAL PATHWAY FOR TOTAL HIP REPLACEMENT: SKIN AND TISSUE FUNCTION

Nursing Dx/Problem	Outcome DOS/Day 1	Outcome Days 2–3	Outcome SNF Days 4–6	Outcome Home Care 3 Weeks (6 Visits)
Impaired skin integrity, RF shearing forces/pressure	Skin on heels, sacrum, unaffected; trochanter intact, pink	Same	Same	Same
Implementation	**DOS/Day 1**	**Days 2–3**	**SNF Days 4–6**	**Home Care 3 Weeks (6 Visits)**
Assessment	Skin over all bony prominences q position change	Same	Same	Same
Tests/Consults				
Medications/Treatments	Overbed frame c̄ trapeze	Same	Same	
Psychosocial				
Teaching			Incisional care	
Activity/Safety/Self-care	Bedrest Turn 2qh toward affected side only	Stand @ bedside c̄ pt & walker Same	Ambulate c̄ walker Same	Ambulate within activity guidelines
Nutrition	Clear liquids	Balanced diet with increased protein, vitamins A & C, zinc, calcium	Same	Same
Transfer/Discharge Coord./ Case Manager		Communicate outcomes achieved, problems/ interventions to SNF	Communicate outcomes achieved, problems/ interventions to Home Health	Communicate outcomes achieved, problems/ interventions to MD & prepare for discharge

See inside back cover for abbreviations.

postpartum hygiene and their newborns' hygiene needs is another example.

Many people are poorly informed about proper oral hygiene. Although most people brush their teeth at least daily, incorrect brushing technique, selecting an inappropriate toothbrush, and failure to include flossing are common errors. Teaching about effective oral hygiene is appropriate whenever oral assessment implies ineffective hygiene practices. Procedure 27–1 provides guidelines.

Prevention and Treatment of Minor Skin Injuries. Parents of young children benefit from information about protecting their youngsters from accidental injury. Bath water that is too hot is a common cause of burns and scalds. Children's natural curiosity and exploration of the environment also contribute to burn accidents. Keeping containers of hot liquids, such as beverage cups, out of reach, turning the handles of cooking pans inward, testing bath water with the wrist or elbow while filling the tub and before putting a child in it, and recognizing that toddlers' mobility expands rapidly are simple but effective ways to prevent burns, falls, and other accidents.

All children experience cuts and scrapes as part of growing up; however, supervising their use of sharp tools and setting good examples for their safe use is a way of avoiding potentially serious injuries.

Basic first aid for minor injuries, such as gentle cleansing of cuts and scrapes with mild antiseptics, application of antibacterial ointment, and covering with a Band-Aid to keep the wound sur-

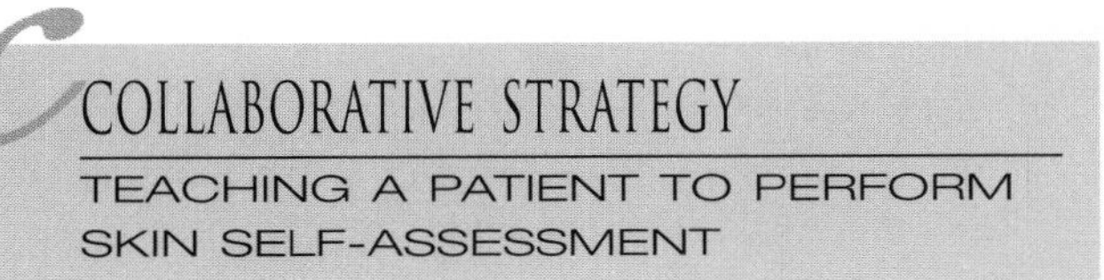

Lesions are a common finding as people age and the skin changes. It is therefore important that patients do skin self-assessments. Nurses can help patients by teaching them to regularly examine their integument for lesions. Patients should be taught to use a mirror to examine their oral cavity and all skin over difficult areas to see like the scalp, neck, back, shoulders, upper arms, buttocks, genitals, and back of the legs.

PROCEDURE 27–1. TEACHING ORAL HYGIENE

PURPOSE: To promote oral health in patients of all ages, through maintaining oral hygiene.
EQUIPMENT: Toothbrush, dental floss, and model teeth (optional).

ACTION 1. Discuss the importance of regular oral hygiene: Oral care helps prevent tooth decay and plaque, stimulates the gingiva, prevents halitosis, and maintains moisture of oral mucosa.

ACTION 2. Discuss oral care supplies that are most effective for maintaining a healthy mouth:

Toothbrush: A lightweight toothbrush with soft straight bristles of equal length is most effective. Hard bristles damage gum tissue. Replace a toothbrush when bristles no longer maintain the original shape of the brush. Electric or battery-operated toothbrushes are easy to use and are as effective as manual brushing in removing food particles and plaque.

Toothpaste: Toothpaste is not required to clean teeth, prevent decay, or remove plaque. Water is sufficient to accomplish this. Sodium bicarbonate is an inexpensive product that is effective in removing stains from the teeth. Toothpastes with fluoride provide protection against cavities and are especially recommended for children (but should not be swallowed).

Dental floss: Use of dental floss is an important means of removing food particles between the teeth, which promote plaque. It is available waxed, unwaxed, and flavored; all are equally effective if used correctly.

Mouthwash: Mouthwash is not essential to oral health. Recent claims that it is effective in preventing plaque have not been substantiated, but it is refreshing.

Mechanical irrigation devices: These devices generate an intermittent stream of water that, when directed against teeth and interdental spaces, is effective in removing debris and organisms as well as stimulating the gums. It cannot remove existing plaque, but is effective in preventing it.

Toothpicks: Round or beveled-edge toothpicks have been found to be effective for cleaning interdental spaces and preventing plaque and gum disease.

ACTION 3. Describe and demonstrate correct brushing technique, using model teeth and brush, or brush only:

a. Hold the brush against the teeth at a 45 degree angle, so the bristles are pointing at the gumline. This allows the bristles to clean under the gum margin.

b. Move the brush back and forth lightly over 2 to 3 teeth at a time, to the count of 10. Repeat until all of the inner and outer surfaces of all the teeth have been brushed. Following a regular order (eg, all outer surfaces of upper teeth, then all outer surfaces of lower teeth, then all inner surfaces) will facilitate reaching all teeth. Using the brush as shown will make cleaning the front teeth easier.

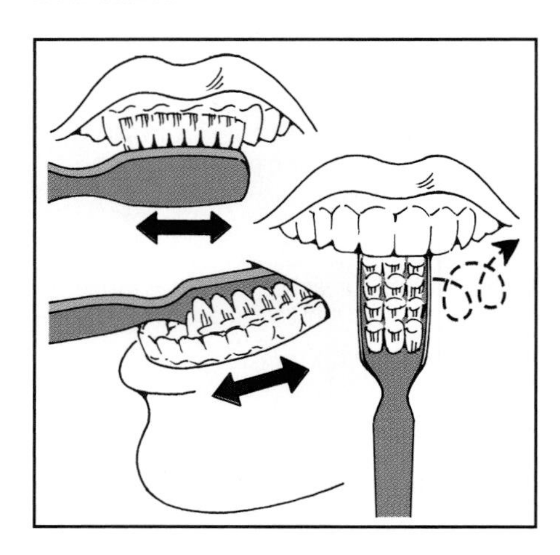

c. Brush the chewing surfaces by placing the brush flush against the teeth and using short back-and-forth strokes. Long strokes tend to contact only the highest points of the teeth.

d. The tongue and the roof of the mouth may be brushed, if desired, to remove thickened saliva that may have collected there.

e. Rinse the mouth as needed, moving water vigorously around the teeth and tongue so additional particles are loosened.

f. Experts recommend brushing for 5 minutes to adequately remove plaque and food particles. It is better to brush thoroughly once a day than ineffectively several times.

ACTION 4. Describe or demonstrate on model teeth the correct flossing technique:

a. Remove a 12- to 15-inch length of floss; wrap one end around index or middle finger of each hand until the length of floss between your fingers is 1½ inches.

Procedure 27–1. (continued)

b. Hold floss taut and slip it between two teeth with a gentle sawing motion, moving the floss downward toward the gums. Curve the floss around the edge of the tooth like a "C," then move the floss below the gumline until resistance is felt.

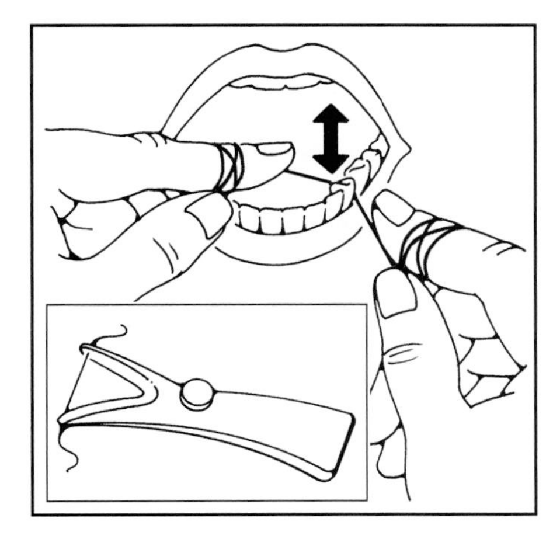

c. Move the floss up and down along the edge of the tooth from gumline to crown several times. Repeat between all teeth. It is helpful to follow a regular pattern (eg, starting at the center, then working toward the back teeth on each side of the mouth, repeating for lower teeth, or starting at the back of one side of the mouth and working toward the other side). When floss becomes frayed expose a new length by unwinding a portion from around one finger.

d. Floss handles are available and are especially useful for patients who lack dexterity needed for the above technique (see figure above).

e. Rinse vigorously after flossing to remove loosened particles. Bleeding may indicate flossing was too vigorous or that gums are inflamed (gingivitis) because of plaque.

f. Flossing should be done at least once a day.

ACTION 5. Provide additional information for parents to promote dental health in children:

a. Avoid putting infants to bed with a bottle of milk or juice as both promote tooth decay. If a bottle is needed, use water.

b. Fluoride treatments or vitamins with fluoride significantly decrease tooth decay in both erupted and unerupted teeth.

c. By the time children are 2 years old, they have all their deciduous (baby) teeth; these teeth should be brushed by parents and teaching of self-brushing should begin as soon as the child can control a toothbrush.

d. Assisting children to establish a habit of brushing teeth after every meal will significantly reduce cavities.

e. Two to three servings of milk or dairy products per day provides calcium needed for strong teeth.

f. Sweets and soft foods adhere to the teeth and promote tooth decay. Limit ingestion of these foods and encourage brushing or at least rinsing with water after sweet snacks.

ACTION 6. Emphasize the importance of regular dental checkups every 6 to 12 months for adults and children, beginning at age 2½ to 3 years.

HOME HEALTH ADAPTATION: Working in the home environment provides nurses with an excellent opportunity to teach proper oral and dental care. Part of the nurse's role is to identify whether the family members have the appropriate equipment and supplies for oral hygiene and to assess whether they have the knowledge and habit patterns that promote oral health.

face moist and clean, aids healing and prevents infections. Minor burns need not be covered, but application of antiseptics or topical anesthetics is soothing.

Protection from Sun Exposure. Teaching about the hazards of ultraviolet (UV) rays is an important means of preventing skin cancer. Recent evidence suggests that sun damage is cumulative, and that damage during childhood and adolescence is particularly harmful. This means that avoiding sunburn by using effective sunscreens throughout one's life must start in childhood and continue through adulthood. Even though children do not usually develop skin cancer, individuals who have been sunburned during the first 20 years of their lives are at greater risk of developing skin cancers as adults. To understand how to protect themselves from the harmful effects of sun exposure, individuals must grasp the meaning of SPF, or sun protection factor, which indicates the degree of protection a sunscreen provides. SPF indicates the length of time a person can stay in the sun without burning while using the sunscreen, compared to the time of sun exposure that would cause a burn on unprotected skin. Therefore, a person who would get sunburned in 15 minutes with no sun protection, using a sunscreen with an SPF of 4 could stay in the sun four

INSIGHTS FROM NURSING LITERATURE

IMPROVING ORAL HYGIENE

Pearson LS. A comparison of the ability of foam swabs and toothbrushes to remove dental plaque: implications for nursing practice. J Adv Nurs. *1996:62–69.*

Foam swabs are widely used by nurses as the primary tool for giving mouth care. Recognizing that oral hygiene helps prevent gingivitis (gum inflammation) and is therefore an important responsibility of the nurse, the researcher studied whether toothbrushes or foam swabs were more successful in removing dental plaque, and used her own mouth and that of a volunteer to study the effects of both. The researcher focused her observations on the gingival crevices and tooth surfaces of the upper and lower front eight teeth. The protocol called for precleaning the mouth to establish a baseline plaque measurement. The researcher then used plaque disclosure tablets to identify plaque. The top teeth were brushed, while the bottom teeth were subjected to a variety of swabbing treatments. The results showed that after 6 days, plaque had accumulated on the crevices of the lower buccal surfaces, and on the apex of one upper incisor, possibly as a result of a change in brushing technique necessitated by the experimental protocol. The researcher's results suggested that foam swabs are ineffective at removing dental plaque from some areas.

times longer—in this case, for an hour—before burning. If that same person used a sunscreen with a 25 SPF, he or she would not burn in 6 hours of exposure. Reapplications are not as effective as initial applications, so that a person could not expect 6 more hours of sun protection from the second application of 25 SPF sunscreen. Also, most products require application at least 30 minutes before sun exposure and reapplication after swimming for maximum effectiveness.

Teaching Self-assessment of the Skin. Stress the importance of regularly inspecting the skin with a good source of natural light. Advise patients to look for new lesions that do not seem to heal. They should also carefully inspect existing moles for changes in size, shape, or general appearance. Using a mirror for areas that are hard to see, such as scalp, shoulders, and legs, is a good idea. Since bathing promotes vasodilation, which may make some lesions difficult to notice, suggest that patients perform the inspection before, rather than immediately after, bathing. Advise them to report lesions that do not heal and moles that change in appearance to their primary care provider.

Screening

Screening for skin changes that suggest actual or potential skin problems is part of the nurse's responsibility in preventive care, even when a skin problem is not a patient's primary concern. Of particular concern are lesions that suggest malignancy, described under *Mucosal Disruptions*, on page 797. Other skin alterations that indicate a need for follow-up are unusual dryness, scratch marks, edema, atypical color, unhealed lesions, and thin, shiny, hairless skin. Each of these could signal problems, as discussed in *Altered Skin and Mucosal Integrity* earlier in the chapter, and in Chap. 17.

Home Health Care

Working in the home provides nurses with an excellent opportunity to promote skin health. Because home nurses often care for patients for weeks, months, or even years, time is available to assess by direct observation family knowledge, resources, routines, and habits. Based on such assessments home nurses are able to engage the patient and family members in a program of health education tailored to their needs and circumstances. The information and skills outlined above are important components of such a program. All members of the family old enough to understand can be taught preventive measures related to the care of the integument and how to do skin and oral self-assessments, with the goal of promoting health and maintaining their integument in good condition.

SUPPORTIVE CARE

Nurses provide supportive skin and tissue care for patients with mild skin problems that are acute or self-limiting. One common problem for which nurses often provide supportive care is pruritus, an irritating itching sensation that individuals commonly attempt to relieve by scratching. Although this brings temporary relief, the increased blood flow caused by scratching enhances the itchy sensation, causing more scratching—setting up a continuous cycle. Pruritus may be a manifestation of a skin or systemic disease, a reaction to drugs or allergens, or a result of dry skin. Supportive care focuses on increasing comfort, protecting the skin from injury, alleviating causal factors when possible, and teaching patients strategies for prevention.

Therapeutic Baths

Although frequent bathing exacerbates pruritus, preparations such as the colloidal oatmeal preparation, Aveeno, or oils such as Alpha-Keri or Lubath are often soothing. Bran, starch, and gelatin added in a proportion of 1 or 2 ounces to a gallon of water also can be used to relieve itching.[27]

Emollients

Emollients are fatty or oily substances that soothe or soften dry skin or mucous membranes. Petroleum jelly, lanolin, vitamin A and D ointment, and vitamin E are examples. There are also many water-based lotions available that eliminate staining of clothing. Patients should apply emollients several times a day and especially after bathing as a preventive measure against dry skin, often a precursor to pruritus. Chemicals such as menthol and phenol are added to lubricating lotions to control puritis.[15]

Topical Antipruritics

Antipruritic agents are available in the form of ointments, pastes, and lotions. For localized itching, cool compresses using normal saline, potassium permanganate, aluminum acetate (Burow's solution), or boric acid are effective (Procedure 27–2). Calamine lotion and 0.5 to 1 percent hydrocortisone ointment provide good relief as well.

(continued on page 823)

PROCEDURE 27–2. APPLYING WARM OR COOL COMPRESSES

PURPOSE: To promote circulation and enhance healing, to promote suppuration, to soften dried wound exudate, and to apply medicated solution (eg, to relieve pruritus).

EQUIPMENT: Material for compress: gauze 4 × 4s or 2 × 2s, eyepads, combipads, washcloths, or towels, depending on the size and location of the application; container to moisten compresses; prescribed solution. For warm compresses: petroleum jelly, cotton-tipped applicators or tongue blades, insulating material: plastic, towels, or dry dressing materials; waterproof underpad; gauze strips or tape. External heat source such as aquathermia pad may also be used. If compresses are used on open wounds, sterile supplies, including sterile gloves and a moistureproof bag will be needed. Prepackaged sterile wet dressings are often used in this case.

ACTION 1. Verify medical order for solution, location, and duration of heat therapy. Gather supplies.

RATIONALE. In most health care agencies, heat therapy is not an independent nursing implementation.

ACTION 2. Discuss the procedure with the patient, including the expected benefits, usual sensations, and desired participation.

RATIONALE. The patient will be less anxious and more likely to participate if this information is shared.

ACTION 3. Wash your hands.

RATIONALE. Washing removes transient microorganisms, therefore preventing their transfer by direct contact.

ACTION 4. If order is for warm compresses, warm prescribed solution or place prepackaged sterile wet dressings in dressing heater. For clean compresses, place pads/towels, etc in a basin of hot water. Preheat aquathermia pad. Sterile solution may be warmed by placing its container in a basin of very hot water.

RATIONALE. Heat transfer takes time. Remaining preparation can be carried out while these materials are warming.

ACTION 5. Screen patient, assist with positioning, drape if necessary. Place waterproof underpad under or adjacent to body part to which compresses are to be applied.

RATIONALE. Screening shows respect for patient's needs for privacy and comfort.

ACTION 6. Assess for skin integrity: general condition of skin and tissue (eg, lesions, edema); and for sensory or circulatory impairment: response to light touch, pinprick, unilateral coolness of extremity.

RATIONALE. Assessment provides baseline for evaluation of effectiveness of compresses. Patients with sensory or circulatory impairment or thin/damaged skin are at greater risk for thermal injury; extreme caution is required when applying heat therapy.

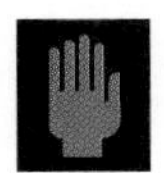

Caution is also necessary when using heat therapy with elderly, very young, or unresponsive patients.

ACTION 7. If compress is for wound, don gloves and remove existing dressing (see Procedure 27–16). Discard in moistureproof bag. Assess condition of wound and drainage.

RATIONALE. Gloves and bag are barriers preventing transmission of organisms to nurse or environment. Assessment provides baseline to evaluate effectiveness of moist heat therapy.

ACTION 8. Apply petroleum jelly to skin to be covered by warm compress. If treating an open wound, clean wound as ordered (see Procedure 27–15), then apply petroleum jelly to surrounding skin with sterile applicator or tongue blade. Skin protection is not needed for cool (room temperature) compresses to treat pruritus.

RATIONALE. Application provides a barrier, protecting skin from burns, maceration, or irritation, while allowing heat to penetrate deeper tissue layers.

Continued

ACTION 9. Quickly wring out compress material so it is damp, but not dripping. Test temperature of clean compress with your inner wrist. If too hot, cool by exposing to air.

RATIONALE. Excess moisture will damage skin and leak from compress. Skin on inner wrist is sensitive to temperature. If this area can tolerate temperature of compress it is likely to be tolerable to patient as well.

ACTION 10. Place compress lightly on prescribed area. If tolerable to patients for several seconds, mold compress closely to skin surface and apply adequate compresses to cover prescribed area with 2 to 4 layers of material.

RATIONALE. Skin is sensitive to sudden change in temperature, so evidence of intolerance will be prompt. Molding excludes air, which is a poor conductor of heat. Extra layers will prolong heat retention and penetration.

ACTION 11. If compress is to be applied to a wound, aseptically place sterile gauze pads in a sterile basin (see Procedure 25–2). Check temperature of solution (41–45C or 105–114F). Pour warm sterile solution to cover gauze. Don sterile gloves (see Procedure 25–3) to prepare and apply compresses as above. If prepackaged sterile wet dressings are used, follow manufacturer's directions.

RATIONALE. Sterile supplies prevent transfer of microorganisms from environment to wound.

ACTION 12. Apply insulating layer such as plastic or dry towels over warm compresses. Use a sterile barrier towel over sterile compresses before additional insulating material is used. When applying compresses to an extremity, maximum insulation is achieved by wrapping insulating layer around extremity.

RATIONALE. Insulation delays heat transfer to environment by convection and conduction. Moistureproof material is preferred to keep bed linens dry. Sterile barrier towel is moistureproof, so prevents contamination of wound by capillary action.

ACTION 13. External heating device such as an aquathermia pad may be wrapped around or placed under insulating layer to extend the therapeutic effect of the compresses.

RATIONALE. Warm compresses become too cold to be therapeutic within 5 to 10 minutes without an external heat source because heat is lost to the environment by conduction and convection.

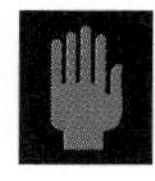

Replace warm compresses every 5 minutes if no external heat source is used.

ACTION 14. Secure compresses, aquathermia pad, and insulating layer with tape or ties.

RATIONALE. If patient movement dislodges compresses, heat will no longer be directed to affected area.

ACTION 15. Explain to the patient that within a few minutes, the compress will feel cooler, because the body's heat receptors adapt to new temperatures rapidly, but that the compress will not actually have cooled significantly in this time period.

RATIONALE. This explanation will prevent the perception that the compress is too cool to be therapeutic and the request for a hotter compress, which could cause a burn.

ACTION 16. Assess patient in 10 to 15 minutes for generalized vasodilation. If the patient feels warm, provide ventilation or remove some covers. If in distress, remove the compress.

RATIONALE. Vasodilation in untreated areas of the body (consensual response) is a reflex response. It is more likely when heat therapy is applied to a large area.

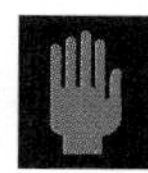

This response may cause a drop in blood pressure in patients with circulatory, pulmonary, or cardiac problems.

ACTION 17. Discontinue compress in 20 to 30 minutes.

RATIONALE. Maximum increase in skin circulation occurs after 20 to 30 minutes of heat therapy. Prolonged heat (30 to 45 min) results in tissue congestion, followed by vasoconstriction, which prevents heat dissipation.

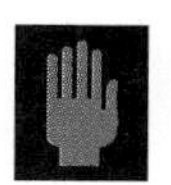

If compress was applied to a wound, use aseptic technique for removing and disposing of compress.

Procedure 27–2. (continued)

ACTION 18. Assess the condition of the skin and/or wound. Report signs of burns or deteriorating skin condition to the physician.

RATIONALE. Assessment is needed to document therapeutic effect.

ACTION 19. Wipe off remaining petroleum jelly; apply wound dressing if needed (see Procedure 27–16). Assist patient to comfortable position; dispose of or store materials according to hospital policy.

RATIONALE. This shows respect for patient needs for comfort and safety.

Recording:
Note length and type of application; condition of skin before and after therapy; and systemic reaction or other problems, if any, and action taken to correct problems.

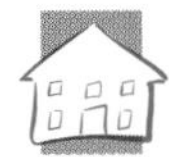

HOME HEALTH ADAPTATION: Prepare basin in which to wet compresses by disinfecting with a solution of sodium hypochlorite (household bleach) in a dilution of 10 parts water to one part bleach. Clean compresses may be dampened and slipped into a resealable plastic bag for heating in a microwave oven. Carefully check temperature before handling. Open bag slowly, allowing steam to escape. Test compress temperature on your own wrist before applying to patient. Double-wrap soiled compresses in plastic bag before discarding into household trash.

Measures to Prevent Pruritus

Eliminating the use of harsh, highly alkaline soaps is one way to prevent or minimize pruritus. Decreasing the frequency of bathing, or avoiding all soap except on the face, axilla, and perineal area, is also helpful. Thorough rinsing is important regardless of the type of soap used.

Some pruritus is the result of sensitivity to cosmetics, deodorants, or laundry products. Avoiding highly perfumed lotions and soaps and experimenting with different laundry products often eliminates itching. Sometimes extra rinsing of bed linens is helpful. Some people are sensitive to fibers used in clothing, particularly wool. Often these people can wear wool garments as long as they avoid direct contact between the wool and skin. Anyone with a sensitivity to wool also should avoid products with lanolin.

Maintaining hydration by increasing daily fluid intake to 3000 mL and raising environmental humidity via room humidifiers also improves pruritus that is secondary to dry skin.

Topical Antifungals

Nurses can offer supportive care to patients experiencing fungal skin and mucosal infections, such as vaginal candidiasis and athletes' foot. These infections often flare up in hot weather or under conditions that increase perspiration. More frequent bathing, thorough drying, and loose-fitting clothing that allows air circulation can prevent flare-ups of fungal infections.

Candida albicans is a common cause of vaginitis. It produces a curdy white, cottage-cheese-like discharge, itching, and vaginal erythema. Vaginal application of nystatin is the most common treatment, and is available over the counter. Nurses recommending its use should caution patients to seek additional care if symptoms do not disappear after the recommended course of the drug. Inform patients that drying labial skin folds thoroughly after bathing or showering (a hair dryer works well), wearing cotton underwear, and avoiding tight-fitting pants are effective preventive measures and promote treatment of active infections.

Athletes' foot responds to topical applications of preparations such as Tinactin, Enzactin, or Desinex in ointment, powder, or spray form. Patients should wash the affected area with mild soap and water and dry well before applying medication. Wearing sandals or leather shoes with absorbent cotton socks enhances evaporation of perspiration. Patients should avoid vinyl or plastic shoes because they trap moisture.

Sitz Bath

Sitz baths (Procedure 27–3) are soothing for patients with hemorrhoids and perineal wounds, such as episiotomies. They enhance healing by cleansing action and promoting circulation. Patients can use their bathtubs for self-administered sitz baths at home.

Eye Irrigation

Although tears naturally cleanse the eyes, occasionally irritants such as debris or chemicals require removal by irrigation, as described in Procedure 27–4. Lubricants or artificial tears provide protection when tear production is diminished, or to reduce irritation from dust or contact lenses.

Ear Irrigation

Some individuals produce excessive cerumen, which may collect in amounts sufficient to interfere with hearing. Irrigating the ear (as discussed in Chap. 32) is a safe means of removing built-up wax. Caution patients against attempting to remove ear wax with cotton-tipped applicators, as they can damage organs of the middle ear.

Home Health Care

Because of advancing age or other factors, patients may have difficulty caring for themselves and may be at risk for mild skin and tissue injury and wounds. Therefore, the supportive role of the home health nurse is to assess the patient's integument, identifying what the patient is and is not able to do independently, and to teach the patient and the patient's caregivers information and skills needed to support the patient's integumentary health. Therapeutic baths and sitz baths, for example, are important skills that, when taught, not only provide protection for the patient's skin and mucosa, but help the family caregiver to provide soothing, comforting care. Families with elders should also be taught to avoid

PROCEDURE 27–3. ASSISTING WITH TAKING A SITZ BATH

PURPOSE: Application of local heat to the perineal/rectal area to reduce inflammation, enhance suppuration, and soften and remove exudates, thereby promoting healing and comfort.

EQUIPMENT: Portable sitz bath, disposable sitz bath kit, or permanently installed sitz bath, towels, and bath blanket (optional), thermometer.

ACTION 1. Review medical order.

RATIONALE. Heat application is not an independent nursing action in some health care facilities.

ACTION 2. Discuss the procedure with the patient, including the expected benefits, usual sensations, and desired participation.

RATIONALE. Patients will be more likely to participate and less anxious if this information is shared.

ACTION 3. Fill the sitz bath ⅓ to ½ full of warm water, depending on the size of the tub and the size of the patient; 105 to 115F (40.5–46C) is preferred if a thermometer is available. If a portable unit is used, fill the bag as well, then clamp the tubing and place the unit on the toilet as shown.

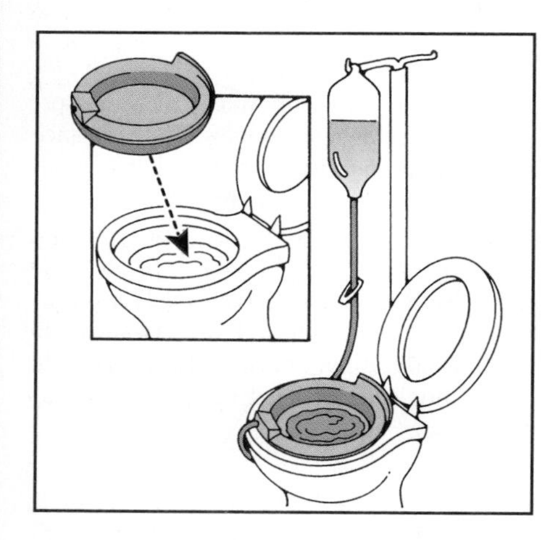

RATIONALE. When the patient sits in the tub, water will be displaced so the water level will rise. Because portable units are small, the water cools more quickly. The bag provides a reservoir of warm water to replace the cooled water in the tub.

ACTION 4. Assist patient to bathroom area, if necessary. Most alert mobile patients need no further assistance for sitz bath if clear explanation is given.

RATIONALE. Bathing and related activities are considered private in most cultures.

ACTION 5. If perineal dressings are present, don gloves to remove and discard in waterproof bag.

RATIONALE. Heat is most effective if applied directly to the skin. Dressings would have an insulating effect.

ACTION 6. Assess affected area for swelling, redness, drainage.

RATIONALE. Assessment provides baseline for evaluating effectiveness of treatment.

ACTION 7. Provide level of assistance patient requires to sit in the tub, show patient how to use clamp to control flow of warm water from the bag.

RATIONALE. Safety is a primary concern, but most patients who are able prefer to perform bathing-related activities independently.

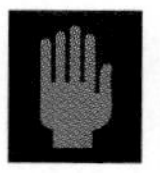

Patients with cardiac, respiratory, or circulatory problems should not be left unattended during heat therapy. See Action 9.

ACTION 8. Provide bath blankets to drape over shoulders and legs if desired

RATIONALE. Some patients may feel chilled when part of the body is warmed by heat therapy.

ACTION 9. Show patient the location of nurse call button. Return to assess patient response to therapy within 5 minutes. Assess for weakness, vertigo, pallor, tachycardia, or shortness of breath.

RATIONALE. These indicate inability to tolerate sitz bath. This is an unusual response in otherwise healthy patients, but assessment of all patients is prudent to prevent injury.

ACTION 10. Return in 15 to 20 minutes to discontinue treatment. Alert mobile patients are able to independently discontinue treatment.

RATIONALE. Maximum increase in skin circulation occurs after 20 to 30 minutes of heat therapy. Prolonged heat (30 to 45 min) results in tissue congestion, followed by vasoconstriction, which prevents heat dissipation.

Procedure 27–3. (continued)

ACTION 11. Assess affected area as in Action 6. Replace dressings if ordered (see Procedure 27–16).

RATIONALE. Evaluation of effectiveness of treatments is a nursing responsibility.

ACTION 12. Clean/disinfect portable or permanent sitz bath according to agency policy. Patients can reuse disposable units as needed.

RATIONALE. Cleaning/disinfecting removes and kills microorganisms, preventing transfer to other patients.

Recording:

Note completion of treatment; condition of affected area before and after treatment; patient's response; and problems, if any, and action taken to correct them.

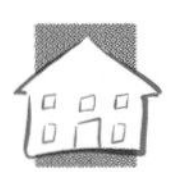

HOME HEALTH ADAPTATION: Clean and disinfect tub with 10% bleach solution before and after patient use to prevent the spread of infection.

CLINICAL GUIDELINE 27–2

ASSISTING PATIENTS WITH HYGIENE

1. Encourage independence in personal care to the extent possible considering patient's physical condition and necessary restrictions related to medical and nursing treatment plans. Self-care promotes self-esteem and reduces feelings of dependence and powerlessness. Large muscle activity during self-care activities stimulates circulation and maintains muscle tone and joint mobility.
2. Adhere as closely as possible to patients' usual hygiene routines, in terms of timing, techniques, and special toilet articles or products used. Loss of control over personal routines is a significant stressor associated with illness and hospitalization.
3. Collaborate with patient and physician to select the least restrictive modification given patient's condition (eg, cover incision and IV site with plastic so ambulatory postsurgical patient can take a shower rather than a sponge bath, use a shower chair for an alert but slightly weak patient).
4. Protect safety during independent hygiene activities by using "occupied" signs rather than locks on showers or tub rooms, instructing patient on the location and use of the call light, and checking on patient at least every 5 minutes. For some patients, remaining outside the door or curtain is advisable.
5. When assisting with hygiene procedures, maintain privacy at all times: close door, pull curtains around bed, and keep all parts of body covered except part being cleaned. Hygiene activities are considered private in most cultures. Body exposure is threatening and demeaning to most individuals and also causes discomfort because of chilling.
6. Wash your hands before and after assisting with hygiene to avoid transfer of microorganisms among patients, nurse, and environment. Gloves may be indicated for some procedures (see specific procedures).
7. Apply principles of body mechanics such as raising the bed to your waist level and moving patient close to the side of the bed on which you are working when assisting patient with hygiene. Extra precaution is needed to avoid bending and stooping when caring for patients in stationary, low beds, which are common in the home setting. Refer to Chap. 33 for more information about body mechanics.

using harsh laundry products when cleaning the clothes and linens used to care for them.

Finally, cerumen accumulation may contribute to hearing difficulty in people of all ages. Another important function of the home nurse, therefore, is to assess the patient's external ear canal for waxy buildup. It is not uncommon for home patients prone to cerumen buildup to require an ear irrigation to remove dry, impacted earwax.

RESTORATIVE CARE

Patients with wounds, skin diseases, or health problems that interfere with the ability to perform self-hygiene and skin care need restorative skin and tissue care. Restorative skin and tissue care includes general hygiene: oral hygiene, bathing (including eye, ear, hair, nail, and perineal care), and care of lesions and wounds. General guidelines for assisting patients with hygiene are summarized in Clinical Guideline 27–2. Each of the individual elements of restorative skin and tissue care is discussed below. Health care facilities that provide inpatient care have routine times for providing hygiene related to usual daily activities. Early morning care, morning care, and hour of sleep care are the most common.

Early morning care is offered at the time of awakening. It enhances well-being and readies patients for breakfast. Early morning care includes assisting with elimination, washing hands and face, oral care, and combing or brushing hair. Patients who need glasses or hearing aids usually desire to put them on after washing their face. If these aids need cleaning (see Chap. 32), it may be done now or later with the bath. Some patients also desire to shave and apply cosmetics or makeup at this time.

Morning care (AM care) is given sometime after breakfast. It includes assistance with elimination, oral care, shower or bath, linen change, and shaving and hair care if not previously done. Often, range of motion and other in-bed exercises or ambulation (see Chap. 33), are considered part of morning care. Hour of sleep (HS) care readies patients for sleep. It encompasses helping with elimination, washing hands and face, oral care, skin care, and straightening or freshening bed linens. Chapter 31 discusses HS care in greater detail.

PROCEDURE 27–4. IRRIGATING EYES

PURPOSE: To cleanse eye of irritants or discharge.
EQUIPMENT: Sterile irrigating solution (normal saline is most common; IV solution, container, and tubing may be used); sterile irrigation set (or sterile basin and toomey syringe); curved (emesis) basin; waterproof pad; and sterile gauze pad (4 × 4) and clean glove.

ACTION 1. Review the medical order. Wash your hands. Discuss the procedure with the patient, including the usual sensations, and desired participation.

ACTION 2. Request or assist the patient to a sidelying position with the affected eye lowest. Place the waterproof pad so pillow, sheet, and clothing are protected. Place an emesis basin with the concave curve against the cheek to collect returned solution. The patient may wish to hold the basin for closer contact.

ACTION 3. If using an irrigation set, fill the syringe with sterile irrigant at room temperature. If using an infusion set, attach and fill the tubing (no needle is used). Do not allow anything unsterile to contact the tip of the syringe or tubing.

ACTION 4. Don a clean glove on your nondominant hand, then retract the upper and lower lids of the affected eye to expose conjunctival sac. Administer solution so it flows from the inner canthus to the outer canthus to prevent fluid from flowing into the unaffected eye or the nasolactimal duct of the affected eye. Flush the cornea and conjunctival sac. Fifteen minutes of flushing is needed for some chemicals. Avoid contacting the cornea with the syringe or tubing tip as this will injure the cornea.

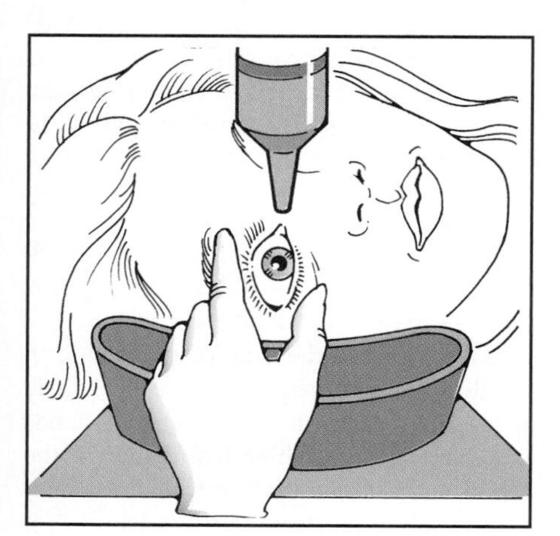

ACTION 5. When the prescribed amount of irrigant has been administered, or the returned solution is clear, gently blot the eye from inner to outer canthus with a sterile 4 × 4 and dry the patient's cheek. Remove and discard used equipment according to agency policy.

Recording:
Note the appearance of the sclera, conjunctiva, and surrounding tissue. Describe discharge, if any. Note the amount and type of irrigant and the patient's response to the procedure.

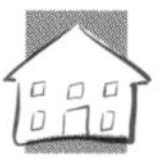

HOME HEALTH ADAPTATION: Commercial sterile normal saline prepackaged for use by contact lens wearers can be substituted for the irrigation solution and syringe since commercial containers are fitted with a nozzle suited to the task.

Oral Hygiene

Most patients prefer to perform oral self-care, even if they cannot get out of bed. If patients need assistance, follow the guidelines in Procedure 27–1. Bring toothbrush, toothpaste, curved basin (also called a kidney or emesis basin), dental floss, water for rinsing, and a disposable waterproof underpad. The most recent infection control guidelines from the Centers for Disease Control and Prevention specify the use of clean latex gloves when doing oral care (see Chap. 25).

Hospitalized patients who have dentures often require help to clean them. Procedure 27–5 outlines denture care.

Oral care is especially important for unconscious patients (Fig. 27–7). They are often mouth breathers, thus promoting drying of the oral mucosa and tenacious oral secretions that accumulate on the tongue and teeth. Procedure 27–6 details oral care for unconscious patients. Many unconscious patients need oral care every 2 hours.

Hair Care

Hair care includes shaving, beard and mustache care, and combing and shampooing scalp hair. Facial hair requires daily care. Most men are uncomfortable if they are unshaven, and some may need to shave twice a day to maintain a desired appearance. Usually men prefer to shave themselves, but if they are unable, shaving is part of daily nursing care. Refer to Procedure 27–7.

Hair care is another aspect of hygiene that most patients prefer to do independently. However, clean, combed hair contributes to well-being and positive feelings about self-presentation, so patients who are unable to manage it usually appreciate help. Refer to Procedures 27–8 and 27–9. In acute care settings, time constraints may preclude shampooing a patient's hair; however, any patient confined to bed for several days benefits from a shampoo.

Bathing Patients

A daily bath or shower is part of most individuals' hygiene habits. Although some may feel that their relative lack of activity when in a hospital makes daily bathing unnecessary, in fact being in bed under covers increases perspiration. Bathing removes accumulated perspiration, skin oils, dead skin cells, and bacteria, and prevents body odor. It also enhances circulation and promotes relaxation and feelings of well-being. Bathing a patient provides a nurse with an excellent opportunity to assess skin condition thoroughly and initiate early treatment of any lesions related to bed rest. Procedure 27–10 describes how to give a bed bath. Some patients, particularly older patients, require special care to prevent dry skin, such as use of moisturizing soap or emollients, or using soap sparingly. Foot and nail care (Procedure 27–11) and perineal and Foley catheter care (Procedure 27–12) are part of the bath and are repeated as necessary throughout the day.

Shower. When possible, most patients prefer to shower. Even patients receiving intravenous fluids or with surgical incisions can shower as long as they can stand independently. Usually, nurses can cover dressings or venipuncture sites with plastic wrap taped on all edges. This prevents wetting the dressing as long as water does not flow directly on the tape. Confer with the patient's surgeon to be sure there are no contraindications to showering. It is a good idea to remain outside the shower area for a short time to be sure patients are not experiencing problems and to check on them periodically. Inform patients of the location of the call light.

A shower chair is a good choice for patients able to tolerate being out of bed but unable to stand safely in a shower. They receive the benefit and enjoyment of a shower without risking accidents.

Assisted Bath. Many patients confined to bed are able to wash themselves if provided with a basin of warm water, soap, and towels. Offer to change the water as necessary and wash their backs, feet, or other areas they find hard to reach. Most patients with indwelling urinary catheters may need assistance to cleanse around the catheter adequately.

Sink Bath. For ambulatory patients unable to shower, a sink bath is often preferable to a sponge bath in bed. They will need help with their backs and feet.

Tub Bath. Some health care facilities have tubs available as another alternative for hygiene. Washing and rinsing are easier in a tub than with a bed bath and many patients prefer a tub bath to a sponge bath or shower. Special precautions are necessary to prevent injury getting into and out of the tub.

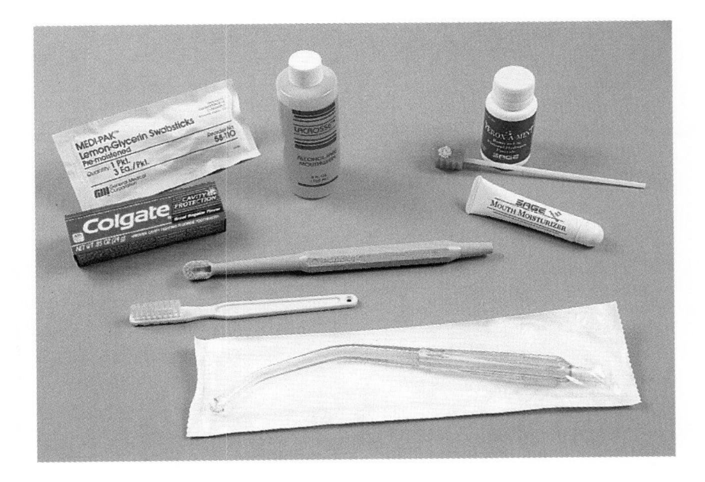

Figure 27–7. Supplies to provide oral hygiene for the unconscious patient: Lemon-glycerine swabs, toothpaste, mouthwash, foam swab, moisturizer, toothbrush, electric toothbrush attachment, and yankauer suction tip.

Linen Change

Having a clean wrinkle-free bed in which to rest makes a significant contribution to patients' will-being, particularly with patients whose activity is limited. Procedures 27–13 and 27–14 contain detailed instructions for changing linen. The decision to make an occupied or unoccupied bed may rest with patient and nurse, or medical orders may specify bed rest, necessitating an occupied bed. Although many nurses believe that making an occupied bed conserves patients' energy, studies have shown that getting patients out of bed for bedmaking results in minimal energy cost and cardiac stress for patients.[28] Because early mobilization is beneficial to most patients' recovery, encourage patients who are able to get out of bed and sit in a chair during bedmaking. Elevate the lower legs of postoperative patients to avoid popliteral pressure venous stasis, decreasing the risk of pathologic clotting (see Chap. 30).

(continued on page 848)

PROCEDURE 27–5. CARING FOR DENTURES

PURPOSE: To remove trapped food particles from dentures and oral cavity, to maintain oral mucosal integrity, and to promote comfort and a sense of well-being.

EQUIPMENT: Denture brush, soft brush or toothette, clean gloves, denture cup or emesis basin, washcloth, gauze, or paper towels, and cleaning agent of patient's preference.

ACTION 1. Discuss patient's preferences for denture care. Most patients prefer to care for dentures independently and many are embarrassed to be seen by others without dentures in place. If assistance is necessary, encourage patients to direct the process as much as possible.

ACTION 2. Wash your hands. Assemble equipment at the bedside. Put clean washcloth, gauze, or paper towel in bottom of basin to cushion dentures if they fall. Ask the patient to remove dentures. If patient is unable to do so, don gloves and use gauze or a paper towel to prevent slipping when grasping the denture to remove it. Grasp the front of the lower plate, lift it, and tip it slightly, using care not to bump it on the upper plate as you take it from the mouth. Place it in the denture cup or emesis basin. Grasp the front of the upper plate, rock it gently from side to side to break the vacuum seal, and then tip it downward slightly to pull it out of the mouth. Put it in the cup or basin.

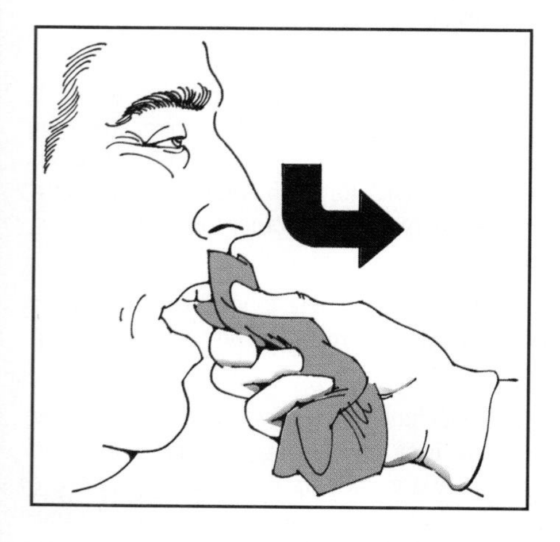

ACTION 3. Wearing gloves, brush all surfaces of both plates at the sink, using a stiff denture brush and cleaning agent of patient's choice. Placing a washcloth or several paper towels in the sink will prevent chipping the dentures if they are dropped during cleaning. Rinse dentures thoroughly with running water. Do not use hot water because this may warp the dentures. Stained dentures may be soaked in denture cleaner or a solution of 5 to 10 mL of vinegar in 240 mL of water.

ACTION 4. Clean patient's tongue and gums with a soft toothbrush, inspecting gums and palate for signs of irritation from the dentures. Offer water or mouthwash to rinse mouth and a towel or cloth to wipe mouth.

ACTION 5. Give dentures to patient for reinsertion. Some patients use denture adhesive, which is applied in a thin layer on the undersurface of each plate. If assistance is needed, insert the plates one at a time, upper and then lower, exerting slight pressure to facilitate adherence to the gums. If dentures are not reinserted, they should be stored in liquid in a marked denture cup.

ACTION 6. Store patient's oral hygiene materials as patient desires.

Recording:
Not usually required. May be noted on checklist. If mucosal lesions are noted, describe lesions and action taken.

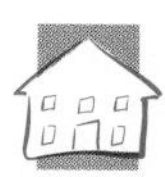

HOME HEALTH ADAPTATION: This procedure adapts well to the home setting.

PROCEDURE 27–6. PROVIDING MOUTH CARE FOR AN UNCONSCIOUS PATIENT

PURPOSE: Cleansing oral cavity, maintaining integrity and hydration of oral mucosa, and preventing oral infections and lesions.

EQUIPMENT: Gauze-padded tongue blade or bite block; soft toothbrush; toothette or lemon-glycerine swabs; clean gloves; cleaning agent: ½-strength hydrogen peroxide, baking soda, or mouthwash; water; 50-mL syringe; emesis basin; suction apparatus with tonsil suction tip; waterproof pad; and emollient such as petroleum jelly, A & D ointment, or commercial lip balm.

ACTION 1. Discuss the procedure with the patient, including the expected benefits, usual sensations, and desired participation.

RATIONALE. Even apparently unresponsive patients may be able to hear and understand. The patient will be less anxious and more likely to participate if this information is shared.

ACTION 2. Gather equipment at bedside, close door, or pull bedside curtains.

RATIONALE. Personal care is considered a private activity in most cultures. Unconscious patients are deserving of the same respect as alert patients.

ACTION 3. Position patient on the side, with head on the edge of the pillow, a curved basin below the mouth, and a waterproof pad under the head and basin.

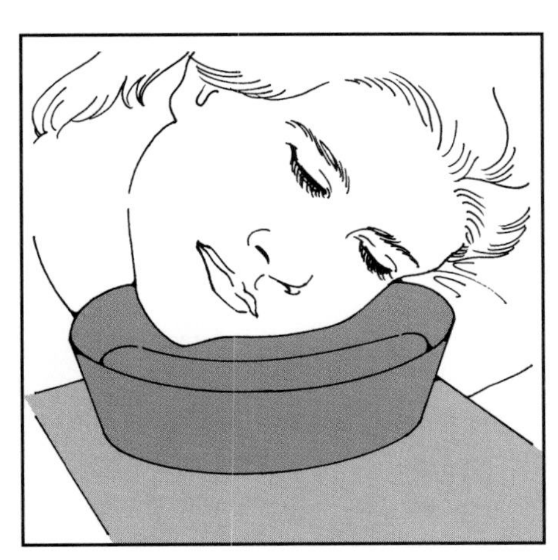

RATIONALE. Unconscious patients often lack a gag reflex, so are at risk for aspiration. This position facilitates flow of liquid out of the mouth by gravity. Basin and pad protect bed linen.

ACTION 4. Place a padded tongue blade edgewise between the back molars on one side of the mouth. A bite block may also be used.

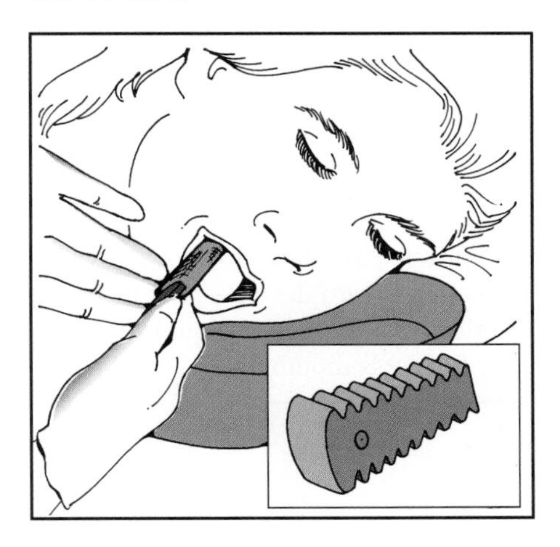

RATIONALE. Keeps the mouth open so oral care and assessment can be carried out. Gloves prevent transfer of microorganisms from patient's saliva or oral mucosa to nurse.

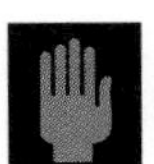

Some unconscious patients bite reflexively when an object is placed in their mouths. Do not try to force the mouth open or place your fingers in the mouth.

ACTION 5. Turn the suction unit on to low suction. Be sure tonsil suction device is attached.

RATIONALE. Tonsil suction apparatus can be used to quickly remove cleaning solution or saliva, which may flow into the throat if patient suddenly changes positions.

Continued

Procedure 27–6. Providing Mouth Care for an Unconscious Patient (continued)

ACTION 6. Moisten the toothbrush with dilute H_2O_2 or mouthwash. Do not use regular toothpaste, as it is hard to rinse. Brush all surfaces of the patient's teeth and tongue as described in Procedure 27–1. Assess the condition of oral mucous membranes as you brush. Dentures of unconscious patients should not remain in their mouths as they can be aspirated; however, oral hygiene is still needed.

RATIONALE. Unconscious patients are often mouth breathers, which contributes to drying of mucosa and formation of crusts, both of which may promote mouth lesions. H_2O_2 is particularly effective in removing organic matter and is antibacterial, so it promotes healing.

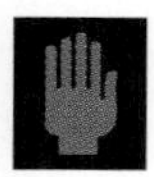

Lemon-glycerine swabs or toothettes may be used as short-term substitute for brushing, but are not as effective as brushes in removing debris.

ACTION 7. Rinse the mouth thoroughly with water from the syringe. Direct the water toward the sides, not the back, of the mouth. Use suction to remove any liquid that does not flow into the basin. Reassess mouth.

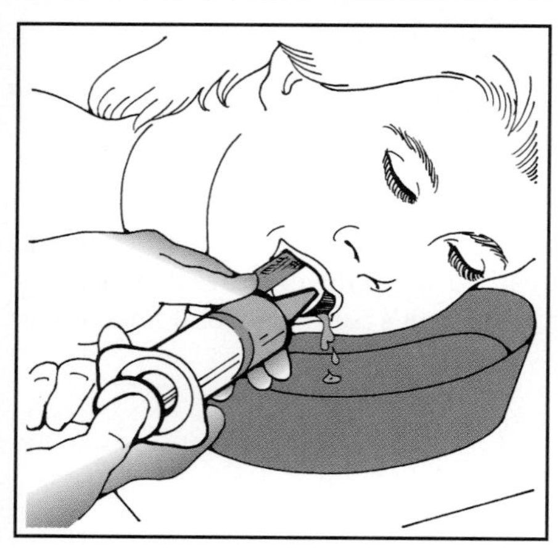

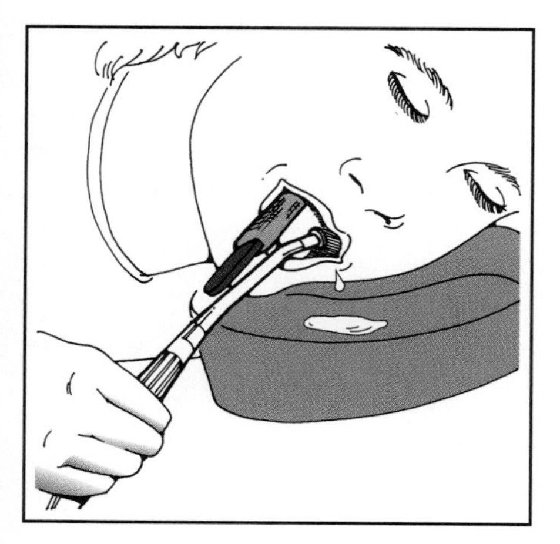

RATIONALE. Rinsing in this manner reduces risk of aspiration while removing loosened debris.

ACTION 8. Dry patient's face. Apply emollient to lips.

RATIONALE. Emollients minimize loss of moisture from tissues and contain additional moisturizing agents.

ACTION 9. Reposition patient. Raise siderails. Remove equipment; clean and store according to agency policy.

RATIONALE. These actions promote patient comfort and safety.

ACTION 10. Repeat every 1 to 2 hours, or more frequently if needed.

RATIONALE. Buildup of dried secretions in the oral cavity occurs rapidly in unconscious patients because of mouth breathing and the lack of activities such as chewing and swallowing, which ordinarily contribute to oral hygiene.

Recording:
Note procedure; condition of oral cavity before and after; problems, if any, and action taken in response.

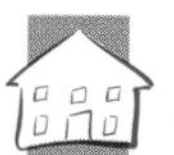

HOME HEALTH ADAPTATION: Suction equipment is not always available in the home setting. To remove the excess liquid that accumulates during mouth care, wrap clean gauze pad around a tongue blade and gently insert to oral cavity, patting surfaces to absorb. Teach family members how to provide oral hygiene and to observe oral cavity for debris and lesions. Inspect patient's mouth on each visit. Check for lesions, hydration, and adequacy of oral care. If the patient is unable to control oral secretions, instruct family to position patient to minimize the risk of aspiration (see Chap. 30, Oxygenation).

PROCEDURE 27–7. SHAVING AND BEARD CARE

PURPOSE: Removal of facial hair to promote comfort and improve appearance.
EQUIPMENT: Razor with sharp blade, shaving cream, basin, washcloth, towel, and clean gloves. Aftershave lotion (optional). Comb for beard or mustache, scissors if trim is desired. Mirror if desired by patient. Electric shaver preferred by some patients.

ACTION 1. Discuss patient's preferences for time and type of shave. Some patients may prefer family member to assist. Some black patients cannot tolerate shaving because it causes skin irritation and/or ingrown hairs; often dipilatory preparations are used instead. Use of an electric shaver is recommended for patients on anticoagulant therapy, taking high doses of aspirin, or with bleeding disorders.

ACTION 2. Assemble equipment and prepare area. Raise bed to nurse's waist height with patient's in Fowler's position; place towel over patient's chest to collect drips and hair. Provide privacy if patient desires.

ACTION 3. *If using a razor:* Soften the beard by applying a moist, warm washcloth to the face and neck for several minutes. Apply an even layer of shaving cream to face and neck. Don gloves. Holding the razor at a 45 degree angle, use firm short strokes in the direction of hair growth to remove facial and neck hair. Pulling skin taut with your other hand in opposite direction of strokes will reduce the likelihood of accidental cuts. Rinse razor frequently in basin of warm water. Some prefer to shave against the direction of hair growth—this results in a closer shave, but is more likely to cause skin irritation. When shave is complete, wipe excess lather with warm, damp cloth; dry face and neck.

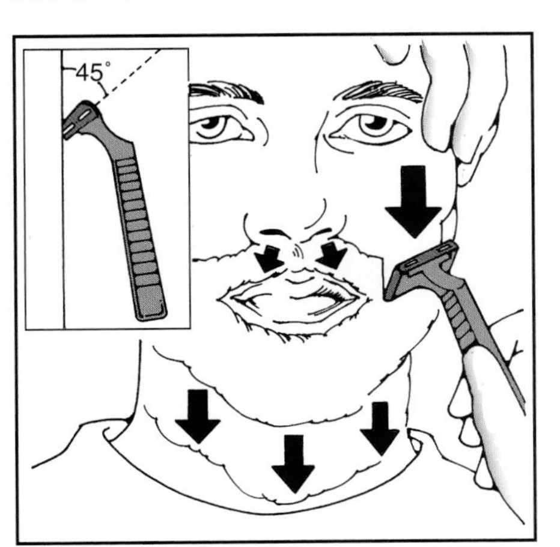

ACTION 4. *If using an electric shaver:* No lather or gloves are needed. If shaver has a flat straight head, use short up-and-down strokes on face, and strokes in the direction of hair growth on sensitive areas (eg, neck). Rotary head shavers work best if circular strokes are used. Hold skin taut while shaving as with razor.

ACTION 5. Use sharp scissors with blunt tips to trim beards and mustaches if patient desires. Beards and mustaches should be combed daily and washed several times per week using facial soap, rinsed well and dried.

ACTION 6. Provide aftershave lotion if desired, remove soiled linen, store personal items according to patient preference. Clean accumulated hair from electric shaver before storing; discard disposable razor in sharps container. Razor, linen, or gloves soiled with blood require special precautions. See agency policy.

Recording:
Routine daily care is not generally recorded, but may be noted on a daily care flow sheet.

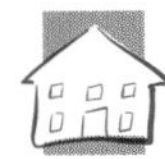

HOME HEALTH ADAPTATION: Using the patient's own shaving supplies and equipment, this procedure adapts well to the home setting and caregiver instruction.

PROCEDURE 27–8. CARING FOR HAIR

PURPOSE: To maintain integrity of hair and scalp and promote sense of well-being.
EQUIPMENT: Comb or brush, and special products desired by patient. For hair matted with blood or excessively tangled: hydrogen peroxide, alcohol, or oil. Gloves if blood is present.

ACTION 1. Discuss patient's preferences for nature and timing of hair care. Most patients prefer to carry out these activities independently, but may be unable due to illness or activity restrictions.

Daily care: Brush or comb hair at least once a day, working from scalp to ends. Style according to patient's preference. Long hair may be more easily managed if parted and groomed in sections; braiding prevents tangling. While caring for hair, assess the scalp for flaking, sores, irritated areas, or areas of hair loss; and note hair luster, texture, thickness, dryness, oiliness, or unusual loss of hair with combing.

Special hair care for black patients: Black patients commonly have thick, curly hair that is more fragile than straight hair; scalp and hair tend to be dry. A comb with widely spaced teeth is recommended. Comb from the scalp outward with a lifting, fluffing motion. Hair-lubricating products are preferred by most black patients. Mineral oil or petroleum jelly may be used for this, if commercial products are not available. If hair is braided in cornrows, these need not be unbraided, even for shampooing.

Tangled or matted hair: Tangles may be loosened by applying a small amount of oil, petroleum jelly, or alcohol. Comb out tangles in a small section of hair toward the scalp. Stabilize a short length of hair with your hand to avoid scalp trauma and comb toward the ends of the hair. If hair is matted with organic substances such as blood, wiping matted areas with gauze or cotton soaked in hydrogen peroxide is effective to clean and untangle hair strands. Wear gloves if blood is present. Badly tangled or matted hair may be infested with lice, so careful inspection for lice and nits (usually found near the root of the hair shaft at the nape of the neck or behind the ears) is indicated. If lice or nits are present, combing with a fine-tooth comb and a shampoo with products containing gamma-benzene-hexachloride is indicated (see Procedure 27–9). Removing tangles can be a difficult and painful process, so may need to be completed in several short sessions rather than all at once.

Recording:
Describe special care given, noting condition of scalp and hair before and after care. Routine daily care is generally not documented, but may be noted on a daily care checklist.

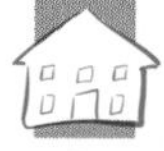

HOME HEALTH ADAPTATION: If the hair is shampooed for lice, instruct the caregiver to wash in hot water all bedding and clothing recently used by the patient. Inspect family members for lice. If found, inform members that treatment is necessary to prevent reinfection of the patient

PROCEDURE 27–9. SHAMPOOING

PURPOSE: To remove oil, dirt, or other substances, or to apply medicated solutions to hair and scalp.
EQUIPMENT: Shampoo, special preparations desired by patient, towels, and hair dryer (optional). If bed shampoo: shampoo trough or bath blanket and waterproof sheet, extra towels, two basins, and pitcher or graduate (an irrigating bag, such as an enema bag, suspended from an IV pole may be used instead), thermometer (optional).

ACTION 1. Discuss preferences for location and timing of shampoo. Most patients prefer to carry out this activity independently, but may be unable due to illness or activity restrictions. Options for location of shampoo include the bed, sink, tub, or shower. A chair or gurney may be used, depending on space limitations. Dry shampoo is available if conditions prevent a wet shampoo. In some agencies, a medical order is required for a wet shampoo.

Shower shampoo: This is most feasible if the shower is equipped with a hand-held device. The patient can sit in a shower chair or, if space permits, lie on a gurney protected with a waterproof sheet (if a sheet is unavailable, one or more large trash bags work well for this, or make a protector, such as described below for bed shampoo).

Tub shampoo: If the patient is able to sit in a bathtub, the hair can be washed and rinsed as part of the tub bath. The shampoo must be done rapidly, however, to avoid chilling the patient.

Procedure 27–9. (continued)

Bed shampoo: If the above locations are too difficult for the patient, the bed can be protected with a plastic shampoo trough or an improvised device to channel and collect the water. To make an improvised trough: fold a bath blanket into quarters lengthwise, then form into a long roll; place the roll on the edge of a plastic sheet (or several overlapping trash bags, if no sheet is available) and continue rolling the blanket tube several turns into the plastic; curve the plastic-covered tube into a horseshoe shape and position it under the patient's head so the remaining plastic can be gathered into a trough and draped into a basin to catch the water.

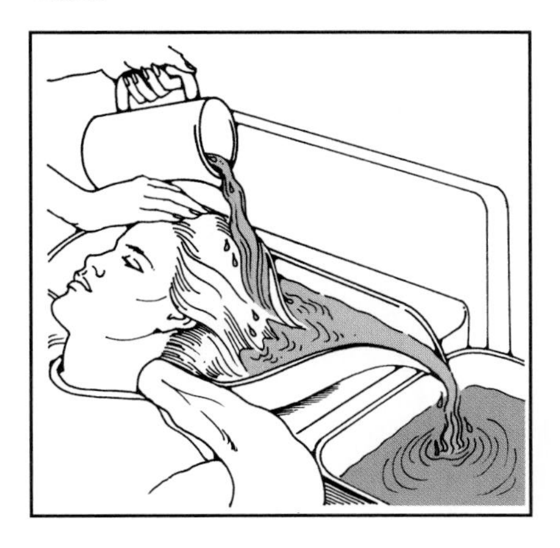

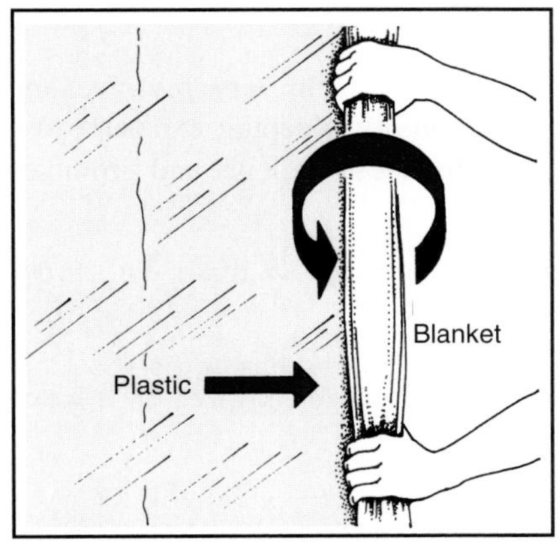

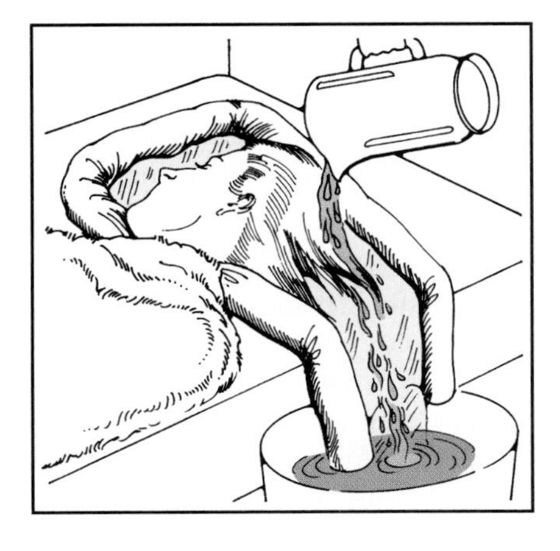

Sink shampoo: This is easiest if the patient is seated in a chair, with the back to the sink (if a chair of suitable height is not available, a bedside commode may be substituted). The head rests on the edge of the sink, which is padded with a towel. A pitcher, graduate, or irrigating bag may be needed to wet and rinse the hair. A bath blanket can be placed over the patient to prevent chilling. It is possible to perform a sink shampoo with the patient lying on a gurney if space permits.

ACTION 2. Position patient and bed, chair, or gurney so nurse's access to patient's hair is optimal. Place a rolled towel around the patient's neck and another around the shoulders. Many patients also desire to hold a small towel or washcloth over their eyes and to be covered with a bath blanket. Position protector for bed or gurney as described above.

ACTION 3. Gather equipment at location selected for shampoo. For bedside shampoo, fill a large basin with warm water (105–110F, 40–41C, or warm to the inner wrist) and obtain a smaller container to pour water; or fill irrigating container with attached tubing, clamp tubing, and hang container from an IV pole at bedside. If running water is used, adjust water temperature as above before directing water over patient's hair.

ACTION 4. Wet hair completely. Cover patient's ear with your free hand to avoid water flowing into ears. Apply a small amount of shampoo and work into a lather with both hands. Massage the scalp with pads of your fingers. Rinse thoroughly with clear water. Repeat lather and rinse if necessary. Apply conditioner if desired and rinse again. Squeeze excess moisture from hair.

ACTION 5. Wrap the patient's head with a dry towel. Reposition if necessary so bed protector can be removed. Blot the hair dry with the towel; comb as described in Procedure 27–8. Apply special products as desired by patient and blow dry hair if situation permits.

ACTION 6. Assist patient as necessary to comfortable bed position. Pillow and patient's shoulders may be covered with a towel if hair is not completely dry.

ACTION 7. Clean and store equipment according to agency policy.

Recording:
Note condition of hair and scalp before and after shampoo; patient's response; and problems, if any, and action taken in response.

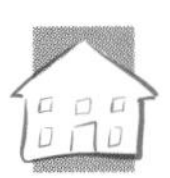

HOME HEALTH ADAPTATION: This procedure adapts well to the home setting using available shampoo supplies and clean containers.

PROCEDURE 27–10. GIVING A BED BATH

PURPOSE: To clean the skin, promote circulation, relax muscles, and promote comfort and well-being. Provides good opportunity for complete integumentary assessment.

EQUIPMENT: Basin, soap in soap dish, washcloth(s), 2 or 3 towels, bath blanket thermometer, deodorant (if patient desires), lotion, clean linen and gown, and linen hamper.

ACTION 1. Mutually select the optimal time for bath and associated hygiene. Typically, patients prefer to wash their face, shave, brush their teeth, and comb their hair before breakfast, and bathe at a later time. Further early morning care consists of offering a bed pan or urinal (see Chap. 29) or helping patients to bathroom or bedside commode. Refer to *Clinical Guideline 27–2,* for general guidelines for hygiene and Procedures 27–1 and 27–5 through 27–9 for shaving, oral, and hair care. Patient may prefer that a family member assist.

RATIONALE. Mutual decision making communicates respect for the patient. Rigid conforming to schedules is often condoned in institutions, for the sake of efficiency, but it is not always most efficient or effective to do so.

ACTION 2. Discuss the procedure with the patient, including the expected benefits, usual sensations, and desired participations.

RATIONALE. The patient will be more likely to participate and less anxious if this information is shared.

ACTION 3. Assemble equipment. Screen patient and raise bed. Lower siderail on near side of bed. Remove positioning aids, pillows except for pillow under head. HOB can be flat or slightly raised.

RATIONALE. This procedure conserves nurse's energy, and promotes body mechanics. See Chap. 33.

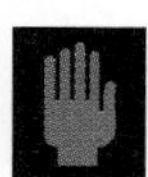

If patient has been incontinent, clean thoroughly before beginning bath. If bath basin is used for this, disinfect it before using it for bath.

ACTION 4. Remove and fold bedspread. Cover top linen with a bath blanket. Ask patient to hold top of bath blanket, then pull top sheet out without exposing patient. If top sheet is to be reused, fold and place on chair. Place soiled linen in hamper. Top sheet may be left in place if no bath blanket is available. Place an additional blanket on top if patient is cold.

RATIONALE. Bathing promotes evaporation of moisture from the skin, which lowers skin temperature. Flannel bath blanket absorbs more moisture and is warmer than a sheet.

ACTION 5. Remove gown with minimal exposure. If patient has an IV, remove opposite sleeve first, then sleeve on arm with IV. Take the IV container off the pole and slip sleeve over tubing and container, rehang, and check flowrate. If an IV controller or pump is in use, adjust screwclamp, remove tubing from machine, remove gown as above, and replace tubing in machine.

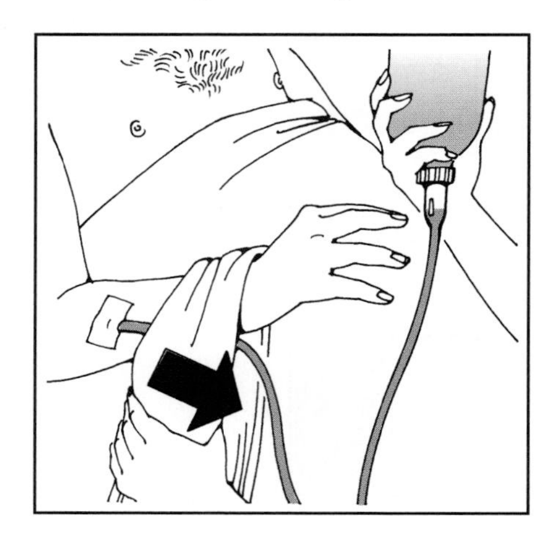

RATIONALE. Removal of gown feels very invasive and generates feelings of vulnerability. Keeping exposure to a minimum shows empathy for these feelings and promotes trust.

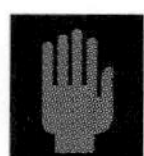

Never separate IV tubing to remove the gown. Disruption of this closed system could allow microorganisms to enter the bloodstream and cause serious infection. Many facilities use gowns with snaps at the shoulders to simplify changing the gown when IV therapy is ongoing.

ACTION 6. Obtain water in basin; 110 to 115F (43–46C) is preferred. If there is no thermometer, use water as hot as is comfortable for your hands. Use slightly cooler water for very young or elderly patients. Test patient's tolerance by lightly touching cheek with washcloth dampened in the water and wrung out. Water should be changed whenever it is cool or soapy.

RATIONALE. Water in open basin cools rapidly by convection, conduction, and evaporation. If too cool at the start, bath will be uncomfortably cold or water will need changing more frequently to keep from chilling the patient. Elderly people have thinner skin and diminished sensory perception, so are at greater risk for thermal injury. Testing patients' tolerance will prevent discomfort or burns.

ACTION 7. Place a towel under the patient's head. Wring out cloth and make a mitt as shown. This "mitt" technique is used throughout the bath. The towel will be used to protect bed throughout bath. Use a second towel to dry patient.

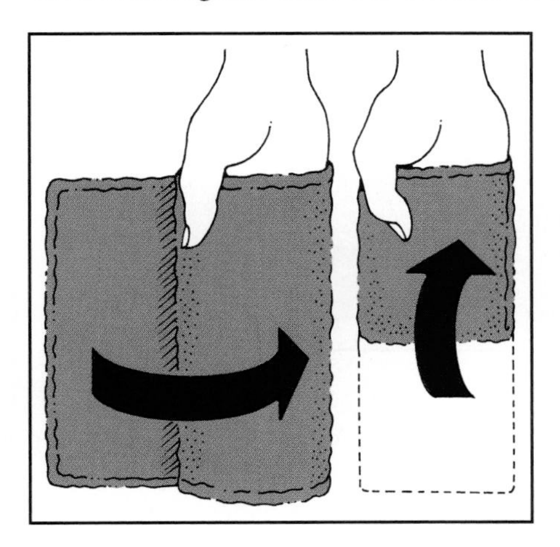

RATIONALE. Towel is used to absorb moisture, protect bed linen. Mitt prevents edges of the cloth from brushing against the skin. This may produce a tickling sensation and may feel cool.

ACTION 8. Using no soap, clean patient's eyes, washing from inner to outer canthus, and shifting the cloth so you use a fresh part with each wipe. Rinse cloth before cleaning second eye. If lids are caked with discharge, let the warm cloth rest on the lid for a few seconds to soften exudate.

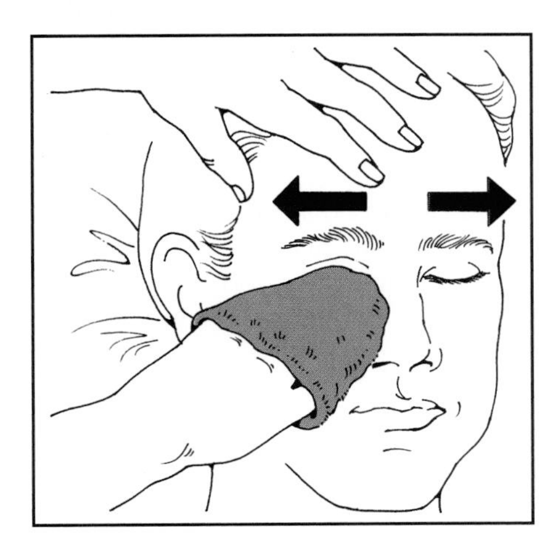

RATIONALE. Soap is irritating to the eyes. Considerable discharge may be present on the eyelids, because the cleansing action of blinking ceases during sleep. Cloth is rinsed to avoid transferring organisms from one eye to the other.

ACTION 9. Clean face, neck, and ears. Use little or no soap depending on skin condition and patient's preference. Some patients use special soaps or cleansers on the face.

RATIONALE. Facial skin may range from very oily to very dry. Oily skin is cleaned more effectively with soap because soap acts to reduce surface tension in water droplets and emulsifies oils; soap makes dry skin drier.

ACTION 10. If soap is used, do not leave soap in basin between uses. Rub a small amount on the cloth and return soap to soap dish.

RATIONALE. Adequate rinsing is difficult when giving a bed bath. Soapy water compounds the problem.

ACTION 11. Rinse as needed. Dry thoroughly with second towel. Use special care in skin folds (eg, on the neck).

RATIONALE. Soap residue is irritating and drying to skin and may alter the skin pH. If skin is not dried, evaporation will result in chilling. Moisture in skin folds causes maceration and possible breakdown and infection.

ACTION 12. Uncover one arm. Move protective towel under the arm. Using soap, wash hand, arm, shoulder, and axilla with firm long strokes from distal to proximal. If skin is dry or thin, use gentler strokes. Pay particular attention to hands and axilla. Rinse, repeat as necessary. Dry thoroughly. Provide nail care, if needed (see Procedure 27–11). Repeat for other arm. Some nurses soak patient's hands in the basin to facilitate cleaning nails. Nail care may be deferred until after bath.

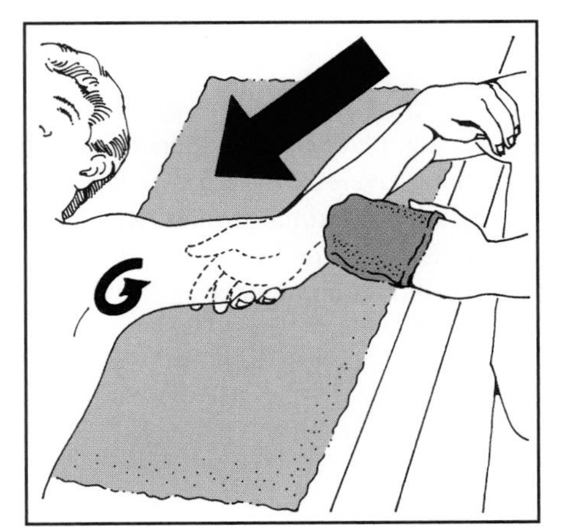

RATIONALE. Firm strokes create friction, which removes bacteria, dead skin cells, and other substances; excessive friction can damage skin. Axilla and hands generally have more bacteria. Distal to proximal strokes stimulate circulation, facilitating venous return to the heart.

Continued

Procedure 27–10. Giving a Bed Bath (continued)

ACTION 13. Expose one side of a female patient's chest and wash it. Lift the breast to clean underlying skin. Note condition of skin under breast. Rinse well and dry. Repeat for other side of chest. For a male patient fold down the bath blanket to expose the chest and abdomen at the same time. Wash, rinse, and dry.

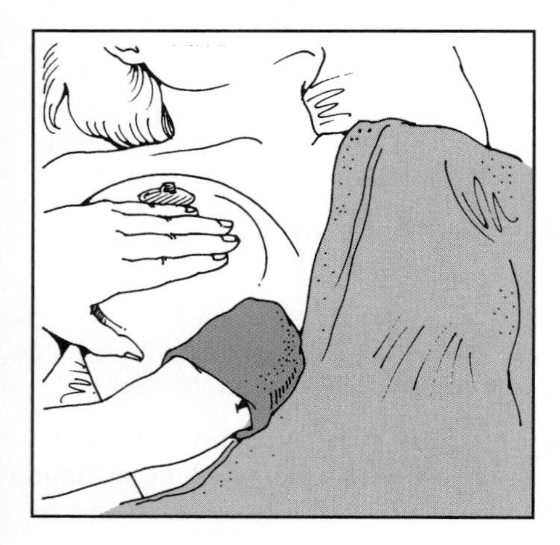

RATIONALE. Most women feel uncomfortable when breasts are exposed. Exposing only the area being cleaned is less threatening. Skin fold under heavy breasts is vulnerable to excoration, especially if patient perspires a lot.

ACTION 14. Cover the chest with the towel, then pull down the bath blanket to expose the abdomen. Keep the pubic hair covered. Wash, rinse, and dry the abdomen as above. Cover the chest, arms, and abdomen with the bath blanket.

RATIONALE. See Action 13.

ACTION 15. Expose one leg; place towel under it, leaving leg flexed. Keep perineum covered. Wash foot, leg, and groin, using firm long, distal to proximal strokes. Rinse and dry. Repeat for other leg. Lotion may be applied if skin is dry, but vigorous massage should be avoided.

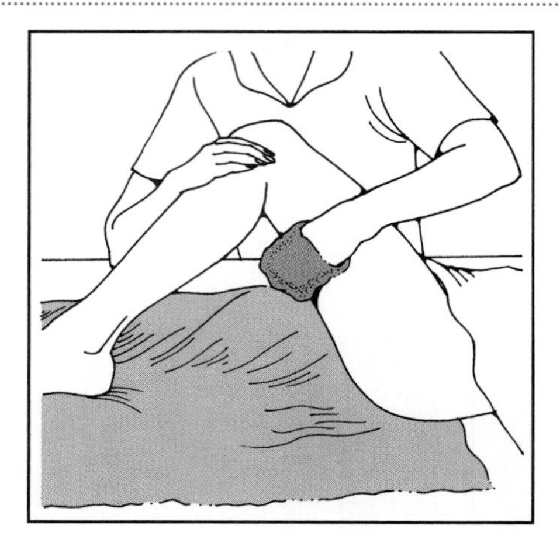

RATIONALE. See rationale for Action 12. Vigorous leg massage is thought to increase the risk of freeing pathological venous clots. Because debilitated patients on bed rest have increased risk of pathologic clotting in the legs, caution is advised, even when no diagnosis of thrombophlebitis has been made.

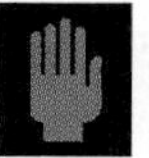

Foot may be soaked in basin, if desired. Patient may prefer to soak feet while seated in a chair as nurse makes the bed.

ACTION 16. Cover legs. Roll patient so back is toward you. Expose back and buttocks. Place towel next to back. Wash, rinse, and dry neck, back, and buttocks as above. Apply lotion, massaging skin over bony prominences. If reddened areas or broken skin is noted, institute appropriate decubitus care in collaboration with the physician. If entire back cannot be exposed when patient turns away, clean exposed part, and then turn patient toward you to expose and clean remaining part.

RATIONALE. Many patients spend most of their time in bed on their backs. The back has many potential pressure areas. Massage stimulates circulation, so prevents skin breakdown. If skin integrity is already disrupted, more aggressive measures are needed.

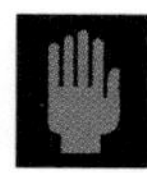

Some nurses prefer to provide perineal care for patients unable to complete it independently before turning the patient for back care. This is efficient, particularly if making an occupied bed is necessary. Use a clean wash cloth for back care if you use this approach.

ACTION 17. Return patient to back. Offer option of independent cleansing of genitals and perineal area. It is important that the patient understand what is being asked. Use commonly understood terms like "private parts" or "between your legs."

RATIONALE. Genitalia are considered the most personal parts of one's body. Genital exposure is embarrassing to most people. Having one's genitals cleaned by another makes many patients feel like they are being treated like small children.

ACTION 18. If patient has a Foley catheter, is confused, or lacks mobility or strength, perineal cleaning must be done by the nurse (see Procedure 27–12).

RATIONALE. The perineal area tends to be dark, warm, and moist. Because of normal secretions, skin folds, and the bacterial population in the vaginal and anal area, odors, skin breakdown, and infection are likely if the perineum is not thoroughly cleaned. A Foley catheter provides a direct route for bacteria to enter the bladder; therefore, meticulous cleaning is essential.

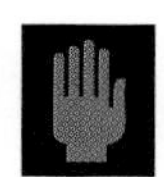

Patients having had rectal or vaginal surgery or childbirth, or who are incontinent, are at greater risk for infection and irritation. Frequent perineal care is needed.

ACTION 19. Provide clean gown and assist patient as needed to put it on. IV container and tubing should be slipped into the sleeve of the gown before the hand and arm. Reassess IV flowrate. Make occupied or unoccupied bed, as appropriate for patient's activity level (see Procedures 27–13 and 27–14). Dispose of soiled linen in hamper, clean and store bath equipment and personal hygiene items, rearrange patient's personal effects as desired. Place call bell in reach. Raise siderail.

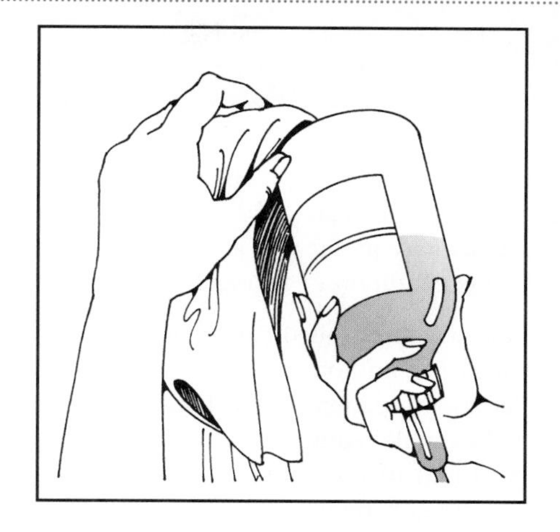

RATIONALE. See Action 5. Clean gown and linen and an orderly environment promote relaxation and well-being. Personal belongings, arranged according to patient's wishes, promote a feeling of personal territory. In an unfamiliar environment such as a hospital, even a small amount of personal territory diminishes feelings of alienation.

Recording:

Routine bathing is usually be recorded on a checklist. Skin or mucosal lesions noted during bath should be described, including appearance, size, location, and drainage, if any. Document nursing action taken. Note any other problems and action taken.

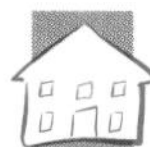

HOME HEALTH ADAPTATION: To avoid back strain and injury, utilize good body mechanics when bathing patient in a low stationary bed. When teaching a family member how to bathe a bedbound person, inform member about the importance of observing the skin over the bony prominences for redness or breakdown, the actions to take if skin changes are observed, and the rationale for and importance of washing the perineal area last.

PROCEDURE 27–11. CARING FOR FEET AND NAILS

PURPOSE: To maintain cleanliness and integrity of nails and surrounding tissue, to promote comfort.
EQUIPMENT: Basin, towel, washcloth, moistureproof pad, nail clippers or scissors, orange stick, and lotion or other emollient.

ACTION 1. Discuss previous foot and nail problems with the patient, usual foot and nail care, and preferences for assistance. Some patients may prefer that a family member provide nail care. Assess condition of feet and nails.

ACTION 2. Determine whether a medical order is needed to cut nails. (This policy is common because of risks associated with accidental cuts in patients with diabetes or circulatory disorders.) Assemble equipment. Foot and nail care is usually done as part of the bath, but may be done separately as needed. Screen patient.

ACTION 3. *Fingernails:* If dirt or other debris is trapped under nails, soaking hands in a basin of warm water for 5 to 10 minutes will facilitate cleaning. A soft nailbrush may be needed to loosen impacted soil. For routine care, soaking of fingernails is not usually needed, although unusually thick nails will be easier to cut if softened by soaking. If nails are long, obtain patient's consent to cut them. Use a nail clipper, cutting straight across the nail, even with the tops of the fingers. If one is available, use an orange stick to clean under the nails. Apply or provide lotion to moisturize skin and cuticles. Cuticles may be pushed back with orange stick.

ACTION 4. *Feet.* Feet commonly require more care because they are subject to trauma from ill-fitting shoes and they are more likely to be poorly perfused or edematous due to circulatory impairment secondary to disease or aging. Patients with diminished vision or flexibility may find self-care difficult, even though they are alert and oriented. Elderly patients' toenails are often thick and difficult to cut without soaking. Feet may be soaked with the patient seated in a chair or by placing a basin in the bed (see Procedure 27–10). Dry feet thoroughly, especially between the toes to prevent maceration or fungal infections. When cutting toenails, use special care to cut straight across the nail to prevent ingrown toenails and to avoid cutting cuticles. A toenail clipper is best for this as it has a larger cutting surface. Do not cut corns or calluses. Clean under nails and apply lotion as in Action 3. If any breaks in the skin, corns, ingrown nails, or other lesions are noted, notify the patient's physician.

Recording:

Routine nail care is not recorded in all agencies. May be noted on a checklist. If lesions are noted or problems are encountered, describe condition and action taken.

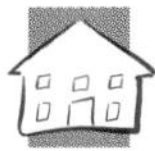

HOME HEALTH ADAPTATION: An important comfort measure in the home setting is to lightly massage the patient's feet after cleansing. If patient finds foot massage relaxing, encourage family members to periodically provide this mutually beneficial measure. Small comfort measures give family members the opportunity to express caring, and the patient the experience of being comforted.

PROCEDURE 27–12. CARING FOR PERINEAL AREA AND FOLEY CATHETER ("PERICARE")

PURPOSE: To promote cleanliness and comfort, and prevent odors, skin irritation, and infection. Perineal care is always part of the daily bath; however, it is done more frequently for patients who are incontinent, who have had rectal or vaginal surgery, and after childbirth.

EQUIPMENT: Basin, soap in a dish, washcloths, towel, disposable gloves, thermometer (optional), bath blanket, and waterproof pad. Irrigation container and bedpan may be used when giving perineal care to a woman.

ACTION 1. Discuss the procedure with the patient, including the expected benefits, usual sensations, and desired participation.

RATIONALE. The patient will be more likely to participate and less anxious if this information is shared.

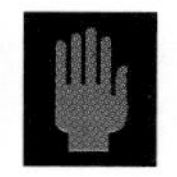

A calm, matter-of-fact approach during the explanation and the care will reduce the discomfiture of patient and nurse about perineal care. The nurse must strive to view the genitals simply as body organs, mentally deemphasizing their sexual function (which is usually the root of the nurse's anxiety), but remain sensitive to patient's feelings of embarrassment.

ACTION 2. Assemble equipment. Fill basin with warm water. Screen patient and raise bed. Lower siderail on near side of bed. Remove positioning aids and pillows except for pillow under head. HOB can be flat or slightly raised.

RATIONALE. See Clinical Guideline 27–2. Also, this method conserves nurse's energy, promotes good body mechanics. See Chap. 33.

ACTION 3. Cover patient's torso with a bath blanket. Fold top covers down to waist. Place a towel or waterproof underpad under patient's buttocks. Ask patient to spread legs. Female patient should also flex thighs (dorsal recumbent position). Pull top covers down to expose genitalia, drape bath blanket over lower abdomen. For a female, bath blanket should cover flexed legs; top covers cover feet only.

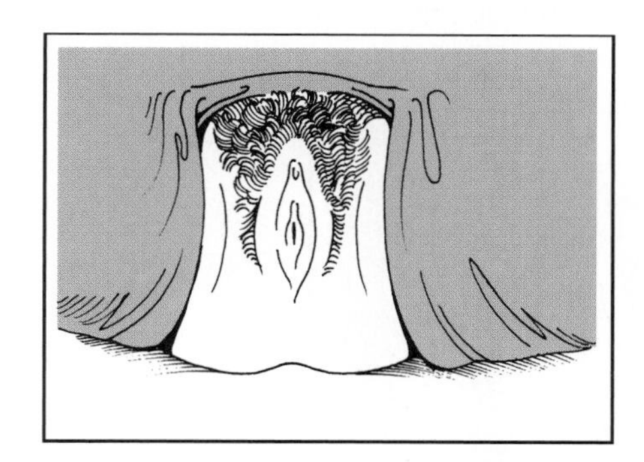

If doing pericare as part of the bath (top covers removed) drape the male patient by lowering bath blanket below genitalia and covering chest and abdomen with a towel.

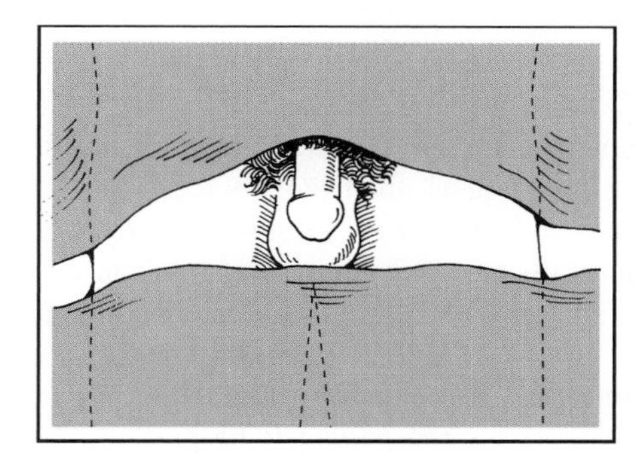

RATIONALE. Receiving such personal care from another often causes feelings of dependency, vulnerability, and embarrassment. These feelings are diminished somewhat by exposing only the part of the body that is to be cleaned.

Continued

ACTION 4. Don gloves. Wash perineum using a small amount of soap and a washcloth as follows.

Female patient: Spread labia majora. Wash from the mons pubis, downward over the urethral and vaginal openings to the base of the labia. Using a different portion of the cloth, wash folds of labia minora and majora on one side, then the other. Rinse and repeat as necessary to remove visible secretions. Clean perianal area in similar manner. Rinse all remaining soap, dry well. If desired, patient can be placed on a bedpan and the perineum rinsed by pouring warm water over it. This technique may be ordered after vaginal surgery.

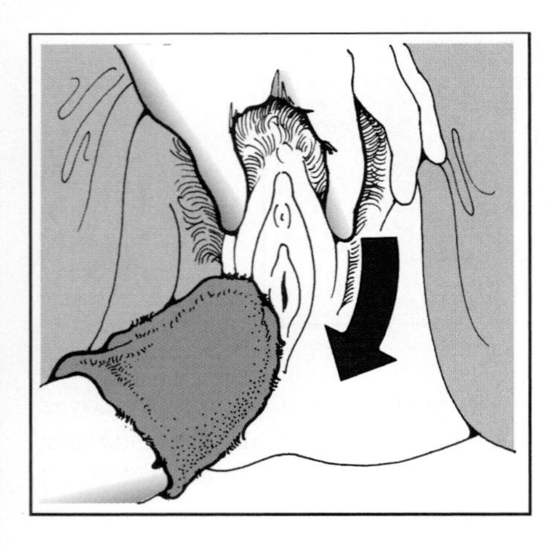

Male patient: Holding the penis by the shaft, wash the glans with a circular motion. If patient is uncircumcised, retract foreskin (1), clean glans, then replace foreskin (2). Clean the penile shaft and anterior scrotum with downward strokes. Cup the scrotum gently in your hand to clean lateral and posterior surfaces and perianal area. Rinse and repeat as necessary. Dry well. An erection during pericare is uncommon (see Note), but if it should occur, acknowledge that it has happened and ask the patient if he prefers that you complete the care or give him a moment of privacy.

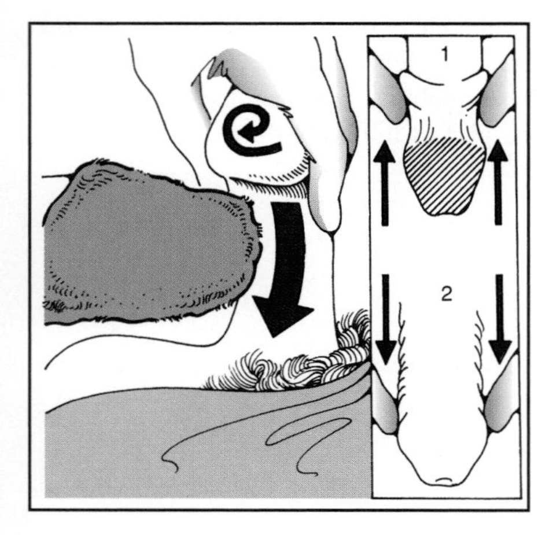

RATIONALE. Gloves act as a barrier, preventing transmission of organisms from patient to nurse. Washing genitalia as described proceeds from cleanest area to area with largest numbers of organisms, thereby minimizing transfer of organisms to cleaner area. Whitish secretions called smegma are normal in labial folds and under glans, but should be removed to decrease likelihood of growth of pathogens. Soap residue irritates skin and mucous membranes, causing itching and excoriation. Moisture, especially between labia and thighs or scrotum and thighs, promotes maceration, skin breakdown, and fungal infections. Scrotum is handled gently to avoid pressure on sensitive testicles. Ignoring an erection, should it occur, belittles the patient and is likely to increase, rather than decrease, patient and nurse embarrassment. Providing the patient with an option for dealing with the situation shows respect.

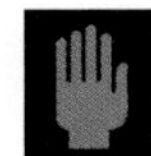

Many beginning nurses are personally embarrassed to give perineal care. For many, this is related to concerns about sexual connotations associated with handling the genitals (see Action 1) and especially, the fear that a male patient will have an erection during care. This is highly unlikely. Most patients feel embarrassment, which suppresses psychic stimuli needed for an erection. Composure on the part of the nurse will increase patient's comfort.

ACTION 5. If patient has an indwelling catheter, clean the portion of the catheter just distal to the urinary meatus prior to cleaning parianal area. Use the same washcloth and a small amount of soap. Hold the catheter steady to prevent its moving back and forth into the urethra as you clean it. Spread the labia of a female so the catheter can be thoroughly cleaned. Use a firm twisting motion, wiping from the meatus outward, 1 to 2 inches. Rinse well.

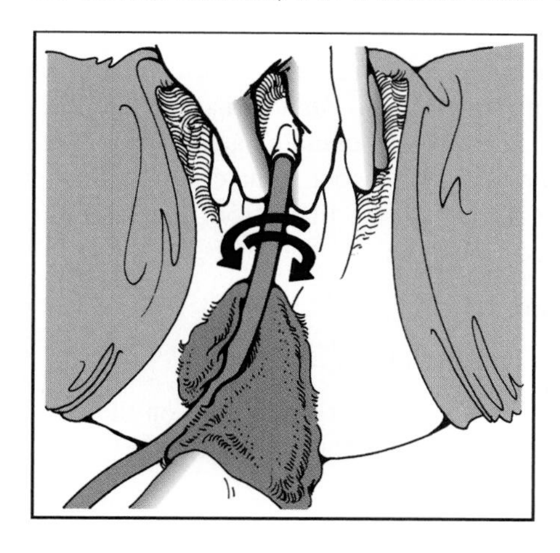

RATIONALE. The catheter acts as a mucosal irritant; therefore, mucus frequently collects around the portion of the tube that exits the meatus. This mucus can be a medium for bacterial growth, increasing the risk of a urinary tract infection. Friction physically removes mucus and bacteria. See also rationale for Action 6.

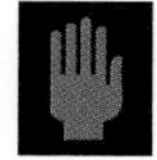

Formerly, antibacterial soaps and ointments such as povidone iodine, and sterile catheter care kits, were recommended for Foley care. Studies have shown soap and water are equally effective, as well as cheaper and less irritating to mucosa.

ACTION 6. If you are unable to thoroughly clean perianal area when patient is supine, ask the patient to turn to the side, facing away from you. Rearrange the bath blanket so only buttocks are exposed. Raise the top buttock and clean the anal area, starting near the genitalia and washing backward. Rinse and repeat as necessary; remove all soap residue and dry well.

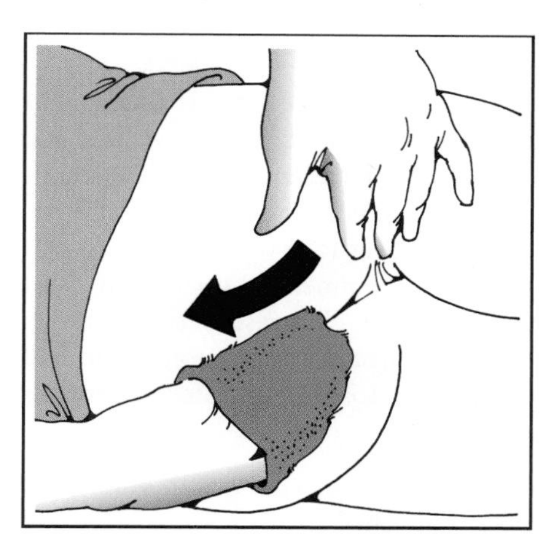

RATIONALE. The anal area contains organisms such as *Escherichia coli,* which can cause vaginal or urinary tract infections. Cleaning from cleanest area to area with most organisms reduces this possibility.

ACTION 7. Remove gloves, discard in waterproof receptacle. Remove underpad and drape, reposition and cover patient, return bed to low position. Dispose of linen, clean and store equipment according to agency policy; or continue with bath.

RATIONALE. This routine promotes patient comfort and safety.

Recording:

Routine perineal care may be documented on a checklist or in narrative charting. In some agencies it is not specifically charted unless problems are encountered. A narrative entry is necessary to document perineal lesions or unusual discharge and describe nursing action taken.

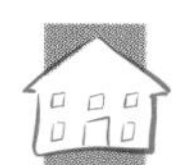

HOME HEALTH ADAPTATION: Teach family caregivers how to provide perineal care and what to observe for and report to the home health professional. Early identification and treatment of lesions will limit the severity of tissue breakdown.

PROCEDURE 27–13. MAKING AN UNOCCUPIED BED

PURPOSE: To promote patient comfort and relaxation.

EQUIPMENT: Top and bottom sheet, pillowcases, drawsheet (optional), waterproof underpads (optional), mattress pad, blanket and bedspread (change only if soiled), and linen hamper (varies with agency policy). Clean gloves if linen is wet with body secretions.

ACTION 1. Discuss need and timing of procedure with patient. Linen is usually changed while patients are showering/bathing, after a bed bath, or when a patient is off the unit for treatments or tests.

ACTION 2. Obtain clean linen as needed. In some facilities, top sheet is reused if it is not soiled. Drawsheet and waterproof pads are needed for patients who are incontinent, have draining wounds, and/or who receive treatments such as wet compresses or wet-to-dry dressings. A pull sheet (folded drawsheet) is recommended for patients who need assistance with position changes. The minimum amount of foundation linen necessary to protect the bed should be used when special foam "eggcrate" mattresses are in use (see Chap. 33).

ACTION 3. Lower head of bed; raise the bed to your waist level. Remove call bell, if attached to linen. To strip the bed of soiled linen:

a. Don gloves if linen is wet with drainage. Loosen linen and lower siderails all around the bed.

b. If spread is clean, fold it before removing it from the bed: fold the top edge so it's even with the bottom edge, grasp at the center of the fold and the doubled bottom edge and raise the spread from the bed, creating a second fold. Continue to fold until it can be easily hung on bedside chair without touching the floor. Fold and remove the blanket in the same manner. Fold top sheet in same manner if it is to be reused.

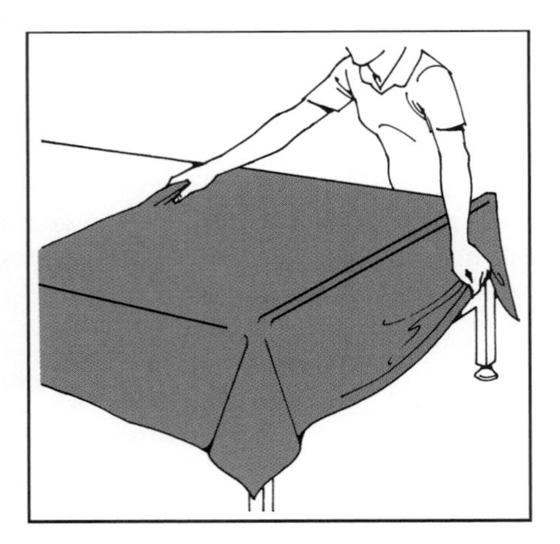

c. Remove all pillowcases; place pillows on chair.

d. Remove disposable waterproof underpads and dispose in waterproof trash receptacle. Gather remaining linen into a ball, rolling edges toward the center, and place in portable hamper, taking care to avoid contacting your uniform with soiled linen. Do not place soiled linen on the floor, as it is grossly contaminated with organisms. It is likely you would contaminate your uniform when retrieving the bundle of linen from the floor for disposal in the central chute.

e. Remove gloves.

ACTION 4. Place foundation linen as follows:

a. If a mattress pad is on the bed, align it on the mattress and smooth wrinkles. Replace if soiled.

b. Place bottom sheet in the center of the bed with folded edge facing the central long axis of the bed. Unfold the sheet toward the head and foot of the bed, allowing the sheet to extend about 1 in. (2.5 cm) over the bottom edge of the mattress, hem down, and the remaining length to extend over the top edge of the mattress. Unfold the sheet toward each side of the bed and smooth wrinkles on the side nearest you. The linen on the far side of the bed can remain partially folded until the first side of the bed is made. Bed linen is unfolded in this way to minimize air currents created if linen is unfolded by waving it in the air. Air currents facilitate spread of microorganisms.

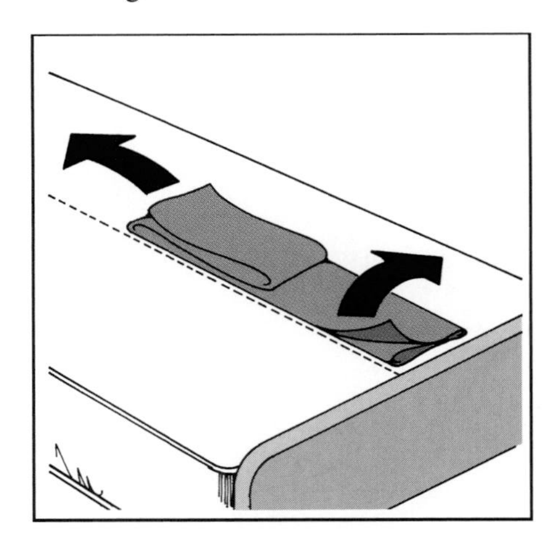

c. Tuck the sheet under the top end of the mattress, pulling the entire length of the tucked portion well under the mattress to firmly secure it. Extra length is needed at the head of the bed to keep the sheet in place when the head of the bed is raised.

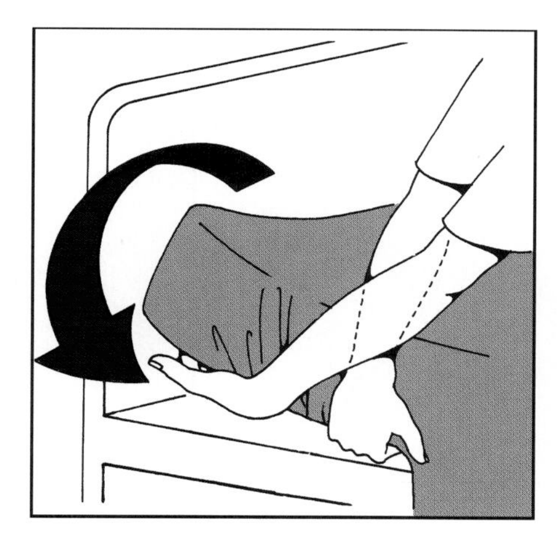

ACTION 5. Miter the corner as follows:

a. Lift the sheet (i) to form a right triangle on the mattress (ii). The triangle's base is along the side edge of the mattress; the side forming the right angle is parallel to the top edge of the bed. Place your other hand as shown to keep the sheet smooth as you form the triangle. The sheet should look like (iii).

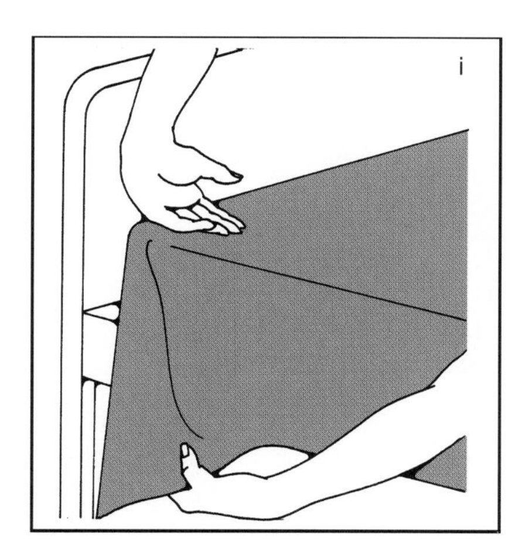

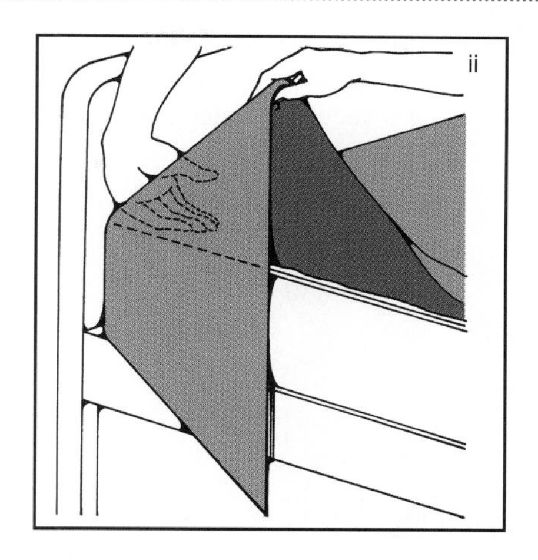

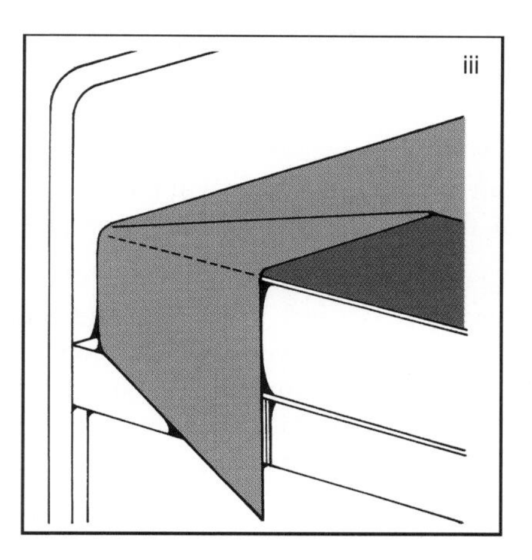

b. Tuck the lower portion of the sheet securely under the side of the mattress without disturbing the triangular fold.

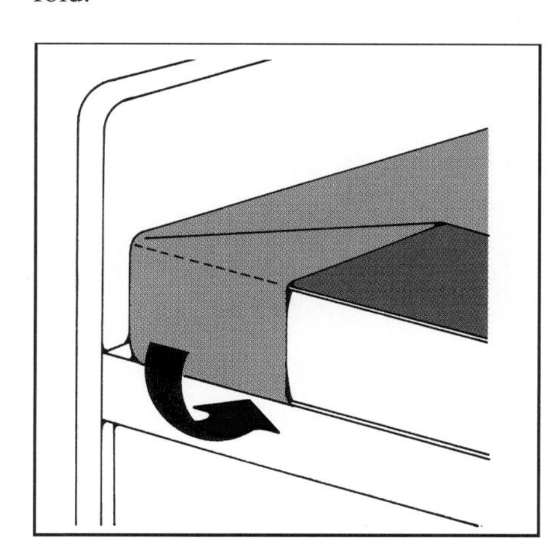

Continued

c. Hold the sheet secure at the edge of the mattress with one hand while bringing the tip of the triangle over your hand, then tucking it securely under the mattress.

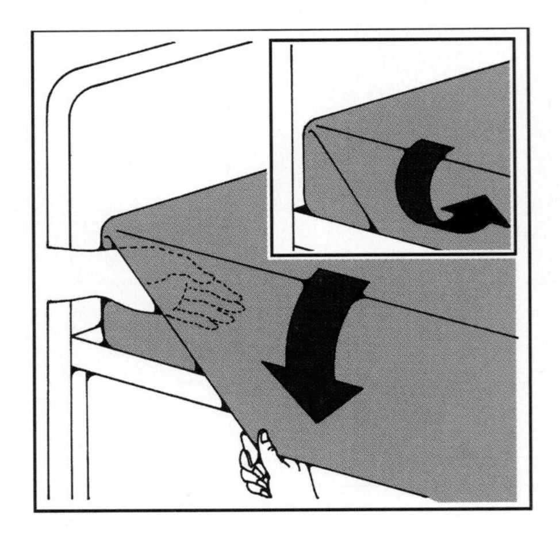

d. Secure the rest of the sheet by tucking it well under the mattress. If not securely tucked, it will pull out when the other side of the bed is made, or when the patient moves in bed.

ACTION 6. If a drawsheet is used, place it so the center fold lies along the center of the mattress. The top edge should be 12 to 15 inches (30–17 cm) from the head of the bed. Unfold toward each side as with the bottom sheet. Tuck in the excess drawsheet so it extends as far under the mattress as possible (see Action 5d).

ACTION 7. Place the top linen as follows:

a. Align the sheet with the fold along the center of the bed and unfold, as with foundation linen. The top edge of the sheet should be even with the top edge of the mattress, hem facing up. Smooth wrinkles.

b. Place the blanket (if used), then the spread over the top sheet, centering, unfolding, and smoothing as above, with the top edges about 6 inches (15 cm) from the head of the bed. Fold the top sheet down to make a cuff over the blanket and spread.

c. Tuck all of the top linen under the foot of the bed at one time. Make a mitered corner using all layers of linen, as in Action 5, except do not tuck the tip of the triangle under the mattress.

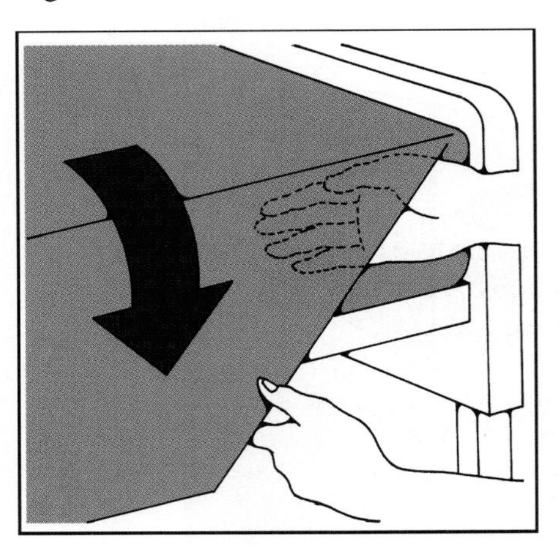

ACTION 8. Move to the opposite side and finish the bed as follows:

a. Fold or roll the top linen away from you to expose the foundation linen.

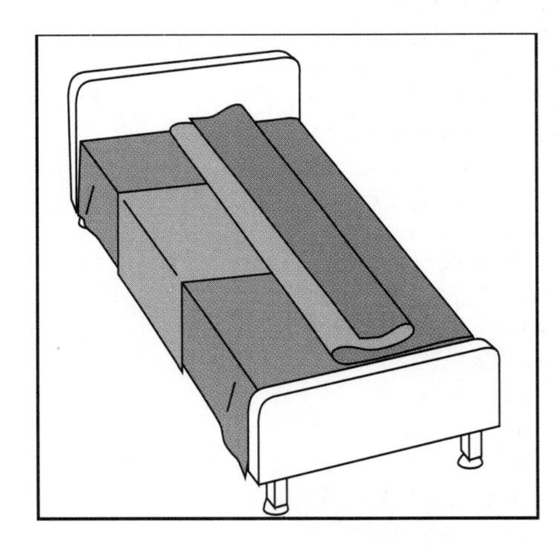

b. Smooth the bottom sheet and tuck it in at the head of the bed, mitering the corner as in Action 5. Tuck in the rest of the sheet in sections, pulling each section firmly with both hands, so the sheet is taut and secure.

c. Smooth the drawsheet, pull the center section tightly with both hands, then tuck it securely as far under the mattress as you can. It may be helpful to brace your knee against the bedframe for more leverage or shift your weight backwards as you pull. Tuck in the top and bottom sections the same way. The foundation should now be tight and free of wrinkles. Adjust any loose areas as necessary. Wrinkled or loose foundation linen causes patient discomfort and creates pressure areas.

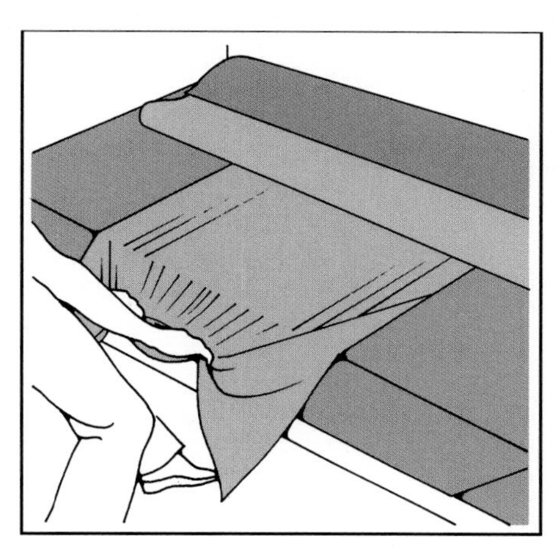

d. Smooth the top sheet, blanket, and spread, one at a time, then tuck in at the foot of the bed and miter as a unit, as in Action 7. Adjust cuff at head of bed, if necessary.

e. Make a toe pleat in the top linen to prevent pressure on the patient's feet: stand at the foot of the bed, reach over the bedframe, and grasp the top linen as a unit about 6 inches (15 cm) from the foot of the bed, and lift the linen toward you—creating a fold across the entire width of the bed.

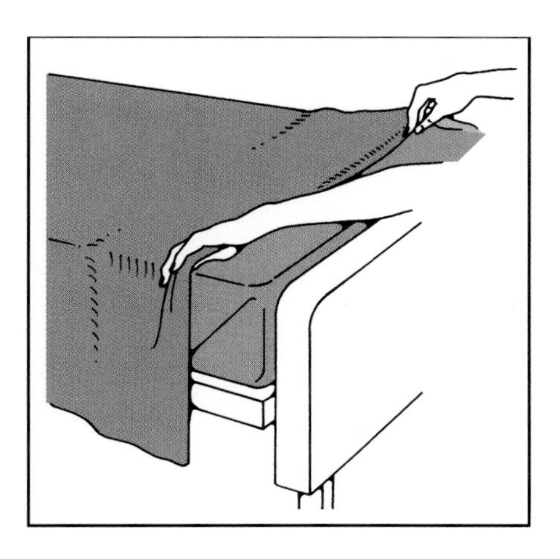

ACTION 9. Replace the pillowcases:

a. With one hand, hold the pillowcase in the center of the closed end.

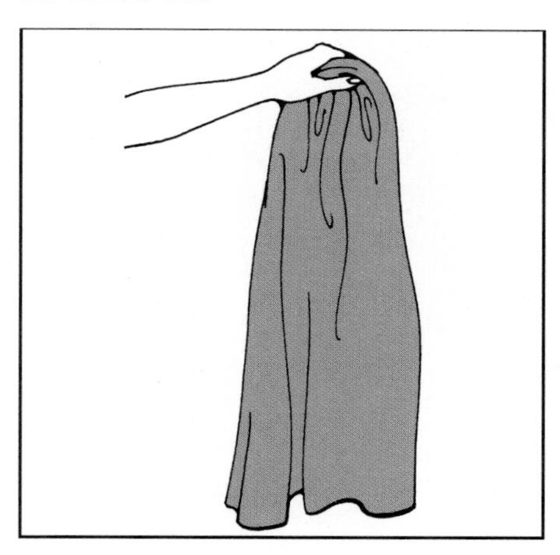

b. With your other hand, gather up the case and invert it over the first hand and forearm.

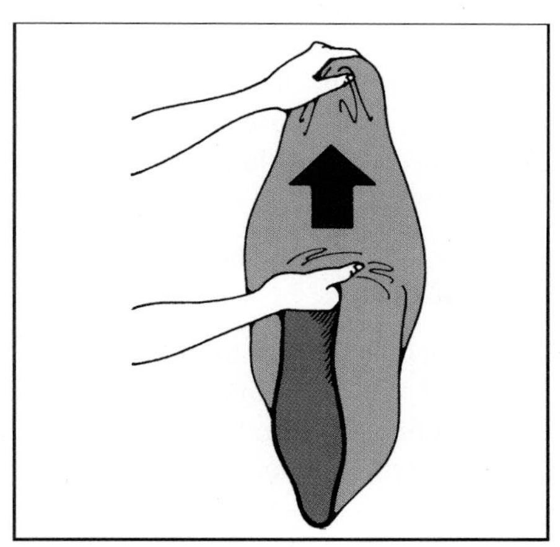

c. Still holding the pillowcase, grasp the center of one end of the pillow with the first hand.

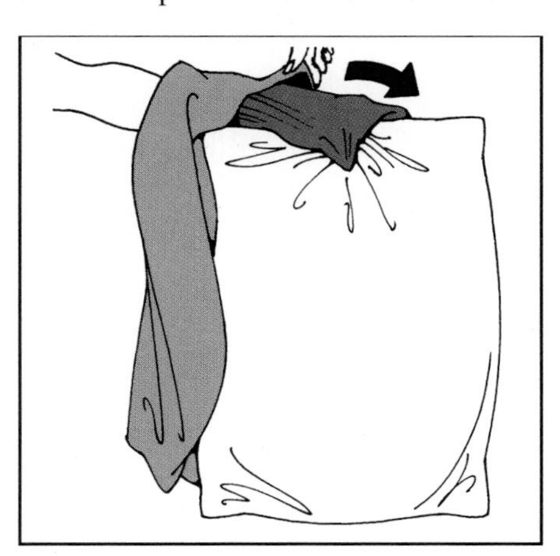

Continued

Procedure 27–13. Making an Unoccupied Bed (continued)

d. Pull the pillowcase over the pillow, aligning corners of case and pillow.

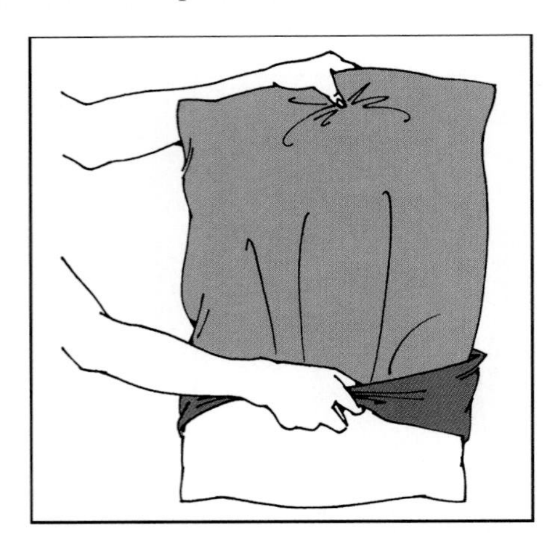

e. Place pillows on the bed according to patient's preference.

ACTION 10. Prepare the bed for the patient: Fanfold top linen to the foot of the bed. Place waterproof pad(s) as needed over the drawsheet. Attach the call light so the patient can reach it when in bed. Raise siderail on one side of the bed. Return bed to lower position unless patient will return to bed via a gurney.

ACTION 11. Rearrange furniture and personal items according to patient's preference.

ACTION 12. Assist patient into bed as needed. Discard soiled linen in central chute or remove portable hamper. Use care to avoid contacting your uniform while carrying soiled linen. Contact transfers microorganisms.

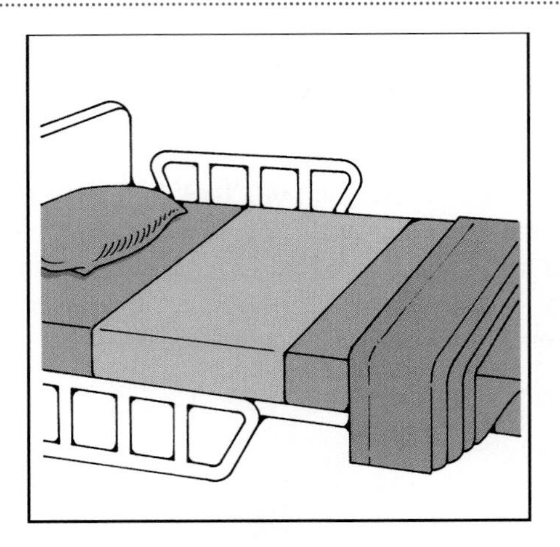

Recording:

May be noted on a checklist. In some agencies bedmaking is not documented.

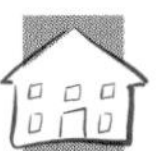

HOME HEALTH ADAPTATION: Place soiled linen inside pillow case for transport to laundry. Bedmaking in the home is adapted to available linens and to the personal preferences of the patient. Lack of convenient laundry facility or service influences decisions on frequency of linen changes. Bed can be freshened by smoothing wrinkled linens, straightening covers, and fluffing pillows. Disposable, plastic-lined underpads serve as moistureproof barriers and reduce need for frequent changes but are expensive. Topping the underpad with a spare sheet folded in half and placed lengthwise across the bed conserves underpads and provides the caregiver with a useful draw sheet.

PROCEDURE 27–14. MAKING AN OCCUPIED BED

PURPOSE: To promote patient comfort and relaxation for patients whose condition or treatment plan precludes their getting out of bed.

EQUIPMENT: Top and bottom sheet, pillowcases, drawsheet (optional), waterproof underpads (optional), mattress pad, blanket and bedspread (change only if soiled), and linen hamper (varies with agency policy). Two pairs of clean gloves if linen has fresh bloody drainage. Because linen change is usually done after the bed bath, equipment for both procedures can be gathered at the same time.

ACTION 1. Obtain equipment. Discuss need and timing of procedure and the desired patient participation with patient. Linen is usually changed immediately after a bed bath, but some patients may prefer a brief rest period prior to changing the linen. A complete linen change may also be necessary after spills, emesis, excessive diaphoresis, or incontinence.

ACTION 2. Screen the patient, close door, if desired. Raise bed to waist height. With far siderail up, ask or assist patient (see Procedure 33–9) to roll as close to the opposite edge of the bed as possible facing away from you. Remove all pillows, except one under the head; move it to the opposite side of the bed. This provides space to change the foundation linen on the near half of the bed.

ACTION 3. Lower near siderail. Don gloves to handle linen wet with drainage. If linen change is done immediately after the bath, patient will be covered with a bath blanket, which can remain in place until the foundation linen has been changed. If top linen is in place, remove and refold spread and blanket as in Procedure 27–13, Action 3b, if both are clean. If soiled, place in hamper. Top sheet may be used to cover patient while foundation linen is changed unless it is wet or very soiled, in which case it should be replaced with a bath blanket as in Procedure 27–10, Action 4. Loosen foundation linen at the head and sides of the bed. Remove soiled disposable underpads and discard in waterproof trash container. If pads are under patient, roll them with soiled foundation linen into a tight roll that extends the length of the bed. Push the roll of soiled linen as close to the patient's back as possible to allow room for the clean foundation linen. Remove gloves. Discard in waterproof trash receptacle.

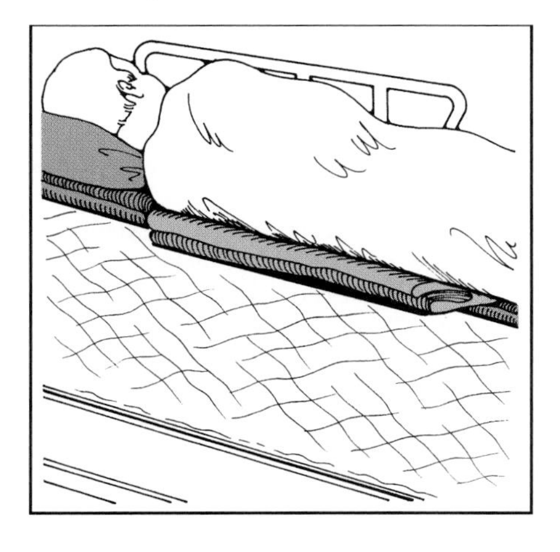

ACTION 4. Replace foundation linen:

a. Smooth the mattress pad, if clean. Replace if necessary: with pad folded in half lengthwise, align it over the mattress on the near side of the bed, then fanfold the excess toward the patient, pushing it as close to the rolled soiled linen as possible.

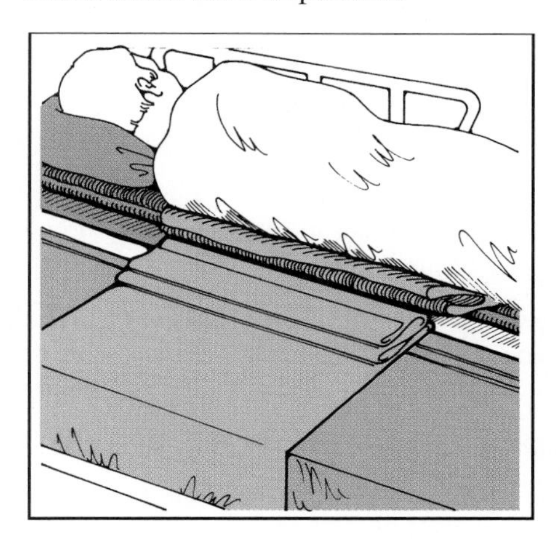

b. Place the clean bottom sheet in the center of the bed and unfold as in Procedure 27–13, Action 4b. Fanfold the excess next to the rolled foundation linen as shown. Miter corner at the head of the bed and tuck in the sides as in Procedure 27–13, Action 5.

c. If a drawsheet is needed, position it as in Procedure 27–13, Action 6. Tuck in the near side, fanfold the excess as above. If disposable underpads are needed, place them over the drawsheet in the same way.

ACTION 5. Remove the pillow under the patient's head and change the pillowcase as in Procedure 27–13, Action 9. Place the freshly changed pillow on the clean foundation linen. If the patient cannot tolerate having no head support, replace the case on another pillow and place it on the clean side of the bed.

ACTION 6. Ask the patient to roll toward you, over the rolled linen. Assist if necessary (see Procedure 33–9). The patient should now be facing you, lying on his or her side on the clean foundation linen. Raise the near siderail.

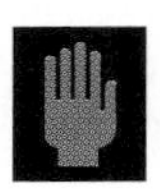

If the used foundation linen is not wet, some nurses place the clean top linen over the patient at this time so the bedmaking can be completed more efficiently (see Action 10).

Continued

Procedure 27–14. Making an Occupied Bed (continued)

ACTION 7. Complete the foundation on the opposite side of the bed:

a. Don clean gloves, if needed. Loosen soiled linen. Roll it into a ball toward the center of the bed. Place in hamper, avoiding contacting your uniform.

b. Unroll and smooth clean linen, one layer at a time. If patient is large, part of the roll may be under the patient, but can usually be pulled free without difficulty. In some cases, it may be necessary to have a second nurse assist by holding the patient as close to the opposite side of the bed as possible, while you free the linen.

c. Securely tuck in the bottom sheet and drawsheet as in Procedure 27–13, Actions 8a to 8c. It is usually necessary to brace your knee on the bedframe for leverage or shift your weight backwards as you pull the sheets to eliminate wrinkles and achieve a taut foundation (see Procedure 27–13, Action 8c).

d. Ask or assist the patient to return to a supine position in the center of the bed.

ACTION 8. If extra pillows have been in use, change the pillowcases as above. Reposition patient, if necessary (see Chap. 33).

ACTION 9. Replace top linen:

a. Place the clean top sheet over the bath blanket covering the patient. Unfold as in Procedure 27–13, step 7a. Ask the patient to hold the top edge of the sheet as you pull the bath blanket toward the foot of the bed. It may be folded for reuse or put with the soiled linen.

b. Place the blanket, if desired, and the spread over the sheet, unfolding, aligning, and smoothing as in Procedure 27–13, Action 7a. Make a cuff over the top edge of the blanket and spread with the top sheet.

c. Tuck in and miter the corner of the top linen as a unit at the foot of the bed, as in Procedure 27–13, Action 7c. Raise siderail.

d. Repeat on other side of the bed.

e. Make toe pleat as in Procedure 27–13, Action 8e.

ACTION 10. Lower the bed, rearrange furniture and personal belongings according to the patient's preference. Remove soiled linen and other supplies; store or discard according to agency policy.

Recording:

May be recorded on a checklist. In some agencies linen change is not routinely recorded unless unusual events occur during the procedure. Rarely, a narrative entry describing the procedure and patient's response is required, even for a routine linen change.

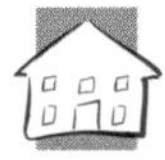

HOME HEALTH ADAPTATION: Making an occupied bed puts the patient at some risk, especially if the bed is narrow. If the patient is in danger and is falling out of bed during the procedure, place one or two straight-backed chairs next to the bed, and move to the opposite side before the patient is rolled over. If a family caregiver is available, ask for assistance in stabilizing the patient's position during the linen change. Teach family caregivers how to make an occupied bed safely.

Wound Care

Wound care includes cleaning and dressing wounds, managing drainage systems, obtaining wound cultures, special procedures such as wound irrigation, wet-to-dry dressings, and application of proteolytic enzymes. Traditionally, it has been standard protocol to use sterile technique when caring for surgical wounds. However, a 1995 pilot study that involved 30 patients with wounds healing by secondary intention found no difference in the healing rate among patients receiving wound care with clean technique and those whose wound care was done with sterile technique.[29] Additional research to replicate these results will be needed before current recommendations are changed. The AHCPR has recently recommended clean technique for pressure ulcer care, as discussed later in this chapter.[30] Although care of uncomplicated surgical incisions is straightforward, wounds that do not heal optimally can present many nursing care challenges. Moreover, wounds are difficult for most patients—not only are they painful, but they are sometimes disfiguring and debilitating. Nurses' recognition that having a wound represents a potential threat to patients' perceptions of their wholeness, ability to function, and physical appearance is an important factor in determining the effectiveness of care.

Cleaning Wounds. Nurses usually clean wounds with significant amounts of drainage and wounds that are healing by secondary or intention as part of a dressing change. Effective cleaning requires correct technique. Procedure 27–15 describes how to clean a wound. Sometimes wound cleansing requires that the wound be first debrided. **Debride** means to remove foreign material or dead or damaged tissue. General guidelines for wound cleansing are described in Clinical Guideline 27-3.

Common solutions are listed in Table 27-9. Sometimes physicians' orders or agency policy specifies a solution or the nurse giving care may select one based on the type and status of the wound. Nurses should be aware that each of these solutions is contraindicated in some types of wounds and that all of them are cytotoxic in

CLINICAL GUIDELINE 27–3

CLEANSING SURGICAL WOUNDS

- Do not routinely clean all surgical wounds with every dressing change. Check agency policy and surgeon preference.
- Refer to the agency policy manual or physician's order sheet in the patient's chart to determine specific solution for cleansing. If no solution is specified, use sterile normal saline.
- Use sterile equipment to clean surgical wounds, even if the wound is infected.
- Use a sterile container (sterile specimen cups are an inexpensive and conveniently sized choice for most wounds) to hold sterile solution and gauze 2 × 2s or 4 × 4s. Gauze may be held in a sterile-gloved hand or with a sterile thumb forceps or a hemostat. Large cotton-tipped applicators (swabs) in foil packets containing antiseptic are available in some agencies. See also Clinical Guideline 25–10.
- Wounds must be cleansed from the cleanest area to the least clean area to avoid transfer of microorganisms. The following facts apply:
  - –The incision line or wound has fewer endogenous organisms than the skin surrounding the incision.
  - –In a vertical incision, especially one that is draining, the highest end of the incision is drier and therefore has fewer endogenous organisms.
  - –A localized area of purulent drainage (eg, oozing from a small part of the incision) contains many organisms.
  - –A drain site separate from the incision has more organisms than the incision and the peri-incisional skin.
- Refer to Procedure 27–15, which describes and illustrates several cleansing methods.
- Record wound cleansing on a checklist or in a narrative note. Describe the location, size, and appearance of the wound, the solution used to clean it,

certain concentrations. The AHCPR 1994 clinical guidelines recommend normal saline because it is physiologic and does not harm fragile tissue.[30]

Applying Dressings

Ideally, dressings should create an optimal environment for wound healing. In reality, dressings sometimes interfere with healing, especially if caregivers select incorrect materials or apply them improperly. Dressings should protect the wound from microbial contamination and trauma, absorb drainage, and yet maintain a sufficiently moist environment to promote healing. Some kinds of dressings also mechanically debride wounds, maintain hemostasis, and promote wound contraction. Covering wounds is also helpful to patients' adaptation to the emotional stress of wounds, because it enables patients to decide when they wish to look at the wound. Many products are available for dressing and caring for wounds. Some are illustrated in Fig. 27–8 and listed in Table 27–10. The choice of supplies depends on the wound, patient situation, and

TABLE 27-9. COMMON WOUND CLEANING SOLUTIONS AND PRODUCTS

Solution	Purpose	Comments
Povidone–iodine	Kills bacteria, spores, viruses, and fungi Surgical scrub To clean infected wounds (1%)	Systemic toxin if used in concentrations of 10% or greater.
Hydrogen peroxide	Mild germicide Mechanically debrides surface wounds Removes blood clots	Breaks down too quickly for sustained action. One-half to one-quarter strength recommended.
Sodium hypochloride (Dakin's solution)	Germicide Inhibits blood clotting Debridement (0.5%) Disinfectant for utensils (5%)	Local irritant to intact skin and granulation tissue.
Acetic acid	Effective against pseudomonas, trichomonas, and candida (0.12% solution)	Irritating to tissue. Toxic to cells in 0.25% or greater solution.
Isotonic solutions, sterile normal saline, Ringer's lactate	Removes exudate and and moisturizes wound surfaces without damaging tissue	Has no bacterial properties.
Proteolytic enzymes	Sloughs necrotic tissue Removes granulation tissue Maintains moist wound surface	Available in sheets and granules. Useful for fragile wounds and skin.

PROCEDURE 27–15. CLEANING A WOUND

PURPOSE: To remove dead tissue and bacteria from wounds and promote healing.
EQUIPMENT: Cleansing or antiseptic solution, receptacle for solution, sterile gloves, sterile gauze squares, sterile forceps, and waterproof bag for disposal of used swabs. May substitute commercially packaged antiseptic swabs according to medical order or agency policy.

ACTION 1. Remove dressings as described in Procedure 27–16. Prepare solution, gauze sponges, and forceps or commercially packaged swabs.

PREPARING SOLUTION, GAUZE SQUARES, AND FORCEPS:

a. Pour solution (Clinical Guideline 25–9), open forceps and gauze packages (Clinical Guideline 25–10), use sterile field, if desired (Procedure 25–2). Some nurses prefer to hold sterile sponges in their sterile–gloved hand rather than forceps.

b. Don sterile gloves (see Procedure 25–3) and pick up the forceps with dominant hand.

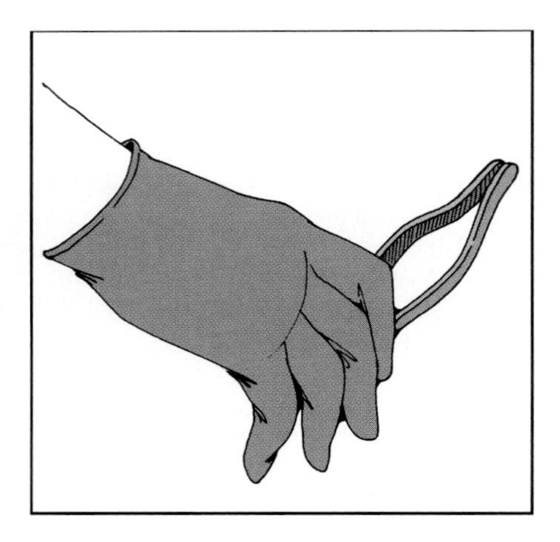

c. Fold a sterile gauze square in quarters with nondominant hand; transfer to forceps with folded edge out.

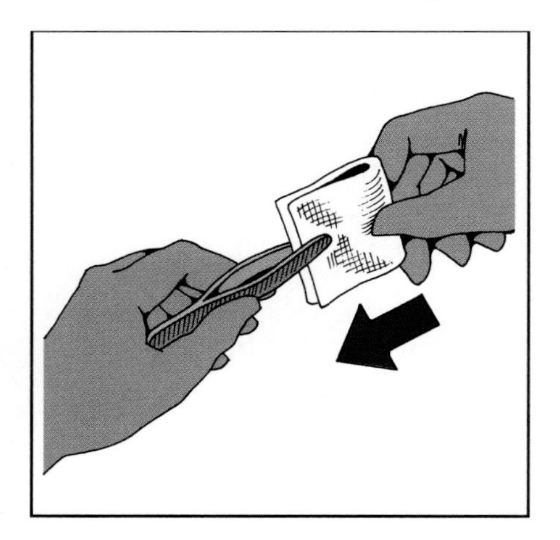

d. Dip gauze in solution until it is wet, but not dripping, keeping tip of forceps pointing down at all times, because gravity causes movement of liquid. If hand is lower, liquid may contact hand, then flow back to tip, which would contaminate tip.

e. When discarding gauze swabs, use care not to touch trash receptacle with forceps, which will be used for entire procedure.

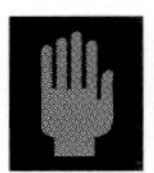

The nondominant hand may be ungloved at nurse's preference providing the option of touching unsterile items (eg, pouring additional solution) during the procedure, which would contaminate a glove if both hands were gloved.

PREPARING COMMERCIALLY PREPARED ANTISEPTIC SWABS: Open packet, remove one swab by grasping handle. Keep wet end of swab pointed downward at all times. A glove is not needed, since the swab's handle prevents the nurse's hand from contacting the wound. Some nurses prefer to wear a clean glove to protect their hand from possible splashes of wound drainage.

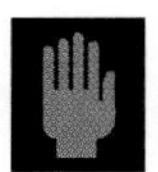

The accompanying illustrations show gauze and forceps for some steps and commercial swabs for other steps. A nurse would select one or the other for the entire procedure. The choice depends on physician's orders and/or agency/policy.

ACTION 2. Cleaning vertical incision.

a. Cleanse the incision line first. For vertical incision, cleanse from the top of the incision downward. Use more than one swab if the wound is long.

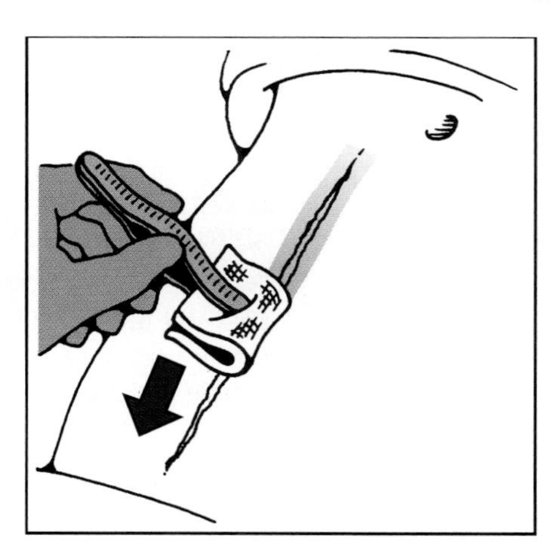

Procedure 27–15. (continued)

b. Cleanse the proximal skin on either side of the incision, working away from the incision, cleaning 3 to 4 in. of surrounding skin, and using a new swab for each stroke. This method prevents inoculating the incision with normal skin flora (because of the surgical skin prep, the incision has the lowest bacterial population, and drainage that harbors microorganisms flows downward).

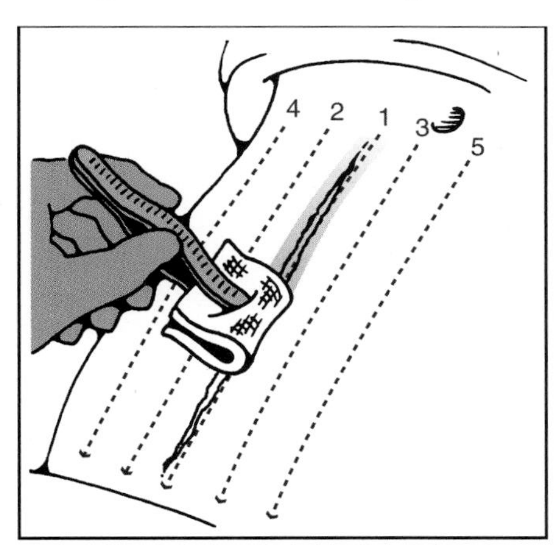

ACTION 3. Cleaning a large horizontal incision.

a. Cleanse the incision first from one end to the other or for a large, deep incision, from the center of the wound outward to either end. Use separate swabs for each stroke to avoid introducing microorganisms.

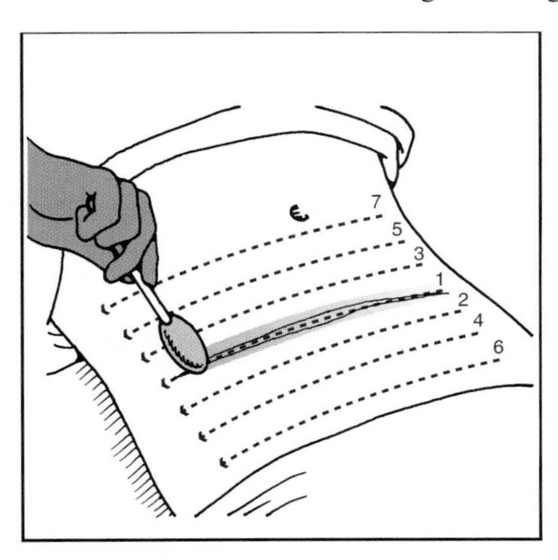

b. Clean the skin above the wound, cleansing from the center outward, or from one side to the other, depending on the amount of drainage. Use a fresh swab for each stroke.

c. Clean the skin below the wound in the same way.

ACTION 4. If the wound has a drain, clean around it last to avoid possible inoculation of the wound with organisms that may be present near the drain. Cleanse the skin around the drain, using circular strokes, working outward from the drain. Use fresh swabs as needed, depending on the amount of drainage.

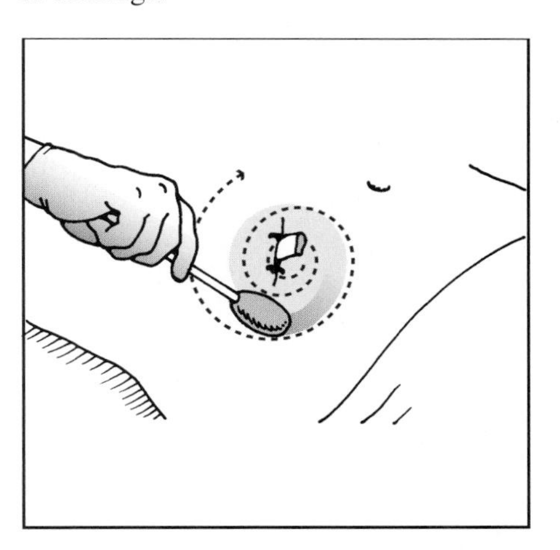

ACTION 5. Cleanse circular or irregularly shaped wounds, such as pressure ulcers, in the same manner: Cleanse from the center outward, using fresh swabs as needed. Clean wound and surrounding skin 3 to 4 inches around wound (or more if drainage is copious).

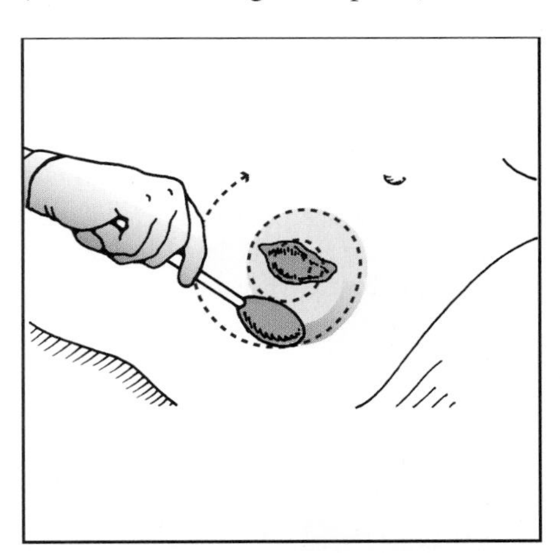

HOME HEALTH ADAPTATION: This procedure adapts easily to the home environment. Double-wrap in plastic bags all contaminated items before placing in patient's trash container.

TABLE 27-10. COMMON SUPPLIES USED FOR WOUND CARE

Solutions	Povidone–iodine	Semi-occlusive:	Semipermeable polyurethane film	Miscellaneous	Sterile gloves
	Hydrogen peroxide	Nonadhering:	Petrolatum gauze		Sterile container (basin, cup)
	Dakin's solution		Telfa		Sterile barrier towel
	Acetic acid		Medicated fine mesh gauze		Sterile tongue blades
	Sterile normal saline	Synthetic:	Spray-on		Sterile swabs
	Ringer's lactate		Semipermeable polyurethane film		Sterile applicators
Instruments	Dressing scissors		Hydrocolloid		Antibiotic ointments
	Thumb forceps		Hydrogels		Skin protectant (petroleum jelly, zinc oxide)
	Straight hemostat		Hydrophilic gels		Moistureproof trash bag
	Kelly clamp (optional)	Absorptive:	Debrisan		
Dressings			Hydra-Gran		
Nonocclusive:	Filled sponges	Debriding:	Elase		
	Gauze sponges (unfilled)		Travase		
	Drain sponges	Tape	Cotton-backed		
	Fluffs		Rayon taffeta		
	Roller gauze		Paper		
	Combination pads (ABDs)		Plastic		
Occlusive:	Petrolatum gauze		Elastic foam		
	Furacin gauze		Waterproof		
	Telfa		Montgomery straps		
	Hydrocolloid				

physician's choice. No single dressing produces an optimal healing environment for all types of wounds or for all stages of healing of one wound.[15] For example, dry sterile dressings are a good choice for closed surgical wounds that are healing well (Procedure 27–16). Wet-to-dry dressings are sometimes used for mechanical debriding (Procedure 27–17). Hydrocolloid dressings, discussed in a later section, enhance healing of pressure ulcers. Sometimes improvising may be necessary to achieve the best environment for healing. Nurses' personal experience, collaborating with experts such as clinical nurse specialists or enterostomal therapists (whose expertise with skin problems associated with stoma care is often applicable to problem wounds), and consulting recent professional literature are good resources for answers to difficult wound-care problems.

Dressings must be properly secured over wounds with tape or bandages to allow air circulation and prevent slipping or dis-

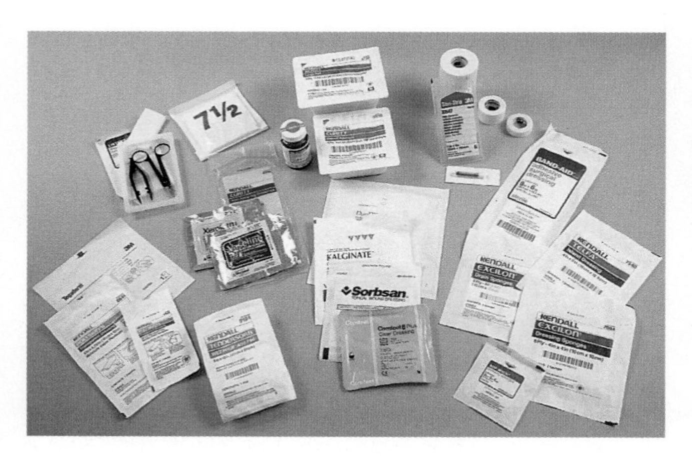

Figure 27–8. A variety of supplies available for wound care.

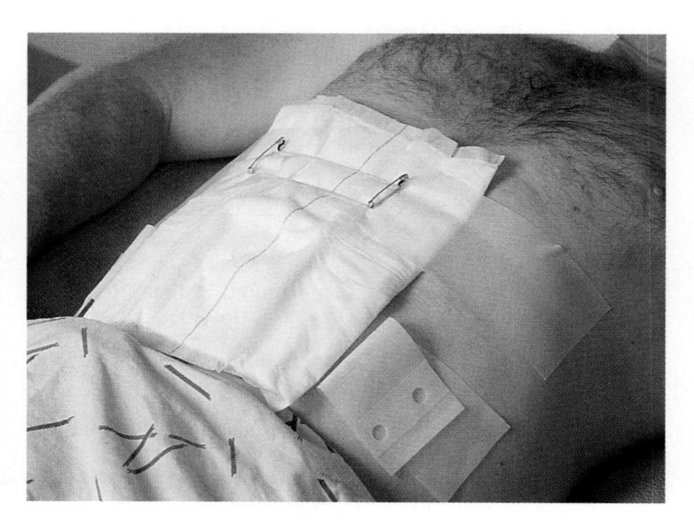

Figure 27–9. Montgomery straps with dressing.

CLINICAL GUIDELINE 27–4

TAPING DRESSINGS

1. Use porous hypoallergenic tape to prevent skin irritation. Occlusive tapes (eg, adhesive tape) trap moisture and cause maceration.
2. Width of the tape should be sufficient to prevent its coming loose with movement, but not so wide that it interferes with air circulation through the dressing. One-inch tape is generally effective; 2-inch tape may beneeded for large dressings.
3. Use the minimum amount of tape that will secure the entire dressing and prevent it from moving over the surface of the wound. Length of the tape extending beyond the edge of the dressing should be approximately one third the width of the dressing. Apply strips of tape near both ends of the dressing. Use additional strip(s) of tape in the center if dressing is large or is applied over a joint.
4. Apply tape so air circulation is not occluded, unless occlusive dressing is ordered. Taping around the edges of a dressing occludes air circulation. Taping too tightly may compromise circulation and cause tension blisters.
5. Rotate sites where tape is applied whenever possible.
6. A skin sealant such as Skin-Prep or Protective Barrier Film before applying tape, or a solid skin wafer barrier around the wound edges (tape is applied to wafer), prevents skin damage from excessive drainage. Do not use sealants on damaged skin, as the alcohol will sting raw skin. Do not use tincture of benzoin. It is drying and causes irritation. Petrolatum-based ointment can also be used to protect wound edges, but apply only to edges to prevent interference with tape adherence.
7. If dressing must be changed frequently, securing the dressing with Montgomery straps will decrease skin irritation from repeated tape removal (Fig. 27–9):
   - Cut straps of appropriate width (material comes in 8 × 10-inch sheets).
   - Remove protective film from adhesive portion and apply to skin adjacent to dressing. Apply a second strap on the opposite side of the dressing.
   - Apply a sufficient number of paired straps to hold dressing in place (see above).
   - Secure straps over dressing with twill tape or rubber bands and safety pins.
8. If tape is used to secure a dressing over a joint, apply tape in the opposite direction of body movement: across the joint, not lengthwise. Elastic tape may secure dressing over joints more effectively than standard tapes; tubular roller bandages may be preferable (see Table 27–11).
9. Do not apply tape around the entire circumference of an extremity.
10. Support skin while removing tape to prevent injury. If hair is present, peel tape in the direction of hair growth. Adhesive remover may be used, but residue should be washed off.

lodging with movement. Guidelines for the correct taping of dressings are described in Clinical Guideline 27–4. Bandaging is illustrated in Table 27–11. Montgomery straps, which enable replacement of dressings without removing tape, are useful for situations requiring frequent dressing changes (Fig. 27–9). Elderly patients are especially vulnerable to skin damage from tape removal, which can actually cause extension of a wound.

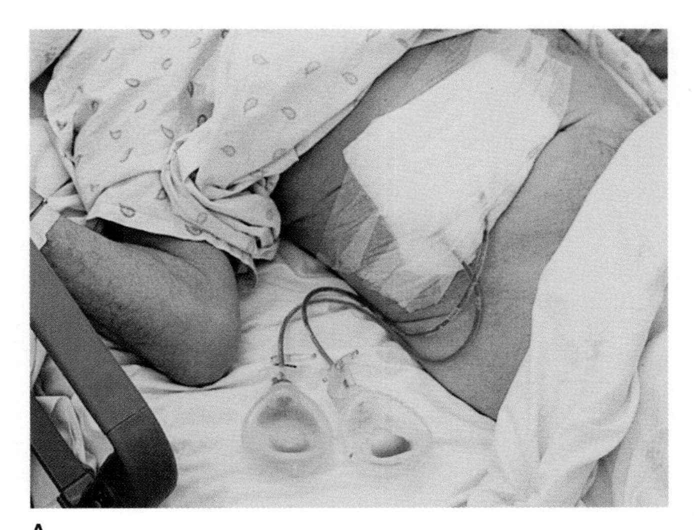

A

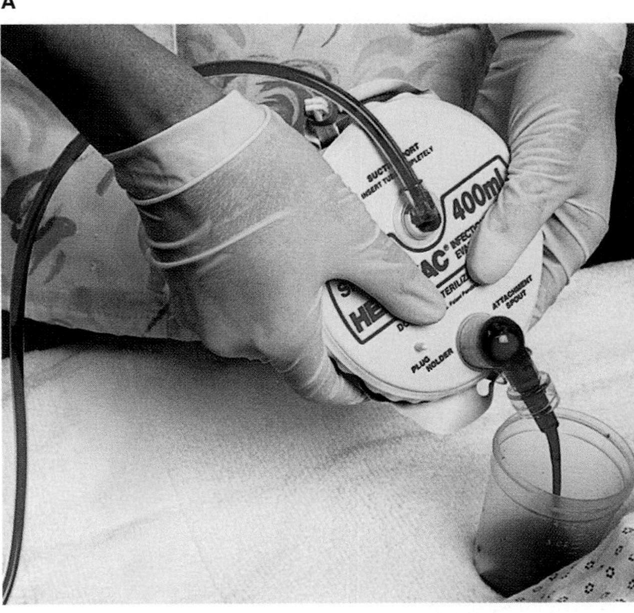

B

Figure 27–10. Wound drainage systems. **A.** Two Jackson-Pratt devices compressed to facilitate collection of exudate. **B.** Nurse emptying drainage from Hemovac drainage system.

Special Wound Care Procedures

Some wounds require care in addition to cleansing and dressing. For example, many surgical wounds have drainage systems that nurses must manage. Wounds with thick eschar and necrotic tissue may need chemical debriding. These and other special procedures are discussed below.

Wound Drainage Systems. Wound drainage is a source of complications of healing. It creates dead space between wound edges, delaying healing, and provides an excellent medium for microorganism growth. To avoid these complications, surgeons often place soft latex drains called Penrose drains or self-contained drainage systems such as the Hemovac or Jackson-Pratt to facilitate evacuation of wound exudates (Fig. 27–10). One end of the drains is placed near the surgical site. The tubing is brought out of the body

TABLE 27-11. TECHNIQUES FOR BANDAGING

Illustration	Instructions	Use
Circular Turns 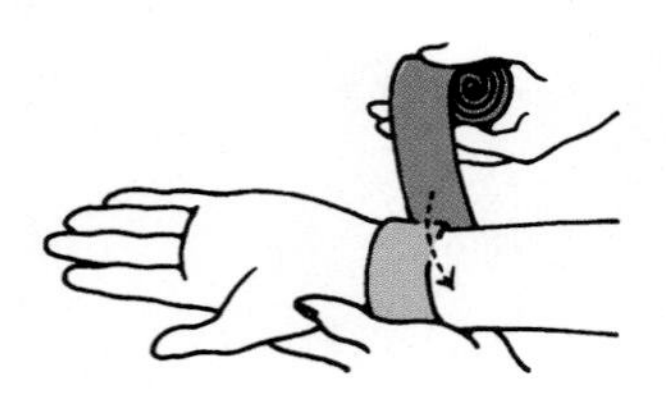	Place flat surface of bandage against extremity; anchor with thumb. Wrap two overlapping layers of bandage over same area.	To cover small cylindrical areas and to anchor bandage for other types of wraps.
Spiral Turns 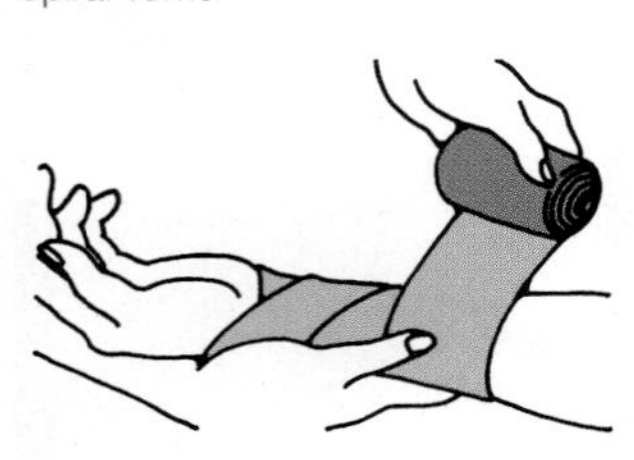	Anchor bandage with circular turns. Wrap bandage on ascending angle, with each turn overlapping previous by $\frac{1}{2}$–$\frac{2}{3}$ of bandage width. Overlap $\frac{2}{3}$ of the previous turn to secure each layer.	To secure dressing or wrap to an extremity whose contour does not vary significantly.
Spiral Reverse Turn 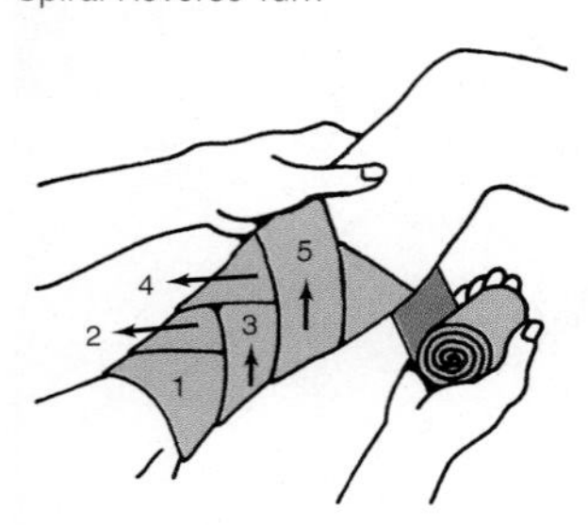	Anchor bandage with circular turns. Wrap with alternating ascending and descending turns in "figure 8" pattern. Overlap $\frac{2}{3}$ of the previous turn to secure each layer.	To secure dressing or wrap to an extremity that has a significantly larger circumference at one end than at the other.
Figure-eight Wrap 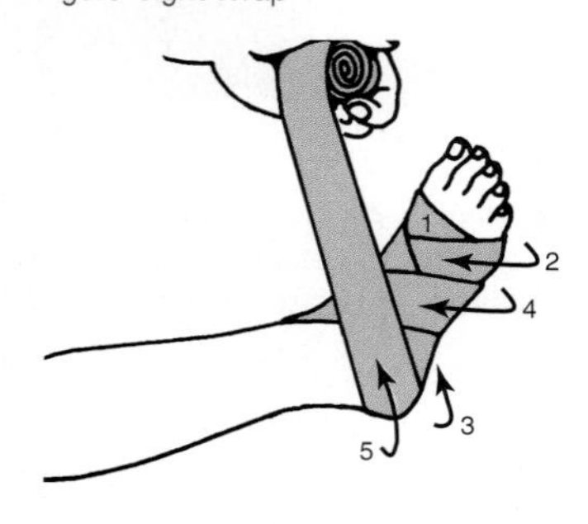	Anchor bandage with circular turns. Wrap around joint in alternately ascending and descending turns, as if to draw an "8".	To secure a dressing or wrap to an extremity on or near a joint.

through a separate incision adjacent to the surgical incision to reduce the risk of wound infection. Procedure 27–18 discusses management of wound drainage systems.

Wound Culture. A wound culture should be obtained whenever a nurse is suspicious that a wound infection is developing. Cleanse the wound before taking a culture specimen so the sample is of fresh drainage. Drainage that has been in contact with the skin for some time is likely to have high populations of skin flora, which may mask the causative organism of an infection. Procedure 27–19 outlines the procedure for obtaining the sample.

Wound Packing. Wound packing is a means of debriding and disinfecting contaminated wounds. Sterile wide-mesh gauze soaked in physiologic or antibacterial solution is placed into a wound cavity so it contacts all wound surfaces. If used as a wet-to-wet dress-

TABLE 27-11. CONTINUED

Illustration	Instructions	Use
Recurrent Bandage (Scalp Wrap) 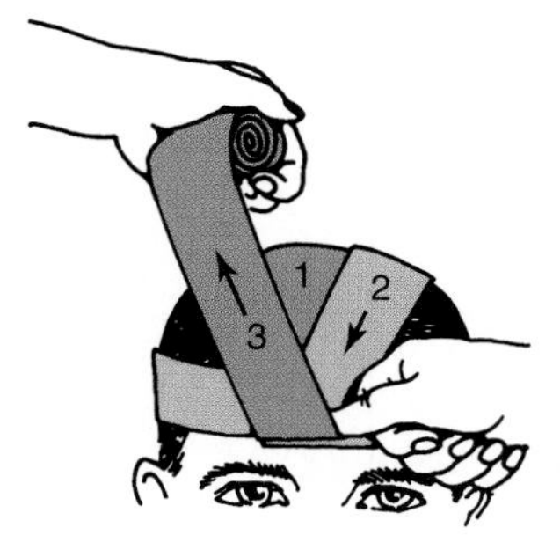 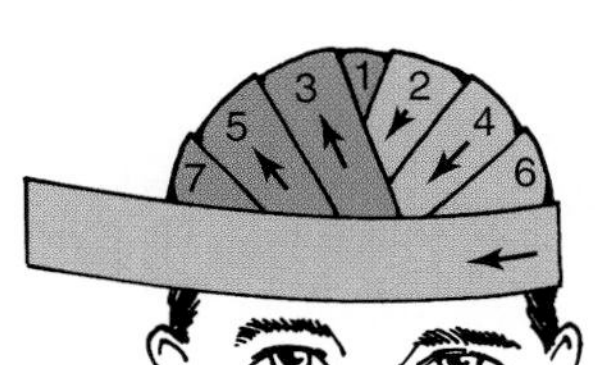	Anchor bandage with circular turns. At center front, make a perpendicular turn, bringing the bandage over the center of the head, until it meets the circular wrap at the back of the head. Reverse directions, bringing the next turn over the head from back to front. Continue wrapping in alternating directions until the head is covered, and then secure with circular turns. Note: Assistance in holding turns will be needed from patient or another nurse. Circular turns may be interspersed with perpendicular turns to secure wrap. For this wrap, kling bandage (self-adhering but without the adhesive) is easier to apply and remains in place longer than regular roller bandages.	Secure dressings on the scalp.
Stump Wrap 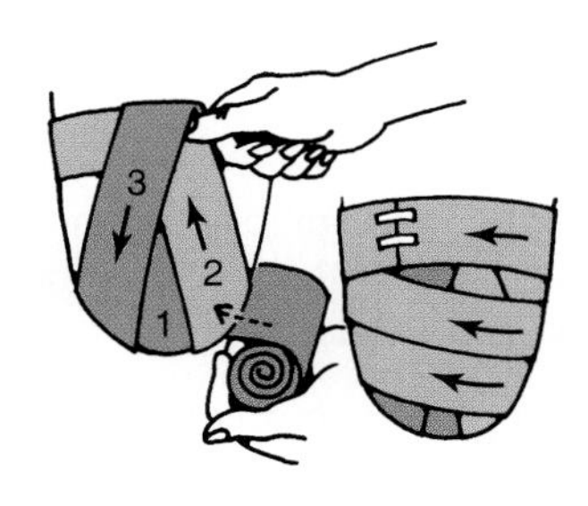	Anchor with circular turns at about 6–12 in. above the tip of the stump. Wrap as for scalp above, except after 4 to 5 lengthwise turns, finish with spiral turns in an ascending direction.	Secure dressings or provide compression for stump.

ing, wound packing maintains a moist environment and dilutes viscous exudates, but does not debride a wound. When allowed to dry before removal, the packing acts as a debriding agent, but care should be taken not to traumatize local tissue or damage granulation tissue (see Procedure 27–17). When no more necrotic tissue remains, wounds healing by second intention are often packed with fine-meshed gauze. This maintains a moist environment and absorbs exudate, but does not damage granulation tissue when removed.[10]

Wound Irrigation. Irrigation is another means of removing exudate and necrotic tissue from a wound cavity to create an environment for optimal healing. It is detailed in Procedure 27–20.

Pressure Ulcer Care

Pressure ulcers, an all too common nursing problem, are a challenge to care for. More than 95% of pressure ulcers develop over bony prominences—the sites most vulnerable to the pressure, friction, and shearing forces that accompany bedrest. Pressure ulcers occur most often in patients who are immobilized, bedridden, and debilitated.

Once a pressure ulcer is apparent, the wound is staged according to the system described above, and monitored frequently for signs of healing or deterioration. Signs of deterioration include increased exudate in the wound site, edema of surrounding tissue, loss of granulation tissue, and a purulent discharge indicating infection.[30] Occasionally, there may be systemic signs such as fever, hypotension, tachycardia, or mental confusion, which signal deterioration in the patient's overall physical state.

Many studies identify malnutrition as a factor that contributes to pressure ulcer formation. Thus, screening patients for nutritional deficiencies and monitoring them for weight loss is an important part of a pressure ulcer care plan. A goal of nursing care is to supply the nutrients needed for positive nitrogen balance—see Chap. 28. Another aspect of care is pain management. Because

(continued on page 863)

PROCEDURE 27–16. CHANGING A DRY STERILE DRESSING

PURPOSE: To protect a wound from injury and microorganisms, absorb drainage, and promote healing.
EQUIPMENT: Sterile gloves, clean gloves, dressing materials, tape, waterproof bag for soiled dressings, and sterile barrier (optional). If wound cleansing is ordered, see Procedure 27–15.

ACTION 1. Verify medical order; check operative report or nursing and medical progress notes to determine if a surgical drain is in place and current condition of wound. Gather supplies.

RATIONALE. Wound care requires a medical order; many surgeons specify solutions or dressing materials desired. Information about wound status assists in the selection of supplies (type and amount), if none are specified in the order. Refer to Table 27–10.

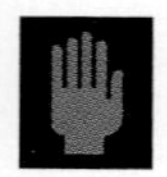

Many surgeons prefer to do the initial dressing change.

ACTION 2. Discuss the procedure with the patient, including the expected benefits, usual sensations, desired participation, and the timing of the procedure. Determine the need for prior pain medication.

RATIONALE. The patient will be likely to participate and less anxious if this information is shared. The procedure may be painful or emotionally traumatic so it is advisable not to plan it just prior to meals, scheduled therapy, or expected visitors.

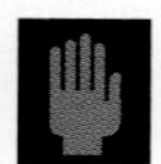

Some patients are anxious or fearful about looking at their surgical incision. Consider this when discussing and planning care. If medication is desired, administer so peak effect can be expected at the time wound care is planned. (See Chap. 25.)

ACTION 3. Wash your hands. Screen patient and close door. Raise bed to waist level. Ask or assist patient to assume a comfortable position that allows exposure of dressing. Fold back covers so they cannot contact wound or surrounding skin when dressing has been removed. Provide additional drapes if necessary for warmth or modesty. If wound is to be cleansed and/or is draining profusely, protect the bed with a waterproof pad.

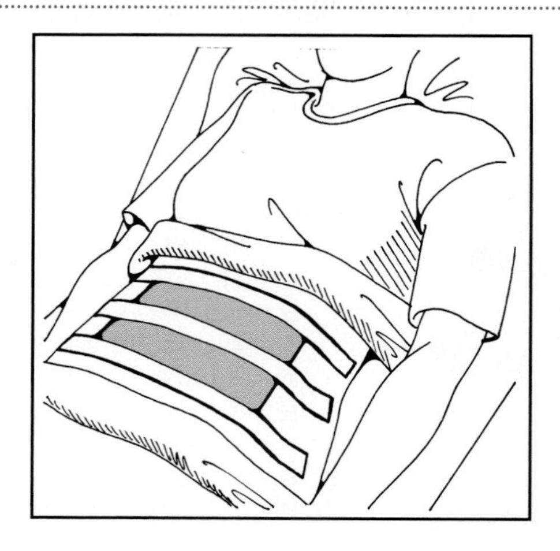

RATIONALE. Screening and draping show respect for patient's needs for privacy; closing door also minimizes air currents, which could transmit airborne organisms to exposed wound. Hand washing and moving covers away from dressing prevent wound contamination by direct contact.

ACTION 4. Prepare a work area large enough to accommodate all sterile supplies and located so it will not be at your back while you cleanse and dress the wound:

RATIONALE. All items needed for a sterile procedure must be available in one area, which is in view at all times. Because one would be unaware of contamination of items out of one's view, they must be considered contaminated.

a. Create a sterile field using a sterile barrier towel (see Procedure 25–3).

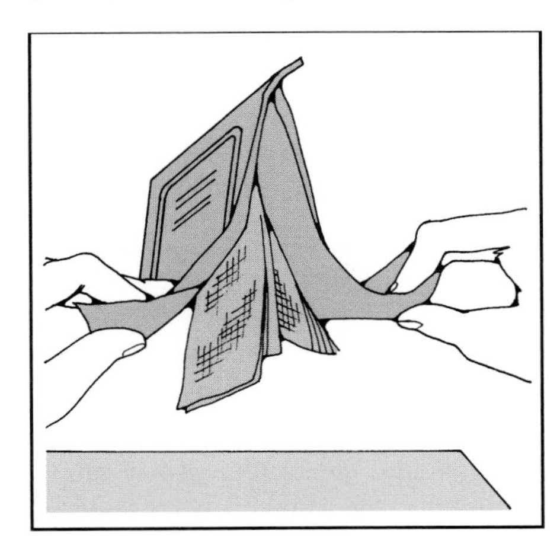

b. Open sterile supplies and place them on the sterile field (Clinical Guideline 25–9).

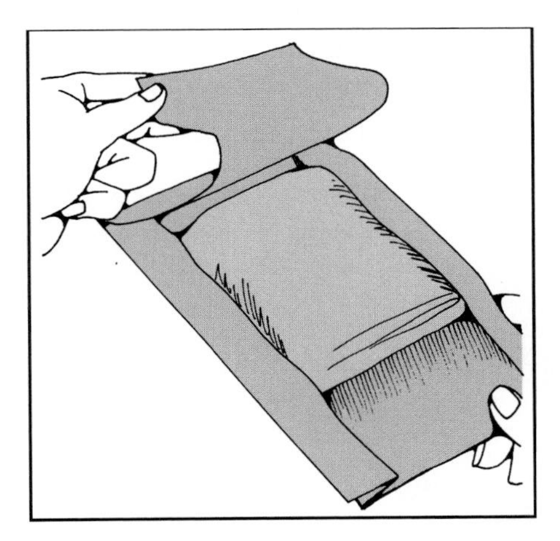

RATIONALE. A sterile field creates a barrier between a clean surface and sterile items, preventing contact with microorganisms.

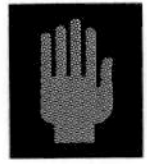

A simple dressing change may be accomplished without a separate sterile field. The wrappers of sterile items may be used to make a sterile field if items are opened carefully. The opened wrappers and their contents are placed directly on the work area.

c. Pour sterile solution for wound care if ordered (see Clinical Guideline 25–10).

d. Make a cuff at the top of the waterproof bag and place it so used dressing materials can be discarded without reaching over opened sterile supplies. It may be taped to the siderail for convenience.

RATIONALE. Moving soiled items over a sterile field can contaminate the field because microorganisms on the items are aerosolized when they are manipulated. A cuff protects the outside of the trashbag so it is not contaminated by items that touch its top edge as they are being discarded. The outside of the bag must remain free of organisms from the wound to prevent transmitting them to the environment.

ACTION 5. Loosen the tape holding the dressing in place. Pull the tape toward the wound while stabilizing the skin under the tape. Wetting the adhesive surface of the tape with an alcohol swab as you lift the tape facilitates removal. Adhesive remover may also be used, if necessary. Montgomery straps (see Fig. 27–9) are not removed unless wet. Release tie or band closure and fold straps away from the dressing.

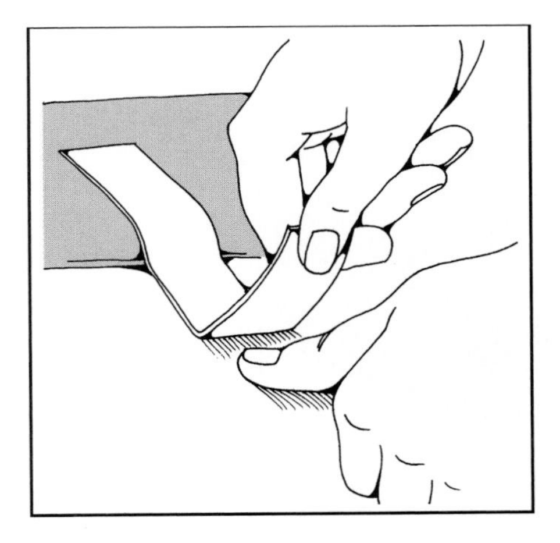

RATIONALE. Pulling toward the wound prevents disruption of healing. Stabilizing the skin reduces discomfort as the tape is removed. Leaving Montgomery straps in place reduces damage to epithelium caused by frequent removal and replacement of tape.

Continued

ACTION 6. Remove the dressing carefully. If the dressing is dry, it may be removed with the bare hand. Don a clean glove to remove a dressing that is damp. All dressing layers may be removed at once if inner dressing does not adhere to the wound and if there is no drain in place. Remove one layer at a time when a drain is present. Use a clean glove to remove inner dressings that do not come off with the outer dressing.

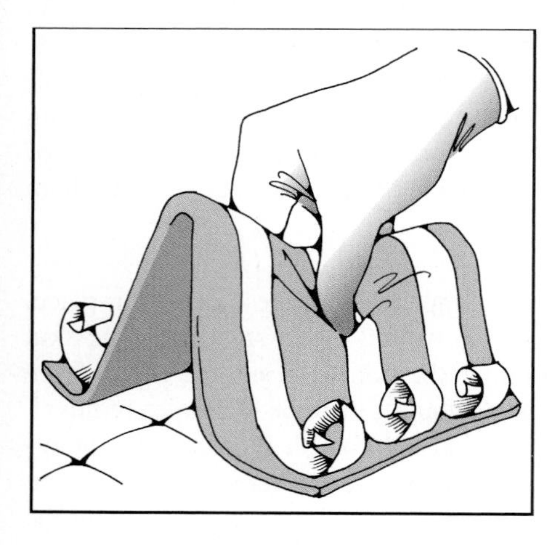

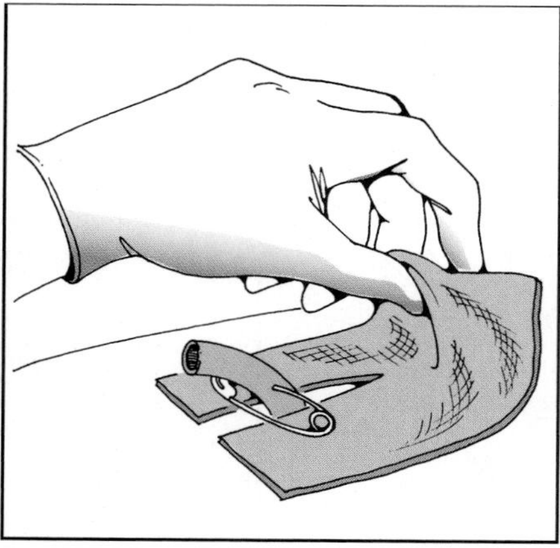

RATIONALE. The outside of a dry dressing is clean, not sterile nor contaminated; therefore, no protection is needed to remove it. A wet dressing contains body fluids; the clean glove prevents contact. Layer-by-layer removal of dressings around a drain reduces the possibility of dislodging the drain.

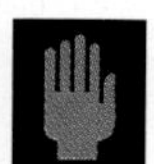

If the inner dressing adheres to the wound, moisten with sterile normal saline to prevent disruption of healing.

ACTION 7. Note the amount, odor and character of drainage as you remove the dressing. Discard dressings and glove, if used, in bag.

RATIONALE. Changes in the amount and character of drainage are cues to nursing action. Gloves that have contacted the soiled dressing are not sterile and cannot be used to cleanse wound or apply new dressing.

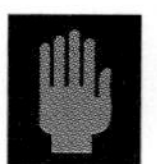

Report purulent, foul-smelling drainage or increased amount of drainage. Obtain culture (see Procedure 27–19).

ACTION 8. Inspect the wound (see also Clinical Guideline 27–1). Note approximation of wound edges, presence of granulation tissue, amount, character, and location of drainage. If the skin next to the wound appears taut and red or puffy, don 1 sterile glove (see Procedure 25–3) on dominant hand; palpate wound site. Note areas that are warm or tender or have increased drainage. Palpate drain site last. Discard glove. Palpation is not necessary if wound appears dry with well-approximated edges. Report signs of infection or delayed healing. Obtain culture if infection is suspected. (See Procedure 27–19.)

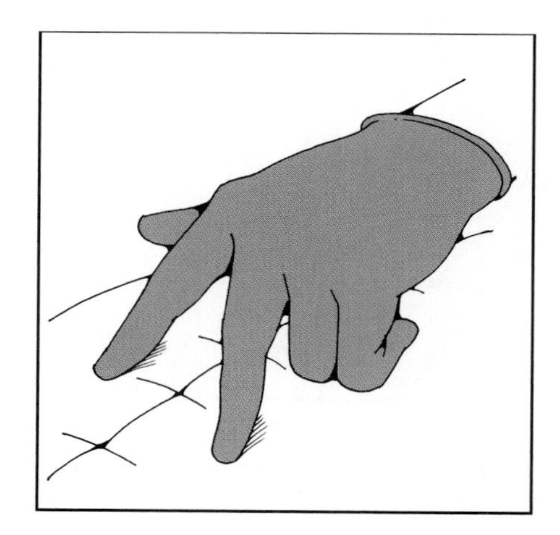

RATIONALE. Approximation of edges of a surgical wound or granulation tissue in an open wound indicate healing. Warmth, tenderness, or gaping areas may indicate infection. See also Action 7. Drain site is assessed last because accumulated drainage there increases the possibility that microorganisms may be present.

ACTION 9. If necessary, cleanse the wound as described in Procedure 27–15, following physician's order or agency policy.

RATIONALE. Wounds are cleaned to remove exudate, dead tissue, and bacteria. Wounds that are healing well may not need cleaning.

ACTION 10. Don sterile glove on dominant hand. Cover wound with gauze squares, fluffs, and/or nonadhering dressing as appropriate. Apply sufficient absorbent dressings for the drainage being produced. If copious drainage is produced and patient is ambulatory, place extra dressings at the lowest portion of the wound.

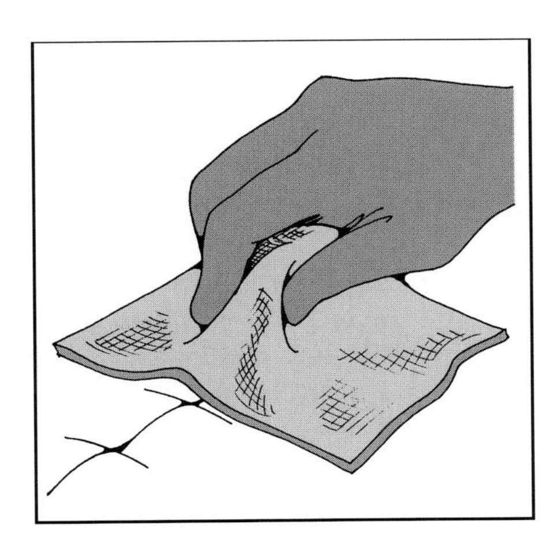

RATIONALE. Nonadhering dressings prevent disruption of healing in wounds that produce sticky exudate, which often causes gauze to adhere to the wound site. Nonadhering dressings neither absorb drainage nor wick it away from the wound, so absorptive dressings must also be added. Wicking is important to prevent drainage accumulating at the wound surface, which macerates skin and slows healing. Gravity will pull drainage toward the bottom of the wound site when patient ambulates. Placing extra absorbent materials there prevents drainage leaking onto gown or floor.

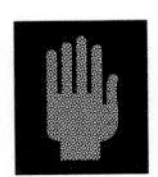

Use the minimum amount of dressing materials that will accomplish the purpose for which the dressing is being applied. An unnecessarily bulky dressing is uncomfortable and using excessive supplies is not cost effective.

ACTION 11. If there is a drain, don a second sterile glove and place 2 drain sponges around the drain in opposite directions.

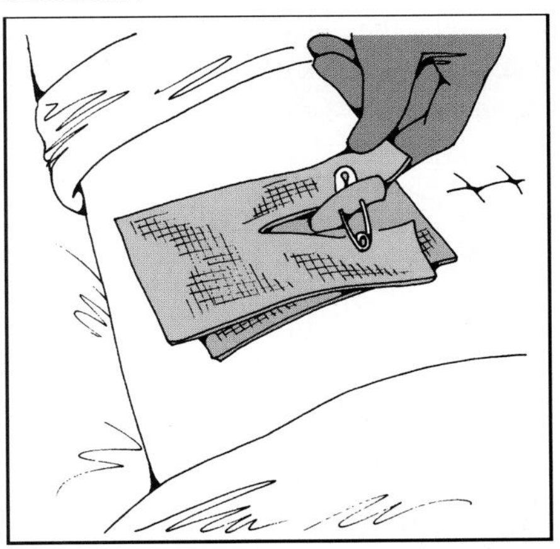

If drain sponges are not available, fold 2 4 × 4s as follows:

a. Unfold to 4 × 8 size.

b. Fold at right angle, place next to drain.

c. Place second folded sponge on other side of drain with right (90 degree) angle in opposite direction.

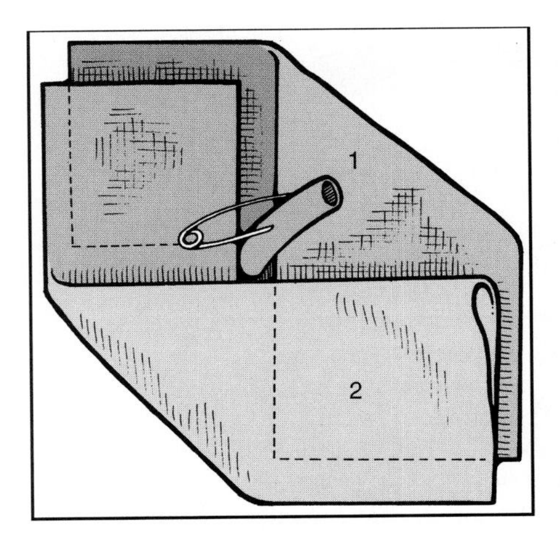

Cover with necessary amount of absorbent dressings.

RATIONALE. Drainage is irritating to skin and slows healing. This arrangement of sponges protects skin around drain. Drain site is dressed last because it is more likely to be contaminated (see Action 8 above).

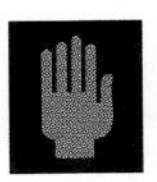

Cutting 4 × 4s to fit around a drain is not recommended, because cut fibers may adhere to or be imbedded in healing tissue.

Continued

Procedure 27–16. Changing a Dry Sterile Dressing (continued)

ACTION 12. If needed, place an outer dressing, such as a combipad over all layers of inner dressings. If glove is wet from touching drain, remove and discard it before placing outer dressing. Touch only the outside of the pad with ungloved hands. Wounds with little drainage may require only a topper(s) over gauze square(s).

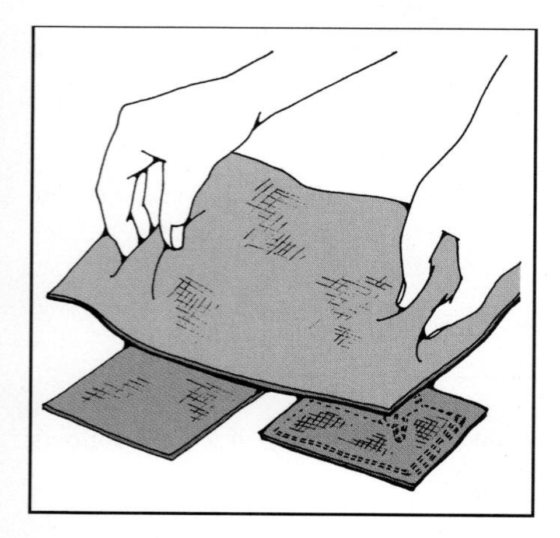

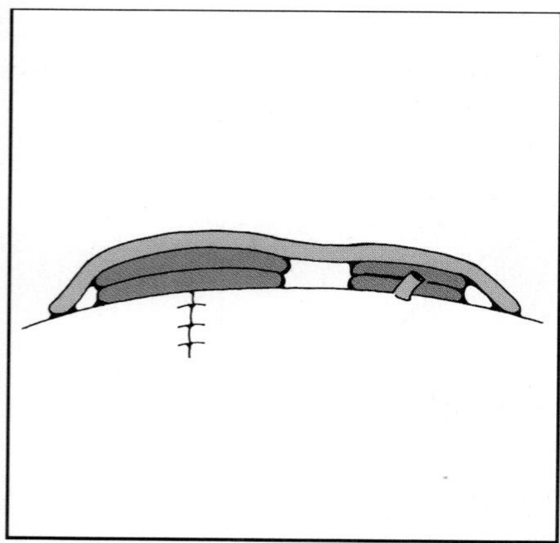

RATIONALE. A single thick absorbent pad wicks and absorbs drainage, and holds all dressing materials in place with a minimum of tape. Glove is removed to prevent transferring potentially pathogenic organisms from drain site to outside of the dressing and, hence, the environment. Touching only the outside of the dressing maintains the sterility of the wound site.

ACTION 13. Tape the outer dressing in place as described in Clinical Guideline 27–4.

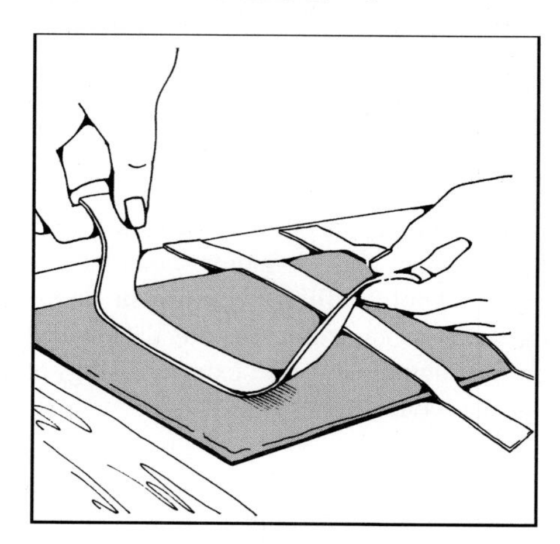

RATIONALE. Correct taping secures the dressing while allowing air circulation to evaporate moisture from dressing, preventing maceration and delayed healing.

ACTION 14. Rearrange patients gown and covers. Assist patient with repositioning if needed and place bed in low position. Be sure all disposable items used in wound care are in waterproof waste bag. If items are too bulky to fit, they can be discarded in room trash container, if plastic-lined. Liner and contents must then be removed. (Dry wrappers may be left in trash can.) Close waste bags securely and dispose according to agency policy. In many agencies, a covered waste container for disposal of biohazardous waste, such as soiled dressings, is placed in each patient room rather than transporting the wastes to a central disposal site after each procedure.

RATIONALE. This shows respect for patient's comfort and personal space. Soiled dressings and items used in wound care provide a medium for bacterial growth and create unpleasant odors. Removing from patient's room and disposing in sealed waste containers reduces environmental hazards, both in and outside of hospital.

Recording:

Note initial appearance of dressing, condition of wound; amount, location, and nature of drainage; specific wound care provided; problems encountered, if any, and action taken to correct them; and patient's response to care.

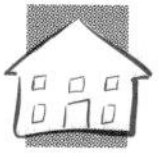

HOME HEALTH ADAPTATION: This procedure adapts easily to the home environment. Double-wrap in plastic bags all contaminated items before placing in patient's trash container.

PROCEDURE 27–17. APPLYING WOUND PACKING OR WET-TO-DRY DRESSINGS

PURPOSE: To promote wound healing by debriding and to control bacterial growth in infected wounds. Packing or wet-to-dry dressings are commonly used on traumatic wounds, pressure ulcers, or infected surgical wounds.

EQUIPMENT: Clean gloves; sterile gloves, sterile barrier towel; wound-cleansing supplies, if ordered (see Procedure 27–15) or sterile irrigation kit, if ordered (see Procedure 27–20); unfilled wide-mesh gauze squares to pack and cover wound (roller gauze, plain or impregnated with antibacterial agent such as nitrofurazone may be ordered for packing); wetting solution as ordered; sterile basin; tissue forceps or sterile applicators (for small wound); tape or Montgomery straps; and waterproof trash bag.

ACTION 1. Verify medical order; check operative report or nursing and medical progress notes to determine current condition of wound. Gather supplies.

RATIONALE. Wound care requires a medical order; many surgeons specify solutions or dressing materials desired. Information about wound status assists in the selection of supplies (type and amount), if none are specified in the order. Refer to Clinical Guideline 27–3.

ACTION 2. Discuss the procedure with the patient, including the purpose and benefits, usual sensations, desired patient participation, and timing of the procedure. Determine the need for prior pain medication.

RATIONALE. Patients will be less anxious and more likely to participate if adequate information is provided for informed decision making. The procedure may be painful or emotionally traumatic, so it is advisable not to plan it just prior to meals, scheduled therapy, or expected visitors.

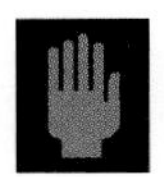

If pain medication is desired, administer so its peak effect can be expected at the time wound care is planned (see Chap. 25).

ACTION 3. Position patient and prepare sterile field as in Procedure 27–16, Actions 3 and 4. In a sterile basin, place sufficient gauze squares or roller gauze to pack and/or cover the wound. Pour ordered wetting solution over gauze so that it is completely saturated. Plastic container in which gauze is packaged may be used as sterile basin. Place it next to the sterile field, not on it, as the outside is contaminated.

RATIONALE. See Procedure 27–16. Surgical asepsis is practiced even when wound is infected, to prevent additional infection by other organisms. Clean technique is acceptable for pressure ulcers.

ACTION 4. Loosen tape or Montgomery straps as in Procedure 27–16, Action 5. Don clean gloves. Carefully grasp the outer dressing and underlying packing material. Cue patient of possible discomfort. Pull dressing and packing away from the wound, pulling toward the center if the wound is large. Dressing will stick, but do not moisten unless dressing sticks to pink granulation tissue. If any packing remains in wound, use a sterile glove or forceps to remove it.

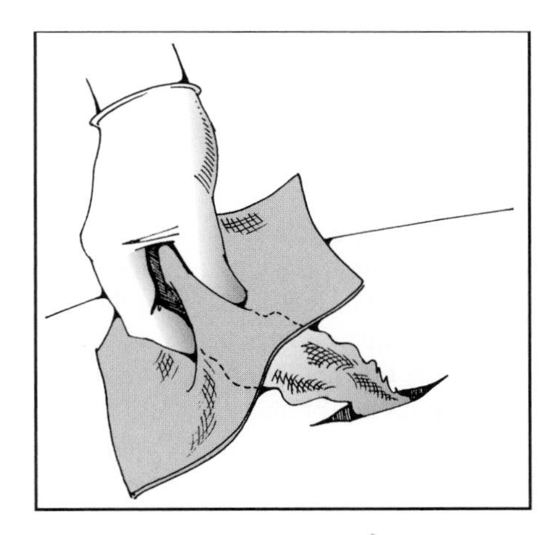

RATIONALE. See Procedure 27–16, Actions 5 and 6. Necrotic tissue interferes with granulation and epithelialization. Moistened gauze traps superficial necrotic tissue in its mesh as it dries. Necrotic debris is then removed with the dried gauze. Some associated discomfort is unavoidable, but is better tolerated if patient is warned. Premedication will decrease pain. More often, packing is used to maintain a moist environment or deliver local medication. For those purposes, packing is not expected to dry between dressing changes.

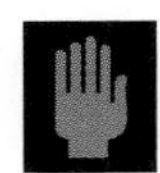

It is not unusual for a small amount of bleeding to accompany the removal of the packing. If a wound is deep, all packing cannot be removed by grasping through outer dressing.

Continued

ACTION 5. Inspect the dressing, packing, and wound as in Procedure 27–16, Actions 7 and 8, noting also presence of necrotic debris on dressing and in wound. Discard dressings and glove in bag. Don sterile glove to remove any remaining packing material; inspect and discard as above. Discard glove.

RATIONALE. See Procedure 27–16, Actions 7 and 8. Assessment provides information about the effectiveness of the treatment and amount of healing. Necrotic tissue is gray to black. When most of the wound surface is covered with fresh pink granulation tissue, debridement is complete. Consult with physician regarding change in wound care.

If the dressing is dry, but with little trapped debris, it was probably too dry when applied. If it is very wet, outer dressings or tape may have been too thick to allow drying.

ACTION 6. Cleanse wound (Procedure 27–15) or irrigate (Procedure 27–20), if ordered.

RATIONALE. Loosened necrotic debris may be removed by cleansing or irrigation. Irrigation is more common for deeper wounds.

ACTION 7. Don sterile gloves. Designate one hand "contaminated," to be used for packing the wound; designate the other "sterile" to be used to obtain materials from the sterile field. Remove one gauze square and squeeze out excess moisture. It should be wet, but not dripping. Unfold the gauze (use both hands, but do not bring hands into contact with one another) (i) and place it into the wound cavity (ii). If wound is small, a sterile applicator or forceps may be used to pack gauze into crevices (iii). For a large wound, add additional squares until packing contacts all wound surfaces and cavity is filled. Some clinicians stipulate that roller gauze rather than several gauze squares be used to pack large wound cavities to prevent individual pieces of packing material being left in the cavity inadvertently. If roller gauze is used, unroll as wound is packed rather than placing roll in cavity (iv). Packing should be slightly fluffed to fill cavity, and completely, but not tightly, packed.

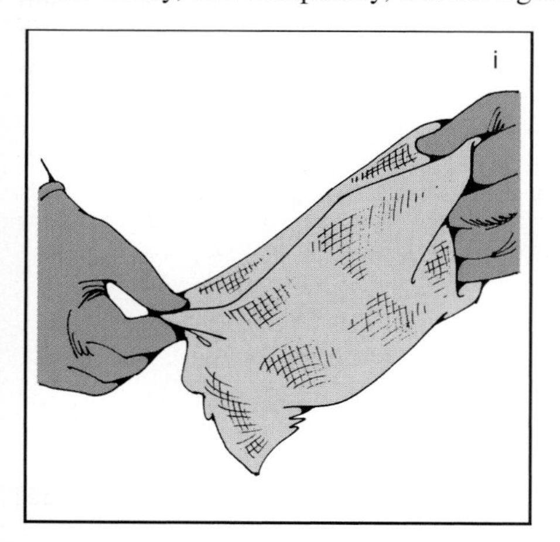

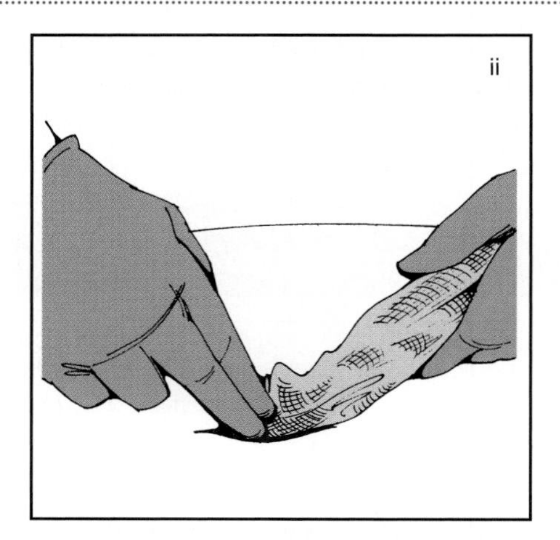

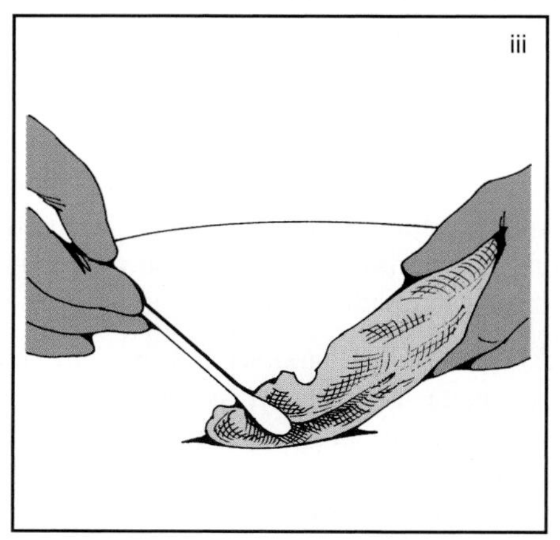

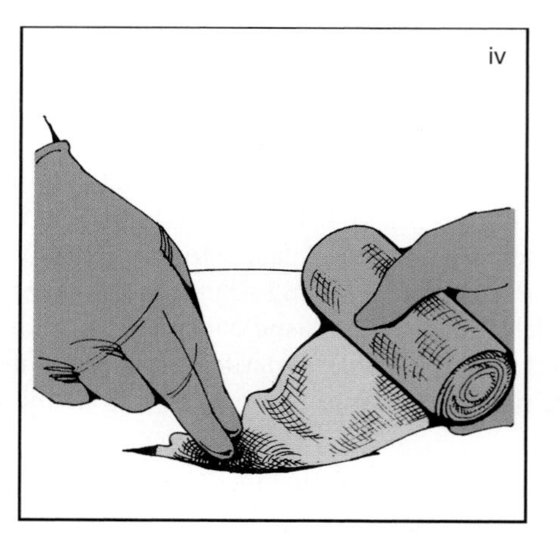

RATIONALE. Touching the sterile field with the hand that has contacted the wound transfers organisms to the field. Debridement occurs only if there is direct contact between tissue and moist gauze; therefore packing must touch all wound surfaces. Saturated packing creates excessive wetness. Tightly packed gauze may interfere with perfusion.

ACTION 8. Using "sterile" hand, cover wound and packing with a sufficient number of dry sterile gauze squares to keep outermost dressing from becoming wet. Remove and discard gloves. A final unfolded gauze square may be applied to provide a continuous surface for taping the dressing. Do not touch inner surface with bare hands.

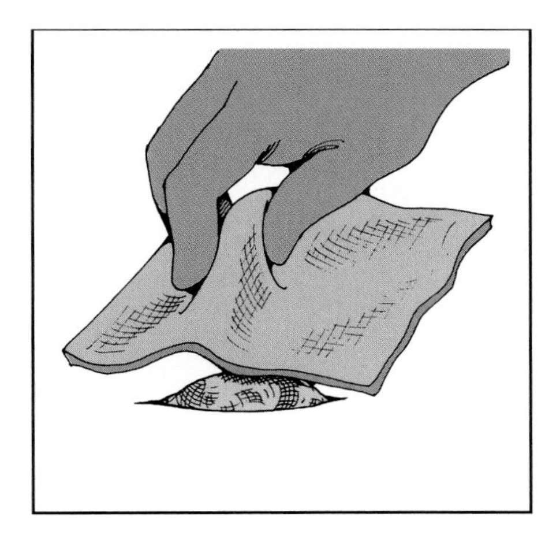

RATIONALE. Using hand that has contacted wound cavity to place outer dressings would transfer organisms to the outside of the dressing and to the environment. If outermost dressing becomes wet, cross-contamination between the wound and the environment is possible by capillary action.

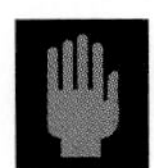

Use of thick outer dressings like combipads is contraindicated if order is for wet or dry dressing, because thick dressings prevent air circulation and drying of packing.

ACTION 9. Secure dressings as described in Clinical Guideline 27–4 or in Table 27–11. Montgomery straps are often used for wet-to-dry dressings because they are usually changed every 4 to 6 hours.

RATIONALE. A correctly secured dressing will protect the wound without retarding healing.

ACTION 10. Reposition patient, remove equipment and replace patient's personal belongings as in Procedure 27–16, Action 14.

RATIONALE. See rationale for Action 14, Procedure 27–16.

Recording:
Note initial appearance of dressing, condition of wound, including amount of necrotic and granulation tissue; amount, location, and nature of drainage; specific wound care provided; problems encountered, if any, and action taken to correct them; and patient's response to care. In some agencies, it is recommended that the number of gauze squares used to pack a large wound be included in nurse's note.

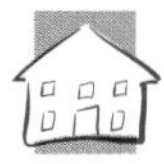

HOME HEALTH ADAPTATION: This procedure adapts easily to the home environment. Double-wrap in plastic bags all contaminated items before placing in patient's trash container.

some patients are unable to articulate their pain, the nurse may have to rely on observations of patient reactions to care activities.

A particularly important part of caring for pressure ulcers is to manage the **tissue load.** Tissue load refers to the distribution of pressure, friction, and shear on the tissue overlying bony prominences. The goal is to create wound tissue conditions conducive to healing. Those conditions include a reduced tissue load and levels of moisture and temperature that promote tissue health. Since pressure is a factor in ulcer development, it follows that reduction of pressure is important to promote healing. The patient is encouraged to assume positions that reduce contact between the ulcer area and the support surface and to change position frequently, ideally every 15 minutes, to shift the pressure points.[30] For patients unable to move, hourly repositioning is advisable, giving attention to proper postural alignment and stability.[30] Patients who cannot assume a variety of positions or who have stage 3 or 4 ulcers on multiple turning surfaces may require a **dynamic support surface,** a bed surface engineered to automatically alter the pressure over skin contact points. Alternating-air mattresses, mattresses with interconnecting air cells that cyclically inflate and deflate to produce alternating high- and low-pressure intervals, are an example of such devices. Such surfaces, although helpful, are no substitute for frequent turning and observation by the nurse, however. Static support surfaces such as foam wedges and pillows may also be helpful in relieving pressure over pressure points, but ring cushions, a variety of static support surface known to cause venous congestion and tissue edema, may raise the risk of ulcer formation.[30] Support surfaces may cause excess moisture to accumulate and macerate intact skin. Attention should be given to provide for airflow over the skin—an important aspect of ulcer prevention.

PROCEDURE 27–18. MANAGING WOUND DRAINAGE SYSTEMS

PURPOSE: To maintain functioning of closed wound drainage systems and assess quantity and quality of drainage.
EQUIPMENT: Clean gloves, antiseptic swabs, measuring receptacle, and waterproof pad. For irrigation, solution and syringe to fit tubing.

ACTION 1. Assess amount of drainage in portable closed wound suction systems at least every 4 hours. Suction is significantly reduced and potential for clogging of tubing increased when device is more than 1/3 full, so it should be emptied whenever fluid approaches this level. Note presence of clots or kinks in tubing. Correct kinks by repositioning reservoir. See Action 5 for clot removal. Fig. 27–10 illustrates wound drainage from closed drainage systems. A Penrose drain does not contain drainage, so dressings must be assessed frequently and changed when wet.

ACTION 2. To empty collection reservoir: Don gloves to protect your hands from exudate. Place waterproof pad on bed under reservoir. Unpin tubing from patient's gown. Open reservoir port that is not connected to drainage tubing and pour contents into measuring receptacle. A medicine cup, disposable drinking glass, or any appropriately sized graduated container may be used. Capacity of graduate should be similar to that of reservoir.

ACTION 3. To reestablish suction:

a. *Disc-shaped unit:* Place unit on a firm surface with port open. Compress unit completely with palm of your hand. Close port before releasing pressure.

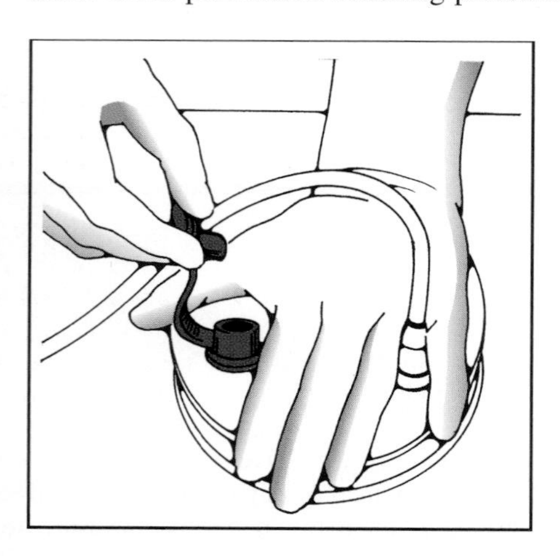

b. *Bulb-shaped unit:* With port open, squeeze unit with one or both hands until all air is evacuated. Close port. Reattach unit to patient's gown below level of wound with safety pin.

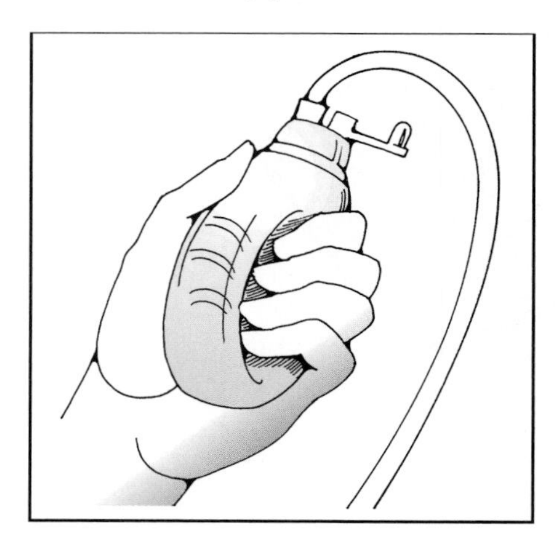

Either system will now exert mild negative pressure, pulling wound exudate into reservoir.

ACTION 4. If tubing is occluded by clots, check agency policy or physician's order for irrigation. Milking or stripping tubing to dislodge clots is usually contraindicated.

ACTION 5. To irrigate:

a. Obtain syringe that will create a seal with tubing attached to unit. Tubing varies in size with size of unit. For very small units, a blunt needle may be required to connect syringe snugly to tubing.

b. Obtain ordered solution. Sterile normal saline is the usual solution. Fill syringe aseptically.

c. Place waterproof pad on bed under unit. Clean junction of tubing and reservoir with firm twisting motion.

d. Detach tubing. Disc-shaped unit can remain on bed; bulb-type unit must be held upright to prevent contamination. Hold tubing in nondominant hand, attach filled syringe.

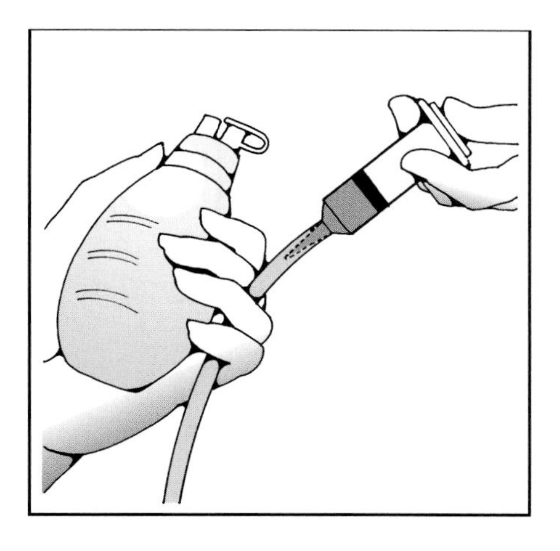

e. Inject fluid slowly until clot is dislodged. If additional fluid is needed, refill syringe and repeat.

f. Reestablish suction as in Action 3 above.

g. Reattach unit to patient's gown as above.

Recording:

Routine emptying is recorded on Intake and Output record. Note character of drainage in narrative notes. If irrigation is necessary, state reason for irrigation, amount and type of solution used, and functioning of unit after irrigation. Record irrigating solution as intake, return as output.

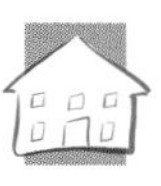

HOME HEALTH ADAPTATION: This procedure adapts easily to the home environment.

The pathophysiology of pressure ulcers involves tissue necrosis, and so debriding by wound packing, wet-to-dry dressings, irrigation, or whirlpool baths is a common aspect of care. Chemical debridement using proteolytic enzymes is another alternative for debriding pressure sores. Hydrophilic products in the form of beads, gels, and powders also aid the debriding process.[13]

Microorganisms can always be cultured in pressure ulcers.[24] If the organisms are allowed to proliferate, this may lead to complications such as *cellulitis* (infection in adjacent tissue), *osteomyelitis* (infection of bone), or *bacteremia* (bacteria in the bloodstream). Synthetic semi-occlusive dressings, in particular the hydrocolloid type, are very effective in promoting phagocytosis, enhancing healing, and also may be used to debride wounds.[15] These dressings promote liquefaction of necrotic tissue. They absorb exudate and maintain a moist wound environment. This characteristic may be mistaken for signs of a wound infection by caregivers who are not familiar with hydrocolloid dressings. Thorough cleaning or irrigation of the wound when changing the dressing will help to rule out this possibility. Application procedure and duration of application vary with specific products, so it is important to follow manufacturers' directions. Clinical Guideline 27–5 provides guidelines for the selection of approaches for the care of pressure ulcers.

A combination of sterile and nonsterile methods for dressing changes of pressure ulcers is now being used.[31] This no-touch procedure saves both time and costs. See Procedure 27–21.

Researchers are testing various other treatments for pressure ulcers, such as topical application of cell-specific growth factors,[32] electrical stimulation,[33] ultrasound/ultraviolet-C and lasers,[34] silicone implants over bony prominences, mechanical tension,[35] nitric oxide[36] (experimental), and ibuprofen (animal model.)[37] Hyperbaric oxygenation also is used to promote healing. Although these are not nursing measures, nurses may assist in their application and assess the results.

The best treatment for pressure ulcers is prevention. Promoting mobility; supporting nutrition and fluid intake; preventing pressure, friction, and shearing; and controlling moisture (eg, from diaphoresis or incontinence) are important preventive measures. They are discussed in greater detail in Chap. 33.

Measures to Support Healing

Supportive care that promotes comfort and well-being enhances healing of wounds of all types. Hygiene measures such as oral care, baths, and shampoos; comfort measures such as positioning and massage; stress reduction techniques such as music therapy, imagery, and meditation; and exercise contribute to healing and support natural defenses against infection. Promoting intake of protein, vitamins A and C, zinc, and adequate fluids is critical to these efforts. Emotional support including active listening and discussion of treatment options and progress of healing is important. Soliciting patient input in planning and carrying out treatment also supports well-being and therefore enhances healing.

Home Health Care

The restorative care of patients in the home often focuses on the healing of acute and chronic wounds. Indeed, as hospital stays grow shorter, patients routinely leave the hospital before their wounds are completely healed. One of the most important functions of the home nurse, therefore, is to perform wound assessment and wound care. Many of the procedures described in this chapter, in fact, are regularly performed in the home. Surgical dressing changes, for example, are done by home nurses.

The prevention of pressure ulcers is another concern in home health nursing. Nurses in the home setting are responsible for identifying patients at risk for pressure ulcers and for instructing caregivers on how to prevent pressure ulcers. Elderly patients who are undernourished, ill, immobile, or incontinent are especially

(continued on page 872)

PROCEDURE 27–19. OBTAINING AN AEROBIC OR ANAEROBIC WOUND CULTURE

PURPOSE: To detect and identify wound pathogens so that definitive therapy can be instituted. Culture is usually obtained during wound care when suspicious drainage or appearance is noted.

EQUIPMENT: Culture tube with rayon- or polyester-tipped swab and culture medium (aerobic and anaerobic tubes are available) and/or sterile syringe with needle for anaerobic culture; plastic bags for specimens; supplies to cleanse and dress the wound.

ACTION 1. Discuss the procedure with the patient, including the purpose and benefits, usual sensations, desired patient participation.

RATIONALE. Patients will be less anxious and more likely to participate if this information is provided.

ACTION 2. Position patient and prepare sterile field as in Procedure 27–16, Actions 3 and 4. Culture tubes or syringes may be removed from peel pack and placed on sterile field with other supplies or placed adjacent to the field on opened wrappers.

RATIONALE. See Procedure 27–16. Culture may be obtained before or after donning sterile gloves.

ACTION 3. Assess and cleanse the wound (see Procedure 27–15). If exudate does not flow spontaneously from the wound, don a sterile glove and press gently on the wound to express fresh drainage. Remove and discard glove.

RATIONALE. Wound is cleansed to remove skin flora. Fresh drainage is most likely to be uncontaminated by skin flora and contain the causitive organism. Glove would contaminate outside of culture tube.

ACTION 4. If exudate seems to be coming from deep within the wound, or a sinus tract is in evidence, obtain anerobic culture first. Don clean gloves. Remove needle from syringe, withdraw fresh exudate, expel air from syringe, and quickly replace and tape needle. Place in bag; seal. If anaerobic culture tube is used, follow manufacturer's directions. Systems used to remove air vary.

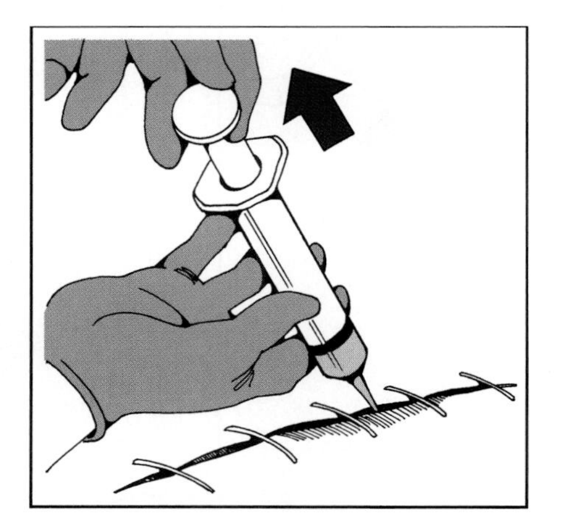

RATIONALE. Organisms growing in deep wounds or poorly perfused tissue are most likely to be anaerobes and so must be protected from air. Taped, capped needle and syringe plunger act as plugs, keeping air away from specimen. Bag protects environment from organisms on syringe.

ACTION 5. Also obtain aerobic culture:

RATIONALE. Aerobes may also infect wounds.

a. Remove cap and attached swab from aerobic culture tube without touching swab.

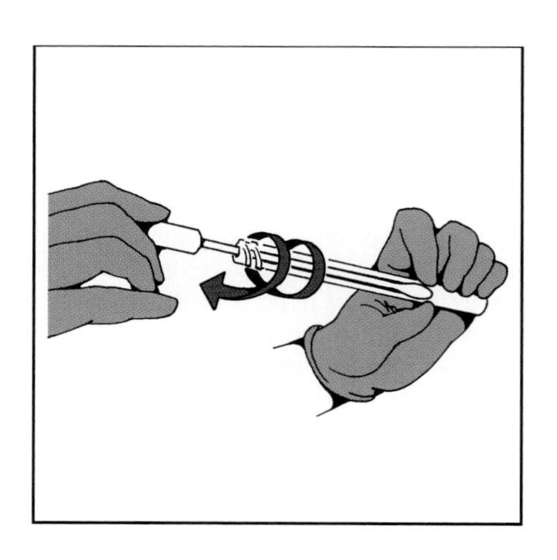

Procedure 27–19. (continued)

RATIONALE. Contact between the swab and nurse's hand transfers organisms to the swab and the wound.

b. Roll the tip of the swab in fresh exudate.

RATIONALE. Rolling coats swab with exudate.

c. Replace it in the culture tube without touching the outside, close tightly, and crush the ampule at the base of tube to release culture medium. Place tube in bag, seal.

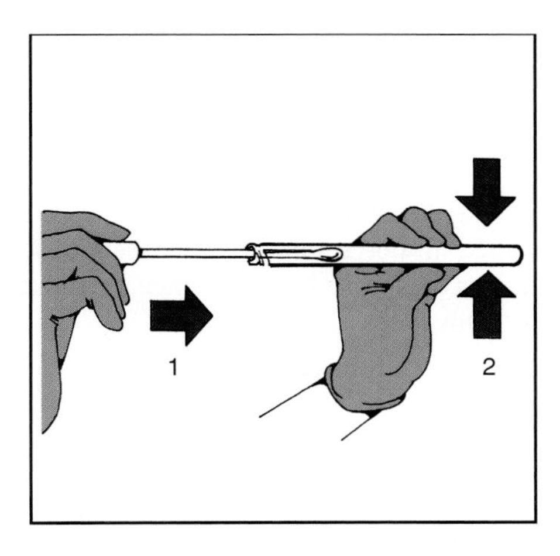

RATIONALE. If the swab with exudate touches the outside of the tube or the tube is not closed correctly, environmental or specimen contamination could result.

ACTION 6. If a wound has a combination of inflamed, necrotic, and/or purulent areas, obtain additional specimens from each area in a separate tube. Insert swabs as deeply as possible into wound crevices, abscess pockets, or eroded areas to obtain best specimen. Remove and discard gloves.

RATIONALE. Organisms with different sensitivity to antibiotics may be present within the same wound. All pathogens must be identified to successfully treat the infection.

ACTION 7. Complete ordered wound care; dress wound, reposition patient, and dispose of supplies as in Procedure 27–16.

RATIONALE. See Procedure 27–16.

ACTION 8. Label each specimen with patient's name, room number, diagnosis, source of specimen, and test desired. If antibiotic therapy has been initiated prior to specimen, note name of drug.

RATIONALE. Facilitates prompt and accurate results. Lab personnel can take measures to prevent undergrowth of culture because of antibiotic in the specimen, if drug is identified.

ACTION 9. Assure that the specimen is delivered to the lab within 20 minutes.

RATIONALE. Some organisms die quickly and others multiply rapidly, creating a potential for false diagnosis of the actual causitive organisms if lab cannot assess specimen promptly.

ACTION 10. Inform patient that test results take 48 hours or more. Inform patient and physician of test results as soon as they are available.

RATIONALE. Positive identification of causitive organisms can only occur after sufficient number have multiplied. Physicians need accurate information to plan therapy. Patients have a right to information about their health status. Correct information facilitates positive coping.

Recording:
Note conditions in wound that prompted obtaining culture, number, and type of specimens obtained, and disposition of specimen. See also Procedure 27–16.

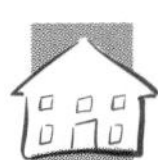

HOME HEALTH ADAPTATION: Place specimen container, labeled *biohazard,* in a plastic bag or pouch. Transport to laboratory in insulated carrier filled with artificial ice or ice from the patient's refrigerator. Request laboratory to phone or fax results to the physician and the home health agency. Note the date and time the specimen is delivered to the laboratory.

PROCEDURE 27–20. IRRIGATING A WOUND

PURPOSE: To clean and debride a wound to promote healing. Irrigation is commonly used for traumatic wounds, pressure ulcers, or infected surgical wounds.

EQUIPMENT: Sterile irrigation set or sterile syringe, sterile basin and clean curved basin; irrigation solution as ordered; waterproof pad(s); clean gloves; equipment for wound packing (Procedure 27–17), if ordered; equipment for sterile dressing change (Procedure 27–16); and extra sterile glove and gauze squares to dry skin around wound. For deep wounds, a sterile catheter, additional sterile glove, and moisture-impervious gown may be added; if irrigating solution is used, add sterile tongue blades, sterile protective ointment, additional irrigation set, and sterile normal saline for rinsing.

ACTION 1. Verify medical order; check operative report or nursing and medical progress notes to determine current condition of wound. Gather supplies. Check expiration date on irrigating solution.

RATIONALE. Wound irrigation requires a medical order; information about wound status assists in the selection of dressing supplies (type and amount), if none are specified in order. Refer to Table 27–10. Many irrigation solutions have a short shelf life. Some must be refrigerated.

ACTION 2. Discuss the procedure with the patient, including the purpose and benefits, usual sensations, desired patient participation, and timing of the procedure. Determine the need for prior pain medication.

RATIONALE. Patients will be less anxious and more likely to participate if adequate information is provided for informed decision making. The procedure may be painful or emotionally traumatic, so it is advisable not to plan it just prior to meals, scheduled therapy, or expected visitors.

If pain medication is desired, administer so its peak effect can be expected at the time wound care is planned (see Chap. 25).

ACTION 3. Wash your hands. If work area is large enough, prepare sterile field with supplies for dressing (Procedure 27–16, Action 4) and, if ordered, packing the wound (Procedure 27–17, Action 3), leaving adjacent space for irrigation equipment. If space is limited, defer sterile field until irrigation is complete; prepare trash bag as in Procedure 27–16, Action 4d.

RATIONALE. Preparing all equipment to complete wound care in advance limits the amount of time the wound is exposed to the environment, decreasing the possibility of airborne contamination and chilling the patient, but if workspace is limited, sterile field is likely to be contaminated while irrigation equipment is being used. See also Procedures 27–16 and 27–17.

If rinsing with sterile normal saline is ordered, a second irrigation setup will be needed. Rinsing is not common, unless irritating irrigation solution is used (eg, Dakin's).

ACTION 4. Loosen cover on irrigation solution. Unwrap irrigation set. Take solution container out of collection basin. Remove container cover and syringe as a unit, being careful not to touch syringe below cover. While holding syringe and cover, pour irrigation solution into container. (Amount depends on the size of the wound.) Remove protective tip from end of syringe and replace cover and syringe on container. If not using irrigation set, unwrap sterile basin and pour solution. Leave syringe in package until after donning gloves (see Action 7).

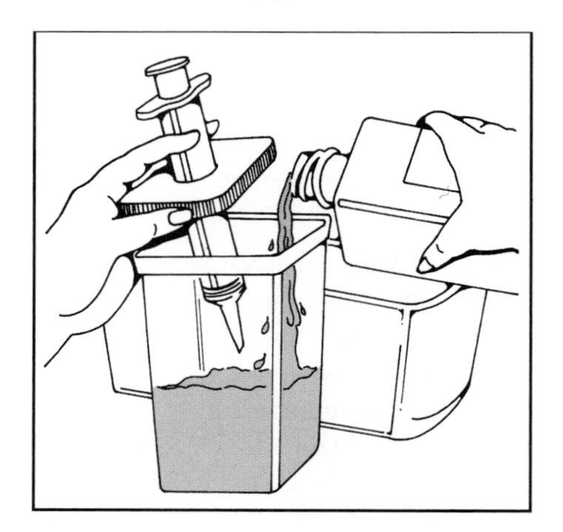

RATIONALE. Irrigation equipment is ready for use. Solution and distal end of syringe remain sterile, having contacted nothing unsterile, and are protected by cover. Outside of container and proximal end of syringe need not remain sterile, as they will not contact wound.

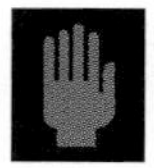

Irrigation solution may be warmed by placing the bottle in a basin of hot tap water for 10 to 15 minutes before pouring into irrigation container. Warm solution promotes comfort and causes local vasodilation, and hence facilitates healing.

ACTION 5. Position patient and expose dressing as in Procedure 27–16, Action 3. Remove dressing; assess wound and dressing as in Procedure 27–16, Actions 5 to 8. Palpatory assessment is usually not necessary.

RATIONALE. See Procedure 27–16. Palpatory assessment is used to detect healing or complications in a sutured incision. Wounds needing irrigation are usually not sutured, but are healing by secondary intention.

ACTION 6. Assist patient to turn, if necessary, so solution will run by gravity to collection basin with least possible contact with intact skin. Tuck waterproof pad(s) under patient, extending to edge of bed; place collection basin next to patient on pad. If irritating solution is used, apply sterile protective ointment to wound edges with sterile tongue blade.

RATIONALE. Solution flowing out of wound will contain debris and microorganisms. Minimizing its contact with skin and bed limits possibility of contamination. Protective ointments create a barrier over skin, so solution cannot contact and damage it. Wound healing is enhanced when surrounding skin is optimally healthy.

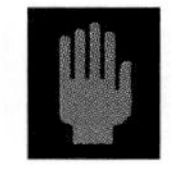

If back splashing of a returning solution is anticipated, don moisture impervious gown before proceeding with irrigation.

ACTION 7. Don clean gloves. Fill irrigating syringe and flush wound with steady pressure from highest to lowest part of the wound. Do not touch wound with syringe. Direct stream so all crevices and wound surfaces are contacted by irrigant. (For deep wounds, see Action 8.) Refill syringe and continue to flush wound until all areas have been cleansed. If possible, hold the collecting basin tightly against the skin below the wound with the nondominant hand while irrigating. Some patients may desire to help by holding collection basin.

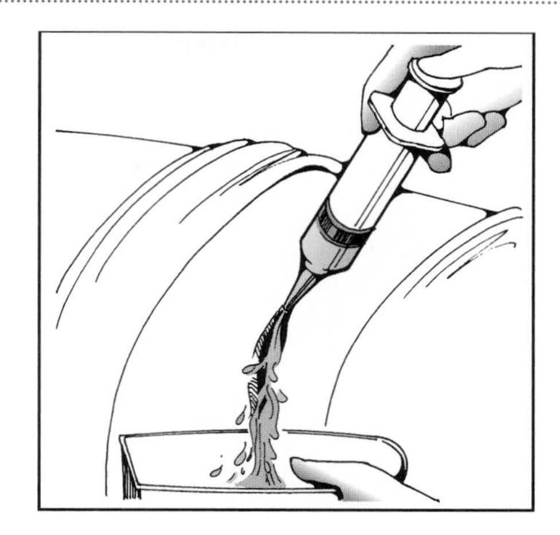

RATIONALE. Gloves protect nurse's hands from organisms in irrigation return. Sterile gloves are not needed at this time because nurse's hands do not contact wound. Pressure of the flowing liquid physically removes superficial debris from wound so all surfaces must be flushed to completely clean the wound. Some solutions also have antibacterial action. Body contours make collecting return in a basin difficult, but close contact with the body will minimize spilling.

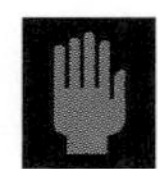

Greater pressure is generated if a syringe with a small tip is used. This is preferable if debris is tenacious. Still greater pressure can be achieved by attaching a blunt needle to the syringe.

ACTION 8. If wound is very deep, or has pockets that cannot be reached with fluid flowing from syringe, attach sterile catheter to syringe:

a. Open peel pack containing catheter; allow catheter to rest on sterile package. Don sterile gloves. Attach catheter to syringe. Fill Syringe.

Continued

b. Direct irrigant to wound pockets or crevices by moving catheter tip.

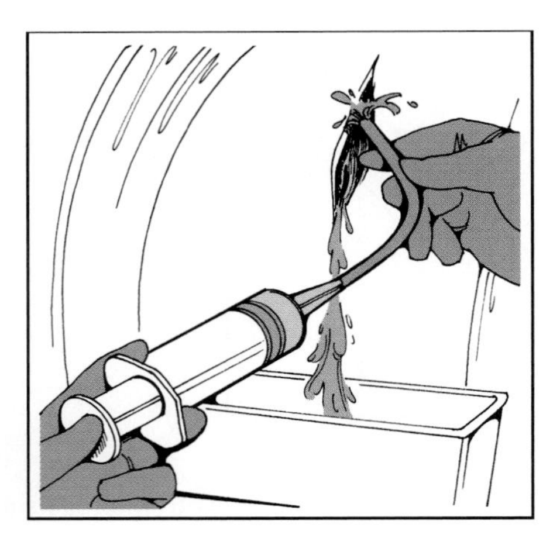

c. Repeat as needed; discard catheter and glove, unless rinse is ordered.

RATIONALE. Debris cannot be removed from a deep wound unless stream of liquid can be focused on all wound surfaces. Catheter acts as an extension of the syringe. Contact with wound and/or adjacent skin during irrigation contaminates glove, so it cannot be used to dress the wound.

ACTION 9. Repeat Actions 7 or 8 using normal saline if Dakin's solution is used to irrigate wound. Remove and discard gloves.

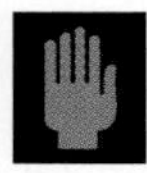

If rinse is required, prepare a second sterile irrigation set and fill container with sterile normal saline before donning gloves and beginning irrigation.

RATIONALE. Dakin's solution (0.5% sodium hypochlorite) is an effective debriding agent, but is irritating to healthy tissue and delays the clotting process, so residual solution must be removed.

ACTION 10. Don sterile gloves. Blot residual irrigant from skin around wound.

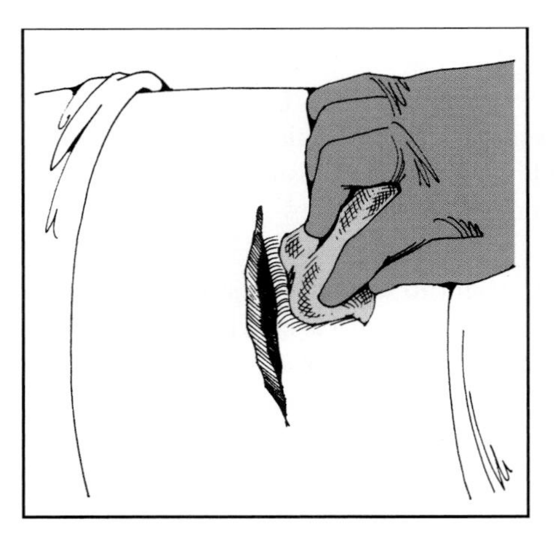

RATIONALE. Excessive moisture causes maceration, which interferes with healing.

ACTION 11. Pack and/or dress the wound as described in Procedures 27–16 and 27–17.

RATIONALE. See Procedures 27–16 and 27–17.

ACTION 12. Reposition patient, remove equipment, and replace patient's personal belongings as in Procedure 27–16, Action 14. Irrigation set may not be reused for a subsequent procedure.

RATIONALE. See Procedure 27–16, Action 14. Liquid (even an antibacterial solution) in irrigation set may support growth of microorganisms.

Recording:

Note initial appearance of dressing; condition of wound before and after irrigation, including amount of necrotic and granulation tissue; amount, location, and nature of drainage; specific wound care provided (including type of irrigation solution); problems encountered, if any, and action taken to correct them; and patient's response to care.

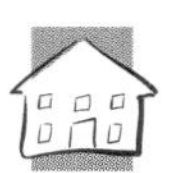

HOME HEALTH ADAPTATION: This procedure adapts easily to the home environment.

CLINICAL GUIDELINE 27–5

WOUND CARE OF PRESSURE ULCERS

Wound	Suggested Care	Action	Tips/Comments
Stage 1	a. Transparent dressing.	a. Traps exudate containing macrophages and leukocytes against wound, promoting natural defenses (autolysis).	a. Adhesive backed; change when loose or fluid builds up; some advise not to use on infected wounds.
	b. Hydrocolloid dressing.	b. Maintains moist environment, promotes autolysis, absorbs exudate.	b. Adhesive may be hard to remove; water resistant; patient can bathe.
	c. Antibiotic, saline, or Vaseline impregnated dressing.	c. Maintains moist environment.	c. Absorptive outer dressing needed.
	d. Relieve pressure.	d. Turn frequently.	d. Prop patient with pillows. Use written schedules.
Stage 2	a. Same as stage 1 if wound is not draining.	a. See stage 1.	a. See stage 1.
	b. Absorptive wound fillers (pastes, granules).	b. Absorbs exudate, nonocclusive, used with other dressings.	b. Do not use on deep, tunneled wounds; may remain in place several days unless excessive exudate.
	c. Hydrogels.	c. Stimulates cellular activity, provides moist environment, debrides, protects new tissue from damage.	c. Change daily; dries out; may macerate surrounding skin; must be secured in place; do not use with undermined wounds.
	d. Polyurethane foam.	d. Absorbs exudate.	d. Used with wound fillers, do not use if minimal exudate.
	e. Irrigate as per physician order (usually normal saline solution).	e. Cleanses ulcer.	e. Warm to body temperature. See Procedure 27–20.
	f. System support • Low air loss and air fluidized beds • Fluid and electrolyte balance • Increase protein, fats, and carbohydrates • Administer vitamin C, iron, zinc, and copper, as per physician order • Physical therapy • Discuss pressure ulcer treatment with patient	f. Collaborative health team effort.	f. Enhances holistic care. Crosses areas of expertise.
Stage 3	Same as stage 2.		
Stage 3, 4, yellow	High-pressure irrigation, hydrocolloids, hydrogels, fillers	Keeps wound clean and moist.	Document changes in color, depth, diameter of wound.
Stage 3, 4, pink to red	Transparent films, hydrocolloid, hydrogel. Same as Stage 2.	Protects from trauma, promotes continued healing.	See stage 3, 4, yellow.
Stage 4, black	Proteolytic enzymes, whirlpool, high-pressure irrigation, surgical debridement, wet to damp gauze.	Softens and /or removes dead tissue.	Use only until eschar is gone.

Sources: Adapted from Braden BJ, Bryant R. Innovations to prevent and treat pressure ulcers. Geriatr Nurs. 1990;11:189–191. Fowler E, Cuzzell JZ, Papen JC. Healing with hydrocolloid. Am J Nurs. *1991;91:63–64. Stotts NA. Seeing red and yellow and black: the three color concept of wound care.* Nursing 90. *1990;20:59–61. Stotts NA. Wound healing. In: Kinney MR, et al. AACN's* Clinical Reference for Critical Care Nursing. *3rd ed. Philadelphia: Lippincott; 1993. Pressure Ulcer Guideline Panel. Pressure ulcer treatment.* Am Fam Phys. *1995;51:1207–1222.*

PROCEDURE 27–21. NO-TOUCH DRESSING CHANGES FOR PRESSURE ULCERS

PURPOSE: To promote healing, to cut costs, and to save steps without compromising the quality of care.
EQUIPMENT: Disposable underpad, 2 pairs of nonsterile gloves, sterile saline, curved basin, sufficient number of packages of sterile 4 × 4 gauze for cleansing, and dressing ulcer tape. Special dressings may be substituted per agency policy or medical order.

ACTION 1. Verify medical order.

ACTION 2. Gather equipment and supplies.

ACTION 3. Follow Actions 2 and 3 as in Procedure 27–16.

ACTION 4. Place clean pad under patient.

ACTION 5. Don glove(s). Remove old dressing and discard.

ACTION 6. Remove and discard soiled glove(s).

ACTION 7. Assess the wound. (See Clinical Guideline 27–1.)

ACTION 8. Wash hands. Open sterile supplies using sterile technique. (See Clinical Guideline 25–9.)

ACTION 9. Don second pair of nonsterile gloves.

ACTION 10. Pour saline from bottle over wound to cleanse.

ACTION 11. Carefully pick up 4 × 4, touching the corners only. Use the 4 × 4s sterile center to slough off necrotic tissue. Begin at the center of the wound and work out. (See Procedure 27–15, Action 5.) Use additional sponges as needed. Dispose of soiled 4 × 4s as per agency policy.

ACTION 12. Dress wound with sterile 4 × 4s or other dressing. Secure with tape if necessary.

ACTION 13. Wash hands.

ACTION 14. Reposition patient keeping off of the area of the pressure ulcer.

ACTION 15. Record data. Refer to Process of Wound Healing and Clinical Guideline 27–1.

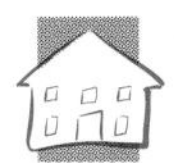

HOME HEALTH ADAPTATION: The procedure adapts easily to the home setting as written.

vulnerable to pressure ulcer development. Home nurses address these problems in their efforts to prevent pressure ulcers and assist family caregivers to provide adequate nutrition and skin care.

As another preventive measure, home nurses assess the need for adaptive appliances such as pressure-reducing water or foam mattresses, gel pads, or foam cushions. Home nurses also plan pressure ulcer care. In cases where a patient has developed ulcers, nurses assess the need for pressure-relief devices such as dynamic support systems that require hospital bed frames. Such appliances are expensive but make care easier for home caregivers. Home nurses also teach family caregivers how to turn and position patients and how to maintain the patient's nutrition and hygiene to support healing. Finally, home nurses monitor the needs of family caregivers. Pressure ulcer prevention and care requires 'round-the-clock effort and can be exhausting for caregivers.

REHABILITATIVE CARE

Rehabilitative skin and tissue care involves supporting adaptation to chronic skin conditions and encouraging self-care or family member care of slow-healing or chronic wounds.

Chronic skin diseases are often debilitating because of their impact on appearance. Skin condition has considerable influence on self-concept and body image. Lesions on exposed parts of the body, especially the face, generate self-consciousness and lack of self-regard. Often individuals with skin alterations become extremely sensitive to others' responses and may even avoid social situations. The anticipation of stares or revulsion from others may be so emotionally stressful that patients perceive actual interactions as too difficult to deal with.

Skin diseases also alter communication. Fearing rejection because of their lesions, patients may limit communication through touching, thereby depriving themselves of a primary means to convey caring, intimacy, and sexuality.

Supporting adaptation to skin alterations begins with listening and encouraging expression of feelings. Many patients feel anger, frustration, and powerlessness. Venting these feelings is an effective prelude to learning about treatment alternatives and participating in planning management of the disease and related problems. Using touch, eye contact, and accepting facial expressions—important aspects of effective care in most situations—are especially meaningful to patients with disfiguring skin lesions, because of the positive regard these behaviors convey.

As with any chronic condition, successful adaptation involves progress toward self-acceptance and periods of apparent regression and discouragement. Patients unable to adapt constructively often benefit from a referral to a psychiatric clinical nurse specialist or other mental health professional.

Rehabilitative management of lesions involves many of the same approaches used in preventive, supportive, and restorative care. Good hygiene, maintaining healthful nutritional and fluid intake, regular exercise, and stress-management strategies contribute to general health and well-being and support healing of lesions. Therapeutic baths and other measures to reduce pruritus provide symptomatic relief of discomfort. Some conditions require special skin care and dressings.

Patients with chronic or slow-healing surgical wounds are often candidates for home care. These patients need a holistic approach to care that takes into consideration social and financial variables, in addition to the physical care of the wound. Establishing a trusting relationship through effective communication is pivotal. Teaching basic asepsis and techniques for wound assessment and care promotes transition to self-management of the wound. Attention to nutritional status is of primary importance. A study of patients receiving home care for wounds found many indicators of nutritional deficiencies. Nearly all the patients had insufficient calorie intake for optimum healing, over half had less than the recommended daily allowance of protein, many had inadequate intake of vitamin C, and more than two thirds had lost weight.[38] Significantly delayed healing is a certain consequence of nutritional deficiencies such as this.

Despite the challenges patients with serious wounds and chronic skin diseases must face, sensitive nursing care with an emphasis on collaborative management can make a significant difference in patient outcomes.

EVALUATION

Evaluating outcomes of patient care is a collaborative responsibility. Clear and reasonable outcomes with measurable or observable evaluation criteria make evaluation straightforward and uncomplicated. Nurse and patient can easily evaluate progress toward healing during the course of care using measurements of wound or lesion size and depth as criteria. Other concrete evidence such as a change in tissue color from black (necrotic tissue) or yellow (fibrous debris or viscous exudate) to red (healthy granulation tissue) is also useful for evaluation. Making a chart or graph keeps visual evidence of progress at hand. The need for changes in approaches as well as satisfactory improvement will be apparent.

The many variables (eg, nutrition, hydration, perfusion, immune status, infection, presence of dead or damaged tissue) that influence healing create the need for a multifaceted approach to care, making altering the plan when progress is unsatisfactory a potentially complex undertaking. Assuring that implementation addresses as many variables as possible and revising one element of the plan at a time is effective.

COLLABORATIVE STRATEGY
PROMOTING WOUND HEALING

The expertise of many health professionals is sometimes needed to promote healing of chronic wounds. Nurses, enterostomal therapists, surgeons, diabetologists, social workers, and infectious disease specialists are among the many providers who may be involved in developing approaches to resolve difficult wounds. A holistic program emphasizing nutrition, exercise, hygiene, and stress management as well as innovative wound care strategies can achieve success.

SUMMARY

Skin, mucosa, and associated appendages are important to health and well-being. They carry out many important functions, including protection, temperature regulation, sensation, excretion, and lubrication.

Factors such as age, nutritional status, sun exposure, personal hygiene, and general health status alter skin and mucosal integrity. Skin lesions, pigmentation changes, wounds, and mucosal disruptions result from mechanical, chemical, biologic, and thermal trauma. The process of healing altered skin and tissue includes inflammation, proliferation, and maturation. Clotting, phagocytosis, fibroplasia, angiogenesis, collagen synthesis and lysis, and epithelialization occur to a greater or lesser degree, depending on whether a wound is healing by primary or secondary intention. Many of the same variables that affect skin integrity also influence healing. Complications such as hemorrhage, infection, and wound separation delay healing.

Assessment of integumentary health encompasses a history and examination of skin and mucosa in all parts of the body, as well as attention to cardiovascular functioning and nutritional, hydration, and emotional status.

Patient and nurse collaboratively address nursing diagnoses including impaired skin integrity, impaired tissue integrity, altered oral mucous membranes, and risk for impaired skin integrity through care planning and management strategies.

Collaborative nurse–patient management of skin and mucosal problems focuses on hygiene, comfort measures, wound care, and measures that support healing and general health such as optimal nutrition, fluid intake, regular exercise, and stress reduction. Teaching and effective communication contribute to positive outcomes. Evaluation of progress toward outcomes is also a mutual responsibility.

LEARNING OUTCOMES

Upon completing this chapter, the student should be able to:

1. List at least three functions of skin and mucosa.
2. Identify at least four factors that influence skin and tissue integrity and describe their effects.
3. Discuss three examples of altered skin and mucosal integrity.
4. Describe the difference between primary and secondary skin lesions and list three examples of each.
5. Describe four types of wounds.
6. Discuss two processes in each of the phases of wound healing.
7. Compare and contrast healing by primary and secondary intention.
8. Discuss a collaborative approach to a health history specific to skin and tissue.
9. Describe the main elements of a skin and tissue examination.
10. Formulate five skin and tissue nursing diagnoses using the taxonomy of nursing diagnosis.
11. Discuss three nursing implementations for impaired skin and tissue integrity for each of the following levels of care: preventive, supportive, restorative, and rehabilitative.
12. Discuss the importance of collaborative nurse–patient management of skin and tissue integrity.
13. Discuss four general nursing approaches to enhance wound healing.
14. Discuss nursing implications for the prevention or treatment of pressure ulcers.

REVIEW OF KEY TERMS

abrasion
caries
collagen
contaminants
contraction
contracture
contusion
cyanosis
debride
dehiscence
dermatitis
dermis
desquamation
dynamic support surface
ecchymosis
epidermis
epithelialization
erythema
eschar
exudate
gingivitis
granulation tissue
hematoma
incision
inflammation
ischemia
jaundice
keloid
lacerations
lesion
leukocytes
macrophages
neoplasms
normal flora
pallor
penetrating wound
perforating wound
petechiae
phagocytosis
pharyngitis
pilomotor activity
plaque
pressure ulcers
primary intention healing
primary lesions
pruritus
puncture wound
rhinitis
secondary intention healing
secondary lesions
shearing
stomatitis
subcutaneous fat
tartar
tertiary intention healing
thrombus
tissue load
urethritis
vaginitis
wound

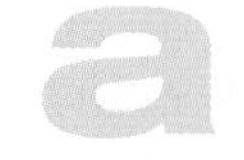

Having Read the Chapter, consider again the opening scenario, page 791, and the following responses to the questions.

Mr. Jones, at age 62, shows signs of sun damage caused by years of overexposure to ultraviolet sun rays. He now faces possible treatment for skin cancer, and although treatment may eliminate the risk posed by his current lesion, his age, previous exposure to radiation, pale, thin skin, and love of outdoor activity puts him at risk for future malignant skin changes. He will benefit from information on the risk factors of skin cancer, self-screening techniques, and preventive measures to limit further damage.

Mr. Jones should be instructed on these factors and the fact that prior sun exposure raises his risk of future lesions. However, the nurse can reassure Mr. Jones that early cancerous changes can be detected by regularly doing skin self-examination. The nurse can also teach Mr. Jones to perform regular exams, using a mirror to inspect hard-to-see areas like the shoulders, legs, face, and scalp. Mr. Jones should be taught to look for new lesions, particularly ones that do not heal, and observe for changes in size, shape, color, margins, or general appearance of old lesions that might suggest a malignancy. The nurse will also want to reinforce the importance of having regular professional checkups and reporting any observed skin changes, such as unhealing sores, to the physician as quickly as possible.

Mr. Jones may already understand how to avoid further exposure to harmful sun rays. The nurse should, however, begin by identifying what Mr. Jones already knows and what his concerns are. If Mr. Jones understands that sun exposure is a cause of skin cancer, he may worry, for example, that he will have to give up gardening. The nurse can reassure Mr. Jones that taking certain precautions will help to minimize his risk of future disease. Mr. Jones should be taught to:

- Apply sun screen with a high SPF to all exposed skin areas 30 minutes before going outside on sunny or overcast days
- Wear long pants, a long-sleeved, high-collared shirt, and a hat to shade his arms, shoulders, face and neck when gardening
- Garden before 10 AM and after 2 PM, when the sun's rays are not at peak strength, and avoid exposure between 10 AM and 2 PM.

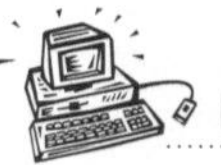

INTERNET RESOURCES

Web Site

Perioperative nursing resources:
http://www.aorn.org/nsgtoday/ internet/links.htm

Treatment of pressure ulcers, clinical practice guideline:
http:// www.AHCPR.gov/guide/

Assessment information:
http://www.merck.com/

REFERENCES

1. Williams PL, ed. *Gray's Anatomy.* 38th ed. New York: Churchill Livingstone; 1995.
2. Wysocki AB. A review of the skin and its appendages. *Adv Wound Care.* 1995;8:53–70.

3. Margolis DF. Definition of a pressure ulcer. *Adv Wound Care.* 1995;8:28-8–28-10.
4. Bergstrom M, Chair. *Quick Reference Guide for Clinicians. Pressure Ulcer Treatment.* Rockville, MD: US Dept HHS; 1994.
5. Bergstrom N, Allman RM, Alvarez OM, Bennett MA, et al. Pressure ulcer treatment: quick reference guide for clinicians. *Adv Wound Care.* 1995;8:22–44.
6. Mayhall CG, ed. *Hospital Epidemiology and Infection Control.* Baltimore: Williams & Wilkins; 1996.
7. Sams WM, Lynch PJ, eds. *Principles and Practice of Dermatology.* 2nd ed. New York: Churchill Livingstone; 1996.
8. Timby BK. *Fundamental Skills and Concepts in Patient Care.* 6th ed. Philadelphia: Lippincott; 1996.
9. Lewis SM, Collier IC, Heitkemper MM. *Medical Surgical Nursing.* 4th ed. St. Louis: Mosby; 1996.
10. Messer MS. Wound care. *Crit Care Nurs Q.* 1989;11:17–27.
11. Hollingsworth H. The healing process. *Nurs Times.* 1994; 90:85–86.
12. Smith SF, Duell DF. *Clinical Nursing Skills.* 4th ed. Stamford, CT: Appleton & Lange; 1996.
13. Jones PL, Millman A. Wound healing and the aged patient. *Nurs Clin North Am.* 1990;25:263–277.
14. Dirkesen SR, Lewis SM, Collier IC. *Clinical Companion for Medical-Surgical Nursing.* St. Louis: Mosby; 1996.
15. Habif TP. *Clinical Dermatology.* 3rd ed. St. Louis: Mosby; 1996.
16. Flanagan M. Assessment criteria. *Nurs Times.* 1994;90:76–88.
17. Stotts NA. In: Kinney MR, Packer DR, Dunbar SB. *AACN's Clinical Reference for Critical Care Nursing.* 3rd ed. St. Louis: Mosby; 1993.
18. Flynn JB, Bruce NP. *Introduction to Critical Care Nursing.* St. Louis: Mosby; 1993.
19. Young ME. Malnutrition and wound healing. *Heart Lung.* 1988;17:60.
20. Sheffield PJ. Tissue oxygen measurements. In: Hunt TK, Davis J, eds. *Problem Wounds: The Role of Oxygen.* New York: Elsevier; 1988.
21. Berk WA. Demystifying treatment of simple lacerations. *Emergency Med.* 1993;25:26–35.
22. Iverson-Carpenter MS. Impaired tissue integrity. *J Gerontol Nurs.* 1988;14:25–29.
23. Demling RH, Way LW. Burns and other thermal injuries. In: Way LW, ed. *Current Surgical Diagnosis and Treatment.* Norwalk, CT: Appleton & Lange; 1991.
24. Dimant J, Francis ME. Pressure sore prevention and management. *J Gerontol Nurs.* 1988;14:18–25.
25. Vasconez LO, Vasconez HC. Plastic and reconstructive surgery. In: Way LW, ed. *Current Surgical Diagnosis and Treatment.* 10th ed. Stamford, CT: Appleton & Lange; 1994.
26. Hay WW, Groothuis JR, Hayward AR, Levin MR, eds. *Current Pediatric Diagnosis and Treatment.* 13th ed. Stamford, CT: Appleton & Lange; 1996.
27. McHenry LM, Salerno E. *Pharmacology in Nursing.* 19th ed. St. Louis: Mosby; 1995.
28. Lane LD, Winslow EH. Oxygen consumption, cardiovascular response, and perceived exertion in healthy adults during rest, occupied bedmaking, and unoccupied bedmaking. *Cardiovasc Nurs.* 1987;23:31–36.
29. Stotts NA, Barbour S, Griggs K, Bouvier B, et al. Sterile vs. clean technique in wound care of patients with open surgical wounds in the post–op period: a pilot study. *J of Wound, Ostomy, Continence Nurs.* 1997; 24(1):10–18.
30. Agency for Health Care Policy and Research. *Clinical Practice Guideline, No. 15: Treatment of Pressure Ulcers.* Rockville, MD: US Department of Health and Human Services. AHCPR Publication No. 95-0652; 1994.
31. Krasner D, Kennedy ML. Using the no-touch technique to change a dressing. *Nurs 94.* 1994;24(9):50–52.
32. Vande Berg JS, Robson MC, Mikhail RJ. Extension of the life span of pressure ulcer fibroblasts with recombinant human interleukin-1β. *Am J Pathol.* 1995;146:1273–1282.
33. Wood JM, Evans PE 3rd, Schalbreuter KU, Jacobson WE, et al. A multicenter study of the use of pulsed low-intensity direct current for healing chronic stage II and stage III decubitis ulcers. *Arch Dermatol.* 1993;129:999–1009.
34. Nussbaum EL, Bieman I, Mustard B. Comparison of ultrasound/ultraviolet-C and laser for treatment of patients with spinal cord injury. *Phys Ther.* 1994;74:812–823.
35. Golstein B, Sanders JE, Benson B. Pressure ulcers in SCI: does tension stimulate wound healing? *Am J Phys Med Rehabil.* 1996;75:130–133.
36. Lyons CR. Emerging roles of nitric oxide in inflammation. *Hosp Pract.* 1996;31:69–86.
37. Salcido R, Donofrio JC, Fischer SB, LeGrand EK, et al. Evaluation of ibuprofen for pressure ulcer prevention: application of a rat pressure ulcer model. *Adv Wound Care.* 1995;8:30–55.
38. Stotts NA, Whitney JD. Nutritional intake and clients in the home with open surgical wounds. *J Commun Health Nurs.* 1990; 7: 77–86.

28

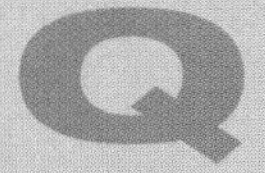

Beryl Jacks is a 72-year-old widow recovering from a right total hip replacement. It is her fifth postoperative day, and she will be discharged tomorrow. Mrs. Jacks has lived alone in a single-story home since her husband's death 5 years ago. Her son, his wife, and a granddaughter live 50 miles from her home. She is particularly fond of her daughter-in-law. Although her son and daughter-in-law work full time, her daughter-in-law plans to spend a week with her after her discharge. When Mrs. Jacks was admitted to the hospital, she was 15 pounds under her ideal weight for her height. She said that she doesn't have much of an appetite, eating only a midday meal and a piece of fruit at bedtime. She will be given a prescription for Tylenol #3 for her surgical pain.

What information and observations are important in the nursing assessment of Mrs. Jacks' current nutritional status? Why?

What should her nurse teach Mrs. Jacks about nutrition before she is discharged?

How might her nurse include Mrs. Jacks' daughter-in-law in the plan of care?

What community resources might benefit Mrs. Jacks' nutritional needs?

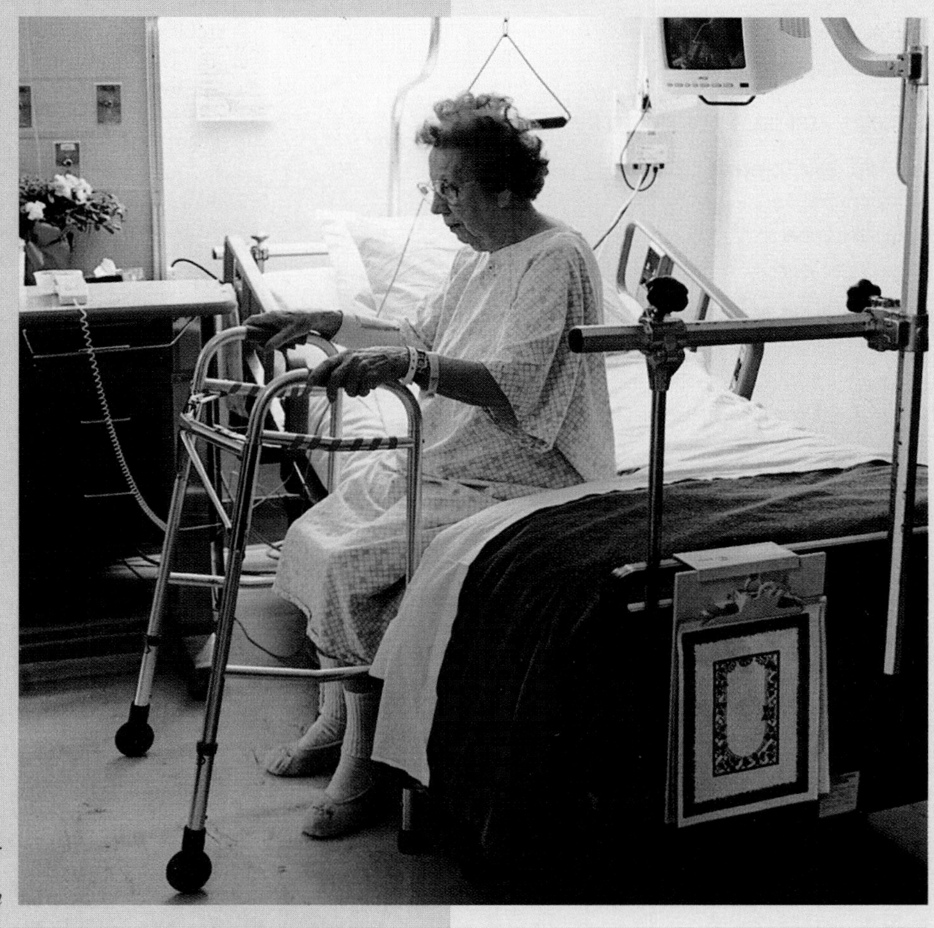

Nutrition

Barbara J. Sarter and Victoria Orton

CHAPTER OUTLINE

Nutrition is the process by which the energy and chemical compounds necessary to create, maintain, and restore body cells are made available to the body from food. The quality of a person's nutrition and his or her state of health are intimately related. Consequently, nutrition is an important focus of nursing care. Nurses collaborate with patients, dietitians, pharmacists, and physicians in planning care to meet patients' nutritional needs, which vary with specific problems. Nurses' participation in this collaboration is central, for it is usually nurses who are primarily responsible for implementing the plan of nutritional care. In addition to the biologic importance of food as a source of nutrients and energy, food also has cultural meaning. Eating is a source of great pleasure for human beings. It is sensory stimulation, a social activity, and psychological reward.

SECTION 1

UNDERSTANDING NUTRITION

Nutrition plays a major role in promoting, maintaining, and restoring health. No matter what a patient's particular health care need, nutrition is always relevant. When a patient's status is on the wellness side of the health–illness continuum, nutritional counseling can help to maintain or increase wellness. When patients are experiencing illness, dietary factors may be the primary cause of the problem, or if not, they are important in restoring health.

The role nutrition plays in attaining optimal health has been repeatedly acknowledged. Although the body can easily adapt to less-than-ideal nutritional states, low-quality nutrition takes a subtle toll on people. There is a direct and causal relationship between the quality of one's nutritional intake and overall sense of well-being.

Dietary factors also are linked to a multitude of diseases. For example, heart disease, certain cancers, cerebral vascular disease, and diabetes all are leading causes of death among North American adults. All of these have proved associations with dietary habits. For example, research has clearly linked a diet high in animal fat with heart disease, hypertension, and cerebral vascular disease.[1] Because of increasing public awareness of the nutritional basis of many serious diseases, more consumers desire information about healthful eating. Nurses have many opportunities to provide accurate, current information.

Perhaps in no other area of health care is a collaborative process so clearly necessary as in nutrition. Because of the highly individualized meanings, habits, and preferences that surround eating, patients' input in nutritional planning is critical. Dietitians, of course, are key figures in this process, as are nurses. A dietitian is formally educated and licensed to provide nutrition-related services such as dietary assessment, teaching, and planning. Physicians may determine what kind of diet is appropriate as a primary or supportive therapy for a medical condition. Nurses must be able to provide ongoing assistance in the implementing a dietary regimen.

OPTIMAL NUTRITIONAL STATUS

Ingestion and digestion, absorption and metabolism, and the social aspects of eating influence nutritional status. This section concerning nutritional science examines energy balance in the body, the basic nutrients involved in nutritional processes, and the phases of the process that begins with food ingestion and ends with the use of nutrients for energy production and cellular metabolism.

ENERGY BALANCE

The concept of energy balance is fundamental to an understanding of nutrition. Energy is the power to do work. A fuel is a source of energy. Human beings can be viewed as energy systems in continuous interaction with the environment, which is a larger energy system. The human organism requires a constant input of energy to maintain its life processes and support its physical activities. **Energy balance** refers to the amount of energy input in relation to the amount of energy output in a given system:

Energy balance = energy input − energy output.

A positive energy balance occurs when input exceeds output. A negative energy balance occurs when input is less than output.

Energy Input

Food provides the fuel for the human energy system. The energy of food, stored in the chemical bonds of protein, fat, and carbohydrate molecules, is measured in kilocalories (kcal) or joules. A calorie is a unit of heat energy. A **kilocalorie** is the amount of heat needed to raise the temperature of 1 kg of water by 1 degree C. Although some people use the words *kilocalorie* and *calorie* interchangeably, kilocalorie is the correct term when referring to nutritional energy.

The body stores energy in the forms of glycogen, fats, and protein. When food is not available, the body draws on its own energy stores to maintain its life processes. Glycogen is the stored form of carbohydrates and is most readily available. It is stored in liver and muscle tissue. Fats are the next most easily recovered energy stores. They are stored in the body's adipose tissue. Proteins are the last source of energy to be drawn upon when carbohydrate stores are exhausted and fat is being used. To use protein as a fuel, the body must break down its own tissues, principally muscles.

Energy Output

Energy output is the energy the body uses. The energy used in the body to support tissue and organ functions is drawn from the high-energy phosphate bonds of adenosine triphosphate (ATP) molecules, which are generated by metabolic pathways. The amount of energy a person uses is primarily determined by two factors: the basal metabolic rate and the amount of physical activity. Energy expended for food digestion, absorption, and transport (the thermic effect of food) also plays a role. To maintain a daily energy balance, the energy intake in the form of food must equal the energy expenditure from basal metabolism, physical activity, and the thermic effect.

Basal Metabolism. Basal metabolism refers to the chemical reactions occurring when the body is at rest. The **basal metabolic rate (BMR)** is the amount of energy required to maintain the resting body's internal activities after an overnight fast. General formulas have been developed to calculate the BMR of the average man and woman (Clinical Guideline 28–1).

Other Energy Expenditures. Table 28–1, which lists the average energy used during some common daily activities, is a tool for estimating daily activity expenditure. The amount of energy used in processing ingested food can be calculated by taking 10 percent of the total kilocalories of food consumed. A patient's total daily energy expenditure (energy output) can then be determined using the formula is Clinical Guideline 28–1.

CLINICAL GUIDELINE 28–1

ESTIMATING DAILY ENERGY EXPENDITURE

CALCULATING BASAL METABOLIC RATE (BMR)

Women:

BMR = 0.9 kcal/kg body weight/hour

Men:

BMR = 1.0 kcal/kg body weight/hour

CALCULATING DAILY ENERGY EXPENDITURE

Daily energy expenditure = (BMR × 24) + (0.1 × daily kcal consumption) + energy of daily activities

Energy Balance and Body Weight

The relationship between energy input and output is reflected in a person's body weight. If a state of energy balance or equilibrium exists (input = output), the body weight remains stable, unless a factor such as fluid imbalance causes a weight change. If a positive energy balance exists (input > output) over a period of time, weight increases. If a prolonged negative balance occurs (input < output), a person experiences weight loss (Fig. 28–1). Many factors

TABLE 28-1. AVERAGE ENERGY EXPENDITURE OF MEN AND WOMEN DURING COMMON DAILY ACTIVITIES

Activity	kcal/hour/kg	
	Men	*Women*
Very Light Dressing, washing, using a computer, writing, standing	1.5	1.3
Light Housekeeping, gardening, walking slowly on level surface	2.9	2.6
Moderate Digging, sexual activity, walking (small hills), stair climbing	4.3	4.1
Heavy Shoveling snow, climbing steep hills, jogging, swimming	8.4	8.0

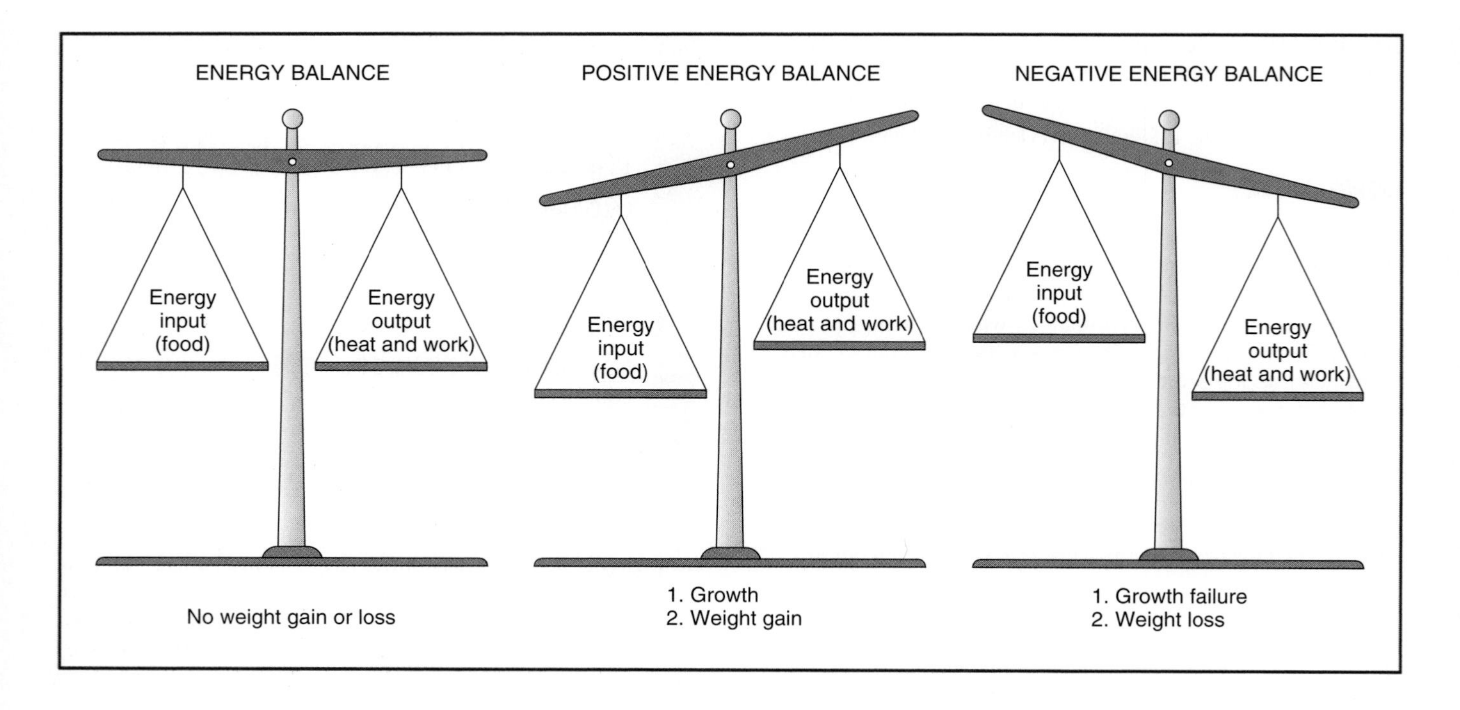

Figure 28–1. Concepts of energy balance. *(From Lewis CM.* Nutrition and Nutritional Therapy in Nursing. *Norwalk, CT: Appleton & Lange; 1986.)*

cause predictable changes in individuals' basal metabolic rate, and thus change their energy requirements. These factors include age, the relative amounts of muscle and fat tissue in the body, endocrine influences, climate, illness, activity level, and malnutrition. The role of each is discussed in a later section.

BASIC NUTRIENTS

The six major classes of **nutrients,** the chemical compounds necessary for body functioning, are carbohydrates, proteins, fats (lipids), vitamins, minerals, and water. Carbohydrates, proteins, and fats are called "energy nutrients" because they provide kilocalories from food. Vitamins, minerals, and water are vitally important substances for the building, maintenance, and metabolic regulation of body tissues. **Essential nutrients** cannot be manufactured by the human body; therefore, they must be supplied by food.

Carbohydrates

The two broad categories of **carbohydrates**—simple and complex—are the most readily available and most efficiently metabolized source of energy for the body.

Simple carbohydrates include monosaccharides (glucose, fructose, galactose) and disaccharides (maltose, sucrose, lactose). Sucrose (table sugar) is the principal ingredient of candies, cakes, and other concentrated sweets. Lactose is the principal carbohydrate found in milk. Some people lack the ability to digest lactose, particularly people from Native American, Asian, African, Mediterranean, and Middle Eastern populations.

Complex carbohydrates, or polysaccharides, are composed almost entirely of glucose molecules bonded together in varying ways. Some examples are glycogen, starches, and fiber. **Glycogen** is not found in food, but is the body's stored form of glucose. **Starches** consist of molecules of 300 to 1000 glucose units. Starches are found in plant foods such as seeds, grains, potatoes and other roots, and legumes (beans). **Dietary fiber,** such as cellulose and pectin, is composed primarily of cell wall constituents of plant foods. In the digestive tract, food fibers absorb water, bind minerals and lipids, and exercise the intestinal muscles by adding bulk.

Increasing attention is being paid to the importance of dietary fiber in the management of a variety of digestive tract disorders and diseases (constipation, diarrhea, hemorrhoids, colon cancer), as well as in lowering elevated glucose and blood lipids. Insoluble fibers, found in fruits, vegetables, and bran, are thought to help prevent colon cancer. Soluble fiber in legumes and oat bran appears to lower blood cholesterol levels. There is no standardized recommendation for the optimal daily intake, but some recent sources suggest a daily intake of 20–35 g of dietary fiber[2] (Table 28–2).

That carbohydrates (starches in particular) are fattening is a misconception. Actually, 1 gram of carbohydrate provides 4 kcal of energy, far less than fats. Carbohydrate foods are easily digested, absorbed, and metabolized; they are economical, tasty, and readily available. The most important reason for ensuring an adequate intake of carbohydrates is that a constant source of glucose is needed for brain and nerve function: a minimum of 100 g of carbohydrate per day is essential. Approximately 55 to 60 percent of the daily kilocaloric intake should come from complex carbohydrates.

Proteins

A **protein** is a complex, long molecular chain made up of large molecules called **amino acids** (or peptides). Human proteins contain 22 different amino acids, in an astronomically large number of possible combinations. Most proteins are polypeptides containing 100 to 300 amino acids, folded and coiled elaborately. The human

TABLE 28-2. FIBER CONTENT OF SELECTED FOOD PORTIONS

Food Portion	Fiber (g)
Fruits	
1 small apple	2
1 small banana	2
1 small orange	2
1 small pear	4
Breads/Cereals	
Whole-wheat bread, 1 slice	2
Dry oatmeal, 3 Tbsp	2
Corn flakes, ⅔ cup	2
Wheat bran, 1 Tbsp	2
Grape Nuts, 6 Tbsp	4
Shredded wheat, 2 biscuits	8
All Bran, 6 Tbsp	12
Vegetables	
Lettuce, raw, 1 cup	1
Carrots, ⅓ cup	2
Celery, 1 cup	2
Brussel sprouts, 4	2
Baked beans, canned, ½ cup	8

body contains tens of thousands of proteins, only a small fraction of which have been identified.

Differences in body proteins distinguish one human chemically from any other. Some of the major body proteins are enzymes, antibodies, and transport proteins. The latter help move molecules in and out of cells or carry molecules from organ to organ through body fluids. All body tissues and organs are made of proteins. Proteins also help to maintain fluid balance by increasing osmotic pressure, attracting water, and buffering acids.

Protein in food supplies the body with the amino acids it needs to make its own proteins. Although the body can make some amino acids itself, there are nine amino acids, called **essential amino acids,** that it cannot make. Because amino acids are not stored, a cell must have available at the same time all the amino acids it needs to synthesize a particular protein. Thus, dietary sources of protein should supply all nine of the essential amino acids in a single meal. A **complete protein** is one containing all the essential amino acids in amounts that are adequate for use in the body. Amino acids that cannot be used for synthesis are converted to fat. The essential and nonessential amino acids found in human proteins are:

Essential Amino Acids
- Histidine
- Isoleucine
- Leucine
- Lysine
- Methionine
- Phenylalanine
- Threonine
- Tryptophan
- Valine

Histidine is essential for infants, and may be essential for adults.

Nonessential Amino Acids
- Alanine
- Arginine
- Aspartic acid
- Citrulline
- Cysteine
- Cystine
- Glutamic acid
- Glycine
- Hydroxylysine
- Hydroxyproline
- Proline
- Serine
- Tyrosine

One gram of protein yields 4 kcal of energy. As mentioned earlier, however, dietary protein is not efficiently metabolized for energy; it takes more energy input to metabolize than either carbohydrate or fat. Having ample carbohydrate and adequate fat in the diet avoids the breakdown of amino acids for energy production. If amino acids are metabolized for energy, they cannot be used to build vital body proteins. Approximately 10 percent of daily caloric intake, or 0.8 g/kg of body weight, should come from protein.

Fats

Fats, also called **lipids,** are a classification that includes fats, oils, and sterols. Fats yield more energy per gram than either carbohydrates or proteins—9 kcal. They insulate the body and protect vital organs and tissues, facilitate nerve conduction, transport other molecules, and are necessary components of many hormones. Fats are composed of triglycerides, which in turn consist of three **fatty acids** combined with glycerol. Fatty acids consist of a chain of carbon atoms with hydrogen attached.

Much attention has recently been focused on the various types of fatty acids and their relation to cardiovascular disease. A **saturated fatty acid** has a chain in which every available carbon bond is holding a hydrogen atom. If only one point on the chain is missing a hydrogen atom, the molecule is called a **monounsaturated fatty acid. Polyunsaturated fatty acids** have more than one point of unsaturation.

Dietary saturated fats play a major role in the development of cardiovascular diseases such as hypertension, coronary artery disease, stroke, and cerebral vascular disease. All animal foods contain saturated fats, red meats having the highest proportion. Most vegetable fats and oils (except coconut and palm oils) are unsaturated. No more than 10 percent of total fat intake should consist of saturated fats.

Phospholipids and sterols (compound fats) combine simple fats with other compounds. They contribute about 5 percent of total dietary fat. Lecithin and cholesterol are of particular nutritional significance. Lecithin, a phospholipid, is an important constituent of cell membranes and helps to keep other fats dissolved in body fluids. Cholesterol, a sterol, is manufactured by the liver from either carbohydrate or fat.

Cholesterol is transformed into sex or adrenal hormones or into bile. It can be combined with proteins and lipids (lipoproteins) for use by body tissues. It is sometimes deposited in arterial walls, contributing to atherosclerosis. Two kinds of cholesterol-carrying lipoproteins are associated with coronary heart disease. High-density lipoproteins (HDLs) lower the risk of this disease, whereas low-density lipoproteins (LDLs) increase the risk.

In general, high blood cholesterol levels are associated with an increased risk of heart attacks. Some people may have a genetically determined high level of endogenous cholesterol, which persists despite severe limits on dietary cholesterol intake. Foods that

TABLE 28-3. ESSENTIAL INFORMATION ON VITAMINS

Vitamin	RDI	Food Sources	Actions	Deficiency Symptoms	Toxicity Symptoms
Fat-soluble Vitamins					
A	5000 IU	Dairy fats, yellow fruits and vegetables, dark green vegetables, tomatoes, liver, kidney, egg yolk.	Adaptation of eyes to light; skin and mucous membrane integrity; normal growth and bone development; role in reproduction.	Night blindness, thick, dry skin, dry eyes, retarded growth, sterility, decreased salivation, diarrhea, susceptibility to infection.	Hypervitaminosis A: *Early:* fatigue, anorexia, irritability, nausea, vomiting, inflamed and cracked lips, dry skin, itching. *Late:* liver and spleen enlargement, headache, subcutaneous swellings, bone pain, hair loss, ascites.
D	400 IU[a]	Fortified milk, eggs, butter, sunlight.	Essential for calcium and phosphorus metabolism.	*Children:* skeletal deformities (rickets), decreased muscle tone, constipation, decreased blood Ca^{++} *Adults:* soft bones	Hypervitaminosis D: elevated blood calcium, calcification of arteries and organs.
E	30 IU[a]	Polyunsaturated oils, whole grains, dark green, leafy vegetables, nuts, legumes.	Antioxidant; cell membrane integrity.	*Infants:* hemolytic anemia, edema, skin lesions. *Adults:* muscular weakness.	Depression, fatigue, diarrhea with cramps, blurred vision, headaches, dizziness, increased clotting time, increased blood lipids, decreased thyroid levels.
K	No Daily Value	Dark green leafy vegetables, liver, eggs, cheese, wheat bran.	Essential for normal blood clotting.	Abnormal bleeding, hemorrhage.	*Infants:* anemia, hyperbilirubinemia, brain damage.
Water-soluble Vitamins					
C	60 mg	Citrus fruits, papaya, cantaloupe, strawberries, cranberry juice, broccoli, brussel sprouts, cauliflower, cabbage, dark green leafy vegetables, tomatoes, baked potatoes, green peppers.	Synthesis and maintenance of collagen: bone and teeth formation; blood vessel integrity; wound healing. Antioxidant: protects other nutrients; facilitates iron absorption; activates folic acid; synthesis of norepinephrine during stress; inflammation; resistance to infection.	Scurvy; skin hemorrhages; swollen, bleeding gums; soft tissue and joint hemorrhage; bone malformations; poor wound healing; weight loss; anemia; depression.	Increased urinary uric acid; kidney stones, anemia; coagulation disorders; false-positive test for sugar in urine; diarrhea; rebound scurvy if massive doses suddenly withdrawn.
Thiamine (B_1)	1.5 mg	Brewer's yeast; wheat germ; whole grains; meat, especially pork; legumes; enriched cereals; nuts; enriched rice.	Essential for energy metabolism, especially of glucose; transmission of nerve impulses; conversion of tryptophan to niacin.	Beriberi; anorexia; muscle weakness; calf tenderness; palpitations; polyneuropathy (tingling and numbness of extremities, foot and wrist drop); constipation. "Wet beriberi": peripheral edema; hypertension; tachycardia; cardiac enlargement; heart failure; elevated blood pyruvic acid and lactic acid.	Unknown.

TABLE 28-3. CONTINUED

Vitamin	RDI	Food Sources	Actions	Deficiency Symptoms	Toxicity Symptoms
Water-soluble Vitamins (continued)					
Riboflavin	1.7 mg	Brewer's yeast, organ meats, milk, dairy products, meats, poultry, fish, breads, pasta, enriched rice.	Energy metabolism; activates vitamin B_6; protein metabolism; formation of red blood cells; gluconeogenesis; glycogen formation; healthy skin and eyes.	Ariboflavinosis: dermatitis; cracks at corners of mouth; sore tongue; photophobia; corneal reddening.	Unknown.
Niacin	20 mg NE[b]	Organ meats, brewer's yeast, meats, poultry, fish, peanuts, coffee, enriched grains; can be formed from tryptophan.	Energy metabolism; synthesis of carbohydrates, protein, fat; healthy skin, nerves, digestive tract; lowers cholesterol levels.	Pellagra: dermatitis; diarrhea; dementia.	Unknown.
Pyridoxine (B_6)	2 mg	Wheat, corn, wild rice, chicken (light meat), meat, liver, green beans, potatoes, bananas.	General metabolism of nutrients; synthesis of nonessential amino acids; converts tryptophan to niacin.	Anemia, weakness, dermatitis, gastrointestinal upset, irritability, convulsions.	Unknown.
Folic acid	400 μg	Liver, meat, green leafy vegetables, whole grains; peanuts.	General metabolism of nutrients, especially amino acids; maturation of red blood cells; prevents certain birth defects and heart disease.	Megaloblastic anemia: weakness; shortness of breath; sore tongue; diarrhea; edema; gastrointestinal upset.	Unknown.
Cobalamin (B_{12})	6 μg	Liver, meat, milk, cheese, eggs.	General metabolism of nutrients.	Megaloblastic anemia (see folic acid), pernicious anemia (symptoms similar to megaloblastic anemia), numbness and tingling of hands and feet.	Unknown.
Pantothenic acid	10 μg	Liver, eggs, milk, whole grains, legumes.	General metabolism of nutrients; synthesis of cholesterol.	Weakness, nausea, irritability.	Unknown.
Biotin	300 μg	Egg yolk, liver, milk, whole grains, legumes.	General metabolism of nutrients.	Dermatitis, muscle weakness, depression.	Unknown.

[a] IU = International Unit
[b] NE = niacin equivalent (includes niacin the body can make from free tryptophan in foods)
Sources: Adapted from Lutz CA, Przytulski KR. Nutrition and Diet Therapy. *2nd ed. Philadelphia: FA Davis; 1997; and from Cataldo CB, Debruyne LK, Whitney EN.* Nutrition and Diet Therapy. *4th ed. St. Paul, MN: West; 1995.*

contain large amounts of cholesterol are red meats, dairy products, and eggs.

Because of the risks associated with saturated fats and cholesterol, unsaturated fats should comprise two thirds of dietary fat intake. Polyunsaturated fats vary widely in their degree of unsaturation. A particular class of polyunsaturated fatty acids called omega-3 fatty acids (found primarily in fish oils) may be of particular benefit in preventing and/or managing heart disease, cancer, arthritis, and asthma. Monounsaturated fatty acids (found in canola oil and olive oil) tend to reduce blood cholesterol while maintaining optimal HDL levels. Thus, one third of dietary fat should be monounsaturated and one third polyunsaturated.

A polyunsaturated fatty acid, linoleic acid, is the only essential fatty acid—that is, the only one that cannot be produced by the body. Linoleic acid must be obtained from dietary sources such as vegetable oils. It enhances skin and capillary integrity, lowers serum cholesterol levels, and prolongs blood clotting time.

Vitamins

Vitamins are organic nutrients indispensable in the metabolic processes that produce energy, manufacture red blood cells, and build and repair body tissues (Table 28–3). Vitamins are classified according to their solubility in fat or in water. The fat-soluble vitamins are vitamins A, D, E, and K. They are found in dietary fats and oils and stored in body fat tissues. Because they can be stored, an excessive intake of fat-soluble vitamins can lead to serious toxic effects.

The water-soluble vitamins include the B vitamins and vitamin C. They are found in the water portion of foods and are carried into water-filled body tissues. They can be readily excreted in the urine if their blood concentration rises too high, although toxic effects may still occur if taken in excessive amounts. The eight B vitamins play specific roles as parts of coenzymes, which combine with inactive proteins to make active enzymes.

Minerals

Like the vitamins, **minerals** do not provide energy but are essential chemical elements in maintaining numerous body processes (Table 28–4). Calcium, potassium, and sodium are minerals that are so critical to vital body functions that they are carefully monitored and regulated in acutely ill patients. Other minerals may also need careful adjustment in seriously ill persons with specific deficiencies or excesses.

Water

Water is more than a medium of transport for nutrients. It is so essential to life that without it, the body can survive only a few days. A minimum of 4 to 6 cups of water is needed daily. Water is part of the molecules that form body cells, tissues, and organs. It is part of numerous chemical reactions, a solvent for many molecules and nutrients, a lubricant and shock absorber, and it plays a role in temperature regulation. Fluid and electrolyte balance is influenced by water intake. With water excretion, metabolic waste products are eliminated from the body. Water is also a by-product of metabolism. Complex renal and hormonal mechanisms adjust water excretion in accordance with water intake so that an appropriate balance is maintained.

Effects of Storage, Processing, and Cooking

Food storage and preparation affect its nutritional value. In general, the longer fruits and vegetables are stored before being eaten, the greater the loss of vitamins. When storage is necessary, temperatures should be kept as low as possible without freezing food, moisture in the produce should be maintained, and exposure to light should be minimized. The more a food is divided or cut, the more surface area is exposed to oxygen in the air. Vitamin C is readily oxidized and rendered nutritionally inactive. Fruits and vegetables, therefore, should be cut as little and as close to eating time as possible. The peels of fruits and vegetables have the most concentrated supplies of vitamins, so trimming or peeling will reduce their vitamin value. Thoroughly washing fruits and vegetables to remove pesticide residues is important.

In canning fruits and vegetables, approximately 50 percent of vitamins are lost, whereas freezing lowers losses somewhat, particularly in fruits. Drying causes losses of vitamins A, C, and B_1 (thiamine). Boiling causes significant losses of minerals, vitamin C, and vitamin A. Steaming reduces these losses by about 50 percent, and pressure cooking greatly minimizes nutrient losses.

DIGESTION, ABSORPTION, AND METABOLISM

The processes that enable the body to convert ingested food into energy are digestion, absorption, and metabolism. Digestion and absorption occur in the organs of the gastrointestinal tract. Metabolism occurs in the cells of the body.

Digestion

Digestion is the breakdown of foods into smaller compounds that can be absorbed into body fluids. Digestion involves mechanical and chemical activity.

Mechanical Digestion. Mechanical digestion involves neuromuscular processes that move food through the digestive tract. Tonic muscle contractions create a continuous muscle tone that facilitates the passage of food and periodic, rhythmic contractions, called **peristalsis,** move intestinal contents through the gastrointestinal tract.

Chemical Digestion. Chemical digestion is accomplished by four types of secretions produced in the gastrointestinal tract:

- Enzymes specific for the breakdown of particular nutrients
- Hydrochloric acid and buffers
- Mucus
- Water and electrolytes

The secretions of the gastrointestinal tract are controlled by neural and hormonal mechanisms.

Absorption

The small intestine is the major site of nutrient **absorption,** where the end products of digestion are transferred from the lumen of the intestine into the circulatory system. The large molecules of proteins, fats, and carbohydrates must be broken down to their smallest components before absorption can occur. Proteins are absorbed in the form of amino acids; fats as fatty acids or glycerides; and carbohydrates as monosaccharides, such as glucose or fructose.

TABLE 28-4. SELECTED ESSENTIAL MINERALS

Mineral	RDI/RDA	Food Sources	Actions	Deficiency Symptoms	Toxicity Symptoms
Major Minerals					
Calcium	1000 mg	Milk, cheese, dark green vegetables, legumes.	Bone and tooth formation; blood clotting; nerve transmission; muscle activity; enzyme activator.	Stunted growth, muscle spasm, osteoporosis, altered thyroid function, hypertension.	Renal stones, constipation, blocks absorption of iron, zinc.
Phosphorus	800 mg (age 18–24: 1200 mg)	Milk, cheese, meat, poultry, fish, whole grains.	Bone and tooth formation; acid–base balance; component of coenzymes.	Weakness: demineralization of bone.	Muscle spasm, skeletal deformities (rickets).
Magnesium	300 mg F: 280 mg M: 350 mg	Whole grains, green leafy vegetables, nuts.	Component of enzymes; regulates nerve and muscle activity.	Tremors, muscle spasms, muscle weakness, seizures, hypertension.	Sedation.
Sulfur	No RDI/RDA	Component of some amino acids and several B vitamins found in dietary proteins.	Component of cartilage, tendon, hair, nails.	Does not occur unless severe protein deficiency present.	Toxicity from nutritional intake unknown.
Sodium	2400 mg (DRV)[a]	Salt, milk, cured meats, pickles, canned soups, cheese, eggs.	Fluid balance; cell membrane permeability; muscle irritability.	Muscle cramps, nausea, anxiety.	Fluid retention, elevated blood pressure.
Potassium	3500 mg (DRV)[a]	Meats, milk, fish, whole grains, oranges, bananas, winter squash, legumes, potatoes.	Fluid balance; transmission of impulses; muscle contraction.	Muscular weakness, paralysis, loss of reflexes, heart block, hypertension.	Nausea, diarrhea, muscular weakness, dyspnea, cardiac arrest.
Chloride	No RDI/RDA	Salt, processed foods.	Fluid balance; acid–base balance; component of gastric juice.	Muscle cramps, anorexia.	Vomiting.
Trace Minerals					
Iron	18 mg	Liver; lean beef; legumes; whole grains; green leafy vegetables; dried fruit.	Constituent of hemoglobin and enzymes.	Iron-deficiency anemia: weakness, pallor, fatigue.	Acute poisoning: shock, death. Overload: liver damage, heart disease.
Iodine	150 μg	Saltwater fish and shellfish, iodized salt.	Constituent of thyroid hormones.	Goiter (enlarged thyroid).	Iodide goiter, skin lesions.
Fluoride	No RDI/RDA	Drinking water, tea, fish.	Strengthens tooth and bone structure.	Dental caries.	Mottling of teeth, bone deformation.
Zinc	15 mg	Meats, seafood, whole grains, legumes, nuts.	Cofactor for more than 70 enzymes; factor in protein metabolism; necessary for WBC functioning.	Growth retardation, impaired immune function, skin lesions, poor healing, poor eyesight.	Anemia, vomiting, diarrhea, muscle pain, renal failure.
Selenium	F: 55 μg M: 70 μg	Seafood, meat, whole grains.	Component of enzyme that functions as antioxidant.	Muscle pain, heart enlargement, heart failure.	Loss of hair, skin lesions, nerve damage.
Copper	2 mg	Shellfish, grains, nuts, legumes, meats.	Component of enzymes for energy production and hemoglobin synthesis; tissue maintenance.	Anemia, bone demineralization, decreased immunity.	Liver and central nervous system damage, kidney malfunction.
Cobalt	No RDI/RDA	Liver, meat, milk, cheese, eggs.	Constituent of vitamin B_{12}.	Not reported except as vitamin B_{12} deficiency.	Malformation of red blood cells.

Continued

TABLE 28-4. CONTINUED

Mineral	RDI	Food Sources	Actions	Deficiency Symptoms	Toxicity Symptoms
Chromium	No RDI/RDA	Brewer's yeast, liver, oysters, wheat products, legumes.	Facilitates glucose uptake by cells; decreases serum cholesterol and triglycerides.	Impaired glucose metabolism.	Toxicity from nutritional intake unknown.
Manganese	No RDI/RDA	Nuts, wheat bran, leafy green vegetables, seeds, dried legumes.	Enzyme activator; catalyst for metabolic reactions.	Weight loss, skin lesions.	Inhalation of dust causes tremors; muscle weakness.
Molybdenum	No RDI/RDA	Organ meats, legumes, grains, dark green leafy vegetables.	Constituent of enzymes that catalyze oxidative reactions.	Deficiencies unknown.	Goutlike symptoms (joint inflammation).

[a] Daily reference value.

Sources: Adapted from Lutz CA, Przytulski KR. Nutrition and Diet Therapy. *2nd ed. Philadelphia: FA Davis; 1997; and from Cataldo CB, Debruyne LK, Whitney EN.* Nutrition and Diet Therapy. *4th ed. St. Paul, MN: West; 1995.*

Vitamins and minerals are absorbed through the wall of the small intestine. The inner mucosal lining of the small intestine is designed to provide maximum surface area for absorption. Mucosal folds have microscopic projections (villi and microvilli) that increase the inner surface area of the intestine several hundredfold.

The primary function of the large intestine is the absorption of water, although minerals and electrolytes are also absorbed. It normally takes from 8 to 72 hours for food to reach the rectum. The bacteria of the colon serve a number of important functions. They synthesize vitamin K and some of the B vitamins, break down bilirubin into bile pigments, and break down undigested proteins and carbohydrates.

Metabolism and Storage

Metabolism refers to the cellular processes by which absorbed nutrients are used for cell maintenance and energy production. The ultimate biologic purpose of food ingestion is to support these metabolic processes, which are essential to the life of the organism. Anabolism and catabolism are the two basic metabolic activities. In **anabolism** body substances are synthesized, and in **catabolism** substances are broken down, leading to energy release.

Carbohydrate Metabolism. As noted earlier, carbohydrate metabolism is the primary source of energy for the body. The glucose available to body cells is obtained from dietary starches and sugars, certain amino acids, and glycerol. Excess glucose is stored as glycogen in limited amounts in the liver. After the body's energy requirements are met, any excess glucose is converted to fat and stored in adipose tissue. Blood glucose levels must be maintained within normal limits for the brain to function properly. Extreme alterations of blood glucose lead to convulsions, coma, and death.

Insulin is the major hormone involved in regulating blood glucose levels. Insulin lowers blood glucose. When it is absent, blood glucose levels increase. Six other hormones can cause blood glucose levels to rise by directly or indirectly stimulating glycogenolysis or gluconeogenesis in the liver. **Glycogenolysis** is the breakdown of glycogen into glucose, which is then released from the liver into the bloodstream. **Gluconeogenesis** is the synthesis of glucose from amino acids or lipid breakdown products by the liver.

Protein Metabolism. Individual cells synthesize proteins they need from amino acids. Protein catabolism occurs primarily in the liver by a process called *deamination,* in which the nitrogen unit is removed from an amino acid, resulting in ammonia and a carbon skeleton (or keto-acid). Ammonia is converted to urea and excreted via the kidneys. Keto-acids can be used to make other amino acids, produce energy via the Krebs cycle, or make fatty acids for storage.

Nitrogen balance is the equilibrium between protein anabolism and catabolism. Nitrogen is the element that distinguishes proteins from carbohydrates and fats. Nitrogen is ingested in protein and excreted in the by-products of protein catabolism (urea, creatinine, uric acid, ammonia salts). When a person is in a state of nitrogen balance, the intake of nitrogen (or protein) is equal to its output. A person who is healthy, ambulatory, not rapidly growing or replenishing tissue, and is consuming a diet adequate in essential amino acids and calories is in nitrogen balance. A **positive nitrogen balance,** however, exists when protein intake is greater than output; it facilitates periods of rapid growth or tissue replacement. A **negative nitrogen balance** exists when protein output exceeds intake. The condition occurs when a diet contains inadequate essential amino acids or calories and during periods of immobility or severe physical trauma.

Fat Metabolism. Fat metabolism and storage occur primarily in the liver and in adipose tissue. When fat is absorbed from the intestine or released form storage in adipose tissue, glycerol, one of the components of fat, is converted to pyruvate, and fatty acids, the other fat component, are converted to acetyl coenzyme A (acetyl-CoA) in the liver. From either of these points, the Krebs cycle may begin, producing energy.

Metabolic Interconversions. Metabolic interconversions are necessary because food intake is variable and intermittent. It is important that all foods be convertible to the same intermediate metabolites and that metabolism continue in the absence of food. This is

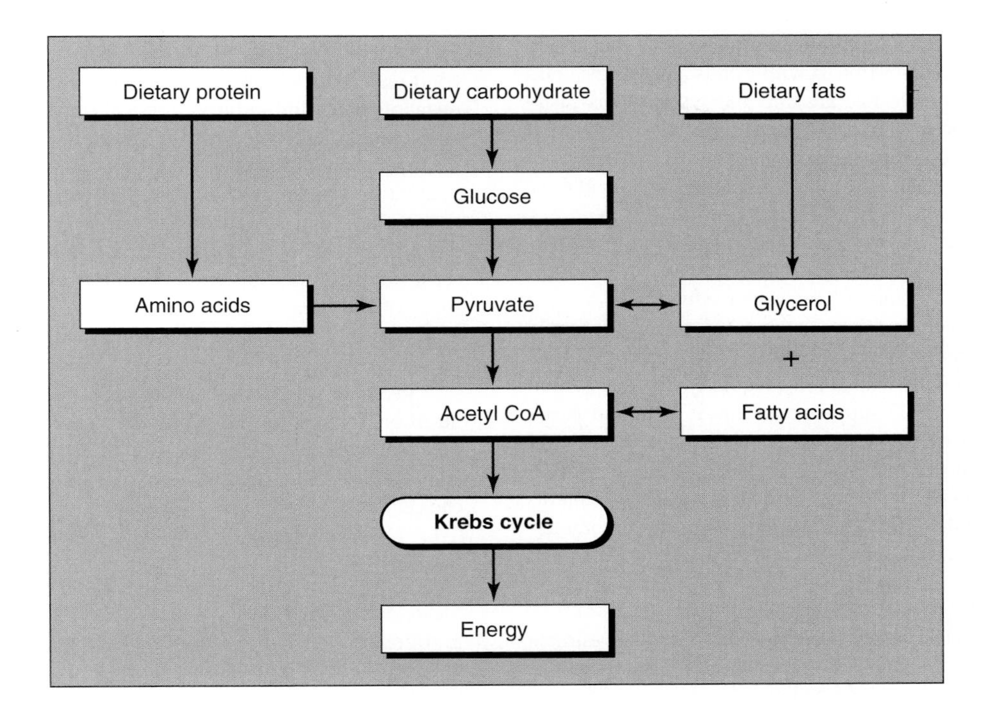

Figure 28–2. Pathways of energy metabolism.

indeed the case. Figure 28–2 illustrates the central pathways of energy metabolism. Because brain cells do not store glucose and require a continuous supply for adequate energy and proper functioning, it is crucial that a minimum blood glucose level be maintained at all times. It is undesirable for amino acids and glycerol to be used for glucose synthesis because toxic metabolites (ketones) accumulate and protein tissue is depleted. Therefore, the importance of adequate dietary intake of carbohydrate cannot be overemphasized.

FACTORS AFFECTING NUTRITIONAL STATUS

BASAL METABOLIC RATE AND ENERGY REQUIREMENTS

Many factors can cause changes in an individual's basal metabolic rate. In a cool environment, for example, metabolic rate increases to generate more heat to maintain normal body temperature. In a warm environment the metabolic rate is lowered to decrease heat production. When an individual has a fever, the metabolic rate increases by about 7 percent for each increase of 1 degree Fahrenheit (0.83 degree C) in body temperature. A person with a higher than normal proportion of muscle to fat tissue will have a higher metabolic rate. Developmental stages marked by rapid body growth (infancy, early childhood, puberty, and pregnancy) are characterized by an increase in metabolic rate. Aging, however, is associated with a decreased rate. Many diseases also alter the metabolic rate. For example, cancer and hyperthyroidism increase metabolic rate; hypothyroidism and malnutrition cause a significant decrease.

When metabolic rate increases, energy requirements also increase to maintain an individual's weight. If energy intake is not increased by adding calories, weight loss will occur. Conversely, if metabolic rate has decreased and energy intake is not decreased, weight gain occurs.

AGE

In addition to variations in metabolic rate and hence energy requirements, different age groups have varying requirements of specific nutrients. If these age-specific nutrient needs are not met, growth and development may be severely retarded or serious health problems may develop.

Infants

The first year of life is a critical period nutritionally. For example, brain development continues through the tenth month after birth. Rapid growth and metabolism require a large amount of energy and nutrients in relation to body weight.

Human breast milk is clearly superior to man-made formulas. It provides carbohydrate and protein in the form of lactose and lactoalbumin, both of which infants can easily digest. Its fat contains a generous proportion of linoleic acid. It contains ample amounts of vitamins and minerals and factors to facilitate their absorption. Breast milk also contains maternal antibodies that protect infants from serious infections until their own immune systems mature. Another component stimulates the development of the infant's gastrointestinal tract and its colonization with normal bacteria.

When a woman chooses not to breast-feed or is unable to, prepared formula feedings provide adequate nutrition. National and international standards exist. The Infant Formula Act of 1980 requires that the standards established by the American Academy of Pediatrics be met by commercial formulas. When an allergy to cow's milk is present, soy-based formula is often recommended.

Solid foods should be introduced into the infant's diet at 4 to 6 months of age. Rice cereal fortified with iron is a good first solid food, as allergic reactions to rice are rare and the starch is easily digestible. Then barley or oatmeal can be tried, followed by vegetables, and then by fruits. Egg yolk can be given at 6 months, but egg whites should be the last food added due to their allergic potential. Meats should be introduced late as well.

Water is vitally important for infants. Infants require proportionally more water in relation to body weight than do adults. Water should be offered frequently between feedings.

Nutritional supplements for newborn infants are generally not needed, with three possible exceptions: vitamin D, fluoride, and iron. Breast-fed infants who are not regularly exposed to sunlight will require vitamin D supplementation. If an infant is not receiving fluoridated water, appropriate supplementation should be provided after 6 months of age. Starting at around 6 months of age, an iron supplement may be prescribed for breast-fed infants until adequate iron intake from solid foods can occur. If commercial formulas are used, they should be iron-fortified.

Children

During childhood lifelong food habits are established. Desirable habits are encouraged with a child's exposure to a wide variety of foods. Concentrated sweets should be limited, a balanced diet consumed, and regular eating times established.

After the age of 1 year, body fat decreases and muscle and bone mass increase. Growth typically comes in spurts, and food intake naturally increases. Protein, calcium, phosphorous, magnesium, and zinc are important nutrients during childhood. Milk is still the most important food in the diet. For growing children, 3 cups of milk per day should be provided. For children over the age of 2, the use of low-fat or nonfat milk leaves more kilocalories available for consumption in the form of foods rich in other essential nutrients, such as iron. School-age, preadolescent children experience a latent period of growth, with a relative decline in energy needs.

Adolescents

The growth spurt in adolescence requires additional calories, protein, minerals, and B vitamins. Iron deficiency can easily develop in girls due to blood losses from menstruation. Fad foods and fad diets are popular with adolescents. A high intake of fast foods at the expense of other foods results in serious nutritional imbalances: an excess of kilocalories, fat, salt, and sugar and deficiencies of vitamins, minerals, and complex carbohydrates. Fad diets to lose weight or change one's figure may precipitate severe malnutrition. Severe forms of this problem are the eating disorders anorexia nervosa and bulimia.

Young and Middle-aged Adults

Body maintenance and repair, rather than growth, drive nutritional needs during adulthood. Notable exceptions to this are during pregnancy and lactation. For example, it has been conclusively established that folic acid supplementation will help prevent the development of neural tube defects in the fetus.[3,4] Caloric requirements are generally significantly lower once adult growth is completed, and they tend to steadily decline with age due to decreases in basal metabolic rate. The calories that are consumed, therefore, must be rich in essential nutrients so that adequate intake can be maintained.

Older Adults

Food requirements for the elderly are influenced by reduced basal metabolic rates and reduced physical activity. Excessive fat should be avoided due to a decreased absorption capacity. Calcium intake for women should be at least 1200 mg daily to prevent the development of osteoporosis. Iron supplementation may also be necessary because decreased stomach acid production and antacid use decrease iron absorbed from foods. Loss of teeth, diminished senses of smell and taste, and reduced saliva production reduce some of the pleasure associated with eating and may influence food choices. Digestive disorders and medications sometimes suppress appetite.

Personal and social factors also influence elderly people's nutritional status. Living alone may decrease motivation to prepare well-balanced meals and eliminates the social pleasure associated with eating. Financial resources often limit affordable food choices.

HEALTH STATUS

Major deviations from or threats to health usually create specific nutritional needs and serious nutritional problems if the needs are not met. Serious and chronic illnesses, surgery, injury, and emotional stress are some of the health-related factors influencing nutritional needs of patients.

Serious Illness

Acute major illnesses such as serious infections increase energy and specific nutrient requirements, due, in part, to the generalized stress response that is initiated. An extreme stress response can produce a hypermetabolic state in which protein catabolism to meet energy requirements may reach such intensity that a state of exhaustion and death may occur.

Chronic Illness

Individuals with chronic illnesses require consistently adequate diets to maintain a maximum quality of life. Loss of appetite is a common problem that makes it particularly difficult to maintain optimum intake. Lack of energy or ability to prepare or eat food is another complicating factor. Immobility causes significant losses of calcium from bones and stimulates protein catabolism.

Surgery

Food and fluids are generally withheld for at least 8 hours before surgery, and for many patients (particularly those undergoing gastrointestinal surgery) it may be several days or even weeks after surgery before a regular diet can be resumed. Loss of blood and body fluids during and after surgery can create severe fluid and electrolyte imbalances, as well as shock. Protein is the nutrient used most by patients recovering from surgery. It plays a pivotal role in antibody formation and wound healing. There is also a general increase in energy (calorie), zinc, and vitamin A, K, and C requirements.[5]

Emotional Stress

Emotional stress creates the same generalized stress response as physical stress. Therefore, prolonged emotional stress can deplete protein stores and lower immunity by reductions in proteins available for antibody and white blood cell production. Loss of appetite may make replacement of protein stores difficult.

SOCIOCULTURAL INFLUENCES

Culture of Origin

Diverse food habits develop as a result of the cultural home environment, the acculturation of an individual to the dominant culture, and economic realities. Moreover, the symbolic meaning of foods and dietary habits may be intermingled with the culture's religious traditions, social organization, and history (see Chap. 10). It is essential that the nurse be familiar with the cultural dimensions of a patient's dietary practices. The inclusion of cultural preference in the dietary plan often enhances patient compliance. Encouraging the family to bring the patient's favorite cultural foods from home can facilitate this. For a collaborative relationship to exist, the nurse must realize the role culture plays in a patient's plan of care.

Religion

The influence of a patient's religion on dietary habits may take the form of certain traditional ritual foods on specific days while including specific prayers or rituals with the meal. One example is the Passover seder for the Jewish faith (in which certain foods take on symbolic meaning). Some religions impose food restrictions for their faithful. Catholics traditionally abstain from meat on Ash Wednesday and the Fridays of Lent, as well as fast on Ash Wednesday, Good Friday, and an hour before the reception of Communion. These practices, however, are not enforced when a patient is ill. Many faiths engage in prayer (to give thanks) before and after mealtime. Moslems and Jews (especially Orthodox) permit only kosher meats, which have had the blood drained. Jewish kosher laws prohibit serving meat and dairy products at the same meal or on the same set of dishes. Mormons, Moslems, and Seventh-Day Adventists do not allow alcoholic beverages. Many Seventh-Day Adventists are vegetarian, as are virtually all Hindus and Buddhists. Nurses can support the spiritual needs of their patients by helping them fulfill their religious dietary practices.

Knowledge About Nutrition

Many people may base their food habits on beliefs acquired through competitive product advertising, peer groups, or family and cultural traditions, rather than expert information.

Extremes in dietary habits or food fads can lead to severe nutrient deficiencies. Individuals with severe or chronic health problems are particularly vulnerable to promises of instant cures, as are adolescents or young adults who are dissatisfied with their bodies.

The best defense against food faddism is an informed consumer. The Internet offers numerous resources for nutritional education, diet analysis, consumer information, and information about nutrition-related topics, such as obesity and eating disorders. Nurses also have an important role to play as providers of information about diet. Individuals who understand basic nutritional principles should be able to make choices that are personally satisfying and nutritionally appropriate.

Lifestyle

Lifestyle influences what one eats, where one eats, with whom one eats, whether one cooks for oneself, how frequently food purchases are made, and how much time is allowed for eating. Drug and alcohol abuse significantly damages a person's nutritional status. Drugs, including tobacco, disturb appetite and can either raise or lower the basal metabolic rate. Alcohol abuse causes serious long-term nutritional effects and potentially fatal liver disease.

Personal Preference

Many people make conscious decisions regarding how and what they will eat on the basis of their personal philosophy, beliefs, and values. Vegetarianism is an example. Nurses must understand the many different forms a vegetarian diet may take and the nutritional implications. Table 28–5 describes various types of vegetarian diets and nutritional considerations. Guidelines for vegetarian meal planning are discussed in the following section.

Economic Situation

In the United States more and more families and individuals are living below the poverty line. For many, hunger and malnutrition are serious problems. People may not have the time, space, or equipment necessary for the most basic cooking. Although the problem requires large-scale social planning, nurses can help people with limited food-purchasing power to obtain the greatest possible nutritional return for every dollar spent on food. Strategies for purchasing economical and nutritious meals are discussed in Section 3.

TABLE 28-5. TYPES OF VEGETARIAN DIETS

Type	Description	Nutritional Considerations
Vegan or strict	Includes only foods derived from plants. No meat, dairy products, or eggs.	Requires careful planning to provide complementary proteins. Requires vitamin B_{12} supplement, possibly vitamin D.
Lactovegetarian	Includes dairy products along with plant foods. No eggs.	Dairy products complement plant products and provide important minerals such as calcium. Careful planning to include iron, vitamin B_{12}.
Ovolactovegetarian	Includes dairy products, eggs, and plant foods.	All nutrients can be provided in sufficient quantities.
Ovovegetarian	Includes eggs and plant foods.	All nutrients can be provided in sufficient quantities.

GUIDELINES AND STANDARDS FOR NUTRITION

Numerous government and private organizations and groups have developed guidelines for healthy eating. Nurses must understand what population a set of guidelines is for, what its stated purpose is, and who developed the guidelines (for example, were the guidelines written to promote a particular industry's product?). The following guidelines and standards are widely recognized and have relevance for the general population of healthy people.

HEALTHY PEOPLE 2000

Guidelines created by the Department of Health and Human Services contain a national strategy for improving the health of the nation for the next decade. They focus on preventing chronic illnesses, injuries, and infectious diseases.[1] The following are risk reduction strategies addressing nutritional needs:

- Reduce dietary fat intake to an average of 30 percent of calories or less and average saturated fat intake to less than 10 percent of calories among people aged 2 and older.
- Increase complex carbohydrate and fiber-containing foods in the diets of adults to 5 or more daily servings for vegetables (including legumes) and fruits, and to 6 or more daily servings for grain products.
- Increase to at least 50 percent the proportion of overweight people aged 12 and older who have adopted sound dietary practices combined with regular physical activity to attain an appropriate body weight.
- Increase calcium intake so at least 50 percent of youth aged 12 through 24 and 50 percent of pregnant and lactating women consume 3 or more servings daily of foods rich in calcium, and at least 50 percent of people aged 25 and older consume 2 or more servings daily.
- Decrease salt and sodium intake so at least 65 percent home meal preparers prepare foods without adding salt, at least 80 percent of people avoid using salt at the table, and at least 40 percent of adults regularly purchase foods modified or lower in sodium.
- Reduce iron deficiency to less than 3 percent among children aged 1 through 4 and among women of childbearing age.
- Increase to at least 85 percent the proportion of people aged 18 and older who use food labels to make nutritious food selections.

RECOMMENDED DIETARY ALLOWANCES

The **Recommended Dietary Allowances (RDAs)** are guidelines for the intake of specific nutrients for normal, healthy people living in the United States. These recommendations are provided by the

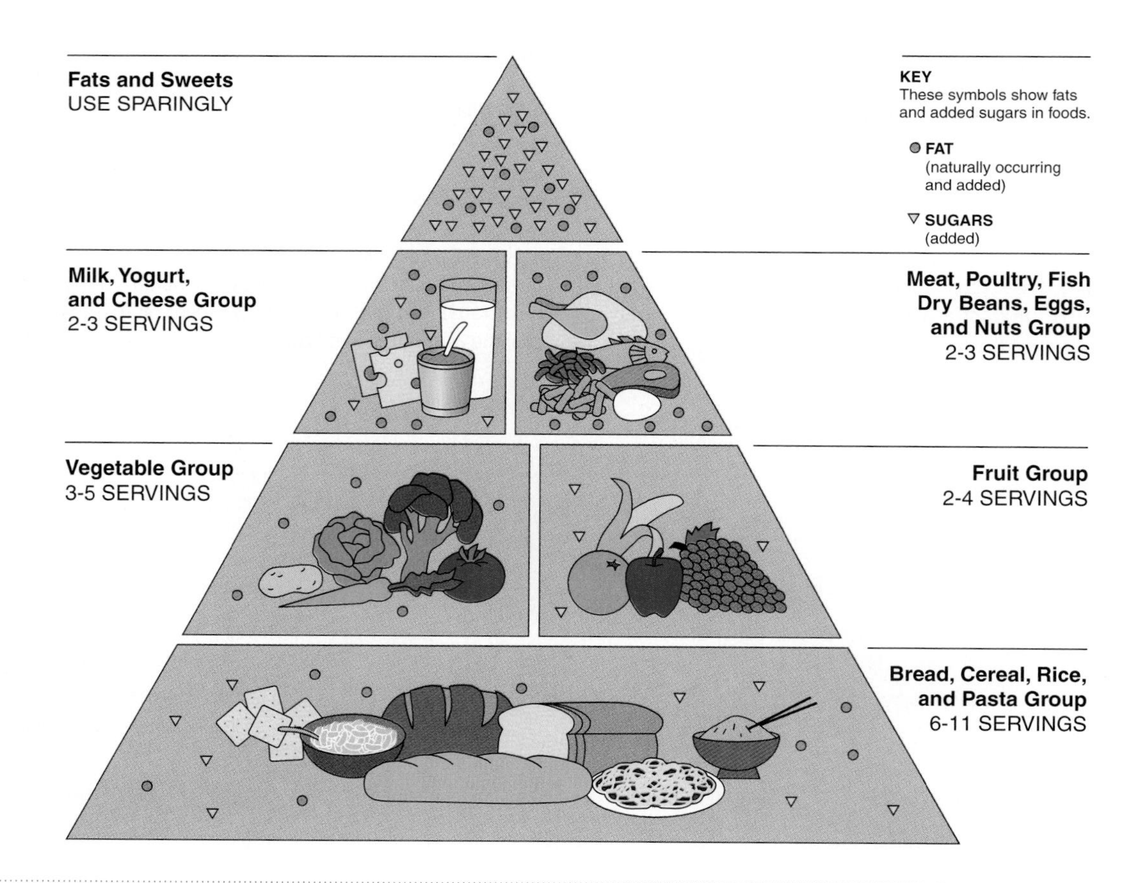

Figure 28–3. The US Department of Agriculture (USDA) Food Guide Pyramid.

Food and Nutrition Board, National Academy of Sciences, and National Research Council and are periodically updated in accordance with ongoing research.

The RDAs are used by the health team as standards for assessing and planning individual dietary intake, parenteral and enteral formulas, and food supplementation programs. To use the RDAs in determining the nutritional quality of a diet, one must first use a table of food composition listing the nutrient and energy content of foods, and then add up the amount of individual nutrients consumed during a 24-hour period. The totals are then compared to the RDAs for the person's age and gender, adjusting, if needed, for diverse weights or heights. Many computerized diet analysis programs are available for performing these calculations.

DAILY FOOD GUIDE

The US Department of Agriculture issued a revised edition of its Basic Four Food Groups Guide in 1991. It is called *The Guide to Daily Food Choices,* and emphasizes a high-complex-carbohydrate, low-fat diet. A graphic form, The Food Guide Pyramid, was released the following year (Fig. 28–3). The **food pyramid** illustrates the relative amounts of each food group that should be consumed in a healthy diet. This figure is available to nurses and other professionals without charge to use for nutritional counseling.

CANADA'S GUIDELINES FOR HEALTHY EATING

Canadian guidelines were published in 1990 to provide general approaches for a healthy diet for persons older than 2 years. Similar to the US Daily Food Guide, the guidelines emphasize a high-carbohydrate, low-fat diet along with regular physical activity.

VEGETARIAN DIETARY GUIDELINES

Vegetarian diets, if planned carefully, can be among the most healthful. They automatically reduce dietary risk factors for cancer and heart disease (particularly saturated fats) and provide generous amounts of fiber, vitamins, and minerals. For vegetarians who do not eat milk products, vitamin B_{12} supplements are recommended.

To ensure high-quality, complete protein intake, the concept of **complementary proteins** can be used. Research has identified specific combinations of plant foods that provide complete protein intake in a single meal:

- Legumes plus grains
- Legumes plus seeds
- Leafy vegetables plus grains

Table 28–6 provides a daily food guide for vegetarians to be used in meal planning.

STANDARDS FOR FOOD LABELING

The Nutrition Labeling and Education Act of 1990 revised the requirements for food label information to meet growing consumer interest in healthy eating. With a few exceptions, all new food labels must have an information panel entitled

TABLE 28-6. DAILY FOOD GUIDE FOR VEGETARIANS

Food Group	Suggested Daily Servings	Serving Sizes
Breads, cereals, and other grain products	6 or more	1 slice bread ½ bun, bagel, or English muffin ½ c cooked cereal, rice, or pasta 1 oz dry cereal
Vegetables	4 or more[a]	Approximately 1 c cooked or raw
Fruits	3 or more	1 piece fresh fruit ¾ c fruit juice ½ c canned or cooked fruit
Legumes and other meat alternates	2 to 3	½ c cooked beans 4 oz tofu or tempeh 8 oz soy milk 2 tbs nuts or seeds 1 egg or 2 egg whites
Milk and milk products	2 to 3 servings[b]	1 c low-fat or skim milk 1 c low-fat or nonfat yogurt 1½ oz low-fat cheese

[a] Include 1 cup of dark greens daily to help women meet iron requirements.
[b] If not using milk or milk products, use soy milk fortified with calcium and vitamin B_{12}.

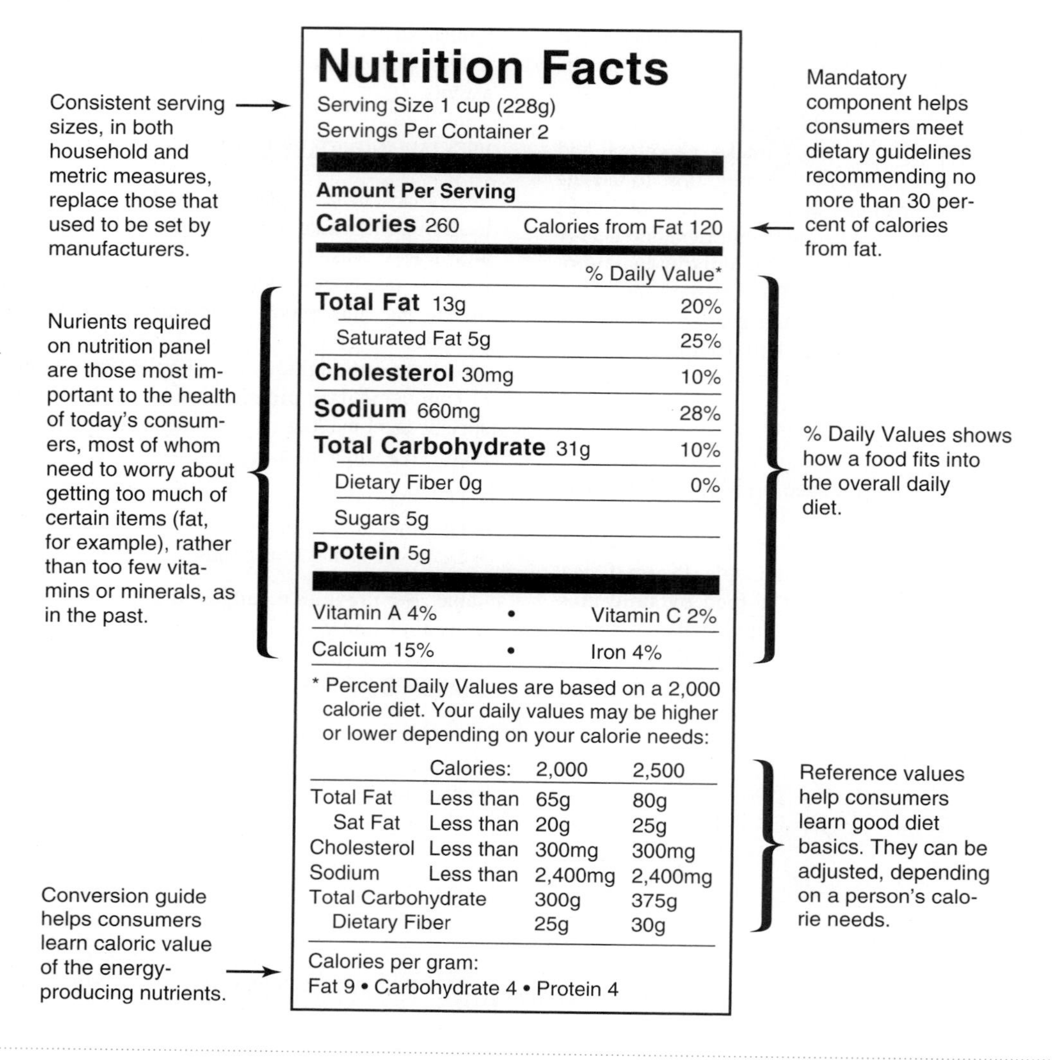

Figure 28–4. Nutrition label format.

Nutrition Facts (Fig. 28–4). This panel must provide information about:

- serving size
- number of servings per container
- total kilocalories per serving
- fat per serving with breakdown of saturated fat and cholesterol
- sodium per serving
- total carbohydrate, fiber, sugars, and protein per serving
- percentage of Daily Values for a person requiring 200 kcal/day of total fat, saturated fat, cholesterol, sodium, total carbohydrate, fiber, sugars, protein, vitamin A, vitamin C, calcium, and iron

The **Daily Values** (Fig. 28–5) are standard values developed by the Food and Drug Administration (FDA) for use on food labels. They consist of two sets of reference values. The **Reference Daily Intakes (RDI)** are for protein, vitamins, and minerals and are based on the RDA. The **Daily Reference Values (DRV)** are for important nutrients that do not have an established RDA.

ALTERED NUTRITION

NUTRITIONAL DISORDERS

Nutritional disorders are among the world's most serious health problems. It is nurses' responsibility to recognize the early signs of such disorders to enable prompt intervention. Nutritional disorders tend to run an insidious, progressive course. In many cases, however, if treated early, the disorder can be completely cured.

Protein–Calorie Malnutrition

Protein–calorie malnutrition (PCM), or protein–energy malnutrition (PEM), results from an overall lack of quality and quantity of food. It is the most prevalent and most serious of the world's primary malnutrition syndromes. PCM is also the most common serious nutritional problem faced by patients in health care facilities. There are three categories of PCM: (1) protein deficiency state, (2) cachexia, and (3) mixed state.

Reference Daily Intakes (RDI)

Nutrient	Amount
Protein[a]	50 g
Thiamin	1.5 mg
Riboflavin	1.7 mg
Niacin	20 mg NE
Biotin	300 μg
Pantothenic Acid	10 mg
Vitamin B_6	2 mg
Folate	400 μg
Vitamin B_{12}	6 μg
Vitamin C	60 mg
Vitamin A[b]	5000 IU
Vitamin D[b]	400 IU
Vitamin E[b]	30 IU
Calcium	1000 mg
Iron	18 mg
Zinc	15 mg
Iodine	150 μg
Copper	2 mg

[a]The RDI for protein varies for different groups of people: pregnant women, 60 g: nursing mothers, 65 g; infants under 1 year, 14 g; children 1 to 4 years, 16 g.
[b]The RDI for fat-soluble vitamins are expressed in International Units (IU), an old system of measurement. The current RDA and tables of food composition use a more accurate system of measurement. Equivalent values are as follows: for vitamin A, 875 μg RE; for vitamin D, 6.5 μg; for vitamin E, 9 mg α-TE.

Daily Reference Values (DRV)

Food Component	DRV	Calculation
Fat	65 g	30% of kcalories
Saturated fat	20 g	10% of kcalories
Cholesterol	300 mg	Same regardless of kcalories
Carbohydrate (total)	300 g	60% of kcalories
Fiber	25 g	11.5 g per 1000 kcalories
Protein	50 g	10% of kcalories
Sodium	2400 mg	Same regardless of kcalories
Potassium	3500 mg	Same regardless of kcalories

Note: The DRV were established for adults and children over 4 years old. The values for energy-yielding nutrients are based on 2000 kcalories a day.

Figure 28–5. Daily Values for food labels. NE = niacin equivalent (defined on Table 28–3). RE = retinol equivalent. TE = alpha tocopherol equivalent.

Protein Deficiency State. **Protein deficiency state** occurs in patients experiencing short-term but severe disorders or stressors such as a major injury or surgery. Nutritional support is often given in the form of intravenous fluid, glucose, and electrolytes. Because 1 liter of most standard intravenous solutions provides only 170 calories and are totally without amino acids, protein malnutrition can develop after about 10 days if no other caloric source is provided. Clinical signs of this form of PCM include fatigue, apathy, edema, decreased serum protein levels, mild to moderate weight loss, and muscle weakness. Because the body breaks down the most readily available protein sources first, blood proteins and enzymes are depleted, and even intestinal microvilli may be damaged. Therefore, lab values such as serum albumen, serum transferrin, and WBCs are low in patients with protein deficiency state. Protein deficiency may impair wound healing and decrease immunity.

Cachexia. A second type of PCM is generalized **cachexia,** which develops from a more gradual but prolonged period of having insufficient food. The result is a syndrome of emaciation, tissue wasting, severe underweight, and sometimes diarrhea.

Mixed State. The third type of PCM is a mixed state in which a cachectic person is subject to an acute stress, for example, a person with cancer who develops pneumonia. A life-threatening situation can result due to severe depletion of vital nutrients, such as the B-complex vitamins, iron, or vitamins A and C. Physiologic changes in the gastrointestinal mucosa may impair nutrient absorption and further aggravate malnutrition. Aggressive nutritional support may be needed to save the patient's life. Clinical signs of this form of PCM include symptoms of specific nutrient deficiencies as well as symptoms associated with the underlying PCM.

Nurses play a critical role in the prevention of PCM. An assessment of every patient's nutritional status is essential. Patients at high risk for developing PCM should be identified—for example, those scheduled for major surgery; those who are unable to ingest foods; those scheduled for multiple procedures requiring pre-fasting; those suffering from nausea and vomiting; and those experiencing major physiologic or psychological stresses. Early interventions such as careful diet planning and use of supplements should be initiated for those at high risk. Continuous monitoring

INSIGHTS FROM NURSING LITERATURE

IDENTIFYING NUTRIENT DEFICIENCIES

Stephens D, Jackson PL, Gutierrez Y. Subclinical vitamin A deficiency: a potentially unrecognized problem in the United States. Pediatr Nurs. *1996;22:377–389.*

The authors note that vitamin A deficiency in its subclinical form—mild deficiency undetectable at physical examination—is a world health problem probably underrecognized in the United States. They note that vitamin A deficiency is associated with measles morbidity. Thus, the American Academy of Pediatrics recommends that supplements be given children 6 to 24 months of age who are hospitalized with measles. Children at risk for deficiency are (1) young children who do not eat sufficient fruits (2 to 4 servings per day) and vegetables (3 to 5 servings per day); (2) children living at or below the poverty line; (3) children with inadequate health care/immunizations; (4) recent immigrants or refugees from countries with a high incidence of vitamin A deficiency; and (5) children with diseases of the pancreas, intestines, or liver or with ineffective fat digestion, which reduces absorption of fat-soluble vitamins, including vitamin A. The authors caution that children considered high risk for vitamin A deficiency are often at risk for other nutritional and health problems as well.

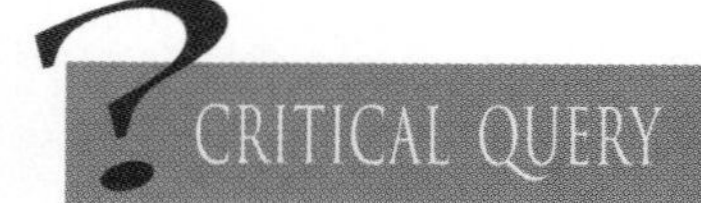

Stephens and associates[6] warn that when children are placed on vitamin supplements, the parents must be told that "more is not better," and to consider vitamins as medications to be kept in a safe place away from children. What advice about safety should the nurse give to parents of preschool children?

of nutritional status and collaboration with dietitians and physicians to initiate enteral or parenteral feeding early rather than late are also essential.

Vitamin and Mineral Deficiencies

Primary nutritional deficiencies are due to an inadequate intake of a nutrient. Secondary nutritional deficiencies result from the body's inability to absorb or metabolize specific nutrients and are encountered in a wide variety of disease states and situations. For example, surgical removal of a part of the gastrointestinal tract can easily lead to a secondary nutritional deficiency. The symptoms of a secondary deficiency of a specific nutrient are the same as a primary deficiency. Table 28–7 lists nutritional deficiency disorders and their symptoms.

OBESITY

Obesity is defined as an excess of total body fat and a body weight of 20 percent above the ideal weight. Latest estimates from the National Health and Nutrition Examinations Surveys indicate a national average prevalence of obesity of 33 percent of women in the United States, and as high as 50 percent in certain ethnic and regional subgroups.[7]

Of concern is the high incidence and prevalence of obesity among Mexican-Americans and Native Americans. Low income is associated with obesity among Mexican-American children and adults,[8] while further research is needed to determine the genetic environment and cultural prevalence of obesity among African-Americans, Asian, and Pacific-Islander Americans and Native Americans.[9,10]

The most commonly used standard of "ideal" weight is the Metropolitan Life Insurance Company's Height and Weight Tables (Table 12–2). The desirability of such tables is often debated, as they were not derived from a representative sample of the North American population.[9]

There are numerous methods for determining the amount of body fat. Measurement of skin fold thickness (using standardized calipers) is useful in assessing body fat; however, the technique is often less reliable in individual patients than are direct measurements of height and weight. Hydrodensometry (underwater weighing) and bioelectrical impedence techniques are also used, but require expensive equipment. Because the **body mass index (BMI),** calculated by dividing the weight in kilograms by the height squared in meters, has the highest correlation with actual measurements of body fat,[7,9] it is the method most commonly used in current research.

Research is ongoing to determine the ideal weight for most people. It appears that there may not be a single ideal body frame; the more likely case is that every person has a unique ideal weight at which he or she feels best, functions optimally, and is physically most healthy.

Despite the controversy about precise determinations of ideal weight, it is apparent that many Americans of all ages, especially

TABLE 28-7. NUTRITIONAL DEFICIENCY DISEASES

Disorder	Nutrient Deficiency	General Symptoms
Vitamin Deficiencies		
Ariboflavinosis	Riboflavin	Dermatitis, eye lesions
Beriberi	Thiamine	Neuromuscular dysfunction
Hypovitaminosis A	Vitamin A	Corneal damage, blindness, night blindness, eye infections
Megaloblastic anemia	Folic acid	Weakness, shortness of breath, sore tongue, diarrhea, edema
Pellagra	Niacin	Gastrointestinal disturbances, mouth sores, dermatitis, neurologic changes
Pernicious anemia	Folic acid, vitamin B_{12}	Weakness, pallor, fatigue, diarrhea, sore tongue
Rickets	Vitamin D	Bone deformities
Scurvy	Vitamin C	Tissue and joint hemorrhages, impaired or delayed wound healing, anemia
Mineral Deficiencies		
Endemic goiter	Iodine	Enlarged thyroid gland
Iron deficiency anemia	Iron	Weakness, pallor, fatigue, headache, palpitations
Osteoporosis	Calcium	Curved spine, easy fracturing

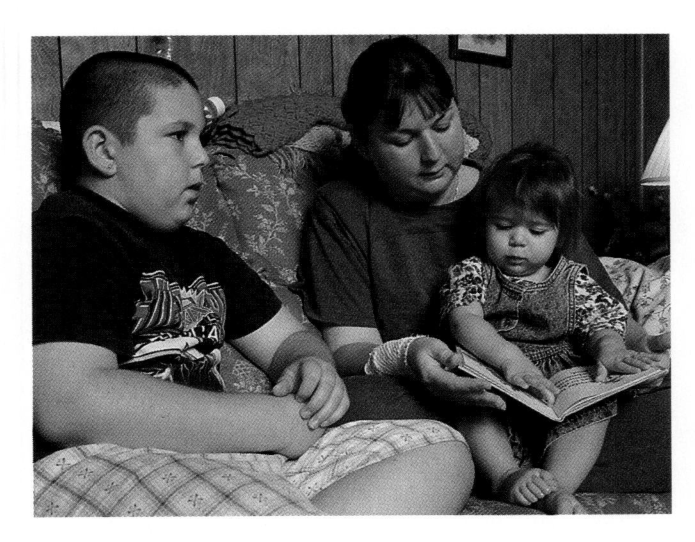

Figure 28–6. **Obesity in children and middle-age adults is associated with medical risks.**

children, adolescents, and middle-aged adults, are **overweight** (body weight 10 percent above ideal) or obese (Fig. 28–6). Of concern to health care professionals are the numerous medical risks associated with excess body fat.

Data published from a follow-up study in the Framingham study show that obesity is an independent risk factor for premature dying.[11] Other research links obesity with cardiac risk factors, such as hypertension, diabetes, hyperlipidemia, renal[12] and pulmonary problems,[13] osteorthritis,[12,13] and birth defects.[7,12,13] Obese patients are also higher surgical risks.

Genetic, psychological, social, and physiologic theories are under investigation to better understand the etiology of obesity. It appears that genetics influence a person's chances of becoming fat more than any other single factor. One genetic theory, the "fat cell theory," maintains that each person has a certain number of fat cells and tends to keep the fat cells filled. The number of fat cells is influenced by genetic factors and eating patterns, especially during infancy and childhood.

Eating is a highly symbolic experience with considerable emotional and social overtones. Hence, psychological variables, such as persons' views of themselves and others' views of them affect eating behaviors and attempts to lose weight.

Physiologically, the "set point theory" postulates that each person has a set point for a certain amount of body fat. To maintain this set point, an "appestat" functions like a thermostat and causes dieting to lower the basal metabolic rate (BMR). This results in more efficient use of calories, and, therefore, makes weight loss progressively more difficult. Increasing the amount one exercises at the same time calorie intake is reduced can increase BMR to a degree. Experts agree that this is the most effective means of weight control. Exercising 20 minutes a day, three times a week and eating three meals a day and low-calorie snacks based on the food pyramid achieves a gradual but consistent weight loss.

INSIGHTS FROM NURSING LITERATURE

THE IMPORTANCE OF FOOD CHOICES IN CHILDHOOD COMPLICATED BY ILLNESS

Purdy KS, Dwyer JT, Holland M, Goldberg DL, Dinardo J. You are what you eat: healthy food choices, nutrition, and the child with juvenile rheumatoid arthritis. Pediatr Nurs. *1996; 22:391–398.*

Ill children have nutrition-related needs. The authors of this article focus on children with rheumatoid arthritis, a chronic inflammatory disease of the joints resulting in various degrees of joint pain, swelling, and stiffness. The goal of nutritional therapy is to provide a diet that promotes normal growth and to prevent obesity while assuring that children consumes an enjoyable diet appropriate for their age. They note that children with arthritis are at risk for many problems, including anorexia, drug/nutrient interactions, physical inactivity, mechanical feeding difficulties, and susceptibility to food fads and quackery as remedies for the disease and weight problems. Such children may suffer from poor linear growth, undernutrition and muscle wasting, excessive weight gain and obesity, and pain in the jaw and upper extremities, which causes difficulty chewing and using utensils. The role of nurses entails nutritional screening and ensuring that families' nutritional concerns are addressed by answering basic nutrition questions and providing general nutrition guidance to the patient and family members.

CRITICAL QUERY

Purdy and associates[14] stress that nurses are in an important position to encourage healthful food choices and impress on children that ultimately they "are what they eat." Considering principles of cognitive and emotional development, identify some strategies the nurse might use to communicate that message to teenagers.

OTHER EATING DISORDERS

Both anorexia nervosa and bulimia are severely destructive eating disorders. Common to both is a deep-rooted insecurity, low self-esteem, dissatisfaction with one's body image, and extreme and pervasive fear of fatness. The behaviors associated with each of these disorders differ. Many individuals, however, manifest behaviors associated with both of these syndromes. Often individuals with eating disorders devise ingenious methods to hide their illness from others. The physical effects of the disorders are often the first clues that a serious problem exists.

Anorexia Nervosa

Anorexia nervosa is, virtually, self-imposed starvation. It occurs primarily in adolescent and young adult females, but is also seen among women in their middle years. Usually, people with anorexia nervosa do not have any loss of appetite, but rigorously control their intake of food. The physiologic effects of this long-term, slow starvation are drastic and frequently life-threatening. Brain shrinkage, endocrine disturbances such as amenorrhea, and severe nutritional deficiencies and metabolic imbalances result. Death is not unusual in prolonged, extreme cases.

Bulimia

Bulimia is characterized by a behavior pattern of uncontrollable binge eating of enormous amounts of food, followed by self-induced vomiting and use of laxatives or diuretics to control weight. The preferred foods are usually sweet, rich, and fatty. Most bulimic individuals maintain a thin appearance but do not lose weight; this factor makes their eating practices more difficult to detect. The most common associated problems are tooth decay, menstrual irregularities, and severe electrolyte imbalances that lead to life-threatening cardiac arrythmias.

SECTION 2
ASSESSMENT OF NUTRITION

NUTRITIONAL DATA COLLECTION

The importance of the assessment phase of nursing process for nutritional planning and implementation cannot be overemphasized. Because of the psychosocial meanings associated with food and eating, it is essential that nurse and patient develop a trusting collaborative relationship. Patients must feel free to reveal the details of their eating habits and nutritional state; nurses must offer support, respect, and confidentiality. Nutritional assessment includes a nutritional history, physical examination, and a review of relevant laboratory and diagnostic test results.

NUTRITIONAL HISTORY

A nutritional history elicits subjective data concerning a patient's eating habits, family and social eating patterns, past nutritional problems, current or potential nutritional problems, and attitudes and knowledge about foods and nutrition. This information is essential to determine needs for and to plan any changes.

Primary Concern

The history reveals whether or not a patient's primary concern is related to nutrition. Some patients may refer directly to appetite, eating problems, body weight, or recent gains/losses in weight as their primary concern; however, many other stated concerns such as fatigue, skin problems, gastrointestinal problems, or generally diminished well-being may be nutrition related. Obtaining information about eating habits and nutritional status determines whether a patient's primary concern can be corrected by nutrition-related approaches. The following example presents a nutrition-related primary concern.

> Debbie Ryan, a 15-year-old girl, comes to an outpatient clinic seeking help for her "horrible skin." The nurse notes that Debbie is quite obese and recognizes that the skin and weight problems could both be related to nutritional habits. The nurse acknowledges Debbie's concerns and works with her to identify strategies that will both improve her skin and reduce her weight.

Current Understanding

In this portion of the history, a nurse determines whether a patient believes that a current health problem is interfering with nutritional needs. Illness or injury can interfere with a patient's ability to meet nutritional needs. Similarly, treatments can cause nutritional problems, as illustrated by the following example.

> Mrs. Anderson, a patient undergoing chemotherapy after a modified radical mastectomy, complains that nausea has drastically reduced her food intake and caused her to lose 20 pounds in 3 months. The nurse asks Mrs. Anderson for specific information about the degree of nausea; when exactly she experiences it in relation to the chemotherapy and how long it lasts; whether she has associated symptoms such as vomiting, diarrhea, and abdominal cramps; what makes the nausea better or worse; and what Mrs. Anderson has done to control the nausea. The nurse knows that cancer chemotherapy itself can cause nausea, and that people often experience anticipatory nausea prior to administration of chemotherapy. Talking with the patient about her current understanding of the problem helps the nurse determine if this is anticipatory nausea, which will require different management than post-chemotherapy nausea.

Past Health Problems/Experiences

The nurse also needs to know if a patient has experienced health problems in the past that have altered nutritional status. Note the date, duration, treatment, and residual effects of any nutritional problems. Identify medications currently in use that could affect nutritional status, such as antibiotics or diuretics.

Personal, Family, and Social History

A family history of obesity, eating disorders, food allergies, diabetes, hypertension, heart disease, cancer, colitis, or ulcers is associated with genetic etiologies and, if present in the family history, would alert nurses to the need for further evaluation and preventive measures. In addition, without a full understanding of the personal and sociocultural meaning of food for a patient, planning will be ineffective. Answers to the questions in Table 28–8 will help a nurse understand relevant aspects of the patient's life. It should be emphasized that discussion of culture and lifestyle is approached in a empathic, nonjudgmental manner. The following example demonstrates the relevance of personal, family, and social history to health.

> Mr. Costello, a 46-year-old investment executive, is being treated for chest pain of cardiac origin. The nurse asks Mr. Costello if anyone in his family has heart disease and if so at what age it was diagnosed. Because of the association of heart disease with a high-fat diet and stress, the nurse also pays special attention to Mr. Costello's personal and social nutritional history. Mr. Costello states that his father died of a heart attack at the age of 43. He describes frequent business lunches of steak and french fries, and often similar dinners. His wife works also, and when they eat at home they often heat up commercially prepared frozen foods in the microwave.

TABLE 28-8. NUTRITIONAL HISTORY: PERSONAL, FAMILY, AND SOCIAL HISTORY QUESTIONS

A. Vocational
1. What type of work do you do?
2. What hours do you work?
3. Does your work involve any physical activity?
4. Does your work ever cause you to skip meals or influence what you eat or drink?

B. Home and Family
1. Do you live alone or with someone?
2. Does your family eat most meals together?
3. Do you like to cook?
4. Who buys food and cooks meals at home?
5. Do you eat alone much? Does that change what you cook? Does it affect how much you eat?

C. Social, Leisure, Spiritual, and Cultural
1. What kind of leisure activities do you enjoy?
2. Do you have time for leisure activities every week?
3. Do you eat with your friends often? What and where?
4. What kinds of foods do your friends prefer?
5. Do you eat out often?
6. Does your religion or culture of origin influence your food habits and preferences?

D. Habits

Exercise
1. Is your lifestyle active or sedentary?
2. Do you have a program of regular exercise? If so, what is it?
3. What kind of physical activity do you do in an average week?

Diet
1. Please write down everything that you have eaten or drunk in the last 24 hours. Is this a typical day's diet for you? If not, describe your usual pattern, if any.
2. Do you have regular mealtimes?
3. What times of the day do you eat?
4. Is your pattern at work the same as at home?
5. Under what conditions do you usually eat (noisy, relaxed, rushed, clean, dirty, etc)?
6. What special foods do you particularly enjoy?
7. What foods do you dislike?
8. How is your food prepared?
9. Do you eat out frequently?

Beverages
1. Do you usually drink liquids with meals? What type? How much?
2. What sorts of beverages do you drink between meals?
3. Do you drink alcohol?
4. Does alcohol intake ever influence what you eat?
5. Do you ever miss meals because of drinking?

Tobacco
1. Do you smoke? Use other forms of tobacco? Have you recently quit?
2. Do you notice a change in your appetite since you quit using tobacco?
3. Do you feel using tobacco changes the taste of foods you eat?

Other Substances
1. Do you take any drugs not prescribed by a doctor? Any recreational drugs?
2. Have you noticed any change in your eating habits since you began taking _______?
3. Do you ever miss meals because of taking _______?

E. Psychological

Coping
1. What kind of situations either increase or decrease your appetite?
2. Do you ever eat when you aren't hungry? For example, because you are nervous? Stressed? Angry? Other reasons?
3. Do stress or emotions ever keep you from eating?
4. What is your overall feeling about food?

Self-image
1. Are you satisfied with your current weight?
2. Is there anything you would change about your body?
3. Do you ever skip meals or limit what you eat, even though you are hungry?
4. Have you ever made yourself vomit after eating?

The fast pace and pressures of Mr. Costello's life become clear. The nurse realizes his risk for a heart attack because of his family history and lifestyle. The nurse knows that low-fat, low-salt meals are important dietary changes that Mr. Costello should make and discusses with him low-fat foods that can be ordered at a restaurant. Mr. Costello is advised of the benefits of low-salt frozen foods and fresh fruits and vegetables. The nurse also discusses a program of regular exercise and relaxation techniques as stress-reducing measures.

Subjective Manifestations

Nurses' questions about subjective manifestations will help to identify related or hidden problems and to gain a comprehensive view of a patient's situation. Table 17–10 presents sample questions about subjective manifestations, some of which are relevant to nutritional status. Querying patients about skin and gastrointestinal symptoms may generate information useful for identifying problems related to nutrition as well. Nurses use these findings in designing care plans that address all the nutritional problems and concerns.

NUTRITION EXAMINATION

The patient's general appearance, skin, mucous membranes, abdomen, and muscles reveal much about nutritional status.

Certain physical measurements are also useful sources of data. Following are specific assessments that will help determine nutritional status.

Measurements

Measures of height, weight, and other anthropometric indicators are essential in judging a patient's nutritional status. A change in weight is an important indicator of diminished nutritional health. Severe weight loss is associated with complications of surgery, such as malnutrition, infections, and respiratory problems. Height and weight are measured consistently using reliable scales. Compare the patient's measurements to standard height and weight tables for the patient's age and sex (see Table 12–2). Height and weight can also be used to compute body mass index (BMI), an index of a person's weight in relation to height. BMI is calculated by dividing weight in kilograms by the square of the height in meters. It is considered a more reliable indicator of obesity than weight alone. The desired range for women is 19.1 to 27.3, and for men 20.7 to 27.8. Obesity-associated health risks occur when BMI is in the range of 27 to 32; if BMI is more than 44.8, the individual is considered morbidly obese.

Other anthropometric measurements that dietitians use to make inferences about body fat and protein stores include the midarm circumference (MAC, MUAC) and the triceps skinfold (TSF). These two values can be used to compute the midarm muscle circumference (MMC). Although not routinely used by nurses, they are useful in collaborative assessment of high-risk patients.

Objective Manifestations

Use the physical examination techniques described in Chap. 17 to complete a nutritional assessment. Physical findings that provide data about the patient's nutritional status—good and poor—are summarized in Table 28–9.

DIAGNOSTIC TESTS

Laboratory tests, x-ray studies, and endoscopic exams are the most commonly used approaches for diagnosing nutritional problems. Nurses must be able to explain to patients the purpose of the procedures and tests, ensure that patients are appropriately prepared, and monitor the results so that abnormalities are incorporated into the plan of care.

Laboratory Tests

Among the laboratory tests, lymphocyte count, albumin, hemoglobin, and transferrin are especially useful for nutritional assessment. Blood and urine tests may require that the patient refrain from eating for a specified amount of time, or observe certain dietary specifications. Table 28–10 describes laboratory tests that may be ordered to assess nutritional status. No single patient will be subject to all of the tests; the physician will determine which are needed.

X-ray Studies

For abdominal x-rays and scans, a regimen of bowel cleansing and ingestion of a special radiopaque substance is often needed. Patients must understand that following the preparatory regimen is absolutely essential to the success of the test. Nurses play a key role in providing patients with a complete explanation of x-rays to be done and the specific self-preparation requirements.

Endoscopic Examinations

Endoscopic examinations are invasive procedures in which a tube with a light and magnifying lens on the distal end is inserted into the digestive tract, through either the mouth or the anus. Any portion of the digestive tract may be examined. Gastroscopy and colonoscopy are two common examples. Endoscopic procedures require that patients provide informed consent.

NURSING DIAGNOSIS OF NUTRITIONAL STATUS

The collaborative gathering of subjective and objective data provides the foundation for developing a nursing diagnosis of a patient's nutritional status. It may be relatively easy to determine an excess or deficiency of calories or specific nutrients, but determining the etiology of a problem requires the utmost skill on the part of nurses and honesty on the part of patients. Patients need to be fully informed regarding the reasons for the assessment questions and diagnostic tests. The significance of the information gained from assessment must also be explained.

Formulating the nursing diagnosis is a collaborative process. The nurse and patient review assessment data together and, if possible, develop the diagnosis and its etiology together. At the very least, nurses' diagnostic judgments should be shared with patients or family so that the plan of care may be mutually developed and effectively implemented. Initiating changes in a person's dietary regimen is always a challenge; however, it becomes more difficult if the problem-solving process is not a collaborative one.

The National Conference Group for Classification of Nursing Diagnoses (NANDA) has identified three nursing diagnoses related to nutrition: altered nutrition: less than body requirements (specify excess); altered nutrition: more than body requirements (specify excess); altered nutrition: risk for more than body requirements. These diagnoses are elaborated in Table 28–11, Sample Nursing Diagnoses: Nutrition. Other nursing diagnoses that can contribute to or result from altered nutritional status are listed at the end of Table 28–11.

In addition to identifying the general nursing diagnosis, the specific excess or deficit must also be determined. Nurses must draw upon comprehensive knowledge of the signs of specific nutritional deficiencies and indicate whether the alteration is related to calories, protein, carbohydrates, fats, particular vitamins, or minerals. For example, generalized overweight or underweight indicates an alteration in caloric intake. Inadequate muscular development or tone indicates a protein deficiency, as do the more severe signs of protein–calorie malnutrition discussed previously. An excess of carbohydrates may manifest as excess body weight, whereas a deficit will result in depletion of protein and fat reserves and gradual weight loss.

Inadequate intake of fats may lead to dry skin and hair and, if severe, hormonal alterations. Refer to Tables 28–3 and 28–4 for signs of specific vitamin and mineral deficits, which may also accompany calorie and/or protein deficiency. The patient's report about dietary patterns is crucial to accurate diagnosis of the specific deficiency or excess.

ALTERED NUTRITION: LESS THAN BODY REQUIREMENTS

This nursing diagnosis indicates that there is an insufficient intake of nutrients to meet metabolic needs. It may result from condi-

(continued on page 902)

TABLE 28-9. CLINICAL SIGNS OF NUTRITIONAL STATUS

Body Area	Signs of Good Nutritional Status	Signs of Poor Nutritional Status
General		
Appearance	Alert, responsive, physically fit.	Listless, apathetic, cachexia (thin, muscle wasting).
Vitality	Endurance, energetic, sleeps well, vigorous.	Easily fatigued, no energy, falls asleep easily, looks tired, apathetic, irritable.
Odors	Fresh breath, no significant body odor.	Foul or fruity breath, unusual body odor.
Weight	Normal for height, age, body build.	Overweight or underweight.
Integument		
Hair	Shiny, lustrous, firm, healthy scalp.	Dull and dry, brittle, loss of color, thin and sparse.
Face	Uniform skin color; healthy appearance, not swollen.	Dark skin over cheeks and under eyes, flaky skin, facial edema (moon face), pale skin color.
Skin	Smooth, good color and turgor, slightly moist, no sign of rashes, swelling, or color irregularities.	Rough, dry, flaky, swollen, poor turgor, pigmented, lack of fat under skin, fat deposits around joints (xanthomas), petechiae (pinpoint capillary hemorrhages), bruises, rashes.
Nails	Firm, pink.	Spoon shaped (koilonychia), brittle, pale, ridged.
HEENT		
Eyes	Bright, clear, moist, no sores at corners or eyelids, membranes moist and healthy pink color, no prominent blood vessels, no exudate.	Pale eye membranes, inflamed membranes, exudate, dry eyes; increased vascularity, cornea soft, small yellowish lumps around eyes, dull or scarred cornea.
Lips	Good pink color, smooth, moist.	Swollen and puffy, cracks in corners of mouth, fissures, scars (stomatitis), chapped lips.
Tongue	Deep red, surface papillae present.	Smooth appearance, beefy red or magenta colored, swollen, hypertrophy or atrophy, sores, lumps.
Gums	Firm, good pink color, no swelling or bleeding.	Spongy, bleed easily, marginal redness, recessed, swollen and inflamed, sores related to dentures.
Teeth	All present, in good repair. If dentures, intact with good fit.	Loose or missing teeth, caries, plaque, ill-fitting or absent dentures.
Glands	No enlargement of thyroid, face not swollen.	Enlargement of thyroid (goiter), enlargement of parotid (swollen cheeks).
Cardiovascular	Normal heart rate and rhythm, no murmurs, normal blood pressure for age.	Cardiac enlargement, tachycardia, elevated blood pressure.
Gastrointestinal	No palpable organs or masses (liver edge may be palpable in children).	Enlarged liver or spleen.
Abdomen	Flat. Bowel sounds present.	Ascites (abnormal fluid), distention, hypo- or hyperactive bowel sounds.
Musculoskeletal		
Skeleton	Good posture, no malformations.	Poor posture, beading of the ribs, bowed legs or knock-knees, prominent scapulas, chest deformity, deformity at diaphragm.
Teeth	Straight, no crowding, no cavities, no pain, bright, no discoloration, well-shaped jaw.	Cavities, mottled appearance (fluorosis), malpositioned, missing teeth.
Muscles	Well developed, firm, good tone, some fat under skin.	Flaccid, poor tone, wasted, underdeveloped, difficulty walking.
Extremities	No tenderness or swelling.	Weak and tender, presence of edema.
Neurologic	Normal reflexes, psychological stability.	Decrease in or loss of ankle and knee reflexes, psychomotor changes, mental confusion, depression, sensory loss, motor weakness, loss of sense of position, loss of vibration, burning and tingling of hands and feet (paresthesia), tremors.

TABLE 28-10. LABORATORY TESTS OF NUTRITIONAL STATUS

Test	Findings/Implications: Normal	Findings/Implications: Abnormal	Patient Preparation
Red blood cell count (RBC)	Male: 4.6–6.1 million/mm^3 Female: 4.2–5.4 million/mm^3	Decreased with iron deficiency, vitamin B_{12} deficiency. Mean cell volume (MCV) increased with B_{12} deficiency and decreased with iron deficiency. Mean cell hemoglobin concentration (MCHC) decreased with iron deficiency.	None
Hemoglobin (hgb or hg)	Male: 14–18 g/dL Female: 12–16 g/dL	Decreased if inadequate protein or iron intake.	None
Hematocrit (hct)	Male: 40–54% Female: 37–47%	Decreased if inadequate protein or iron intake.	None
Iron	50–150 g/dL	Decreased if inadequate iron intake and with protein malnutrition.	None
Total iron-binding capacity (TIBC)	250–450 μL/dL	Increased in iron deficiency anemia, decreased in protein deficiency. Sensitive indicator of protein malnutrition. 150–200: mild; 100–149: moderate; less than 100: severe.	None
Lymphocyte count	1700–3500/μL 25–35% of total WBCs	Decreased if inadequate protein intake. Sensitive indicator of nutritional state.	None
Protein serum urine	 6–8 g/dL 0–5 mg/dL	Decreased if inadequate protein intake or malabsorption syndrome.	No fatty meal prior to test
Albumin	3.5–5 g/dL	Decreased if inadequate protein intake; level of depletion implies degree of undernutrition. 2.8–3.4: mild; 2.1–2.7: moderate; less than 2.1: severe.	No fatty meal prior to test
Transferrin	20–50% saturation	Increased if iron stores low, decreased in protein malnutrition. TIBC is a quantitative measure of transferrin.	None
Calcium	4.5–5.5 mg/dL	Decreased if malabsorption or vitamin D deficiency.	None
Phosphorus	2.5–4.5 mg/dL	Decreased if vitamin D deficiency, undernutrition, starvation.	None
Fasting blood glucose	60–100 mg/dL	Increased if diabetic, in some infections.	Overnight fast
Fatty acids	25 mg/dL	Increase indicates high risk of heart disease.	Overnight fast
Cholesterol	120–220 mg/dL	Increase indicates high risk of heart disease: 200–240: moderate risk; greater than 240: high risk.	Overnight fast
HDL cholesterol	29–77 mg/dL	Less than 25: extreme risk for coronary heart disease (CHD); 26–35: high risk for CHD; 46–59: low risk for CHD.	Overnight fast
LDL cholesterol	60–160 mg/dL	Greater than 160: high risk for CHD; 130–159: moderate risk for CHD.	Overnight fast
Lipids	400–1000 mg/dL	Increase indicates high risk of heart disease.	Overnight fast
Triglycerides	20–190 mg/dL	Increase indicates high risk of heart disease.	Overnight fast
Creatinine serum urine	 0.5–1.5 mg/dL 85–135 mL/min	Decreased if inadequate protein intake, decreased in catabolic states when muscle mass depleted.	None
Urea nitrogen serum urine	 5–25 mg/dL varies with intake	Increased in catabolic state. 24-hour urine test can be compared to protein intake to assess nitrogen balance.	None

Adapted from: Cataldo CB, DeBruyne LK, Whitney EN. Nutrition and Diet Therapy. *4th ed. St. Paul, MN: West; 1995; Eschelman MM.* Introductory Nutrition and Nutritional Therapy. *3rd ed. Philadelphia: JB Lippincott; 1996; and Watson J, Jaffe MS.* Nurse's Manual of Laboratory and Diagnostic Tests. *2nd ed. Philadelphia: FA Davis; 1995.*

TABLE 28-11. SAMPLE NURSING DIAGNOSES: NUTRITION

Nursing Diagnosis	Defining Characteristics/Manifestations: *Subjective Data*	Defining Characteristics/Manifestations: *Objective Data*	Etiology
Altered nutrition: more than body requirements for calories *1.1.2.1.*	Reports chronic or sudden weight increase Reports sedentary lifestyle: "I usually don't like exercise."	Weight more than 20% above ideal Increased subcutaneous fat: triceps skin fold greater than norms	*Physical:* Excessive intake in relation to metabolic need: sedentary lifestyle
Altered nutrition: less than body requirements for calories *1.1.2.2.*	None	Weight 20% below ideal 24-hour food intake less than 70% of RDA Not oriented to person, place, time, or situation Progressive weight loss Poor muscle tone	*Cognitive:* Inability to ingest food: confusion
Altered nutrition: less than body requirements for calories and protein *1.1.2.2.*	States does not have enough money to buy food Reported food intake is less than RDA	Weekly food expenditures indicate inadequate money for food Steady weight loss Weight 20% below ideal 24-hour food intake less than 70% of RDA Poor muscle tone	*Sociocultural/Life Structural:* Inability to ingest food: insufficient income
Altered nutrition: less than body requirements for protein *1.1.2.2.*	Reported intake of protein foods is less than RDA Unable to state importance of protein in diet Unable to list foods high in protein	Decreased muscle mass Poor muscle tone Generalized edema Decreased RBC count Decreased serum protein or albumin Decreased lymphocyte count	*Cognitive:* Inability to ingest protein: knowledge deficit

Nursing Diagnosis	Risk Factor
Altered nutrition: risk for more than body requirements for calories *1.1.2.3.*	*Sociocultural/Life Structural:* Social/occupational situation encourages overeating and drinking

OTHER NURSING DIAGNOSES RELATED TO NUTRITION

PHYSICAL
Activity intolerance
Constipation
Diarrhea
Impaired physical mobility
Ineffective breathing pattern
Fatigue
Fluid volume deficit
Risk for fluid volume deficit
Altered oral mucous membranes
Self-feeding deficit
Impaired skin integrity
Risk for impaired skin integrity
Impaired swallowing
Impaired tissue integrity

COGNITIVE
Altered health maintenance
Knowledge deficit
Altered thought processes

EMOTIONAL
Anxiety
Ineffective individual coping
Anticipatory grieving
Dysfunctional grieving
Spiritual distress

SELF-CONCEPTUAL
Body image disturbance
Self-esteem disturbance

SOCIOCULTURAL/LIFE STRUCTURAL
Ineffective family coping: compromised or disabling
Diversional activity deficit
Altered family processes
Impaired home maintenance management
Social isolation
Impaired social interaction

Source: The nursing diagnoses and etiologies on this table and the definitions of nursing diagnoses in the body of the text not credited to other sources are from Nursing Diagnosis: Definitions and Classification, 1997–1998. *Philadelphia: North American Nursing Diagnosis Association; 1996. Manifestation categories for etiologies and specifications of general etiologies on these tables are authors' original work.*

tions that interrupt the supply or use of nutrients or that increase the body's demand for nutrients. The nutritional deficit may be calories, protein, fat, specific vitamins or minerals, or a combination. Height and weight tables will help determine if a general caloric deficit exists. A body weight of 20 percent or more below the ideal is a major defining characteristic of this diagnosis. More specific assessment data are necessary to determine deficits of individual nutrients. The general etiologies of a nutritional deficit are briefly discussed below, along with more specific defining characteristics. Although the NANDA taxonomy does not specifically list risk for altered nutrition: less than body requirements as an approved diagnosis, astute nurses are aware that a risk state for insufficient intake to meet body requirements can be recognized and treated by nurses before an actual deficit exists. Any of the etiologies discussed below can be risk factors for this diagnosis.

- *Etiology: inability to ingest foods.* A patient may have difficulty ingesting foods for a variety of reasons; for example, the oral cavity may be deformed (cleft palate), or a medical problem, such as cancer of the throat or an esophageal hernia, can interfere, as can absent or poor teeth. Such physical limitations are often associated with protein deficiency because of the difficulty encountered in eating meat. Psychological factors such as an obsessive fear of being poisoned or of becoming fat may be the cause of a severe limitation of food ingestion. Social and economic factors may place serious limits on the quantity and quality of food intake.
- *Etiology: inability to digest foods.* Problems digesting foods also have a variety of causes; for example, one or more organs involved in digestion may be missing due to congenital or surgically induced conditions. Or a disease process, such as cancer or cystic fibrosis, may alter the gastrointestinal tract's secretion of enzymes or hormones essential for digestion. Psychological factors, such as anxiety, may interfere with digestion by causing severe diarrhea or vomiting. An inability to digest foods may be either complete or specific for certain foods. For example, the patient with celiac disease has particular difficulty digesting fats. Many people are allergic to particular foods, such as milk due to lactose intolerance.
- *Etiology: inability to absorb nutrients.* Structural alterations, disease processes, and other pathologic processes may be responsible for problems with nutrient absorption. For example, a patient who has undergone a total gastrectomy (removal of the stomach) will lack intrinsic factor, which is essential for the absorption of vitamin B_{12}. In addition, inflammatory or infectious disease may alter the mucosal lining of the intestines so that absorption is impaired. Psychological or physical factors can cause diarrhea, which interferes with nutrient absorption because rapid peristalsis decreases contact time between the food and the mucosal lining.
- *Etiology: knowledge deficit.* Knowledge deficits are among the most common etiologies of inadequate nutritional intake. Many, perhaps most, people base their eating habits on peer pressure, personal preferences and aversions, or sociocultural traditions. Nutrition education, even when provided, is not effective unless a person is motivated to learn and the information is presented in a way that is easy to grasp. Knowledge deficits can lead to deficits in total energy or to deficits or excesses of any specific nutrient.

ALTERED NUTRITION: MORE THAN BODY REQUIREMENTS

This nursing diagnosis indicates that there is an excessive caloric or nutrient intake relative to metabolic need. A body weight of 20 percent or more over the ideal is the general defining characteristic. The fundamental etiology of this alteration is a food intake that is greater than energy expenditure.

- *Etiology: excessive intake in relationship to metabolic need.* This imbalance may result from a low energy expenditure due, for example, to a sedentary lifestyle or a hypometabolic state that may occur in certain diseases such as hypothyroidism. Or the imbalance may be caused by a large food intake due to compulsive eating, overfeeding, or social factors. A number of dysfunctional eating patterns have been associated with the development of obesity, such as pairing food with other activities (eg, studying, watching television), eating in response to external cues (eg, social situations), or eating in response to internal cues (eg, anxiety or depression). Usually, the excessive intake will be fats and sugars rather than protein.

ALTERED NUTRITION: RISK FOR MORE THAN BODY REQUIREMENTS

Because of the importance of preventive approaches to obesity, the diagnosis altered nutrition: risk for more than body requirements is included in the taxonomy. This diagnosis is defined as the presence of risk factors for excess caloric intake relative to metabolic need. The presence of any of the risk factors discussed in the following paragraphs, particularly when combined with a sedentary lifestyle and dysfunctional eating patterns, are predictive of a high risk for obesity.

- *Risk factor: hereditary predisposition.* Research has documented that obesity tends to occur in persons who have overweight family members, particularly one or both parents. Controversy exists, however, as to whether this pattern is due to genetically controlled metabolic factors or to a family's attitudes toward food and its eating patterns. Body build and certain rare genetic disorders are clearly hereditary and may exert a powerful influence in the development of obesity.
- *Risk factor: excessive energy intake during late gestational life, early infancy, and adolescence.* The determination of this etiology is based on research regarding the development of adipocytes (fat cells) during the life span. Certain critical periods occur during which the adipocytes are most susceptible to proliferation or growth in size. These critical periods are the last half of pregnancy,[15] the first 2 years after birth, and the adolescent years. If nutritional intake, especially of fats and sugar, exceeds energy requirements during these critical periods, fat tissue will be synthesized or increased and will be extremely difficult to remove or decrease afterward.
- *Risk factor: frequent, closely spaced pregnancies.* Women who have numerous pregnancies with only a short interval between them will have difficulty returning to their normal nonpregnant weight. Each subsequent pregnancy therefore occurs at a higher baseline weight, compounding the overall weight gain and the problems associated with losing the excess weight.
- *Risk factor: dysfunctional psychological conditioning in relationship to food.* Dysfunctional conditioning means that food becomes a

replacement for the usual means of meeting human needs. Because of the tremendous symbolic importance of food in relation to human needs such as love, care, comfort, taste, variety, and prosperity, it is not surprising that food can easily become a substitute source of fulfillment. Once such a cycle starts, it can be a very complex process to reverse.

- *Risk factor: membership in lower socioeconomic group.* Nutritionally imbalanced diets often occur among populations that must buy inexpensive foods, many high in fat and low in protein. Fresh fruit and vegetables, dairy products, and lean meats tend to cost more than starchy, fatty "junk foods." Excessive calories and inadequate nutrients are the typical content of low-cost diets. In addition, in families where both parents work, children are often unsupervised, free to consume high-calorie snacks. Moreover, many individuals in lower socioeconomic groups are uninformed about their nutritional needs.
- *Risk factor: knowledge deficit.* The earlier discussion of knowledge deficit as an etiology of inadequate nutritional intake applies to this diagnosis as well.

STATING THE NUTRITIONAL DIAGNOSIS

Nursing diagnosis of a patient's nutritional status is the basis for mutual planning to correct nutritional problems. A diagnostic statement that is most useful for planning clearly identifies not only the problem but also its specific etiology and the major defining characteristics that the patient exhibits.

The taxonomy of nursing diagnoses lists general etiologies that underlie excessive or inadequate calories or nutrients for body needs. These etiologies have been discussed above. To be useful in a clinical situation, these general etiologies must be refined—that is, the specific contributing factor(s) need to be identified, not only so nurses can ascertain whether nursing therapy can correct the problem but also so specific nursing implementation can be determined. A patient whose inability to ingest food is related to a biologic factor (eg, ill-fitting dentures) can benefit from nursing measures to facilitate ingestion as a temporary measure until the biologic factor (eg, denture problem) is corrected.

Multiple defining characteristics listed in the taxonomy may indicate a nutritional problem. No one patient would experience all of these signs and symptoms at the same time. Stating those that a given patient exhibits in the diagnostic statement facilitates later recognition of resolution of the problem, when these defining characteristics should no longer be evident. The following are examples of complete nursing diagnostic statements of a nutritional problem:

- Altered nutrition: less than body requirements for calories related to ill-fitting dentures, as evidenced by inability to ingest desired foods "because my upper plate slips" and "I can't chew right—makes me choke"; sore inflamed buccal cavity, and body weight 20 percent less than ideal for height and frame.
- Altered nutrition: more than body requirements for calories related to maintaining usual eating patterns while suspending regular exercise program; as evidenced by recent weight increase to 10 percent above ideal for height and frame; reports unable to attend exercise class because of schedule change, and description of typical daily intake "same as before," which is 500 kcal per day greater than calculated needs for current activity level.
- Altered nutrition: risk for more than body requirements for calories and fat. Risk factors: 8-month-old child at 95th percentile of weight for age and height; mother reports continued intake of 30 ounces of formula daily while increasing intake of solid foods.

SECTION 3

NURSE-PATIENT MANAGEMENT OF NUTRITION

PLANNING FOR OPTIMAL NUTRITION

After the assessment and diagnosis of nutritional status has been accomplished, nurse and patient collaborate to plan desirable outcomes of care, strategies to attain these outcomes, and evaluation criteria to determine the extent to which the outcomes are achieved.

The more desired outcomes reflect a patient's wishes and expectations, the greater the chance a plan will succeed. The causes of nutritional alterations are complex and stem from all aspects of the person. Therefore, the desired outcomes of care must comprehensive. At the same time, evaluation criteria should be specific, with target dates for accomplishment.

Short-term outcomes are helpful, as they are steps toward meeting the long-term outcomes. For example, a goal of increasing weight by 20 pounds for an anorexic will seem frightening and overwhelming. Identifying weekly goals of 1 or 2 pounds of weight gain will be less threatening. Weight is often used as an outcome measure in nutritional planning.

After determining specific desired outcomes for each nursing diagnosis, the next step in collaborative planning is to determine effective measures to correct the diagnosed alteration. A goal in planning care is for patients to maintain as high a level of independence as possible while promoting maximal nutritional benefits. Table 28–12, Nurse–Patient Management of Nutrition Problems, shows sample desired outcomes, nursing implementation, and evaluation criteria for the nursing diagnoses listed in Table 28–11. Interdisciplinary planning also is carried out for patients who have medical diagnoses with nutritional implications. Table 28–13, Partial Critical Pathway for Total Hip Replacement: Nutrition, and Table 28–14, Partial Critical Pathway for Congestive Heart Failure: Nutrition, illustrate partial critical pathways—interdisciplinary plans that incorporate concepts from this chapter.

NURSING IMPLEMENTATION TO PROMOTE OPTIMAL NUTRITION

Assessment data, desired outcomes, and/or critical pathways direct patients and nurses to a general level of care and to certain nursing approaches. Teaching activities and dietary counseling usually are an important part of a nutritional care plan. When patients cannot obtain foods or eat independently, more direct assistance—sometimes including specialized technical procedures—is required to provide a source of nutrition. These approaches are discussed in the following sections.

(continued on page 906)

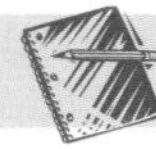

TABLE 28-12. NURSE-PATIENT MANAGEMENT OF NUTRITION PROBLEMS

Nursing Diagnosis	Desired Outcomes	Implementation	Evaluation
Altered nutrition: more than body requirements for calories R/T excessive intake in relation to metabolic need: sedentary lifestyle *1.1.2.1.*	1. Ideal body weight for height attained	1a. Review 24-hour food diary to identify patterns of excessive intake 1b. Teach principles and guidelines for good nutrition 1c. Provide food guide for use in menu planning 1d. Collaborate with patient to plan a balanced and appealing low-calorie diet 1e. Teach techniques to maintain diet plan: prepare small portions; eat slowly and chew thoroughly; eat low-calorie snacks only at scheduled times; plan for a small weekly "splurge"; drink plenty of water	1a. Weight loss of 1–2 lb/week until ideal body weight attained 1b. Ideal body weight maintained
	2. Daily diet meets all RDAs	2a. Review 24-hour food diary to identify deficits of specific nutrients 2b. Teach principles and guidelines for good nutrition 2c. Provide food guide for use in menu planning 2d. Collaborate with patient to plan a balanced and appealing low-calorie diet	2a. 24-hour diary shows all RDAs met 2b. Physical exam: good muscle tone; skin, mucous membranes, and hair appear healthy; no edema; serum protein normal for age
	3. Engages in regular exercise	3a. Teach patient ways that exercise promotes healthy weight loss 3b. Collaboratively develop a plan for increasing activity level and regular exercise that patient enjoys	3. Patient participates in aerobic exercise at least 30 min 3–4 times per week
Altered nutrition: less than body requirements for calories R/T inability to ingest food: confusion *1.1.2.2.*	1. Caloric and nutritional intake will meet RDAs	1a. Nurse, family, or significant other to feed patient. Meals planned by computing daily calorie and nutrient needs. 1b. Offer and assist with quality snacks between meals based on computation of daily calorie and nutrient needs	1a. 80% or more of each meal is ingested 1b. Progressive increase in or maintenance of weight at ideal value 1c. Progressive improvement in nutritional status as evidenced by: erect posture; good skin turgor; clear skin, eyes, and mucosa; firm muscles; prompt healing; mental alertness
	2. No injury related to eating or ingestion	2a. Speak clearly to patient when feeding, naming foods, describing texture and temperature 2b. Ensure upright positioning of patient during eating	2. Patient chews and swallows foods presented without aspiration

TABLE 28-12. CONTINUED

Nursing Diagnosis	Desired Outcomes	Implementation	Evaluation
Altered nutrition: less than body requirements for proteins and calories R/T inability to ingest food: insufficient income *1.1.2.2.*	1. Knowledge of low-cost foods with quality nutritional value	1a. Teach principles of good nutrition and shopping: • Avoid convenience foods • Use nonmeat protein sources • Buy in bulk when possible • Buy fresh, not canned, fruits and vegetables in season • Read labels for nutrient value of foods • Use complex carbohydrates rather than simple sugars • Compare prices 1b. Provide food guide for use in shopping	1a. 80% or more of each meal is ingested 1b. Progressive increase in or maintenance of weight at ideal value 1c. Progressive improvement in nutritional status as evidenced by: erect posture; good skin turgor; clear skin, eyes, and mucosa; firm muscles; prompt healing; mental alertness
	2. Caloric and nutrient intake meets RDAs	2a. Provide food guide for use in menu preparation 2b. Collaborate with patient to select healthful, inexpensive menus that are appealing	2. 24-hour food diary shows balanced, adequate nutrient intake
	3. Knowledge of options to increase income	3. Consult with social worker to facilitate access to public assistance sources such as: programs for women and children, food stamps, and job counseling	3. Patient identifies and contacts community agencies for assistance
Altered nutrition: less than body requirements for protein R/T inability to ingest protein: knowledge deficit *1.1.2.2.*	1. Knows importance of protein for optimum health	1a. Teach importance of protein for health 1b. Teach foods high in protein 1c. Provide food guide for use in menu planning; collaborate with patient to select menus that are appealing	1. Patient correctly states roles played by protein in body functions
	2. Daily protein intake meets RDAs	2. Teach importance of protein for health	2a. Lists foods high in protein 2b. 24-hour food diary shows protein intake meets RDAs
	3. No signs of protein deficiency	3. Teach importance of protein for health	3. Physical exam shows good muscle tone, no edema, hair strong and shiny; serum protein RBCs and lymphocyte values normal for age

Continued

TABLE 28-12. CONTINUED

Nursing Diagnosis	Desired Outcomes	Implementation	Evaluation
Altered nutrition: risk for more than body requirements for calories. Risk factor: social/ occupational situation encourages overeating and drinking *1.1.2.3.*	1. Caloric intake and metabolic demand are balanced	1a. Use 3-day food diary to assess current diet 1b. Teach principles of good nutrition 1c. Collaboratively develop a low-fat diet plan and an exercise plan that are pleasing to patient's needs and preferences	1. Achieves and maintains ideal weight
	2. Daily food intake meets RDAs	2a. Use 3-day food dairy to assess current diet 2b. Teach principles of good nutrition 2c. Provide food guide for use in menu planning	2. Food diary shows diet meets RDAs
	3. Knowledge of strategies to avoid excessive intake in social situations	3. Discuss strategies to avoid intake related to social pressure including: • Choosing low-calorie menu selections and nonalcoholic beverages for business lunches/socializing • Limiting snack intake in social settings—eat nutritious low-calorie snack before event, drink water with lemon or lime during event • When eating with family, eating small portions of high-calorie dishes, select larger portions of vegetables and salads • Avoiding social activities involving meals when possible • Joining support groups such as Weight Watchers	3. Identifies at least 3 strategies being used to decrease intake in social settings

Source: See Table 28–11.

PREVENTIVE CARE

Individuals requiring preventive care are healthy, experiencing no obvious nutritional alterations; however, as mentioned earlier, high-level wellness depends on optimal nutrition and is an appropriate goal of first-level nursing approaches. Identifying people at risk for nutritional alterations, either less than or greater than metabolic need, and nursing implementation designed to prevent nutritional alterations from occurring are also important goals of preventive care.

Lifestyle Analysis

Lifestyle analysis provides an important adjunct to the complete nutritional history and assessment for identifying individuals at risk for nutritional alterations. A person's lifestyle provides important clues to potential nutritional problems. For example, a high-pressure, fast-paced career often predisposes an individual to caffeine and alcohol abuse, consumption of junk foods, and inadequate relaxation for proper digestion. A sedentary lifestyle places a person at risk for nutrition intake greater than metabolic need. The etiologies for alterations in nutrition provide important clues about risk factors in apparently healthy individuals.

Lifestyle Counseling

Lifestyle counseling is indicated if, after a lifestyle analysis, a person decides to follow a healthier lifestyle. Counseling helps patients define their needs and explore alternative solutions. It is the patient who determines the need for change and develops the plan of action. The nurse in the counseling role is a facilitator, not a manager.

TABLE 28-13. PARTIAL CRITICAL PATHWAY FOR TOTAL HIP REPLACEMENT: NUTRITION

Nursing Dx/Problem	Outcome DOS/Day 1	Outcome Days 2–3	Outcome SNF Days 4–6	Outcome Home Care 3 Weeks (6 Visits)
Altered nutrition: less than body requirements for protein/calories R/T inability to eat following surgery	Hydration and calories for basal metabolism met through IV therapy	Tolerates oral fluids and foods of choice high in fiber, protein, vitamins A and C, zinc, calcium Absence of nausea	Eats 6 small meals daily high in fiber, protein, vitamins A and C, zinc, calcium Same	Same; progresses to 3 regular meals and 3 snacks high in fiber, protein, vitamins A and C, zinc, calcium
Implementation	**DOS/Day 1**	**Days 2–3**	**SNF Days 4–6**	**Home Care 3 Weeks**
Assessment	Tissue turgor, oral membranes for hydration Nausea/vomiting I and O q shift	Same Same Same	Same Same	Same
Tests/Consults				
Medications/Treatments	Monitor IVs Sips of water	Wean to oral fluids Advance to regular diet high in protein, zinc, calcium, vitamins A and C, fiber		
Psychosocial				
Teaching		Need for small, frequent intake of food and fluids high in protein, vitamins A and C, zinc, calcium and fiber	Food choices high in protein, vitamins A and C, zinc, calcium and fiber	
Activity/Safety/Self-care				
Nutrition	Clear liquids	Assist c̄ food selection high in protein, fiber, calcium, vitamins A and C, zinc	Same	
Transfer/Discharge Coord./Case Manager		Communicate outcomes achieved, problems/ interventions to SNF	Communicate outcomes achieved, problems/ interventions to Home Health	Communicate outcomes achieved, problems/ interventions to MD and prepare for discharge

See inside back cover for abbreviations.

Values Clarification

Values clarification is another useful nursing approach for people at risk for nutritional alterations. Values are deep-seated, enduring beliefs about what is important in one's life. Patients will need to look within and at their own behavior to determine what kind of value they place on good nutrition in relation to other personal values. Does a patient place more value on convenience or social conformity than on carefully prepared healthful meals? How important is personal health in a patient's scale of values? Does a patient's spending patterns suggest that he or she values new clothes more than healthful food? These and many other similar questions will help patients to recognize what value they place on healthy eating. If patients realize that there is a contradiction between their stated values and their behavior they may be motivated to plan a change in lifestyle so that actions are congruent with values. Or through discussion with a nurse, a patient may decide to change priorities and make good nutrition a valued goal.

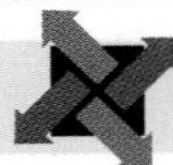

TABLE 28-14. PARTIAL CRITICAL PATHWAY FOR CONGESTIVE HEART FAILURE: NUTRITION

Nursing Dx/Problems	Outcome Primary Care Visit	Outcome Home Care Week 1 (3 Visits)	Outcome Home Care Week 2 (3 Visits)	Outcome Home Care Weeks 3–4 (3 Visits)
Altered nutrition: more than body requirements for calories R/T excessive intake in relation to body need	Verbalizes need & desire to lose weight	Verbalizes endorsement of diet plan	Loses 1 lb/week until ideal weight achieved	Ongoing
Implementation	**Primary Care Visit**	**Home Care Visit Week 1**	**Home Care Visit Week 2**	**Home Care Visit Weeks 3–4**
Assessment	Weight	Weight Hydration, fatigue Analyze eating patterns	Weight Same Same	Weight Same Same
Tests/Consults	Refer to Home Health			
Medications/Treatments				
Psychosocial	Reflective listening	Explore feelings about weight	Same	Explore feelings about progress toward weight loss goals
Teaching		Disease process Care plan Diet plan, balanced nutrition, food pyramid, high-fiber foods, foods to avoid	Review, reinforce as needed Techniques to maintain plan	Same Reinforce as needed Relationship between exercise, diet, and weight
Activity/Safety/ Self-care	Bedrest, HOB 30–45 degrees c̄ BSC or BRP		Progressive activity	Same
Nutrition	1500 cal, low fat 2 g Na, fluid 1 L/d	Develop diet plan c̄ pt	Same	Pt to plan diet for 1 week
Transfer/Discharge Coord./Case Manager		Communicate outcomes achieved, problems to MD	Same	Same Prepare for discharge

See inside back cover for abbreviations.

Health Education

Nurses often provide basic nutrition education to help individuals achieve and maintain optimal health. In addition to direct teaching, nurses also provide written information and audiovisual resources (Fig. 28–7). Numerous nutritional education resources are available for consumers from such groups as the USDA, National Cancer Institute, American Heart Association, and the American Diabetes Association. Food tables list the nutrient values of foods. Patients with special risk factors for a particular disease can be given special meal-planning guides published by various groups and agencies, such as the American Heart Association and the American Cancer Society. Collaborating with a dietitian will help nurses gain access to a multitude of meal-planning resources. The Internet is also a resource. Every search engine has *nutrition* listed in its index. There are research news sites, nutritional analysis programs, companies marketing nutritional supplements, newsgroups, and discussion groups. A specific topic may also be searched, for example, "weight reduction." For health professionals, numerous information sources will keep one up to date on the latest research and clinical practices. Figure 28–8 is an example of a web site that presents topics on nutrition and health.

Age-related Approaches

Preventing health problems related to nutritional imbalances is important at every stage of the life cycle. The potential problems and issues vary considerably for each age group. Some points to help nurses provide age-appropriate nutritional counseling are listed in Clinical Guideline 28–2.

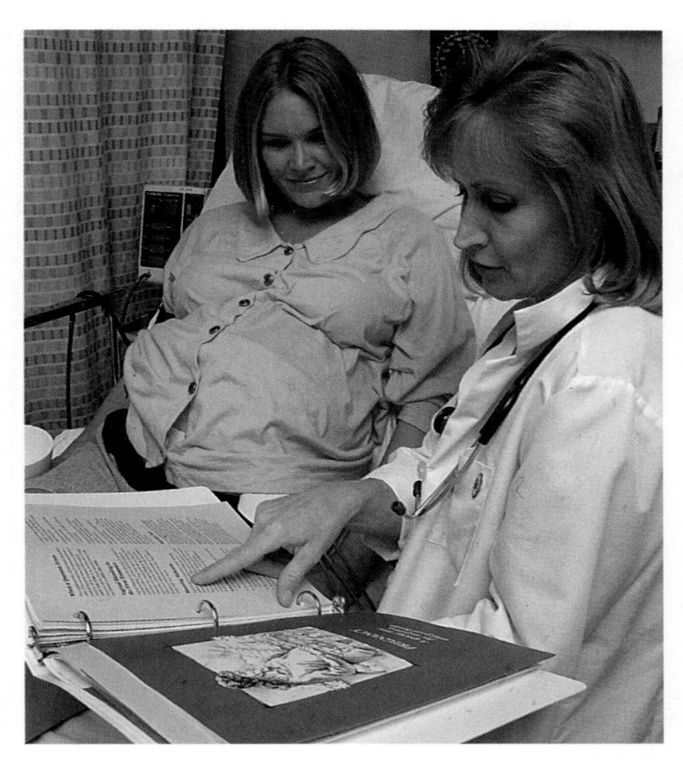

Figure 28–7. Nurses are a source of nutrition information for pregnant women.

CLINICAL GUIDELINE 28–2

AGE APPROPRIATE NUTRITION COUNSELING

Inform patients of the following approaches:

INFANCY AND TODDLERHOOD

- Offer new foods one at a time.
- Decrease amount of breast feeding or formula/milk intake as solid food intake increases.
- Limit fruit juices by diluting with water and offering plain water at least some of the time.
- Offer fruits and vegetables rather than highly sweetened or salty foods as snacks.

CHILDHOOD

- Offer variety and give freedom in selection of foods.
- Nutrition education should begin in the preschool years.
- Stress prevention of obesity in childhood.

ADOLESCENCE

- Emphasize healthy meals and snacks as a method of weight control.
- Discourage skipping meals, then bingeing.

MIDDLE YEARS

- Emphasize easy-to-prepare meals for working persons.
- Encourage exercise as a means of weight control.
- Encourage moderate fat intake.

OLDER ADULTS

- Suggest freezing leftovers in individual portions if cooking only for oneself.
- Encourage socializing during mealtime.
- Use social service programs for nutritional support.

Home Health Care

Home care measures to prevent nutritional deficiencies are directed primarily toward individuals with an injury or disease who may be immobilized to some extent, temporarily or permanently. Since these patients are at risk for choking, teaching home caregivers how to correctly execute the Heimlich maneuver is important (see Procedure 30–8). Healthy children and adults in the same household may also need nutrition information. Interventions are primarily educative, emphasizing the value and availability of nutrition centers, nutritional screening programs, nutritional counseling hotlines, employee wellness programs, and other services to meet the nutritional needs of women, infants, and children (eg, WIC) in the community is also part of preventive home care. Nurses providing home care have a particularly valuable vantage point. They have an opportunity to make first-hand observations of usual food selections and even food preparation. By examining food storage areas with patients, home health nurses can determine whether patients' food selections are generally healthful; identify problem areas, if any; and can also assess the adequacy of food storage, including refrigeration, and provide related teaching as appropriate.

SUPPORTIVE CARE

In providing supportive care nurses focus on patients showing early signs of altered nutrition, either more than or less than body requirements. Such individuals may require hospitalization or may attempt to manage their problems while maintaining as normal a lifestyle as possible. The nurse's role in supportive care is to help patients assess the extent of the nutritional problem, determine its probable cause, choose appropriate interventions to restore optimum nutritional status or to prevent further alteration.

Nursing implementation involves the same approaches used for preventive care. Lifestyle analysis and counseling, values clarification, teaching, and daily meal planning will assist patients to cope with nutritional problems. Other appropriate measures are described below.

Nutritional Supplements

Nutritional supplements may help patients with early nutritional alterations. A physician or dietitian usually prescribes the supplement; nurses monitor their use and effectiveness. General nutritional supplements may add kilocalories to the diet, or specific vitamins or minerals may be supplemented. For example, a patient with alcoholism would need a thiamine supplement.

Teaching

Teaching should include "smart shopping"—how to read food labels (see Fig. 28–4, page 892) to determine kilocalories and nutrient values. Specific areas for teaching will depend on the etiology of a patient's nutritional problem.

Exercise

Exercise is a key part of an overall program for weight reduction. Exercise should be individually planned in accordance with a

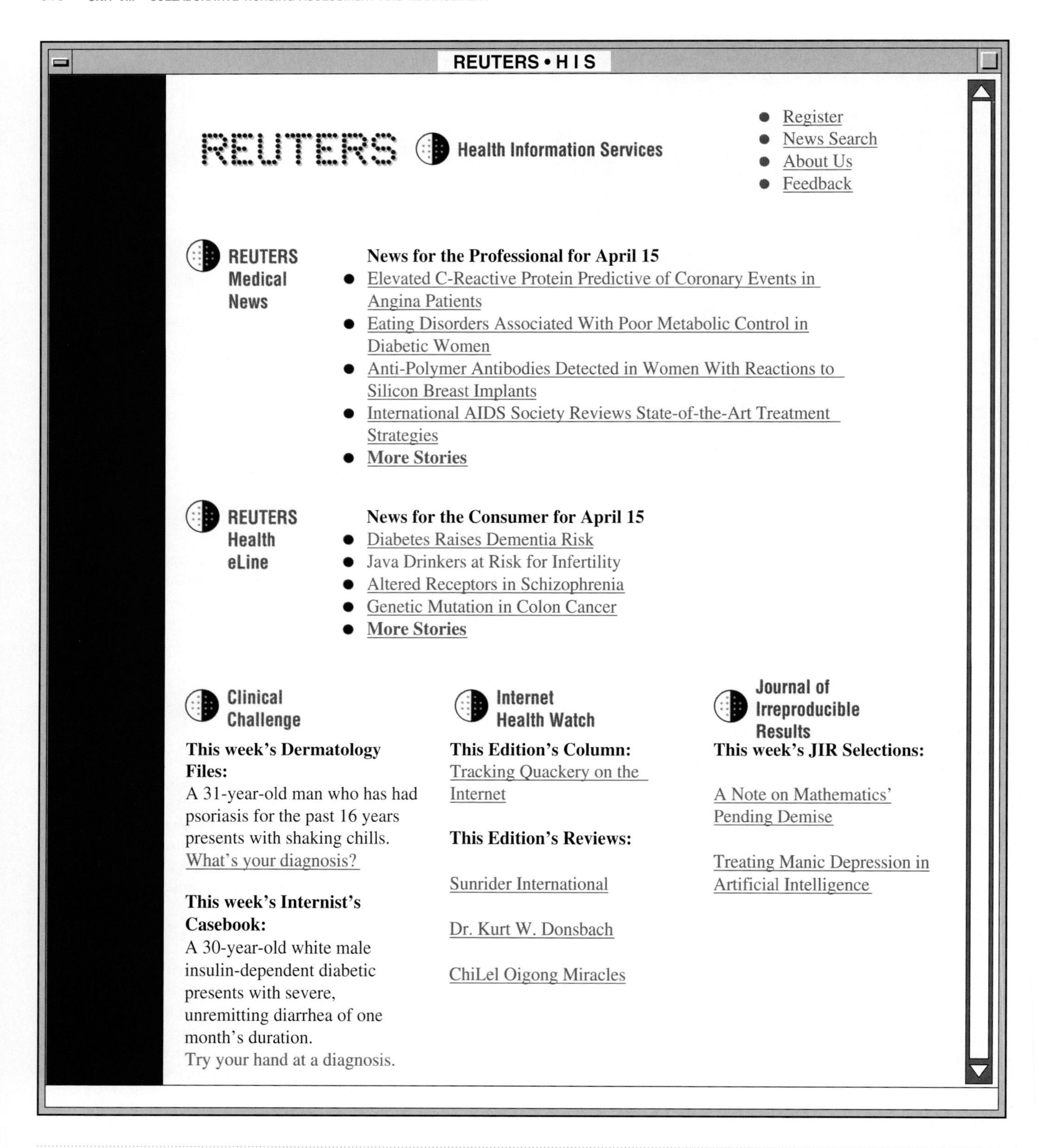

Figure 28–8. A web site on health and nutrition.

patient's capacity, body characteristics, interests, environment, and lifestyle. With aerobic exercise that maintains heart rate at 75 percent of the maximum rate for a 30-minute period, the body will consume its fat stores for energy and excercise of lower intensity will also influence energy balance. A realistic schedule and type of exercise should be planned. Planning exercise sessions three times a week initially is recommended. Setting aside a regular time for exercise makes it easier to incorporate it into one's schedule of activities.

Enhancing Eating Pleasure

If a patient receiving supportive care is hospitalized, nurses should prepare an environment conducive to eating. Patients receiving outpatient care can be counseled about environmental influences on intake. A relaxed, clean, and neat environment with social interaction and adequate time will help make meals enjoyable. Noxious smells and sights should not be present. Offer hospitalized patients an opportunity to wash hands and face before eating and a towel to protect clothing and sheets if desired. Attractive food presentations with manageable portions and needed utensils will make a meal more appetizing.

Assisting with Menu Selection

A patient may need assistance from nurses to select nutritious meals from a hospital menu and may also need assistance in obtaining a special menu, such as one for kosher or vegetarian diets. Nurses can use this opportunity to provide individualized nutrition education as well as to ensure that high-quality foods are selected.

Home Health Care

Home health care at the supportive level attempts to minimize the consequences of a nutritional deficit or excess or assist with food selection and preparation for special diets. This often involves emphasizing limiting the use of commercially prepared foods and teaching how to use food labels for effective food selection. Also, specific nutrient needs and their food sources for patients taking certain drugs are emphasized—for example, the importance of potassium-rich foods such as orange juice and bananas for patients taking diuretics or potassium supplements. Many of the approaches used in preventive care also are appropriate as supportive implementation. Other nursing interventions include support groups for the patient and caregivers, along with Meals-on-Wheels for homebound patients.

RESTORATIVE CARE

Acute nutritional problems requiring complex nursing implementation are the focus of restorative care. Such problems may be related to severe primary nutritional deficiencies such as starvation or may be due to a wide variety of disease processes. Continuous assessment is necessary due to the unstable nature of acute nutritional alterations. Often nurses will serve as the primary providers of nutrition. The physician or dietitian may prescribe therapeutic diets; the nurse's role is administering and evaluating. Table 28–15 describes standard and commonly ordered therapeutic diets. Procedures 28–1 through 28–5 present additional nursing techniques that may be carried out in restorative care.

Tray Presentation/Preparation

Food should be served at the temperature intended: hot foods hot, cold foods cold. The tray should not be overly crowded, and all items should be within the patient's reach. If a patient cannot cut the food, nurses should assist, but it is important that this is not done in a manner that is demeaning. Many adults find dependency of this kind humiliating.

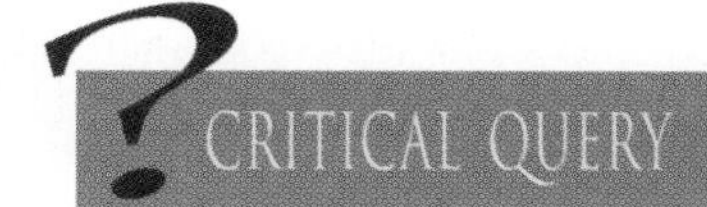

Kayser-Jones,[16] who studied mealtime in nursing homes, identified a need on the part of institutionalized elders for individualized care to promote adequate food intake. She concluded, "Food is such an important part of our lives. It is tragic that in the last months or years of their lives, many nursing home residents are denied one of life's greatest pleasures" (p. 31). What are some strategies the nurse can use to identify the individualized preferences and needs of elderly patients in regard to eating?

Positioning for Safe Eating

Elevate the patient's head as high as possible to minimize the risk of aspiration and provide access to the tray (Fig. 28–9). If at all possible, patients should eat in a sitting position, either on the side of the bed or in a comfortable chair.

Assisting Patients with Dysphagia

Patients who have difficulty swallowing need foods that are easily swallowed. Bites should be small. Highly textured foods stimulate swallowing more than smooth foods. Lightly sweetened and seasoned foods are more easily swallowed. Foods to be avoided are milk, pulp fruits, hamburger patties, onions, thick soups, white bread, custards, crackers, and bitter or acidic foods. Provide ample time for swallowing each bite. Nurses may need to remain with the patient in case choking occurs.

Feeding

Feeding patients who are unable to self-feed is a skill and an art that takes diligence, patience, and a calm, pleasant atmosphere for maximum effectiveness. Perhaps in no other nursing care situation do patients feel so directly dependent on a nurse for a function of such great symbolic importance. Feeding is a nurturing activity that should ideally take place within the context of a carefully developed therapeutic nurse–patient relationship. Otherwise patients may have great difficulty in accepting a dependent role and may claim not to be hungry. Refusal to eat may have complex etiologies that require professional intervention. Procedure 28–1 describes the steps to be followed when feeding a patient.

Use of Special Appliances and Utensils

Special appliances and utensils have been developed for people with specific physical disabilities that interfere with ingestion. Specially shaped spoons, forks, and knives allow easy grasping. Closed cups with no-spill straws and splints for support of hands or arms are also available. Nurses should consult with dietitians or occupational therapists when a special utensil is needed. Figure 28–10 illustrates some assistive devices.

Enteral Feeding

Enteral feeding is an important means of feeding patients whose intake is less than body requirements. **Enteral** means, literally, "via

TABLE 28-15. STANDARD AND THERAPEUTIC HOSPITAL DIETS

Diet	Indications for Use	Comment
Regular	Used for patients requiring no particular modification.	Some hospitals may offer a prudent regular diet as a health-promoting measure (a prudent diet offers food low in saturated fat and cholesterol with substitution of polyunsaturated fat).
Soft		
Traditional	May be used during the transition phase in the progression from a liquid to a regular diet, in the convalescent phase of acute infections, and with mild gastrointestinal disturbances.	Modified in texture so as to include foods that are low in fiber and thus easy to chew, and foods that are simply prepared, mild in flavor, and easily digested.
Mechanical or dental soft	May be used for patients who have chewing problems, mouth sores, or difficulty swallowing.	
Liquid		
Clear	May be used before and after surgery or during acute gastrointestinal illness.	
Full	May be used before and after surgery, in infectious diseases, in situations where chewing and swallowing problems are present, and with gastrointestinal problems.	
High fiber	May be used for patients with irritable bowel, constipation, elevated blood lipids, diabetes. Helps reduce risk of cancer.	Adds volume and weight to stool, speeding transit of undigested materials through the intestine.
Low residue	May be used before and after intestinal surgery or for patients with inflammatory bowel disease.	Reduces fecal mass; low in fiber; milk and meat limited; vitamin and mineral supplements may be necessary.
Bland	May be used for patients with severe heartburn or ulcers.	Eliminates alcohol, caffeine, spices, acidic foods.

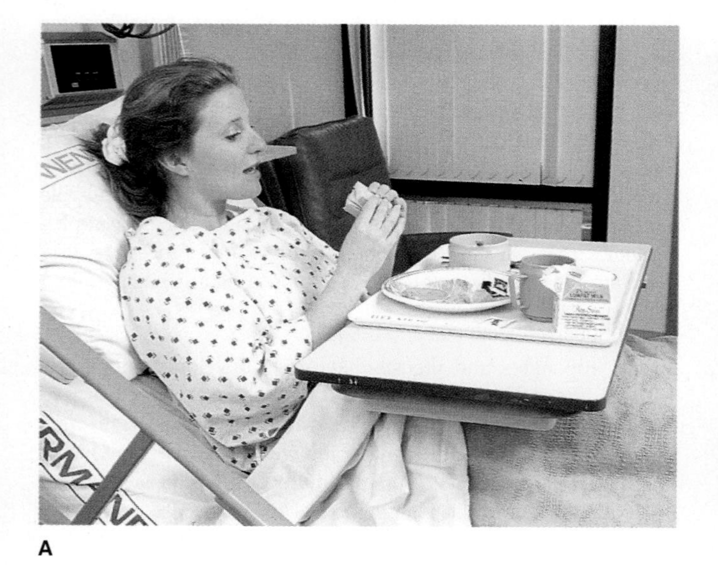

A

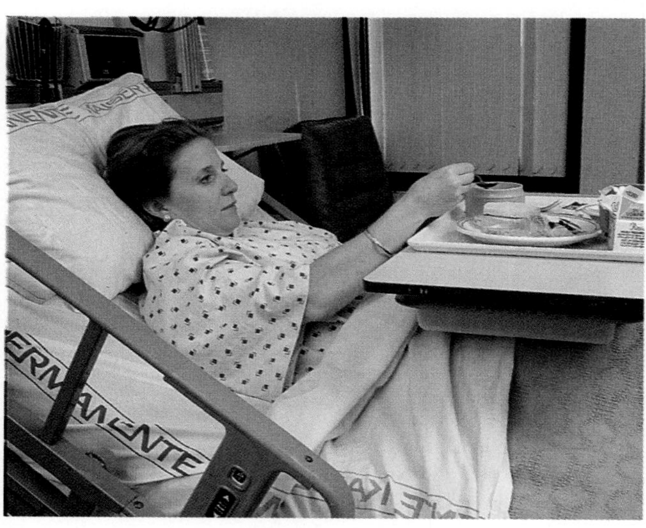

B

Figure 28–9. **A.** A patient is more comfortable eating while sitting upright. **B.** A patient who is left to eat with the head of the bed in a low position is at risk for aspirating food.

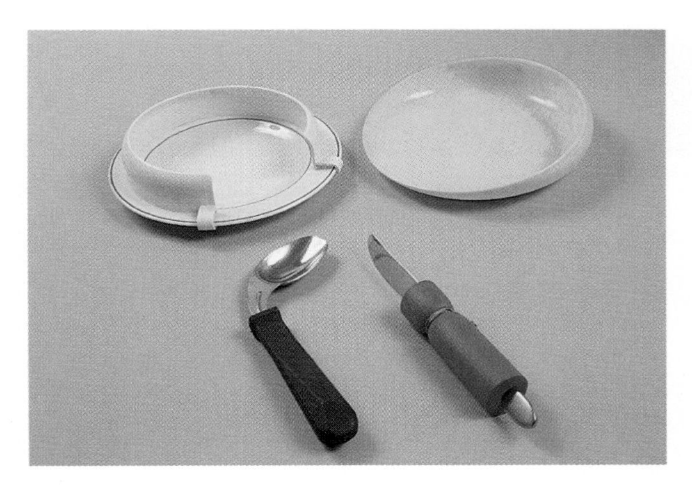

Figure 28–10. Eating devices assist patients to maintain sufficient nutrition independently. Plates facilitate scooping; spoon and knife facilitate grip.

the gastrointestinal tract" rather than by mouth. The types and number of enteral formulas have dramatically increased in the last few years. Table 28–16 (page 925) presents information about common types of enteral formulas. Equipment available for enteral feedings and routes of administration have also become more sophisticated (Fig. 28–11, page 925). Enteral tubes are used to administer a liquid formula directly into the stomach, duodenum, and in some cases, the jejunum. The formulas are usually highly concentrated solutions of carbohydrates, fat, amino acids, vitamins, and minerals. Diarrhea is a common side effect of tube feedings.

To correct the diarrhea, less concentrated solutions can be used, or the solution can be diluted and administered at a lower rate. Another possible cause of diarrhea is a specific intolerance of one or more of the nutrients, such as lactose intolerance.

One way of preventing diarrhea is to administer continuous, rather than intermittent, feedings. A small amount of the formula is infused continuously, its rate maintained constant by use of a feeding pump. When intermittent feedings are used, a large quantity of formula is administered in a short time interval. The larger volume in the intestines is more likely to result in diarrhea.

Inserting a nasogastric feeding tube is usually a nursing responsibility. A number of different types and brands of tubes are available. It is best to use tubes made of soft flexible material, with as small a diameter as possible, to minimize patient discomfort.

For patients with a nasogastric feeding tube, mouth care is particularly important because there are no liquids being ingested orally to lubricate the oral mucosa. Also important is protection of the skin surrounding the tube from pressure or other irritation. Tubes that are inserted surgically, such as jejunostomy tubes, require special skin care and occasionally dressings at the insertion site to prevent irritation or infection. Procedures 28–2 through 28–4 discuss the management of enteral feeding tubes. Procedure 28–5 describes discontinuing an NG tube. Clinical Guideline 28–3 (page 925) and Table 28–17 (page 926) address problems and precautions that a nurse must be aware of when monitoring patients receiving enteral feedings.

Total Parenteral Nutrition

When a patient's digestive tract is unable to absorb nutrients, an alternate route for nutrient administration must be provided. **Total parenteral nutrition (TPN)** is the administration of a nutritionally complete solution intravenously. This process has revolutionized the nutritional care of many patients who would die of malnutrition were TPN not available. Any patient who is unable to tolerate foods or fluids in the digestive tract should be considered a candidate for TPN if it is expected that the intolerance will persist for more than 1 or 2 weeks. If short-term nutritional support is expected, the solution can be given through a peripheral vein; if long-term support is anticipated, it must be given through a central vein, such as the subclavian. A full discussion of TPN and related nursing care is beyond the scope of this text.

Home Health Care

Home health in the restorative mode addresses nutritional deficits and prepares patients for self-management of nutritional needs. Home nurses provide direct assistance as well as teaching patients and families how to meet nutritional needs. Many of the preventive and supportive home care implementations are appropriate for restorative care as well. Patients needing home restorative care may be receiving tube feedings. They will need to use the same guidelines and monitoring for tube feedings addressed previously. Emphasize the importance of supplemental water. Patients with dysphagia also receive home care. They and their families need to know how to select and prepare appropriate foods, how to stimulate and evaluate swallowing, and when to withhold oral foods pending professional evaluation. How to manage choking episodes is also critical teaching for these patients and family caregivers. (See Procedure 30–8.)

REHABILITATIVE CARE

Nutritional rehabilitation is the focus of this level of care. Here the aim is to maximize patients' nutritional status after an acute nutritional alteration and to facilitate self-care ability. Nurses use strategies similar to those used in preventive and supportive care. Supporting lifestyle changes, counseling, and referral to support groups assume particular importance in the rehabilitation process.

Supporting Lifestyle and Habit Changes

After an acute nutritional alteration, a patient is often highly motivated to implement lifestyle changes that will hasten recovery and prevent further problems. Patients will need specific guidelines and practical suggestions regarding new eating patterns and habits. They also require encouragement and support as they initiate changes in previous patterns. Close follow-up and reinforcement are necessary.

(continued on page 926)

PROCEDURE 28–1. FEEDING A PATIENT

PURPOSE: To provide adequate nourishment to patients unable to feed themselves.
EQUIPMENT: Food selected by patient, if possible; napkin or towel; instruments for cutting and eating; water; washcloth; towel; cup; and basin.

ACTION 1. Wash hands.

RATIONALE. Protect patient from hospital-acquired infection.

ACTION 2. Check tray: Foods ordered by patient are delivered? Foods within prescribed diet?

RATIONALE. Patient involved in meal selection increases satisfaction; restricted foods may seriously harm patient.

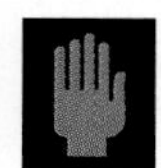

If patient unable to select foods, try to engage family/friends in selection. Use food selection as focus for teaching regarding healthy diets.

ACTION 3. Create a clean, quiet, and pleasant environment.

RATIONALE. A cluttered, dirty, malodorous, or rushed atmosphere will decrease appetite.

ACTION 4. Assist patient to sitting position unless contraindicated. If patient cannot sit, elevate head and shoulders.

RATIONALE. Reduces risk of aspiration, facilitates swallowing.

ACTION 5. Place a napkin or towel under patient's chin.

RATIONALE. Protects patient and bed. Spilling is more likely when patient is being fed by another.

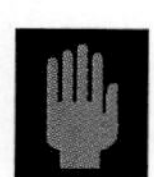

Many patients will feel demeaned by resemblance to bib. Acknowledge this and explain reason.

ACTION 6. Place tray where patient can see and smell food. Encourage patient to indicate what food is wanted for each bite. Serve hot and cold foods at intended temperatures.

RATIONALE. Olfactory stimuli enhance appetite. Active participation reduces patient's feelings of helplessness and/or loss of dignity.

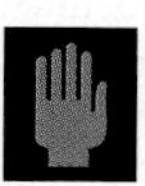

Conversing with the patient about pleasant topics may stimulate appetite and ease anxiety.

ACTION 7. If patient is unable to select foods, give a variety. Offer high-calorie, high-protein foods first.

RATIONALE. If entire meal is not eaten, the most nourishing foods will have been ingested.

ACTION 8. Offer quantities that can be easily chewed. Allow time for patient to eat at own pace.

RATIONALE. See rationale for Action 4.

ACTION 9. Offer liquids periodically.

RATIONALE. Stimulates saliva, allowing improved digestion and easier swallowing.

ACTION 10. When finished, offer materials for washing and mouth care and assist as needed. Leave in a position of comfort.

RATIONALE. Hygiene and positioning enhance comfort and promote relaxation, which facilitates digestion.

Recording:
Record type of diet patient selects or is prescribed. Record percentage of meal consumed, patient's response to eating, and any difficulties with chewing or swallowing. In many facilities, this information is recorded on a checklist rather than in narrative notes.

HOME HEALTH ADAPTATION: This procedure is easily adapted to the home setting. Family caregivers may need teaching about feeding techniques, as well as approaches to diminish their loved one's feelings of helplessness when being fed.

PROCEDURE 28–2. INSERTING A NASOGASTRIC TUBE (FEEDING OR DECOMPRESSION TUBE)

PURPOSE: To provide a route for administration of liquid food or for removal of gastrointestinal fluid and air.
EQUIPMENT: Feeding tube (preferably small diameter, soft, plastic) or NG tube (usually a Levin or Salem sump tube); water-soluble lubricant or lidocaine jelly; waterproof pad or towel; tissues; emesis basin; glass of water and straw, or ice chips; hypoallergenic adhesive tape, 50-mL syringe; bowl of ice; stethoscope; penlight.

ACTION 1. Wash hands.

RATIONALE. Prevents the transfer of microorganisms from the nurse's hands to the patient.

ACTION 2. Discuss the procedure with the patient, including its purpose and benefits, nurse's actions, desired patient participation, and sensations commonly experienced.

RATIONALE. Patient will be less fearful and more willing to participate if the purpose, benefits, and procedure of the tube are clear.

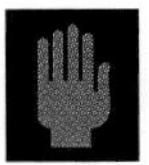

If patient is unconscious, explain procedure to family, if present. Tell family tears are produced when nasal mucosa is irritated and do not indicate patient is in distress.

ACTION 3. Gather all equipment on overbed table. Raise bed to nurse's thigh level and lower siderail.

RATIONALE. Provides for efficient performance of procedure with minimal strain to nurse and patient.

ACTION 4. Screen patient. Place in high Fowler's position and place towel across chest.

RATIONALE. Privacy is needed for invasive procedures. Tube will pass more easily in high Fowler's position because of gravity and patient's effective swallowing.

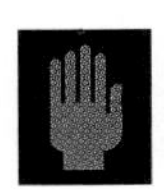

If patient cannot sit up, lateral position may be used.

ACTION 5. Arrange a signal for patient to indicate if feeling discomfort. Place tissues and emesis basis within patient's reach.

RATIONALE Stimulation of throat may cause gagging or trigger emesis. Patient will be less fearful if aware that nurse will respond to signal.

ACTION 6. Determine the appropriate insertion length for the tube by measuring the distance from the patient's nares to the earlobe and from the ear to the tip of the sternum. Mark this distance from the tube's end with a piece of tape. Many tubes are premarked to aid in noting distance to insert. The marks do not replace measuring as described, but eliminate need for marking with tape.

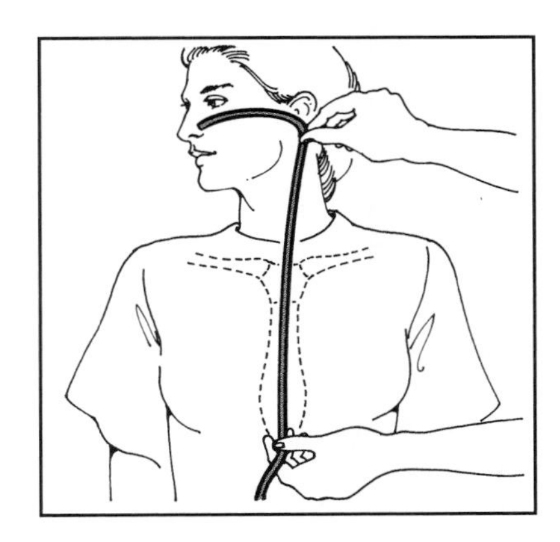

RATIONALE. The tube must extend into the stomach to decrease risk of aspiration of tube feeding formula or to remove gastric contents. This measurement approximates the distance from the nose to the stomach cavity. Marking the length will decrease risk of the tube not being inserted far enough.

Continued

Procedure 28–2. Inserting a Nasogastric Tube (continued)

ACTION 7. If inserting a small-bore feeding tube, lubricate *inside* of lumen (included in kit). Insertion stylet may have been placed inside feeding tube by manufacturer. If not, insert stylet now and secure with luer-lock connector. If no stylet, place the first 10 cm of tube in bowl of ice so that the first 6 cm are gently curved.

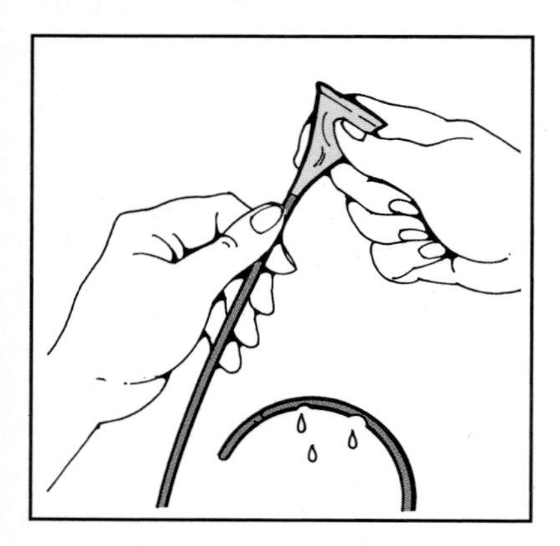

RATIONALE. Small-bore tubes are very soft and flexible. Stylet provides stiffness necessary for insertion of tube. Liquid reduces friction inside the small tube, facilitating stylet insertion and removal. If no stylet, the ice will stiffen the tube and the curve will help the tube to pass through the nose.

ACTION 8. Inspect nostrils to determine which one is most patent. Ask patient about previous nose fracture or deviated septum.

RATIONALE. Previous trauma to the nose may leave scar tissue, making the canal too narrow for the tube. Attempt to introduce tube in other nostril.

ACTION 9. If patient is not allergic to lidocaine or Cetacaine®, spray the nostril and posterior pharynx with anesthetic spray. Wait 3 to 4 minutes for anesthesia to take effect. Lubricate the first 15 to 20 cm (6–8 in.) of the outside of the tube with lidocaine jelly or a water-soluble lubricant.

RATIONALE. Anesthetic will make insertion of tube less uncomfortable. Lubricant reduces friction and irritation to mucosa. Water-soluble lubricant will dissolve without causing respiratory irritation if the tube accidentally enters the trachea.

ACTION 10. Gently insert the tube into nostril, with curve aiming down. Ask the patient to open mouth. Slight pressure may be needed to advance tube.

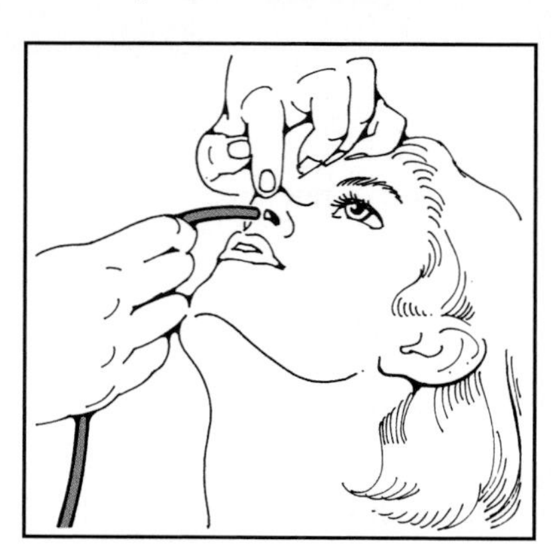

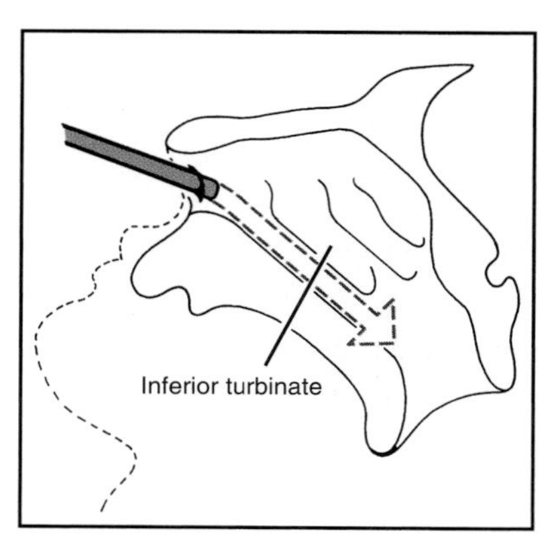

RATIONALE. This direction follows the natural contour of the nasal passage, thereby decreasing mucosal irritation. Open mouth will help to keep the nares open.

ACTION 11. If resistance is met, slightly withdraw the tube and readvance until it reaches the nasopharynx. If obstruction persists, relubricate tube and try the other nostril.

If the tube coils up or advances into the mouth, withdraw it back into the nasopharynx.

Procedure 28–2. (continued)

ACTION 12. Advance the tube 6 to 10 cm, then rotate 180 degrees and continue to advance while asking patient to swallow sips of water through a straw. Advance the tube with each swallow until premarked length is reached. Inserting tube too rapidly or out of synchrony with swallowing may cause tube to coil in oropharynx. If patient gags, suggest panting for a few breaths.

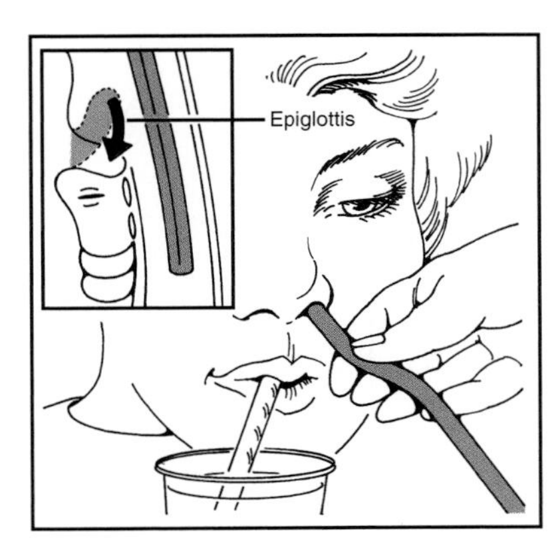

RATIONALE. Rotating tube directs the tube toward the esophagus and away from the trachea. Swallowing closes the epiglottis and assists passage of tube over the glottis and into the esophagus. Panting suppresses the gag reflex, a common response to the passage of the tube.

ACTION 13. If the patient coughs or gasps for air, the tube has entered the trachea. Immediately withdraw the tube back into the nasopharynx.

RATIONALE. The cough reflex is stimulated by the presence of a foreign body in the trachea. The tube will continue to interfere with O_2 exchange until it is removed.

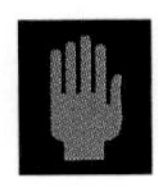

Some comatose patients may not retain this cough reflex. See Action 14.

ACTION 14. Confirm placement of tube in the stomach by either *(left)* aspirating gastric contents and testing pH or *(right)* injecting 5 to 10 cc of air from the syringe into tube, and listening with stethoscope over the epigastric region for the sound of air entering the stomach.

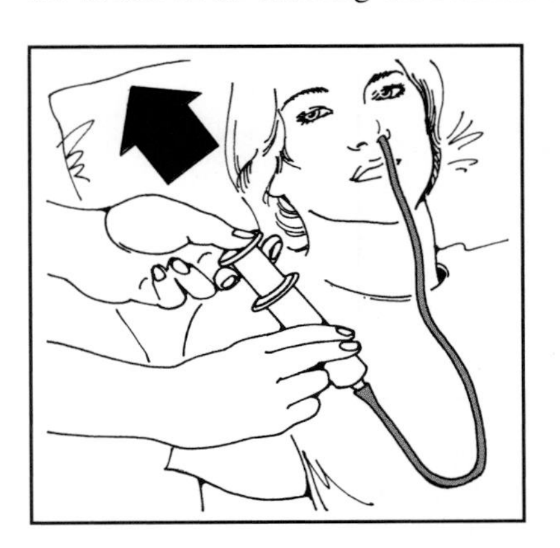

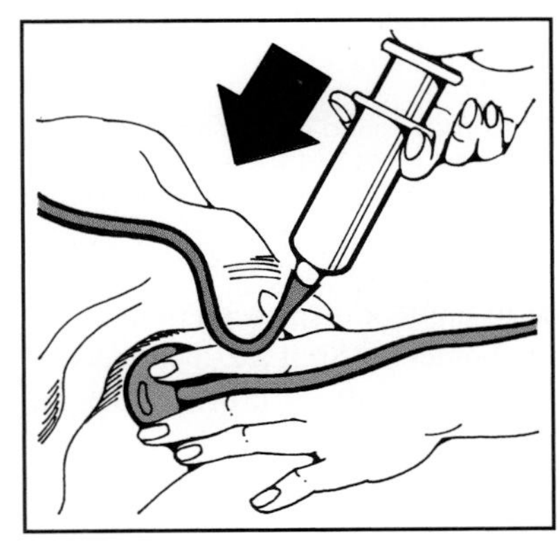

RATIONALE. Placement in stomach must be confirmed to avoid risk of aspiration of liquid into the lungs. Tube placement can be definitively confirmed by either x-ray or assessing pH of tube aspirate. Mean gastric aspirate pH is 3.02, compared with 6.57 for intestinal and 7 or greater for lung aspirates. Auscultating air movement is the least reliable method of determining tube placement.

Continued

ACTION 15. If tube inserted is small-bore feeding tube, remove stylet prior to testing for placement.

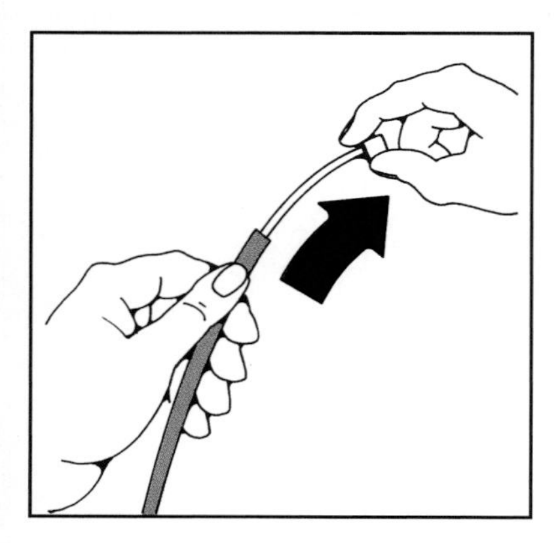

RATIONALE. Lumen of these tubes is very small and is nearly obstructed by the stylet. Also the luer-lock device securing the stylet prevents attachment of a syringe for aspiration or instillation of air.

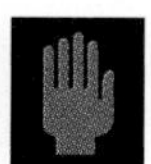

Small-bore soft tubes may make aspiration impossible because negative pressure causes them to collapse. If gastric contents cannot be aspirated, x-ray confirmation of feeding tube placement should be obtained.

ACTION 16. Secure tube to prevent displacement and rubbing, which can erode nasal mucosa: Split a 2-inch piece of 1-inch wide hypoallergenic tape halfway down its length. Attach unsplit end of tape to nose and wrap split ends around tubing in opposite directions. For small-bore tubing, tape need not be split.

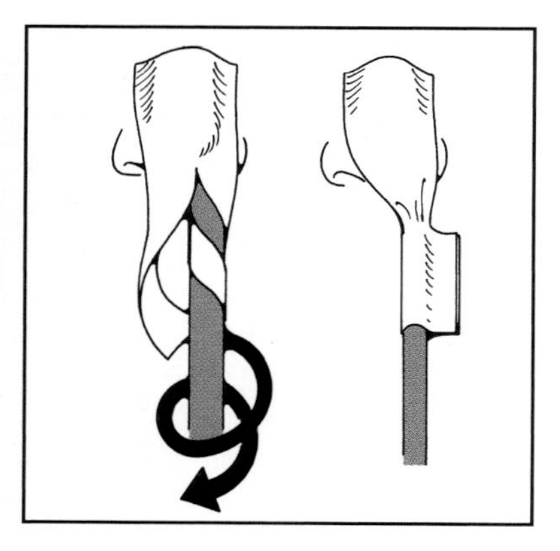

RATIONALE. Displacement increases risk of aspiration. Rubbing against nasal and pharyngeal mucosa or traction from the tube being inadvertently pulled are very uncomfortable.

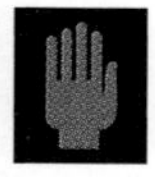

Tape may need daily replacement as skin oils decrease adhesion. Clean residual adhesive from nose before applying new tape (acetone, nail polish remover, or tape remover can be used). Recheck placement after retaping.

ACTION 17. Anchor tubing to patient's gown with tape or rubber band and safety pin, taking special care to keep the tube from rubbing against nasal mucosa.

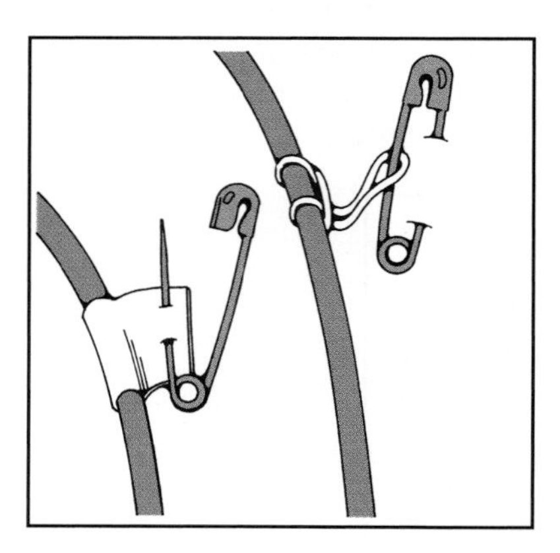

RATIONALE. Pressure of tubing can cause tissue ulceration and necrosis as well as discomfort.

ACTION 18. Connect distal end of tubing to suction machine (see Procedure 25–4) or to tube feeding apparatus (see Procedure 28–3) as ordered or plug end with catheter plug.

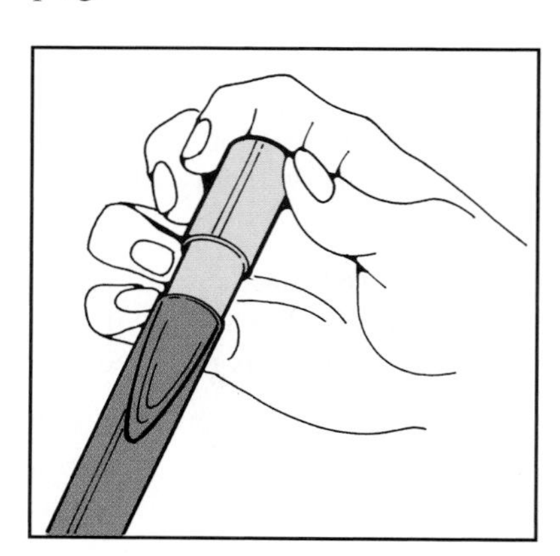

RATIONALE. Intubation is ordered for a specific purpose, which should be promptly carried out. Gastric contents may leak from proximal end of tubing if it is not plugged or connected to appropriate apparatus.

ACTION 19. Provide oral hygiene with mouthwash and/or lemon glycerine swabs q2–3 hours. Lip balm may be applied. Clean nares at least q shift with moist cotton-tip applicator. Apply water-soluble lubricant to nostril prn.

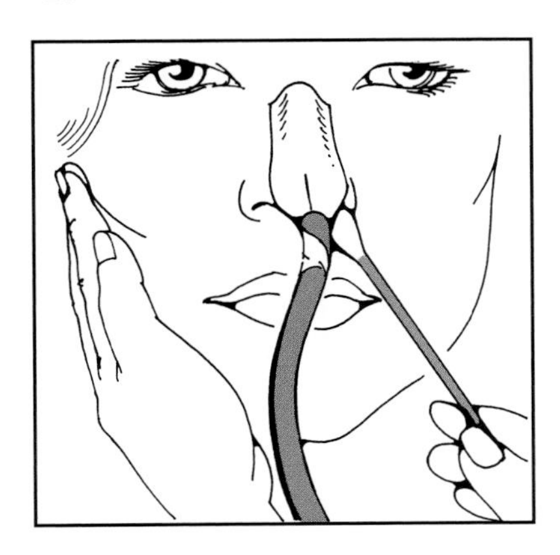

RATIONALE. NG tubes often stimulate mouth breathing, which causes oral mucous membranes to become dry and uncomfortable. Nasal mucus production is stimulated by the tube and may become encrusted around tube.

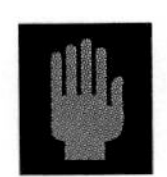

If NG tube is being used for decompression (see Procedure 25–4), some physicians allow ice chips, hard candy, or chewing gum to stimulate saliva and lubricate mouth.

Recording:

Chart the time of insertion, which nostril was used; the quantity and pH of fluid returned, if any; problems encountered, if any; associated actions taken; and patient's response to the procedure.

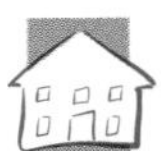

HOME HEALTH ADAPTATION: Although placing an NG tube in a home setting is unusual, the insertion procedure does not vary with the setting. A portable in home x-ray can be arranged to verify placement if aspiration of gastric contents is impossible or if auscultation of air is inconclusive to confirm placement of tubing in the stomach. If the patient is confused, collaborate with the family to use an appropriate restraining device to prevent displacement or removal of the tubing.

PROCEDURE 28–3. ADMINISTERING ENTERAL FEEDING

PURPOSE: To provide nourishment to the patient unable to ingest food by mouth.
EQUIPMENT: Feeding solution; feeding pump or drop regulator, or catheter-tip 60-mL syringe; cup of water.

ACTION 1. Verify physician order for type, quantity, rate, and frequency of feeding.

RATIONALE. Tube feeding formulas are considered medications. Nurses may not administer medications without a physician's order.

ACTION 2. Discuss procedure with patient, including purpose, anticipated benefits, nurse's actions, and desired patient participation. Gather all equipment at bed- or chairside.

RATIONALE. Patient will be less fearful and more willing to participate if the purpose, benefits, and procedure of tube insertion are clear.

ACTION 3. Elevate head of bed 20 to 30 degrees.

RATIONALE. Facilitates gastric emptying; prevents regurgitation or aspiration.

ACTION 4. Verify placement of the feeding tube (see Procedure 28–2, Action 14).

RATIONALE. End of tube must be in the stomach. Aspiration pneumonia can occur if the formula is introduced into the trachea or flows there because of reflux from the esophagus.

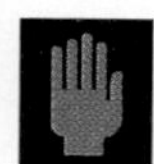

Soft feeding tubes collapse when negative pressure is applied. Use air instillation method or x-ray verification of placement.

ACTION 5. If residual from previous feeding is obtained, measure and record. Reinstill residual to stomach.

RATIONALE. Residual formula is mixed with gastric secretions. It is returned to prevent electrolytic depletion.

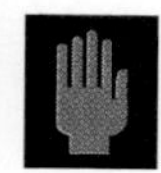

Residual of more than 150 mL suggests poor motility and absorption. Postpone feeding and notify physician. Note: Aspiration of residual not feasible unless rigid NG tube or gastronomy tube is used.

ACTION 6. **Continuous feedings.**

a. Place a 4-hour supply of formula in feeding bag of bottle. Label container with date and time solution was added. Some institutions add food coloring to formula to aid in early detection of aspiration (mucus becomes colored if formula enters respiratory tract).

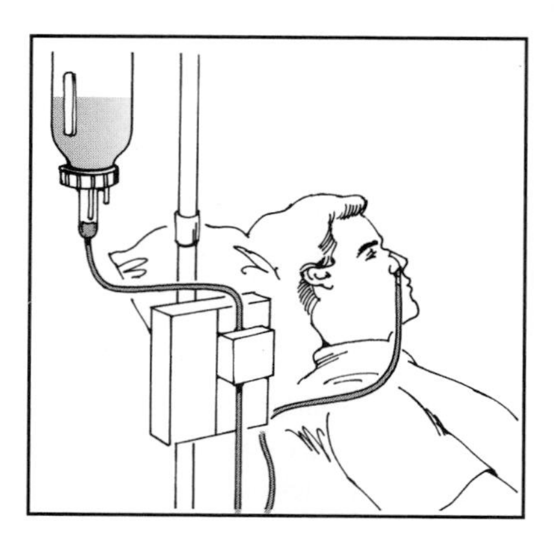

RATIONALE. Milk-based formula is an excellent medium for bacterial growth. Potential increases with greater time at room temperature.

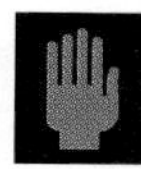

Some agencies use prefilled, sealed containers, which can remain in use for 24 hours without risk of bacterial growth. Ice may also be used to slow bacterial growth, but not all patients tolerate iced formulas.

b. Hang container on IV pole, and clear air from tubing by allowing solution to flow through.

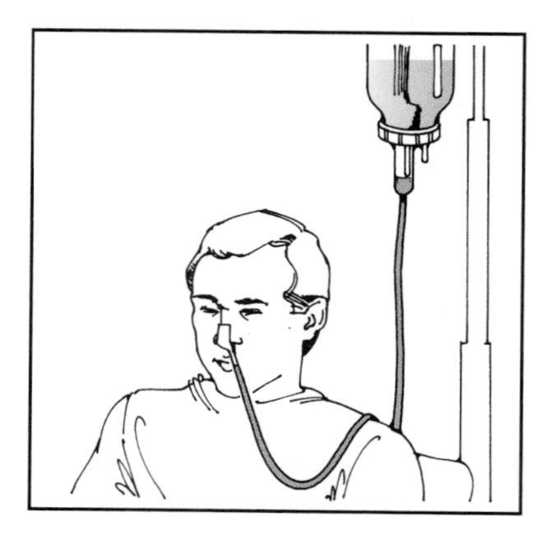

RATIONALE. Air distends stomach, causing discomfort and possible vomiting.

Procedure 28–3. (continued)

c. Regulate the infusion with the flow clamp or with an automatic pump.

RATIONALE. Continuous slow drip is used to prevent complications related to highly concentrated formulas. Rapid uncontrolled infusion may cause diarrhea or vomiting. Small-bore tubes limit rate attainable by gravity drip, so positive peristaltic pumps must be used.

d. Assess lungs and abdomen every shift.

RATIONALE. Lung congestion suggests aspiration. Check the placement. Distended abdomen or decreased bowel sounds suggest formula is not being absorbed. Consult with physician and/or dietitian.

e. HOB should remain elevated to 20 to 30 degrees during infusions. If patient care (such as linen change, chest physiotherapy) requires patient to be flat, turn off feeding at least 30 minutes prior to positioning patient flat.

RATIONALE. Presence of tube affects efficiency of cardiac sphincter of stomach. Placing patient flat while formula is infusing may allow reflux via esophagus to pharynx, causing aspiration.

f. Calculate 24-hour fluid requirements on all patients receiving continuous tube feedings. Interrupt feeding to administer water in 30–60 mL bolus via syringe attached to end of feeding tube (see Action 7). Frequency varies with amounts of additional fluid required by patient, but once per shift is common. Water may be given by mouth if patient is conscious and able to swallow.

RATIONALE. Continuous tube feeding orders are based on calorie needs, but may not supply adequate fluids.

g. Replace feeding bag and tubing at least every 24 hours.

RATIONALE. See Action 6a.

ACTION 7. **Intermittent feedings**

USING A PREFILLED BOTTLE:

a. Open the bottle and replace the cover with the tubing/screw-cap unit. Hang from IV pole and clear air from tubing as in Action 6b.

RATIONALE. Displacing air from the tubing prior to attaching it to the feeding tube prevents gastric distension and vomiting.

b. Attach tubing to feeding tube, open clamp and regulate flow as ordered with screw clamp or feeding pump.

RATIONALE. Careful regulation of flow prevents complications and discomfort. If bolus is given too rapidly, diarrhea, abdominal cramps, or vomiting may occur. If this happens, slow the rate of administration.

c. At completion of feeding, flush feeding tube with water as described under "Using a Syringe," below.

RATIONALE. Flushing tubing helps prevent clogging and bacterial growth in tubing and provides fluid.

USING A FEEDING BAG:

a. Add ordered amount of solution to feeding bag. Prepare and regulate flow as in steps 6a and b.

b. At completion of feeding, flush feeding tube with water as described under Using a Syringe.

RATIONALE. Flushing tubing helps prevent clogging and bacterial growth in tubing and provides fluid.

c. Rinse bag and tubing thoroughly and store for reuse. Discard and replace after 24 hours.

RATIONALE. Rinsing removes residue of formula, which is a medium for bacterial growth. Reusing equipment for more than 24 hours increases risk of contamination and related complications.

USING A SYRINGE:

a. Attach 50-mL syringe, without plunger, to clamped feeding tube.

RATIONALE. Keeping tube clamped until syringe is filled with solution prevents air from entering stomach. (See Action a, Using a Prefilled Bottle.)

Continued

b. Pour feeding solution into syringe, unclamp, and regulate flow of solution to approximately 30 mL/min by raising or lowering syringe. Refill syringe as necessary until ordered quantity has been administered. Do not allow syringe to empty completely before adding additional formula. If fluid does not flow by gravity, replace plunger and administer using positive pressure at no more than 30 mL/min.

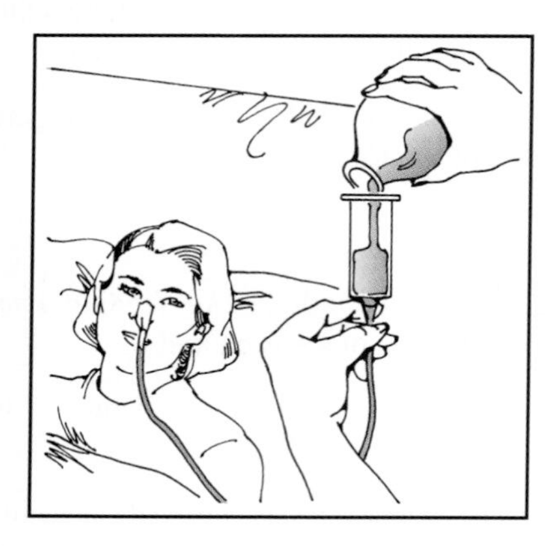

RATIONALE. Research has shown that this rate is tolerated by most patients. Refilling before syringe is empty prevents air from entering stomach.

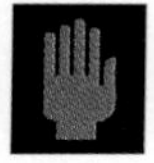

Syringe administration is used most often for infants and children. It is an impractical method for the volumes required by adults.

c. When formula level reaches tip of syringe, flush feeding tube with 50 mL or prescribed amount of water; clamp tube before detaching syringe.

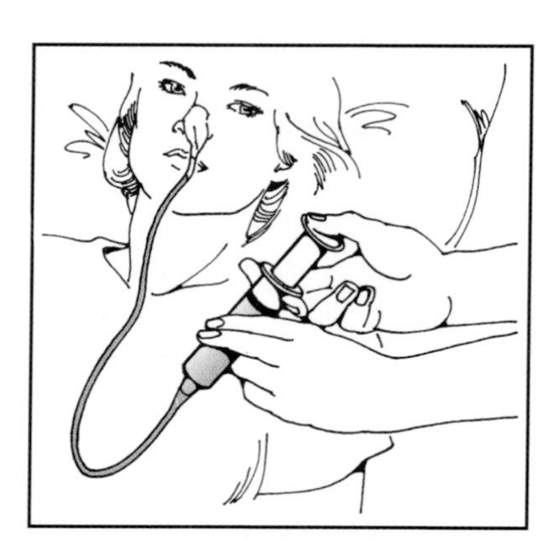

RATIONALE. Flushing tubing helps prevent clogging and bacterial growth in tubing and provides fluid. Clamp prevents air from entering stomach or gastric contents from leaking out.

d. Position patient or request patient to keep head of bed elevated to 30 degrees for 30 to 60 minutes after feeding.

RATIONALE. Facilitates gastric emptying; prevents regurgitation or aspiration.

Recording:

Commonly charted on flowsheet. *Continuous feeding:* Document placement check, lung and abdominal assessment, type, concentration and rate of formula infusion. Note untoward effects and action taken. *Intermittent feeding:* Document placement check, residual obtained. Note the time of feeding, amount of formula and water instilled, and patient response.

HOME HEALTH ADAPTATION: It is essential to confirm placement before beginning any feeding and to document the findings. If there is any question about placement, request an in-home x-ray to be taken. Family members who are conscientious and capable of learning how to safely administer tube feedings can be taught the technique. Allow ample opportunity for them to practice with assistance and supervision until they can demonstrate proficiency and verbalize confidence. All family caregivers should be instructed, however, to observe for adverse signs and symptoms and to report them promptly. If long-term enteral feeding is anticipated, it is likely that the physician will surgically place a jejunostomy tube to administer feedings with minimal aspiration risk.

PROCEDURE 28–4. CARING FOR A GASTROSTOMY OR JEJUNOSTOMY TUBE SITE

PURPOSE: To prevent skin breakdown or infection and accidental tube removal.

EQUIPMENT: Catheter plug; 4 × 4-inch gauze dressing; tape; petrolatum; zinc oxide or other skin barrier; hydrogen peroxide; betadine or mild soap.

ACTION 1. When tube is not in use for decompression or feeding, keep it sealed with a cap or clamp.

RATIONALE. Prevents leakage of gastric or intestinal contents.

ACTION 2. Check site of tube entry at least once per shift. Cleanse any leakage around the site as ordered and dry the skin. Use care not to disturb the suture securing the tube to the skin. Betadine, hydrogen peroxide, or soap and water are commonly ordered for skin care.

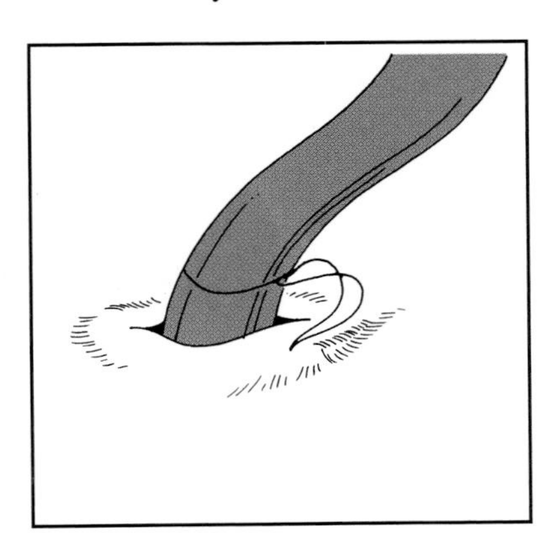

RATIONALE. Leakage of gastric contents causes skin excoriation and possible subsequent infection.

ACTION 3. Apply petrolatum or other skin barrier and cover with a 4 × 4-inch gauze dressing.

RATIONALE. These substances are insoluble in water, and so will not dissolve in GI secretions and will therefore minimize skin irritation.

ACTION 4. Tape tube to the outside of the dressing. Tube may be connected to feeding apparatus or, less commonly, to suction apparatus or gravity drainage.

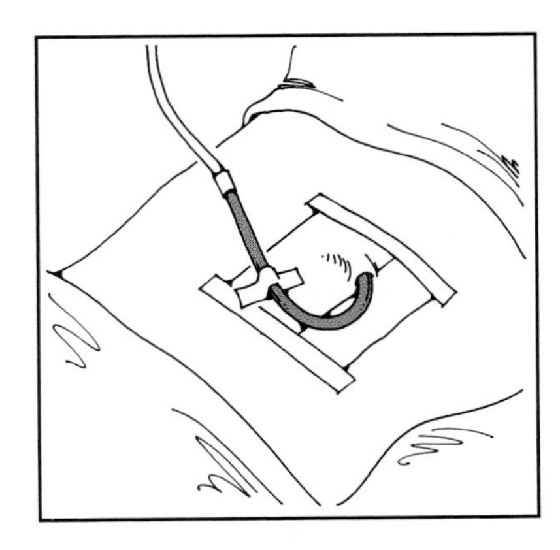

RATIONALE. Prevents tension on the tube causing possible widening of skin opening and/or accidental removal of tube.

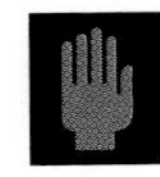

If tube is accidentally pulled out, cover the opening with a sterile petrolatum dressing until tubing can be reinserted.

Recording:

Record date and time of site check and/or dressing change. Record skin condition, any leakage of fluid or formula, skin care provided, and type of dressing applied.

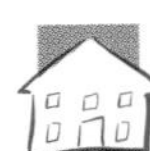

HOME HEALTH ADAPTATION: Teach family caregivers how to clean around the tube insertion site, change dressings as necessary, and to look for adverse signs and symptoms and report them. If the patient is confused, collaborate with the family to use an appropriate restraining device to prevent displacement or removal of the tube.

PROCEDURE 28–5. REMOVING A NASOGASTRIC TUBE

PURPOSE: Discontinuing decompression or tube feeding.
EQUIPMENT: Waterproof pad, clean gloves, mouth care preparations of choice, fresh water, adhesive remover.

ACTION 1. Verify orders for removal of tube.

RATIONALE. Medical order is required to discontinue a medically ordered treatment.

ACTION 2. Assess abdomen for bowel sounds. If not audible, consult with physician.

RATIONALE. Decompression NG tubes are used postoperatively and are left in place until bowel sounds return. If removed before peristalsis resumes, pooled gastric secretions may cause nausea and vomiting.

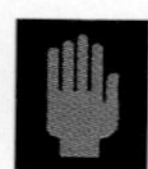

If used for administering liquid feedings, tubes are discontinued when patient is able to resume oral intake. Bowel sounds should have been present throughout therapy.

ACTION 3. Discuss procedure with patient. Provide information about desired participation and usual sensations associated with removal:

a. Patient should be in Fowler's position.

b. Tube will be removed rapidly to minimize gagging.

c. Exhaling as tube is removed will relax pharynx (decreasing irritation and preventing aspiration).

d. Slight irritation of throat and nostril may accompany withdrawal. Eyes may water.

e. Slightly bitter aftertaste is common; mouth care will relieve this effect.

RATIONALE. A clear understanding of the procedure will increase the effectiveness of patient participation and reduce apprehension.

ACTION 4. Free tubing from gown, carefully remove tape from nose, moving tube as little as possible.

RATIONALE. Movement of tube creates friction and erosion of mucous membranes of nose and throat. After several days of intubation, there is sufficient irritation that even a small amount of movement of the tube is painful.

ACTION 5. Place waterproof pad over patient's gown. Don clean gloves.

RATIONALE. Protects nurse and patient from contact with secretions in or on tube.

ACTION 6. Disconnect tube from suction machine or feeding pump. Firmly pinch tube or fold it back on itself to prevent fluid leaking.

RATIONALE. Leaking fluid from the tube during removal may cause aspiration.

ACTION 7. Cue the patient, then withdraw the tube steadily and rapidly while patient exhales.

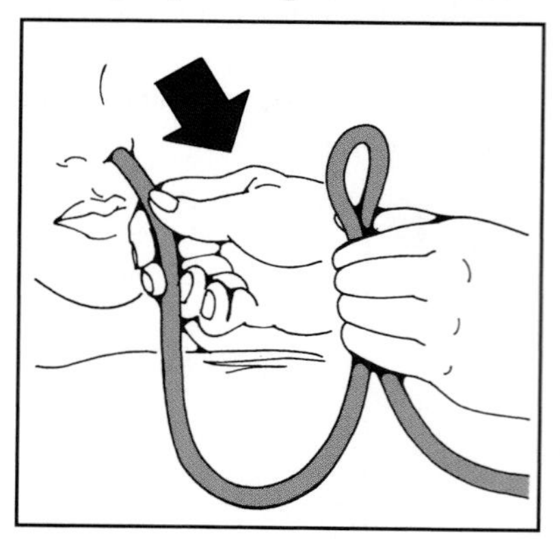

RATIONALE. Avoids startling patient, enhances relaxation.

ACTION 8. Wrap tube in waterproof pad; remove gloves; dispose of all according to agency policy.

RATIONALE. Prevents transfer of microorganisms to environment.

ACTION 9. Provide tissues to blow nose; mouthwash, toothbrush, or lemon-glycerine swabs to freshen mouth. Provide opportunity (or assist) to wash face.

RATIONALE. Promotes comfort.

ACTION 10. Offer fluids—encourage sipping, not rapid intake.

RATIONALE. Patient with NG tube has been npo or receiving fluids by slow drip. Patients may be eager to drink, but rapid intake may cause nausea and vomiting.

Recording:
Note completion of procedure, patient's response, amount of drainage in suction container if tube was used for decompression, and complications (if any) and action taken.

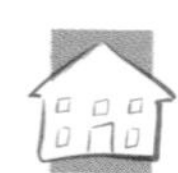

HOME HEALTH ADAPTATION: Removal of nasogastric tube does not vary with the setting.

TABLE 28-16. COMMON TYPES OF ENTERAL FORMULAS

Type	Content/Use
Standard or intact	Blended natural foods or protein isolate formulates (containing a protein that has been separated from a food).
Hydrolyzed formulas (monomeric)	Contain broken-down protein molecules (amino acids or short peptide chains).
Modular formulas	Made by combining "modules" of single nutrients to construct individualized formulas.
Special-use formulas	Designed to meet the needs of patients with specific dietary needs because of nutritional alterations or diseases.
Low-residue formulas	Well tolerated; useful following GI surgery or in early stages of recovery from GI disease.
High-residue formulas	Have added fiber; help to maintain GI integrity in prolonged enteral feeding. May benefit persons with diarrhea or constipation.

CLINICAL GUIDELINE 28–3

MONITORING PATIENTS RECEIVING TUBE FEEDINGS

PARAMETER	FREQUENCY
Placement of nasogastric tube	Each time intermittent feeding is initiated At least every shift when feeding is continuous
Tolerance	
Nausea	At least every shift*
Abdominal distension	At least every shift*
Urine glucose and acetone	q8h, may discontinue after 48 hours if consistently negative in nondiabetic patient
Residual feeding in stomach	Before starting intermittent feeding, every shift for continuous feeding*
Hydration	
Urine specific gravity	Every shift
Intake and output	Every shift
Weight	Daily
Skin turgor, moisture	Every shift
Nutrition status (See Table 28–9)	Every 7–10 days
Lung sounds	Every shift

*Check q4h when continuous feeding first started or when rate is changed.

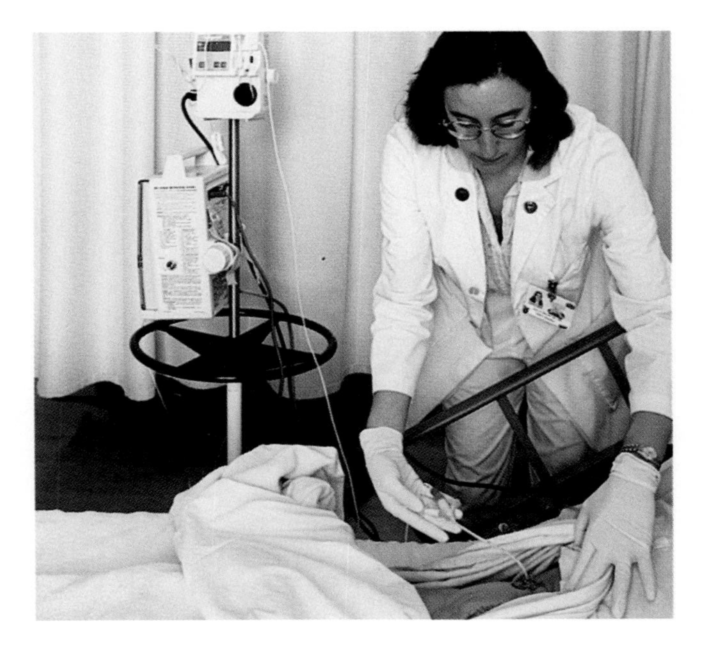

Figure 28–11. Gastrostomy feeding tube is inserted directly into the patient's stomach. *(From Smith S, Duell D.* Clinical Nursing Skills: Nursing Process Model; Basic to Advanced Skills. *4th ed. Norwalk, CT: Appleton & Lange; 1996:464.)*

INSIGHTS FROM NURSING LITERATURE

OPTIMIZING NUTRITION FOR INSTITUTIONALIZED ELDERS

Kayser-Jones J. Mealtime in nursing homes: the importance of individualized care. J Gerontol Nurs. *1996;March:26–31.*

Noting that eating problems often arise from complex interacting factors, the researcher designed a study to identify the factors that influence eating among patients in nursing homes. Her methodology was participant observation and in-depth interviews. She talked to physicians, nursing staff, nursing home residents, and their families. Findings showed themes related to (1) providing food individuals like and enjoy and (2) helping those who need assistance in a safe manner that preserves their dignity.

Many subjects complained that food was served cold and not seasoned to their liking. Food refusal was frequently associated with mild swallowing problems or the subject's desire, despite a lack of motor skill, to eat unassisted. Such problems, the researcher noted, are easily compensated for by giving subjects adequate time for eating. Some staffers, furthermore, failed to recognize that subjects' desire for independence could be supported with minimal assistance, such as by opening containers.

TABLE 28-17. COMMON PROBLEMS ASSOCIATED WITH ENTERAL FEEDINGS

Problem	Possible Cause	Prevention/Treatment
Nausea, vomiting, abdominal distension	Administration too rapid, delayed gastric emptying	Avoid bolus feedings, administer by slow continuous drip. Dilute formula, gradually increase concentration.
Diarrhea, abdominal cramps	Intolerance to hypertonic formula	Dilute formula, gradually increase concentration.
	Bacterial contamination	Refrigerate open containers of formula. Use medical asepsis when handling formula and equipment. Change bag and tubing at least q24h, rinse equipment used for intermittent feeding with each use.
	Rapid administration of formula	Use slow continuous drip administration via feeding pump.
	Lactose intolerance	Use lactose-free formula in high-risk patients.
Clogged feeding tube	Medications not adequately flushed through tubing	Use liquid forms of drugs when available. Finely crush tablets and mix with water. Flush tube with water before and after medications.
Dehydration	Diarrhea	See above.
	Insufficient fluid intake	Calculate fluid needs, administer supplementary fluids to match needs.
	Osmotic diuresis related to high carbohydrate concentration	See Hyperglycemia.
Hyperglycemia	High carbohydrate concentration	Assess blood and urine glucose, change to lower carbohydrate formula, dilute formula or reduce rate of administration. Physician may consider giving insulin.
Aspiration pneumonia	Incomplete closure of gastroesophageal sphincter; delayed gastric emptying.	Use gastrostomy, jejunostomy tubes, or small-diameter nasoenteric tubes; elevate head of bed during and 30 min after feeding; administer by slow continuous drip; check gastric residual.
Constipation	Low-fiber formula Lack of exercise Drugs	Increase fluids. High-fiber formulas. Encourage activity. Give laxatives or enemas as needed.

Counseling

The same principles of counseling discussed earlier can be applied to rehabilitative care. Patients' needs for optimism are particularly significant during the process of rehabilitation. Progress may be slow, and discouragement is common. Nurses can provide a climate of realistic hope to support patients through these low points.

Referral to Support Groups

Adolescents, parents with children requiring prolonged dietary changes, and the elderly may find support groups particularly helpful in maintaining lifestyle changes. Dietitians may be of help in identifying local groups. In our society, support groups exist for almost every health problem. Discussion groups on the Internet provide readily available support and current information.

EVALUATION

The evaluation of nurse and patient actions to promote optimal nutrition can only be as good as the outcomes that have been identified. If goals are specific and realistic, evaluation criteria, which also must be specific and measurable, easily flow from them. Many of the assessment criteria for nutritional status can be used as individual evaluation criteria. Clinical indicators of nutritional status—such as physical findings, anthropometric measures, and lab tests—are appropriate evaluation criteria. Nurses should attempt to be as specific and as individualized as possible when selecting criteria for the evaluation of nutritional care. Progress toward desired outcomes is monitored during the course of care as well as on specified target dates.

SUMMARY

Nutrition involves processes that are complex and elaborately regulated so as to maintain a constant supply of nutrients to the cells of the body. The nutrients obtained from food are digested, absorbed, and metabolized to produce the energy necessary to sustain all the life processes and to build and repair body tissues. Nursing diagnoses related to altered nutrition describe problems of food intake, digestion, absorption, or metabolism.

Nutritional assessment must focus on all aspects of patients' nutritional activities and status, not only the physical dimensions. Because nutrition is intimately associated with emotional, social, and cultural factors, all of these must be thoroughly assessed. The entire process, including assessment and management of nutritional problems, must involve a fully collaborative relationship between patient and nurse to be effective. Nutritional alterations cannot be corrected without a patient's active interest, motivation, and effort, and these can only be manifested in a collaborative relationship.

Nursing implementation to promote nutritional well-being may involve any of the four levels of care. The spectrum of nursing skills ranges from teaching and counseling to complete responsibility for feeding a patient. Feeding techniques include oral, enteral, and parenteral measures. The insertion of a tube into the alimentary tract is a means of providing nutrition to patients unable to orally ingest food.

The nurse's role in a collaborative interprofessional effort is of utmost significance. The primary caring relationship between nurse and patient often places nurses in the highly nurturing role of feeding patients. Even if this is not necessary, the nurse's continuous and intimate concern with the patient's nutritional needs places the nurse–patient relationship in a central position.

LEARNING OUTCOMES

Upon completing this chapter, the student should be able to:

1. Discuss the role of nutrition in preventing illness, restoring health, and promoting high-level wellness.
2. Calculate the total daily energy requirement for an individual.
3. Describe the processes of digestion, absorption, and metabolism.
4. Discuss the cultural dimensions of nutritional needs.
5. Describe current guidelines and standards used in nutritional assessment and planning.
6. Describe the etiology and symptoms of selected nutritional deficiency diseases.
7. Outline the components of a comprehensive nutritional history for patients across the life cycle.
8. Identify physical findings indicative of good as well as compromised nutritional status.
9. Identify diagnostic tests useful in nutritional assessment.
10. Describe at least three nursing diagnoses from the North American Nursing Diagnosis Association (NANDA) taxonomy that relate to nutritional problems.
11. Describe nursing measures and procedures for promoting optimal nutritional health across the life cycle.
12. Describe the roles of the interdisciplinary team members in collaborating for optimal health.

REVIEW OF KEY TERMS

absorption
amino acid
anabolism
anorexia nervosa
basal metabolic rate (BMR)
body mass index (BMI)
bulimia
cachexia
carbohydrate
catabolism
complementary protein
complete protein
complex carbohydrate
Daily Reference Values
Daily Values
dietary fiber
digestion
energy balance
enteral
essential amino acid
essential nutrient
fat
fatty acid
food pyramid
gluconeogenesis
glycogen
glycogenolysis
insulin
kilocalorie
lipid
metabolism
mineral
monounsaturated fatty acid
negative nitrogen balance
nitrogen balance
nutrient
nutrition
obesity
overweight
peristalsis
polyunsaturated fatty acid
positive nitrogen balance
protein
protein–calorie malnutrition (PCM)
protein deficiency state
Recommended Dietary Allowances (RDA)
Reference Daily Intake (RDI)
saturated fatty acid
simple carbohydrate
starch
total parenteral nutrition (TPN)
vitamin

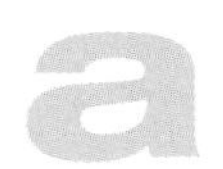

Having Read the Chapter, consider again the opening scenario, page 877, and the following responses to questions about nutrition assessment and teaching prior to discharge of Mrs. Jacks after her total hip replacement.

Assessment of Mrs. Jacks' nutritional status includes obtaining a nutritional history and performing a physical examination to determine other indicators of compromised nutritional status besides her weight loss. Mrs. Jacks, her son, and her daughter-in-law are sources of data needed for Mrs. Jacks' nutritional history. The following is important information for her nurse to gather:

- Has Mrs. Jacks' weight been stable at the current level for some time or does current weight reflect a recent weight loss?
- Is Mrs. Jacks concerned about her current weight?
- Are there other stressors (eg, economic or emotional) that may be contributing to her being under the ideal weight?
- A 24-hour food diary to identify risks for specific nutritional deficiencies that may be related to her being underweight.

- Data about favorite foods and recipes and her plan to meet the increased nutrient needs related to the recent metabolic stressor: healing a significant surgical incision.
- Data about Mrs. Jacks' social support system for resources to help with shopping and cooking for several weeks after her daughter-in-law leaves.

Her nurse should note the following in the nutrition examination:

- Condition of her integument and mucous membranes with particular attention to edema or lesions, such as those listed in Table 28–9.
- Muscle tone and strength, evidence of subcutaneous tissue loss
- Hemoglobin, hematocrit, and serum protein levels

This information is needed so Mrs. Jacks' nurse can determine the existence of additional risk states or deficiencies and effectively plan post–discharge dietary intake with Mrs. Jacks and her son and daughter-in-law.

Mrs. Jacks needs to know about basic nutrient needs and how to meet them, but more importantly the nutrients critical to enhance bone and tissue healing: protein; vitamins A, K, and C; zinc; and calcium. Since she is under her ideal weight, addressing available calorie-dense nutritional supplements would also be appropriate. Constipation may be a problem because of limited exercise, so fiber-rich foods are also important.

Mrs. Jacks' daughter-in-law should have the same information about Mrs. Jacks's needs. A joint teaching session that also addressed obtaining groceries and assistance Mrs. Jacks may need to prepare foods would also be effective. Since the distance between their homes is too great for daily visits, preparing and freezing multiple, single-meal–sized portions of foods Mrs. Jacks enjoys would also help.

Community resources such as Meals-on-Wheels would be helpful in this situation.

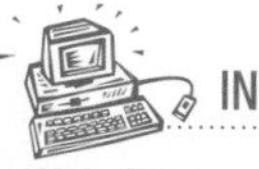

INTERNET RESOURCES

Web Sites

Nutrition (information on nutritional value of foods):
http:// www.fsci.umn.edu/tools.htp

American Diabetes Association:
http://www.diabetes.org

Internet FDA (Food and Drug Administration):
http://www. fda.gov

Koop Cyberkitchen:
http://www.shapeup.org

Clinical and applied nutrition information:
http://arborcom.com

REFERENCES

1. Rimm EB, Ascherio A, Giovanucci E, Spiegelman D, Stampfer MJ, Willett WC. Vegetable, fruit, and cereal fiber intake and risk of coronary heart disease among men. *JAMA.* 1996; 275:447–451.
2. Lutz CA and Przytulski KR. *Nutrition and Diet Therapy.* 2nd ed. Philadelphia: FA Davis, 1997.
3. Centers for Disease Control and Prevention. Recommendations for use of folic acid to reduce number of spina bifida cases and other neural tube defects. *JAMA.* 1993;269:1233, 1236, 1238.
4. Spencer JP. Practical nutrition for the healthy term infant. *Am Fam Phys.* 1996;54:138–144.
5. Cataldo CB, De Bruyne LK, Whitney EN. *Nutrition and Diet Therapy.* 4th ed. St. Paul, MN: West; 1995.
6. Stephens D, Jackson PL, Gutierrez Y. Subclinical vitamin A deficiency: a potentially unrecognized problem in the United States. *Pediatr Nurs.* 1996;22:377–389.
7. Prentice A, Goldberg G. Maternal obesity increases congenital malformation. *Nutr Rev.* 1996;54:146–152.
8. Olvera-Ezzell N, Power TG, Cousins JH, Guerra AM, Triyillo M. The development of health knowledge in low-income Mexican-American children. *Child Dev.* 1994;65:416.
9. Broussard BA, Johnson A, Himes JH. Prevalence of obesity in American Indians and Alaska Natives. *Am J Clin Nutr.* 1991;53 (Suppl.):1535.
10. Kumanyika SK. Special issues regarding obesity in minority populations. *Ann Intern Med.* 1993;119:650–654.
11. Hubert HB, Feinleib M, McNamara PM, Castelli WD. Obesity as an independent risk factor for cardiovascular disease; a 26 year follow up of participants in the Framingham heart study. *Circulation.* 1983;67:968.
12. Muller DC, Elahi D, Pratty RF. An epidemiological test of the hyperinsulinemia-hypertension hypothesis. *Endocrinol Metab.* 1993;76:544.
13. Zerah F, Harf A, Perlemuter L, Louno H, Lorinok AM, Atlan G. Effects of obesity on respiratory resistance. *Chest.* 1993;103: 1470–1475.
14. Purdy KS, Dwyer JT, Holland M, Goldberg DL, Dinardo J. You are what you eat: healthy food choices, nutrition, and the child with juvenile rheumatoid arthritis. *Pediatr Nurs.* 1996;22: 391–398.
15. Hachey DL. Benefits and risks of modifying maternal intake in pregnancy and lactation. *Am J Clin Nutr.* 1994;59 (Suppl.): 4545–4645.
16. Kayser-Jones J. Mealtime in nursing homes: the importance of individualized care. *J Gerontol Nurs.* 1996; March:26–31.

29

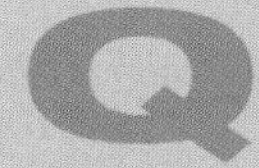

Georgette Briggs is 36 years old, married, and has two children. She holds a middle management position in a large manufacturing company. Her job is stressful. She often skips lunch, and she works late several nights a week.

In the last 6 months, Mrs. Briggs has had four episodes of watery diarrhea, associated with pain, fever, appetite and weight loss, and abdominal fullness. Her diagnosis is ulcerative colitis, which is a stress-related condition in which the lining of the colon becomes inflamed. A week ago, she was admitted to the hospital with bloody diarrhea, for which her doctor, fearing possible hemorrhage, advised surgery. Mrs. Briggs underwent a colon resection, and is now well along in her recovery. Her intravenous and Foley catheters are to be removed this afternoon, and if all goes well she will be discharged soon.

How should her nurse prepare Mrs. Briggs for the removal of the Foley catheter?

What is the procedure for removing a Foley catheter?

What observations should her nurse make in relation to Mrs. Briggs's urinary and bowel functions?

How can her nurse assist Mrs. Briggs to regain and maintain her urinary and bowel health?

How might Mrs. Briggs' lifestyle be contributing to her illness?

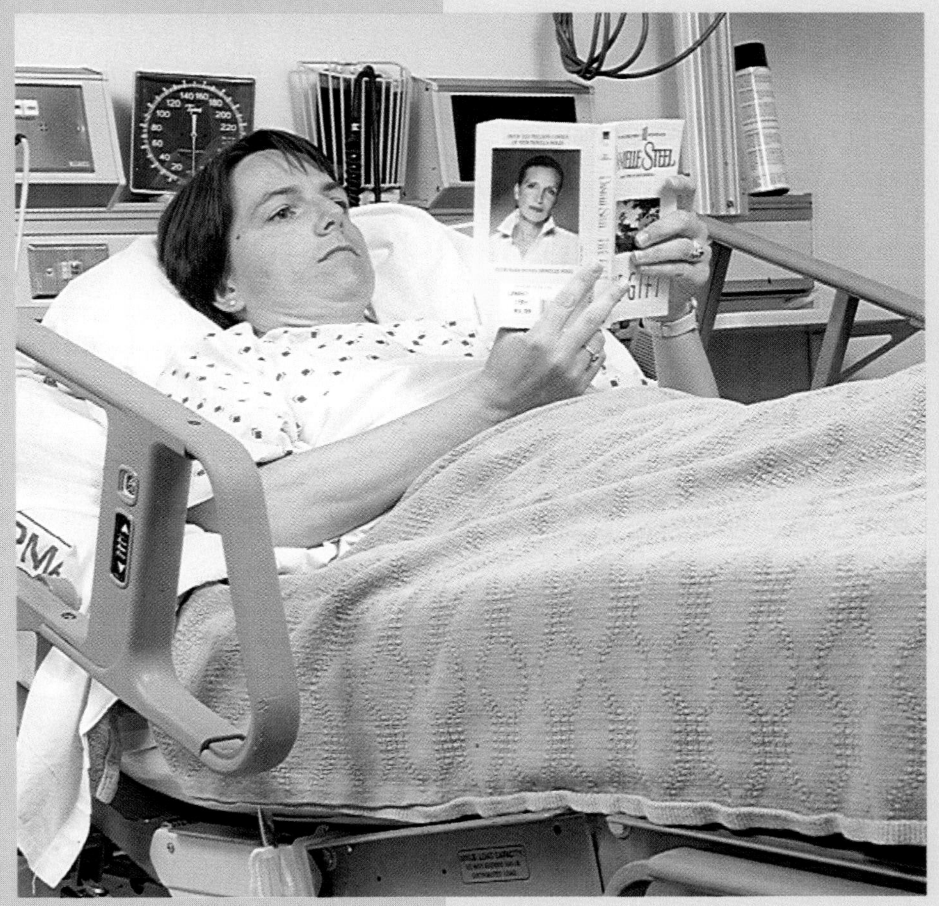

Elimination

Carol A. Sedlak, Margaret O'Bryan Doheny, and Nancy L. Bradley

CHAPTER OUTLINE

Removal of body waste via the intestinal and urinary tracts—**elimination**—is a complex function that is vital to health. Elimination involves intricate physiologic and psychological interrelationships and is affected by an individual's lifestyle, health status, and emotional state. Both bowel and urinary elimination are discussed in this chapter. Alterations in elimination influence well-being and may indicate a change in health status. Examples of commonly experienced alterations in elimination are constipation when traveling away from home and urinary frequency at times of stress.

Nurses need to acquire skill in collecting data about urinary and bowel function to identify alterations that can be corrected by nursing implementation planned in collaboration with other members of the health care team, the patient and family, from whom comprehensive information is elicited. For effective data collection, nurses need to apply knowledge of basic anatomic structures and physiologic functions related to elimination as well as communication and physical assessment techniques. Analysis of a comprehensive elimination database may yield nursing diagnoses of altered elimination. Once nursing diagnoses are established, nurse and patient together plan approaches that will promote optimal elimination.

This chapter provides a basis for the understanding of elimination function, assessment of elimination, and management of common elimination problems.

SECTION 1

UNDERSTANDING ELIMINATION

Healthy individuals often take for granted their ability to control elimination. Depending on a catheter for urinary drainage or soiling the bed with feces may embarrass a patient and affect body image. An approach that demonstrates sensitivity and understanding is essential when caring for persons who are unable to manage elimination processes. A working knowledge of anatomy and physiology is basic to understanding elimination.

OPTIMAL BOWEL ELIMINATION

The function of bowel elimination is to rid the body of undigested waste once nutrients and water have been absorbed for use by the body. These functions are mainly carried out in the lower gastrointestinal (GI) tract, which consists of the colon, rectum, and anal canal. Although the large intestine is primarily responsible for bowel elimination, the entire gastrointestinal tract plays a role.

COLLABORATIVE STRATEGY

UNDERSTANDING THE PERSONAL AND SOCIAL MEANING OF ELIMINATION

Although elimination is a natural and normal body function, strong social mores surround both the products and process of human elimination. Individuals as members of society can be expected to share the conflicts of society and fear a loss of control over their elimination process. This fear is a powerful motivator and may significantly affect the patient's capacity to collaborate when the health problem involves elimination. The nurse's sensitivity to the human emotions surrounding elimination is therefore essential to caring for persons who are unable to manage their own elimination.

ANATOMY AND PHYSIOLOGY

Upper GI Tract

The entire gastrointestinal tract is essential to the process of bowel elimination. Following ingestion of food, nutrients are mechanically and chemically broken down by enzymes in the mouth and stomach. The partially digested food then moves along the tract to the small intestine, where most nutrients are absorbed.

Colon

The colon is a tubular structure of muscle lined with mucous membrane extending 1.5 m (5 ft) from cecum to anal canal. It consists of the cecum; ascending, transverse, and descending colon; sigmoid colon; rectum; and anus. The functions of the colon are (1) absorption of water and nutrients (2) fecal elimination.

The colon absorbs large quantities of water (as much as 2.5 L) in 24 hours. Up to 55 milliequivalents (mEq) of sodium and 23 mEq of chloride are absorbed daily. The speed at which the colonic contents move determines how much water is absorbed from the chyme.

Fecal elimination is accomplished by moving the chyme—normally a soft, formed prefecal mass—along the colon into the rectum and anal canal. **Peristalsis,** a wavelike muscular contraction along the length of the colon advances the colon contents. Mass peristalsis occurs about 1 hour after a meal. This knowledge should aid the nurse in planning elimination implementations for a patient.

Colonic mucus is secreted to protect the lining of the colon. The mucus also serves as a binding agent to hold the fecal material together. Mucus secretion is stimulated by parasympathetic nerves. An extreme emotional reaction can cause overstimulation of these nerves and therefore an overproduction of mucus, resulting in stringy mucoid stools with little or no feces.

Rectum and Anal Canal

Waste products, feces, enter the sigmoid colon and are stored there until just before defecation (the act of having a bowel movement). The rectum is normally empty of feces until just before defecation. Rectum length varies according to age. In the adult, rectal length is about 10 to 15 cm (4 to 6 in.). The distal portion of the rectum (3 to 5 cm or 1½ to 2 in. long) is called the anal canal.

The rectum contains vertical and transverse folds of tissue that help retain feces. Each vertical fold contains a vein and an artery. The veins, when repeatedly distended either by pressure exerted during straining to defecate or by increased intra-abdominal pressure associated with pregnancy or heavy lifting, can become permanently dilated. This condition is called **hemorrhoids.** Hemorrhoids can make defecation painful and may cause varying amounts of blood loss (Fig. 29–1).

The anal canal contains internal and external sphincter muscles. The internal sphincter is involuntarily controlled by the autonomic nervous system. Although the external sphincter is influenced by the internal sphincter, it is usually voluntarily controlled. When sensory nerves in the rectum are stimulated by the entrance of the fecal mass, the individual becomes aware of the need to defecate.

Defecation

Defecation is influenced by reflexes but is also under voluntary control. The **gastrocolic** and the **duodenocolic reflexes,** which occur in response to distension of the stomach and the duodenum, contribute to defecation by stimulating *mass peristalsis* along the entire length of the GI tract.[1] Mass peristalsis is most predominant within 15 minutes after eating breakfast.

The intrinsic defecation reflex occurs when feces distend the rectum, initiating the peristaltic waves in the descending and sigmoid colon and the rectum and forcing feces toward the anus. As

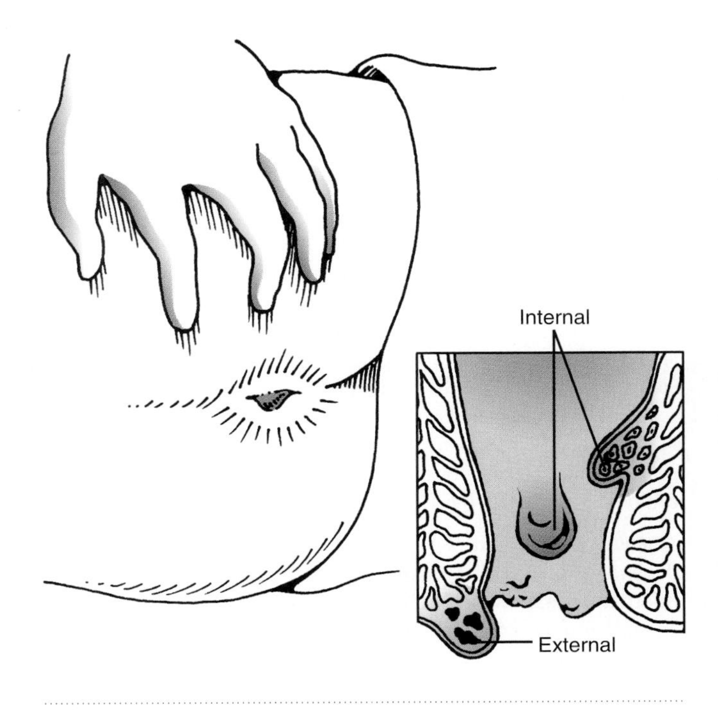

Figure 29–1. Hemorrhoids.

these peristaltic waves approach the anus, the internal sphincter is inhibited from closing. The parasympathetic defecation reflex, triggered by the presence of feces in the rectum, intensifies the intrinsic defecation reflex. Signals are sent to the spinal cord and back to the colon and rectum to intensify the peristaltic waves and relax the internal anal sphincter.

Voluntary neuromuscular control can be used to delay or facilitate defecation. As the feces move into the anal canal and the internal anal sphincter relaxes, the individual feels the urge to defecate. Defecation is initiated by relaxing the external anal sphincter while contracting the abdominal muscles and the diaphragm. The increased abdominal pressure moves feces down the anal canal. The levator ani muscles of the pelvic floor are also voluntarily contracted to aid in fecal expulsion. The **Valsalva maneuver**—holding one's breath while exerting expiratory effort against a closed glottis, and then contracting the abdominal muscles—is also often used to help expel feces.

When an individual ignores the urge to defecate or consciously contracts the external sphincter muscles to delay defecation, the urge to defecate may disappear for several hours before reoccurring. Repeatedly ignoring the urge to defecate over a period of months or years can result in an abnormally enlarged rectum and loss of rectal sensitivity. The individual's perception of the need to defecate becomes dulled, creating the potential for constipation, discussed as follows.

NORMAL BOWEL ELIMINATION

Normal Patterns

Normal patterns of bowel elimination vary widely. Some individuals defecate one to two times a day; others, two or three times a week. There are many techniques that individuals use to assist with bowel function, such as drinking a cup of hot water before breakfast, or prune juice at night, or reading while using the toilet. Such measures may support physiologic processes. Drinking warm fluids on arising, for example, stimulates the gastrocolic reflex and can create a desire to defecate.

Characteristics of Normal Stool

The nurse should observe feces for consistency, amount, color, shape, odor, and the presence of any unusual matter.

Consistency. Consistency refers to stool firmness or density. Dietary intake and the quantity of fluid intake directly affect the stool's consistency; however, normal stool is soft and formed. Speed of peristalsis will determine the liquid content and the shape of the stool. Decreased peristalsis results in small, hard, dry stools; increased peristalsis causes liquid, unformed stools.

Softer-than-normal stools are variously described as "soft," "semiformed," or "loose," if they are liquid with some solid material. "Liquid stools" consist of colored fluid only. Very solid stools can be described as "hard" or "constipated."

Amount. The amount of fecal material passed each day will vary depending on the dietary intake. Patients are the best source of information about their customary amounts of stool. The nurse should also observe and note any increase or decrease in the amount of stool.

Color. The color of adult stool is normally brown, because of the presence of bile pigments. If there is lack of bile or an obstruction to its flow, a clay-colored or white stool results. Formation of gallstones, which obstruct the biliary tract, is a common cause of clay-colored stools. Malabsorption syndrome also causes a pale-colored stool. Black stools may be a side effect of iron supplements or may be caused by upper gastrointestinal bleeding. Bright red blood in the stool is most commonly associated with bleeding hemorrhoids, but may also indicate lower GI bleeding. **Melena** is the term used to refer to blood in the feces.

Shape. The shape of a normal stool reflects that of the rectum. If an intestinal obstruction is present, the stool may become pencil-thin or ribbon-shaped as it squeezes by the obstruction. Pencil-thin stool can also be caused by rapid intestinal motility.

Odor. Stool usually possesses a characteristic fecal odor. Some foods may alter the stool odor. Foul-smelling stools are associated with malabsorption syndrome. Blood in the feces or intestinal infection may also change stool odor.

Components. Normal stool components include the end products of digestion. There should be no visible blood or mucus or any other unusual matter, such as undigested food or worms. Worms are common in some areas of the world and may occur occasionally in the United States. Pinworms, which resemble fine white threads, or tapeworms, which are ⅛ to ¼ inch wide and may grow 5 to 20 feet long, may be visible to the naked eye. Their eggs (ova) may be easily detected by microscopic survey of a strip of clear plastic tape that has been placed briefly over the anal opening. Tapeworms or segments of the worm can also appear in the stool.

FACTORS AFFECTING BOWEL FUNCTION

Many factors may affect bowel function. Some common factors include age, life-style, health status, and emotional state. These factors produce the individual variation seen in bowel elimination.

Age

Fecal elimination patterns change throughout the life cycle. Changes are caused by continued physiologic development, then by age-related losses of function.

Infants. Infants (birth to 1 year) are unable to control defecation due to lack of neuromuscular maturity. Stool frequency and characteristics depend upon feeding method. Breastfed infants have loose, seedy, golden yellow stools, often after every feeding. The stools are not irritating to the infant's skin. Stools of formula-fed infants are pale yellow, firmer, and irritating to the skin. Formula-fed infants usually have only one to two stools a day.

Toddlers. Toddlers (ages 1 to 3 years) become physically ready to control bowel elimination between 18 and 24 months of age; however, cognitive and psychosocial readiness, also essential, frequently is achieved later. Daytime bowel control, therefore, is usually accomplished around 30 months. Attempting to toilet train toddlers before they are ready, or punishing them for "accidents," may create significant stress and delay control. If toddlers are hospitalized, they often regress and temporarily lose control of elimination.

Preschool and School-aged Children. Preschool (ages 3 to 5) and school-aged (ages 6 to 12) children exhibit a variety of defecation patterns, usually establishing an individual pattern that is characteristic. Constipation is a common problem in both age groups. It may be related to dietary changes, febrile illness, or emotional or environmental changes. Parents should be cautioned against indiscriminate use of laxatives to treat constipation; increasing fluids, fruits, vegetables, and grains is preferable.

Adolescents. Adolescents (ages 13 to 18) experience a period of rapid growth. Both the stomach and the colon enlarge to accommodate the greater food intake that accompanies this growth spurt, and stools often increase in size and number.

Young and Middle-aged Adults. Young (ages 18 to 35) and middle-aged (ages 35 to 65) adults establish characteristic individual bowel elimination patterns that vary with dietary, life-style, and other variables discussed later.

Older Adults. Older adults (over age 65) frequently experience constipation. This can be attributed to several factors. Many elderly adults must take several medications (discussed below) for treatment of chronic diseases. Difficulties in chewing associated with loss of teeth or poorly fitting dentures lead to choosing soft foods, which decreases bulk in the stool. Diminished thirst sensation and reduced mobility contribute to limited fluid intake as well as to less activity. All of these factors, plus the loss of colon and abdominal muscle tone that frequently occurs with age, increase risk for constipation.[2] Many older individuals rely on laxatives to correct constipation, but laxative use often compounds the problem and may even result in dependency. Increasing exercise, fluids, and bulk-producing foods will reduce constipation risk and make laxatives unnecessary.

Loss of muscle tone may also affect the internal anal sphincter, and even though the external sphincter is still intact, some elderly persons experience difficulty controlling defecation. Older adults also may become less aware of the need to defecate because of impaired nerve impulse transmission.[3]

Life-style

Bowel function can be disrupted by a chaotic life-style of irregular meals, changing schedules, and increased stress. A sedentary life-style increases the risk of constipation, because peristalsis is stimulated by exercise. A regular pattern of intake and elimination is health promoting. Nurse–patient collaboration can often help patients establish healthier patterns.

Diet. Diet plays an essential role in promoting healthy elimination. Eating meals at regularly scheduled times will help establish regular bowel patterns. Adequate intake of dietary fiber provides bulk that will keep the stool soft and increase the speed of passage through the intestines. This in turn limits the amount of water that is absorbed from fecal matter, thus producing a soft, formed stool. Foods that are valuable sources of fiber include whole grains (breads and cereals), fresh fruits (apples, oranges), root vegetables (carrots, turnips, celery), greens (lettuce, spinach), legumes (dried beans, peas), and cooked fruit (apricots, prunes).[4] These high-fiber or bulk-producing foods stretch the bowel wall, stimulating peristalsis and initiating the defecation reflex. Some foods, such as beans, onions, and cabbage, are gas producing; the gas distends the bowel and may cause cramping or excessive bowel activity.

Certain foods are difficult for some people to digest and may cause digestive upsets or watery stools (diarrhea). Foods that promote normal elimination in one person may create constipation or diarrhea in another. For example, milk and milk products should be avoided by people who are lactose intolerant. Milk contains lactose, a simple sugar, that is broken down in the body by the enzyme lactase. Individuals with lactose intolerance do not produce the enzyme lactase and are therefore unable to digest foods containing lactose. This can result in abdominal cramping, nausea, gaseous distension, and diarrhea.

Exercise. A sedentary life-style decreases peristalsis. Conversely, regular general exercise contributes to regular elimination patterns. Some exercises help maintain the tone and strength of the abdominal and pelvic floor muscles that are used in defecation.

Weak muscles may result from severe illness, prolonged immobility, or neurologic disease that impairs nerve function. Individuals with these conditions may benefit from special conditioning exercises to strengthen the muscles of the abdomen and pelvic floor to facilitate healthy elimination.

Elimination Habits. Toilet training, the type of toilet facility, daily schedule, and attitude toward one's body influence elimination habits.

Bowel elimination is a private matter and most people prefer to use their own toilet facilities. Establishing a bowel pattern that permits use of home facilities at a convenient time is advantageous. Busy and changing work schedules can cause disruption of regular habits and increase risk for constipation.

A change in environment such as hospitalization often disrupts established elimination habits. Lack of privacy, change in routines, altered intake of food and fluids, diminished activity, and ingesting multiple medications all contribute to altered elimination patterns.

Health Status

An individual's elimination patterns may be influenced by a variety of health factors: hydration, pain, tissue integrity, and medications. Diagnostic procedures that require fasting or enemas can also affect elimination.

Hydration. Adequate hydration is crucial to healthy elimination. Six to eight glasses (1400 to 2000 mL) of fluid per day is the normal requirement for an adult. Fluid is necessary for efficient movement of intestinal contents and for the absorption of nutrients and electrolytes. Fluids also enter the intestine from saliva, gastric secretions, pancreatic juices, and bile.

The gastrointestinal tract contributes to maintaining fluid balance. If alterations in other body systems cause a fluid loss or deficiency, the intestine will absorb more fluid, helping intra- and extracellular fluid volumes remain relatively constant. However, the resulting decrease in the amount of fluid within the intestine slows peristalsis and hardens the feces. Therefore, when assessing bowel function, nurses must be alert to any condition that causes fluid loss.

Pain. Pain may also influence bowel function. Hemorrhoids, rectal and perineal surgery, or abdominal surgery can cause discomfort during defecation. As a result, patients may suppress the urge to defecate and become constipated. Nurses should also be alert to other conditions that could create discomfort for patients during defecation. Position on the bedpan, pressure ulcers, and pelvic and hip fractures are other possible causes of pain.

Tissue Integrity. Impaired tissue integrity of the bowel and external anal area makes elimination painful and may lead to constipation.

For example, hemorrhoids sometimes ulcerate and bleed and ulcers and fissures sometimes develop in the anal area, causing excoriation and irritation.

Medications. Many medications can alter bowel function. For example, antibiotics can produce diarrhea and abdominal cramping; narcotic analgesics and opiates decrease peristalsis with resulting constipation. Diuretics, which cause the body to eliminate fluid, may predispose individuals to constipation. Iron preparations may also cause constipation. When patients have diarrhea or constipation it is important to evaluate the side effects of any medication they are taking.

Some medications aid in bowel elimination or relieve constipation. They are called **laxatives** or **cathartics.** These drugs act by softening the stool or by promoting peristalsis. Overuse of these drugs can cause dependency. Severe diarrhea can also result from overuse of laxatives, creating electrolyte imbalance and dehydration. Nurses should carefully assess patients' use of these medications, because they are readily available over the counter. Children may take large doses of gum or candy laxatives (such as Ex-Lax) if they are not kept out of reach, resulting in serious poisoning.

As discussed above, appropriate hydration, diet, and exercise make laxatives unnecessary. If a laxative is necessary, bulk laxatives or stool softeners are preferable.[5] These medications can be purchased over the counter or prescribed. Advise patients who use laxatives to carefully follow directions on the label to avoid any complications.

Anesthesia. Anesthesia and surgery also affect bowel elimination. General anesthetics produce temporary slowing or cessation of peristalsis, whereas regional or spinal anesthesia affects bowel activity minimally or not at all. Handling the bowel during surgery often leads to temporary loss of peristalsis. This is called **paralytic** or **adynamic ileus.** It can last for 24 to 48 hours, although some patients experience paralytic ileus for a longer period of time. Most surgeons order n.p.o. status (nothing by mouth) for postoperative patients until bowel sounds return. Therefore, auscultation for bowel sounds is an important aspect of care for all postoperative patients.

Diagnostic Procedures. Diagnostic procedures to evaluate gastrointestinal function usually require that the bowel be empty. Patients are expected not to eat or drink after midnight of the day preceding the examination and may be required to have a cathartic and an enema. After clearing the bowel for these tests, normal defecation will usually not occur until the patient has resumed eating. If barium is used as a contrast medium for these procedures, constipation or fecal impaction may occur unless the barium is effectively cleared from the GI tract. Therefore, a posttest cathartic or enema is usually ordered.

Emotional State

Emotional stress can affect the function of all body systems; the GI system is particularly susceptible. Anxiety, fear, and anger accelerate the digestive process and increase peristalsis to provide nutrients for body defense. This acceleration can lead to gaseous distension and diarrhea. In contrast, some individuals experience sluggish peristalsis when under stress and may become constipated.

The symptoms and the course of diseases of the GI tract can be affected by emotional stress. Ulcerative colitis, gastric ulcers, and Crohn's disease all worsen with emotional stress, even though the primary cause of these diseases has been shown to be physiologic.

Early toilet training can interfere with a child's later bowel elimination patterns. Spanking or making a child sit on the potty chair for a long time will make training extremely stressful. Continuous battles between parent and child may lead to chronic constipation in the child. Positive reinforcement and a relaxed atmosphere about toileting help reduce the child's emotional stress.

Some individuals are overly concerned, even preoccupied, by the need to have a daily bowel movement. Disruptions in regular habits related to illness or diagnostic tests may create significant concern. Nurses need to accept the level of anxiety that these individuals experience. Explanations of the physiologic basis for the delay in bowel function may allay anxiety.

Patients reveal clues about their emotional state and elimination concerns in various ways. For example, some directly express concerns about elimination; others make multiple requests for laxatives or prune juice. Collaborative assessment and planning are effective in resolving bowel elimination problems.

ALTERED BOWEL ELIMINATION

Constipation, diarrhea, incontinence, flatulence, and fecal impaction are types of altered bowel elimination. These problems may arise from physiologic or psychological factors. Surgical alteration of the intestine also affects bowel elimination.

CONSTIPATION

Constipation is the passage of small, hard, dry stool, or the passage of no stool, for an unusually long period of time for that person. It is a common problem that nurses can help to prevent. Difficulty passing stool and straining accompany constipation. However, it is important to remember that some individuals defecate several times a week, others one to two times a day. Careful assessment of elimination habits, therefore, is necessary before making a diagnosis of constipation.

Constipation has many causes, including insufficient exercise, irregular defecation habits, overuse of laxatives, disease processes, inappropriate diet, medications, and increased emotional stress. Pregnant women may suffer from constipation because of increased progesterone levels, which cause smooth muscle relaxation and slow peristalsis. In fact, any condition that leads to slowing of intestinal peristalsis or causes excess absorption of water may result in constipation.

Constipation affects healthy and ill individuals. The person who is constipated will have various complaints. Uncomfortable symptoms such as nausea, heartburn, back pain, headache, or distress in the rectum or intestines may be reported. The patient will state that bowel elimination has been less frequent than usual or that there have been no stools. A feeling of abdominal distension or bloating is often described. Feelings of rectal fullness, pressure in the rectum, and a palpable mass may also be reported. Activities of daily living and appetite may be impaired. Patients often express difficulty in passing stools. Straining during defecation may lead to development of hemorrhoids and rectal bleeding.

Other threats to health occur with constipation when the patient has had recent abdominal or rectal surgery. Sutures may rupture and wounds may open from the stress of straining at defecation, but this is a rare occurrence. Straining during defecation is accompanied by breath holding (the Valsalva maneuver), which can cause additional problems for the patient with heart disease, brain injury, or respiratory disease. Breathing and exhaling through the mouth while straining can reduce the hazard, but it is best to avoid any straining.

DIARRHEA

Diarrhea is the rapid movement of fecal matter through the intestine, resulting in frequent evacuation of loose and watery stools. The stools often contain mucus and may be blood streaked.

Food poisoning or intolerance, infection, disease, and antibiotics and other drugs are among the causes of diarrhea. In addition, diarrhea can be caused by severe emotional stress. Some surgical procedures may result in diarrhea. The rapid passage of intestinal contents does not allow for the usual absorption of fluid and electrolytes, often resulting in serious fluid and electrolyte imbalances. This can be life-threatening, especially in infants or elderly and debilitated patients. Several causes of diarrhea, along with the body's physiologic response, or alteration, are listed in Table 29–1.

The person with diarrhea is often disturbed and embarrassed at having increased stool frequency and liquid stools. The odors and sounds of liquid stools and gas, and the possibility of not being able to get to the toilet, bedpan, or commode in time, increase the anxiety. Frequent watery stools, abdominal cramps, and general weakness are the major symptoms reported. Nausea and vomiting often accompany diarrhea.

Diarrhea limits activity and causes discomfort, loss of appetite, and weakness. Frequent trips to the bathroom may predispose weakened patients to injury from slipping or falling. Frequent, irritating liquid stools can cause skin breakdown in the anal and perineal areas and on the buttocks.

FECAL INCONTINENCE

Fecal incontinence is the loss of the voluntary ability to control the elimination of gas and feces. Comatose or confused patients are often incontinent of feces. Some neuromuscular diseases, spinal cord trauma, and tumors of the anal sphincter muscles interfere with the functioning of the anal sphincter or its nerve supply and cause fecal incontinence. Mental disorders such as dementia, Alzheimer's disease, schizophrenia, and severe depression may make the patient unable to recognize the need to defecate.

TABLE 29–1. DIARRHEA: CAUSES AND PHYSIOLOGIC RESPONSES

Cause of Diarrhea	Physiologic Alteration or Response
Food poisoning/intestinal infection (streptococcal or staphylococcal enteritis)	Increased mucus secretion and rapid intestinal motility.
Food or fluid allergies	Food or fluid not digested completely.
Food intolerance (eg, lactose intolerance)	Increased mucus secretion and rapid intestinal motility.
Chemicals: medications, laxatives	Irritation of intestinal tissue and/or increased intestinal movement.
Antibiotics	Intestinal mucosa inflamed and irritated due to superinfection. Antibiotics suppress the normal bacterial flora and allow other bacteria normally limited by the presence of normal flora to multiply. Some of these bacteria are hydrophilic (water-attracting). They cause an influx of fluid into the colon, which stimulates excessive peristalsis.
Other chemicals ingested, or foreign substances (eg, food preservatives)	Irritation of intestinal mucosa.
Iron preparations	Irritation of intestinal tissue in some individuals.
Colon diseases	
Crohn's disease, colitis	Ulceration, inflammation of intestinal walls, rapid intestinal motility.
Malabsorption syndrome	Fluid and nutrient absorption reduced.
Surgical procedures	
Gastrectomy	Stomach cannot hold as much food and food enters duodenum too rapidly for proper absorption.
Resection of colon	Loss of colon fluid absorption because colon length is reduced.
Emotional stress (anxiety)	Rapid intestinal motility.
Tapeworm	Irritation of intestinal tissue with increased motility of intestine.

Fecal incontinence can be severely damaging to an individual's body image. Odor, cleanliness, and staining are potential sources of embarrassment, and the person may not want to get out of bed or venture out of the house, causing social isolation.

Tissue breakdown in the perianal area may also result from incontinence. Acidic feces that contain digestive enzymes can cause excoriation, bleeding, and pain around the anal area. The patient may then suffer physical discomfort as well as the psychosocial discomfort.

FLATULENCE

Flatulence is an accumulation of excessive amounts of gas in the gastrointestinal tract. Expulsion of gas via the rectum is called *flatus*. If flatulence is accompanied by increased motility, *borborygmus* (the sound made by the gas rumbling and being propelled through the intestines) results. When intestinal motility is decreased, gas accumulates and stretches and distends the bowel wall, causing abdominal fullness, pain, and cramping.

Normally gas formed in the GI tract by bacterial action on the chyme, and gas diffusing from the bloodstream, are expelled through the mouth or anus. It is not uncommon for an adult to form up to 10 liters of intestinal gas in 24 hours. However, certain foods (beans, cabbage, onions, and cauliflower) increase gas production and create flatulence. Carbonated beverages are another common cause of flatulence, as is swallowing large amounts of air. Air swallowing is sometimes associated with anxiety; gum chewing and using drinking straws also promote air swallowing.

Any of the factors that reduce intestinal activity have the potential for increasing flatulence, because the gas is not propelled out of the body. Narcotics, anesthetics, abdominal surgery, immobility, and tight-fitting clothing are some examples.

Patients with flatulence and flatus complain of "gas pains" and "passing a lot of gas." They also may complain of fullness or a bloated feeling. *Eructation* (belching) is often present, along with the characteristic odor of gas that is expelled from the rectum, both of which may cause considerable embarrassment.

If gas accumulates and the bowel distends, cramping and pain may become pronounced and may limit activities of daily living. The resultant decrease in activity often exacerbates the problem. Some individuals also experience difficulty breathing and shortness of breath. This results when flatulence causes severe abdominal distension. Lung expansion is reduced because the diaphragm is pushed upward by the distension.

FECAL IMPACTION

A **fecal impaction** is a collection of putty-like or hard stool in the rectum that cannot be expelled. In severe cases the impacted feces may extend into the sigmoid colon. The stool must be removed to prevent serious illness.

In the well population, the elderly, children, and those with poor bowel habits are the most likely to develop fecal impaction. Others at risk for impaction include comatose, confused, or debilitated individuals and individuals who do not pass the barium contrast material after a barium enema.

Fecal impaction may cause great discomfort. People with a fecal impaction do not feel well; they often complain of a feeling of malaise. In spite of a frequent urge to defecate, people with an impaction are not able to do so. There may be diarrhea, caused by liquid feces draining around the impacted mass. Abdominal cramping, rectal pain, abdominal pain, and loss of appetite with nausea and vomiting may also occur.

FECAL ELIMINATION VIA AN OSTOMY

The term ostomy refers to an artificial opening. When cancer, other diseases, or trauma create conditions that will not allow the passage of fecal matter through the intestines and anus, an ostomy or **stoma** may be constructed surgically in the abdominal wall (Fig. 29–2).

Description and Location of Ostomies

Ostomy procedures such as *gastrostomy* (opening through the abdominal wall into the stomach) and *jejunostomy* (opening through the abdominal wall into the jejunum) are often performed to provide an alternative route for draining gastric secretions or for administering entral feedings (see Chap. 28). Bowel-diversion ostomies are performed to provide an alternative route for fecal elimination. There are two types: *ileostomy* (opening into the ileum); and ascend-

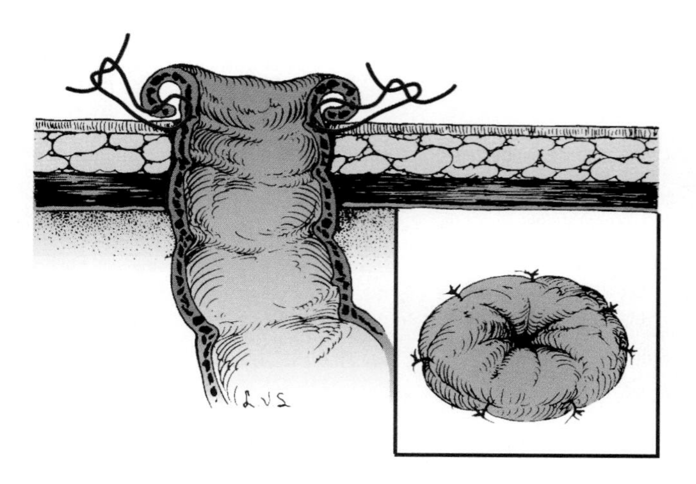

Figure 29–2. Cross-section and top view of an intestinal stoma, showing the opening through the abdominal wall to the intestine (single-barreled end colostomy). *(From Way LW, ed.* Current Surgical Diagnosis and Treatment. *10th ed. Stamford, CT: Appleton & Lange; 1994.)*

COLLABORATIVE STRATEGY

ASSISTING THE PATIENT WITH FECAL INCONTINENCE

A difficult problem for nurse and patient to manage is fecal incontinence. Strong social taboos surround it. Even in the hospital, where the patient has every right to expect tolerance and support for the problem, interpersonal messages too often reflect the attitudes of society. The nurse will help by communicating an understanding of and sensitivity to the patient's situation, and then by establishing a plan to assist the patient with personal hygiene and self-presentation until the patient is able to resume self-care.

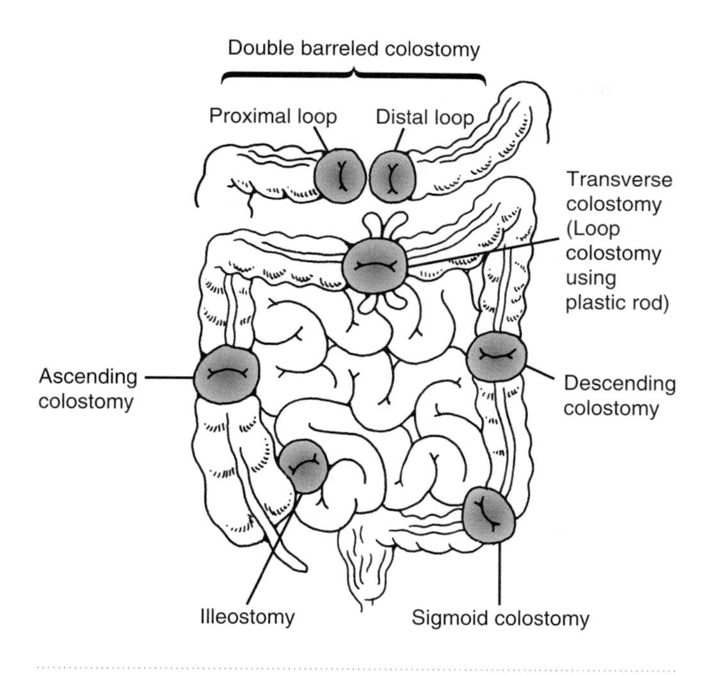

Figure 29–3. Ostomy locations.

ing, transverse, and sigmoid *colostomies* (opening into the ascending, transverse, or sigmoid colon) (Fig. 29–3). Colostomies are further categorized according to (1) whether they are permanent or temporary and (2) the method of constructing the stoma or ostomy.

A temporary colostomy is often performed to allow the distal end of the bowel to rest or heal from injuries caused by trauma or disease. When the injury is healed, the colostomy is reanastomosed (the bowel is surgically sewn back together) and the regular fecal route is restored. When the rectum or anus is not functioning as a result of a birth defect or a disease, such as cancer of the bowel, a permanent colostomy is done. Diseased or injured bowel may or may not be removed when a permanent colostomy is created.

Variations in the Characteristics of Stool

The site of the stoma determines the consistency of stool that is excreted. With an ileostomy, almost no water is absorbed because intestinal contents are excreted before they reach the colon. This results in frequent liquid stools. Liquid stools are also produced by an ascending colon colostomy for the same reason, but transverse colostomies have more solid formed stools. The stool from a sigmoid colostomy is very similar to that typically passed rectally (Table 29–2).

Variations in the Patterns of Elimination

Different ostomy sites result in varying patterns of elimination. A regular bowel elimination pattern cannot be established with ileostomies and ascending colostomies, because there is continuous drainage of liquid stool. Therefore, a bag or pouch must be worn all the time, and the bag must be emptied and washed several times a day. Skin care at the time the bag is changed, or when leakage occurs, is essential to prevent serious skin breakdown at the stoma site.

Descending and sigmoid colostomies generally allow a person to regain a regular bowel pattern. The patient is taught to irrigate the colostomy, a procedure that is similar to an enema (see Procedure 29–8). This establishes a regular pattern of bowel emptying and eliminates the need to wear a pouch. Regulating the diet with selected foods at specific times also contributes to predictable bowel movements, usually once or twice a day. However, many patients choose to continue the use of a pouch in order to feel secure.

Effect on Well-being

A person with a stoma for fecal elimination must adapt to a change in body image along with greatly altered bowel elimination patterns. Problems in self-presentation (see Chap. 26) become para-

TABLE 29–2. ILEOSTOMY AND COLOSTOMY COMPARISONS

Ostomy	Drainage Type	Odor	Regulation	Skin Breakdown
Ileostomy	Semiliquid to liquid	Minimal	None—must wear plastic stoma bag or dressing[a]	Skin easily irritated because of high level of potent digestive enzymes
Ascending colostomy	Liquid to semisoft or soft	Need to use deodorant in bag	None—must wear plastic stoma bag or dressing[a]	Same as ileostomy
Transverse colostomy	Soft	Very strong odor	None—must wear stoma bag or dressing[a]	If exposed to stool, skin breakdown can occur
Sigmoid colostomy	Formed to soft	Odors usually can be controlled	May achieve control with irrigation—may not need bag or dressing over stoma	Same as transverse colostomy

[a]It has been reported that a few patients have achieved some control for these ostomies. The length of time an ostomy is in place may help the stool become more formed because the remaining colon compensates by increasing water absorption.

mount. Loss of self-esteem and an overwhelming sense of powerlessness may be caused by spillage of liquid stool, foul odors, and inability to control and regulate bowel movements. Sexual functioning is often a major concern.

The patient and significant others must deal with new equipment, odor control, scheduling bathroom time, and emotional and sexual concerns in adapting to and coping with an ostomy. Resources are often available to provide support and encouragement. For example, an enterostomal therapist, a nurse with additional education in stomal care, can help with teaching and coordinating care. Members of the United Ostomy Association can visit the patient to explain how to live with an ostomy. Patients can join this organization and meet others who are dealing with ostomies. The American Cancer Society provides ostomy equipment and supplies for patients with financial need.

OPTIMAL URINARY ELIMINATION

The purpose of urinary elimination is to replace fluid balance and rid the body of the end products of metabolism. This work is carried out primarily in the kidneys, where urine is formed, the end-products of metabolism are excreted, and control of fluid and electrolytes takes place. Each kidney contains over 1 million nephrons, the structures that collectively rid the body of wastes. The nephron is the functional unit of the kidney.

Although the kidneys are crucial to the filtration process, three other urinary tract structures—the ureters, bladder, and urethra—are vital to effective urinary elimination. Once urine is formed, it is drained by the ureters, which join the renal pelvis to the bladder. The bladder is the hollow organ that stores urine and serves as the organ of excretion. From the bladder, urine is transported to the outside of the body via the urethra.

Urine formation and elimination depend on a number of physiologic, sociocultural, and developmental factors. Blood volume and flow, and fluid and food intake affect the formation of urine. The urine elimination process, also called voiding, micturition, and urination, is affected by a person's neuromuscular status, position for voiding, privacy, cleanliness of surroundings, and age.

ANATOMY AND PHYSIOLOGY

Kidneys

The kidneys are positioned behind the peritoneum in the posterior aspect of the upper abdominal cavity, one on either side of the vertebral column. They lie in front of the 11th and 12th ribs and are well protected by the abdominal muscles, intestines, and a layer of fat. The medial margin of the kidney is concave; the other edges and surface areas are convex. The hilum originates from the medial side, and it is from the hilum that the ureters, lymphatics, nerves, and renal blood vessels enter and leave the kidney.

The *nephron* is the working unit of the kidney. The processes of filtration, reabsorption, and secretion are carried out by the nephrons. *Filtration* occurs in the glomerulus, a group of capillary loops that allows water and electrolytes to exit but not larger molecules. Glomerular filtrate is the term for the fluid that is filtered by the nephron unit. The **glomerular filtration rate** (GFR) indicates the amount of filtration that occurs within a given time. The average GFR for a normal adult is 125 mL per minute. An average of 180 L of glomerular filtrate is formed every day. Composition of the glomerular filtrate is basically the same as plasma, but without

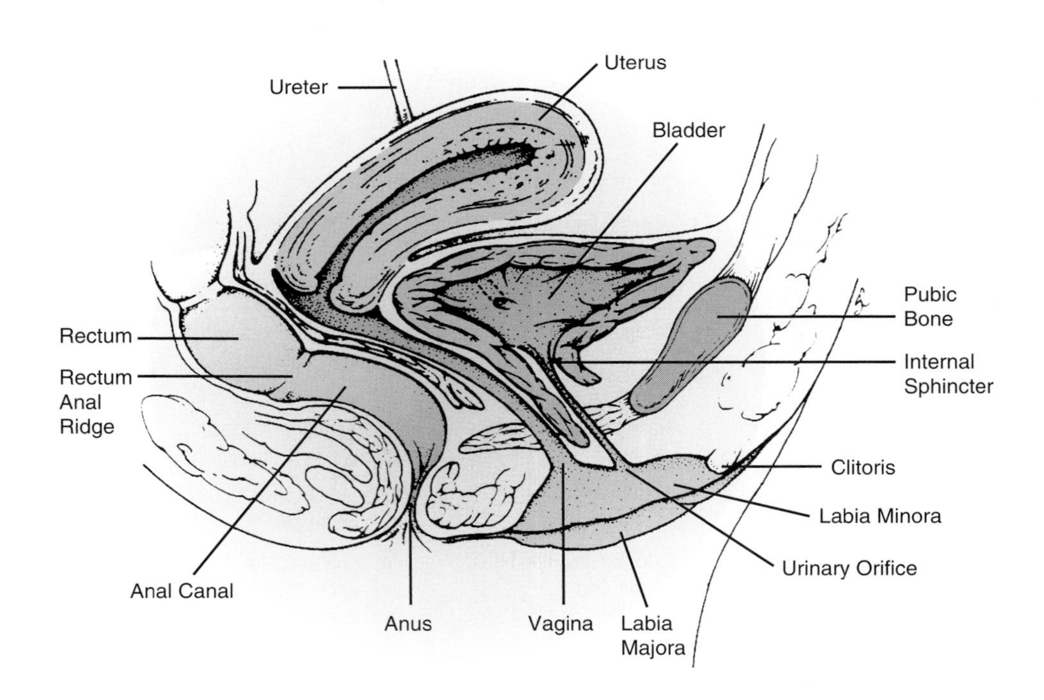

Figure 29–4. Normal position of the bladder in the female. *(From Smith S, Duell D.* Clinical Nursing Skills: Nursing Process Model, Basic to Advanced Skills. *4th ed. Stamford, CT: Appleton & Lange; 1996.)*

significant amounts of proteins. The appearance of protein in the urine, **proteinuria,** is often a sign of glomerular injury, although small amounts may normally appear after prolonged standing or heavy exercise.

Although the kidneys filter 180 L of fluid a day, the average urine output is only 1.2 to 1.5 L (1200 to 1500 mL) a day. This difference is explained by the *reabsorptive* functions of the renal tubular system, where approximately 99 percent of the filtrate, including water, electrolytes, and other compounds such as glucose, is reabsorbed.

In the tubular system, substances are also *secreted* and therefore excreted in urine. Some of these play a major role in the regulation of acid–base balance: potassium ions, hydrogen ions, and ammonia.

The usual composition of urine is 95 percent water and 5 percent solutes, which include electrolytes and organic solutes. The usual production of urine is 50 mL per hour; an hourly output of 30 mL or less suggests inadequate blood perfusion to the kidneys or kidney damage.

The rate of urine production is influenced by various factors: circulatory status, fluid intake, metabolic diseases such as diabetes, autoimmune diseases such as glomerulonephritis, congenital disorders and infections, drug or alcohol ingestion, and prescribed medications such as diuretics.

Ureters

Once urine is formed, it passes from the renal pelvis to the bladder via the ureter. The ureters are tubular structures that are 26 to 30 cm (10 to 12 in.) long in the adult. The distal ends of the ureters connect to the bladder floor. A small flaplike fold at the junction of the ureters and bladder prevents the reflux of urine back into the kidneys. Small amounts of urine drain continuously from the kidneys into the ureters.

Bladder

The *bladder,* which lies posterior to the symphasis pubis, usually holds 300 to 600 mL of urine. However, it is capable of holding twice that capacity because of folds in the lining and elasticity of the walls. When distended, the bladder may extend past the symphysis pubis and, in extreme cases, to the height of the umbilicus. The bladder is located anterior to the uterus and vagina in women (Fig. 29–4); in men it can be found posterior to the prostate gland and anterior to the rectum (Fig. 29–5).

The bladder is composed of two main parts: the fundus or body, in which urine collects; and the neck, which is an extension of the urethra. At the base of the bladder is a triangular area called the *trigone,* where the ureters enter the bladder posteriorly and the urethra leaves the bladder. The muscle within the bladder neck is frequently referred to as the *internal sphincter.* The tone of this muscle keeps the neck empty until the pressure in the fundus of the bladder rises. The internal sphincter is under the control of the autonomic nervous system.

Urethra

The *urethra* is the passageway through which urine leaves the body. It extends from the bladder to the urinary opening on the outside of the body *(urinary meatus).* Within the urethra is the second sphincter that controls urination, the *external sphincter,* which is under the control of voluntary skeletal muscle. The urethra contains a mucous lining that is continuous with that of the bladder and ureters. This lining is susceptible to trauma and infection, which can readily extend to the bladder, ureters, and kidneys.

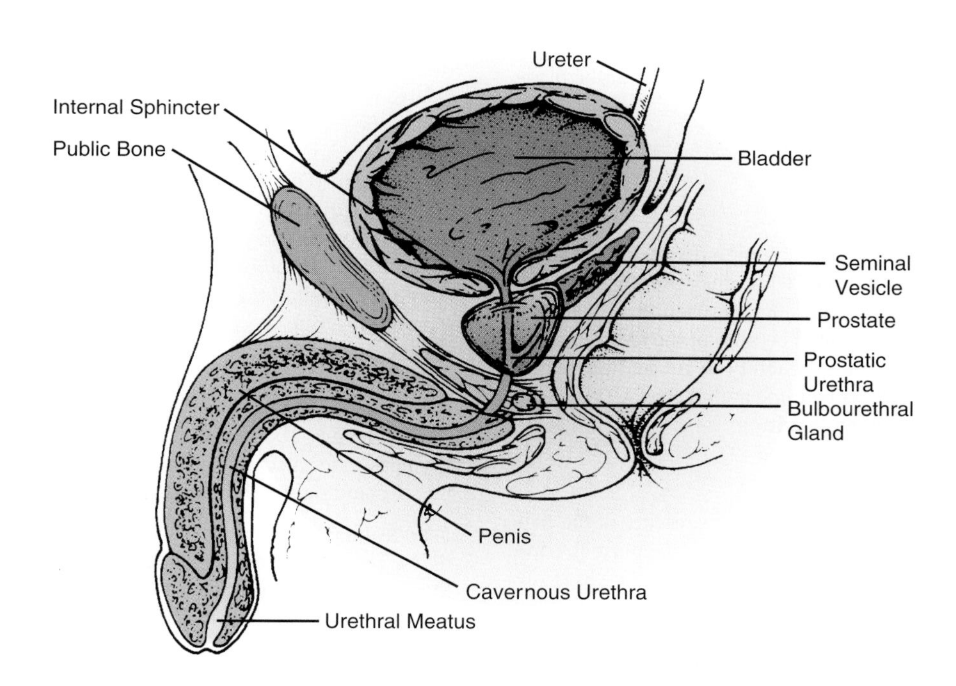

Figure 29–5. Normal position of the bladder in the male. *(From Smith S, Duell D.* Clinical Nursing Skills: Nursing Process Model, Basic to Advanced Skills.*4th ed. Stamford, CT: Appleton & Lange; 1996.)*

Women are more prone to these problems because the female urethra is very short, measuring about 3.7 cm (1½ in.). Bacteria from the vaginal and anal areas can easily travel this short distance to the bladder, where they colonize and produce infection if natural defense mechanisms are not functioning optimally. In men, the urethra is approximately 20 cm (8 in.) long. The male urethra also functions as a passageway for semen.

In women, the urinary meatus is located between the labia minora, below the clitoris, and above the vaginal orifice. In men, the opening is located at the distal end of the penis.

Micturition Reflex

The bladder is primarily innervated through pelvic nerves that connect mainly with the cord segments S-2 and S-3. The sensory nerves of the bladder send impulses to the spinal cord at the level of the second to fourth sacral vertebrae, where the micturition center is located. The stretch receptors in the bladder neck are particularly strong and are mainly responsible for starting the reflexes that control bladder elimination. Both the detrusor muscle and the internal sphincter are under parasympathetic control, which contracts the detrusor muscle and relaxes the internal sphincter in response to the signals sent to the micturition center. Unless the reflex is interrupted at this point by voluntary muscular control of the external sphincter, urination will occur.

Voluntary Neuromuscular Control

When a person is ready to void, the centers in the cortex can help initiate a micturition reflex and inhibit the contraction of the external sphincter. Voluntary urination usually occurs as follows: the abdominal muscles are contracted, which increases pressure in the bladder. Simultaneously, the muscles of the pelvic floor are relaxed, which allows more urine to enter the neck of the bladder, further stretching its walls. The micturition reflex is then initiated and the external urethral sphincter is relaxed. Under these conditions the bladder is emptied. Usually, no more than 10 mL of urine remains in the bladder after voiding. Urine that is left in the bladder after voiding is called *residual urine.*

NORMAL URINATION

Normal Patterns

Patterns of urinary elimination vary among individuals, but most people void about five times a day while they are awake. They usually void initially upon waking, after meals, and at bedtime. Normally, voiding at night is minimal because of the reduced renal blood flow during rest, the kidney's ability to concentrate urine, and the decreased fluid intake as bedtime approaches. Urination is considered a private matter in most cultures.

Characteristics of Normal Urine

Color. Urine is usually light yellow due to the presence of the pigment urochrome. Depending on the specific gravity, normal urine may range from pale to deep yellow. Urine should be clear; the waste products are not usually visible, unless the urine is alkaline, which causes some phosphates and urates to settle out. Factors causing a change in urine color and clarity include disease, dietary intake, and hydration status.[6] Medications, disease, diet, and fluid intake may alter the color and clarity of urine.[7] Many drugs can alter the color of urine; among these are multivitamins, iron preparations, and some diuretics. Color changes may range from pink, red, or orange to dark brown or black.

Odor. Freshly voided urine should have a slightly aromatic odor; a foul odor may be a result of drugs, food, or urinary tract infection. Stale urine smells of ammonia because bacteria convert urea to ammonia.

Amount. Daily urine production varies with age, fluid intake, and health status. Infants and children excrete large volumes of urine in relation to their size. A 6-month-old infant excretes between 400 to 500 mL of urine daily. In comparison, an adult normally voids 1200 to 1500 mL of urine a day, usually voiding 150 to 600 mL at a time. Urine output of less than 30 mL per hour should be reported immediately to a physician. Urine production of more than 55 mL per hour in an adult or more than 2000 mL a day is excessive. It may be caused by increased fluid intake, certain kidney disorders, endocrine diseases, or the use of diuretics.

FACTORS AFFECTING URINATION

Among the factors that affect urinary elimination are fluid intake, age, health status, medications, and emotional state.

Fluid Intake

Because the kidneys provide the main control for fluid homeostasis, fluid intake influences urine production and thus micturition. Water-induced diuresis occurs when an individual drinks a large amount. The fluids increase the circulating plasma volume and thus the amount of glomerular filtrate, resulting in increased urine production. Decreasing fluid intake decreases urine output. Patients who complain of urinary frequency (voiding an increased number of times during the day or night) often cut back their fluid intake so as to decrease the need for urination. However, this requires patient teaching on the nurse's part, because decreasing fluid intake can cause problems such as dehydration.

Certain fluids, such as alcohol and caffeine-containing drinks, inhibit the release of antidiuretic hormone (ADH), thereby directly influencing urine output. Cells in the renal tubules do not reabsorb water when ADH release is inhibited. Cola, cocoa, tea, and coffee all increase diuresis and micturition. Additionally, some foods high in water content, such as fruits and vegetables, may also increase urine output. If the body becomes depleted of fluid through perspiration, respiration, or digestion, water is reabsorbed by the glomeruli, urine becomes more concentrated, and output is decreased.

Age

Age influences both urinary production and urine excretion. Changes associated with age occur in the kidneys, bladder, and muscles and nerves that affect micturition.

Infants. Infants (birth to 1 year) cannot concentrate urine effectively. Therefore, they excrete large volumes of urine in relation to their size. The kidneys start excreting urine in utero between the 11th and 12th week of development, but the placenta carries out fetal regulatory and excretory function until birth.

Children. Between 1 and 2 years of age, a child's kidneys can concentrate as much urine as an adult's and urine takes on the characteristic yellow-amber color. Control of urination begins between

2½ to 3 years of age, but nighttime control may not be achieved until age 4 or 5. Girls are often able to gain urine control sooner than boys. During childhood, the kidneys and bladder grow in proportion to the rest of the body.

Adolescents and Adults. Renal filtration of the blood and micturition are usually maintained at full capacity through age 50. Diseases of the urinary tract and metabolic and cardiovascular problems can alter kidney function in the adult, as can other factors discussed below.

Older Adults. Adults older than 65 years frequently experience changes in urinary elimination. Age-related changes in the kidney result in a decreased adaptive capacity. Changes in the nephrons, proximal and distal convoluted tubules, and renal blood vessels produce diminished renal blood flow and glomerular filtration rate, as well as decreased ability to concentrate urine. The elderly therefore require greater amounts of fluid intake to excrete a given amount of metabolic waste. In healthy elderly people, control of fluid volume and excretion is usually effective, in spite of these changes. However, older adults are susceptible to kidney and urinary problems when stressed by injury or disease.

The ureter, bladder, and urethra also reflect the aging process.[8] Urination often becomes a concern for the elderly, because decreased bladder capacity, combined with poor ability to concentrate urine, leads to more frequent urination. This can disrupt sleep patterns and create risks for injury when elderly people walk to the bathroom in semidarkness or when not fully awake. Vision or mobility problems, also common among older individuals, compound the problem.

Elderly women are also at risk for bladder infections and stress incontinence because relaxation of perineal support structures interferes with complete emptying and external sphincter control. Periodic dribbling of urine may also be related to these changes. In men, *prostatic hypertrophy* (enlargement) often causes difficulties initiating urination. Incontinence does not occur because of aging, although some diseases may compromise urinary control. Other urination problems in the elderly are related to chronic diseases of other body systems. For example, arthritis may make getting to the bathroom and getting on and off the toilet difficult.

Health Status

Disease, surgical procedures, medications, and diagnostic examinations often alter urinary elimination patterns.

Diseases. Pathology involving the urinary system may affect urinary elimination or urine production. Hereditary anomalies, infection, cancer, and obstruction can all occur in the renal system. They may produce changes ranging from production alterations, such as release of large amounts of poorly concentrated urine, to blockages that result in obstruction of urinary outflow.

Cardiovascular, respiratory, and neuromuscular system pathology may alter urine production or affect a person's ability to void or to get to the toilet. Neuromuscular diseases may lead to loss of bladder tone and inability to control urination. Cardiovascular disease such as hypertension may cause changes in the blood flow to the kidneys, which can lead to decreased production of urine. Because the respiratory system and the renal system together maintain acid–base balance, diseases of the respiratory system affect the renal system. If both systems are impaired, acid–base balance may be severely compromised. (See Chap. 34 for discussion of acid–base balance.)

Surgery. Surgery alters urinary elimination in several ways. First, surgery initiates a stress response in which vasopressin (ADH), epinephrine, and renin levels are increased. These hormones increase vascular resistance, promote fluid retention, and therefore decrease urine output. Surgery also contributes to reduced urine output for two reasons: hypovolemia resulting from the npo (nothing by mouth) state prior to surgery, and blood and fluid loss during surgery. Anesthetics, anticholinergics, narcotics, and sedatives used before, during, and after surgery may interfere with voiding in the postoperative period. Anesthesia and other drugs such as narcotics and sedatives, which alter levels of consciousness, may make it difficult for an individual to realize the bladder is full, resulting in retention or incontinence. These same medications may also make it difficult to get on a bedpan or stand to void in a urinal.[9] To help reduce these problems, an indwelling (Foley) catheter is often placed before surgery.

Surgical or diagnostic procedures that involve instrumentation of the urinary tract, lower abdomen, or pelvic region may impair urination because of trauma and inflammation to tissues. Aftereffects of surgery include obstruction of urine flow, interference with the relaxation of sphincters and muscles, pain during voiding, and bleeding from the urinary tract.

Medications. A number of medications can alter normal urinary function, causing, for example, changes in urine characteristics, production, and elimination from the bladder. **Diuretics** are medications that increase urine excretion.

Because of its waste excretion, the kidney is especially vulnerable to toxicity from drugs. Although some drugs rarely cause nephrotoxicity, antibiotics (especially aminoglycocides, tetracyclines, sulfonamides, and vancomycin); diuretics; and anesthetics are frequently toxic to the kidney.[10] Signs of nephrotoxicity include increased blood urea nitrogen (BUN) and serum creatinine levels, decreased urine output, edema, weight gain, hematuria, and albuminuria.

Emotional State

Individuals under acute stress often experience urinary urgency and frequency. The sympathetic nervous system, which is active during stress, promotes internal sphincter relaxation, therefore stimulating the urge to void even though the bladder is not full. Paradoxically, acute stress may also interfere with relaxation of the external sphincter and perineal muscles. When this occurs, complete emptying of the bladder is difficult or impossible, despite the frequent urge to void. If stress is prolonged (for several hours, for example), urine production is suppressed because of decreased circulation to the kidneys. In this situation, the urge to urinate may be delayed until the stress is resolved.

For some individuals, lack of privacy or anxiety associated with illness and hospitalization may disrupt normal voiding patterns. Incomplete emptying of the bladder or inability to initiate voiding is common.

▲ ALTERED URINARY ELIMINATION

Alterations in urination comprise a broad category of problems, such as incontinence, retention, dysuria, anuria, and oliguria.

Some alterations in elimination result from alterations in urine production. These include conditions such as anuria and oliguria, which nurses monitor but for which the physician prescribes specific treatments.

URINARY INCONTINENCE

Urinary incontinence is the loss of control over voiding. The individual is unable to stop the passage of urine from the bladder. The problem may be temporary, as in the acutely ill patient who is unconscious, or it may be permanent because of neuromuscular damage. The flow of urine may be almost continuous or it may occur sporadically. Incontinence can be treated and in most cases controlled through nursing and medical interventions. The impact of incontinence is immense; it affects not only the patient and family but also health care workers and the health care industry as well.

There are several types of incontinence, each with a different etiology (see the discussion of nursing diagnoses for Altered Patterns of Urinary Elimination in Section 2 of this chapter). Risk factors include infection of or trauma to the urinary tract; change in tissue and muscle tone after childbirth, with aging, and after weight loss or gain; neuromuscular conditions that interfere with the transmission of sensory or motor impulses for urination; medications that increase urinary frequency or change sensory input; and psychological factors such as anxiety, fear, confusion, or disorientation.

Incontinence can be devastating to patients and their families personally, socially, and financially. Patients may suffer from embarrassment, social isolation, depression, anxiety, or impaired skin integrity. The family responsible for the physical care of an incontinent family member often experiences physical strain and mental worry. If the patient is institutionalized, the family may be torn about the decision, and the patient may feel betrayed.

Although incontinence can affect individuals at any age it is most often seen in the elderly. Urinary incontinence is prevalent in older women; at least 50 percent of residents in nursing homes suffer from incontinence.[11] Certain conditions, such as impaired mobility and impaired cognition, are often associated with incontinence.[12] Many patients who have suffered strokes are incontinent, especially when cortical function is impaired. However, although incontinence affects the elderly more than other groups, it is not invariably associated with the aging process.

ENURESIS AND NOCTURIA

The involuntary loss of urine beyond the age when bladder control is usually achieved, is called **enuresis.** Enuresis is further defined as nocturnal, diurnal, or both.[13]

Nocturnal enuresis is the loss of urine during sleep after the age of 4 or 5, when most children can avoid nighttime voiding. This condition may continue into the teen years and, rarely, into adulthood. Diurnal enuresis is the loss of urine during the day. This latter condition often occurs because a child delays voiding too long because of play or other distractions, but may be secondary to pathology.

Nocturia, in contrast, is excessive voiding at night; the individual is aware of the need to urinate and gets up to void. It is not unusual for some people to get up once at night to void, but when an individual's pattern changes, so that awakening for urination repeatedly occurs several times per night, the change should be assessed.

Age, stress, disease, and medications can play a role in both enuresis and nocturia. Heredity seems to play a role in enuresis because there is an increased incidence among close relatives of those who have experienced it. Other physiologic, psychological, and environmental factors thought to contribute to enuresis include food allergies, small bladder capacity, urinary tract infection, fluid intake after dinner, and inaccessibility to toilet facilities. Common causes of nocturia include pregnancy, urinary tract infections, stress, diuretics and increased fluid intake. In men older than 50 years, prostate enlargement contributes to nocturia. It is also felt that decreased bladder tone, chronic diseases such as congestive heart failure and diabetes, and use of diuretics play a significant role in nocturia that occurs with aging.

Safety is a concern for both adults and children who awake at night to go to the bathroom. Many accidents occur when sleepy individuals get up to go to the bathroom. Additionally, enuresis is often a source of embarrassment. Bedwetting may create feelings of isolation and altered self-concept. It is important that the family be understanding of the alteration, because it can be a source of frustration, anxiety, isolation, and behavioral problems for the child.

FREQUENCY, URGENCY, AND DYSURIA

Normally, urination occurs painlessly and effortlessly about five times a day, and most people can hold about 150 mL of urine in the bladder without feeling a strong desire to void. **Urinary frequency** refers to urination at more frequent intervals. The amount voided may be either large or small; the term refers only to the number of times one voids in 24 hours. **Urgency** is a sudden strong desire to urinate. The urge to void may be so strong that it leads to incontinence. **Dysuria** means difficult or painful urination. Individuals may complain of discomfort during, before, or immediately after voiding. Frequency, urgency, and dysuria may occur separately or in combination.

Pregnancy, increased fluid intake, diuretics, and urinary tract infections are common causes of frequency. Urgency is a common complaint during stress or urinary tract infections, when it is associated with weak external sphincter control. Dysuria is common in any condition that causes trauma or inflammation of the bladder or urethra. When individuals complain of any of these symptoms, it is important to question them about other concerns, such as hesitancy (difficulty in initiating voiding), hematuria (blood in the urine), and pyuria (pus in the urine).

Frequency, urgency, and dysuria may cause minor problems for a patient or they may be a main source of concern. These problems may disrupt activities of daily living and lead to embarrassment. Patients often attempt to reduce fluid intake to control these problems, but usually this does not solve the problem and may even make it worse.

OLIGURIA, ANURIA, AND POLYURIA

Oliguria is urine production of less than 30 mL an hour. **Anuria** refers to producing less than 100 mL of urine in a day. Oliguria and anuria are signs that the kidneys are not working or are not adequately perfused. **Polyuria** is the production of large amounts of urine in relation to fluid intake; it does not refer to the frequency or time interval of urination. Polyuria, however, may accompany frequency.

A variety of metabolic, urologic, and cardiovascular disorders manifest themselves as disturbances in the normal output of urine. Kidney disease, heart failure, severe burns, and shock can cause anuria or oliguria. Oliguria may also be present in dehydration. Causes of polyuria include diabetes mellitus, diabetes insipidus, kidney disease, diuretics, and increased fluid intake, especially fluids containing alcohol and caffeine.

Persons experiencing anuria or oliguria are often acutely ill. Fluid and electrolyte and acid–base imbalances, along with retention of metabolic wastes, cause edema, respiratory difficulty, and confusion. Renal failure may be present or impending. Shock or dehydration may also be present. The individual in shock appears pale and weak; the skin is usually cool and clammy. In dehydration, the skin feels hot and dry with decreased turgor. Anuria is a grave sign indicating that death may ensue if circulatory status or waste product removal is not improved.

The individual with polyuria may appear healthy or may have few complaints, but the nurse should assess for thirst and weight loss and determine whether excessive fluid intake is a factor.

RETENTION

Urinary retention is a state in which the individual cannot initiate or complete evacuation of accumulated urine from the bladder. Urinary retention may be acute or chronic. Chronic retention may persist over a period of months and may be irreversible. Chronic retention is sometimes referred to as "overflow incontinence" or "paradoxical incontinence," because patients are unable to void until the intra-abdominal pressure increases to such a degree that urine is involuntarily voided.

Acute retention may occur after surgery, diagnostic procedures involving the urinary tract, delivery of a baby, and with obstruction in the urinary system. Medications that may cause retention include anesthesia, opiates, sedatives, antihistamines, and anticholinergics. Social factors or emotion may also play a part in retention. Fear, stress, and pain may produce anxiety and tension, resulting in urinary retention.

Chronic retention is classified according to one of two causes: (1) weak or absent detrusor contraction or (2) bladder outlet obstruction. Factors that contribute to altered detrusor muscle contraction include chronic bladder distension, as with prostate enlargement, or impairment of the sensory and motor branches of reflex arc, as found after spinal cord damage. Factors that contribute to bladder outlet obstruction include strictures and prostatic hypertrophy.

Urinary retention can be a significant threat to well-being. In some cases of chronic retention, bladder-training programs can restore near-normal elimination patterns; however, some patients with chronic retention require a permanent indwelling catheter or must learn intermittent self-catheterization. These latter interventions may create significant body-image alterations.

Nurses' understanding of bowel and bladder elimination is essential to providing quality care and to effective collaboration with patients. Helping patients understand elimination aids collaboration.

SECTION 2

ASSESSMENT OF ELIMINATION

ELIMINATION DATA COLLECTION

Elimination data is collected about the process and products of elimination as well as factors that may influence elimination. An individual's elimination habits are a personal, private concern. To lessen embarrassment during the assessment, privacy is provided. The nurse must avoid demonstrating embarrassment and be able to discuss openly a patient's elimination needs and problems. Most beginning nursing students will find this difficult, because of their own socialization about the privacy of elimination. Sharing these concerns in small groups or clinical conferences may help students develop a more relaxed, open attitude about this body function.

ELIMINATION HISTORY

The elimination history should focus on the many factors that may affect this vital function. For example, normal elimination patterns may be altered by the home environment, number of bathroom facilities, number of family members, and any condition that might impair a patient's ability to eat regularly, maintain a healthy fluid intake, or walk to the bathroom. Special dietary requirements, work schedules, and medications also may impede establishing regular elimination patterns.

Elimination problems have an impact on patients' life-style, self-concept, and activities of daily living. Information related to any change in bowel habits is especially significant because the change may be a warning sign of cancer. Changes in urine characteristics and patterns signal possible urinary tract, metabolic, cardiovascular, or neuromuscular problems.

Primary Concern

Explore the patient's primary concern to determine whether it is related to or has affected elimination patterns. Some complaints—such as constipation, diarrhea, burning, and dribbling—are directly related to elimination. Other complaints—such as headache, nausea, and abdominal pain—may also be related to elimination. Abdominal trauma may affect elimination. Circulation or breathing problems may cause weakness and decreased mobility, which can interfere with elimination. Therefore an elimination assessment is necessary both for patients whose primary concern involves urination or bowel elimination, and for those whose complaint suggests that elimination may be affected.

Current Understanding

If the primary concern is altered elimination, it is helpful to obtain information about the nature of the problem, what the patient believes may have caused it, what makes it better or worse, and what the patient has done to correct it. If another health problem has contributed to altered elimination, find out how the problem interferes. Often this information suggests possible nursing diagnoses and topics for later health teaching. The following example illustrates current understanding.

Mrs. Elias, age 63, is being treated for joint pain and stiffness, especially in her hips and knees. She reports that sitting on the toilet is painful, so she has decreased her fluid intake "so I don't have to urinate so often." The nurse realizes that limiting fluid intake increases Mrs. Elias' risks of constipation and urinary tract infection and makes a note to discuss this further with her before she leaves the clinic.

Past Health Care Experiences/Problems

Determine whether past health care experiences have caused short-term or residual effects on bowel or urine elimination. Explore whether the patient routinely takes medications that may alter urinary elimination (eg, antihypertensives, steroids, or cardiac medications) or influence bowel elimination (eg, laxatives or iron). If radiologic studies of the urinary tract are planned, determine whether the patient has a history of allergy to iodine, as many contrast materials used in these studies contain iodine. The following example illustrates a past health care experience.

Monica Flynn has delivered her second baby and is being admitted to the postpartum unit. She says, "I hope I don't have the same trouble I had with my first baby. It hurt so much to have a bowel movement because of my hemorrhoids and my stitches, that I kept holding back—and then I became constipated and it hurt even more." Monica's nurse resolves to encourage fluids and to teach Monica how high-fiber foods will contribute to soft, formed stools that are easier to pass.

Personal, Family, and Social History

Life-style affects elimination. Regularity of meals, fluid intake, and exercise routines are some examples. Besides personal activities, elimination patterns may be related to vocational or home and family factors. Conversely, alterations in elimination patterns affect feelings of well-being and therefore interfere with the quality of daily life. See Table 29–3 and the following example.

Jeannette James is a young professional woman who seeks health care for urinary burning and frequency. She states that she feels like she has to empty her bladder often, but that "very little urine comes out." When the nurse questions her about her usual urinary patterns and fluid intake, Ms. James responds that she doesn't drink much water because she rarely leaves her desk except for lunch. Many days she empties her bladder only at lunch and after work. The nurse recognizes that these symptoms suggest a urinary tract infection and that Ms. James' habits increase the risk that the condition will be a recurrent problem.

Subjective Manifestations

A review of subjective manifestations helps nurses identify patients' usual patterns and recognize actual or potential abnormalities.

The following case illustration provides an example of the nurse's use of subjective manifestations data in planning patient care.

Mr. Jones, 75 years old, comes to the clinic because of abdominal pain. He states that his last bowel movement was 3 days ago and describes the stool as hard, formed, dry, and dark brown. He also states that he can't understand why he hasn't gone to the bathroom as he took a double dose of the laxative he usually uses. Upon further questioning, Mr. Jones

TABLE 29-3. ELIMINATION HISTORY: PERSONAL, FAMILY, AND SOCIAL HISTORY QUESTIONS

A. Vocational
1. What type of daily activities do you engage in (work, school)?
2. Do your working hours influence your urine or bowel elimination?

B. Home and Family
1. Describe a typical day.
2. Do you ever have to suppress elimination urges due to lack of facilities, time, or privacy?
3. Are there any family members with past or current health problems affecting elimination?

C. Social and Leisure
1. What are your favorite leisure activities?
2. Do your elimination patterns have any effect on your leisure activities?
3. Do your leisure activities affect your elimination patterns?

D. Sexual
1. Has your sexual relationship been satisfactory?
2. Have you noticed any symptoms of urinary problems after sexual intercourse?

E. Habits

Exercise
1. Do you exercise regularly? How often and what types of exercise?
2. Have your elimination patterns influenced your exercising?
3. Has your exercising had an effect on your elimination patterns?

Diet
1. How many meals do you eat per day?
2. Are you on a special diet of any kind? Prescribed by a physician? Someone else? Self?
3. Describe a typical day's menu at home and when you eat out.
4. What are the types and amounts of bulk and fiber foods you eat most every day?
5. Do any foods or fluids cause you elimination difficulties? List these.
6. Do you use any foods and fluids to keep bowels regular?
7. Are there any foods you don't eat? Why?

Beverages
1. How much fluid do you have each day? What types of fluids?
2. Do you use alcohol? How much do you drink in a day? A week?
3. Do you use caffeine? Tea? Coffee? Soft drinks? Do any beverages affect urination or bowel elimination?

Other Substances
1. What medications do you take regularly? Occasionally?
2. Do any medications affect your elimination patterns?

Sleep
1. How many hours do you sleep at night?
2. Are you awakened in the night by the urge to empty your bladder? How often? To have a bowel movement?

F. Psychological
1. Are you experiencing any stress currently?
2. Do your elimination habits change when you become stressed?
3. Has a recent change in elimination patterns been stressful?

reveals that he has used an over-the-counter laxative every day for the last 6 months. The nurse believes that Mr. Jones' constipation may be related to his reliance on laxatives. The nurse then further assesses Mr. Jones' definition of constipation, understanding of bowel function, usual diet, and fluid intake.

ELIMINATION EXAMINATION

Physical assessment data obtained using measurement, inspection, auscultation, and palpation complete the picture of patient elimination status suggested by the elimination history.

Measurements

Measurements that reflect elimination status include intake and output, weight, abdominal girth, and blood pressure. Body surface area is calculated from height and weight.

Intake and Output. Accurate intake and output measurement is vital to determining fluid status and efficiency of kidney function. Comparing intake and output measurements provides clues to abnormalities such as oliguria, polyuria, and anuria. For comparisons of intake and output to be valid, all forms of output—including liquid stool, emesis, and wound and other drainage—must be measured and recorded. When there is excessive fluid loss via abnormal routes, urine output usually decreases to compensate. Refer to Chapter 34 for a more detailed discussion of intake and output measurement.

Weight. Short-term weight changes reflect fluid gains and losses. Patients with severe cardiac or renal disease may demonstrate consistent rapid weight gain over weeks or even months. Daily monitoring of weight provides data about trends and changes in status. For accurate comparisons, it is recommended that daily weights be measured at the same time each day, using the same scale. Many health care facilities schedule daily weights in the morning before breakfast.

Body Surface Area Calculation. Calculation of body surface area (BSA) to determine basal fluid requirements is frequently necessary for patients with compromised elimination, because fluid intake must be restricted to minimize fluid retention or increased to facilitate bowel elimination. Chapter 34 presents instructions for calculating BSA and measuring body weight on various types of scales.

Abdominal Girth. Abdominal girth may be part of the elimination examination, because it is one indicator of abdominal distension. Abdominal girth may increase because of abnormal fluid retention in the peritoneal cavity (ascites) or because of altered bowel elimination, such as constipation, excessive flatulence, or bowel obstruction. The circumference of the abdomen is measured with a tape measure at the level of the umbilicus. The girth may be measured daily or more frequently to detect increases or decreases. Consistent placement of the tape measure is essential for comparison of successive values to be valid.

Blood Pressure. Blood pressure is also related to elimination status, particularly kidney function. When blood pressure is abnormally low, kidney perfusion may be inadequate for efficient filtration, and urine output falls. Elevated blood pressure is usually associated with vasoconstriction, which also reduces renal perfusion and therefore urine output. Moreover, many patients being treated for hypertension are given medications that influence kidney function, and some medications used to treat kidney problems influence blood pressure.

Objective Manifestations

The elimination examination also includes general observations and assessment of the skin, abdomen, genitalia, and perianal area, as well as inspection of urine and feces. If general observations point out problems with mobility or orientation, then mobility and neurological assessment is also relevant.

General Observations

General observation of a patient can provide clues that elimination processes are altered or at risk. The patient's overall appearance (general movement, facial expression, and posture) may indicate the presence of an elimination problem. For example, patients who grimace, hold their stomachs, and curl up in a fetal position often have acute abdominal pain. Abdominal pain is often associated with elimination problems such as diarrhea or intestinal obstruction. Dry skin and mucous membranes imply altered fluid status, which influences both urine and bowel elimination.

Confusion may indicate that a patient is at risk for incontinence or it may be a manifestation of severe kidney failure. Odors may be another indicator of problems. An ammonia-like or feces-like smell may indicate incontinence. The nurse must verify the significance of general observations by collecting additional data relevant to elimination status.

Integument. The integument also provides information suggestive of elimination problems. Dry skin and mucous membranes, coated tongue, ropey saliva, and sluggish capillary refill imply fluid volume deficit. This may be caused by abnormal fluid losses in stool (diarrhea) or urine. Conversely, individuals with fluid volume deficit often become constipated because of increased reabsorption of water by intestinal mucosa.

Edema is another indicator of elimination problems. It often occurs with altered kidney function. The nurse should palpate all tissue, particularly dependent areas, for fluid collection. (Refer to Chap. 34 for technique and grading of edema.) In ambulatory patients, dependent areas are the lower legs and feet, but in bedridden patients, dependent areas include the sacrum and lower back.

Abdomen. Abdominal examination is an important component of the elimination assessment. The examination includes inspection, auscultation, and palpation. If inspection reveals distension (a protuberant abdomen with a rounded contour), consider elimination-related causes. Although there are several causes of abdominal distension that are not related to elimination, generalized symmetrical distension is often caused by intestinal gas or constipation. Asymmetrical distension may be related to bowel obstruction. If obstruction is suspected, observe for the presence of visible peristaltic waves. Sit next to the patient and gaze across the profile of the abdomen for several minutes. Observe for elevated oblique bands starting in the upper left quadrant and moving downward to the right. Distension that is limited to the area between the symphysis pubis and the umbilicus may be caused by a full bladder. Findings during auscultation may support or rule out these possible causes of distension.

Inspection also includes assessment of stomas and peristomal skin in patients who have had urinary or bowel diversion surgery.

The stoma itself should be assessed for color, edema, and bleeding. A well-perfused stoma is deep pink to brick red, whereas a dark red to purple color suggests impaired circulation to the stoma or bowel. Stomal edema or bleeding is abnormal except during the immediate postoperative period. A small amount of oozing in a fresh stoma is not uncommon, but if frank, bright red blood is seen, the cause must be determined and corrected. Common peristomal skin alterations requiring attention include erythema, weeping, edema, erosion, itching, and burning. All of these may be caused by allergic reaction to products used in ostomy care or by irritation from fecal matter or urine.

Crusting, scaly patches, erosion, and bleeding commonly result from mechanical trauma—for example, from vigorous or frequent removal of adhesives used to affix a stoma pouch. Folliculitis, evidenced by reddened, raised hair follicles around the stoma, may also result from traction when adhesives and pouch are removed. Some patients develop a fungal infection around a stoma site, which is manifested by patchy erythematous areas intermixed with dry, scaly itching areas. A bacterial infection may also occur, resulting in large weeping erythematous areas, crusting, and purulent sores. Patients with stomas benefit from teaching by the enterostomal therapist, as many of these complications can be avoided with appropriate stoma care.

When abdominal inspection is complete, auscultate for bowel sounds as discussed in Chapter 17. Absent bowel sounds are expected immediately after surgery, but absent or hypoactive bowel sounds (faint sounds occurring 30 seconds or more apart) in patients who are not postoperative suggest decreased intestinal motility or other pathology requiring further investigation. Borborygmus (loud rumbling, gurgling bowel sounds) are also abnormal and suggest increased motility. The cause may be gastroenteritis or recent laxative use.

Palpate the abdomen after auscultating. Light palpation may detect generalized tenseness suggestive of excessive gas. Soft, boggy rounded masses may be felt across the two upper quadrants or along the left lateral border of the upper and lower left quadrants. These masses are feces within the transverse and descending colon. Although presence of fecal material in the descending colon is not abnormal, in the right transverse or ascending colon it suggests bowel elimination problems. Some patients may complain of cramping after bowel segments are palpated.

A distended bladder may also be confirmed by palpation. Palpate above the symphysis pubis for a smooth, round, rather tense mass. Rarely, it may extend as high as the umbilicus. Often the patient will complain of a desire to empty the bladder because of pressure caused by palpation.

Genitalia. Proceeding in a head-to-foot fashion, the genitalia are assessed next in an elimination examination. Although this part of the examination is often uncomfortable for beginning students, particularly with patients of the opposite sex, it should not be omitted. Carrying out the assessment while providing perineal care may reduce embarrassment. A respectful, matter-of-fact approach is helpful to both patient and nurse (see Chap. 17). Significant findings may include discharge from the urethra (or in the periurethral area in women) and redness, swelling, or excoriation of tissues. A urinary tract infection may be the cause of these symptoms, particularly if the patient history includes complaints of frequency, urgency, and dysuria. Patients with indwelling catheters are at risk for periurethral irritation and discharge, as well as for bladder infections, and so more frequent assessments are warranted.

Perianal Area. Hemorrhoids may be detected in the perianal area. They may cause slight bleeding and pain with defecation. Some patients with hemorrhoids have frequent constipation as a result of suppressing defecation to avoid pain. Redness and excoriation in the perianal area may be caused by incontinence and will be exacerbated if incontinence continues.

Neurologic and Mobility Assessment. Neurologic and mobility assessments are relevant for any patient whose ability to walk independently is compromised. Generalized weakness, poor balance, lower extremity contractures, or a need for assistive devices (canes, crutches, wheelchair) imply difficulty getting to toilet facilities, particularly in a strange environment such as a health care institution. Confusion and disorientation may contribute to mobility problems and increase a patient's risk for incontinence and subsequent skin breakdown related to poor hygiene. Paralysis, whether partial or complete, may compromise urinary and bowel elimination. Many paralyzed patients require indwelling urinary catheters and are incontinent of stool; some benefit from bowel training (see Rehabilitative Care later in the chapter) to facilitate

TABLE 29-4. URINE CHARACTERISTICS AND COMMON ALTERATIONS

Parameter	Usual Character	Common Alterations	Possible Cause
Color	Pale yellow (straw-colored to amber)	Dark amber	Decreased fluid intake, medications
		Colorless, pale	Large fluid intake; diuresis (caffeine, alcohol, other drugs); kidney disease; diabetes insipidus
Clarity	Clear	Cloudy	Infection: bacteria, pus, or white blood cells in urine; diet (increased protein)
Odor	Faint aromatic	Malodorous	Infection, medications, tannins in wine, diabetic acidosis

management of bowel elimination. Comatose patients cannot control urine or bowel elimination and therefore require complete elimination care.

Urine and Stool Characteristics. Assessment of urine and stool characteristics completes the elimination examination. Tables 29–4 and 29–5 summarize usual characteristics of urine and stool, as well as common alterations and their causes.

DIAGNOSTIC TESTS

Diagnostic examinations and laboratory tests provide additional data about the functioning of organs related to elimination. Nurses can use this information to support certain nursing diagnoses. Diagnostic tests include laboratory tests (blood, urine, and feces), x-rays, nonradiologic examinations such as scans and sonography, and direct visualization. Most of these procedures are done in special departments by specially trained personnel. Refer to Tables 29–6 to 29–8. Nurses make independent decisions about performing some diagnostic tests. For example, nurses commonly check for the presence of blood in stool and assess the pH, specific gravity, sugar, ketones, blood, and protein in urine. See Preventive Care later in the chapter.

NURSING DIAGNOSIS OF ELIMINATION STATUS

The final step in the elimination assessment is analyzing the subjective and objective data to generate nursing diagnoses. These diagnoses then form the basis for collaborative planning with the patient to promote optimal urinary and bowel elimination. Tables 29–9 and 29–10 summarize several nursing diagnoses related to elimination. The beginning student will find the taxonomy of nursing diagnoses a helpful guide for clustering data and stating nursing diagnoses. The following sections discuss nursing diagnoses related to bowel and urinary elimination and their etiologies. The diagnoses have been approved by the North American Nursing Diagnosis Association (NANDA).

DIAGNOSES RELATED TO BOWEL ELIMINATION

Three nursing diagnoses related to bowel elimination are addressed here: constipation, diarrhea, and bowel incontinence. Examples of subjective and objective data, defining characteristics, and established or suggested etiologies for these diagnoses are presented in Table 29–9. Other nursing diagnoses that are related to

TABLE 29–5. STOOL CHARACTERISTICS AND COMMON ALTERATIONS

Parameter	Usual Character	Common Alterations	Possible Cause
Color	Brown	Clay or white	Obstruction or absence of bile
		Light green	Enteric infection
		Black or tarry	Iron compounds; upper GI bleeding
		Pale with fatty-appearing substance	Fat malabsorption
		Red/blood-streaked	Lower GI bleeding, hemorrhoids, or some foods such as beets
Consistency	Moist, soft, and formed	Hard, dry	Slowed peristalsis, poor hydration
		Liquid, unformed	Intestinal irritants such as enteric pathogens, some foods, some medications; all promote hypermotility of the intestine and decreased water absorption
Odor	Characteristic pungent fecal odor, affected by food eaten	Aromatic, extremely pungent, foul	Blood or infection in intestinal tract, malabsorption of fat
Shape	Diameter and contour of the rectum	Narrow, pencil-shaped, ribbon-like	Obstruction with resulting hypermotility of the intestine
		Round, small	Poor hydration, slowed peristalsis
Amount	Varies with intake and diet (100–400 g daily)	Bulky (pale, frothy)	Fat malabsorption
Constituents	Dead bacteria, undigested food, fat, bile pigment, remains of digestive enzymes, sloughed intestinal mucosal cells, water	Blood, pus, mucus, foreign bodies, worms	GI bleeding, infection, intestinal parasites, swallowed objects, inflammation, irritation

TABLE 29-6. COMMON LABORATORY TESTS OF URINE AND STOOL

Test/Description	Findings	Nurse's Responsibility
Urine		
Urinalysis Gross and microscopic analysis for diagnosis of urinary tract infections, renal and other metabolic disease.	pH: 4.5–8.0 Specific gravity: 1.003–1.035. Protein: 2–8 mg/dL. Glucose: negative. Ketones: negative. RBCs: 1–2/low-power field. WBCs: 3–4/low-power field. Casts: 3–4/low-power field.	Send a freshly voided, labeled specimen (see Procedure 29–1) of at least 50 mL to the lab in a clean, dry container. Specimen may be refrigerated 6–8 hours. Midstream specimen preferred.
Urine Culture and Sensitivity Analysis for presence of organisms in urine and drugs to treat the infection.	Identifies causative organism of urinary tract infection and antibiotics to which the organism is susceptible.	Send a freshly voided, labeled clean catch specimen (or obtain via catheterization) of 2–10 mL to the lab in a sterile container. Note time specimen was obtained on label.
24-Hour Urine Collection Measures 24-hour urine clearance of specific substances. Creatinine clearance is commonly measured to assess kidney function.	Identification of quantity of specific component(s) excreted in urine in a 24-hour period. Used to diagnose disease states that alter production and/or excretion of specific substances (eg, protein, electrolytes, metabolites).	Have patient empty bladder at the time the test is to begin. Discard specimen and note time. Collect all urine produced for the next 24 hours in a clean container and transfer to collection bottle supplied by lab. Keep bottle cool. Label collection bottle with patient name, time period of collection, and name of test(s) to be completed.
Stool		
Stool Culture Analysis for causative organism of enteric infection.	Identifies organisms other than normal intestinal flora that are present in stool.	Collect fecal sample about 1 inch long. (See Procedure 29–2.) Place in sterile container, label with patient name and suspected organism. Do not administer barium or mineral oil 24 hours prior to test.
Stool for Ova and Parasites (O & P) Analysis for parasites or their eggs in patient's intestine.	Identifies parasites such as protozoa or worms that are growing in intestinal tract.	Send serial specimens collected over a 3-day period. Take all specimens to the lab within 30 minutes. Identify countries patient has visited within 1 year on lab slip. If tapeworm is suspected, send entire stool. Do not administer barium, antacids, or mineral oil for 1 week prior to test.
Stool for Occult Blood	See Procedure 29–3.	

altered bowel elimination but are not covered in detail here are listed at the end of Table 29–10.

CONSTIPATION

Constipation is defined in the taxonomy of nursing diagnoses as a change in normal bowel habits characterized by a decrease in frequency and/or passage of hard, dry stools. There are many possible etiologies for this diagnosis. Therefore, collaboration with the patient is important to determine the most appropriate one.

- *Etiology: less than adequate fluid intake.* If fluid intake is less than body requirements, extra water is absorbed from the colon to meet metabolic needs, and will result in hard, dry feces.
- *Etiology: less than adequate dietary intake.* Excessive dieting, immobility, illness, and lack of interest in food sometimes found among the elderly population are among the reasons for diminished dietary intake.
- *Etiology: less than adequate fiber.* As discussed previously, fiber promotes peristalsis because it increases bulk of intestinal contents. A preference for highly processed convenience foods is a common reason for lack of fiber in the diet.
- *Etiology: less than adequate physical activity; immobility.* As discussed in an earlier section, activity promotes peristalsis.

(continued on page 952)

TABLE 29-7. COMMON DIAGNOSTIC TESTS OF BOWEL FUNCTION

Test/Description	Patient Preparation	Posttest Nursing Care
Upper GI Series X-ray of esophagus, stomach, and small intestine using contrast media such as barium or water-soluble agent such as Gastrographin. Used to diagnose obstructions, changes in mucosa, and altered motility.	Discuss: • Purpose of test. • Need to drink 16–20 oz of contrast media (barium is chalky). • Test may take up to 6 hours. • Discomfort minimal. • Position changes necessary on rotating x-ray table. • npo 8–12 hours before test. • Need for laxative or enema after test if barium used; stool will be light-colored for a few days. Encourage questions. Check/obtain signed consent. Administer contrast media immediately before test.	Do not offer food or fluids until x-ray department verifies all views have been completed. Encourage fluids to 2 L to facilitate elimination of barium. Administer laxatives as ordered; assess stool to verify excretion of barium. If patient not hospitalized, request patient notify physician if barium not excreted within 2 days. Provide opportunities to discuss concerns regarding test results.
Barium Enema X-ray of large intestine after administration of barium or barium and air via rectal tube. Used to diagnose obstructions and changes in bowel mucosa.	Discuss: • Purpose of test. • Colon must be free of fecal material for this test, so a clear liquid diet is required for the 24 hours prior to test, a laxative may be ordered the day before, and cleansing enemas are given before barium is administered. • Increased fluid intake is recommended the day before the test to maintain hydration. • Barium instillation may cause cramping; deep breathing/relaxation may relieve. • Retention of the barium during the test is important but rectal tube may have an inflated portion to assist retention. • X-ray table will be tilted; various positions will be necessary; test takes ½–1 hour. Encourage questions. Check/obtain signed consent. Administer enemas as ordered on day of test.	Assist patient to toilet facilities to expel barium; all barium should be expelled immediately if possible. Encourage fluids to 2 L and administer a laxative to facilitate excretion of any residual barium. Provide opportunities for uninterrupted rest after test; most patients find it extremely tiring. Provide opportunities to discuss concerns regarding test results.
Sigmoidoscopy Visualization of the anus, rectum, and sigmoid colon. Colonoscopy Visualization of the colon. Used to evaluate and/or biopsy suspicious bowel lesions (tumors, inflammation).	Discuss: • Purpose of test. • Nature of test preparation (varies—usually involves clear liquid diet, cathartics, and enemas). • Position for sigmoidoscopy is knee/chest or Sims; for colonoscopy, Sims. • Insertion of well-lubricated flexible tube into the rectum will create pressure, urge to defecate. Air may be insufflated to aid visualization, which may cause cramping during and after the test. Relaxation/deep breathing helps; sometimes sedative given. • Sigmoidoscopy takes 15–30 minutes; colonoscopy, 30–90 minutes. Encourage questions. Check/obtain signed consent. Administer enema, sedative as ordered.	Assess vital signs every 30 minutes for 2 hours. Encourage expulsion of gas; large amounts expected. Provide opportunities for uninterrupted rest. Observe for signs of bowel perforation: rectal bleeding, abdominal pain, fever. Confer with physician if symptoms present (small amount of bleeding is expected if polyp removed). If patient discharged, instruct patient to report these symptoms to physician. Provide opportunities to discuss concerns regarding test results.
CT/CAT Scan See Table 29–8.		

TABLE 29-8. COMMON DIAGNOSTIC TESTS OF URINARY FUNCTION

Test/Description	Patient Preparation	Posttest Nursing Care
Blood Urea Nitrogen (BUN) Assessment of levels of nitrogenous wastes in the bloodstream. Reflects efficiency of glomerular filtration. Normal limits: 5–25 mg/dL.	Discuss purpose of test. No physical preparation required.	No physical care required. Note creatinine values; if both elevated, suggests kidney disorder. If kidney disorder is not suspected, encourage increased fluid intake; dehydration is a possible cause of elevated BUN.
Serum Creatinine Assessment of creatinine, a byproduct of muscle metabolism in serum. Excreted by kidneys; considered a more sensitive indicator of kidney function than BUN. Normal limits: 0.5–1.5 mg/dL.	See BUN, above.	No physical care required. Note BUN value, see above. Assess urine output.
KUB X-ray of kidneys, ureters, bladder. Reveals size, calculi, and bladder masses.	Discuss: • Purpose of test. • No pretest restrictions of food/fluid. • Position for test is supine, table may be tilted. Encourage questions.	No special care required. Provide opportunities to discuss concerns regarding test results.
Intravenous Pyelogram (IVP) X-ray of entire urinary tract after intravenous administration of contrast media. A series of x-rays is taken as kidney clears a contrast media and it is excreted via the bladder. X-ray taken after voiding (excretory urography) determines if residual media is in bladder. Used to detect calculi, masses, changes in kidney size or function.	Discuss: • Purpose of test. • Previous reaction to iodine, contrast dye, or seafood (may contraindicate test). • Need for npo 12 hours before test, laxative, and enema to prevent bowel contents from interfering with visualization. • Transient flushing, metallic taste associated with dye injection. • Supine position for test. • Length of test about 20–30 minutes; requires 5 or more x-rays, possibly one during voiding. Encourage questions. Check/obtain signed consent. Check BUN; confer with physician if over 40 mg/dL. Administer enema. Encourage patient to empty bladder.	Monitor vital signs and urine output. Observe for delayed reaction to contrast media: urticaria (itchy rash), flushing, tachycardia, dyspnea. Confer with physician if allergic reaction or oliguria noted. Observe injection site for irritation, hematoma; apply warm or cold compresses if present. Offer food and fluids. Provide opportunities to discuss concerns regarding test results.
Retrograde Pyelogram X-ray of bladder, ureters, and kidney after contrast media is introduced via a ureteral catheter. Used to detect calculi, masses, and kidney hypertrophy, especially when IVP contraindicated (allergy to media or poor kidney function). May be combined with *cystogram,* in which bladder is filled to capacity with contrast media. This reveals bladder fistulas, tumors, or calculi, and prostate hypertrophy.	Discuss: • Purpose of test. • Need for laxative, enema as for IVP. • Use of cystoscope for placement of catheters (see discussion points on next page). • Lithotomy position for test. • Length of procedure 30–90 minutes. • Need for increased fluid intake before and after test to facilitate excretion of contrast media. Encourage questions. Check/obtain signed consent. Encourage patient to empty bladder. Administer enema, sedatives, analgesics, as ordered.	Assess as for cystoscopy (see below). Assess drainage from ureteral catheters if left in place. Provide food and fluids as soon as recovered from anesthesia. Provide opportunities to discuss concerns regarding test results.

TABLE 29-8. CONTINUED

Test/Description	Patient Preparation	Posttest Nursing Care
Cystoscopy Direct visualization of bladder, urethra, and prostate using a cystoscope. Used to detect calculi, tumors, urethral strictures, and prostate hypertrophy. Can also be used to remove calculi, perform biopsy, and resect excessive prostatic tissue.	Discuss: • Purpose of test. • Liquid diet day of test unless anesthesia planned, then npo. • Use of anesthesia (local or general) or sedatives and analgesia for test. • Possible need for IV. • Possible use of antibiotics to prevent infection. • Use of cystoscope, a thin telescopic tube that is introduced via the urethra. • Patient may feel pressure if not anesthetized. • Lithotomy position for test. • Length of procedure 30–60 minutes (longer if tissue removal anticipated). • Possibility of retention catheter after procedure. • Possibility of swelling, blood in urine (hematuria), burning on urination (dysuria) after procedure. Encourage questions. Check/obtain signed consent. Administer premedications as ordered.	Assess vital signs according to postanesthesia policy. Assess urinary output (amount, character) for 48 hours after procedure. Confer with physician if urinary retention, gross hematuria (bright red urine), tachycardia, hypotension, or fever noted. Provide increased fluids. Provide pain relief measures (see Chap. 32). Provide opportunities to discuss concerns regarding test results.
CT or CAT Renal/Pelvic Scan Uses a narrow x-ray beam to produce multiple-angle views of target organ, resulting in a three-dimensional picture. Used to detect structural bowel or urinary tract abnormalities, tumors, stones, abscesses, and cysts.	Discuss: • Purpose of test. • Use of oral contrast media (about 15 oz) evening before and day of scan for pelvic examination (bowel, bladder) or 1 hour before scan for kidney scan. • Allergies—see IVP earlier in table. • Usually npo status 8 hours before exam. • Possible need for IV. • Scanner is a large circular machine; (doughnut-shaped); patient will be strapped to a narrow table, scanner will surround and revolve around body, making clicking noises. Test is not painful, but may be necessary to hold breath several times during test. • Length of procedure 30–90 minutes. • Encourage questions. • Check/obtain signed consent. • Administer contrast media as ordered.	Assess for delayed allergic reaction to contrast (see IVP earlier in table). Provide food and fluids. Provide opportunities to discuss concerns regarding test results.

TABLE 29-9. SAMPLE NURSING DIAGNOSES: BOWEL ELIMINATION

Nursing Diagnosis	Defining Characteristics/Manifestations: *Subjective Data*	Defining Characteristics/Manifestations: *Objective Data*	Etiology
Constipation *1.3.1.1* *1.3.1.1.2*[a]	Reports decreased frequency of bowel movement. Reports abdominal fullness, rectal pressure. Reports straining at stool. "I don't drink liquids much except with meals."	Hard, dry stools. Abdominal distension.	*Physical:* Less than adequate fluid intake.
Constipation *1.3.1.1* *1.3.1.1.2*	Reports decreased frequency of bowel movement. Reports abdominal fullness, rectal pressure. Reports straining at stool. "It's embarrassing to have a BM when someone else is in the room."	Hard, dry stools. Abdominal distension.	*Emotional/environmental:* Lack of privacy.
Diarrhea *1.3.1.2*	Reports frequent, loose, liquid stools since ingesting meal of "leftovers."	Hyperactive bowel sounds. Watery, brown stool with particles of fecal matter.	*Physical:* Intestinal irritation.

[a] Etiologies and defining characteristics for 1.3.1.1 and 1.3.1.1.2 are combined in this table.
Source: The nursing diagnoses and etiologies on this table and the definitions of nursing diagnoses in the body of the text not credited to other sources are from Nursing Diagnosis: Definitions and Classification, 1997–1998. *Philadelphia: North American Nursing Diagnosis Association; 1996. Manifestation categories for etiologies and specifications of general etiologies on these tables are authors' original work.*

Whether related to general life-style or to illness and its treatment, minimal physical activity promotes constipation. Prudent nurses anticipate this risk factor when caring for patients whose illness or treatment involves limiting activity, and when possible take measures to offset the risk, such as increasing fluids and fiber.

- *Etiology: lack of privacy.* Because most people consider defecation a private activity, they may suppress defecation when private toilet facilities are not available. However, the simple act of providing privacy for elimination when patients are in health care facilities can prevent their becoming constipated.
- *Etiology: emotional disturbance, stress.* As discussed previously, the gastrointestinal system is particularly susceptible to alterations related to emotional status. Often the experience of seeking health care or concerns about the seriousness of a health problem or its treatment creates sufficient stress to interfere with normal bowel elimination. Therefore, constipation may accompany many health alterations.
- *Etiology: chronic use of enemas and laxatives.* The effects of dependency on laxatives have been discussed above. Because a patient's use of laxatives implies that bowel elimination is a real concern, nurses need to be sensitive in their approach to assisting the patient to correct the laxative dependency.
- *Etiology: change in daily routine.* As discussed earlier, the gastrocolic reflex stimulates mass peristalsis approximately 15 minutes after breakfast. Many people, therefore, have a pattern of regular bowel elimination after breakfast. If circumstances prevent elimination at this time, particularly over the course of several days, constipation may result.

DIARRHEA

Diarrhea is the frequent passage of loose, fluid, unformed stool. Diarrhea is usually accompanied by cramping and abdominal pain and frequently limits daily activities. No etiologies for diarrhea have been included in the taxonomy to date; however, three generally accepted etiologies for diarrhea are presented here.

- *Etiology: intestinal irritation.* Toxins, whether produced by contaminated foods or pathogens gaining entry into the GI tract, are irritating to the intestinal mucosa. Some individuals are allergic to certain foods. The natural defense of the body against this irritation is to increase peristalsis to hasten the exit of the offending substance from the body. The outcome is diarrhea and the accompanying loss of fluid and electrolytes. It should be noted that many laxatives are intestinal irritants and therefore can produce diarrhea if used incorrectly.
- *Etiology: emotional stress.* Although for some people, stress produces constipation, others experience parasympathetic dominance of bowel function under stress. This results in increased motility and increased frequency of bowel movements. Often mucus production in the intestines increases as well, so stools may contain obvious mucus.

TABLE 29-10. SAMPLE NURSING DIAGNOSES: URINARY ELIMINATION

Nursing Diagnosis	Defining Characteristics/Manifestations: *Subjective Data*	Defining Characteristics/Manifestations: *Objective Data*	Etiology
Functional incontinence *1.3.2.1.4*	Reports inability to control urine elimination at night: "I just can't find the way to the BR when I wake up in the night. It's only been been a problem since I've been in here."	Newly admitted to skilled nursing facility. Bed or floor near bed wet at night on several occasions since admission.	*Environmental:* Altered environment.
Stress incontinence *1.3.2.1.1*	Reports loss of small amounts of urine when laughs or sneezes.	Weight more than 20% over ideal for height.	*Physical:* High intra-abdominal pressure.
Urinary retention *1.3.2.2*	Reports increasing bladder discomfort. "I got up to go twice, but I can't—I'm afraid it will hurt my stitches." "When you press there (lower abdomen), I really feel like I have to go!"	Spontaneous vaginal delivery 3 hours ago. Midline episiotomy; intact, no swelling. Bladder palpable above symphysis pubis.	*Emotional:* Fear or pain inhibiting reflex arc.

OTHER NURSING DIAGNOSES RELATED TO ELIMINATION

PHYSICAL
- Impaired skin integrity
- Risk for impaired skin integrity
- Risk for infection
- Fluid volume deficit
- Activity intolerance
- Fatigue
- Impaired physical mobility
- Toileting self-care deficit
- Sleep pattern disturbance

COGNITIVE
- Sensory–perceptual alterations
- Pain
- Altered thought processes
- Knowledge deficit
- Dysreflexia

EMOTIONAL
- Anxiety
- Fear

SELF-CONCEPTUAL
- Body image disturbance
- Self-esteem disturbance
- Hopelessness

SOCIOCULTURAL/LIFE STRUCTURAL
- Social isolation

DEVELOPMENTAL
- Altered growth and development

SEXUAL
- Altered sexuality patterns
- Rape-trauma syndrome

Source: See Table 29–10.

- *Etiology: high-osmolality enteral nutrition formulas.* Individuals who are unable to consume solid foods for an extended period of time are often given specially formulated liquids that contain all of the necessary calories for metabolic needs. The formulas may be given orally or via tube feedings. Many of these formulas have a high osmolality (concentration of molecules in a solution), and are therefore hypertonic. When in the intestine, the hypertonic liquid causes water to be drawn into the intestine from the mucosa of the intestines, increasing the volume of the intestinal contents and stimulating peristalsis. (See also Chap. 28 for further discussion of enteral feedings.)

BOWEL INCONTINENCE

The taxonomy of nursing diagnoses defines bowel incontinence as a change in normal bowel habits characterized by involuntary passage of stool. Bowel incontinence is a cause of physical, emotional, and social distress to individuals experiencing it and to their family members.

No accepted etiologies are included in the taxonomy. A review of the physiology of bowel elimination suggests that interference with neurologic functioning, including problems that alter mental status, are most often responsible for bowel incontinence. Most of these cannot be influenced by nursing therapies. However, in some cases, bowel training programs, discussed later under Rehabilitative Care, are effective. Although nurses usually cannot correct bowel incontinence, they can help patients avoid some associated complications, such as skin breakdown, emotional distress, and social isolation.

DIAGNOSES RELATED TO URINARY ELIMINATION

Altered patterns of urinary elimination are also or concern to nurses. Nursing diagnoses related to urinary elimination include urinary incontinence and urinary retention. Although the taxonomy of nursing diagnosis includes five types of urinary incontinence (functional, reflex, stress, total, and urge incontinence), only functional and stress incontinence are addressed here. Table 29–10 presents these diagnoses with sample etiologies and defining characteristics. Other nursing diagnoses related to altered urinary elimination patterns are listed at the end of the table.

FUNCTIONAL INCONTINENCE

The taxonomy of nursing diagnoses defines **functional incontinence** as the involuntary, unpredictable loss of urine. For example, the aged person who has limited mobility because of arthritis and must climb stairs to go to the bathroom may have a problem with this type of incontinence.

- *Etiology: altered environment.* Causes of functional incontinence include barriers that interfere with timely access to toilet facilities. Environmental barriers may include lack of privacy, unfamiliarity with surroundings, or distance to the facilities.
- *Etiology: sensory, cognitive, or mobility deficit.* These might include such variables as fear, anxiety, confusion, leg weakness, or severe pain, any of which may compromise an individual's ability to get to toilet facilities before the urge to void becomes too strong to repress.

STRESS INCONTINENCE

Stress incontinence is defined in the taxonomy of nursing diagnoses as the loss of urine of less than 50 mL that occurs when there is a sudden increase in intra-abdominal pressure. These sudden pressure increases may be caused by sneezing, laughing, lifting, or vomiting. When intra-abdominal pressure is increased, the bladder is compressed. If the urinary sphincters and pelvic floor muscles do not maintain sufficient tone, urine is squeezed out of the bladder. Stress incontinence is most common in women.

- *Etiology: weakness or degenerative changes in pelvic muscles and structural supports.* Degenerative changes in pelvic muscles and structural supports is a common reason for stress incontinence. This is most often related to the aging process, although obesity and pelvic muscle weakness from multiple vaginal births contribute.
- *Etiology: high intra-abdominal pressure.* High intra-abdominal pressure may result from obesity or the increased size of the uterus during pregnancy, or both. With this etiology, muscle tone in sphincters and pelvic floor is adequate to contain urine under usual circumstances, but high baseline intra-abdominal pressure causes loss of urine.
- *Etiology: overdistension.* The individual who ignores the signal to urinate and consistently overdistends the bladder between voidings may develop stress incontinence. When the bladder is overdistended, pressure on the sphincters is increased. It then becomes increasingly difficult to control the external sphincter against leakage of urine with the added activity produced in sneezing, coughing, laughing, or lifting objects.

COLLABORATIVE STRATEGY
DIAGNOSING INCONTINENCE

Several types of urinary incontinence are recognized in the taxonomy of nursing diagnosis. Because the nursing measures needed to assist a particular patient will differ with the type of incontinence, a careful assessment of the specific subjective and objective manifestations is vital. Collaboration with the patient to bring out the subtleties that may differentiate one type of incontinence from another is thus very important.

URINARY RETENTION

Urinary retention occurs when an individual is unable to empty the bladder completely. Typically, residual urine remains in the bladder after attempts to void. Eventually the bladder may become overdistended. Some of the etiologies of urinary retention, such as weak detrusor muscle tone (which causes continual constriction of the external sphincter, because detrusor contraction is the stimulus for sphincter relaxation); inhibition of reflex arc because of neurologic pathology; and urethral blockage (which may be the result of trauma, prostate enlargement, or tumors) are not readily treatable by nursing therapies. Two etiologies can be treated by nursing implementation, and so are addressed here.

- *Etiology: inhibition of reflex arc.* Fear of pain during voiding or generalized anxiety can result in inability to relax the external sphincter, despite signals initiated by contraction of the detrusor muscle as the bladder distends. Even though the individual consciously attempts to relax the perineum and external sphincter, the sphincter remains contracted because of stronger sympathetic nervous system signals limiting relaxation.
- *Etiology: blockage.* The urethra and perineum may become inflamed and swollen due to irritation during urinary diagnostic procedures such as cystoscopy, surgery involving the bladder or prostate, or pressure of the fetal presenting part during

childbirth. This swelling may present a physical barrier to the passage of urine as well as make sphincter relaxation difficult.

STATING THE ELIMINATION DIAGNOSIS

The nursing diagnosis is the basis for a collaborative individualized patient care plan. The more precisely it describes the etiology and defining characteristics a particular patient presents, the more effectively it can guide the selection of nursing implementations. When possible, general etiologies and defining characteristics should be made more specific by using the signs and symptoms in the database.

For example, a patient complains of intermittent difficulty passing stools, stating that he often goes 4 days without a bowel movement and that his stools are hard and marblelike. The nurse also learns that he works long hours at a desk job. He says, "I get a little exercise on the weekends, but I'm usually too tired to do anything after work but have a drink and watch TV. That's often the first liquid I'll have except for breakfast coffee and a soft drink at lunch." An appropriate nursing diagnosis for this patient may be: Constipation related to lack of regular exercise and less than adequate daily fluid intake as evidenced by reported straining at stool; hard, small stools every 4 days; daily fluid intake of less than 1000 mL, and lack of regular physical exercise.

This method of stating nursing diagnoses makes the exact nature of the patient's elimination problem clear to all caregivers and provides guidelines for developing realistic desired outcomes and nursing implementation. When a patient's primary concern is an elimination problem, or the nature of the problem suggests that elimination may be affected, a thorough database that includes subjective and objective elimination data will facilitate nursing diagnosis. Then collaborative nurse–patient management to bring about resolution of the problem can begin.

SECTION 3

NURSE-PATIENT MANAGEMENT OF ELIMINATION

Collaborative management of altered elimination patterns begins with planning strategies that will help meet the patient's elimination needs. Then implementation is carried out and evaluated for effectiveness in meeting the outcomes.

PLANNING FOR OPTIMAL ELIMINATION

The planning phase includes collaborating with patients to establish desired outcomes, identifying implementation that will help accomplish the outcomes, and selecting evaluation criteria. All components of the plan should be congruent with patients' wishes and resources.

Mutual consideration of the nursing diagnosis statement should generate desired outcomes that are realistic and agreeable to the patient. An appropriate outcome for the patient with constipation discussed earlier might be: Bowel elimination pattern of one soft, formed bowel movement at least every other day within 2 weeks. Such specific desired outcome statements help the nurse document progress toward outcome attainment and guide selection of implementations. Table 29–11 provides examples of appropriate outcomes, approaches, and evaluation criteria for bowel and urinary elimination problems. Finally, Table 29–12, Partial Critical Pathway for Total Hip Replacement: Elimination Function, and Table 29–13, Partial Critical Pathway for Congestive Heart Failure: Elimination Function, show collaborative plans of care that incorporate concepts from this chapter.

NURSING IMPLEMENTATION TO PROMOTE OPTIMAL ELIMINATION

Nursing measures to promote elimination are divided into four levels of care:

- *Preventive care*—activities related to promoting healthy elimination, screening, and preventing elimination problems
- *Supportive care*—assisting patients with early signs of elimination problems
- *Restorative care*—assisting with acute elimination problems
- *Rehabilitative care*—facilitating adjustment to chronic alterations in elimination patterns

Descriptions of these nursing measures follow.

PREVENTIVE CARE

First-level nursing implementation for elimination is focused on promoting normal micturition and defecation in healthy patients. The most important first-level nursing activity is teaching patients to take time for elimination. Not taking the time to defecate, or ignoring the urge to void, are common causes of constipation and urinary tract infections. Teaching is thus an important part of preventive care.

Health Education

Areas to consider in patient teaching are dietary habits and regular exercise. It is especially important that patients have an adequate fluid intake. Drinking eight glasses of water a day helps keep both bowel and urine elimination regular and effortless. Tea, coffee, colas, and alcohol have a diuretic effect; their use should be reduced or avoided if frequency or incontinence is a problem. Eating adequate amounts of fiber and eating foods from all the basic food groups is important. High-fiber foods include whole grains and nuts, raw vegetables, and fresh fruits. Gum chewing and drinking carbonated beverages may contribute to flatulence, and patients may be advised to avoid these habits.

Helping a patient determine the time when the urge to defecate usually occurs will help to establish regular bowel habits. Setting aside the same time each day for bowel elimination will help develop a pattern. Advising the patient to avoid tight-fitting clothing may also be helpful. Tight clothing interferes with the ability to bear down using the abdominal muscles and thus hinders elimination.

Urination and defecation in women are promoted by assuming a squatting position. Toilet facilities should help provide an effective position for defecation. A squatting position with the thighs flexed will increase abdominal pressure and aid stool expulsion. Most adults achieve this by leaning forward while sitting on

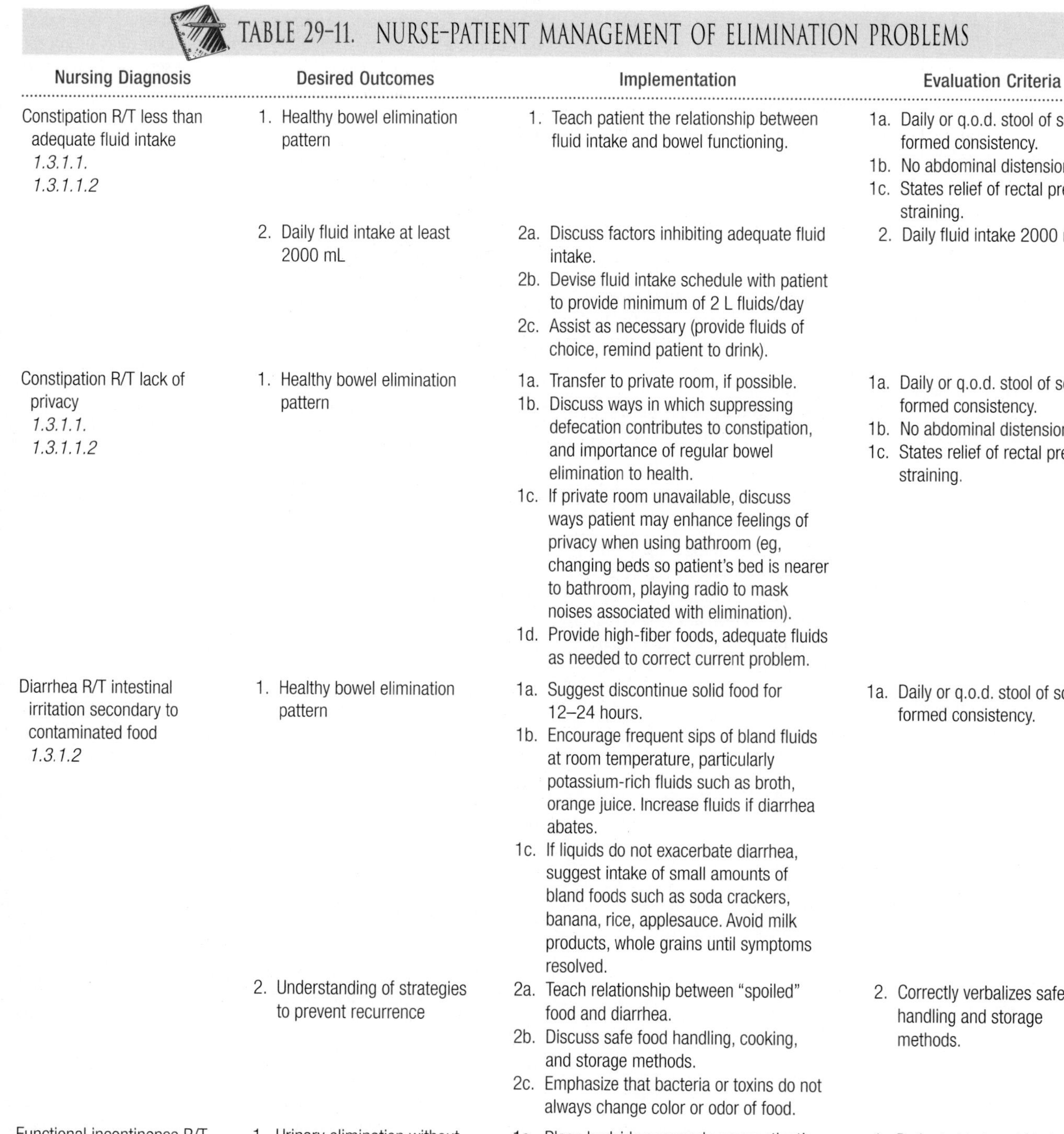

TABLE 29-11. NURSE-PATIENT MANAGEMENT OF ELIMINATION PROBLEMS

Nursing Diagnosis	Desired Outcomes	Implementation	Evaluation Criteria
Constipation R/T less than adequate fluid intake *1.3.1.1.* *1.3.1.1.2*	1. Healthy bowel elimination pattern	1. Teach patient the relationship between fluid intake and bowel functioning.	1a. Daily or q.o.d. stool of soft-formed consistency. 1b. No abdominal distension. 1c. States relief of rectal pressure, straining.
	2. Daily fluid intake at least 2000 mL	2a. Discuss factors inhibiting adequate fluid intake. 2b. Devise fluid intake schedule with patient to provide minimum of 2 L fluids/day 2c. Assist as necessary (provide fluids of choice, remind patient to drink).	2. Daily fluid intake 2000 mL.
Constipation R/T lack of privacy *1.3.1.1.* *1.3.1.1.2*	1. Healthy bowel elimination pattern	1a. Transfer to private room, if possible. 1b. Discuss ways in which suppressing defecation contributes to constipation, and importance of regular bowel elimination to health. 1c. If private room unavailable, discuss ways patient may enhance feelings of privacy when using bathroom (eg, changing beds so patient's bed is nearer to bathroom, playing radio to mask noises associated with elimination). 1d. Provide high-fiber foods, adequate fluids as needed to correct current problem.	1a. Daily or q.o.d. stool of soft-formed consistency. 1b. No abdominal distension. 1c. States relief of rectal pressure, straining.
Diarrhea R/T intestinal irritation secondary to contaminated food *1.3.1.2*	1. Healthy bowel elimination pattern	1a. Suggest discontinue solid food for 12–24 hours. 1b. Encourage frequent sips of bland fluids at room temperature, particularly potassium-rich fluids such as broth, orange juice. Increase fluids if diarrhea abates. 1c. If liquids do not exacerbate diarrhea, suggest intake of small amounts of bland foods such as soda crackers, banana, rice, applesauce. Avoid milk products, whole grains until symptoms resolved.	1a. Daily or q.o.d. stool of soft-formed consistency.
	2. Understanding of strategies to prevent recurrence	2a. Teach relationship between "spoiled" food and diarrhea. 2b. Discuss safe food handling, cooking, and storage methods. 2c. Emphasize that bacteria or toxins do not always change color or odor of food.	2. Correctly verbalizes safe food handling and storage methods.
Functional incontinence R/T unfamiliar environment *1.3.2.1.4*	1. Urinary elimination without incontinence	1a. Place bedside commode near patient's bed. 1b. Keep siderails down at foot end of bed to facilitate getting out of bed. 1c. Keep nurse call light in reach, encourage patient to call for nurse if having difficulty getting up or getting to commode. 1d. If incontinent only at night, encourage spacing fluid intake so daily fluid needs met without fluid intake after 7–8 PM. 1e. Keep night light on when patient asleep.	1. Patient able to void in bedside commode without incidents of incontinence.

TABLE 29-11. CONTINUED

Nursing Diagnosis	Desired Outcomes	Implementation	Evaluation Criteria
Stress incontinence R/T high intra-abdominal pressure *1.3.2.1.1*	1. No involuntary passage of urine	1a. Discuss causes of stress incontinence. 1b. Teach exercises to strengthen pelvic floor muscles. 1c. Discuss benefits of frequent urination to prevent internal bladder pressure from full bladder. 1d. Discuss how obesity increases abdominal pressure. 1e. Collaboratively plan weight-reduction diet (see Chap. 28) and exercise plan (see Chap. 33) if patient desires to lose weight.	1. Patient reports no further incidents of stress incontinence.
Urinary retention R/T fear of pain inhibiting reflex arc *1.3.2.2*	1. Complete emptying without catheterization	1a. Discuss how emotions can inhibit perineal and external sphincter relaxation that is necessary for voiding. 1b. Apply topical anesthetic ointment to stitches, explain how this will prevent urine from irritating stitches. 1c. Explain how fluid intake facilitates bladder elimination. 1d. Encourage fluid intake of 2 L/day. 1e. Explain that you must measure urine to assess for complete emptying: use "hat" collector (Fig. 29–7). 1f. Assist voiding by: Pouring measured amount of warm water over perineum. Providing basin of warm water to immerse hands. Running water in sink next to patient. Encouraging patient to visualize/imagine sight and sound of running water. Providing a glass of water and a straw; ask patient to blow through the straw to produce bubbles in water. Breaking spirits of ammonia ampoule in "hat" collector (Fig. 29–7). 1g. Suggest patient take warm shower and allow urine to flow during shower (subsequent voids must be measured to assess emptying). 1h. Assess abdomen for bladder distension after voiding. 1i. Assess 3 consecutive voids for volume greater than 200 mL. 1j. If unable to void or residual urine suspected, confer with physician for order to catheterize.	1a. Patient voids at least 200 mL 1b. Abdomen nondistended. 1c. Continued independent voiding.

Source: See Table 29–9.

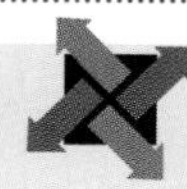

TABLE 29-12. PARTIAL CRITICAL PATHWAY FOR TOTAL HIP REPLACEMENT: ELIMINATION FUNCTION

Nursing Dx/Problem	Outcome DOS/Day 1	Outcome Days 2–3	Outcome SNF Days 4–6	Outcome Home Care 3 Weeks (6 Visits)
Constipation R/T immobility, pain medication, lack of privacy		Bowel movement × 1	Bowel movement qod	Healthy bowel elimination pattern established
Implementation	**DOS/Day 1**	**Days 2–3**	**SNF Days 4–6**	**Home Care 3 Weeks**
Assessment	Bowel sounds	Same Abdominal distension Hydration	Same Same Same Previous pattern & habits Digital check for impaction prn	Same Same Same Same
Tests/Consults				
Medications/Treatments	Stool softener	Pain control measures prior to attempting use of bedpan/commode Provide privacy Stool softeners if needed	Same Same Same	BSC &/or raised toilet seat
Psychosocial				
Teaching		Need to increase intake of water & high-fiber juices Cues to drink	Food choices high in fiber Relationship between pain med, constipation, & need for fluid & high-fiber foods	Methods to establish healthy bowel elimination patterns
Activity/Safety/Self-care		Assistive devices as needed	Same	Same
Nutrition	Fluids to maintain hydration	High-fiber juices	High-fiber foods	Same
Transfer/Discharge Coord./Case Manager		Communicate outcomes achieved, problems/ interventions to SNF	Communicate outcomes achieved, problems/ interventions to Home Health	Communicate outcomes achieved, problems/interventions to MD & prepare for discharge

See inside back cover for abbreviations.

the toilet. Children and short people can gain a more functional position by using a footstool. Elderly patients and those with joint diseases may find it difficult to sit down and rise from a standard toilet seat and will benefit from the use of an elevated toilet seat (Fig. 29–6). Men commonly stand to urinate. All patients should be reminded of the importance of washing hands after elimination, and women should be taught to wipe the perineal area from front to back to avoid carrying microorganisms from the vagina or rectum to the urinary meatus. Those who change infants' diapers may need reinforcement about the importance of washing hands after diaper changes.

Routine Health Screening

Routine screening to detect elimination problems often involves testing of urine and stool specimens. The accuracy of some tests may be affected by collection and storage methods, and so it is helpful to know which tests are planned so that proper techniques

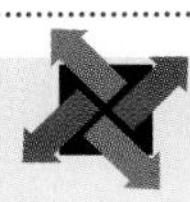

TABLE 29-13. PARTIAL CRITICAL PATHWAY FOR CONGESTIVE HEART FAILURE: ELIMINATION FUNCTION

Nursing Dx/Problem	Outcome Primary Care Visit	Outcome Home Care Week 1 (3 Visits)	Outcome Home Care Week 2 (3 Visits)	Outcome Home Care Weeks 3–4 (3 Visits)
Constipation R/T fluid restriction & lack of high-fiber foods	Verbalizes benefits of high-fiber foods	BM q2–3 day Identifies high-fiber foods	Same Eating high-fiber foods 3 ×/day	Same Same
Implementation	**Primary Care Visit**	**Home Care Visit Week 1**	**Home Care Visit Week 2**	**Home Care Visit Weeks 3–4**
Assessment	Bowel sounds	Same Bowel elimination pattern Abdominal distension Digital exam for impaction prn	Same Same Same Oral intake	Same Same Same Same
Tests/Consults	Refer to Home Health			
Medications/Treatments	Stool softeners	Institute daily bowel elimination routine	Reinforce as necessary	Same
Psychosocial	Reflective listening	Sensitivity to personal & cultural habits	Same	Same
Teaching		Disease process Care plan Food & fluids high in fiber Exercise & daily bowel elimination routine Risks of laxative dependence	Review, reinforce as needed Reinforce as needed Reinforce as needed Reinforce as needed	Same
Activity/Safety/Self-care	Bedrest, HOB 30–45 degrees c̄ BSC or BRP	Progressive activity as tolerated	Same	Same
Nutrition	Restrict fluid to 1 L/day High-fiber diet	Same Same	Same Same	Same Same
Transfer/Discharge Coord./Case Manager		Communicate to MD achieved outcomes	Same	Same Prepare for discharge

See inside back cover for abbreviations.

can be used. See Table 29–6 for specific guidelines relating to common urine and stool tests.

Most patients prefer to obtain their own specimens; in some cases, the nurse may assist. Procedures 29–1 and 29–2 provide guidelines for collecting specimens, as well as appropriate patient instructions for self-collection of specimens. Figure 29–7 illustrates a collector commonly called a "fireman's hat" or "top hat" that can be placed under the toilet seat to catch urine or stool. Figure 29–8 shows a pediatric urine-collection bag that is used to obtain urine samples from infants and children not yet toilet trained.

Sometimes nurses test specimens. Table 29–14 lists and describes techniques for urine tests. Measuring urine specific gravity requires a multiple test dipstick that has a special reagent area for specific gravity (more common method) or a urinometer (less common method).

The most common test of stool done by nurses is determining the presence of blood, often an early sign of colon cancer or other

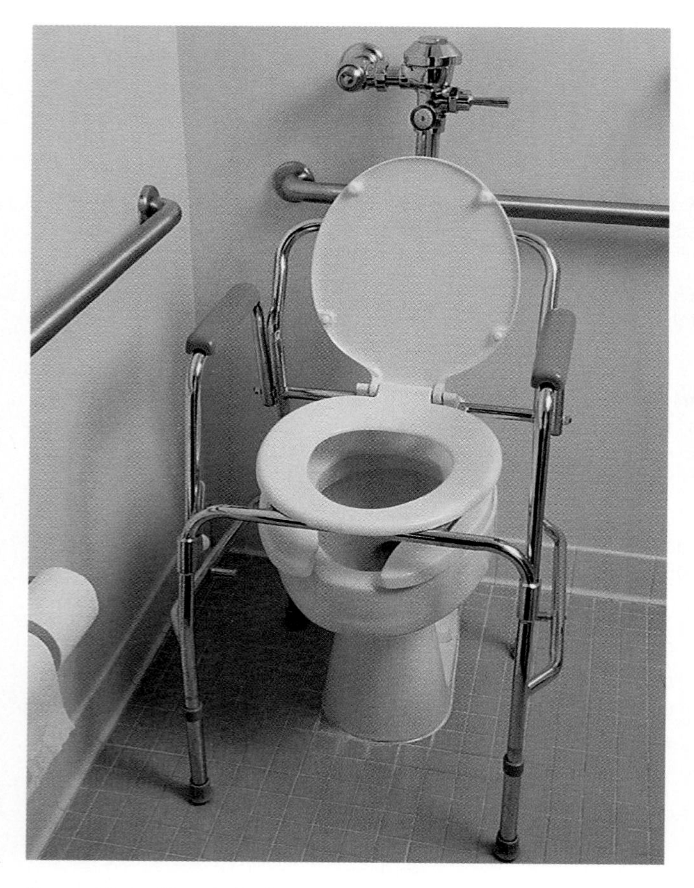

Figure 29–6. Elevated toilet seat.

intestinal pathology. Refer to Procedure 29–3. The Hemoccult slide and developer, one of the methods described in that procedure, is illustrated in Fig. 29–9.

Nurses may also instruct patients how to perform simple screening tests at home. It is particularly important to emphasize

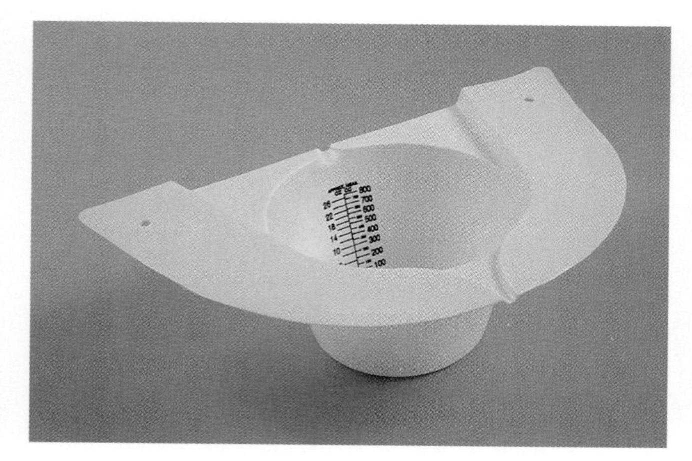

Figure 29–7. Specimen collector, often called "fireman's hat" or "top hat."

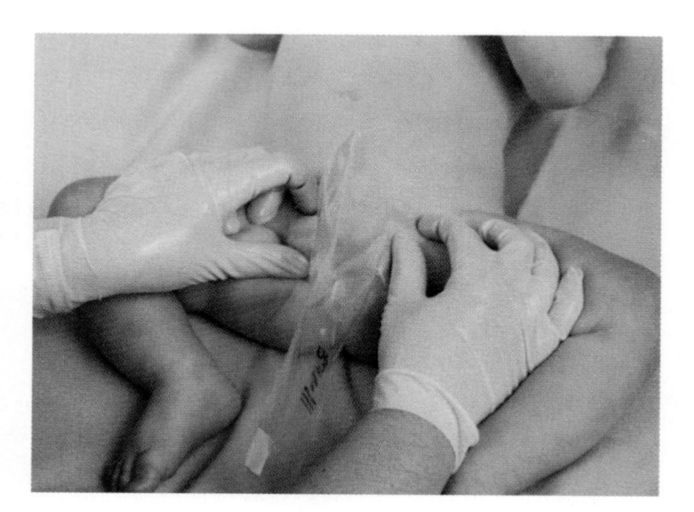

Figure 29–8. Pediatric urine collection bag. *(From Smith S, Duell D. Clinical Nursing Skills: Nursing Process Model, Basic to Advanced Skills. 4th ed. Stamford, CT: Appleton & Lange: 1996.)*

that accuracy depends on use of reagents before the expiration date stamped on the package and on precisely following manufacturers' directions. Sometimes different brands of reagents require slightly different steps to achieve a correct reading.

Home Health Care

The elements of preventive care just discussed, apply to the care of patients in the home. Home nurses encourage healthy bowel and bladder function by teaching family members about the need for

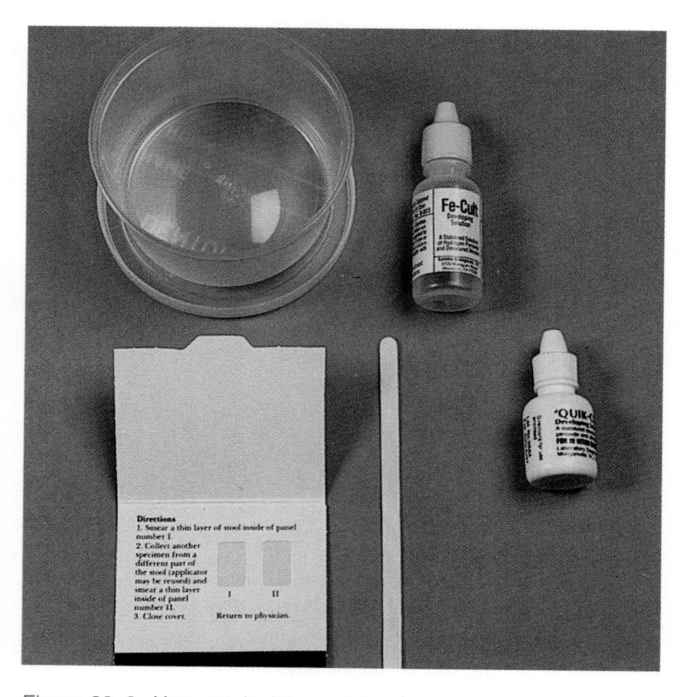

Figure 29–9. Hemoccult slide and developer. *(From Smith S, Duell D. Clinical Nursing Skills: Nursing Process Model, Basic to Advanced Skills. 4th ed. Stamford, CT: Appleton & Lange; 1996.)*

PROCEDURE 29–1. COLLECTING A RANDOM OR CLEAN-CATCH URINE SPECIMEN

PURPOSE: To collect urine for testing.
EQUIPMENT: Clean urinal, bedpan, or specimen hat; specimen container with lid (sterile if specimen is for culture); nonsterile gloves; plastic bag; and twist tie. For clean catch, also need antiseptic wipes or antiseptic solution/sterile cotton balls in sterile cup. (Commercial kits are available for clean-catch specimens.)

ACTION 1. Discuss with the patient the reason for the procedure, desired patient participation, and expected benefits.

RATIONALE. Patient will be more willing to participate and less anxious if reasons and benefits are clear.

ACTION 2. Assist the patient to the bathroom or commode, if needed. Provide specimen container and, if specimen is to be clean catch, antiseptic wipes or antiseptic-soaked cotton balls. Advise patient to remove undergarments and wash and dry hands.

RATIONALE. Ambulatory, alert patients can independently obtain specimens and usually prefer to do so.

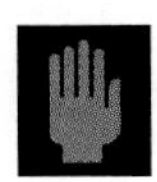

If testing is to be completed by the nurse, specimen can be collected in a urinal or specimen hat rather than a specimen container.

ACTION 3. For a clean-catch specimen, instruct patients to:

a. Clean themselves prior to voiding, using the wipes or antiseptic-soaked cotton. *Male patient:* Clean tip of penis from center outward using a circular motion, repeating three times (if uncircumcised, retract foreskin). *Female patient:* Spread labia minora with one hand, cleanse each side, and then center from front to back, using three separate cotton balls or wipes for each stroke. Keep labia spread during voiding.

RATIONALE. Clean-catch urine is used to detect presence of bacteria inside the bladder. Friction and antiseptic action remove normal flora, which would contaminate specimen, from meatal area.

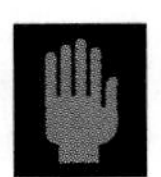

This cleansing is unnecessary for random sample.

b. Initiate voiding, then place the container in the stream of urine, filling it about half full, and then complete voiding into the toilet. Hold collection cup so as to avoid contact with the legs or external genitalia. Avoid touching the rim or inside of the container. (Midstream sample is not needed for random urine.) Discard toilet tissue in toilet, not in specimen hat.

RATIONALE. Initial stream of urine flushes remaining microorganisms from the meatus. Midstream sample is most free of external contamination. Touching inside of the container would contaminate contents with normal flora from patient's hands or genitalia.

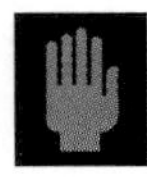

Females may find collecting the specimen is easier when sitting facing the back of the toilet.

c. Cover container tightly without touching inside of cover.

RATIONALE. Prevents contamination of specimen or environment.

ACTION 4. If assisting the patient to obtain a specimen, don nonsterile gloves.

RATIONALE. Body fluids may contain pathogenic organisms. Gloves prevent skin contamination by direct contact.

ACTION 5. Provide privacy and place the female patient on a bedpan (see Procedure 29–4), with legs spread so urine flow does not contact legs. Male patients may use urinal for random (unsterile) sample or void directly into specimen container.

RATIONALE. Elimination activities are considered private in most cultures. Respecting this need promotes trust and minimizes embarrassment.

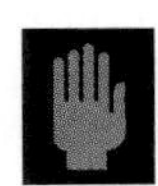

Males unable to stop the flow of urine in midstream can be placed on a bedpan to collect volume of urine greater than capacity of clean-catch container.

ACTION 6. For clean-catch specimen, cleanse labia or penis as described in Action 3.

Continued

Procedure 29–1. Collecting a Urine Specimen (continued)

ACTION 7. Ask the patient to void into the bedpan/urinal. If sample is to be clean catch, obtain a midstream sample as the patient voids.

RATIONALE. See Action 3b.

ACTION 8. Remove bedpan or urinal. Remove gloves to assist to position of comfort, if needed, then reglove to transfer specimen.

RATIONALE. See Procedure 29–4.

ACTION 9. Transfer urine to a specimen container if patient has voided into a bedpan or specimen hat; cover tightly. Discard remaining urine.

RATIONALE. See Action 3c.

ACTION 10. Clean the outside of the specimen container, remove gloves by turning inside out. Discard according to agency policy. Wash hands. Place container in plastic bag and close with twist tie.

RATIONALE. Prevents transfer of organisms from urine to environment.

ACTION 11. Label specimen and send to lab as soon as possible.

RATIONALE. Accuracy of some tests is compromised if urine stands at room temperature.

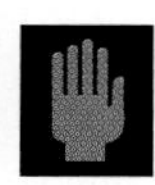

Urine may be refrigerated without affecting some tests. Check with lab personnel.

ACTION 12. When laboratory report is returned to the patient's chart, inform patient of result.

RATIONALE. Patient has a right to information about personal health status.

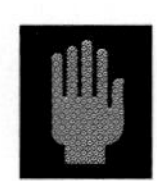

Encourage patient to also discuss test results with the physician.

Recording:
Note date, time, and purpose of specimen; characteristics of urine; and complaints of dysuria, if any.

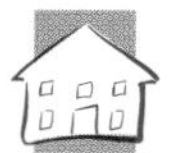

HOME HEALTH ADAPTATION: A large clean bowl or container may be placed in toilet if a bedpan, commode, or specimen hat are not available. After obtaining specimen, wash bowl with warm soapy water, rinse, and soak for 15 minutes in a sodium hypochlorite (bleach) solution of 1 part bleach to 10 parts water. Rinse thoroughly. Place the specimen container in a plastic bag or pouch with the requisition in a separate compartment of pouch. Transport specimen to lab in an insulated container with artificial ice and labeled "Biohazard." Request lab to fax or phone results to physician and home health Agency. Note time that specimen is delivered to lab.

dietary fiber, an adequate fluid intake, and the effects of various medications on bowel and bladder function and consequences of overuse of laxatives and enemas.

Many patients seen in the home are elderly. Although aging is not a cause of bladder or bowel dysfunction, there are changes associated with aging and the elderly are thus at risk for elimination problems. Indeed, problems such as urinary dribbling, often associated with bladder dysfunction and the fecal oozing that accompanies bowel impaction, are common. They may be chronic, or may come on unexpectedly such as when an elderly person becomes ill. Therefore, a thorough assessment of elderly patient's bowel and bladder function, as described earlier, is an important part of a home nurse's role. Attention to contributing factors, which the nurse can help to alter, is an important aspect of the assessment.

Home nurses are careful to document the patient's bowel and bladder habits, fluid and food intake patterns, and medical status and treatment, and to review the medications the patient takes. Patients are also questioned about their functional abilities related to toileting. If elimination problems are suspected a thorough assessment that includes an examination of the patient's abdominal and perineal areas, general cognitive function, strength, coordination, and mobility is warranted.

Another aspect is assessing the home itself. Home nurses are interested in whether the setting is safe, and whether patients have the adaptive appliances they need to support healthy elimination. Is the patient's route to the bathroom unimpeded and free of barriers that may cause accidents? Does the house have safety features such as nightlights and bathroom safety bars? Is the patient able to safely use the existing bathroom fixtures, or

PROCEDURE 29–2. OBTAINING A STOOL SPECIMEN

PURPOSE: To obtain a sample for testing.
EQUIPMENT: A clean dry bedpan or specimen hat, nonsterile gloves, plastic or waxed cardboard specimen cup with lid and/or culture tube, two tongue blades, plastic bag, and twist tie.

ACTION 1. Discuss the procedure with the patient, emphasizing:

a. The reason for the specimen.

b. The importance of preventing mixing of urine with stool.

c. That nurse should be notified as soon as defecation is complete.

ACTION 2. Provide privacy. Assist patient as needed to bathroom or commode or onto bedpan, and to place specimen hat.

Do not obtain a stool specimen directly from the toilet. Chemical cleaners placed in toilet tanks or residue of chemicals used to clean the toilet bowl can alter test results.

ACTION 3. When defecation is complete, assist patient as needed with hygiene and/or returning to bed. (Gloves are needed to clean patient.)

ACTION 4. Don gloves. Assess feces for blood, mucus, or other abnormal constituents.

ACTION 5. Using tongue blades, transfer a midportion of the sample, including any blood or other abnormal constituents, to specimen container and close tightly. If stool culture is ordered, dip applicator swab into feces and place in culture tube according to package directions. Use care not to contact outside of container with fecal matter.

ACTION 6. Empty and clean bedpan or specimen hat and return it to its place (used for one patient only). Specimen hat may be discarded after cleaning if no further samples are needed.

ACTION 7. Remove gloves by turning them inside out over tongue blades and discard in leakage-resistant trash container. Wash hands.

ACTION 8. Place specimen container in plastic bag, close bag, label according to agency policy, and send to lab within 1 hour.

ACTION 9. When laboratory report is returned to patient's chart, inform patient of results.

Recording:
Note date, time, and disposition of specimen; appearance of stool.

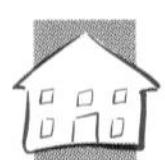

HOME HEALTH ADAPTATION: A large clean bowl or container may be placed in toilet if a bedpan, commode, or specimen hat not is available. After obtaining specimen, wash bowl with warm soapy water, rinse, and soak for 15 minutes in a sodium hypochlorite (bleach) solution of 1 part bleach to 10 parts water. Rinse thoroughly. Place the specimen container in a plastic bag or pouch with the requisition in a separate compartment of pouch. Transport specimen to lab in an insulated container with artificial ice and labeled "Biohazard." Request lab to fax or phone results to physician and home health agency. Note time that specimen is delivered to lab.

are adaptive appliances such as built-up toilet seats or even a bedside commode needed? These are some of the questions that home nurses answer when providing preventive care in the home.

SUPPORTIVE CARE

Patients who require supportive care generally demonstrate early signs of elimination alterations. The nurse will need to help the patient evaluate the extent and nature of the elimination problem and determine whether nursing or medical treatment is indicated. If the problem is treatable by nurses, patient and nurse can discuss various approaches and develop outcomes aimed at restoring healthy elimination patterns and preventing other elimination problems.

Correcting Mild Constipation

Nursing implementation for patients with mild constipation includes some techniques that were discussed under Preventive Care. Other nursing measures focus on dietary and exercise measures.

Diet. Diet and adequate fluids continue to be important at this level of care. For the person who tends to be constipated, an increased intake of high-fiber foods and fluids will be helpful. Mild laxatives or a Fleet enema may be prescribed to correct the immediate problem; however, teaching is an important part of care so that the constipation does not recur and the patient does not learn to rely on laxatives or enemas.

Exercise. Exercise can be an important approach at this care level. Swimming, riding a stationary or regular bicycle, and walking

TABLE 29-14. COMMON URINE TESTS PERFORMED BY NURSES

Name, Range of Normal Limits	Procedure	Additional Information
Specific gravity 1.003–1.040	All urine specimens should be at room temperature. *Multiple-test dipstick:* Dip reagent-impregnated dipstick into 2 mL fresh urine. Read according to manufacturer's specifications. *Urinometer:* Fill the clean calibrated container with urine, twirl the urinometer and allow it to float freely and stop. Read the number at the meniscus at eye level. Electronic monitors requiring only one drop of urine, that are also more accurate, are available in many settings.	Specific gravity of urine is a test of concentration and depends upon hydration status in the healthy person; thus, a dehydrated (and/or a hyperosmolar) patient would have a high specific gravity. A fixed specific gravity indicates that the patient's kidneys do not vary the concentration of urine.
Blood (occult blood, hemoglobin) Negative to 1000 RBC/mL	Follow the manufacturer's directions for dipstick, tablet, or other product.	Hematuria or hemoglobinuria can be detected by tests using a chemical that is sensitive to the presence of RBCs, hemoglobin, or myoglobin.
pH 4.5–8	Dip reagent-impregnated dipstick into freshly voided urine sample or place a drop of urine on test tape. Pay particular attention to (1) the time in which the reagent reacts and should be read, and (2) identification of the particular color chart for the test.	Maximum urine acidity is 4.5; maximum alkalinity is 8–9.
Protein Negative (trace in isolated sample)	Same as for pH, above. Refrigerate 24-hr specimen and record exact start and end time.	Proteinuria or albuminuria merit further investigation; 24-hour quantitative collections are often ordered upon a repeated positive finding. Increase in glomerular permeability is often a cause of albuminuria.
Ketones (acetone, diacetic acid) Negative	Dipstick (see pH, above) is most common method. If using tablets, follow manufacturer's directions	Excessive fat metabolism coupled with starvation state or diabetic ketoacidosis are common causes of ketonuria. Other diseases or ingestion of alcohol or drugs can also cause ketonuria.
Glucose (Clinistix, Diastix, Tes-tape, Clinitest tablets) Negative	Same as ketones, above.	Glycosuria (glucose in urine) occurs when the renal threshold for glucose (180–200 mg/dL) is exceeded. Most common cause is diabetes mellitus. Urine testing is not a precise method for diabetes control. Assessment of blood sugar using electronic monitors or reagent sticks has replaced urine testing in most health centers. Screening for glycosuria is routinely done during pregnancy and may be done on patients receiving hyperalimentation or high-carbohydrate tube feedings.

stimulate peristalsis. People with sedentary employment are usually most in need of regular exercise to regain and maintain regular bowel patterns.

Weakened abdominal and pelvic floor muscles can contribute to difficulty passing stools. Two simple exercises can correct that.

- While lying supine, tighten abdominal muscles as though pushing them to the floor. Hold muscles tight to count of three and relax. Repeat five to ten times as tolerated.
- Flex and contract thigh muscles by raising the knees one at a time slowly toward the chest. Repeat five times for each leg. Increase as tolerated.

These exercises often help people who have been unable to get out of bed and have had to use a bedpan for a considerable time.

Correcting Mild Diarrhea

When mild diarrhea and cramping are present, food intake should be reduced or avoided. The healthy adult with mild diarrhea may

PROCEDURE 29–3. TESTING STOOL FOR OCCULT BLOOD

PURPOSE: To determine if gastrointestinal bleeding is occurring as indicated by hidden blood in the stool.
EQUIPMENT: Materials to obtain stool specimen (Procedure 29–2). Testing products: reagent, hemoccult slide (Fig. 29–9) or hematest tablet, and filter paper.

ACTION 1. Discuss the procedure with the patient, emphasizing:

a. Purpose of the test.

b. That certain medications as well as meat, turnips, and horseradish may cause false-positive results, in which case a repeat test may be necessary after 48 to 72 hours without ingesting these substances.

c. That vitamin C tablets may mask bleeding and must therefore be discontinued for 48 to 72 hours for accurate results.

d. That up to three serial tests may be done.

ACTION 2. Obtain the specimen according to Procedure 29–2.

ACTION 3. Perform test according to manufacturer's directions. For example:
Hemoccult: Open cardboard envelope and smear stool from two different parts of the sample on the circles indicated, close cover, wait 3–5 minutes, then turn over, open as indicated and place 2 drops of reagent on indicated areas.

ACTION 4. Read results. According to package directions, a dark blue reaction is a positive reaction; pale blue indicates a retest on another specimen is desirable; no color change is negative.

ACTION 5. Dispose of used test materials, gloves, and tongue blades in leakage-resistant trash container. Wash hands.

ACTION 6. Inform patient of test results, answer questions regarding significance.

Recording:
Note test performed and result.

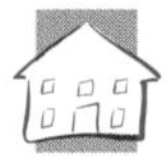

HOME HEALTH ADAPTATION: Notify physician of test result. Record time that physician is notified.

avoid food for 12 to 24 hours with no serious side effects. The diet should be confined to bland, easily digested foods such as bananas, white rice, applesauce, and tea; avoiding foods, such as milk, that are high in fat. Patients should be taught that if symptoms persist for more than 24 hours, especially in children, assessment by a health care provider is necessary.

The patient with recurrent mild diarrhea should avoid foods that exacerbate intestinal irritation and cramping. Limiting foods with high fiber content, such as raw fruits and vegetables, is helpful, because fiber stimulates peristalsis.

Preventing Recurring Urinary Tract Infections

Urinary tract infection (UTI) is relatively common, especially among women. This is because the proximity of the urinary meatus to the anus makes transfer of bowel flora likely and the short urethra allows bacterial migration to the bladder. Supportive care involves helping patients reduce their risks for recurrence. Techniques such as scrupulous hygiene, increased fluid intake, avoiding bladder distension, and urinating after intercourse are useful.

Hygiene. Hygiene practices include washing hands before and after urination. Instructing women to wipe the perineum from front to back is also an important teaching point. Bathing regularly is also important.

Fluid Intake. Fluid intake promotes optimum urine flow, reducing opportunities for bacterial growth. A patient with normal renal and cardiovascular states should drink 1500 to 2000 mL of fluid daily. Individuals prone to UTI may need to increase the fluid intake to 3000 mL daily. The resulting increase in frequency and volume of voiding may wash out any bacteria at the lower third of the urethra, thus reducing the chance of infection. Nurses may also need to suggest strategies to increase daily intake despite a busy work schedule. Fluids should be limited before bedtime to prevent nocturia.

Preventing Bladder Distension and Urinary Stasis. To prevent bladder distension and urinary stasis, nurses should teach patients to act upon the initial urge to void, not to hold the urine. The longer urine stays in the bladder, the more bacteria can multiply. Urinating more frequently helps prevent bacteria from multiplying.

Preventing Nocturia

Behaviors that help prevent nocturia or maturational enuresis include limiting fluids in the evening, avoiding fluids containing caffeine or alcohol, and voiding before bedtime. Sometimes waking a child during the night to void prevents nocturnal bedwetting. This temporary measure can contribute to the child's self-esteem, although it will not directly correct the problem.

Preventing Stress Incontinence

Strengthening the abdominal and perineal muscles helps promote complete bladder emptying and can prevent or correct stress incontinence. Abdominal exercises discussed previously as an aid to correcting constipation will also facilitate complete emptying of the bladder. Additionally, instructing people to use the abdominal muscles during urination will help.

Pelvic muscle exercises, **Kegel exercises,** are suggested to strengthen the voluntary periurethral and pelvic muscles.[11] The exercise entails tightening the perineal muscles for up to 10 seconds (as if to stop urination or defecation), followed by relaxation. The exercise should be performed 30 to 80 times a day. It is useful for both women and men.

If the patient is overweight, a weight-loss program to reduce intra-abdominal pressure may be helpful. Avoiding bladder stimulants, such as alcohol or caffeine, also decreases episodes of stress incontinence.

Home Health Care

Supportive care in the home involves assisting patients who have mild to moderate problems with bowel or bladder evacuation. Occasional urinary dribbling or fecal oozing, or chronic urinary or bowel incontinence that medical treatment cannot improve, are examples of conditions a home nurse confronts.

Monitoring a patient's pattern of evacuation is the first step in supportive home care. Records of urinary and bowel patterns enable a home nurse to pinpoint when a patient is likely to become incontinent, and thus to set up a toileting schedule that anticipates the patient's needs. Scheduled urination or bowel movements may reduce the number of accidents a patient has, and help build the patient's morale. Some nursing actions that may be helpful in the home setting are the following.

- Making sure the toilet is easy to reach, and close enough for the patient to get to quickly. A bedside commode may be helpful.
- Setting up a scheduled toileting program.
- Setting an alarm clock to remind the patient of when it is time to use the toilet.
- Scheduling fluid intake in relation to the patient's sleep time to prevent the need for frequent nighttime toileting.
- Teaching the patient and caregivers the signs of fecal impaction.
- Initiating a program of pelvic exercise.

When a patient is bothered by incontinence, urinary or fecal, the nurse may recommend undergarment liners for mild cases, or disposable incontinence briefs when a patient suffers from frequent incontinence episodes. Incontinent patients and their caregivers are instructed about the importance of checking the briefs frequently and changing them whenever wet or soiled, and about the need to wash and dry the perineal area, and apply protective ointment to protect the skin against urine or fecal irritation, each time the brief is changed.

INSIGHTS FROM NURSING LITERATURE

MANAGING URINARY INCONTINENCE

Beckman NJ. An overview of urinary incontinence in adults: assessments and behavioral interventions. Clin Nurse Specialist. *1995;9:241–247.*

Describing the enormous economic and social impact of urinary incontinence as a human affliction, the author stresses that the goal of care may not be cure, but rather improving the condition, providing comfort, and preventing complications. The nursing assessment of incontinence, according to the author, involves confirming the presence of incontinence and differentiating the type. Acute incontinence is related to an acute illness or its treatment, while chronic incontinence cannot be traced to an acute problem. Assessment also involves identifying contributing factors by gathering information on the time of day, number of continent and incontinent voids, and events precipitating incontinent voids.

The author confirms that the least invasive treatments, namely behavioral interventions, should be tried first. These rely on bladder and habit training programs in which nurses monitor the patient's incontinence status and provide a set voiding schedule incorporating progressive increases in intervals between voiding, prompting to use the toilet, and positive reinforcement techniques to teach patients to request toilet assistance from caregivers when needed.

RESTORATIVE CARE

Restorative care focuses on acute elimination problems. This level of care includes assisting the patient to assume correct positioning on the bedpan, administering enemas and irrigations, inserting urinary catheters and rectal tubes, removing fecal impactions, and providing incontinence care and colostomy care.

Assisting with Elimination

Patients who require restorative care are often confined to bed and may need to use the bedpan and urinal for elimination. Nurses should provide as much privacy as possible and help patients position the pan correctly. Patients are often embarrassed and uncomfortable using the bedpan and may try to avoid its use. Some risk injury or falls to try to get to the bathroom themselves. It is therefore imperative that nurses be acutely aware of patients' elimination needs to avoid accidents or falls. When nurses do not offer a bedpan or urinal frequently to patients who are immobile or confused, accidental soiling of the bed is not unusual.

If a patient is unable to position the urinal, the nurse should position it. Place the urinal between the person's legs, with the head of the penis directed into the urinal. It may be necessary for the nurse to hold the urinal in place. For incontinent bedridden men, the urinal is sometimes propped in place between the legs.

Children who are hospitalized may also need assistance with elimination. Like adults, some children are uncomfortable in strange surroundings and find that they have difficulty with urination or bowel elimination. A change in surroundings may cause children to regress in their toilet habits. See the earlier discussion of toilet training under Health Education in the section on Preventive Care.

Two types of bedpans are available: a standard bedpan and a smaller type called a fracture pan. The fracture pan is used for patients who have musculoskeletal disorders that make it difficult

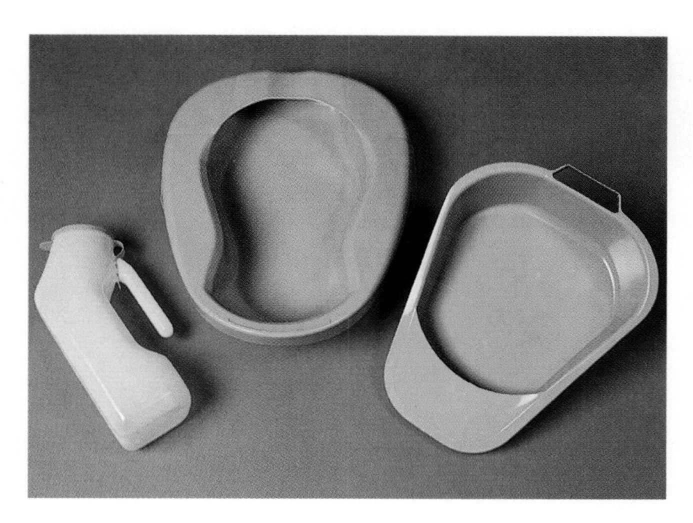

Figure 29–10. *(Left to right)* Urinal, standard bedpan, fracture pan. *(From Smith S, Duell D.* Clinical Nursing Skills: Nursing Process Model, Basic to Advanced Skills. *4th ed. Stamford, CT: Appleton & Lange; 1996.)*

or impossible to raise their buttocks off the bed. Figure 29–10 shows both types of bedpans and a urinal. Procedure 29–4 describes helping a patient to use a bedpan.

Many patients who are unable to get to the bathroom but can bear weight can use a bedside commode. The bedside commode allows the patient to assume a more effective position for elimination than a bedpan and usually is easier for nurse and patient than placing and removing a bedpan. It can be left in place at the bedside, and many people can use it without assistance from a nurse.

Administering Medications

Physicians and advanced practice nurses often prescribe medications to aid bowel and urinary elimination. Nurses administer these drugs and check for side effects in hospitalized patients.

Cathartics and laxatives promote emptying of the bowel and have short-term effects. These medications assist elimination by providing bulk or lubrication, causing chemical irritation, or softening stools. Nurses should teach about the potential harmful effects of these drugs. The action of laxatives ranges from harsh to mild, and these drugs affect different people in different manners; therefore the nurse will need to document in detail how these drugs are affecting the patient.

Suppositories (bullet-shaped cylinders of medication administered into the rectum) are also used to promote bowel evacuation and require a physician's order. Suppositories are helpful in bowel retraining and generally act within 30 minutes. They may act by softening the stool, distending the rectum, or stimulating rectal mucosa nerve endings. Again, the nurse must be aware of any side effects and the action the suppository drug has on the patient.

Antidiarrheal medications are also prescribed by physicians. These medications alleviate diarrhea by protecting irritated bowel mucosa, absorbing toxic substances and gas, or shrinking inflamed and swollen tissues.

Medications used to promote healthy urinary elimination include diuretics and antimicrobials. Diuretics influence water and electrolyte balance. They have a wide variety of mechanisms of action and frequently affect other body functions, such as blood pressure. Careful monitoring for effectiveness and side effects is critical. Antimicrobials are used to treat urinary tract infections. Usually the drug of choice is determined by the organism causing the infection. These drugs also produce side effects that should be monitored.

Administering Enemas

Enemas are used to remove feces and flatus and must be prescribed by a physician. An **enema** consists of a solution that is instilled into the rectum and sigmoid colon for the purpose of stimulating peristalsis and causing defecation to occur. In addition to relieving constipation, enemas have other uses:

- Removal of impacted feces.
- Bowel preparation for x-rays, endoscopic examinations, and surgical procedures.
- Clearing the bowel so that a bowel training program can begin (see Table 29–15 and Procedure 29–5).

Enema equipment is available in disposable prepackaged units, some of which may be reused for the same patient (Fig. 29–11). Some institutions use stainless steel enema cans, which are not disposable.

When the enema order states "Enemas until clear," nurses should repeat the enema until the patient passes only fluid containing no fecal material. The fluid may be yellow-brown. Usually only three consecutive enemas are given. If the return still contains particles of feces after three enemas, notify the physician and request further direction, as repeated enemas can cause serious fluid and electrolyte depletion. If a patient cannot control the external rectal sphincter, the nurse can administer the enema with the patient in low Fowler's position on the bedpan. Administering enemas with the patient seated on the toilet is not effective because the solution does not enter enough of the rectal and colon area, and insertion of tubing when the person is seated can injure the rectal wall.

Because enema administration may be embarrassing, nurses should provide for privacy by draping. If a patient uses the bathroom after the enema has been administered, instruct not to flush the toilet so that the enema results can be assessed and documented.

(continued on page 970)

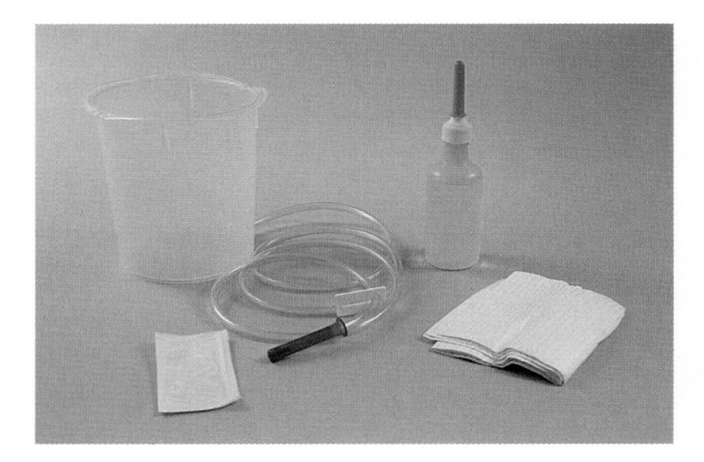

Figure 29–11. *(Left)* Disposable enema set. *(Right)* Prepackaged enema.

PROCEDURE 29–4. ASSISTING PATIENT WITH A BEDPAN

PURPOSE: To facilitate elimination in nonambulatory patients.

EQUIPMENT: Bedpan, toilet tissue, nonsterile gloves, damp washcloth or antiseptic towelette, air freshener (optional), and moisture-impervious apron or gown.

ACTION 1. Discuss with the patient the reason for the procedure, desired patient participation, and expected benefits.

RATIONALE. Patient will be more willing to participate and less anxious if there is an opportunity to clarify concerns and the reasons and benefits for the procedure are clear.

ACTION 2. Close door, pull curtains around bed.

RATIONALE. Elimination activities are considered private in most cultures. Respecting this need promotes trust and minimizes embarrassment.

ACTION 3. Put on nonsterile gloves.

RATIONALE. Body fluids may contain pathogenic organisms. Gloves prevent skin contamination by direct contact.

ACTION 4. Raise bed to nurse's waist level, fold top linen so placement of bedpan can be visualized.

RATIONALE. Prevents nurse backstrain; facilitates correct placement of bedpan.

ACTION 5. Raise head of bed 30 to 40 degrees. Ask patient to flex knees and raise buttocks off bed.

RATIONALE. Use of patient's muscles facilitates maintenance of muscle tone and strength.

ACTION 6. Slide bedpan under buttocks so rounded seat is under buttocks. Avoid pressure on sacrum. Pan may be padded with a small towel to protect bony prominences if patient is very thin.

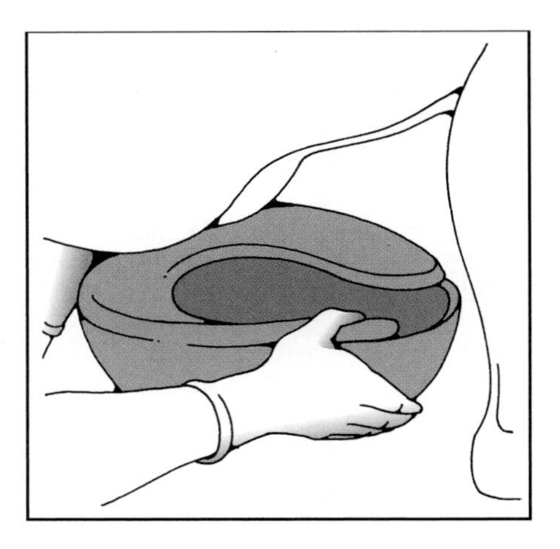

RATIONALE. Correct placement prevents discomfort and skin injury as well as preventing spills.

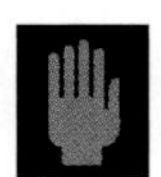

If metal bedpan is used, rinse with warm water prior to placing it, to eliminate discomfort should the bedpan be cold.

ACTION 7. If a patient cannot raise self, assist by placing your hand under patient's lower back, with your elbow on the bed. Your arm can then act as a lever to assist in raising buttocks.

RATIONALE. Leverage produces greater energy output with less effort than lifting directly.

ACTION 8. If patient is very weak or too large to lift, place bedpan by rolling. With bed flat and opposite siderail up, roll patient away from you onto side; place pan against buttocks; roll patient onto back while stabilizing pan. Pan position may need slight adjustment. Some nurses prefer to roll patient toward them. This is also permissible, but may make stabilizing the pan more difficult as the patient rolls. Cornstarch may be used on the pan to promote sliding for repositioning pan.

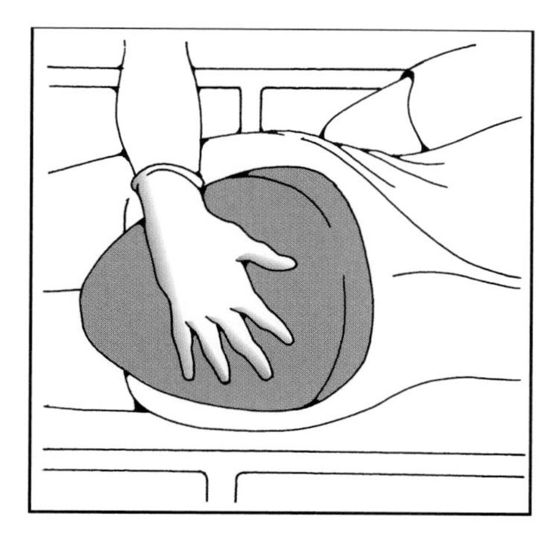

RATIONALE. Lifting a patient unable to assist is likely to cause injury to nurse. Rolling takes less energy and allows one nurse to safely position a large or helpless patient.

ACTION 9. Raise head of bed and knee gatch if not contraindicated. If head of bed cannot be raised, use fracture pan (Fig. 29–10).

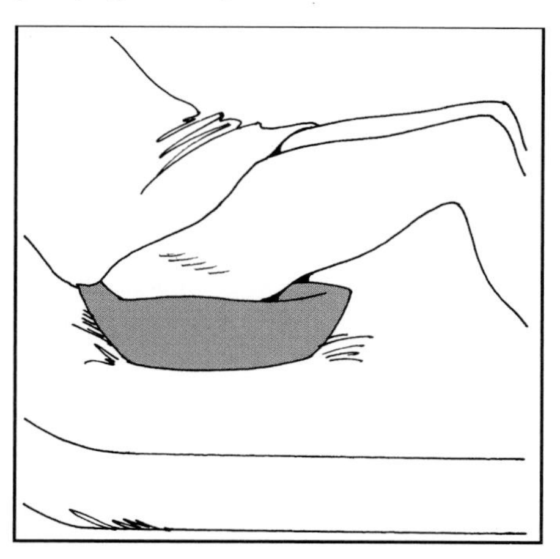

RATIONALE. This position more closely approximates physiologic position for defecation.

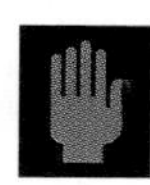

Knee gatch should remain flat for patients with vascular stasis, vascular surgery, or hip injury/repair.

ACTION 10. Replace covers, place tissue and call light in reach, and return bed to low position. Leave alert patient to complete elimination. If specimen is needed or output is to be measured, provide alternate receptacle for discarding tissue. Remove gloves. Wash hands.

RATIONALE. See Actions 2 and 3.

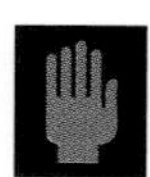

Remain in room or at bedside if there is any question about patient's alertness. Do not leave any patient on pan for more than 15 minutes.

ACTION 11. When patient has finished, provide towelette or warm damp washcloth for handwashing.

RATIONALE. Removes perineal flora from patient's hands, promotes comfort.

ACTION 12. Reglove. Remove bedpan carefully as patient raises buttocks. Note whether perineum was cleaned thoroughly by patient. (See Action 13 if further cleaning is needed.) Take pan to bathroom or dirty utility room to measure contents, obtain specimen, and empty. Some agencies provide bedpan covers—especially recommended if bathroom does not adjoin patient's room.

RATIONALE. See Action 2. Contents of pan may easily spill. Immediate removal of contents reduces patient embarrassment. Self-cleaning is awkward with bedpan and even alert patients may be unable to accomplish it. (See Action 13.)

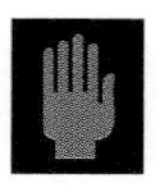

An apron or gown impervious to moisture is needed if splashing of body fluids is likely and therefore should be considered when placing and removing a bedpan for patients with bowel urgency/diarrhea or when emptying a very full bedpan. Dispose of used apron/gown according to agency policy.

Continued

ACTION 13. To assist patient with perineal cleaning, ask patient to roll to side while you stabilize bedpan. Wrap toilet tissue around your gloved hand several times and wipe perineum from urinary meatus toward anus. Repeat as necessary with new tissue until perineum and anus are free of urine and feces. In some situations, warm soapy water may be needed to thoroughly clean after defecation in bedpan.

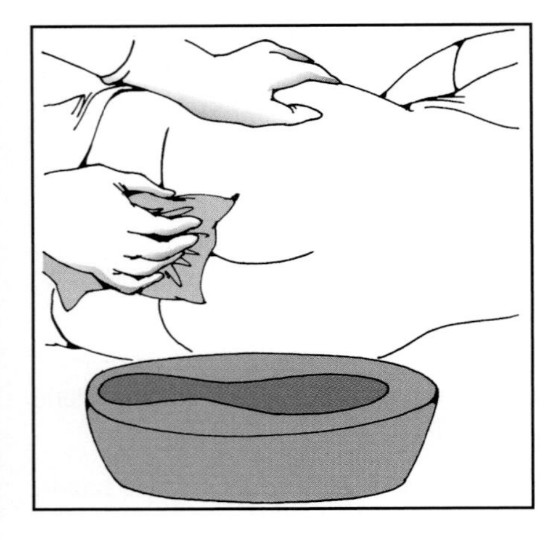

RATIONALE. Urethral contamination with fecal organisms, which promotes urinary tract infection, is prevented by cleaning in this manner. Thorough cleaning is critical to prevent skin breakdown and odor/discomfort from residual feces or urine.

ACTION 14. If patient needs assistance with positioning and replacement of covers, place bedpan on bedside chair or near foot of bed, remove gloves, and assist. Then obtain new gloves to empty pan.

RATIONALE. Gloves are contaminated with perineal and/or fecal organisms that would be transferred to other areas unless gloves are removed.

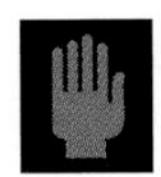

Do not place pan on floor, to prevent transfer of bacteria from floor to bedpan, then to patient's bed.

ACTION 15. Empty bedpan into toilet or hopper and rinse with bedpan flusher. Return to storage. Remove and discard gloves in leak-resistant trash receptacle. Wash hands. Bedpan should not be left on floor of bathroom (see Action 14.)

RATIONALE. Prevents transfer of organisms from urine to environment.

Recording:

Use of bedpan need not be recorded. If output is being measured, record on I&O record. If a specimen has been obtained and/or tested, record the test and results on appropriate flowsheet.

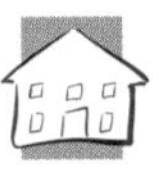

HOME HEALTH ADAPTATION: Because beds in most homes are of a stationary height, home health caregivers must be careful to use appropriate body mechanics to prevent strain and injuries, that is, bend knees and keep back straight. Instruct family members about appropriate body mechanics and how to assist the individual with bedpan use. A fracture pan may be easier for family members to place. Put 2 or 3 pillows under the upper torso after placing patient on pan.

Relieving Flatus

To help expel flatus a rectal tube can be inserted. To insert a rectal tube, provide privacy, position the patient sidelying, and don unsterile gloves. Lubricate a rectal tube of appropriate size (22–24 French for adults, 12–18 French for children), separate the buttocks to visualize the anal opening, and gently insert the tube 4 to 6 inches toward the umbilicus. If hemorrhoids are present, especially cautious insertion is indicated. Enclose the open end of the tube in an absorbent pad or plastic bag and secure with a rubber band. Remove the rectal tube after 20 to 30 minutes and document patient response.

Caring for Fecal Impaction

When enemas and laxatives fail to promote the complete evacuation of fecal material, digital removal of impacted stool is the next alternative. Agency policies may specify which level of health care personnel are permitted to remove stool digitally, and a physician's order may be required. Assist the patient to a side-lying position, screen for privacy, and don clean gloves, lubricating the index finger. Slowly insert the lubricated finger toward the umbilicus and gently break up the fecal mass. Pull out small bits of fecal material with the curved index finger.

This procedure is usually uncomfortable and can create irritation and bleeding. Observe the patient for signs of fatigue, pallor, or change in pulse rate, and stop the procedure if these occur. Digital stimulation can induce the urge to defecate and the nurse may need to assist the patient onto a bedpan or commode. Follow-up measures such as enemas or suppositories may be used for a few days after removal of the impaction to facilitate restoration of the usual defecation pattern.

(continued on page 976)

TABLE 29-15. TYPES OF ENEMAS

Type of Enema	Mode of Action	Undesired Effects	Nursing Responsibilities
Cleansing			
1. Tap water enema (500–1000 mL) *Note:* Do not administer more than three consecutive enemas without consulting physician. "Clear" does not mean without color. Infants and children should not be given tap water enemas because they are at risk for fluid and electrolyte imbalance.	Volume of fluid distends bowel and stimulates peristalsis.	Sodium deficit. Potassium deficit resulting from osmotic transfer of Na and K from cells lining the bowel to the water (hypotonic solution) in the bowel.	Observe patient for symptoms of hyponatremia, hypokalemia, water intoxication, particularly when giving multiple enemas. *Hyponatremia* evidenced by decreased blood pressure, lethargy, stomach cramps. *Hypokalemia* evidenced by generalized muscle weakness, cardiac arrhythmias, shallow respirations. *Water intoxication* evidenced by nausea and vomiting, tachycardia, increased blood pressure, headache, dizziness, confusion.
2. Normal saline (500–1000 mL) Infant (150–250 mL) Toddler (250–350 mL) Child (300–500 mL)	Same as above. Isotonic solution, so minimal disruption of fluid and electrolyte balance.	Minimal.	
Irritant			
1. Bisacodyl or Fleet: (prepackaged 30 mL) 2. Soap solution (500–1000 mL: 5 mL mild soap to 100 mL water)	Hypermotility of the bowel is created by irritating the bowel mucosa. The contact laxative acts directly on the mucosa of colon by stimulating sensory nerve endings to produce peristalsis and evacuation.	Persistent mucosal irritation can last for 3 weeks.	For soap solutions, put water in bag first to prevent soap from foaming; mix gently.
Hypertonic			
1. Magnesium sulfate (Epsom salts)	Water is drawn into the bowel from the extracellular fluid. The bowel becomes distended and produces mechanical stimulation, leading to evacuation of large amounts of fluid and bowel contents.	Magnesium excess. Fluid volume deficit, caused by the hypertonic solution drawing water from interstitial spaces, especially in children and other susceptible persons.	Observe for symptoms of hypermagnesemia: flushing, hypotension, bradycardia, depressed deep tendon reflexes.
2. Sodium biphosphate and sodium phosphate (prepackaged 118 mL)	Same as above.	Increased sodium absorption: Should be avoided for patient requiring sodium restriction, or with impaired renal function. Hyperphosphatemia and hypocalcemia.	Observe for symptoms of hypernatremia, such as red flushed skin, dry sticky mucous membranes, thirst, decreased urine production.
Lubricating			
Oil retention enema (mineral oil, prepackaged 133 mL)	Softens and lubricates hard stool without irritating mucosa of colon. Stimulates normal bowel movement, as only rectum, sigmoid, and part of the descending colon are evacuated.		Instruct patient that holding the enema for 30 minutes to 1 hour will increase its effectiveness.
Carminative			
1. 1-2-3 (30 g magnesium sulfate: 60 mL glycerine: 90 mL water) 2. Milk and molasses (equal parts of 80–100 mL) 3. Mayo (240 mL water: 60 mL sugar: 30 mL sodium bicarbonate)	Carminative enema solutions release gas, distend rectum and colon, and stimulate peristalsis.		

PROCEDURE 29–5. ADMINISTERING A CLEANSING ENEMA

PURPOSE: To empty the lower bowel in patients who are constipated, are being prepared for surgery or diagnostic studies, or who need bowel training.

EQUIPMENT: Enema setup including bag or can with attached rectal tube and clamp, water-soluble lubricant, and waterproof underpad; ordered solution; nonsterile gloves; and bath blanket (optional). If patient cannot ambulate: bedpan or commode, toilet tissue, and damp washcloth or towelette. Prepackaged enema solutions may also be used as ordered (see end of Procedure). Moisture-impervious gown or apron optional.

ACTION 1. Check physician's order.

RATIONALE. Medical order is required for instillation of solutions into the rectum.

ACTION 2. Discuss with the patient the reason for the procedure, desired patient participation, usual sensations, and expected benefits.

RATIONALE. Patient will be more willing to participate and less anxious if there is an opportunity to clarify concerns and the reasons and benefits for the procedure are clear.

ACTION 3. Clamp tubing. Prepare solution as ordered in enema container. Usual amount prepared is 1500 mL. From 500 to 1500 mL may be administered (250–500 mL for children). See Table 29–15 for common additives in cleansing enemas.

RATIONALE. Greater volumes may overdistend the bowel causing cramping pain.

ACTION 4. If tap water is used to make solution, use water from the tap that feels warm (*not hot*) to the inner aspect of the wrist (105–110F). Small-volume commercial solutions are used at room temperature.

RATIONALE. Warm water stimulates peristalsis, hot water will burn bowel mucosa, although patient will not feel burning because bowel has no temperature-sensitive nerves.

ACTION 5. Expel air from tubing by allowing solution to flow to tip. Reclamp.

RATIONALE. Air may cause cramping if introduced into the bowel.

ACTION 6. Identify patient.

RATIONALE. Administering an enema to the wrong patient is considered a medication error. Serious harm to the patient could result.

ACTION 7. Close door and pull curtains around bed.

RATIONALE. Elimination activities are considered private in most cultures. Respecting this need promotes trust and minimizes embarrassment.

ACTION 8. Raise bed to nurse's waist height.

RATIONALE. Prevents backstrain and fatigue from bending to bed in low position.

ACTION 9. Ask/assist patient to assume left lateral position.

RATIONALE. Allows gravity to facilitate the flow of fluid along the curve of the sigmoid colon, and retention of fluid if sphincter is weak.

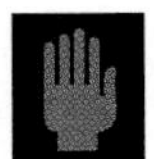

Position is not critical and may be altered for comfort to dorsal recumbent or right side.

ACTION 10. Arrange bed covers or bath blanket so only patient's buttocks are exposed.

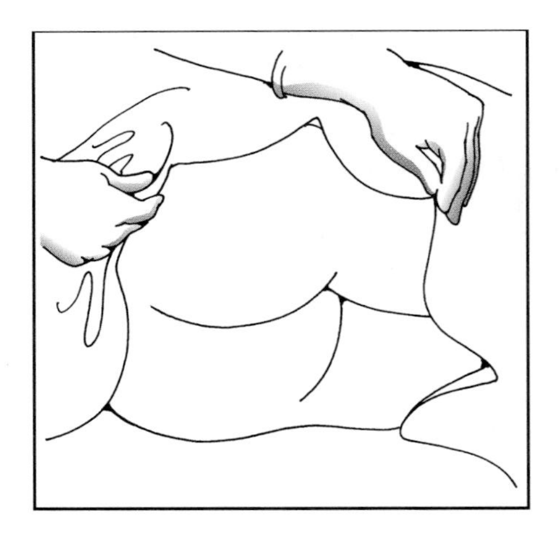

RATIONALE. Unnecessary exposure is demeaning and may chill patient.

ACTION 11. Put on nonsterile gloves.

RATIONALE. Gloves are a barrier preventing contact with fecal material, which may contain pathogens.

ACTION 12. If patient is not ambulatory, place bedpan on bed or bedside commode next to bed. Some ambulatory patients may prefer to have a pan or commode nearby. Patients with very poor sphincter control may be placed on bedpan to give enema.

RATIONALE. Relieves patient's anxiety about soiling the bed if enema cannot be retained.

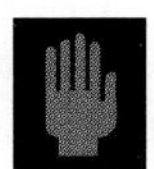

If premature expulsion of enema and resulting splashing is a risk, a moisture impervious gown or apron is indicated.

ACTION 13. Place waterproof pad under buttocks.

RATIONALE. Protects bed linens from leakage that may occur while patient is retaining enema.

ACTION 14. Lubricate distal 8 to 10 cm (3–4 in.) of tube. Lubricate 2 to 5 cm (1–2 in.) for a child.

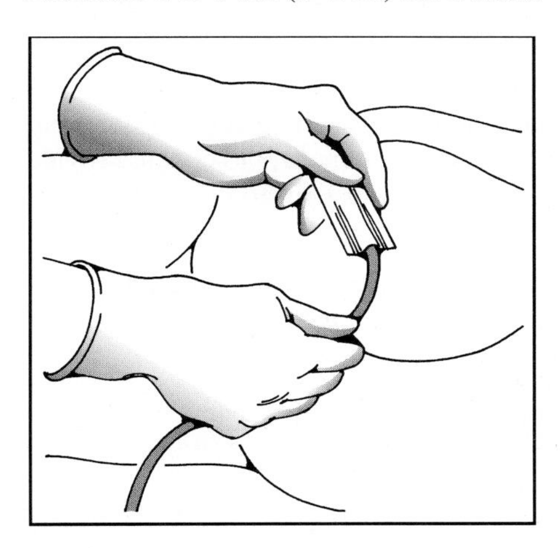

RATIONALE. Reduces friction between tube and rectal mucosa. Friction damages tissue.

ACTION 15. Lift the patient's buttock to expose the anus. Ask patient to take a deep breath and exhale slowly through the mouth while relaxing gluteal and sphincter muscles. Tell patient you will introduce tube during exhalation.

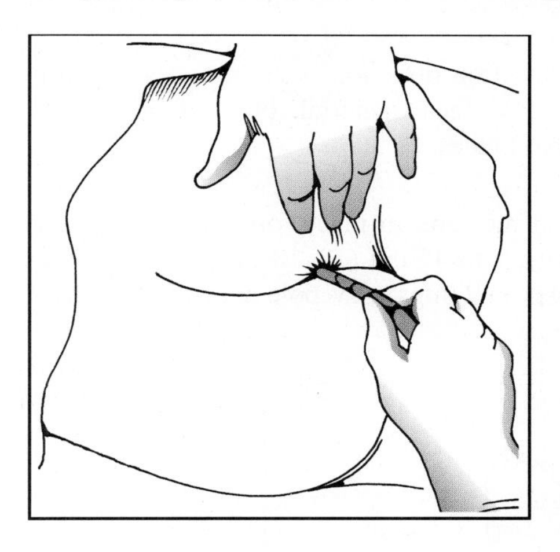

RATIONALE. Breathing facilitates relaxation, thereby reducing discomfort from insertion of the tube. If patient is alerted when tube will be inserted, reflex contraction of sphincter can be inhibited.

ACTION 16. Slowly insert the tube into the rectum toward the umbilicus, advance about 3 to 4 inches (1–2 in. for children).

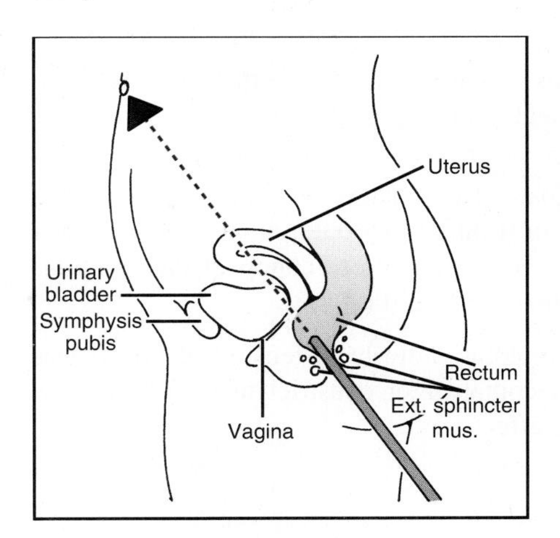

RATIONALE. Follows the contour of rectum, minimizing risk of bowel perforation or abrasion, and locates tip of the tube above internal sphincter so enema can be retained.

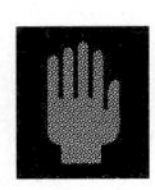

If hemorrhoids are noted, extra gentleness is necessary to reduce discomfort.

Continued

ACTION 17. If tube meets resistance during insertion, recheck insertion direction. If correct, allow a small amount of fluid to flow while attempting to advance the tube. If resistance persists, assess for impaction. DO NOT force tube.

RATIONALE. If insertion direction is correct, resistance is most likely caused by fecal material. Flow of liquid may allow tube to bypass feces.

ACTION 18. Hold the tube in place, open the clamp and raise the container 30 to 45 cm (12–18 in.) above the rectum. Container may be hung on IV pole adjusted to correct height.

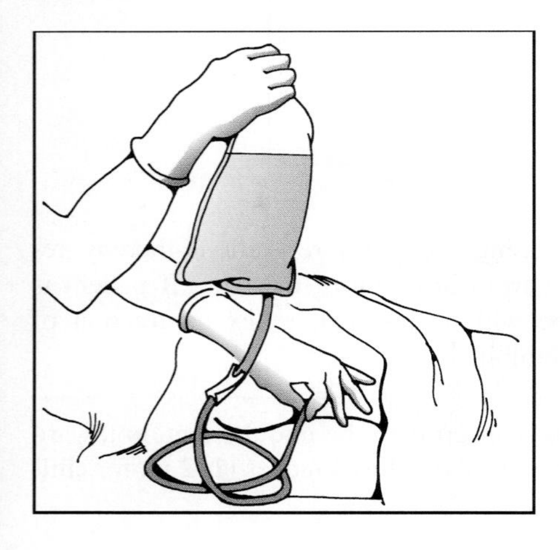

RATIONALE. This height will introduce the fluid slowly so rapid distension and cramping are prevented.

ACTION 19. If patient complains of cramping, an urgent need to defecate, or if fluid flows out around the tube, lower container slightly or partially close clamp. If these actions do not correct situation, stop fluid flow.

RATIONALE. Symptoms indicate distension of bowel was too rapid. Lower container or constrict tube to slow flow and decrease this effect.

ACTION 20. When cramping passes, continue to administer fluid until patient complains of fullness or all solution has infused. Then clamp tubing and remove tube.

RATIONALE. Attempting to administer more fluid than the patient can tolerate will cause premature expulsion.

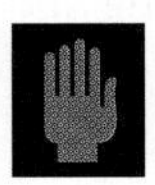

Patients with poor sphincter control cannot retain large amounts of solution.

ACTION 21. Tell the patient that retaining the fluid for 5 to 10 minutes will increase the effectiveness, because the longer the solution is retained, the stronger the resulting peristalsis.

RATIONALE. Patient is more likely to accept moderate discomfort if a clear benefit will result.

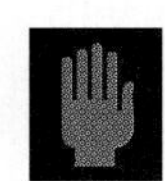

Holding a folded tissue firmly against the anus will assist the patient to retain the enema.

ACTION 22. When patient has a strong urge to defecate, assist as needed to bathroom, commode, or bedpan. Provide tissue and call light, then leave patient to complete expulsion.

RATIONALE. Elimination activities are considered private in most cultures. Respecting this need promotes trust and minimizes embarrassment.

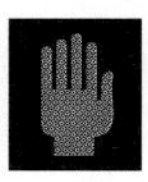

Assess patient for weakness and dizziness before leaving. Stay with patient who shows these symptoms.

ACTION 23. When patient has expelled enema, assess amount and character of output.

RATIONALE. Evaluation of effectiveness of procedure is necessary to determine the need for further treatment.

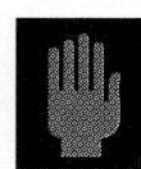

Rarely the enema cannot be expelled and must be siphoned. Reposition patient, reinsert lubricated tube. Introduce about 50 mL of fluid, then lower container below rectum so that negative pressure pulls fluid into container. Repeat until all fluid is returned.

ACTION 24. Assist as needed with hygiene, clean bedpan or commode, and discard enema supplies in leak-resistant trash receptacle. Remove gloves and gown, if used, by pulling them off inside out and discard similarly. Wash hands.

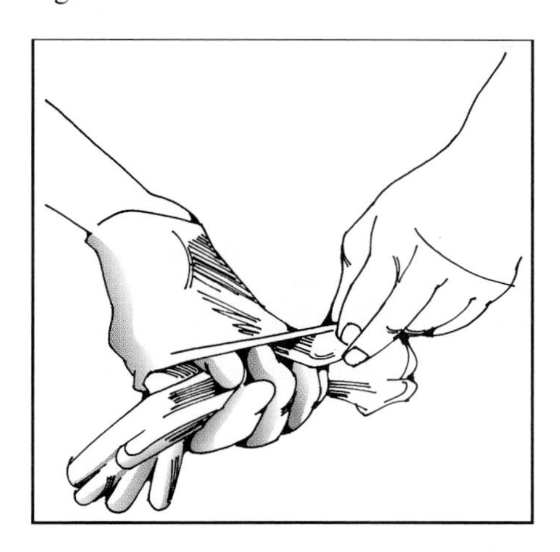

RATIONALE. These activities prevent transfer of fecal organisms to environment.

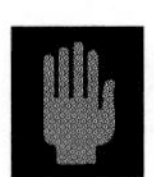

If a series of enemas is needed, equipment may be reused, but should be disposed of correctly when series is complete.

ACTION 25. Assist as needed with repositioning in bed. Replace any soiled or damp linen.

RATIONALE. Promotes comfort and well-being. Enemas are exhausting for most patients.

PREPACKAGED ENEMAS

ACTION 1. Prepare the patient as in Actions 1 and 2 and 6 to 15.

RATIONALE. See Actions 1 to 15.

ACTION 2. Remove cap and insert prelubricated tip into rectum toward umbilicus.

RATIONALE. Follows the contour of rectum, minimizing risk of bowel perforation or abrasion, and locates tip of tube above internal sphincter so enema can be retained.

ACTION 3. Roll container (as with a tube of toothpaste) to expel all of the contents into the rectum.

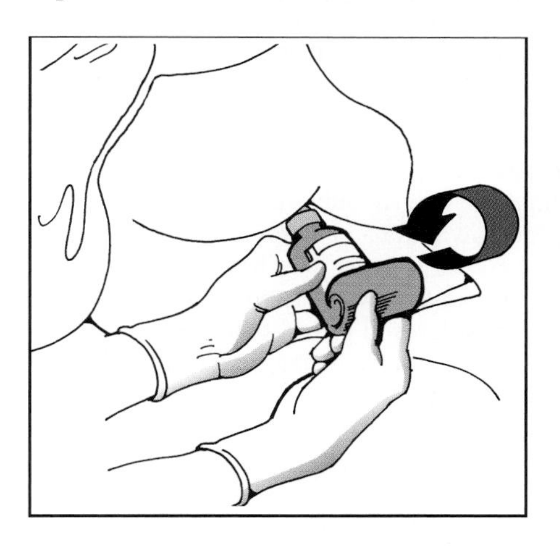

RATIONALE. Prepackaged enemas usually contain 200 mL or less. Because most of them are hypertonic, only small amounts are needed to stimulate defecation (see also Table 29–15).

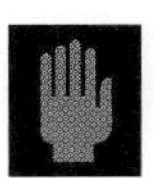

Some patients are able and prefer to self-administer this type of enema.

ACTION 4. Continue with Actions 21 to 25.

RATIONALE. See Actions 21 to 25.

Recording:

Note type of enema and results: amount, color, consistency, any abnormal constituents of return; state of abdomen (soft, distended); patient response and condition of patient after procedure.

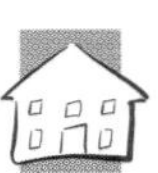

HOME HEALTH ADAPTATION: If a prolonged procedure is anticipated and the patient is in a low stationary bed, place a bath towel or similar protective cushioning on floor for nurse to kneel on. Creative use of available household items (clothes hanger on a floor lamp) may be necessary to securely hold prepared solution during preparation and insertion of tubing. Or, request assistance of family members or other caregivers. If equipment is to be reused, wash tubing with warm soapy water, and rinse.

INSIGHTS FROM NURSING LITERATURE
BOWEL ELIMINATION PATTERNS OF MIDDLE-AGED AND ELDERLY PATIENTS

Ross DG. Altered bowel elimination patterns among hospitalized elderly and middle-aged persons: quantitative results. Ortheped Nurs. *1995;14:25–31.*

The researcher selected two samples of hospitalized patients, including 154 elderly subjects and 149 middle-aged subjects, none of whom had a chronic bowel disease. He then gathered baseline data on their bowel elimination patterns, including use of laxatives, suppositories, enemas, and bran, and asked patients to record their bowel movements in a diary. He also assessed subjects' functional status using the Index of Activities of Daily Living, and cognitive status using the Visual Analog Scale for Confusion.

The findings showed that before hospitalization, the elderly subjects used more laxatives, suppositories, and enemas, and had lower fluid intakes than middle-aged patients. Eighty-nine percent of the elderly subjects and 88 percent of the middle-aged subjects experienced a change in the bowel elimination pattern when hospitalized, some developing fecal impactions. Controlling for gender, illness severity, and functional and cognitive status, the findings showed altered diet and activity were more important factors in the bowel changes experienced by the elderly than in those experienced by the middle-aged subjects.

Assisting Patients Who Are Incontinent of Feces

As discussed in the nursing diagnosis section, most causes of fecal incontinence are not treatable by nurses. Offering a bedpan or assisting the patient to toilet facilities within 20 to 30 minutes after breakfast, when the gastrocolic reflex is most active, may prevent accidental soiling. However, timing of bowel evacuation is difficult to predict in incontinent patients who do not eat regular meals or who are receiving liquid nutrient formulas. Fecal incontinence collectors are used in some health care facilities to alleviate soiling and prevent associated skin irritation. Application and emptying of fecal incontinence collectors are detailed in Procedure 29–6.

Routine Colostomy Care

Ostomy care requires that the nurse be knowledgeable about each type of ostomy, as discussed in Section 1 of this chapter (Table 29–2). Assessment of the stoma and surrounding area, as discussed under abdominal inspection, is essential to maintaining stomal integrity. Early recognition of potential problems assures prompt treatment.

Collaboration in ostomy care helps a patient adjust to changes in defecation patterns, body image, and life-style. The nurse's attitude and knowledge can be an essential component in helping patients adapt. In addition, the expertise of a specialist in this field, the enterostomal therapist, should be used if available (Fig. 29–12). Procedures for changing and fitting ostomy appliances are not addressed in this text, but are included in most textbooks of medical–surgical nursing and nursing procedure books.

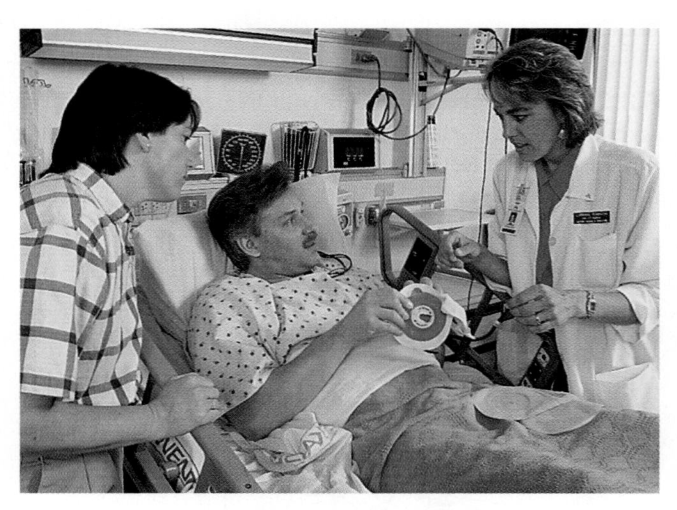

Figure 29–12. Enterostomal therapist teaching a couple about ostomy equipment.

A great many products for ostomy care are on the market. Several examples are shown in Fig. 29–13. These include skin care products, appliances to fit over the stoma, and special irrigating sets. The stoma therapist will know what a particular patient needs and what is available. Selection of proper pouching products is vital for the patient's progress in rehabilitation.[14] Appliances may be either disposable or reusable. Appliances used in hospitals tend to be disposable, whereas patients who have had a colostomy for some time usually use reusable appliances. Temporary appliances are made of transparent plastic with a peel-off adhesive square around the opening. This opening can usually be cut to fit closely around the stoma to prevent leakage and skin irritation. Disposable pouches should be drainable so they can be emptied without being removed (see Procedure 29–7).

Odor control, very important to patients, can be ensured by using the most appropriate type of appliance, emptying it frequently, and cleaning it well before reapplying. Some patients use special odor-absorbing products inside their ostomy appliance.

A colostomy irrigation distends the bowel and stimulates peristalsis, thereby causing bowel evacuation to occur via the stoma. Not all types of colostomies require routine irrigation. Descending and sigmoid colostomies are commonly irrigated, while ileostomies and ascending colostomies are not irrigated because feces are liquid and drain from the stoma continuously.

COLLABORATIVE STRATEGY
MANAGING OSTOMIES IN THE HOME SETTING

Whether or not a patient is able to achieve optimal health after an ostomy will depend on the quality of home management. New patterns necessitated by an ostomy may or may not be easily integrated into family life and daily living. The ability of patient and significant others to manage an ostomy can be enhanced by caring support from the nurse. Collaborating with patients in their own surroundings can help to reduce external barriers and promote confidence that the ostomy need not interfere with valued activities.

PROCEDURE 29–6. APPLYING AND EMPTYING A FECAL INCONTINENCE COLLECTOR

PURPOSE: Used to collect feces when patients have no anal sphincter control, thereby preventing excoriation of skin and soiling of bed.

EQUIPMENT: Fecal incontinence collector, blunt-tip scissors, mild skin cleanser, water, washcloth and towel, waterproof underpad, nonsterile gloves, and spray adhesive or porous tape (optional). Drainage bag and tubing optional for liquid stool. Bedpan or graduate to empty collector.

ACTION 1. Discuss procedure, including purpose and benefits. Explain procedure, even if patient appears unresponsive.

ACTION 2. Screen patient, raise bed to nurse's waist level, assist patient to lateral or Sims' position. Arrange covers so that only buttocks are exposed.

ACTION 3. Don gloves, place underpad beneath patient's buttocks. Thoroughly wash and dry perineal and anal area. Trim hair around anal opening so that none will be under adhesive portion of collector.

ACTION 4. Following manufacturer's directions, prepare collector to fit patient. It may be necessary to cut a larger opening in the collector. Some brands may require use of skin prep or additional adhesive to improve adherence of device.

ACTION 5. Fold adhesive portion in half to facilitate correct positioning on patient, then remove paper backing to expose adhesive barrier.

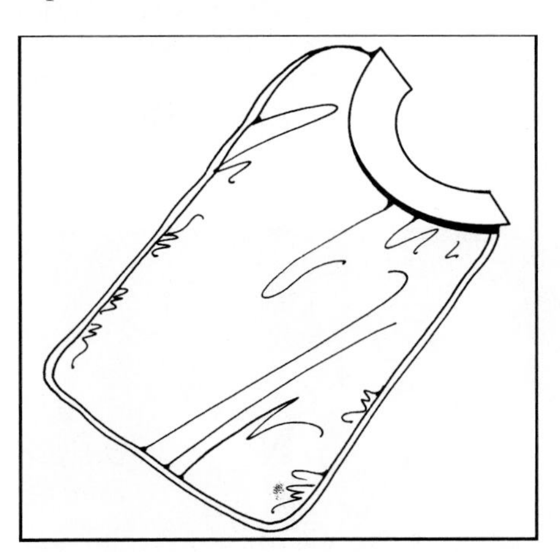

ACTION 6. Lift patient's buttock to expose anus. Press narrowest part of barrier between the anus and scrotum or vaginal opening, opposite end against coccygeal area. Release buttock and press sides of barrier so collector adheres to perianal skin without creating pressure or pulling of tissue.

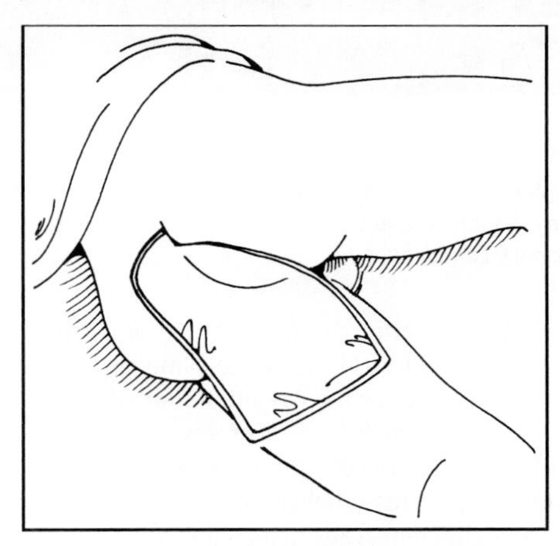

ACTION 7. Check to see that drainage cap is securely closed. If patient has frequent liquid stools, cap may be replaced with drainage tubing and collection bag similar to that used with indwelling catheters. For solid stools, drain may be cut off and bag sealed with pouch clamp (see Procedure 29–7).

ACTION 8. Remove gloves and position patient comfortably. Wash hands. Check collector several times each shift or whenever patient is turned and repositioned. Empty frequently to prevent skin irritation, diminish odors, and prolong adhesive contact.

ACTION 9. To empty collector: don gloves; with patient sidelying, open drainage cap and squeeze contents into bedpan or large graduate. Discard gloves. Wash hands.

ACTION 10. Replace collector whenever seal to skin is broken. Remove carefully and discard as with body wastes.

Recording:
Note that collector is in use, and describe condition of perianal skin and amount and character of output.

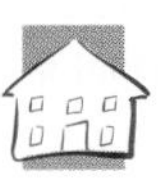

HOME HEALTH ADAPTATION: Instruct family members about the need to check collector frequently and how to apply and empty the bag.

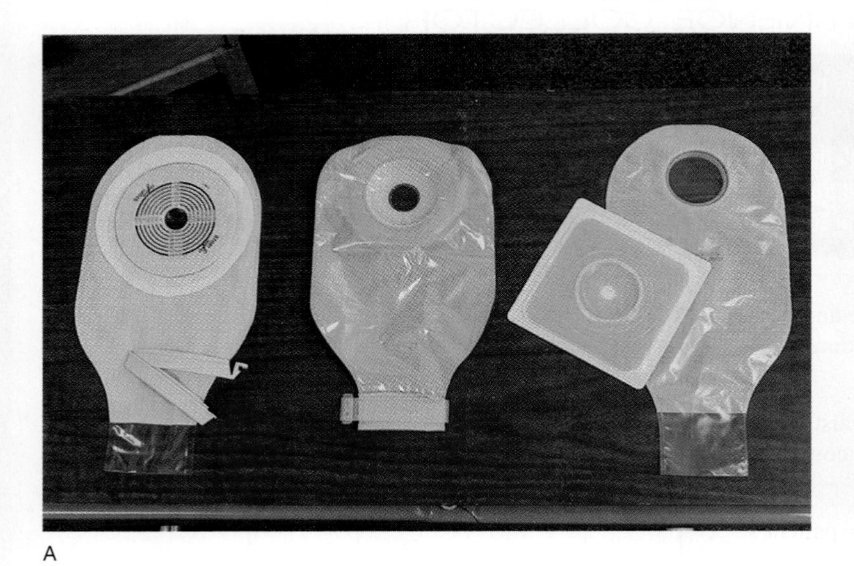

A

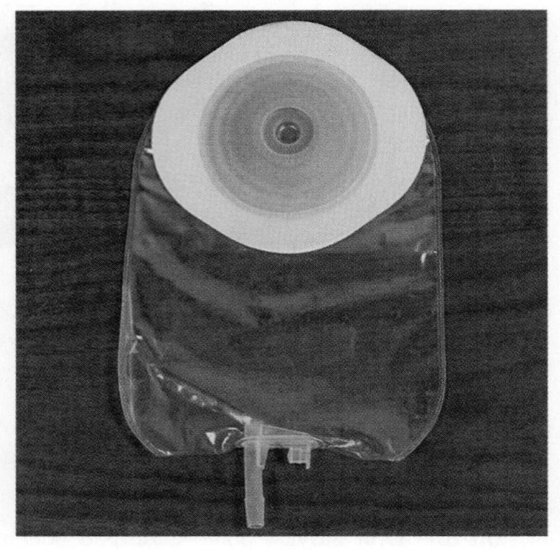

B

Figure 29–13. Examples of colostomy and ileostomy appliances. **A.** Open-ended or drainable pouches for colostomies. **B.** Drainable ileostomy pouch. *(From Smith S, Duell D.* Clinical Nursing Skills: Nursing Process Model, Basic to Advanced Skills. *4th ed. Stamford, CT: Appleton & Lange; 1996.)*

Daily irrigations can sometimes control the time of elimination. Therefore, irrigation should be done at the same time each day. Patients need to select a time for the irrigation that will allow this activity to fit into their schedule. Colostomy irrigation is detailed in Procedure 29–8. Because colostomy irrigation can take up to an hour to complete, patients often decide to control elimination by a rigid dietary regimen instead. Even with the use of irrigations, however, dietary factors are important. Laxative foods should be avoided as they may cause unexpected evacuation; gas-forming foods should also be avoided.

Inserting a Urinary Catheter

Urinary **catheterization** is the passage of a tube into the bladder through the urethra. Catheterization may be done for the diagnosis, treatment, or prevention of problems associated with the urinary tract. Some diagnostic reasons for insertion of a catheter include monitoring urine output and obtaining specimens. Catheterization can also be used to treat such problems as urinary obstruction or retention associated with surgery, medications, or childbirth. Catheters are often inserted before procedures that may result in urinary complications.

The purpose of the procedure determines the type of catheterization. A straight catheterization (intermittent) is often done for diagnostic purposes, such as measuring residual urine (the urine left in the bladder after voiding) or obtaining a sterile urine specimen. This type of catheterization may also be used in cases of simple postoperative retention. Some patients use intermittent self-catheterization as part of a bladder training program (see the section on bladder training later in this chapter).

When a catheterization is performed before surgery or for a urinary obstruction, such as benign prostatic hypertrophy, the catheter is left in place for hours or days. This is called an indwelling (or retention) catheter (sometimes the term Foley catheter is used). An indwelling catheter has a small inflatable balloon near the tip to hold it in place inside the bladder. The balloon is deflated for insertion and removal of the catheter.

The steps for catheterization are essentially the same for both intermittent and indwelling catheters. The technique for inserting a catheter is described in Procedure 29–9. Figure 29–14 shows a complete kit for indwelling catheter insertion.

The purpose of the catheterization, the length of time the catheter will be in place, and the patient's urinary tract anatomy determine the size and type of catheter to use. The most common catheters are straight or retention catheters in sizes 14-18 French gauge for adults and sizes 8-14 French gauge for children.

As with any procedure, catheterization carries risks. Therefore, it should be done only when it is in the patient's best interest.

(continued on page 981)

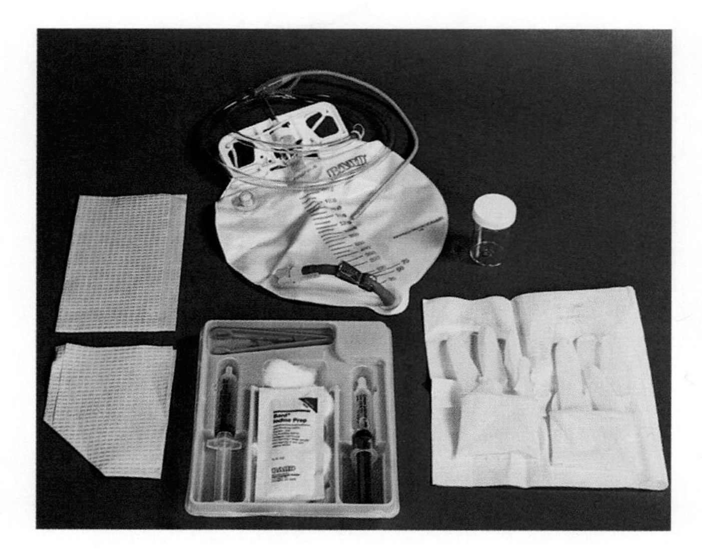

Figure 29–14. Equipment found in disposable kit for insertion of indwelling catheter. *(From Smith S, Duell D.* Clinical Nursing Skills: Nursing Process Model, Basic to Advanced Skills: *4th ed. Stamford, CT: Appleton & Lange; 1996.)*

PROCEDURE 29–7. EMPTYING AN OSTOMY POUCH

PURPOSE: To remove fecal drainage, promote stoma and skin integrity, and reduce odor.
EQUIPMENT: Nonsterile gloves, waterproof underpad, damp cloth, and bedpan or large graduate. Moisture-impervious gown or apron optional.

ACTION 1. Discuss procedure with patient regarding needs for assistance, teaching, and scheduling of procedure. Pouches should be emptied when ⅓ to ½ full of drainage or when full of gas to prevent breaking seal on pouch due to increased weight of contents. With new ostomies, clean disposable pouches are used to more easily assess color of the stoma. Some patients are able to empty ostomy pouches without assistance; others, especially if ostomy is new, will require teaching and support. Ultimately self-care is desirable. The enterostomal therapist is a resource for patients and nurses in the selection of equipment and care of the stoma.

ACTION 2. Screen patient, and adjust bed to nurse's waist height and to semi-Fowler's position. Adjust covers so bag is exposed.

ACTION 3. Don gloves. Place waterproof pad under pouch so patient's body and bed linens are protected from spills. Moisture-proof gown is indicated if splashing of stool is expected.

ACTION 4. Place bedpan or graduate on bed so that clamped end of pouch extends over it. Holding pouch so clamped end is higher than stoma, open pouch clamp (sometimes rubber band may be used to close pouch).

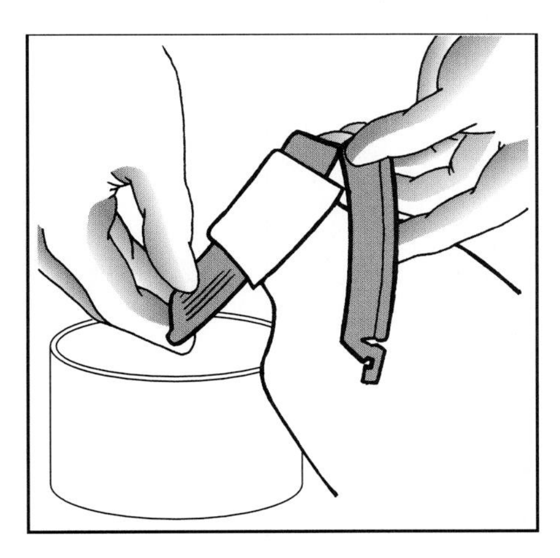

ACTION 5. Unroll pouch end, and then fold back on itself to make a cuff. This will prevent end from contacting fecal drainage, making cleaning it unnecessary before resealing bag. Drain pouch into collection container, flattening so all drainage is removed. Note character and amount of drainage.

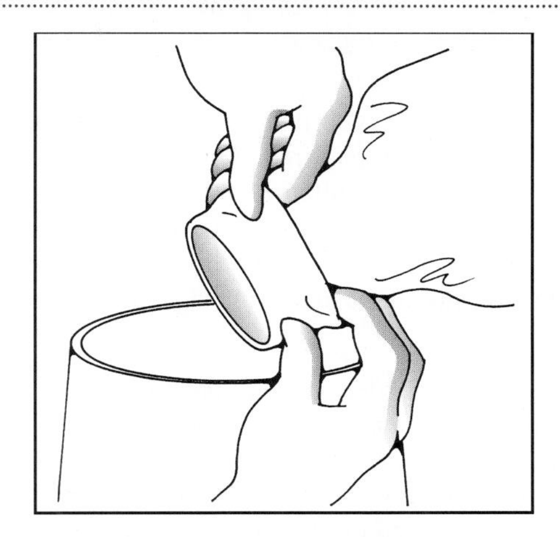

ACTION 6. Raise pouch above level of stoma, unfold cuff, and then reroll end and apply clamp. If desired, rinse disposable pouches after emptying by pouring tepid water from a paper cup into the distal (draining) end. Some patients may desire that the pouch deodorant be placed in the pouch prior to closing it.

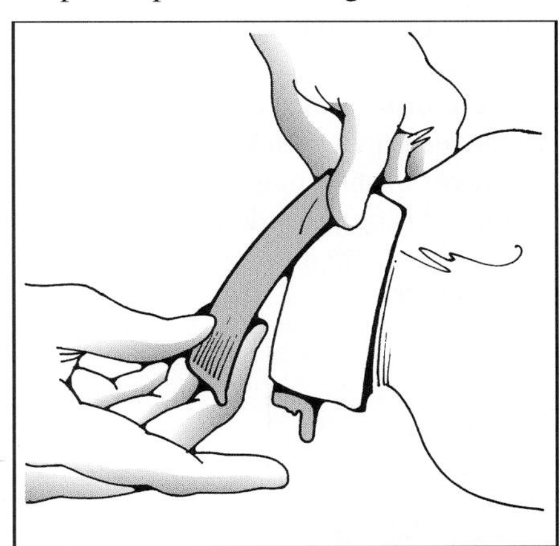

ACTION 7. Discard drainage in toilet. Remove gloves (and gown if used) by turning inside-out and discard according to agency policy. Wash hands.

Recording:
Note character and amount of drainage, condition of stoma (may not be observable if bag is opaque), nature of teaching, and patient response.

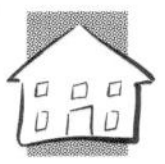

HOME HEALTH ADAPTATION: If a prolonged procedure is anticipated and the patient is in a low stationary bed, consider proceeding while kneeling at the bedside to minimize stooping. Place a towel or similar protective cushioning on the floor to kneel on.

PROCEDURE 29–8. IRRIGATING A COLOSTOMY

PURPOSE: To regulate time of colon elimination, prevent unexpected evacuation or leakage, or cleanse colon in preparation for visualization or surgery.

EQUIPMENT: Colostomy irrigation set including irrigation bag with tubing, cone, clamp, and irrigation sleeve; prescribed irrigant; lubricant; nonsterile gloves, IV pole or wall hook to suspend bag; bath blanket; and bedpan and waterproof pad if patient is to remain in bed. Moisture-impervious gown or apron optional.

ACTION 1. Discuss procedure with patient, including timing and amount of assistance required. Optimal time is within 1 hour after a meal. Consultation with an enterostomal therapist may also be necessary to determine if modifications of equipment or procedure are necessary. Patients with long-standing colostomies usually manage irrigation independently.

ACTION 2. If assistance is needed, prepare patient and 500 to 1000 mL solution as for enema (see Procedure 29–5, Actions 1 to 8, and 12). Patients should be in semi-Fowler's position if irrigation is to be done in bed. Most patients prefer to do irrigation while seated on the toilet.

ACTION 3. Arrange bed covers and gown to expose stoma. Place waterproof pad to protect bottom sheet. Patients seated on toilet may desire blanket to cover knees. Hang irrigating container so bottom is level with seated patient's shoulder (12–18 in. above stoma).

ACTION 4. Don gloves. Remove and empty ostomy appliance, if necessary. Many patients who irrigate their colostomies to regulate elimination need only a gauze pad to cover the stoma between irrigations. Place drainage sleeve over stoma. Karaya washer may be used around stoma to minimize leaking during procedure. Distal end of sleeve should extend between patient's legs into toilet or into bedpan if patient is in bed.

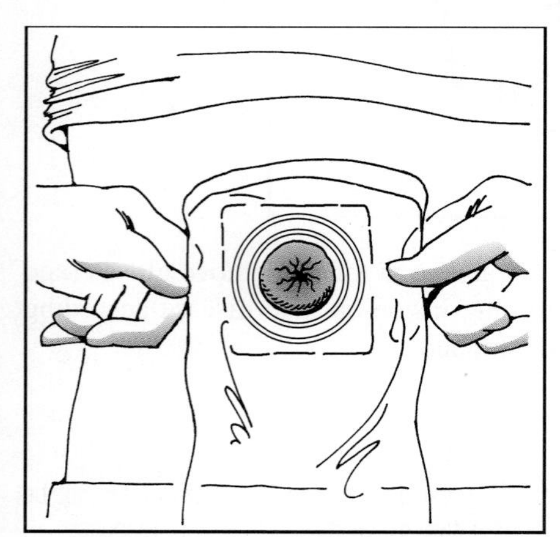

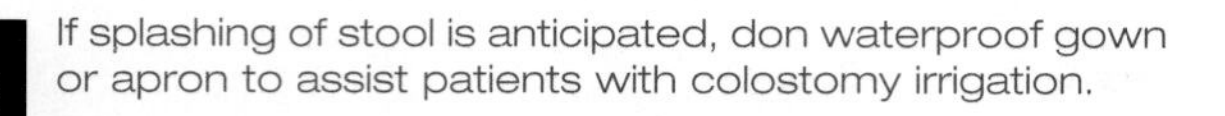

If splashing of stool is anticipated, don waterproof gown or apron to assist patients with colostomy irrigation.

ACTION 5. Lubricate end of cone. Insert cone through opening at top of sleeve, and then into stoma, using rotating motion. Do not force cone or colon perforation or abrasion could occur.

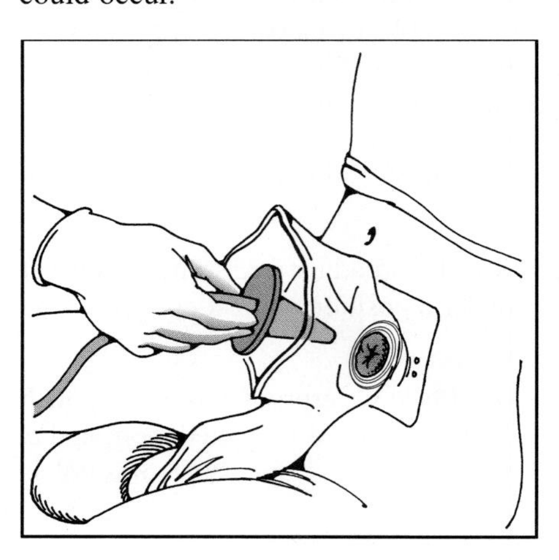

ACTION 6. Open clamp to allow fluid to enter bowel using same precautions as with enema (Procedure 29–5, Actions 19 and 20). Maintain pressure on cone or stoma to prevent backflow out of stoma.

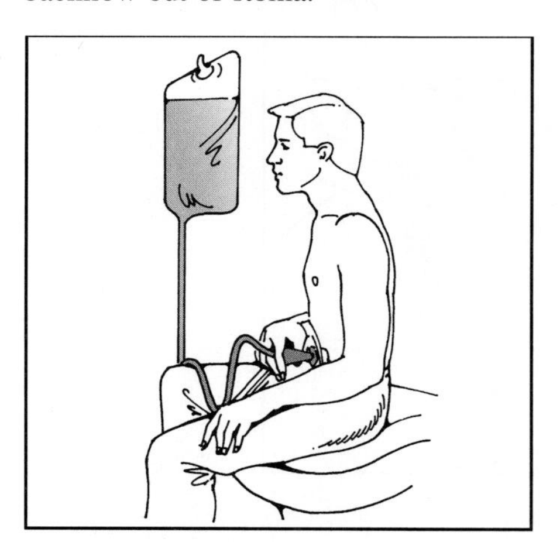

ACTION 7. When fluid has been instilled, remove cone (some prefer to keep cone in place 5–10 minutes). When cone is removed, fluid and feces will flow into toilet or bedpan via sleeve in intermittent bursts.

ACTION 8. After 15 minutes, or when flow of fluid ceases, clean bottom of sleeve, fold to waist, and secure with clamp. Remove and discard gloves (and gown if used) in leak-resistant trash container. Wash hands. Encourage ambulatory patient to move about for 20 to 30 minutes to facilitate elimination of any remaining feces and liquid.

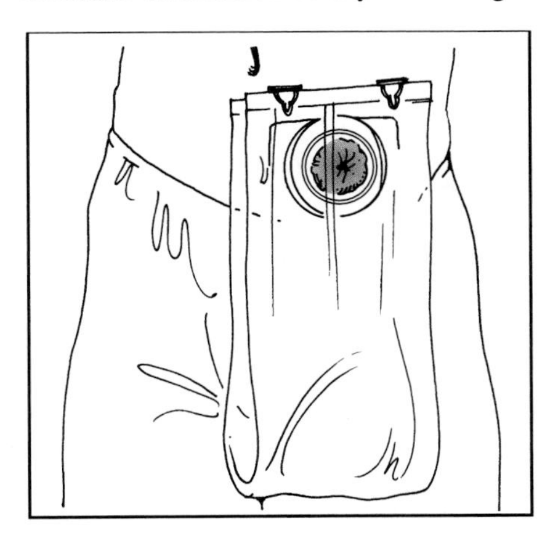

ACTION 9. When evacuation is complete, reglove, and rinse sleeve with tepid soapy water from irrigation container while patient is seated on toilet or bedpan. Cleanser such as Peri-Wash can also be used. Then remove sleeve, store for future use, clean around stoma, dry well, and replace appliance or gauze pad. Remove and discard gloves as in Action 8. Wash hands.

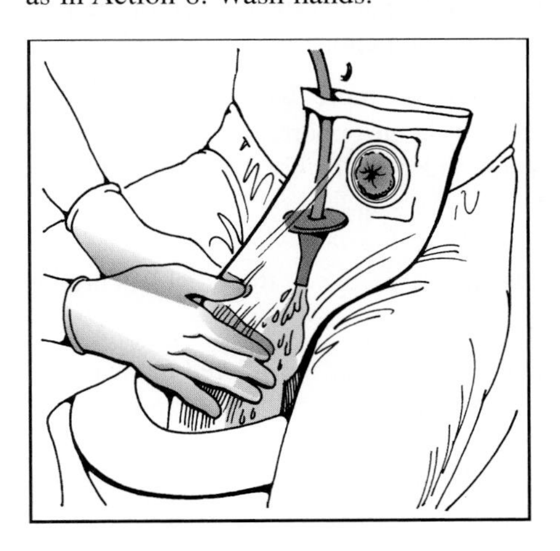

Recording:
Note time of procedure, volume instilled, nature of return, patient response. Describe condition of stoma and peristomal skin, and note replacement of appliance or gauze. If teaching was done, document content of teaching and response.

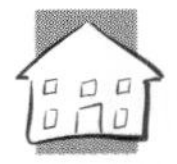

HOME HEALTH ADAPTATION: Creative use of available household items (eg, a clothes hanger on a floor lamp, bathroom cupboard door, or knob) may be necessary to hold an irrigation bag. If irrigation will be a daily procedure, suggest placing a permanent hook on the wall for the patient's convenience.

If bladder control is an issue, it is better to use other methods first to promote bladder function. Complications of catheterization include urinary tract infection, mucosal trauma, and hydronephrosis (collection of urine in the renal pelvis). Urinary tract infections are a major concern. These infections account for 40 percent of all nosocomial infections.

Caring for the Patient With an Indwelling Catheter

The care of the patient with an indwelling catheter is a nursing responsibility. Monitoring for problems and preventing complications are the main nursing roles. Positioning the catheter, maintaining sterility, obtaining specimens, monitoring urinary output,

(continued on page 988)

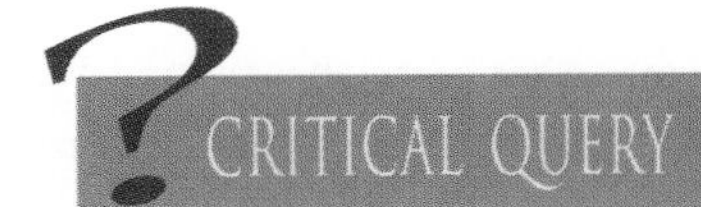

CRITICAL QUERY

Wells and Doughty,[14] authorities on ostomy care, identify the main issues in managing ostomies as skin protection, drainage containment, odor control, ease of application, and cost-effectiveness. One might add patient stress reduction and self-image maintenance. How might the effectiveness of the products used in ostomy care (ostomy pouches, adhesives, odor-absorbing products) contribute to the patient's psychological well-being?

PROCEDURE 29–9. INSERTING A STRAIGHT OR INDWELLING (FOLEY) URINARY CATHETER

PURPOSE: To remove urine from the bladder. Straight catheters are used to relieve retention, measure residual urine, or obtain a sterile urine specimen. Indwelling catheters are used to decompress the bladder during surgery, to maintain drainage in the postoperative period, and as a temporary remedy for incontinence. In some cases indwelling catheters are long term.

EQUIPMENT: Urinary catheterization set, nonsterile gloves, damp washcloth, towel, bath blanket, and extra light source.

ACTION 1. Discuss with the patient the reason for the procedure, desired patient participation, and expected benefits.

RATIONALE. Patient will be more willing to participate and less anxious if there is an opportunity to clarify concerns and the reasons and benefits for the procedure are clear.

ACTION 2. Provide privacy: close door, pull curtains around bed.

RATIONALE. Genital exposure is considered invasive in most cultures. Patient will feel less vulnerable in protected space.

ACTION 3. Wash hands.

RATIONALE. Prevents transfer of transient microorganisms on nurse's hands to patient's environment.

ACTION 4. Raise bed to nurse's waist level.

RATIONALE. Allows nurse to complete procedure with optimal posture, thereby preventing backstrain.

ACTION 5. Assist female patient to dorsal recumbent position, drape with bath blanket: place over patient with one corner directed toward her head, opposite corner over perineum. Wrap the remaining corners, one around each leg over the knee under calf, over ankle. Then anchor the corner under the heel. (Corner over perineum will be folded toward chest during procedure). Male patient should be in supine position with thighs slightly abducted and covers arranged so penis is exposed but legs are covered. Bath blanket can be placed over chest and abdomen if desired.

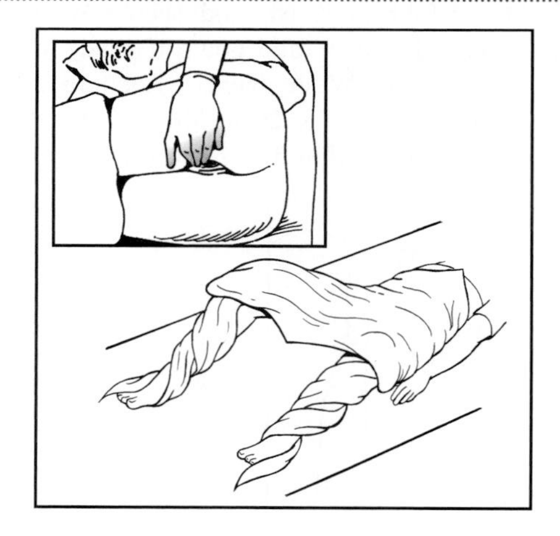

RATIONALE. Position provides access to urinary meatus without straining nurse's back. Draping diminishes feeling of exposure, prevents chilling.

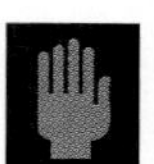

If patient prefers, cover torso only, omit drape over legs. Some elderly or arthritic females are unable to abduct thighs as required in dorsal recumbent position. Side-lying position with upper leg flexed toward shoulder (as in inset) may be used in this case.

ACTION 6. Don nonsterile gloves. Wash perineal area with warm damp washcloth, dry thoroughly. If male patient is not circumcised, retract foreskin during washing. Remove gloves by turning inside-out and discard in leak-resistant trash container.

RATIONALE. Pericare reduces number of microorganisms around meatus. Gloves provide a barrier against perineal organisms, which may be pathogenic.

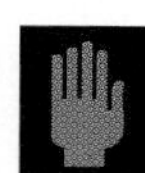

Changes in perineal muscle tone associated with childbirth and aging may alter meatal location in females. Locating meatus during perineal care facilitates correct insertion of catheter.

ACTION 7. Adjust extra light source so beam is directed on perineum. If free-standing lamp is not available, assistant may be needed to hold a flashlight.

RATIONALE. Normal room lights may not provide sufficient focused light to locate female patient's meatus.

ACTION 8. Expose perineum. Place catheter set between patient's legs and unwrap, touching corners only, creating sterile field. (See Procedure 25–2.) Most sets are packaged in a plastic bag, which can be taped to siderail for disposal of used supplies.

RATIONALE. Facilitates carrying out procedure with minimal reaching over sterile field, thereby reducing possibility of contamination.

ACTION 9. Unfold sterile underpad by grasping one corner with fingertips, lifting it away from sterile field and shaking it. Then grasp opposite corner. *Male patient:* slip drape under penis, covering thighs. *Female patient:* Ask patient to raise buttocks, then slide drape about 2 inches under buttocks.

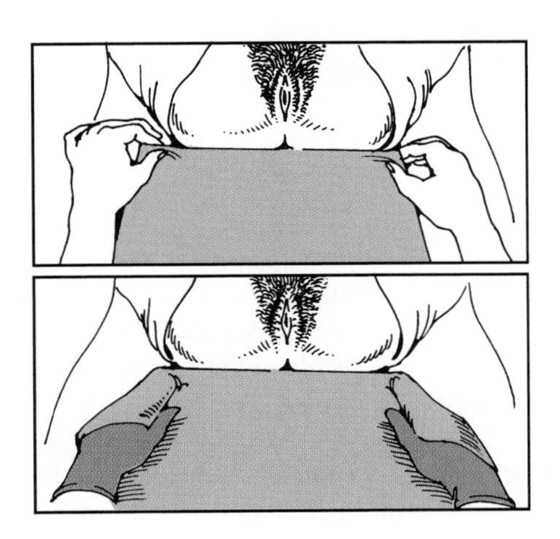

If sterile gloves are packaged on top in the catheterization set, don gloves (see Procedure 25–3). Pick up drape as described, then fold corners over your hands so gloves are covered while placing drape under female.

RATIONALE. Drape and wrapper now create a continuous sterile field that acts as a barrier to microorganisms. Nurse has not touched portion of field on which sterile supplies will be placed.

ACTION 10. Don sterile gloves and prepare sterile field as follows. (For straight catheterization, omit Actions a and b.)

RATIONALE. Sterile gloves act as a barrier preventing transfer of organisms from the nurse's hands to objects that will contact or enter sterile body cavity (bladder). Preparation of field requires two hands, so must be completed before nurse begins cleansing perineum. Gloved hands should touch only sterile items when preparing field.

a. Close clamp at base of collection bag attached to catheter. In most sets, bag and catheter are beneath tray holding lubricant, cotton, etc.

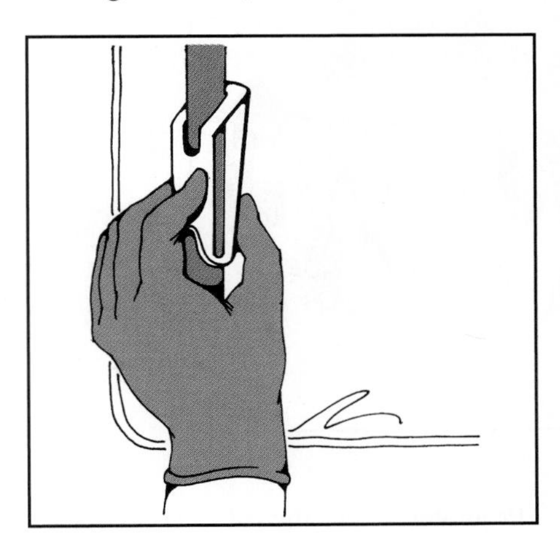

b. Place fenestrated drape so opening exposes labia or penis.

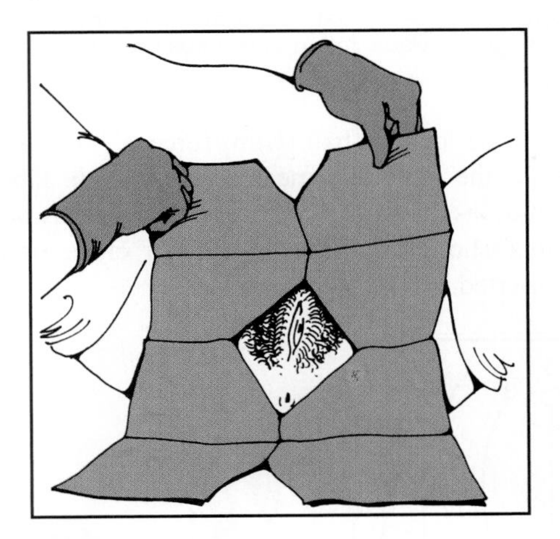

Often omitted as it may slip, risking contamination.

c. Pour antiseptic over cotton balls, squeeze lubricant on tray, open specimen container.

Lubricant is in a syringe in some kits.

Continued

Procedure 29–9. Inserting a Urinary Catheter (continued)

ACTION 11. Cleanse patient as follows.

FEMALE PATIENT:

a. Expose the meatus by spreading labia minora *outward* and *upward*: place the thumb and index or middle finger of your nondominant hand about midway down the labia, between the labia minora; spread your fingers then pull tissue gently upward.

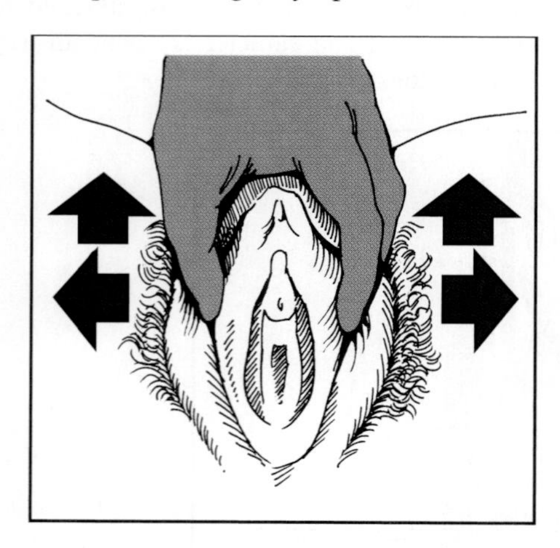

RATIONALE. Promotes cleansing of meatus and surrounding skin folds, reducing possibility of introducing organisms into the bladder.

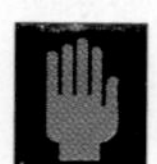

Placing the fingers on the upper half of the labia majora to expose meatus is a frequent error. Poor cleansing and visualization of meatus results.

b. Holding one cotton ball with forceps for each stroke, cleanse the labia and meatus. Clean from labia majora inward, as shown in figure, using downward strokes. Labia should not be allowed to close until catheter is inserted.

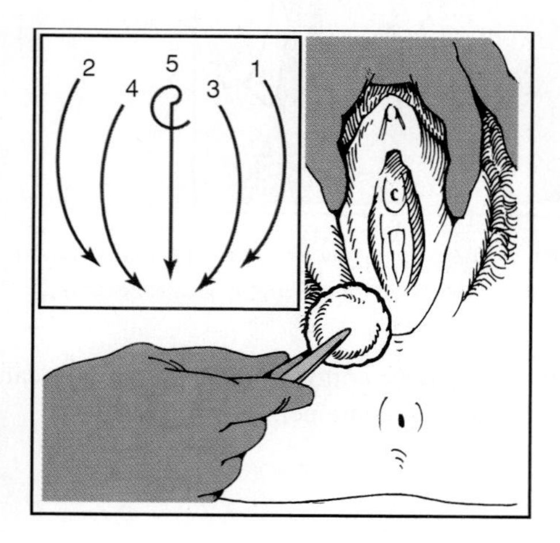

RATIONALE. Friction and chemical action reduce bacterial population around meatus. Using new swab for each stroke and maintaining labia in open position prevent transfer of microorganisms from contaminated to cleaned area.

Using a twisting motion when cleaning over the meatus may cause it to open slightly, facilitating visualization.

MALE PATIENT:

a. Hold the penis up by grasping the shaft just below the glans.

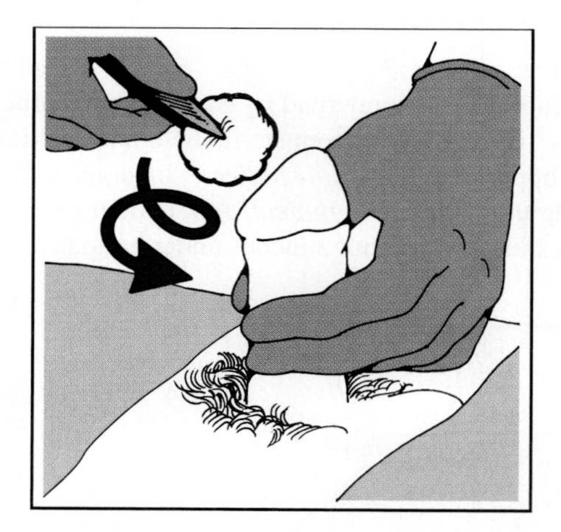

b. Clean the glans in a circular motion from meatus outward. Repeat three times using separate swab for each stroke. Continue to hold penis in this position until catheter has been inserted.

RATIONALE. Friction and chemical action reduce bacterial population around meatus. Using new swab for each stroke and maintaining penis in upward position prevent transfer of microorganisms from contaminated to cleaned area.

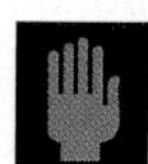

If foreskin has not remained retracted, it must be retracted prior to cleansing to remove organisms beneath it.

ACTION 12. Generously lubricate catheter tip: 2 to 3 inches for female, 6 to 7 inches for male.

RATIONALE. Lubrication reduces trauma to urethra from friction. Male urethra is longer, so more lubrication is needed.

Some experts advocate instilling lubricant directly into the male urethra to improve lubrication.

Procedure 29–9. (continued)

ACTION 13. If inserting a straight catheter, place the collection basin near the meatus and place distal end of catheter in it.

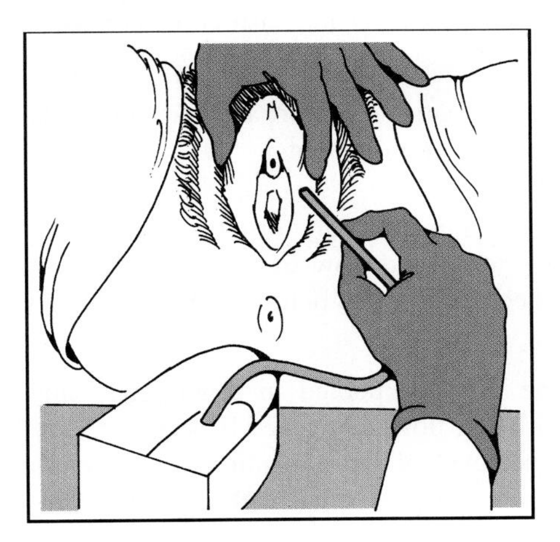

RATIONALE. Urine will flow out of catheter as soon as bladder is entered.

ACTION 14. Tell patient you are ready to insert the catheter, which will create a sensation similar to voiding; or rarely, pressure and mild burning; and that the sensation will cease when catheter is in place. Suggest that patient take a deep breath, then exhale.

RATIONALE. If the patient knows what to expect, anxiety is decreased, trust increased. A deep breath facilitates sphincter relaxation, minimizing irritation.

ACTION 15. As patient exhales, insert the catheter in the direction of the urethra: in females parallel to the plane of the bed, then slightly downward, 2 to 3 inches; in males toward the abdomen, 8 to 9 inches. Slight resistance is commonly felt when catheter passes external and internal sphincters. Twist catheter slightly, and then pause or change the angle of the penis slightly to relax sphincters. Do not try to force catheter.

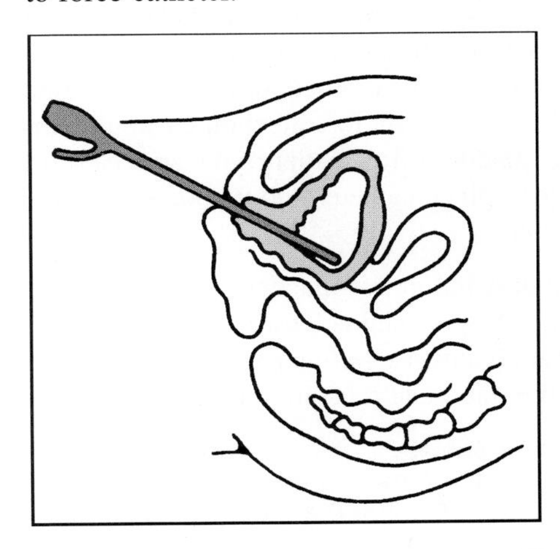

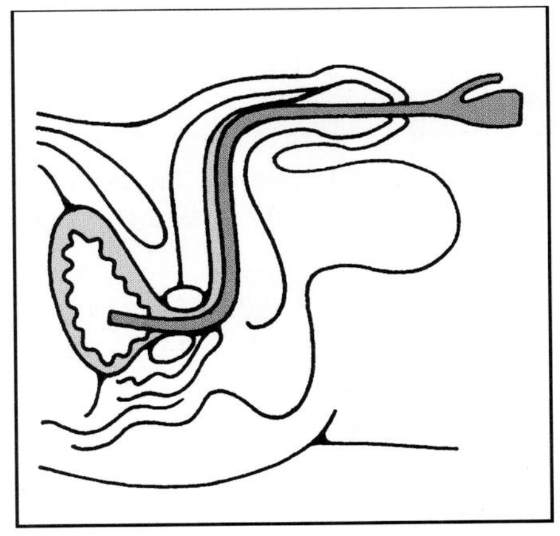

RATIONALE. Following the anatomical direction reduces discomfort and irritation.

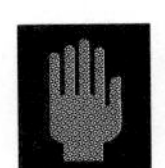

If catheter has been advanced 4 to 5 inches in a female patient with no urine return, it is likely that the catheter is in the vagina. Leave it in place to assist in correct location of meatus, obtain a new catheter set, and begin again. In males, unusual resistance may be caused by strictures, prostate enlargement, or other abnormality. If a smaller diameter-catheter cannot be inserted, consult with physician.

Continued

ACTION 16. When urine flow is noted, advance catheter 1 to 2 inches, then hold it in place with nondominant hand.

RATIONALE. Advancing catheter well into bladder facilitates emptying and prevents trauma to bladder neck when retention balloon is inflated. Forcing catheter may cause urethral trauma.

ACTION 17. For a straight catheter, hold catheter in place until urine flow ceases. (If specimen is required, pinch catheter after several mL have drained, direct flow of urine into specimen cup, then redirect to collection basin to complete emptying of bladder.) Tell patient you are ready to remove catheter, then pinch catheter and withdraw in same direction as insertion.

RATIONALE. Withdrawing in this manner minimizes irritation. Sterile midstream specimen is least likely to be contaminated by perineal organisms. Telling patients before withdrawing catheter will facilitate relaxation (see Action 14).

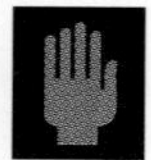

Some sources indicate that no more than 750 mL should be drained from bladder at one time. Rapid decrease in intra-abdominal pressure may cause reflex dilation of pelvic vessels, which decreases venous return to the heart, lowering blood pressure. Follow agency policy. Recent review of the research literature indicates that this practice may be an unnecessary tradition.[15]

ACTION 18. For retention catheter, inject all liquid in syringe to inflate balloon, then tug gently to assure catheter is anchored.

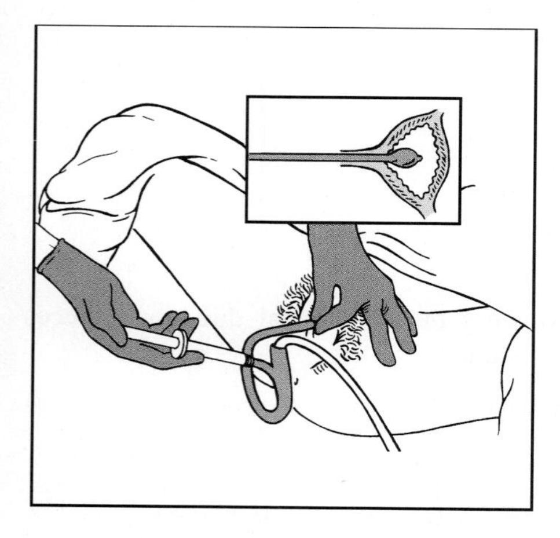

RATIONALE. A 5-mL balloon requires 8 mL of liquid because 3 mL remains in the lumen of the catheter. A partially inflated balloon may traumatize bladder neck.

ACTION 19. Clean patient's perineum of residual lubricant and antiseptic. If foreskin was retracted, replace it over glans. Remove used equipment, including drapes and gloves, and discard in leak-resistant trash container. Wash hands.

RATIONALE. Promotes patient comfort and prevents transfer of microorganisms to environment.

ACTION 20. Hang drainage bag on bedframe. Coil drainage tubing so downward flow of urine to collection bag is facilitated. Secure tubing to bottom sheet with safety pin or clamp.

RATIONALE. Urine that has pooled in tubing may flow back into bladder if urine flow is impeded by kinks or loops in tubing below the level of the collection bag. Bacteria growing in this urine is a cause of catheter-induced urinary tract infections.

ACTION 21. Tape catheter, allowing slack between perineum and tape to allow for changes in position without creating tension on balloon in bladder.

RATIONALE. Pulling on the catheter as a result of movement or tangling will be directed against the tape, not the bladder neck, as would be the case were the catheter not taped securely.

FEMALE PATIENTS:

Tape catheter to inner thigh.

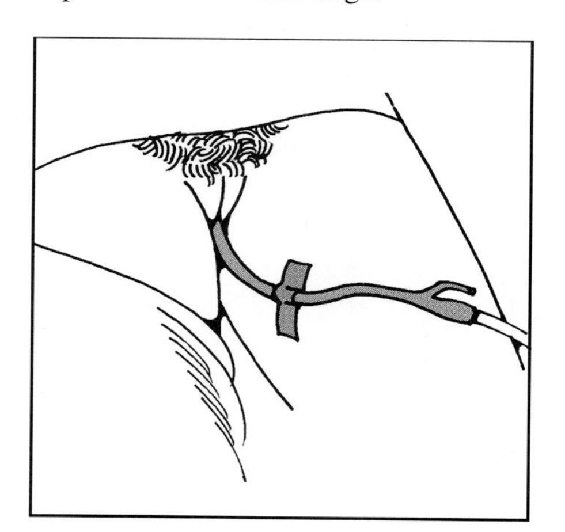

Procedure 29–9. (continued)

MALE PATIENTS:

Tape catheter to abdomen or to anterior thigh depending on agency policy.

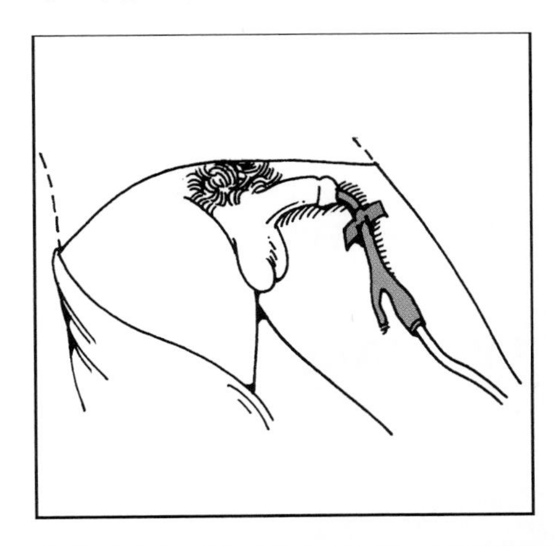

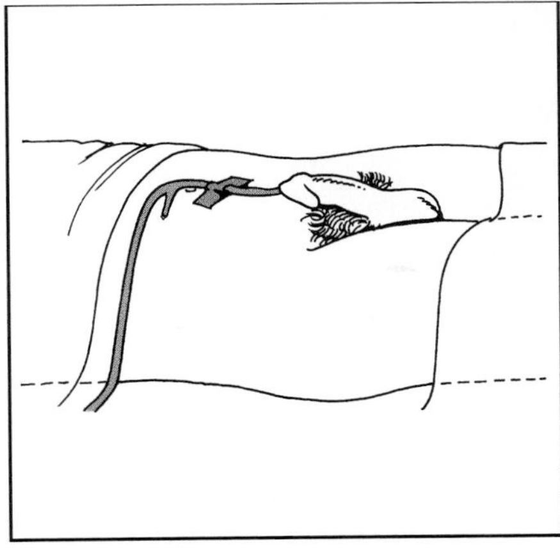

RATIONALE. Pressure at the penile–scrotal junction caused by bending the catheter, which some urologists feel increases potential for tissue necrosis, is eliminated if the catheter is secured to the abdomen.

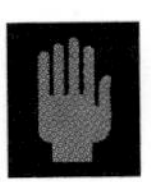

Taping must be rechecked frequently. Some facilities use commercially prepared catheter straps to secure catheters.

ACTION 23. If specimen is needed, it may be obtained from drainage bag. Don nonsterile gloves to obtain specimen. Label and send to lab (see Procedure 29–10).

RATIONALE. Because catheter has just been inserted, bag contains fresh urine. Gloves protect nurse's hands from any organisms in patient's urine.

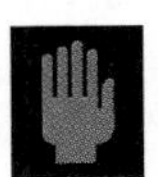

Subsequent specimens must be obtained via special port (see Procedure 29–10).

ACTION 24. Inform patient that lying on drainage tube will impede urine flow, pulling on catheter may cause pain and injury, and raising drainage collector above the level of the bladder is a cause of infections in the bladder.

RATIONALE. An informed patient can assume responsibility for health-related behaviors and can protect self from errors by uninformed providers.

Recording:
Note type (straight or indwelling) and size of catheter inserted; amount and character of urine obtained; problems, if any, and action taken; patient's response to procedure; and type, reason, and disposition of specimen.

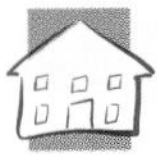

HOME HEALTH ADAPTATION: Have available additional catheter sets, catheters of varying sizes, and sterile gloves. Safely position patient close to side of bed to minimize back strain. Request assistance with positioning from caregiver whenever possible. Drape patient with sheet, blanket, or towels to protect modesty and for warmth. If a freestanding lamp is not available, place pillows at foot of bed and create a crevice in pillow to hold flashlight at appropriate angle for meatus visualization.

and teaching are some of the approaches nurses use with catheterized patients.

Handwashing prior to and after contact with any part of the catheter is mandatory. Research has shown that personnel who fail to wash their hands between manipulating catheters can cause cross-contamination among patients. Gloving alone is not sufficient to prevent this problem. For example, hands should be washed and then gloved before the catheter drainage bag is emptied. Once the emptying is done, gloves should be removed and the hands washed once again. Some experts recommend that patients with catheters not be roomed together because of the high rate of cross-contamination.

Perineal care is recommended at least twice daily when a patient has an indwelling catheter. This care should include cleaning the first 1 to 2 inches of tubing as it leaves the meatus. Secretions are a good medium for bacterial growth and should be removed gently with soap and water (see Chap. 27).

Correct positioning of the drainage bag and tubing is another important aspect of indwelling catheter care. The tubing should hang freely at all times and be kept free of kinks or compression.

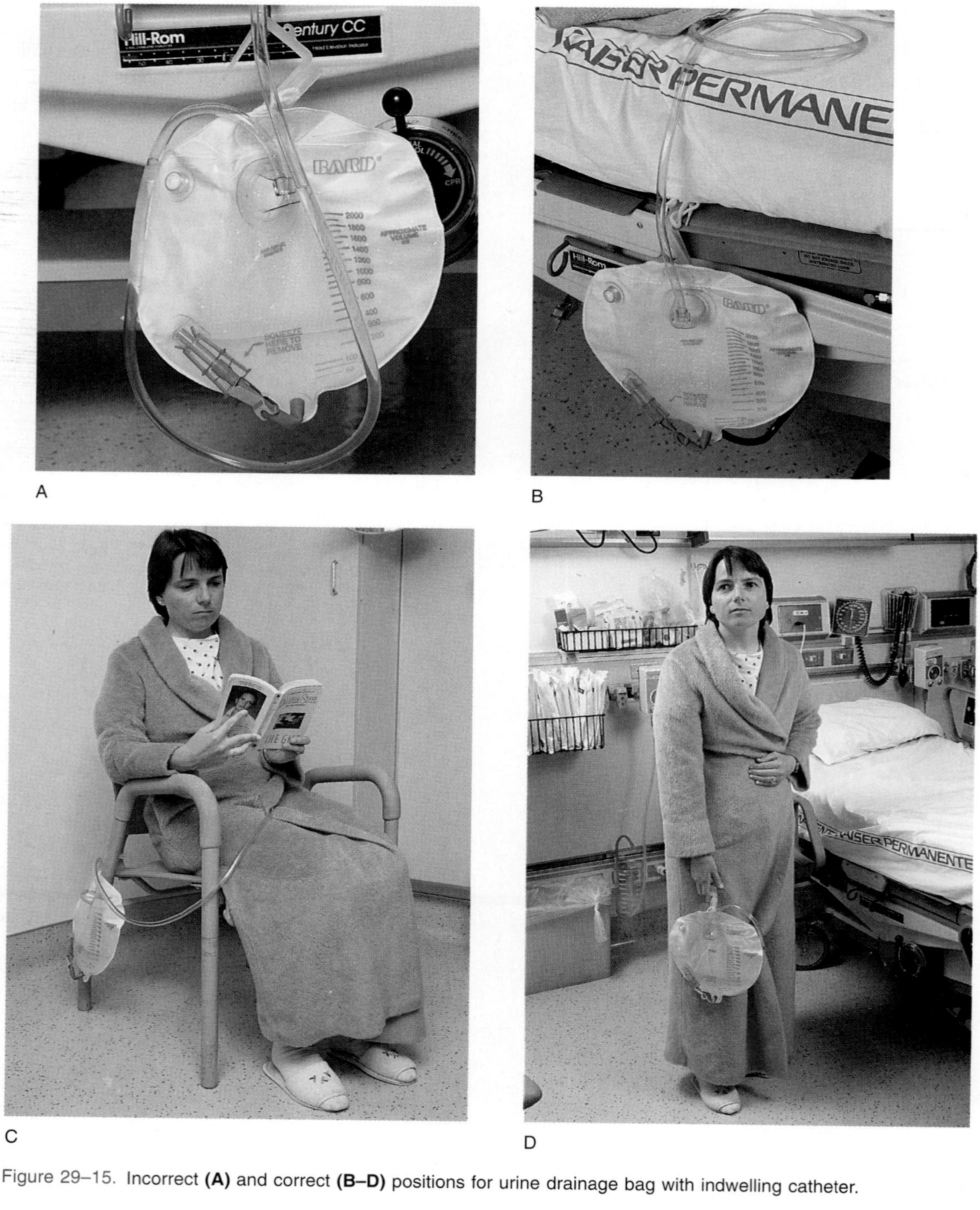

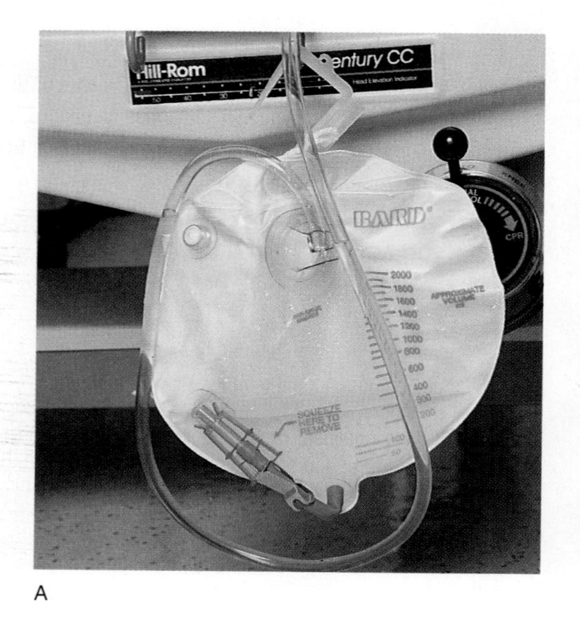

A

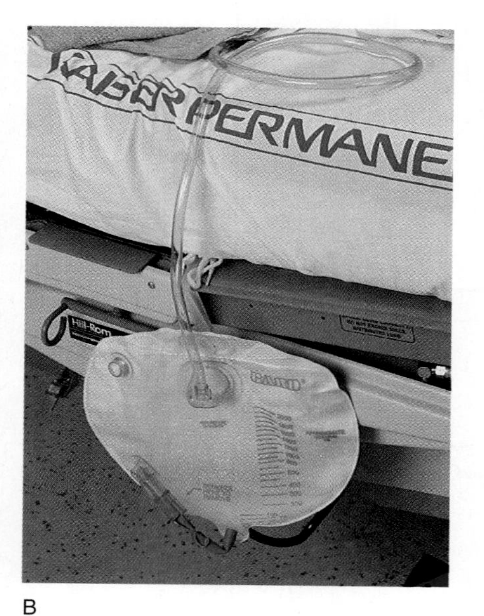

B

C

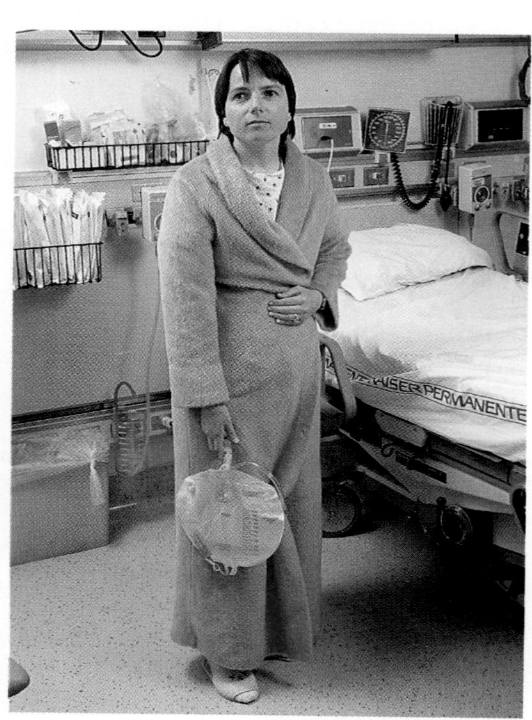

D

Figure 29–15. Incorrect **(A)** and correct **(B–D)** positions for urine drainage bag with indwelling catheter.

The drainage bag should be kept below the level of the bladder at all times, and the drainage tubing should not drape below the level of the bag. Urine in the collection bag is a medium for bacterial growth; reflux of this contaminated urine into the bladder is a cause of urinary tract infections. When the patient is in bed, the bag should hang on the bedframe; when the patient is in a chair, the bag should hang on the side of the chair below the level of the bladder. The bag should be carried below the waist when ambulating, and it should never be placed on the floor. Figure 29–15 illustrates correct and incorrect positioning for the urine collection bag.

Emptying the urine collection bag must be done in such a way that contamination is avoided. At the bottom of the bag is a tube that drains the bag; this is always clamped, except when emptying. This drainage tube is housed in a protective covering that is connected to the drainage bag (Fig. 29–15). The urine should be emptied and measured using a graduated container that is used for urine only and that is used for only one patient. Bags are usually emptied only once every shift unless full.

Monitoring urine output is another nursing responsibility. Urine is monitored for color, amount, clarity, and odor. The frequency of monitoring depends on the patient's condition. Some drainage bags have calibrated auxiliary containers, which allow for relatively precise hourly output readings without opening the system (Fig. 29–16). Nurses should question patients about discomfort, such as pain or burning around the catheter. Urine draining from a catheter should be clear, yellow, and odorless.

If a urine specimen is needed from a patient with an indwelling catheter, it should be obtained from a specific area near the proximal end of the catheter tubing where fresh sterile urine can be aseptically obtained. This portion of the tubing is made of resealable rubber and is often called a cathport. The urine is removed using sterile technique (see Procedure 29–10).

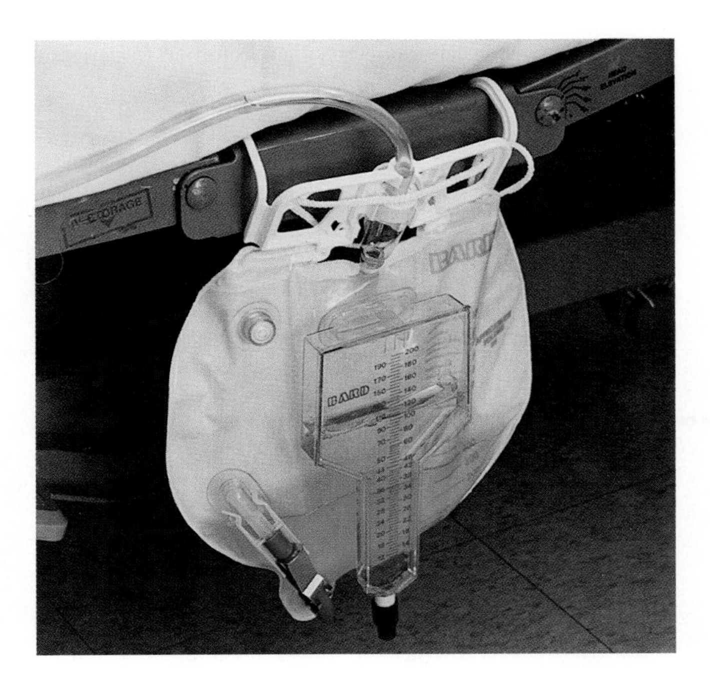

Figure 29–16. **Urinary drainage bag with attached urine meter.** *(From Smith S, Duell D.* Clinical Nursing Skills: Nursing Process Model, Basic to Advanced Skills. *4th ed. Stamford, CT: Appleton & Lange; 1996.)*

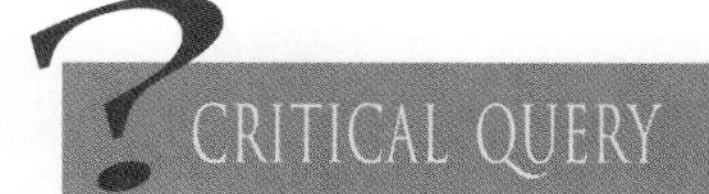

Brooks,[15] who did a study of incontinence in a group of homebound elderly patients, found that home care nurses knew more about methods for treating urinary incontinence than about distinguishing types of incontinence. What implications might this finding have for the care that patients receive?

Removing a Retention Catheter

Removing a retention catheter is a relatively simple procedure. Nurses can reassure patients that discomfort will be minimal.

Remove the tape anchoring the catheter and then place a waterproof pad between the legs of a female patient or over the scrotum and thighs of a male. Don nonsterile gloves and insert the appropriate-size sterile syringe, without a needle, into the valve at the end of the balloon arm. Draw out fluid until negative pressure is felt. (Some types of catheters require that a syringe and needle be used to withdraw the fluid, and some require only that the nurse cut the balloon part and allow the fluid to drain.) Be certain to withdraw the full amount of fluid injected when the catheter was inserted.

Remove the syringe from the valve. Instruct the patient to take a deep breath, and gently withdraw the catheter as the patient exhales. If the catheter does not withdraw easily, do not use force. Notify the physician for further intervention. After the catheter is removed, the nurse should discuss measures to promote normal elimination. Encourage fluid intake and emphasize the importance of responding promptly to the urge to void. Patients are also asked to urinate into a container in which the urine can be measured so urination patterns can be monitored.

An indwelling catheter may be left in place for days, weeks or months, depending on physician's orders. Catheters are not changed on a routine basis, but only as needed. Catheter bags and tubing should be changed if there is an excess of built-up sediment, leakage, or contamination. Sylastic catheters are reported to need changing less frequently than latex catheters and therefore are recommended for people who need long-term catheter placement.

Applying an External Catheter

An external or condom catheter is a device that fits over the penis and is then attached to a drainage collection system. It is most frequently used for patients with total urinary incontinence, although it may be used for bladder training or collection of a urine specimen. External catheters are also called Texas catheters. Although an external catheter can be made from a condom, tape, tubing, and a collecting bag, commercially made catheters are readily available. Figure 29–17 illustrates various samples.

Applying the external catheter is not an invasive procedure, so there tends to be less trauma to the urinary tract and less potential for infection than with an indwelling catheter. However, skin excoriation and necrosis may occur, and external catheters may be difficult to keep in place. Careful monitoring of the catheter and perineum is mandatory, and the catheter should be replaced at least once every 24 hours (see Procedure 29–11).

(continued on page 993)

PROCEDURE 29–10. OBTAINING A SPECIMEN FROM AN INDWELLING CATHETER

PURPOSE: To collect sterile urine for testing when a catheter is in place.
EQUIPMENT: Clamp or rubber band, nonsterile gloves, sterile alcohol wipes, a 3- to 10-mL sterile syringe with a 1-inch 21- to 25-gauge needle (or plastic cannula for needle-less systems), and specimen cup (must be sterile if sample is for culture).

ACTION 1. Discuss the reason for the procedure, including expected patient participation and benefits. Screen patient, and place clamp or rubber band on drainage tubing, just distal to the aspiration port.

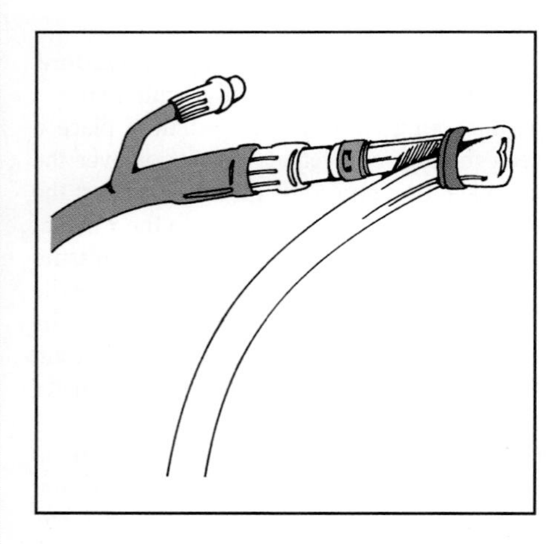

ACTION 2. Return in 10 to 15 minutes, don gloves. Cleanse aspiration port with alcohol swab and insert needle into port at a 30 degree angle (see A and B). If drainage system has no port, cleanse distal end of catheter and insert needle distal to balloon inlet at a 30 degree angle toward drainage tube (C).

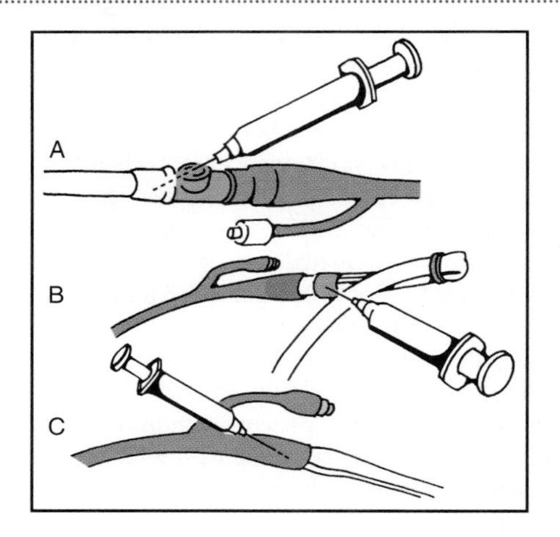

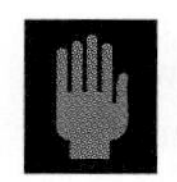

In response to the need for needle safety, some manufacturers produce a sample port on the drainage tubing that is accessed using a blunt cannula to obtain a specimen.

ACTION 3. Withdraw 3 to 20 mL of urine (varies with number and type of tests ordered). Transfer urine to appropriate specimen container, label, and arrange for transport to lab within 30 minutes. May refrigerate sample for up to 1 hour without affecting accuracy of most tests.

ACTION 4. When laboratory result is returned to patient's chart, inform patient of result.

Recording:
Note character of urine, reason for specimen, and date and time sent to laboratory.

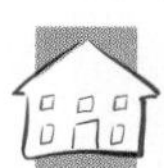

HOME HEALTH ADAPTATION: Obtaining a specimen from an indwelling catheter does not vary with setting.

PROCEDURE 29–11. APPLYING AN EXTERNAL (CONDOM OR TEXAS) CATHETER

PURPOSE: To prevent soiling and skin excoriation from urinary incontinence. To collect a urine specimen from a patient lacking voluntary control of urination.

EQUIPMENT: External catheter with adhesive (cloverleaf or spiral to apply directly to penis, or elastic tape or Velcro strap to apply outside the catheter sheath); nonsterile gloves, warm damp washcloth and towel; drainage collection bag (leg bag or indwelling catheter type); blunt scissors; and skin protector/tincture of benzoin (optional).

ACTION 1. Discuss with the patient the reason for the procedure, desired patient participation, and expected benefits.

RATIONALE. Patient will be more willing to participate and less anxious if there is an opportunity to clarify concerns and the reasons and benefits for the procedure are clear.

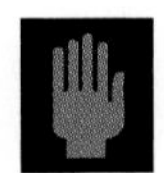

This device is often used on patients who seem unable to comprehend explanation; but explanation should not be omitted, as patients may understand even though they do not respond.

ACTION 2. Close door, pull curtains around bed.

RATIONALE. Genital exposure is considered invasive in most cultures. Patient will feel less vulnerable in protected space.

ACTION 3. Wash hands.

RATIONALE. Prevents transfer of transient microorganisms on nurse's hands to patient's environment.

ACTION 4. Raise bed to nurse's waist level.

RATIONALE. Allows nurse to complete procedure with optimal posture, thereby preventing backstrain.

ACTION 5. Assist patient to supine or semi-Fowler's position with thighs slightly abducted and covers arranged so penis is exposed but legs are covered. Bath blanket can be placed over chest and abdomen if desired.

RATIONALE. Position provides access to urinary meatus without straining nurse's back. Draping diminishes feeling of exposure, prevents chilling.

ACTION 6. Don nonsterile gloves. Wash perineal area with warm washcloth, dry thoroughly. If patient is not circumcised, retract foreskin during washing, then replace. Assess penis and scrotum for skin irritation or edema. Document nature of lesions and action taken.

RATIONALE. Gloves provide a barrier against perineal organisms, which may be pathogenic. Perineal care removes organisms and secretions that may cause skin irritation under catheter sheath.

Catheter should not be applied over irritated skin unless skin barrier type of adhesive such as cloverleaf is used.

ACTION 7. Clip hairs at base of penis. If using adhesive inside sheath apply as follows.

a. *Cloverleaf:* Carefully pull the glans through the opening in the cloverleaf, remove protective backing on underside, press each "leaf" against shaft of penis, taking care to push away any hairs. Remove backing from outside of cloverleaf. Adhesive surface is now exposed to secure catheter.

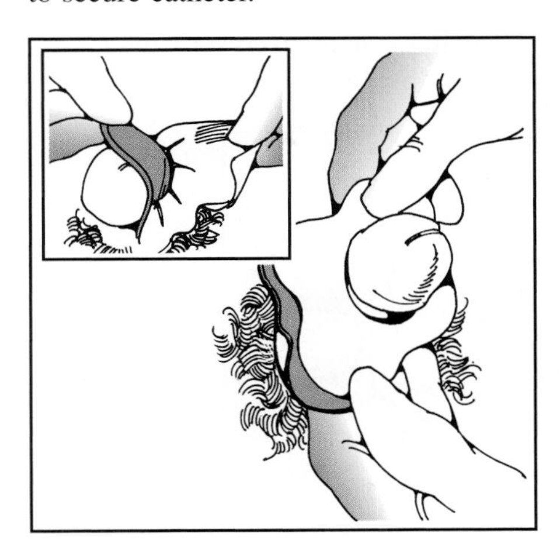

RATIONALE. Hairs easily adhere to adhesive, causing discomfort upon removal. Cloverleaf device is stretchable, so will accommodate changes in size of penis, such as an erection.

Continued

b. *Spiral:* Remove backing from one side of the double-sided foam adhesive strip and wrap it around the shaft of the penis in spiral fashion. Ends of strip should not overlap. Tincture of benzoin or protective skin spray may be used under strip. Remove backing from outside of foam strip.

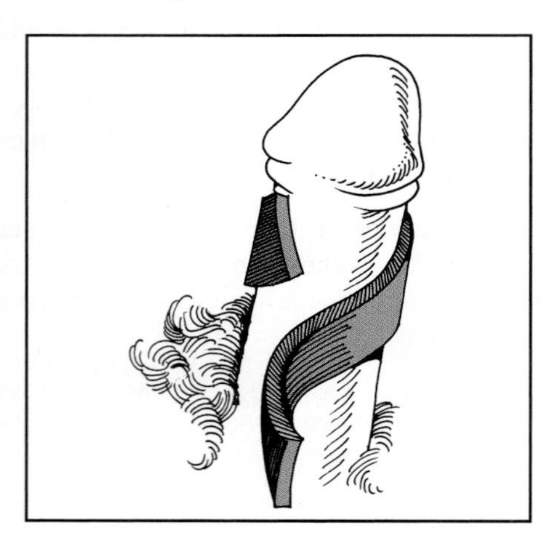

RATIONALE. If ends of adhesive overlap, circulation to penis would be impeded if size of penis increases. Spiral strips are not made from skin-protective barrier material, so benzoin or spray may be needed to protect sensitive skin from adhesive-related irritation.

ACTION 8. If sheath is not rolled, roll the top downward. Some types have an inner flap to prevent reflux, which should be exposed by rolling as in figure.

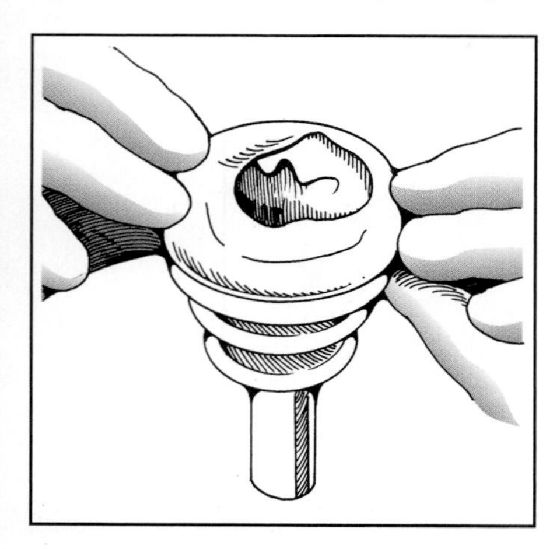

RATIONALE. Rolled sheath is easier to fit smoothly over penis.

ACTION 9. Position sheath so inner flap is centered around meatus. If there is no flap, place sheath over glans so there is a space of 1–2 inches (2.5–5 cm) between the tip of the glans and the tip of the sheath. Roll catheter smoothly up shaft of penis until adhesive is covered. Sheath usually covers ¾ of the length of the penis.

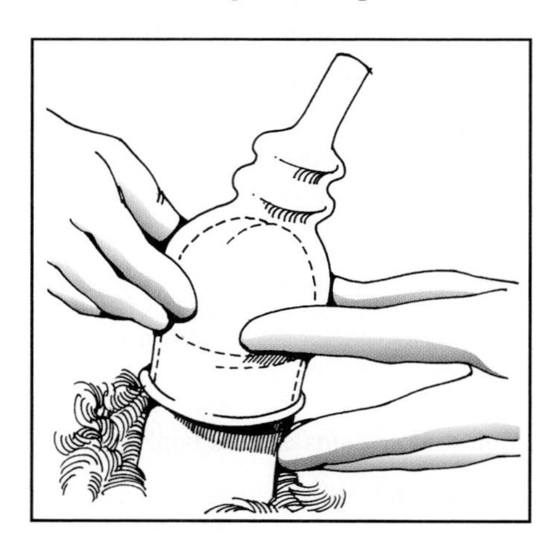

RATIONALE. Inner flap must fit around meatus to prevent reflux. Sheath must be wrinkle free to diminish pressure or pulling on skin. Leaving space at end of sheath prevents irritation due to friction on glans and allows for free drainage of urine.

ACTION 10. If no adhesive was used prior to applying, secure sheath with a strip of elastic tape wrapped over sheath in a close spiral (see illustration, Action 7b) or in a circular fashion with ends abutted, not overlapping. Velcro or rubber strap may be used. Follow manufacturer's directions.

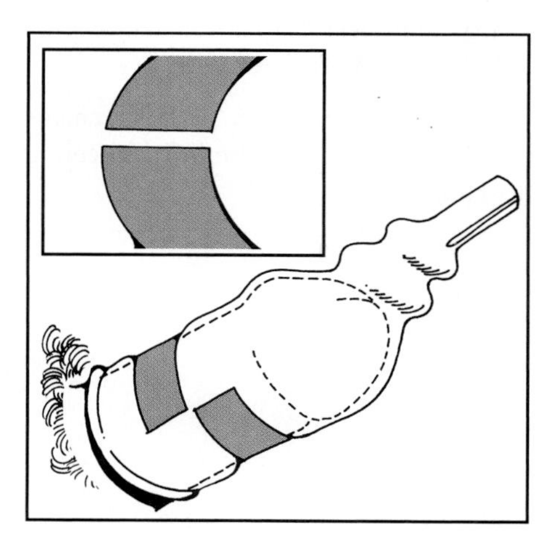

RATIONALE. Overlapping tape will cut off circulation to the penis if increase in size occurs.

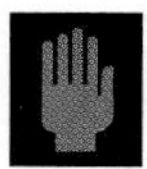

Nonelastic tape should never be used to secure catheter.

ACTION 11. Attach drainage system securely to end of sheath.

RATIONALE. Provides conduit for urine, keeping patient and bed dry.

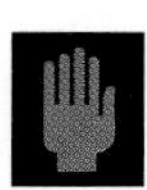

Leg bag is preferred for active patient.

ACTION 12. Hang drainage bag on bedframe. Coil drainage tubing so downward flow of urine to collection bag is facilitated. Secure tubing to bottom sheet with rubber band and safety pin or clamp.

RATIONALE. Urine that has pooled in tubing may flow back toward penis if urine flow is impeded by kinks or loops in tubing below the level of the collection bag. Bacteria growing in this urine is a cause of catheter-induced urinary tract infections. Moisture macerates skin.

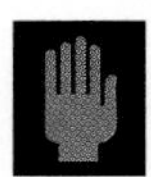

Leg bag has two elastic or rubber straps that secure it to lower leg. Tubing should be long enough to prevent pulling on catheter with movement.

ACTION 13. Assess the condition of the penis 15 minutes after application, then hourly × 2. Routine assessment is necessary whenever position is changed or at least twice per shift.

RATIONALE. If tape is too tight, circulatory stasis will be evidenced by discoloration, then edema. This must be corrected immediately to prevent necrosis. Position changes may cause twisting of the drainage tube, causing pressure on penis.

ACTION 14. Remove catheter daily to assess skin condition and provide peri care.

RATIONALE. Moisture from perspiration or urine that cannot evaporate make skin under sheath particularly vulnerable to breakdown.

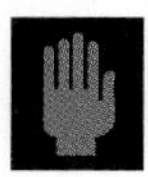

If breaks in skin are noted, an alternative method of applying catheter, or alternative method of collecting urine, is indicated.

ACTION 15. To remove sheath, remove tape and roll or slip sheath off penis. If adhesive was applied directly to penis, use adhesive remover or alcohol swabs to moisten adhesive surface before removing. Protective skin spray peels off readily; benzoin may be washed off.

RATIONALE. If adhesive is not removed carefully, skin may be damaged.

Recording:

Note condition of perineal area, type of device and adhesive applied, and amount and character of urine collected. Document daily replacement of catheter and skin condition at the time catheter is changed.

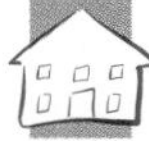

HOME HEALTH ADAPTATION. Teach family members or caregivers how to apply and remove external catheter. Instruct them to inspect penis for discoloration or edema following initial application and to remove catheter promptly and contact the case manager for additional instructions. Also instruct them that each day the external catheter is removed, skin condition is inspected and the catheter is reapplied if no breaks are noted.

Irrigating a Urinary Catheter

Catheter irrigations are usually done to maintain or restore patency when sediment, such as pus or blood, interferes with drainage. Sodium chloride is the most common solution used for urinary irrigation. Use of sterile technique is vital.

When irrigations are anticipated on a regular basis, the *closed irrigation* method should be used (Fig. 29–18). The closed technique is the preferred method of maintaining catheter patency because it minimizes the possibility of introducing microorganisms during irrigation. Closed irrigations may be continuous or intermittent. *Open irrigation* (also called hand irrigation) is sometimes used to restore patency of a urinary drainage system. Hand irrigation involves separating the drainage tubing from the catheter and irrigating the catheter via a syringe (Fig. 29–19). Observe for return of irrigant and repeat with additional fluid per agency policy. Open irrigation is less desirable because there is a high likelihood of introducing microorganisms when the opened system is manipulated. Therefore, infection is more common when open irrigation is done. Irrigant fluid (open and closed) is charted as intake.

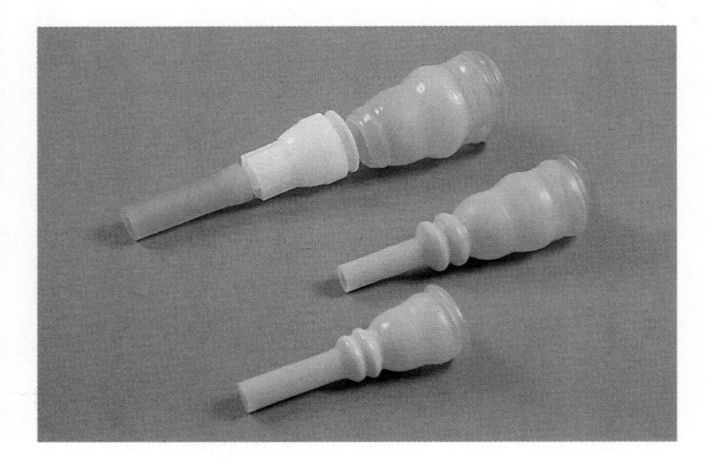

Figure 29–17. Condom catheters of various types and sizes.

INSIGHTS FROM NURSING LITERATURE

INDWELLING URINARY CATHETER IRRIGATION

Getliffe KA. Bladder instillations and bladder washouts in the management of catheterized patients. J Adv Nurs. *1996; 23:548–554.*

According to this article, the most common cause of recurrent urinary catheter blockage is the precipitation of minerals in the urine. Crystal-like precipitates form encrustations in the catheter lumen, which gradually grow to block the flow of urine out of the catheter. This process occurs under alkaline urinary pH conditions, and involves the release of ammonia from urea by urease-producing bacteria in the urine. The author summarizes numerous studies of various treatment methods, most of which involve irrigating the catheter and bladder with acidic washout fluids. These studies, as the author notes, document risks, but show only conflicting results on the benefits of irrigation with saline or various acidic fluid irrigants. Thus, nurses often have to rely on frequent catheter changes to prevent mineral accumulation and catheter blockage.

Home Health Care

Restorative home health care involves caring for patients who have had episodes of illness that result in bowel or bladder dysfunction. With the trend toward shorter hospital stays, it is not uncommon for patients to require IVs, indwelling catheters, and urinary collecting systems in the home. Indeed, home care nurses often teach patients and caregivers how to insert and care for catheters, how to empty and change a urine collector bag, and how to recognize the signs of catheter blockage or urinary infection.

A common home care problem is catheter obstruction. Nurses teach patients and their caregivers the signs of catheter obstruction, and what to do should an obstruction occur. Patients are taught, for example, to make sure that their catheters do not become kinked and are free of external pressure that may obstruct the catheter. Further, they are taught to change their body position. Changing position may alter the way the catheter lies in the bladder; how a catheter lies is sometimes a cause of obstruction. When these measures fail, however, patients are taught to replace their

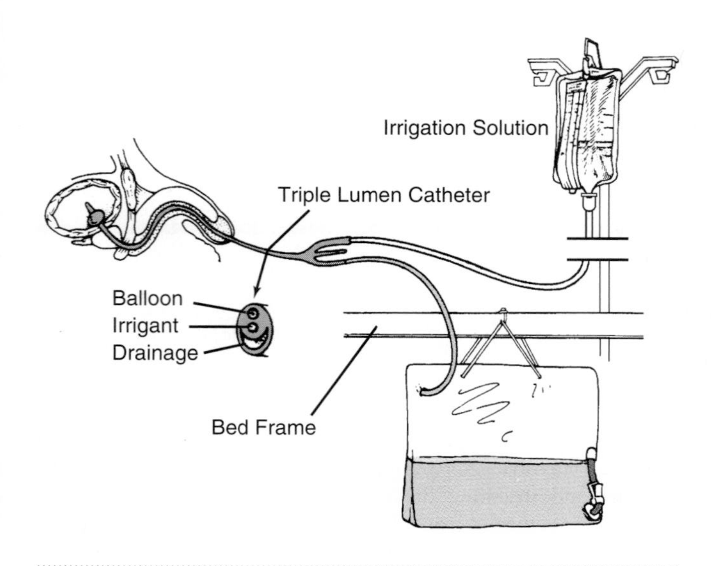

Figure 29–18. Setup for closed bladder irrigation using a triple-lumen catheter. *(Adapted from Smith S, Duell D.* Clinical Nursing Skills: Nursing Process Model, Basic to Advanced Skills. *3rd ed. Norwalk, CT: Appleton & Lange; 1992.)*

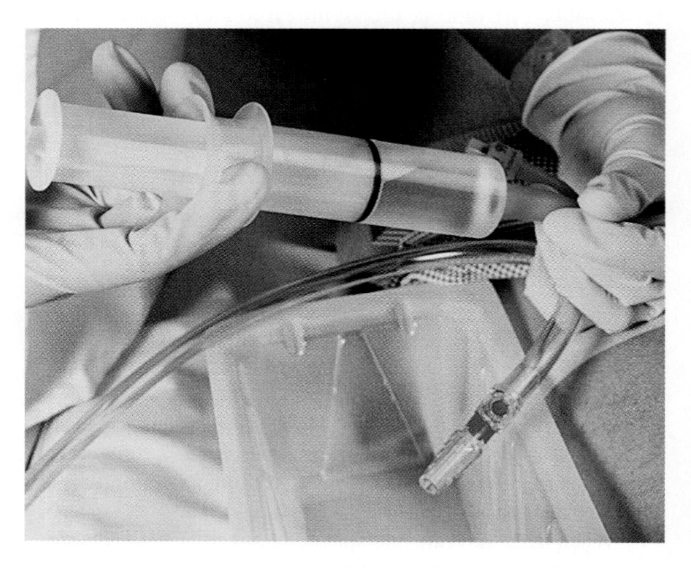

Figure 29–19. To irrigate indwelling catheter, apply gentle but firm pressure to syringe to instill irrigant. *(From Smith S, Duell D.* Clinical Nursing Skills: Nursing Process Model, Basic to Advanced Skills. *4th ed. Stamford, CT: Appleton & Lange; 1996.)*

own catheters, or to instill a sterile acidic solution to clear crystal-like encrustations that may form and block the flow of urine.

The procedures for indwelling catheter insertion, care, and removal are the same for patients in the hospital and at home. Home nurses often find that inserting urinary catheters in a patient's home can be challenging, especially when the patient's bed is in a fixed, low position. That position might require the nurse to bend or stoop during the procedure. Securing adequate lighting or finding space to lay out supplies are other problems that require creative solutions in the home setting.

Another common problem for patients at home is fecal impaction. When preventive and supportive implementations fail, nurses are often called upon to help relieve the condition. Finally, home nurses have an important role in ostomy care, particularly in the postdischarge period when patients with new ostomies are not yet independent in managing their ostomy. The ostomy procedures described earlier apply to patients in the home setting.

REHABILITATIVE CARE

Rehabilitation and the reestablishment of near-normal elimination patterns are the major concerns of fourth-level patient care. This care should be initiated before patient discharge from a health care facility. Home management of care requires the understanding and collaboration of patient, family, and significant others.

Early hospital discharge presents major challenges to home health care nurses. Patients are often sicker and the recovery period may lead to alterations in bowel and bladder function, especially if the patient is inactive.

Nurses collaborate with patients in planning bowel and bladder training or retraining. These programs involve monitoring fluid intake and diet, positioning techniques, muscle strengthening exercises, and habit formation. The goal is to retrain the bladder or bowel to empty periodically after injury or disruption of normal routines. The program can be supplemented by aids such as external catheters, intermittent self-catheterization, electrical stimulation of the micturition reflex, laxatives, or stool softeners.

Bowel Training

Through bowel training, some people who are incontinent of stool can achieve normal defecation. Those who have some control of abdominal muscles and the anal sphincter are most likely to be successful. By setting up a daily routine for elimination and using measures to promote elimination, some patients regain control of bowel reflexes. The components of a bowel training program are as follows.

- Determine what the patient's usual elimination pattern is and document the incontinent episodes.
- Collaborate with the patient to determine the best time to initiate bowel control measures.
- Obtain physician's order for oral stool softener or suppository if necessary to facilitate defecation.
- Determine whether particular fluids normally stimulate defecation and administer before the time for bowel evacuation.
- Provide assistance to the bathroom at the selected times.
- Maintain privacy and limit elimination time to 15 to 20 minutes.
- Instruct the patient to lean forward at the hips while sitting on the toilet, place hands over the left lower abdomen and apply some manual pressure, and bear down without straining to stimulate bowel evacuation.
- Provide acceptance and encouragement even if the patient is not able to defecate at the selected time.
- Collaborate with the patient to develop and carry out an exercise program that is within the patient's ability.
- Work with the patient to develop a plan for regular mealtimes and adequate intake of fiber and fluids which are essential to bowel control.

Home Management of Ostomies

The patient with an ostomy should be given information about the anatomic changes caused by the surgery. The use and care of the ostomy equipment and the use of correct techniques for draining and irrigating ostomies are important considerations for this level of care. Other important areas are odor control, preservation of periostomal skin integrity, maintaining fluid and electrolyte balance, and identifying ways to prevent stoma blockage.

Nurses should inform patients of the signs and symptoms to report to their health care provider. Instructions for appropriate activity levels and precautions related to participation in contact sports are also important. Patients with ileostomies should be informed that they should not take enteric-coated tablets or time-released capsules because absorption may not take place before the medication is excreted.

Information is also needed about available community resources that can help patient and family with home management and adjustment to the changes that result from an ostomy. Some resources include the United Ostomy Association, accessible at the website below, ostomy support groups, community health agencies, enterostomal therapists, home health agencies, the Visiting Nurses' Association, as well as individual, family, and financial counseling services. Resources are available for financial support (food stamps), and the American Cancer Society provides equipment. These resources can help the patient obtain equipment and supplies and work out financial and family problems.

Bladder Training

Bladder retraining is often used for individuals with a reflex bladder. These patients have an intact voiding reflex arc, but no sensory input from the bladder; therefore, the bladder empties without warning when it is full. The principles of bladder training are useful for anyone who is incontinent of urine. The components of a bladder training program are as follows.

- Collaborate with the patient to plan a regular daily fluid intake pattern that includes 2000 to 3000 mL of fluid.
- Identify the patient's usual voiding pattern.
- Plan the voiding schedule with regular attempts to void about 30 minutes prior to usual time bladder empties.

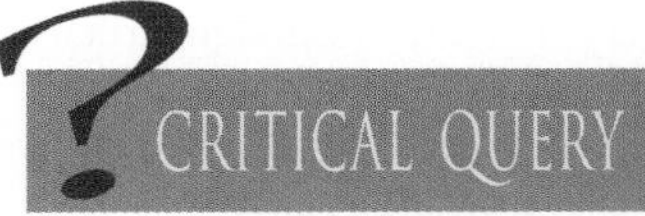

CRITICAL QUERY

Palmer,[16] a nurse researcher, noted that the beliefs that health care professionals hold about a condition often determine the types of interventions they choose to treat that condition. In her survey of a 250 nurses, she found that 48 percent erroneously identified advanced age as a cause of incontinence. How might nurses holding such a belief approach the care of elderly patients? How might understanding that advanced age is not a cause of incontinence enable nurses to be more helpful?

INSIGHTS FROM NURSING LITERATURE

MANAGING THE BOWEL PATTERNS OF ELDERLY REHABILITATION PATIENTS

Gibson CJ, Opalka PC, Moore CA, et al. Effectiveness of bran supplement on the bowel management of elderly rehabilitation patients. J Gerontol Nurs. *1995;21:21–30.*

The researchers focused on the importance of dietary fiber in preventing constipation among patients admitted to a rehabilitation hospital. They studied a convenience sample of 137 subjects assigned to intervention and control groups. On admission, all patients were placed on a bowel management program consisting of daily activity, a set toilet time based on toileting history, a fluid intake of at least 1500 mL per 24 hours, and judicious use of laxatives, suppositories, and enemas. The intervention subjects also received a mixture of all-bran cereal, applesauce, and prune juice each day. The data showed that intervention subjects required significantly less laxative therapy to maintain a functional bowel pattern.

- Assist the patient to develop an association between a particular activity and emptying the bladder. Some effective "tricks" include concentrating, stroking the inner thighs, drinking water, pouring warm water over the pubic area, or exerting manual pressure over the bladder.
- Identify with the patient factors that aggravate incontinence, such as medications or caffeine, and determine whether they can be reduced.
- If the patient is able, teach perineal exercises (see Supportive Care earlier in the chapter).
- Discuss the use of perineal pads or adult diapers to maintain dryness during the development of control.

In the rehabilitative stage of adapting to elimination problems, patients assume progressively greater responsibility for management of elimination. Rather than focusing on direct care or active collaboration, nurses act as consultants. Resources such as those listed above can provide patients with additional support and strategies for maintaining optimum elimination.

Some patients use intermittent self-catheterization as part of a bladder training program. Self-catheterization is scheduled so that continence is achieved and bladder distension is prevented; initially, it is usually performed every 4 hours. Although urinary catheterization is a sterile nursing procedure, studies have demonstrated the effectiveness and safety of clean technique for self-catheterization at home. Important teaching points for self-catheterization include the following:

- Emphasize the importance of clean equipment, proper handwashing, and thorough washing of the perineum before inserting the catheter.
- Discuss techniques and rationale for lubricating the catheter adequately.
- Demonstrate methods for correctly identifying the urinary meatus (women may find a mirror helpful).
- Explain how far to insert the catheter.
- Provide a list of signs and symptoms of urinary tract infection.

EVALUATION

Evaluating patient care to promote optimal elimination patterns is the final component of nurse–patient management. It is based on the desired outcomes and evaluation criteria that nurse and patient developed together. Patient and nurse observe for the behaviors described in desired outcome statements or evaluation criteria. Evaluation of the desired outcome should be done at the time stated in the outcome, but nurse and patient should also monitor progress made toward the goal. If the evaluation indicates that desired outcomes are not being achieved it is necessary to reassess and reconsider outcomes and implementation.

As outcomes are achieved, progress is documented in the patient record. If outcomes are not met, reassessment data and additional plans are also recorded.

Management of elimination concerns is a sensitive, sometimes difficult endeavor, because people often hesitate to collaborate due to the intimate nature of the elimination process. Patients may find speaking about urination and defecation embarrassing or unpleasant. Nurses who demonstrate a concerned, professional approach will gain trust and enhance willingness to collaborate in managing elimination functions. The result will be that patients achieve greater autonomy and more healthful elimination.

SUMMARY

The lower gastrointestinal tract and the kidney with its associated structures are responsible for the excretion of the majority of the body's waste products. Understanding these organs' structures and functions is necessary to carrying out nursing responsibilities to promote healthy elimination.

Collaborative assessment (data gathering, data analysis, and diagnosis) and collaborative management (planning, implementation, and evaluation) of elimination are essential, as is carrying out elimination-related care ordered by physicians.

Elimination, particularly if altered, affects other body functions; therefore, elimination assessment addresses not only the bowel and urinary tract but also selected aspects of integumentary, cardiorespiratory, neuromuscular, and psychological functioning.

The nursing diagnoses detailed in this chapter include only those directly related to elimination. These diagnoses and their etiologies are presented as a basis for identifying, understanding, and providing patient care to promote optimum elimination. The discussion of nursing implementation focuses on independent nursing measures and medically ordered procedures that are directly supportive of elimination. Health promotion and prevention, supportive care, restorative (or acute) care, and rehabilitative care are among the activities of nurses.

Elimination alterations can be disruptive, uncomfortable, and embarrassing to patients. Nurses who are cognizant of this and sensitive to the distress that elimination assessment and implementation may cause can help alleviate patient concerns and facilitate nurse–patient collaboration to correct or minimize the impact of elimination problems.

LEARNING OUTCOMES

Upon completing this chapter, the student should be able to:

1. Name and describe the primary function of the major organs of bowel and urinary elimination.
2. Describe the normal patterns of elimination in an adult.
3. List four factors affecting bowel function and four factors affecting urinary function and describe their consequences.
4. Describe variations in elimination that may occur in the course of the life cycle.
5. Identify six alterations in bowel elimination.
6. Identify five alterations in urinary elimination.
7. List data to be obtained in an elimination history.
8. Identify essential elements of a nursing examination of bowel and urinary function.
9. Identify at least six diagnostic tests used in determining elimination status.
10. List nursing diagnoses describing altered bowel elimination and identify an etiology for each.
11. List nursing diagnoses describing altered urinary elimination and identify an etiology for each.
12. Describe examples of preventive, supportive, restorative, and rehabilitative nursing implementation that promote bowel and bladder function and give the rationale for each.
13. Describe common learning needs of patients with altered elimination.
14. Write a nursing care plan for a patient with altered elimination.
15. Discuss the nurse's role in collaborating with patients to promote optimal elimination function.

REVIEW OF KEY TERMS

adynamic ileus
anuria
cathartics
catheterization
constipation
diarrhea
diuretics
duodenocolic reflex
dysuria
elimination
enema
enuresis
fecal impaction
fecal incontinence
flatulence
functional incontinence
gastrocolic reflex
glomerular filtration rate
hemorrhoids
Kegel exercises
laxatives
melena
nocturia
oliguria
paralytic ileus
peristalsis
polyuria
proteinuria
stoma
stress incontinence
urgency
urinary frequency
urinary incontinence
urinary retention
Valsalva maneuver

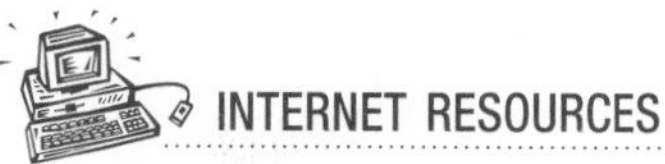

INTERNET RESOURCES

Web Sites

Constipation:
http://www.ayurvedic.org/consti.html

National Institute on Aging—Spry Foundation:
http://www.fortnet.org/SPRY/const.html

United Ostomy Association:
http://www. uoa.org

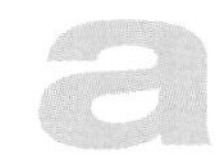

Having Read the Chapter, consider again the opening scenario, page 929, and the following responses to the questions.

After informing Mrs. Briggs, who is preparing for discharge following a colon resection, about the procedure to remove her Foley catheter, her nurse takes time to answer questions and address any concerns that Mrs. Briggs has. She informs Mrs. Briggs that the discomfort of catheter removal is slight. The nurse removes the tape anchoring the catheter, and places a waterproof pad over Mrs. Briggs' thighs. Wearing nonsterile gloves, she inserts a sterile syringe into the balloon port and withdraws 8 mL of fluid from the balloon. The nurse then instructs Mrs. Briggs to take a deep breath, and as she exhales, the nurse puts gentle traction on the catheter, slowly removing it. The nurse notes the time of removal.

When the catheter is out, Mrs. Briggs' nurse encourages her to drink fluids and emphasizes the importance of responding promptly to the urge to void. She instructs Mrs. Briggs to use the specimen collector (fisreman's hat) for her first voiding, so that the urine can be measured.

Her nurse notes that because of Mrs. Briggs' condition and the nature of the treatment she has received, it is important to observe and record the color, clarity, and odor of Mrs. Briggs' urine, and the frequency and volume of her urination. It is also important to note the presence of bowel sounds, passage of flatus, and the color, consistency, odor, and volume of her stool, and the frequency of her defecation.

The nurse decides to talk with Mrs. Briggs about changing her habits to include drinking eight glasses of fluid each day. She also notes the need to discuss with Mrs. Briggs elements of her lifestyle—stressful job, extensive responsibility, working late, not eating regularly—which may promote stress-related body symptoms.

REFERENCES

1. Guyton AC, Hall JE. *Textbook of Medical Physiology.* 9th ed. Philadelphia: Saunders; 1995.
2. Schuster CS, Ashburn SS. *The Process of Human Development: A Holistic Life-Span Approach.* 3rd ed. Philadelphia: Lippincott; 1992:1497.
3. Ignatavicius DD, Workman ML, Mishler MA. *Medical-Surgical Nursing: A Nursing Process Approach.* 2nd ed. Philadelphia: Saunders; 1995.
4. Mahan LK, Strump-Escott S. *Krause's Food, Nutrition, and Diet Therapy.* 9th ed. Philadelphia: Saunders; 1996:614–615.
5. Lemone P, Burke KM. *Medical Surgical Nursing: Critical Thinking in Client Care.* Menlo Park, CA: Addison Wesley; 1996.
6. Malarkey LM, McMorrow, ME. *Nurse's Manual of Laboratory Tests and Diagnostic Procedures.* Philadelphia: Saunders; 1996: 52–60.
7. Jaffe MS, McVan BF. *Laboratory and Diagnostic Test Handbook.* Philadelphia: FA. Davis; 1997.
8. Matteson MA, McConnell ES, Linton AD. *Gerontological Nursing: Concepts and Practice.* 2nd ed. Philadelphia: Saunders; 1997:338–342.
9. Fraulini KE. *After Anesthesia: A Guide for PACU, ICU, and Medical-Surgical Nurses.* Norwalk, CT: Appleton & Lange; 1987: 228–20.
10. McKenny LM, Salerno E. *Pharmacology in Nursing.* 19th ed. St. Louis: Mosby-Yearbook; 1995.
11. Agency for Health Care Policy and Research. *Urinary Incontinence in Adults: Acute and Chronic Management.* Clinical Practice Guideline No. 2 (1996 update). AHCPR pub. no. 96-0682, March 1996.
12. Palmer MH. A health-promotion perspective of urinary continence. *Nurs Outlook.* 1994;42:163–169.
13. Wong DL. *Whaley & Wong's Nursing Care of Infants and Children.* 5th ed. St. Louis: Mosby; 1995:805.
14. Wells JA, Doughty DB. Pouching principles and products. *Ostomy/Wound Management.* 1994;40:50–63.
15. Brooks MJ. Assessment and nursing management of homebound patients with urinary incontinence. *Home Healthcare Nurse.* 1994;13:11–16.
16. Palmer MH. Nurses' knowledge and beliefs about continence interventions in long-term care. *J Adv Nurs.* 1995;21:1065–1072.

30

Oxygenation

Carol J. Archibald

Georgette Jacobson, age 66, a retired school teacher, was admitted to the emergency room two days ago with chest pain radiating to the left arm, shortness of breath, and fatigue. At the time of admission, she was pale, diaphoretic, extremely apprehensive and restless. Her heart sounds were somewhat distant, and a fourth heart sound, typical of heart attack, was present. Subsequent laboratory tests, electrocardiograms, and other procedures confirmed a diagnosis of myocardial infarction, or heart attack. Mrs. Jacobson, a lifelong smoker, but also an avid trail hiker and golfer, is now receiving low-flow oxygen therapy by nasal cannula as she is prepared for heart surgery to bypass a bloodclot in a major coronary artery.

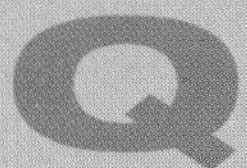

What is the purpose of the oxygen therapy?

What noninvasive clinical procedure may be used to monitor the effect of the therapy as Mrs. Jacobson waits for surgery?

What teaching will Mrs. Jacobson require to prepare her for the immediate postoperative period?

For preventing a recurrence of the disease?

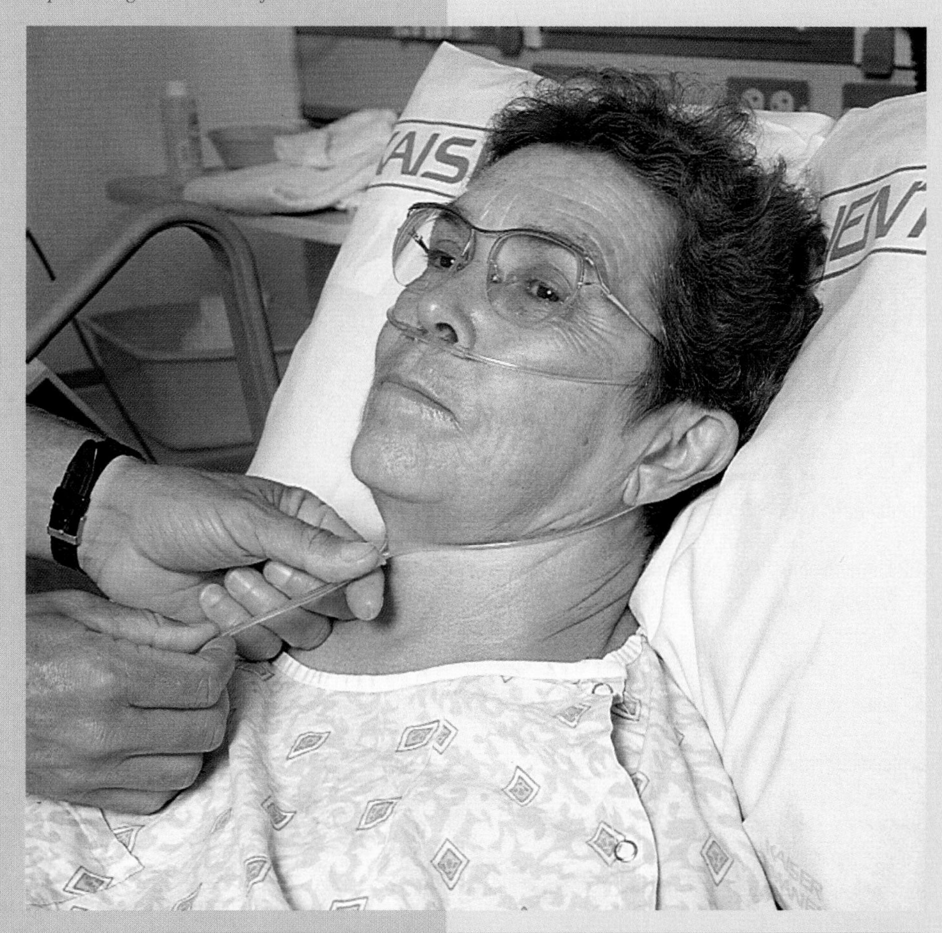

CHAPTER OUTLINE

Oxygen is fundamental to all life processes. Because cells require oxygen to carry out their metabolic processes, a steady supply of oxygen to each cell is a primary bodily need. Maintaining airway, breathing, and circulation are the first priorities for life. Oxygenation, the process of supplying body cells with oxygen, begins when air is inhaled and its oxygen extracted. Oxygen must then be delivered to the cells. In addition, through breathing and circulation, the waste products of cellular metabolism are removed and transported to the proper organs for excretion or chemical breakdown.

Any compromise of oxygenation can be serious. Nurses can prevent some oxygenation problems and teach patients how to prevent others. Nurses must also be able to intervene when oxygenation problems arise. Among those patients at special risk for oxygenation problems are preoperative and postoperative individuals and persons with chronic illness or active respiratory disease. The very old and the very young are also at special risk, as are individuals with cardiovascular disease. People who smoke or are exposed to heavy air pollution or respiratory hazards in the workplace are also among those at risk.

Diseases affecting oxygenation are major causes of disability in North America. In the United States, lung disease is the third leading cause of death. The death rate from lung disease is increasing faster than that of any other disease category,[1] while diseases of the heart and blood vessels are the leading cause of death.[2] In addition to those who die, many more people suffer the consequences of these diseases each year. Death caused by these diseases is often preceded by a long period of disability, suffering, and lowered quality of life.

SECTION 1
UNDERSTANDING OXYGENATION

THE PROCESS OF OXYGENATION

Oxygenation is the process of supplying oxygen to the body cells to support their metabolic processes. The three major components of oxygenation are:

- **Ventilation:** movement of air into and out of the lungs.
- **Diffusion:** the exchange of gas between alveoli and capillaries and between capillaries and tissues.
- **Perfusion:** delivery of blood throughout the body for cellular gas exchange.

Perfusion involves the pumping action of the heart, the vascular delivery system of the blood, and the hemoglobin that carries most body oxygen and carbon dioxide.

The body oxygenates itself by drawing in air from the environment, carrying it through a series of passageways in the lungs, and exchanging the oxygen across an alveolar-capillary membrane to the blood. The heart pumps the oxygenated blood to all body cells to supply their energy and oxygenation needs. The waste product of cellular oxygen metabolism is carbon dioxide, which moves out of the cells and into the blood to be carried to the lungs for excretion.

VENTILATION

Ventilation is accomplished through respiration—the inhaling and exhaling of air via the respiratory tract. The respiratory tract has two divisions: (1) the upper airways and (2) the lower respiratory tract, which lies within the thoracic cavity.

Upper Airways

The upper portion of the respiratory tract consists of the nose, pharynx, larynx, and trachea (Fig. 30–1). They form the passageway for air to enter the body. Because many foreign substances can enter the body with the incoming air, several respiratory defense mechanisms help protect the body (Table 30–1), the first of which is air filtration. This occurs in the upper airway.

Normally, air enters the nose through the nares, moves through the pharynx and the larynx, then the trachea. When air enters through the mouth rather than the nose, the protective functions of the nose are bypassed, and dry, unfiltered air moves into the lungs. Lung tissues may become dry and irritated.

The pharynx allows food as well as air to pass. In the front of the pharynx, at the base of the tongue, is the epiglottis, a small flap that closes over the airway to prevent food or foreign matter from entering the airway during swallowing. Air moves from the pharynx, into the larynx, and on into the trachea. The trachea divides (bifurcates) into the right and left mainstem bronchi at a point called the carina.

Lower Respiratory Tract

The lungs, which lie inside the thoracic cavity, make up the lower respiratory tract. They are separated from each other by the mediastinal structures (the structures that are in the middle of the chest). The right lung is divided into three major divisions or lobes, while the left lung has two lobes. Each lobe is divided into smaller compartments, or lobules, which are further divided into still smaller segments, acini. The final division is comprised of the alveoli (air sacs), which are the site of air exchange.

Air is supplied to the lungs via the trachea and the right and left mainstem bronchi. Each bronchus divides several times to form the lobar, segmental, and subsegmental bronchi, and finally the bronchioles. The most distant bronchioles are called the terminal or respiratory bronchioles, which connect with the alveoli. Each generation is smaller in diameter than the preceding generation, but adds more branches. As a result, the surface area of each successive generation is larger than that of the generation preceding it. The bronchi, which are filled with air with each breath, act solely as passages for air and do not participate in gaseous exchange. The surface area comprising their walls is referred to as **anatomic dead space**, a term for areas where no air exchange occurs. It comprises a volume of about 1 mL/lb normal body weight or about 150 mL in a 150-lb adult.[4]

Thoracic Cavity

The chest wall structures include the rib cage, intercostal muscles, and diaphragm. The chest is lined with parietal and visceral pleura. The pleural membranes are joined at the edges to form a potential space (intrapleural space). Their function is to secrete small amounts of fluid, which lubricates the pleura and causes them to work as a single unit while sliding over each other during respiration. In other words, the lungs stick to the chest wall because of the pleural fluid. Anything (fluid, air, blood, pus) that intervenes in the intrapleural space has the potential to reduce the adhesiveness between the two pleural membranes and to take up space, thereby decreasing lung volume. This then decreases oxygenation.

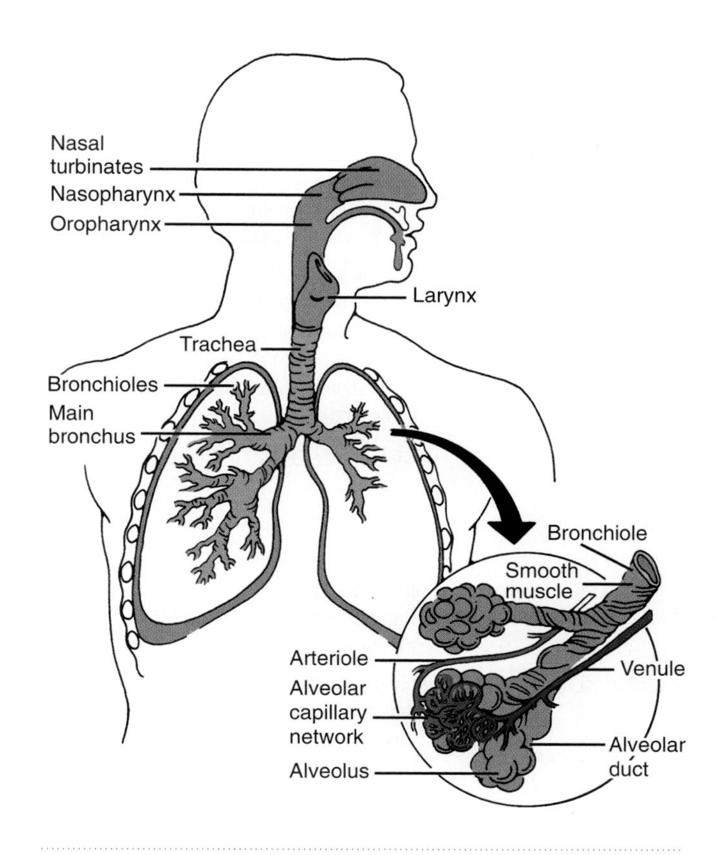

Figure 30–1. The respiratory tract.

The sternum, spine, and 12 pairs of ribs comprise the bony structure of the thorax. Several muscles are attached to the ribs. The major muscle of respiration is the diaphragm, a dome-shaped muscle that separates the chest and the abdomen. When the diaphragm contracts, it descends, increasing the size of the thoracic cavity. The abdominal contents are pushed downward by the diaphragmatic movement. Conditions such as obesity, abdominal distension, and pregnancy limit the downward movement of the diaphragm and thus may limit the depth of respiration. Upward movement of the diaphragm may be impeded by conditions that trap excess air in the lungs (such as asthma). When diaphragmatic action is limited or breathing is labored, the accessory muscles, including the scalene, sternocleidomastoid, and intercostal muscles, are used to increase the size of the chest cavity so that air may enter. The external intercostal muscles and parasternal muscles normally raise the rib cage and increase the size of the thoracic cavity. When a deep inspiration is forced, the scalene muscles and sternocleidomastoid muscles aid in the expansion and raising of the rib cage, thereby increasing the size of the thoracic cavity. Forced exhalation is accomplished by a squeezing action of the intercostal muscles.

Mechanics of Breathing

Breathing consists of two phases: **inspiration** (moving air in) and **expiration** (moving air out). Air movement results by changing

TABLE 30-1. RESPIRATORY DEFENSE MECHANISMS

Mechanism	Description	Factors That Reduce Defense
Air filtration	Nasal hairs, sharp angles of inside of nose, and nasal mucous membrane trap most large foreign particles that are inhaled.	Chronic, prolonged mouth breathing.
Mucociliary clearance	Mucus in the lower airways traps incoming particles and debris. Mucus contains secretory immunoglobulin A (IgA), which helps protect against bacteria and viruses. Many cilia (hairlike projections) beat rhythmically to move the mucus and trapped debris to the mouth for swallowing and expectoration.	Thickened sputum; dehydration; smoking; high oxygen levels; infection; drugs such as atropine, alcohol, anesthetics.
Cough	Clears airway by high-pressure, high-velocity airflow.	Lung disease; neuromuscular disease, intubation, thickened sputum.
Sneeze	Irritation to the nose stimulates trigeminal reflex to clear nose.	
Reflex bronchoconstriction	Inhalation of irritants (dust, allergens, aerosols, fumes, smoke) triggers immediate bronchoconstriction to shut out the irritant. Protection is most effective if the dose of irritant is small and exposure time brief.	Airways may be excessively irritable and overreact to inhalation of irritants, as in asthma.
Alveolar macrophages	Primary defense in alveoli. Macrophages rapidly phagocytize inhaled foreign particles. Debris from phagocytic process is moved to airways or to lymphatic system for removal from body. Nonphagocytized particles may remain in lungs for indefinite periods and stimulate tissue changes. Examples: asbestos, coal dust, silica, debris from smoking.	Smoking cigarettes or marijuana, air pollution, drugs such as alcohol, and steroids.
Immunologic defenses	T and B lymphocytes and certain phagocytes function in complex pattern to defend against foreign invasion. IgA is contained in airway mucus. This helps defend against sinus and respiratory infections.[3]	Certain lung and systemic diseases, such as AIDS; thickened sputum; infection; drugs such as atropine.
Sieve and filtering mechanisms	Pulmonary capillaries filter out large bacteria, blood clots, and fat globules to protect the heart, brain, and other body areas. If particles filtered out are small, they are handled by macrophages or immunologic defenses. If large, they may obstruct a pulmonary vessel and cause clinical symptoms.	

intrathoracic pressures in relation to atmospheric pressure, because gases always flow from an area of greater pressure to one of lesser pressure. When the pressure inside the chest is lower than atmospheric pressure, outside air flows into the chest. When the pressure inside the chest is greater than outside atmospheric pressure, air flows out of the chest.

The body lowers intrathoracic pressure by enlarging the thoracic cavity—the diaphragm contracts (lowers) and the chest wall expands. In quiet respiration, the diaphragm moves only about 1 cm. However, in forced inspiration, the diaphragm can move about 10 cm. To stimulate exhalation, the thorax and diaphragm relax and allow the chest cavity to decrease in size. This increases internal pressure and causes exhalation of air into the atmosphere.

Air movement, and thus ventilation, is facilitated by an upright or seated posture. The airways are larger in the upright position than in the supine. Normally, the bases of the lungs are better ventilated than the apices when a person is in an upright position.[4]

Control of Ventilation

Respiration is one of the few bodily functions that may be under either automatic or partial voluntary control. See Chap. 17 for more on the control of respiration.

Automatic Control. When control of respiration is automatic and unconscious, respiration is precisely regulated to supply appropriate amounts of oxygen to the body cells and to rid them of carbon dioxide (CO_2). Respiratory rate and depth change quickly to accommodate varying metabolic needs. Respiration is ultimately controlled by the respiratory center, a collection of nerve fibers and cells located bilaterally in the medulla and pons sections of the brain. The chemoreceptors in the respiratory center respond to increases in hydrogen ion concentration (decreased, or acid, pH), which stimulate ventilation, or decreases in body acids (increased, or alkaline, pH), which inhibit it.

The carbon dioxide level (P_{CO_2}) in the blood is a primary regulator of ventilation because it affects the pH (acid–base level) of the cerebral spinal fluid and therefore the respiratory center. When a person breathes very rapidly or deeply, more CO_2 is excreted than usual, elevating the pH of the blood. When the respirations are slower or more shallow, CO_2 builds up, reducing blood pH.

Under normal circumstances, P_{CO_2} is much more important than P_{O_2} (oxygen level) in regulating respirations; but if disease has rendered the cerebral chemoreceptors insensitive to higher than usual P_{CO_2} levels, a decrease in P_{O_2} can stimulate respiration via the peripheral chemoreceptors, located in the carotid bodies at the bifurcation of the aortic arch, instead. This is called the **hypoxic respiratory drive.**

Mechanical sensors, located in the lungs, upper airways, chest wall, and diaphragm, also play a part in regulating respiration. Pulmonary stretch receptors, for example, a type of mechanical sensor, activate as the lungs inflate, and protect the lungs and chest from overexpansion. This is called the Hering–Breuer reflex. Other mechanical receptors sense irritants, such as noxious fumes or pollens, and, when stimulated, cause reflexive rapid, shallow breathing and bronchoconstriction, which prevent the irritant from reaching the gas-exchange surface.

The impulses from the mechanical sensors, including the Hering–Breuer reflex, are sent to the brain via the vagus nerve, part of the parasympathetic nervous system. Stimulation of the vagus nerve causes bronchoconstriction (narrowing of the airways), which increases the work of breathing. On the other hand, stimulation of the sympathetic nervous system generally relaxes and opens the airways, resulting in easier breathing.

Pain and emotional stimuli also affect respiration.[5] Typically, breathing becomes more rapid and shallow when a person is experiencing pain or a strong emotion. This response can be overridden by voluntary control, discussed in the next section.

Voluntary Control. Respiration can also occur under voluntary control. If a person wishes to breathe rapidly or slowly, this can be done for a certain period of time. A person cannot, however, voluntarily cease to breathe long enough to cause death. Ultimately, the brain will supersede voluntary control to keep the person alive. Respirations may also be consciously controlled for short periods of time by a person with respiratory problems. These methods of voluntary control can be taught as breathing exercises.

Lung Volumes and Capacities

There are anatomic measurements for the various amounts of air that can be contained in the lungs. The standard terminology for lung volumes and capacities and their definitions are:

- **Tidal volume (V_T).** The volume of gas that is moved with each breath. Composed of the volume entering the alveoli plus the volume remaining in the airway (about 500 mL in an adult).
- *Expiratory reserve volume (ERV).* The maximum amount of gas that can be expired with a forced expiration.
- *Residual volume (RV).* The volume of gas that remains in the lungs at the end of a forced expiration.
- *Inspiratory reserve volume (IRV).* The maximum volume of gas that can be inhaled with a forced inspiration.
- *Inspiratory capacity (IC).* Tidal volume plus inspiratory reserve volume.
- *Functional residual capacity (FRC).* Expiratory reserve volume plus residual volume.
- **Vital capacity (VC).** Inspiratory reserve volume plus tidal volume plus expiratory reserve volume.
- **Total lung capacity (TLC).** Maximum volume of gas that the lungs can contain. Inspiratory capacity plus functional residual capacity or vital capacity plus residual volume. TLC is not a volume of air that can be exchanged.

Anything that affects the volume of air contained in the lung can affect lung volumes and capacities. For example, a person with asthma or emphysema tends to retain air in the chest. This increases the residual volume, which in turn lowers the tidal volume, the inspiratory reserve volume, and the expiratory reserve volume.

Surfactant

Surfactant, a lipoprotein that coats the alveolar membrane, decreases alveolar surface tension and thus increases alveolar stability. The alveolus has a natural tendency to collapse. If the alveoli collapsed or closed at the end of each breath, a very high inspiratory pressure would be needed to force them open again to receive the next breath. Surfactant prevents the alveoli from collapsing with each breath and decreases the pressure needed to inflate the alveoli on the next breath. Surfactant thus reduces the work of breathing.[6] Surfactant is short acting, and so it must be continually replenished. Normal ventilation seems to be the most important factor in replenishment of surfactant. Insufficient air exchange may therefore lead to **atelectasis** (collapse of alveoli, which may be limited to a small area or involve the whole lung) due to the diminished renewal of surfactant. Cigarette smokers are known to have decreased levels of surfactant.

DIFFUSION

Diffusion, the process of oxygen–carbon dioxide exchange, occurs via the alveolar–capillary membrane, located in the lungs.

Alveolar–Capillary Membrane

The respiratory zone of the lung, where air exchange occurs, consists of the most distal respiratory bronchioles and the alveoli. An adult has about 300 million alveoli, with a total volume of about 2500 mL and a surface area for diffusing that is about the size of a tennis court. A membrane one-cell thick separates the alveoli from the alveolar capillary network. It is the actual site of gas exchange[5] (Fig. 30–1). Conditions that increase the distance between the alveolus and the pulmonary capillary reduce gas exchange. Such conditions include pulmonary edema, in which fluid accumulates in the interstitial space between the alveolus and the capillary. An infection such as pneumonia reduces gas exchange because inflammatory exudate inside the alveolus prevents oxygen from getting to the alveolar–capillary interface.

The Lung's Circulation

The lung has two circulatory systems: the *pulmonary circulation,* which provides blood for gas exchange with the alveoli, and the *bronchial circulation,* which supplies the metabolic needs of the pulmonary tissues.

The pulmonary circulation begins with the pulmonary artery, which arises from the right ventricle of the heart and branches so that each alveolus is in direct communication with a pulmonary capillary. This is where gas exchange (diffusion) occurs. The oxygenated blood is then pumped to the left side of the heart for distribution to the body. The pulmonary circulation also serves the oxygenation needs of the bronchi and alveoli.

The other lung tissues are oxygenated by blood from the bronchial circulation, which branches off from the bronchial arteries. These arteries arise from the thoracic aorta. The bronchial circulation supplies the lung's supporting tissues, nerves, and the outer layers of the pulmonary arteries and veins. In the event of interruption of the pulmonary circulation, the bronchial circulation can support the metabolic needs of the alveoli and bronchioles as well. This prevents an obstructed pulmonary capillary from causing the death of these tissues.[3]

Movement of Gases

Dalton's Law states that any gas in a mixture of gases behaves as though it were the only gas present. Therefore, gases other than oxygen and carbon dioxide in the air do not have to be considered when studying the gases of respiration. The respiratory gases are measured as partial pressures, or the pressure exerted by a single gas in a mixture of gases.[5] When the partial pressure of these gases are discussed, the capital letter P is used before the chemical abbreviation for the gas (for example, PO_2). Further definitions are found in Clinical Guideline 30–1.

CLINICAL GUIDELINE 30–1

SYMBOLS FOR PARTIAL PRESSURES OF SELECTED RESPIRATORY GASES

- PO_2 Partial pressure of oxygen in the blood
- PAO_2 Partial pressure of oxygen in the alveoli
- PCO_2 Partial pressure of carbon dioxide in the blood
- $PACO_2$ Partial pressure of carbon dioxide in the alveoli
- PaO_2 Partial pressure of oxygen in the arteries
- $PaCO_2$ Partial pressure of carbon dioxide in the arteries
- PVO_2 Partial pressure of oxygen in the veins
- $PVCO_2$ Partial pressure of carbon dioxide in the veins

As previously stated, the alveolar–capillary membrane is only one cell thick. Oxygen and carbon dioxide move easily across this membrane by diffusion from areas of higher pressure to areas of lower pressure. As the alveoli fill with air on inhalation, the oxygen concentration is higher in the alveoli than in the capillary blood. Therefore, oxygen diffuses into the blood. In contrast, the pulmonary capillary blood returning from the body is high in carbon dioxide, which diffuses into the alveoli for excretion by exhalation. Carbon dioxide is 20 times more diffusible than oxygen, so PCO_2 is a better measure of ventilation, or the amount of air being moved by the lungs, than is PO_2.

The actual PO_2 of inhaled air depends on the barometric pressure of the environment. PO_2 is lower at high altitudes than at sea level. Therefore, living at a high altitude for about 6 weeks will cause the body to manufacture extra red blood cells (mild polycythemia) to compensate for the lower PO_2 in the outside air. The body's oxygen level can be changed by administering oxygen therapy. This increases the amount of oxygen in the inhaled air and thus raises oxygen levels in every area of the body without a change in respiration.

PERFUSION

Perfusion is accomplished via the action of the heart and the circulatory system, as the blood is moved through the circulatory system.

The Heart

The heart is a double pump that keeps the body alive by circulating the blood. It has the ability to adjust the rate and force of its contraction as the body's needs for blood supply change.

Anatomy. The heart is composed of four chambers: the right and left atria and the right and left ventricles (Fig. 30–2). Each side of the heart is composed of one atrium and one ventricle. The *atria* are storage areas and passageways for the blood to reach the ventricles. The *ventricles* are muscular structures that create the pumping force to move the blood: the right ventricle to the lungs and the left ventricle to the rest of the body. Ordinarily, the pressure in the pulmonary vessels is low, and relatively little force is required to move the blood to the lungs. As a result, the right ventricle is a relatively thin and weak muscle. The left ventricle, which must generate considerably greater force to pump blood to the entire body, is a heavier, stronger muscle.

The two atria and the two ventricles are each divided by a heavy wall called a *septum*. The ventricular septum also houses the tissue for conducting the electrical impulses that stimulate the ventricles to contract. Inside the ventricles are bundles of muscle and strong fibers, the chordae tendinae, which are attached to the margins of the valves separating the atria and ventricles. These fibers help the valves to open and close. The four valves of the heart are the openings between the chambers and the portals of exit for blood leaving the heart. All of the valves are supported by strong fibrous tissue called valve rings.

Cardiac Cycle. The job of the heart is to pump blood. For maximal effect, all of the parts of the heart must act in a synchronized, rhythmic fashion. Several complex mechanisms act to achieve this synchronization. The myocardial (heart muscle) cells are positioned in such a way that impulses generated in one cell quickly pass to the others, causing the entire group of cells in the atria or

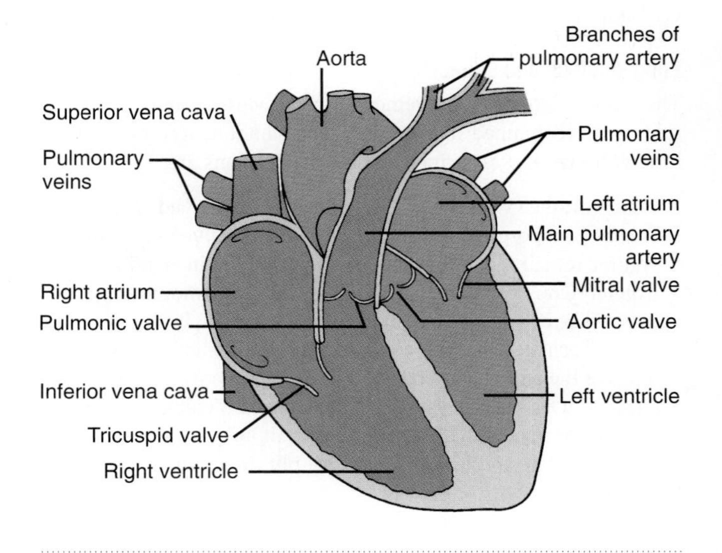

Figure 30–2. Heart chambers and major vessels.

ventricle to contract as a unit. Nowhere else in the body are cells grouped in this manner. Each atrium and each ventricle acts as a separate unit. The atria fill and contract simultaneously to empty blood into the ventricles. After they have filled, the ventricles contract simultaneously to eject blood into the pulmonary artery and the systemic circulation. The mechanical events of the cardiac cycle are called systole and diastole. **Systole** refers to the time of ventricular contraction, when blood is being ejected from the heart to the lungs and the rest of the body. **Diastole** is the time of ventricular relaxation, or rest, repolarization, and refilling.

Control of the Heart. The heart has the property of automaticity, or the ability to contract in a regular rhythm. Cardiac action is regulated by a complex electrical conduction system. Normally, this is paced by the sinoatrial (SA) node, which is located in the right atrium. The SA node is controlled by the vagus nerve, a part of the parasympathetic nervous system. The vagus nerve exerts a slowing action on the SA node to prevent it from discharging electrical impulses too rapidly. The body has other mechanisms for regulating heart activity. These include changes in the systolic blood pressure and changes in blood pH, carbon dioxide, and oxygen levels.

Cardiac function may be affected by sympathetic nervous system stimulation, electrolyte imbalances, drugs, hypoxia, and cardiac injury or disease. These problems may cause the heart to be excitable or irritable, resulting in an irregular or rapid heartbeat. Conversely, the heart may be stimulated too infrequently, resulting in a slow heart rate. A compromised heart may be unable to tolerate excess work or to supply its own oxygen needs and, as a result, may fail.

Circulation

Blood leaves the heart through the arteries. Generally, arteries carry newly oxygenated blood to the tissues, and veins carry deoxygenated blood from the tissues back to the heart and lungs. The pulmonary artery, which carries blood from the heart to the lungs, is the only place in the body where unoxygenated blood is carried by an artery. The pulmonary artery branches into the pulmonary capillary bed for oxygen and carbon dioxide exchange. The oxygenated blood returns from the lungs to the left atrium via the pulmonary vein. This is the only vein in the body that carries newly oxygenated (arterial) blood. Blood leaves the left ventricle via the major artery in the body, the aorta. The aorta branches numerous times into smaller and smaller arteries that supply the entire body with blood. The smallest arterial structures, which branch into the capillary beds, are the arterioles. The junction of the arterioles and capillaries contains precapillary sphincters that can constrict or relax as necessary to control the flow of blood to a specific capillary bed.

Blood circulating through the capillary bed exits via the venules, or smallest veins in the body. Gradually, these drain the blood into larger veins until the superior vena cava and inferior vena cava drain the collected blood into the heart. Veins in the legs and skeletal muscles contain a series of flaps or folds (valves) to prevent backflow of blood due to gravity and thus aid in the movement of blood returning to the heart.

The Blood

Body oxygenation depends on the transport of oxygenated blood to the body tissues. When the blood leaves the tissues, it carries away the waste products of cellular metabolism, especially carbon dioxide. The blood cells that transport oxygen and carbon dioxide are called *erythrocytes,* or red blood cells (RBCs). Erythrocytes are small biconcave discs. The erythrocytes are formed in the bone marrow of long bones and large flat bones and complete their maturation in the circulatory system. There is rapid turnover of erythrocytes and hence a constant need for new cells. Each erythrocyte lives about 120 days.[7] Because of the rapid turnover, a relatively constant supply of nutrients is required to maintain a stable quantity of erythrocytes. The components of a balanced diet that are essential to erythrocyte synthesis include amino acids, iron, copper, vitamin B_6 (pyridoxine), cobalt, vitamin B_{12} (cobalamin), and folic acid.[8]

The **hematocrit** is a measure of the relationship of erythrocytes (or solids) to liquids in the blood. It is found by taking a blood sample and spinning it rapidly in a centrifuge to force the heavier solid elements (RBCs) to collect at one end of the tube and the lighter, liquid portion of the blood to collect at the other. The relationship between the two portions is then measured. If 40 percent of the length of the tube of blood is solids and 60 percent is liquids, then the hematocrit is said to be 40 percent.

The essential component of the erythrocyte for oxygen transport is **hemoglobin,** which is made up of an iron-containing pigment (heme) and a protein (globin). Oxygen is loosely bound to the iron in the heme for distribution to body cells. This combination is called oxyhemoglobin. Each heme molecule can combine with a maximum of four oxygen molecules. A heme molecule that is carrying four oxygen molecules is considered to be 100 percent saturated. When heme is 100 percent saturated, oxygen transfer to tissue is optimal.

If the hemoglobin level is low, or if it is of poor quality and unable to take up normal amounts of oxygen (as in sickle cell anemia), the total amount of oxygen delivered to the tissues will be lower than normal. Normal oxygen transport is also compromised if the iron bound to the heme molecule does not remain in the ferrous state. Certain toxins and oxidizing agents convert ferrous iron to ferric iron, forming methemoglobin, which cannot carry oxygen.

CELLULAR RESPIRATION

Cellular respiration, or internal respiration, consists of the use of oxygen and production of carbon dioxide by cells and the gaseous exchanges between the cells and their fluid medium.[5] All of the processes discussed thus far exist to support cellular respiration.

Plasma-to-cell Transfer

Hemoglobin-bound oxygen is not directly involved in the gas exchange with tissues. Oxygen diffuses from the hemoglobin molecule into the plasma, and then into the interstitial fluid, and finally into cells. For oxygen to be released from hemoglobin, a gradient must be established. This occurs when the small amount of free oxygen dissolved in plasma diffuses out of the bloodstream as the blood flows through the capillaries. The reduction in plasma PO_2 relative to erythrocyte PO_2 causes hemoglobin to release its oxygen to the plasma. Because the PO_2 of plasma is higher than that of the interstitial fluid or the cells, oxygen diffusion is a continuous process.

Several factors affect the release of oxygen from hemoglobin to the tissues. It is facilitated by an increase in $PaCO_2$, greater production of metabolic acids (decreased pH), and an increase in body temperature. Conversely, hemoglobin's affinity for oxygen is greater, and oxygen is therefore less likely to be released, when body temperature falls, pH falls, or $Paco_2$ falls.

The loss of oxygen from the heme molecule increases its affinity for carbon dioxide, for which there is a gradient in the opposite direction. Hence, as oxygen moves into the cells, carbon dioxide moves from cells, to interstitial fluid, to plasma, to erythrocytes for transport to the alveoli, from which it is excreted from the body in the exhaled air.

Oxygen Use

Oxygen is essential to body cells because it is a major component of the reactions that produce cellular energy. The energy, which is produced in the form of adenosine triphosphate (ATP), is essential for the metabolic activities of the body cells. A continuous supply of oxygen is essential if the cells are to be able to carry on their activities.

Cellular oxygen requirements vary according to the demands placed on the cell. The body at rest normally requires about 250 mL of oxygen per minute and produces about 200 mL of CO_2 per minute. Factors that increase oxygen need are fever, exercise, and shivering. Heavy exercise increases muscular oxygen needs and CO_2 production by as much as 20 times. Factors that decrease cellular oxygen need are relaxation and hypothermia.[7]

Anaerobic Metabolism

If the blood is not adequately oxygenated, the diffusion gradient to the tissues is less, so the heme gives up oxygen less readily. A decrease in the oxygen supply to a cell or group of cells leads to a state of partial or total hypoxia. **Hypoxia** is oxygen deficiency at the tissue level. Anaerobic metabolism is the term for the cellular activities that take place when oxygen is not being supplied. Depending on the severity of the hypoxia, the cells may adapt, be injured, or die. When hypoxia occurs, production of ATP is impaired. Glycolysis—the breaking down of glucose—can continue anaerobically for a time, but this produces only very small amounts of ATP. The waste product of anaerobic metabolism is lactic acid, not carbon dioxide. The lungs cannot rid the body of lactic acid, so it builds up in the body and causes metabolic acidosis.[5] The compensatory response by the lungs, hyperventilation, is discussed in a later section. However, respiratory compensation can be sustained only if there is a sufficient supply of oxygen to the body. Without oxygen, death ensues.

FACTORS AFFECTING OXYGENATION IN HEALTH

A person whose body is well oxygenated should be able to carry out the usual activities of daily living without excess fatigue or dyspnea. There is a range of levels of oxygen need both among healthy individuals and within a given individual at different times and circumstances. Many of the factors that affect oxygenation in healthy or relatively healthy individuals could be considered lifestyle factors. Others are physiologic, developmental, or environmental.

GENERAL HEALTH AND LIFESTYLE

Fitness

Exercise and conditioning, which are closely related, contribute to fitness. Exercise increases the metabolic rate of several major organs, thereby increasing their oxygen requirements. During exercise, skeletal muscles demand and receive a much larger blood supply than they do during rest. The heart contracts more rapidly and forcefully and the person breathes more deeply and rapidly to supply the extra oxygen needed for exercise.

Conditioning is the improvement in oxygen utilization that occurs in response to regular exercise. A conditioned muscle requires less oxygen per unit of work than an unconditioned muscle. In other words, the more conditioned a muscle becomes, the less oxygen it needs to accomplish a given task. Hence the cardiopulmonary workload is reduced for all activities when a person is well conditioned. This is why aerobic exercise and conditioning programs are an important part of maintaining good health.

Nutrition

Two nutrition-related factors influence oxygenation: weight and nutrient intake. Individuals who are overweight sometimes experience compromised oxygenation, because the heavy lower thorax and abdomen reduce the capacity of the lungs to expand. This is a problem particularly when the person is lying down. Moreover, the extra muscular work required for body movement when a person is overweight increases oxygen demand. This effect may be magnified if the person is poorly conditioned, which is often the case, as a sedentary lifestyle is a common contributing factor to obesity. It is not unusual, therefore, for an overweight individual to experience shortness of breath with mild physical exertion.

To produce the quantity and quality of erythrocytes needed for optimum oxygen transport, individuals must consume the nutrients needed to synthesize erythrocytes and hemoglobin (see *The Blood,* earlier in this chapter). A well-balanced diet supplies sufficient nutrients for healthy individuals to produce adequate erythrocytes. (See also Chap. 28.)

Smoking

Smoking is a lifestyle choice that is a direct cause of decreased oxygen availability to the body tissues. When a person smokes cigarettes, some of the oxygen in the lungs—and consequently in the blood—is replaced by carbon monoxide from the cigarette smoke. Therefore, bodily oxygenation is reduced. Chronic smokers always have a high level of carbon monoxide in their blood. This is also true of people who live and work with smokers. Smoking in a closed space, such as an automobile, leads to rapid accumulation of carbon monoxide in the enclosed air and a high carbon monoxide level in the blood of everyone inside, whether they are actually smoking or not.

Substance Abuse

Substance abuse is a major problem physiologically, psychologically, and socioeconomically. Various substances can cause diverse oxygenation problems. For example, opiates such as meperidine (Demerol), heroin, and morphine can cause (among other effects) slow, shallow respirations; hypoxia; or even respiratory arrest, hypotension, and cardiac arrhythmias. The use of alcohol impairs the protective reflexes of the airway, which increases the risk of aspiration of food or emesis. Barbiturates produce bradycardia (slowed heart rate), hypotension, changes in respiratory rate and depth, and respiratory paralysis and circulatory collapse. Stimulants such as cocaine, amphetamines, and benzene can cause serious tachycardia (increased heart rate), hypertension, tachypnea (rapid shallow breathing), and even cardiac arrest. Hallucinogens such as LSD and PCP can cause tachycardia, hypertension, respiratory paralysis, and hyperthermia (which elevates metabolism). Withdrawing from drugs has serious consequences for oxygenation. Tachycardia, hypertension, respiratory changes, fever, and cardiovascular collapse have been reported.[9]

Emotional Stress

Stress can affect oxygenation by increasing the body's metabolic rate. When a person is upset or under acute stress, the adrenal medulla releases hormones called catecholamines, which act to prepare the body to protect itself. This increases the oxygen need of many body tissues and therefore increases the work of the heart and lungs, which must pump more oxygenated blood to meet the higher oxygen demands.

DEVELOPMENT

Although the same general principles apply, there are some differences in the anatomy and physiology related to oxygenation of the body at various age levels, particularly at extremes of age.

Premature Infants, Infants, and Toddlers

Oxygenation is often compromised in premature infants for several reasons. *Respiratory distress syndrome* (RDS) is common. RDS occurs because premature infants often lack surfactant, which is necessary to maintain alveolar patency. Not only is the work of breathing increased dramatically in RDS, but insufficient oxygen–carbon dioxide exchange results in hypoxia. Premature infants are also at risk for irregular breathing patterns and apnea.[10]

Infants of diabetic mothers may have delayed lung maturation, which increases their risk for RDS.[11] In the first 3 months of life, infants are obligate nasal breathers due to the large size of the tongue and the shape of the epiglottis.[12] Therefore, it is critical that at least one nostril be kept clear at all times.

There are other anatomic differences. Whereas the adult chest wall can expand downward, so its size is increased by lowering the diaphragm, infants do not have this capability. Instead, their chest walls expand outward or horizontally to enlarge the chest cavity for inspiration. In some cases, an infant's chest wall may be drawn in during inspiration, creating mild retractions (or indentations of the chest wall). This is considered normal in the neonate. Retractions should disappear as the child becomes older and the chest becomes more rigid. Diaphragmatic-abdominal breathing continues until about 5 years of age. If an infant or young child has a respiratory problem, a state of respiratory insufficiency may be reached more quickly than in an older child or adult because the accessory muscles of breathing are not yet well developed.[12]

Infants are susceptible to airway obstruction or collapse because the airway is small and relatively straight and the cartilage that supports it is still soft. The risk of airway obstruction continues through toddlerhood. At this age, aspiration of food or small objects is relatively common as well.

The respiratory rate of infants is rapid, ranging from 30 to 70 breaths per minute; the sleeping respiratory rate is usually less than 40 per minute. An infant's normal pulse is 120 to 160 per minute. A toddler's respiratory rate averages 20 to 30 beats per minute; pulse rate is 100 to 110.

Preschool and School-aged Children and Adolescents

The cardiorespiratory physiologic processes mature throughout childhood. By 7 years of age the transition to thoracic breathing is complete. The normal respiratory and pulse rates decline with age. For example, in a preschool child the respiratory rate is 20 to 30 and the pulse rate 90 to 120, while an elementary school age child has a respiratory rate of 20 to 26 and a pulse rate of 70 to 110. Teenagers' pulse and respiratory rates, and their anatomy and physiology, are the same as that of adults.[12]

Older Adults

As a person ages, connective tissue changes cause some loss of lung elasticity. Some individuals also experience postural changes related to osteoporosis, which decrease the capacity for lung expansion. Normal Po_2 gradually declines with age. Healthy people in their 80s, for example, have some measure of alveolar deterioration, even if they have never smoked. This is called physiological emphysema. As a result, the normal Po_2 for an elderly person is somewhat lower than for a younger adult. The exact Po_2 that is normal for each elderly person is an individual matter, but anything above 80 mm Hg is considered acceptable. A low Po_2 may increase the cardiac workload and reduce exercise tolerance somewhat, but for the healthy aging person, it should not compromise normal activities of daily life. Conditioning and individual factors such as genetics and smoking history affect elderly persons' oxygenation and exercise status far more than do physiologic changes.

ENVIRONMENT

Air Quality

Clean air is essential to optimum oxygenation. Today air pollution is either a continuous or intermittent problem in many urban areas and is even a problem in some rural areas. Air stagnation worsens the effects of pollution. Air pollution interferes with oxygenation because some of the noxious gases in the air take the place of oxygen in the lungs and in the blood.

Altitude

Because barometric pressure decreases as altitude increases, the oxygen content of the environmental air is lower at high altitudes than at sea level. If a person travels to a higher altitude and stays there for 6 weeks, extra red blood cells will be produced in order to carry more oxygen to the body cells. The person will have increased fatigue and a reduced exercise tolerance for about 6 weeks; only after that time will he or she regain the previous energy level. High altitudes may have a particularly detrimental effect on a person with cardiac or pulmonary disease. Such a person's already compromised bodily Po_2 can fall low enough to cause serious respiratory distress.

Climate

Weather extremes also tend to increase bodily oxygen needs. Oxygen consumption increases in very hot weather as well as in very cold weather. Going out into very cold weather is stressful to the body and should be avoided by people with cardiopulmonary compromise. Individuals with oxygenation problems should not attempt to work outside in excessively hot or cold weather.

ALTERED OXYGENATION

INTERRELATEDNESS OF OXYGENATION PROCESSES

The processes that support oxygenation are interrelated. Therefore, a change in one of the processes often affects the others. Without adequate ventilation, for example, diffusion, perfusion, and cellular respiration will not be normal.

Altered oxygenation may be divided into four categories: (1) altered ventilation, (2) altered diffusion, (3) altered perfusion, and (4) altered cellular respiration.

ALTERED VENTILATION

Altered ventilation refers to changes in the movement of air from the atmosphere to the alveoli. There are two types of altered ventilation: hypoventilation and hyperventilation.

Hypoventilation

Hypoventilation is the condition of inadequate movement of air into and out of the lungs. Typically, this is detected by a rise in the P_{CO_2}. It *cannot* be accurately assessed by watching a person breathe. The signs and symptoms of hypoventilation include altered respiration (either slow and shallow or deep and labored due to efforts to move additional air), dyspnea (difficulty breathing), orthopnea (difficulty breathing unless sitting or standing), tachycardia, and anxiety. Neurologic changes, such as altered judgment, coordination, or level of consciousness, also may be present. Factors contributing to hypoventilation may include airway obstruction, lung or chest pathology, inappropriate administration of oxygen, and pain in the thorax or abdomen.

Airway Obstruction. Airway obstruction blocks movement of air into and out of the lungs. As the work of breathing increases, oxygenation may be compromised. Airway obstruction may be caused by a foreign body or by excess secretions, among other factors.

A foreign body is not an uncommon cause of airway obstruction. Children often place small objects or food in their mouths and aspirate them (ie, the object or food goes down the trachea to the lung). Adults aspirate food, fluids, or oral secretions. Once in the lung, the foreign body may partially or completely occlude a small or large airway. The more complete the obstruction and the larger the airway occluded, the more serious the patient's respiratory distress will be.

Excessive respiratory secretions may also obstruct airways when lung pathology is present. For example, a person with pneumonia or chronic bronchitis, both of which cause large amounts of secretions, may be unable to cough effectively to clear the secretions out of airways. If a large airway or many smaller airways are affected, serious respiratory distress and compromised oxygenation can result.

People who are extremely fatigued, generally debilitated, or who have a neuromuscular disease that affects the chest may retain secretions because they are unable to cough well enough to clear them out of the chest. These individuals may also be unable to sustain the increased work of breathing caused by the obstructed airways and so are unable to move air into and out of the lungs effectively. As a result, oxygenation will be compromised.

Decreased Lung Capacity. If lung expansion is restricted, the volume of air that can be exchanged is also limited. Pregnancy is a common cause of decreased lung capacity. As pregnancy advances and the uterus expands, the diaphragm is pushed upward. Therefore, deep breathing is difficult and a subjective sensation of shortness of breath is common. Usually the loss of capacity is not severe enough to cause compromised oxygenation.

A full stomach can compromise respirations in a similar fashion. It is more likely to reduce oxygenation or cause respiratory distress in a person who already has cardiopulmonary disease. This is why those with oxygenation problems are encouraged to eat small meals rather than large ones and to avoid gas-forming foods.

Lung capacity can also be reduced by other circumstances. For example, if a person has pneumonia, many of the alveoli are filled with exudate and are not available for gas exchange. If a person has a chest injury and cannot expand the chest wall normally, lung capacity is diminished. Diseases causing bony deformity of the thorax may limit lung expansion. These are only a few examples of disorders that can reduce lung capacity and increase the risk for hypoventilation.

Inappropriate Administration of Oxygen. Normally, the body is stimulated to breathe by the buildup of carbon dioxide, which stimulates the respiratory center. If a person has a chronically high CO_2 level, the respiratory center can lose its sensitivity to excess CO_2. When this happens, the peripheral chemoreceptors stimulate the body to breathe by their response to hypoxia or a low oxygen level. If a patient who normally retains CO_2 excessively is given a high level of oxygen, the P_{O_2} may not fall to a level low enough to stimulate the peripheral chemoreceptors, and the person may cease to breathe. This sometimes happens to patients with chronic lung disease who turn their oxygen levels up too high in response to dyspnea or respiratory distress.

Hyperventilation

Hyperventilation means that a person moves more air through the lungs than normal. This can be assessed by a low Pa_{CO_2} when the arterial blood gases are measured. It cannot be assessed by watching the patient breathe. A person's breathing may appear to be deep and rapid when, actually, the individual is simply working very hard to move an abnormally small amount of air. That person may have **tachypnea** (rapid, shallow respirations) or **hyperpnea** (increased rate and depth of respirations), but not necessarily hyperventilation. Some possible causes of hyperventilation are anxiety, pain, reduced atmospheric oxygen, lung pathology, and metabolic acidosis. Some of these are discussed below.

Decreased Atmospheric Oxygen. The body responds to reduced atmospheric oxygen on a short-term basis by hyperventilating. For example, if a person moves to a high altitude or is in a closed space with little available oxygen, the tendency is to breathe more deeply and rapidly in order to move more oxygen into the body and improve oxygenation.

Anxiety, Fear, and Pain. Anxiety, fear, and pain are stressors that can cause hyperventilation. Direct stimulation of the respiratory center from the limbic system (activated during strong emotions) may contribute to hyperventilation associated with fear and pain.[5] Conscious voluntary efforts to slow and deepen respirations can overcome stress-induced hyperventilation.

Acid-Base Balance. Metabolic status affects oxygen need in a variety of ways. Body cells must maintain a pH between 7.35 and 7.45 to function correctly. If metabolic acids build up in the body, the cells function less effectively and need more oxygen. In addition, the lungs attempt to reduce the total acid load in the body by eliminating more CO_2 than usual. Hence, hyperventilation can be a physiologic response to metabolic acidosis as the lungs work to reduce the body's acid load. Conversely, in a person with metabolic alkalosis, or too little acid in the body, the lungs attempt to conserve acid by depressing ventilation. (Acid–base balance is discussed in detail in Chap. 34.)

ALTERED DIFFUSION

In altered diffusion, the ability of the respiratory gases to diffuse from the alveoli to the pulmonary capillaries and back again is impaired. Usually, the problem is one of barriers in the diffusion path, either fluid accumulation or excessive secretions, or altered anatomy of the alveolar–capillary structure.

Fluid Accumulation

Many conditions may cause fluid accumulation in the diffusion path. One is failure of the left ventricle. When the left side of the heart cannot pump effectively, the blood then backs up into the pulmonary circulation. The pulmonary capillaries are distensible and can accept a great deal of blood; however, when they reach their capacity, fluid is pushed out into the pulmonary interstitium. This results in a layer of fluid between the alveoli and capillaries, called **pulmonary edema,** which greatly reduces the ability of the gases to diffuse between the alveoli and the pulmonary capillaries. As the condition progresses, fluid seeps into the alveoli as well, so that there are two layers of fluid between the gas in the alveoli and the pulmonary capillaries. As a result, the movement of oxygen and carbon dioxide between the air and the blood is seriously impeded.

Excessive Secretions

Secretions can accumulate in the alveoli for a variety of reasons, such as a chest cold or pneumonia. These secretions cover some of the alveolar surfaces so that the diffusing membrane becomes much thicker. As a result, gaseous movement is hampered.

Alveolar Pathology

Abnormalities of the alveoli may reduce the surface area available for gas exchange. For example, in emphysema, there is destruction of alveolar and capillary tissues. As a result, less surface area is available for gas exchange.

ALTERED PERFUSION

Altered perfusion refers to problems with the delivery of oxygenated blood to the body tissues. A variety of problems can cause altered perfusion. Several of the major ones are discussed here.

Decreased Cardiac Output

The delivery of adequate oxygen to the tissues depends on a normally functioning heart. The left ventricle in particular must pump regularly and energetically to deliver blood to the body. If the functioning of the left ventricle is impaired, the body will not receive an adequate blood supply. This leads to fatigue and impaired organ function. In addition, blood can back up into the lungs, as described above under *Fluid Accumulation.*

Hypovolemia or Low Hemoglobin Level

For gas exchange to take place, adequate blood volume and adequate numbers of red blood cells must be available to carry the oxygen and nutrients. A serious blood loss (hypovolemia), a low hemoglobin level, or a low red blood cell count could leave an individual with too few functioning red blood cells to carry the oxygen needed to nourish the body.

Vascular Occlusions

Delivery of blood to a localized area of the body can be interrupted by a variety of vascular occlusions. The occlusions may be of two types: internal and external.

Internal Occlusions. Internal occlusions are caused by excessive clotting of the blood, stasis of the blood, or excessive viscosity of the blood. If an arterial blood vessel is totally or partially occluded by a clot, the area served by that vessel will not be properly perfused and oxygenated. The effects may be local, such as when the clot is in a leg or an arm, or they may be more widespread, such as when the clot is in the lung or the brain. A clot in the lung *(pulmonary embolism)* could cause hypoxia and its general effects, while a clot in the brain could cause a cerebral vascular accident (stroke).

Conditions of the vessels themselves can also impair the delivery of blood. Conditions involving thickening, loss of elasticity, and calcification of the arterial walls are not uncommon. There may also be deposits of fats, cholesterol, and debris on the inner walls of the arteries. Any of these conditions reduces the size of the involved vessels and hinders their ability to increase in diameter when an increased blood supply is needed in the area. Spasm of the arteries sometimes also occurs. This reduces the blood supply to the area served by the vessel. If it occurs in a vessel that supplies a skeletal muscle, the result is usually pain and reduced exercise tolerance.

External Occlusion. External occlusion of a vessel can result from factors within or outside the body. Either way, the compressed vessel cannot supply the needed amount of blood to body tissues. Within the body, the most common causes of pressure on a vessel are edema (swelling) or tumors. Pressure from outside the body can result from poor positioning (as when one leg is lying directly on top of the other), or from constricting bandages, casts, braces, antiembolism stockings, or clothing (such as garters). Signs and symptoms distal to the compression may include edema, discoloration, discomfort, coolness of the extremity, and diminished pulses. It is always important to check for indicators of external compression if any risk factor exists and to take all possible measures to prevent external compression of the vessels.

ALTERED CELLULAR RESPIRATION

Altered cellular respiration refers to a change in the oxygen-carbon dioxide exchange between the cells and the fluid medium surrounding them. Any of the above alterations may compromise cellular respiration on a local or generalized basis. In addition, fever, edema, toxic substances, or conditions that alter metabolism may influence cellular respiration directly.

Fever

Fever is the most common condition that has a direct effect on cellular respiration. When the body temperature rises, the rate of metabolic activity increases, creating an increased demand for oxygen throughout the body. As previously discussed, more oxygen is released from hemoglobin when body temperature is elevated, thus helping to meet cellular needs.

Other problems that elevate metabolism are drugs such as steroids and adrenalin, and diseases of the adrenal glands or the

COLLABORATIVE STRATEGY

HYPOXIA

Collaborating with a patient who is severely hypoxic can be extremely taxing to the patient and even inappropriate when hypoxia renders the patient breathless or confused. Such manifestations significantly diminish the patient's capacity to participate in a health interview, and it may be necessary to shift the focus of collaboration to the patient's significant others until the patient's condition is improved.

thyroid. Metabolic increases can be particularly damaging to persons who have heart disease or compromised brain tissue. These tissues are easily damaged if their oxygen needs are not met.

Edema

In edema, fluid occupies space in interstitial fluid and thereby increases the distance between the cells and the capillaries that bring them oxygenated blood. The increased distance slows diffusion of oxygen from the capillaries to the cells and carbon dioxide from the cells into the bloodstream. Severe edema can significantly alter cellular respiration and result in cellular hypoxia.

CLINICAL GUIDELINE 30–2

POSSIBLE CONSEQUENCES OF ALTERED OXYGENATION

HYPOXEMIA

- Decrease in blood oxygen concentration (Po_2)
- *Signs and symptoms:* May be absent. May be increased respiratory rate and depth.

HYPOXIA

- The lack of adequate oxygen supply at the tissue level. Reflected in low Po_2.
- *Signs and symptoms:* Increased respiratory rate and depth, impaired judgment, drowsiness, disorientation, headache, tachycardia, hypertension.

HYPERCAPNIA

- Retention of CO_2 in the body. Reflected by high Pco_2.
- *Signs and symptoms:* Initially stimulates respiration. If accumulates, produces central nervous system depression (confusion, diminished sensory acuity, coma, respiratory depression).

HYPOCAPNIA

- Low concentration of CO_2. Reflected by low Pco_2. Usually caused by hyperventilation.
- *Signs and symptoms:* Lightheadedness, dizziness, and altered sensation (paresthesias).

TISSUE NECROSIS

- Tissue death due to low oxygenation.
- *Signs and symptoms:* Pain, darkened color, progressing to white; swelling; liquefaction.

Toxins

Toxic substances may prevent tissues from receiving adequate oxygen, even when perfusion is adequate. For example, carbon monoxide (CO) interferes with oxygen transport, because it binds more readily and tightly to heme, displacing oxygen. Even though the number of circulating red blood cells is adequate, many will be carrying CO, not O_2. CO does not diffuse from RBCs as blood passes through capillaries, so fewer RBCs are available to take up oxygen when the blood returns through the pulmonary circulation. Furthermore, the heme that is carrying oxygen releases it less readily in the presence of carbon monoxide.

CONSEQUENCES OF ALTERED OXYGENATION

The consequences of altered oxygenation may include hypoxia, hypercapnia, hypocapnia, and tissue necrosis (Clinical Guideline 30–2). Further discussion of the signs and symptoms of oxygenation dysfunction is found later in the chapter. Understanding the major causes and pathologies of altered oxygen supply provides a basis for assessment and management of related patient health problems.

SECTION 2
ASSESSMENT OF OXYGENATION

OXYGENATION DATA COLLECTION

Because oxygenation is one of the most basic of human needs, the assessment of oxygenation status is a critical nursing activity. Nurses can obtain many clues to oxygenation status by skillful assessment. This section focuses on aspects of history and physical examination that are pertinent to oxygenation status. It should be used in addition to the other history and physical examination information contained in Chap. 17.

OXYGENATION HISTORY

Although a careful history is a critical component of any assessment, a detailed history may be inappropriate for the newly admitted patient with oxygenation problems. A patient who is severely hypoxic or in severe pain, for example, may be unable to talk except for very brief phrases and remarks. Hypoxic patients also may be too confused to give an accurate history. In these instances, patients' energy is best saved for life processes. A history may be obtained from a family member or deferred until the patient is better able to converse. Only the physical examination would be done at this time. The historical information is organized according to the typical health history format.

Primary Concern

Sometimes a patient states the primary concern as a problem related to oxygenation—for example, "I can't catch my breath" or "I have a lot of congestion in my chest." In this case, immediately proceed with the oxygenation data collection. However, some statements of primary concern may be less direct; for example, "I'm tired all of the time" or "I can't get around like I used to." Such concerns may indicate a variety of problems, but can signal alterations affecting oxygenation. A prudent nurse would conduct an oxygenation assessment to verify or rule out a nursing diagnosis related to oxygenation.

> Ann Seymore, a 35-year-old single professional woman, complains of audible wheezing and tightness in her chest. She states that she has been generally healthy throughout her life with no noticeable allergies or respiratory distress. Within the last few weeks, she has developed a tightness in her chest and her exercise tolerance is reduced. She had been running 2 miles a day. Now, she is unable to complete the 2 miles without one or two rest periods. Her friends have also commented that they can hear her wheezing. She did not notice the wheezing until they pointed it out. She wheezes audibly even at rest in an upright position. She is sleeping poorly at night but cannot point to any particular reason for awakening frequently and having to sit up for a while before she goes back to sleep. She has continued her usual work and household activities, but this is becoming increasingly difficult.
>
> As a result of the discussion about Ms. Seymore's problem, the nurse recognizes that pursuing the oxygenation history and examination is relevant. He notes that Ms. Seymore's regular exercise can be an asset to her overall health status.

Current Understanding

It is appropriate to begin the interview by asking about patients' current understanding of the problem. Ask about the mode of onset, precipitating events, patients' view of the severity of the symptoms, their relation to daily activities or changes in them, and the effect of various treatments. Such questions tell nurses what to look for in the detailed history and physical examination and give an idea of the expectation for care. They also can give clues about patients' understanding of the basis for the problem and possible health teaching that may be indicated.

For example, many smokers deny that they smoke enough to affect their health. They also may feel that they are unable to stop smoking and that as a consequence there is no point in trying. Therefore, heavy smokers commonly either deny that smoking is related to their present symptoms or make statements such as "coughing is normal for me."

Past Health Experiences/Problems

Asking whether patients have had past health problems that have affected oxygenation, such as respiratory infections, allergies, coughs, dyspnea, wheezing, heart problems, or circulatory problems, and if there are residual effects is also helpful. Because many medications influence cardiac or respiratory function, ask patients to list medications they take regularly or intermittently. The following case example illustrates the importance of past health experiences and problems in the oxygenation assessment.

> Interviewing Mrs. Solomon, who was admitted to a medical unit after an acute asthma attack, the nurse learns that Mrs. Solomon has been treated with an iron preparation for "low blood" (ie, anemia) but that she stopped taking the medication because it caused constipation. Checking the patient's current hemoglobin and hematocrit reports, the nurse finds that both hemoglobin and hematocrit are abnormally low. The nurse communicates with Mrs. Soloman's physician about the possible need for iron therapy and devises a teaching plan to help Mrs. Solomon minimize the constipation associated with iron preparations.

Personal, Family, and Social History

Impaired cellular oxygenation can affect nearly all aspects of a person's life. Helping patients to minimize or cope effectively with the deficit is a primary nursing responsibility. The personal and social history provides information about patients' habits and preferences that can be used in collaborative planning of nursing approaches for the current health problem (Table 30–2).

> Mrs. Jenkins, age 48, is referred to the pulmonary clinic after participating in a public health screening program that found her pulmonary function to be below normal limits. During the interview, she states that she has smoked three to four packs of cigarettes a day for about 30 years. She admits to increasingly frequent "colds" accompanied by the production of large amounts of yellow or green sputum. In the last 10 years, she has stopped hiking with her family and now leaves chores such as carrying groceries, bedmaking, and vacuuming to her teenage children. When asked why she has given up these activities, she attributes her loss of exercise tolerance to aging.
>
> As a result of this history, the nurse recommends medical evaluation of Mrs. Jenkins's condition based on data regarding heavy smoking, increasing respiratory infections, reduced pulmonary function, and reduced exercise tolerance. She advises Mrs. Jenkins that with treatment, her condition will probably improve. Particularly important, she explains to Mrs. Jenkins that her problems are not solely due to aging.

Smoking history deserves special emphasis in a discussion related to oxygenation. Tobacco use is one of the most important risk factors for cardiopulmonary disease. If a patient smokes or has smoked in the past, a specific smoking history is essential to the oxygenation assessment. Ask when the patient began smoking, how many years he or she smoked, and how many packs per day. Inquire if the number of packs smoked per day has varied at different times (see Table 30–2). If so, find out how many years the patient smoked each number of packs per day. A pack-year history can then be calculated by multiplying the number of packs per day times the number of years smoked. For example:

$$1 \text{ ppd} \times 10 \text{ years} = 10 \text{ pack-years}$$
$$2 \text{ ppd} \times 10 \text{ years} = 20 \text{ pack-years}$$

Following is a case illustration for calculating a smoking history.

> Mr. Garcia states that he started smoking at the age of 12 and smoked one pack of cigarettes per day until he was 16. At that time, he increased his smoking to one and one-half packs per day for 6 years. At age 22, he increased to three packs per day, and has smoked at that level since. He is now 48. What is his pack-year history?

$$1 \text{ ppd} \times 4 \text{ years} = 4 \text{ pack-years}$$
$$1\tfrac{1}{2} \text{ ppd} \times 6 \text{ years} = 9 \text{ pack-years}$$
$$3 \text{ ppd} \times 26 \text{ years} = 78 \text{ pack-years}$$
$$\text{Total: } 4 \text{ pack-years} + 9 \text{ pack-years} + 78 \text{ pack-years} = 91 \text{ pack-years total smoking}$$

Ask when the patient stopped smoking (if he or she has stopped) and why. People often stop smoking when symptoms become intolerable. A patient's reason for stopping smoking gives an idea of the point at which the patient acknowledged the seriousness of the symptoms.

TABLE 30-2. OXYGENATION HISTORY: PERSONAL, FAMILY, AND SOCIAL HISTORY QUESTIONS

A. Vocational
1. What jobs have you had?
2. When was each and for how long?
3. Were you exposed to chemicals or other breathing hazards in any job (eg, asbestos, formaldehyde, pesticides, silica, etc)?

B. Home and Family
1. Where do you live? How long have you lived there?
2. Where have you lived in the past?
3. Is environmental pollution a problem where you live?
4. Have your breathing problems interfered with your home and family responsibilities? How have you dealt with this?
5. Can you bend over and tie your shoes, carry a bag of groceries, walk uphill, climb stairs, make a bed, and vacuum? If you stopped any of these activities, when and why?

C. Social and Leisure
1. What are your favorite leisure-time activities?
2. Who do you usually share these activities with?
3. Do you belong to clubs or groups?
4. Have you had to limit social or leisure activities because of breathing difficulties?
5. What are your hobbies?
6. Do any of your leisure activities involve exposure to dusts, fumes, or other irritants?

D. Sexual
1. Has your sexual activity been affected by your breathing problems? In what way?
2. If yes, have you and your partner been able to adapt in a way that both of you can accept?

E. Habits

Exercise
1. Approximately how much exercise do you get each week? What exercise do you do?
2. Do you have to stop and rest frequently during the activity?
3. Do you get short of breath or wheeze during exercise?

Diet
1. What do you eat during a typical day?
2. Do any foods cause you particular problems?
3. Are you able to prepare your meals without difficulty?
4. Do you ever skip meals because of breathing difficulty after eating?
5. Do you have any problems obtaining groceries?

Beverages
1. What kinds of beverages do you drink each day?
2. Do you drink caffeinated drinks? How many?
3. Do you use alcohol? How much?
4. How much milk do you drink per day?
5. What would you estimate to be the total number of 8-ounce glasses of all liquids that you drink on most days?

Sleep
1. In what position do you sleep?
2. Can you breathe comfortably when lying flat on your back? If not, how high do you prop up to breathe?
3. Do you ever wake up at night coughing or short of breath?

Tobacco Use
1. Have you ever smoked cigarettes, cigars, or pipes? If so, when and how many?
2. Have you ever used smokeless tobacco (snuff)?
3. If you used any of these and stopped, when and why?
4. If you did smoke, did the amount you smoked change at different times during your life?
5. How many packs per day or cigars per day did you smoke during each of those time periods?

Other Substances
1. Have you used marijuana, cocaine, pills, or other drugs at any time during your life?
2. What did you use and how long did you use it?
3. What symptoms did you get from it?
4. When and why did you stop?

F. Psychological

Coping
1. Have you experienced stress in your life recently?
2. What has been helpful to you in dealing with stress?
3. Has stress caused increased breathing difficulty?

Self-image
1. Has your illness affected the way you feel about yourself?
2. Would you say that your self-respect has been altered?

Sick Role
1. Is there anything that is particularly difficult about being in the hospital (or, being sick right now)?
2. Is there anything that you feel could be done to make this experience easier?

Subjective Manifestations

A thorough review of patients' subjective manifestations, using clues found in the discussion of past health problems and the history of present problems, will help nurses focus on pertinent areas of subjective manifestations. See Tables 17–30 and 17–31 for sample questions to elicit information about subjective manifestations that are relevant to oxygenation. An explanation of the symptoms that frequently accompany oxygenation imbalances also is included in Table 30–3 as a guide in directing these questions.

OXYGENATION EXAMINATION

The oxygenation examination focuses on areas of the body that are particularly affected by cardiovascular or respiratory pathology. It

TABLE 30-3. SUMMARY OF SIGNS AND SYMPTOMS THAT FREQUENTLY ACCOMPANY ALTERATIONS IN OXYGENATION

Symptom	Definition	Explanation
General		
Fatigue	Feeling of tiredness, weariness.	Hypoxia, cardiac insufficiency, faulty dietary habits.
Reduced exercise tolerance (dyspnea on exertion [DOE])	Reduced capacity for activity.	May be due to impaired tissue oxygenation from cardiac or respiratory insufficiency.
Chills	Attacks of shivering, feeling of excessive coldness.	Often accompany infections or fever.
Sudden weight gain	As described.	May be due to fluid retention secondary to heart disease; may compromise ventilation.
Integument		
Coldness of extremities	As described.	May be due to poor circulation to extremity because of lowered cardiac output or vascular compromise.
HEENT		
Pain, itching of eyes or nose, nasal congestion, sneezing	As described.	Often due to allergy; may be due to infection of eyes, nose, sinuses.
Respiratory		
Orthopnea	Must sit or stand in order to breathe comfortably.	May be due to fluid accumulation in the lungs resulting from cardiac failure. May be due to poor diaphragmatic function or to lung pathology.
Dyspnea	Marked shortness of breath, audible, labored breathing, accompanied by distressed expression.	May accompany lung or cardiac pathology. May result from inhaling fumes. May be due to allergy.
Hyperpnea	Increase in the rate and/or depth of breathing.	Exercise, partial airway obstruction, excessive lung secretions, hypoxia, early hypercapnia.
Tachypnea	Rapid, shallow breathing, usually defined as greater than 20 per minute.	Decreased lung capacity (obesity, pregnancy), anxiety, pain, shock, cocaine or amphetamine use, pulmonary disease, neurologic disease, drug withdrawal.
Bradypnea	Decreased respiratory rate.	Hypercapnia, metabolic alkalosis, inappropriate administration of oxygen, opiate use, drug overdose, central nervous system dysfunction.
Apnea	Cessation of breathing.	Cardiac arrest, airway occlusion, injury to respiratory center.
Cheyne–Stokes respiration (periodic breathing)	Episodes of apnea interspersed with periods of rapid, deep breaths and then slow, shallow breaths.	Deep sleep, congestive heart failure, brain disease, drug overdose, renal failure.
Kussmaul respiration	Abnormally deep, often rapid, sighing-type respirations.	Diabetic ketoacidosis, metabolic acidosis.
Ataxic respiration	Short bursts of irregular breathing with periods of apnea.	Brain damage.
Pain during breathing	As described; worsens with inspiration.	May be due to chest wall injury, pleural irritation, or strained chest muscles.
Cardiovascular		
Paroxysmal nocturnal dyspnea (PND)	Sudden attacks of respiratory distress during sleep.	Usually due to cardiac failure.
Chest pain	Pain in the chest that may or may not radiate to the arm, shoulder, or jaw. Does not worsen with inspiration.	Usually due to insufficient oxygenation of the heart muscle.
Intermittent claudication	Pain in legs or hips when walking; relieved by rest.	Inadequate oxygenation of leg muscles on exercise, usually due to cardiovascular disease.
Neurologic/Psychological		
Memory problems, confusion, anxiety	As described.	May be due to insufficient oxygenation to the brain as a result of cardiac or pulmonary insufficiency.

CLINICAL GUIDELINE 30–3

RAPID ASSESSMENT OF OXYGENATION

Because major body organs alter their function quickly in the presence of a low blood supply, assessment of these organs can provide information about oxygenation status.

NEUROLOGIC FUNCTION

- Patient should be alert and oriented, not unduly anxious or restless.
- Altered level of consciousness, irritability, poor judgment, or disorientation may reflect a low blood supply to the brain.

CARDIAC FUNCTION

- Heart rate should be regular, and within normal limits for age and sex.
- Pulses should be present and of healthy quality.
- Continuous monitoring, if available, should reveal no arrhythmias.
- Capillary refill should be prompt.
- Extremities should be warm, dry, of healthy color, and without edema.

BLOOD PRESSURE

- Blood pressure should be within normal limits for age and gender with no abrupt changes related to changes in body position (eg, supine to standing).

RESPIRATORY FUNCTION

- Breathing should be quiet, regular, and unlabored.
- There should be no cough, shortness of breath, or orthopnea.

includes observation and assessment of vital signs, the chest, integument, HEENT (head, eyes, ears, nose, and throat), cardiovascular system, respiratory system, and abdomen. When rapid assessment of oxygenation status is needed, focus on the four areas outlined in Clinical Guideline 30–3.

Measurements

Every physical examination should include measurement of the vital signs, temperature, pulse, respiration, and blood pressure (see Chap. 17). Blood pressure should be measured with a patient supine, standing, and sitting. Height and weight should also be measured and compared with a table of norms. Discuss recent changes in weight.

Objective Manifestations

General observation and examination of the integument, HEENT, chest, cardiovascular system, abdomen, and neurologic system supply data relevant to oxygenation status.

General Observations. Nurses can make some general observations relevant to oxygenation status while taking the health history or getting patients admitted and settled into the hospital. An observant nurse can gain a great deal of information before asking a single question. Is the patient alert, oriented, and behaving appropriately? Confusion or lethargy may be due to hypoxia. Can he or she speak in complete sentences, or does shortness of breath limit expression to very short phrases? Does the patient have frequent coughing, wheezing, swallowing, or sniffing?

Note and describe the patient's general appearance. For example, does the patient appear well groomed and clean, or disheveled, dirty, and unkempt? Poor hygiene may result from a low energy level or poor activity tolerance because of insufficient oxygenation. Does the patient appear generally healthy or unhealthy?

During the initial contact, draw some conclusions regarding patients' apparent age. Oxygenation problems often cause individuals to appear much older than their biologic age. This might be charted as "appears older than stated age."

Patients' posture, movement, and apparent energy level can give more clues to oxygenation status. Patients unable to move about at a healthy pace may have inadequately oxygenated muscles. Often, simple activities of daily living can cause such a person to become dyspneic. Posture can also give clues to possible respiratory problems. If a patient is unable to lie down, the orthopnea should be carefully assessed and noted.

Patients' facial expression can convey a great deal of information. Does a patient's face convey feelings of fear or panic? If a patient's face or body language seems to convey a different emotion than his or her words, ask for clarification: "I notice that you are gritting your teeth and frowning. You look as though you are in pain."

Integument. Integumentary assessment is also relevant to oxygenation. Oxygenation disorders may lead to a variety of changes in skin color. Some people become ashen, pale, gray, or cyanotic (bluish color). Cyanosis may be generalized or it may be limited to certain areas, such as the lips and nailbeds. Document and describe the severity and location of the cyanosis. However, if a person does not appear cyanotic, do not take this as evidence of adequate oxygenation. In order for cyanosis to occur, more than one third of hemoglobin (Hgb) must be unsaturated with oxygen.[13] Some people with pulmonary disease do not move air out of the lungs very well. As a result, they retain carbon dioxide, which is a vasodilator, and have a very pink, red, or ruddy skin color. This red color is also characteristic of carbon monoxide poisoning.

Another abnormality of skin color is the presence of excessive bruising or of purpura, which are tiny purple spots. These are most prevalent on the extremities and usually signal a bleeding disorder or long-term use of steroids.

Inspect the fingers closely. Persons with long-term oxygenation problems (such as cystic fibrosis and lung cancer) often have clubbing of the fingers (Fig. 30–3). In clubbing, the profile of the fingernails flattens out and the base of the fingernail becomes soft and spongy. Discoloration of the fingertips can be a clue to cigarette smoking.

The skin of the feet and lower legs displays characteristic changes in individuals with inadequate circulation. Poor peripheral oxygenation causes thin, darkly discolored, or purplish skin in the lower legs and feet.

Also, inspect the legs for edema or abnormal hair distribution. Individuals with insufficient arterial circulation may have no hair below their knees. They may have breaks in the skin or skin ulcers as well. Observe for varicose veins, which are large gnarled veins that are prominent on the surface of the legs. The feet may also feel much cooler than the rest of the body.

Note capillary refill time by depressing the skin over the sternum and the nailbeds of the fingers and toes and watching for return of the pink color. Normally the refill takes less than one second. Sluggish refill, greater than 1 second, indicates possible

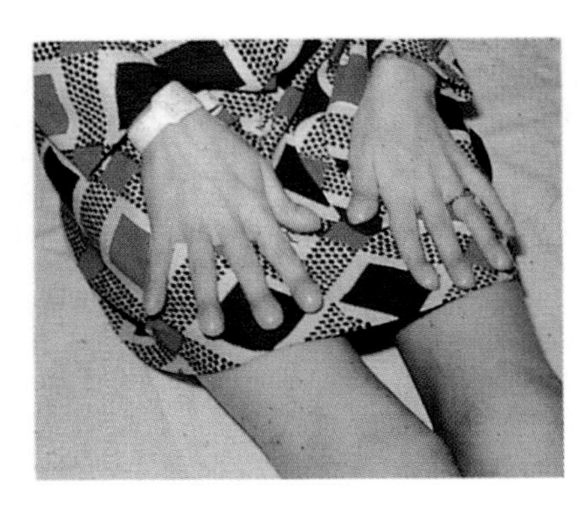

Figure 30–3. Clubbing of the fingers indicating lack of oxygenation to the extremity.

perfusion problems, often related to depletion of body fluid volume. Poor capillary refill in the toes can be related to vascular disease.

HEENT. Several portions of the head, ear, eye, nose, and throat examination can yield important data about oxygenation. Particulars on how to conduct this portion of the examination, as well as more complete information about examination of these organs, may be found in Chaps. 17 and 32.

Check the pupils for size, equality, and speed of reaction to light, which can give clues as to oxygenation of the brain. If there is cerebral edema (swelling of the brain) or lack of oxygen to the brain, the pupils tend to be large and less reactive. One or both pupils that are fixed (nonreactive to light) and dilated signal a neurologic or oxygenation emergency.

Observe the form and symmetry of the nose. Note whether there are changes in the shape of the nostrils during breathing. *Nasal flaring* (enlargement of the nares on inspiration) indicates air hunger, suggesting serious respiratory distress. Carefully inspect the inner surfaces of the nose in good light for signs of inflammation. In healthy people, the nasal mucosa will be pink and moist, with no evidence of edema, bogginess, exudate, drainage, or bleeding. The nasal septum should be straight. There should be no polyps, which are fingerlike projections of nasal mucosa. Asthmatics are especially prone to nasal polyps.

Note the position of the mouth during breathing. Pursed-lip breathing, slow exhalation through puckered lips, is often used by individuals with chronic oxygenation problems to slow and control respiration and achieve better oxygen–carbon dioxide exchange with less respiratory effort. Note also whether this maneuver occurs only on exertion or during quiet sitting as well.

Carefully inspect the interior of the mouth and pharynx. Note the color and moisture of the mucosa. The pharyngeal and oral mucosa should be smooth, moist, and pink with no evidence of exudate, ulcerations, or discoloration. Cyanotic mucous membranes suggest hypoxia.

Inspect the neck for distension of the veins. Venous distension indicates increased venous pressure, often related to reduced myocardial contractility (strength of heart muscle contraction).

Chest and Cardiovascular System. Techniques for examining the chest and descriptions of the landmarks that guide the examination are discussed in Chap. 17. The discussion here addresses changes in the chest examination that suggest oxygenation problems.

Begin with inspection. First, expose the chest and inspect for shape. Some people with pulmonary disease have an increased distance from the front to the back of the chest (increased anterior-posterior [A-P] diameter), or barrel chest. This is a result of air trapping within the lungs; however, not all individuals who trap air have an increased A-P diameter. Some who have chronic obstructive pulmonary disease (COPD) may trap air by flattening their diaphragms. In this case, the chest contours do not change. The diaphragmatic flattening can easily be seen on a lateral chest x-ray.

Inspection also includes observing chest movements during the respiratory cycle to assess respiratory rate, rhythm, depth, quality, and type of breathing. Also consider the following: Are the respirations regular? Labored? Are they associated with use of the accessory muscles, such as the sternocleidomastoid and shoulder girdle? People in respiratory distress often sit upright and lean on their arms or elbows to aid in pushing up on the shoulder girdle. This position of resting on the arms to breathe is called the tripod position (Fig. 30–4). When the diaphragm, the major muscle of respiration, is not moving normally due to air trapping or pushing up from the abdomen, the only way the person can enlarge the chest to lower intrathoracic pressure and take a breath is to raise the shoulder girdle and upper chest. Often, the person who is using

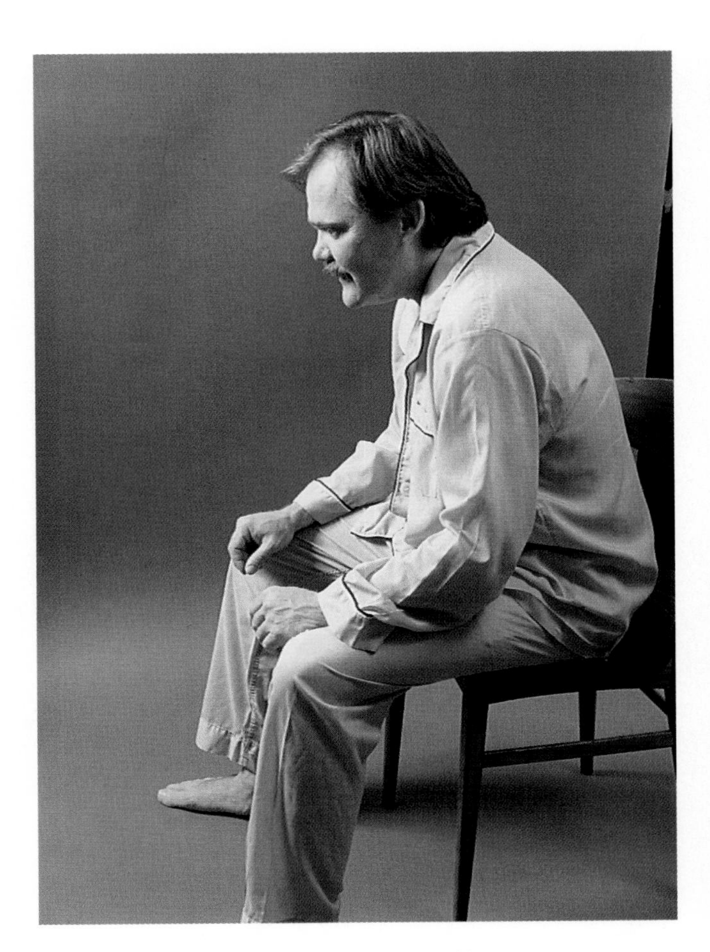

Figure 30–4. Tripod position to assist breathing.

accessory muscles to breathe also purses the lips, as discussed previously. **Dyspnea** is the term used to describe difficult, labored breathing (see Table 30–3).

Retractions, a sign of serious respiratory distress, are another consequence of difficult air exchange. Intercostal retractions are indentations, or pulling in, of the intercostal muscles while breathing in. Retractions are also sometimes evident above the clavicle and below the sternum. Bulging of the intercostal spaces during expiration may accompany retractions. In young infants, substernal retractions are common with only moderately increased inspiratory effort because the chest structures are very pliable.

When breathing is painful, many patients splint their respirations. They attempt to hold the chest as still as possible with each breath. Very little respiratory movement will be observed as the chest is held stiff, still, and rigid.

If a patient is coughing, note whether the cough is productive or nonproductive. A nonproductive cough is often related to upper respiratory irritation or infection, whereas a productive cough often indicates lower respiratory problems. If the cough is productive, note the character of the sputum. Thick yellow-to-greenish sputum may signal an infection that could threaten oxygenation.

Inspect the precordium, the area of the chest just over the heart, for bulging or pulsations. These are abnormal signs that indicate cardiac enlargement or unusually forceful contractions of the cardiac muscle. These signs suggest the potential for perfusion problems.

CLINICAL GUIDELINE 30–4

DESCRIPTIVE TERMS FOR PULSES

PULSE RATE

Tachycardia: Rate persistently greater than 100 beats per minute at rest.
Bradycardia: Rate less than 50 beats per minute at rest.

PULSE VOLUME

Normal: Full, strong, easily palpable.
Thready: Weak throughout stroke.
Bounding: Unusually full, pounding.
Collapsing: Normal upstroke, fades immediately.
Bigeminal: Alternating amplitude: full beat followed by weak beat.

QUANTIFYING VOLUME

4+: Full, bounding, such as during or immediately after strenuous exercise.
3+: Normal.
2+: Slightly weaker than normal, such as in dehydration.
1+: Can be obliterated with pressure.
0: Absent.

PULSE RHYTHM

Regular: Evenly spaced beats.
Irregular: Spaces between beats are of different lengths, may seem to be "regularly irregular" (a pattern can be noted) or completely irregular (spaces between beats erratic, unpredictable).

Next, palpate the precordium for lifts, heaves, or thrills. *Lifts* or *heaves* indicate forceful heart contractions. *Thrills,* which feel like vibrations, are usually caused by turbulent blood flow through the heart valves. These abnormal signs indicate cardiac pathology that could compromise perfusion.

Palpation of peripheral pulses provides information about perfusion of body tissues. (Pulse locations and techniques for palpating pulses are covered in Chap. 17; see Table 17–9.) Weakness or absence of a peripheral pulse implies impaired perfusion to the body parts distal to it. For example, a weak carotid pulse suggests diminished brain perfusion. Assess the femoral, posterior tibial, and dorsalis pedis pulses to evaluate circulation to the legs and feet. Clinical Guideline 30–4 lists and defines descriptive terms for pulses.

Auscultation of the chest is the next step. Breath sounds indicate the movement of air in the lungs, obstructions to air flow, and the presence of secretions. Follow the guidelines for auscultating breath sounds discussed in Chap. 17 *(Conducting an Examination of the Thorax and Lungs).* Abnormal breath sounds and their causes are summarized in Table 30–4.

Heart sounds provide data about cardiac rhythm and blood flow through the heart. See the discussion in Chap. 17 *(Cardiovascular System: Topographic Anatomy).* Auscultate the heart with both the diaphragm and the bell of the stethoscope because some abnormal heart sounds are low pitched and, therefore, more audible through the bell.

Although normally only the S_1 and S_2 heart sounds are heard, it is sometimes possible to hear a third (S_3) or a fourth (S_4) heart sound. S_3 is the sound of rapid ventricular filling and may be heard in some healthy children, teenagers, and adults under 30 during the resting phase of the ventricles (diastole), especially if the chest wall is thin. Many pregnant women develop an S_3 by the 13th week of pregnancy. If a person is over 30 and not pregnant, the S_3 should be investigated as it may be an early sign of heart failure. A nurse can mimic the cadence of the S_1, S_2, and S_3 by silently sounding out "Kentucky" as the heart sounds are auscultated. The presence of an S_4, the sound of atrial contraction, is not by itself diagnostic of heart disease, although it is very often the result of pathology. The sound of "Tennessee" mimics the cadence of the S_4, S_1, and S_2. Other diastolic sounds—OS, the opening snap of the mitral valve, and EJ, the ejection click or clicking sound heard as blood is ejected, particularly from the left ventricle—signal a malfunctioning valve. The extra sounds are evaluated for their timing in the cardiac cycle (systole, diastole) and location of maximum intensity.

A heart murmur is a swishing or whooshing noise cause by partial obstruction of the blood flow by one or more heart valves, increased flow across a valve, backward flow through a valve, or flow through a hole in the septum of the heart. Murmurs are evaluated for their timing in the cardiac cycle, their location (auscultatory area where they are best heard), radiation if any (neck, axilla), intensity (graded on a scale of 1 to 10), pitch (high, medium, low), and quality (musical, rumbling, harsh, blowing, ascending, descending, or plateau).

Auscultation of blood vessels may be part of the oxygenation assessment. If plaque has built up within a vessel so that blood has to rush around it, a swishing noise can be heard on auscultation. This is called a *bruit.* Evaluation of the major arteries such as the abdominal aorta, carotids, and femoral artery includes auscultating for bruits.

TABLE 30-4. SUMMARY OF ABNORMAL BREATH SOUNDS

Sound	Description	Location/Causes
Crackles (formerly called rales)	Diffuse, discontinuous crackling sounds. Usually heard during inspiration and don't generally clear with coughing. Can mimic by listening to soda fizz or by rubbing hairs together beside ear.	Localized or generalized throughout chest. Caused by movement of fluid in small airways or sudden popping open of alveoli or small airways that had been closed/deflated. Sounds that clear after a few deep breaths are known as atelectatic rales (crackles), an early sign of impending atelectasis (collapsed alveoli).
Gurgles and rumbles (formerly called rhonchi)	Heavy, continuous snoring or rattling sounds. Can often clear by coughing or suctioning.	Over-large airways. Sometimes diffuse throughout chest. Caused by air turbulence as air moves through large airways partially obstructed by secretions, swelling, or tumors.
Wheezing	High-pitched, continuous whistling sounds. Usually occur in a specific progression, which gives clues to severity of narrowing of airways. Often may be heard without a stethoscope. Does not clear with coughing.	Air rushing through a narrowed airway. Due to obstruction or bronchospasm (spasm of muscles surrounding the airways; asthma). Heard all over lung fields. Usually more prominent on expiration.
Pleural friction rub	Localized grating or clicking noises, associated with pain on breathing. Rub is not heard if breath is held. Does not clear with coughing.	Localized at any point of pleural irritation. Caused by inflamed pleura and chest wall.
Abnormal spoken breath sounds:		
Egophony (E to A change)	When stethoscope is placed over localized area of consolidation and patient says "E," it sounds like "A" through stethoscope. As the consolidation clears, the sound will become more like "E."	May be heard anywhere in lung fields. Consolidation or presence of infectious debris in alveoli (pneumonia) alters transmission of voice sounds through the chest wall.
Whispered pectoriloquy	Whispered syllables are heard more distinctly than usual through the stethoscope.	As above for egophony.
Absent or diminished	Normal vesicular sounds become distant or disappear.	May occur anywhere in lung fields. Diminished sounds caused by atelectasis; absent sounds by airway obstruction or pneumothorax (collapsed lung).

Blood pressure is evaluated as part of the oxygenation assessment. The techniques for blood pressure measurement and normal values are found in Chap. 17.

Abdomen. Any increase in abdominal contents can cause abdominal organs to push up on the diaphragm and obstruct breathing. These include obesity, pregnancy, fluid accumulation in the abdomen such as ascites (fluid that accumulates due to liver disorders), and large tumors. Conditions such as abdominal surgery incisions and peritonitis (inflammation of the abdominal lining), lead to abdominal guarding, a conscious attempt to limit abdominal muscle movement. They can also affect chest movement and thus interfere with breathing. Abdominal assessment is described in more detail in Chap. 17.

Neurologic/Psychological. Interference with the oxygen supply to the brain can cause confusion, impaired judgment, compromised coordination, and altered levels of consciousness. Patients with difficulty breathing often are anxious or irritable. Increased levels of carbon dioxide in the blood diminish sensory acuity, whereas decreased levels cause abnormal sensations (paresthesias) such as numbness and tingling of the extremities. If any of these are noted, a more complete assessment of mental status, coordination, and sensation may be appropriate. These are detailed in Chap. 17 *(Neurologic System).*

DIAGNOSTIC TESTS

A wide variety of diagnostic tests are used to evaluate oxygenation status. Laboratory tests of blood and sputum, as well as diagnostic examinations, including pulmonary function tests, vascular Doppler studies, and visualization via endoscope, x-rays, and scans, provide information about ventilation and perfusion that may be useful in diagnosing and treating oxygenation problems.

Nurses should understand the reasons for these procedures to be able to prepare patients for them. Nurses must also understand the basic nursing care related to each test. Tables 30–5 and 30–6 present an overview of information needed by the beginning nursing student about common tests of oxygenation. Procedures 30–1, page 1023, and 30–2, page 1025, provide direction for obtaining a sputum sample, needed for some diagnostic tests.

(continued on page 1022)

TABLE 30-5. COMMON LABORATORY TESTS TO ASSESS OXYGENATION

Test/Description	Findings/Implications: *Normal*	Findings/Implications: *Abnormal*	Nurse's Responsibility
Hemoglobin (Hgb or Hb) Measures oxygen-carrying capacity of blood. Used to monitor patient's response to treatment.	Neonate: 14–24 g/dL. Infant 1 month: 11–20 g/dL. 2 months to 1 year: 10–15 g/dL. Child: 11–16 g/dL. Adult male: 14–18 g/dL. Adult female: 12–16 g/dL. Elderly male: 12.4–15 g/dL. Elderly female: 11.7–13.8 g/dL.	*Low* hemoglobin indicates inadequate oxygen-carrying capacity of blood if less than 12 g/dL (male) or 10.2 g/dL (female). Caused by blood loss, RBC destruction, insufficient dietary iron or folic acid. *Effects:* Weakness, dizziness, tachycardia, fatigue, dyspnea. If extreme: cardiac failure.	Discuss: • Purpose of test. • Venipuncture required. • No food/fluid restrictions. Encourage questions. Request patient to maintain pressure to site for 5 minutes after venipuncture. Discuss implications of test results. Teach nutrients necessary to maintain normal hemoglobin levels; food sources; and daily servings needed.
Hematocrit (Hct) Measures percentage by volume of red blood cells in whole blood. Used to evaluate anemia and oxygen-carrying capacity.	Neonate: 50–68%. Infant 1 month: 37–49%. 2 months to 1 year: 29–40%. Child: 31–45%. Adult male: 40–54%. Adult female: 36–46%. Elderly male: 36–56%. Elderly female: 30–54%.	*Increased* hematocrit caused by disease, severe dehydration, high altitude. *Effects:* Elevated hematocrit increases blood viscosity; therefore, creates risk for vascular congestion, elevated cardiac workload, thrombus formation. *Decreased* hematocrit caused by anemia, other diseases, hemodilution, reaction to blood transfusions. *Effects:* Fatigue, shortness of breath, dyspnea, increased cardiac workload.	Same as for hemoglobin. May use fingerstick to obtain. Do not obtain from arm with an IV running—will be diluted. If a tourniquet is on for over a minute, will elevate Hct due to hemostasis.
Red Blood Cell Count (RBC) A determination of the number of circulating erythrocytes in whole blood. Used to diagnose and evaluate anemias.	Neonate: 4.8–7.2. Infant 2 months to 1 year: 4.1–6.4. Child: 3.8–5.5. Adult male: 4.5–6.0. Adult female: 4–5 (all values in millions/μL).	Dehydration may mask anemia. *Increased* RBCs caused by disease, severe dehydration, shock. *Effects:* See Hematocrit, above. *Decreased* RBCs caused by impaired RBC production, increased RBC destruction, dietary deficiency of folic acid, B vitamins, pregnancy. *Effects:* See Hematocrit, above.	Same as for Hemoglobin, above.
Serum Potassium (K^+) Measures circulating K^+. Most K^+ in body is intracellular and cannot be measured. Is essential for maintenance of electrical conduction in heart and function of other muscles.	3.5–5.5. mEq/L.	Life-threatening values: below 2.5 or above 6.5 mEq/L. *Increased* K^+ level caused by acidosis, cell damage, renal failure, excessive K^+ therapy, IV K^+ therapy when urine output is low. *Effects:* Weakness, malaise, nausea, vomiting, muscle irritability, cardiac arrhythmias. *Decreased* K^+ levels caused by diarrhea, vomiting, nasogastric suction, diuretic therapy, IV therapy without K^+ replacement. *Effects:* Decreased reflexes; rapid, irregular pulse; muscle weakness; hypotension; confusion.	Discuss: • Purpose of test. • No food/fluid restrictions. • Venipuncture required. Encourage questions. Avoid prolonged tourniquet. Deliver specimen to lab promptly. Standing leads to hemolysis, which alters K^+ values. Discuss results of test. Teach dietary sources of K^+, number of daily servings. Discuss medications patient takes that affect or are affected by K^+ levels.

TABLE 30-5. CONTINUED

Test/Description	Findings/Implications: Normal	Findings/Implications: Abnormal	Nurse's Responsibility
Arterial blood gases (ABGs) Implies effectiveness of gas exchange in lungs. Assessment for disturbances of acid-base balance in body. Po_2: Amount of oxygen dissolved in blood. Pco_2: Amount of CO_2 dissolved in blood. pH: Measure of acid concentration in blood. HCO_3: Measure of bicarbonate or base in blood.	Po_2: 80–100 mm Hg. Pco_2: 35–45 mm Hg. Do not vary significantly with age except Po_2 is lowered in those over 80 and those living at high altitudes. pH: 7.35–7.45. HCO_3: 22–28 mEq/L.	*Low* Po_2, *high* Pco_2, caused by conditions that impair respiratory function: neurological, respiratory, or muscular disease; drug overdose; airway obstruction; lung damage. *Effects:* Respiratory distress, tachycardia, reduced level of consciousness, restlessness, anxiety. May result in cyanosis or death. *Low* Pco_2: Hyperventilation, fever, asthma. *Effects:* Tingling fingers and face, tachycardia, anxiety, dizziness, diaphoresis, tetany. *Low* pH (<7.35) indicates acidosis. May be caused by impaired oxygenation, or metabolic conditions (diabetes, severe diarrhea). *High* pH (>7.45) indicates alkalosis. May be caused by extreme anxiety, fever or metabolic conditions (severe vomiting, K^+ loss). *Low* HCO_3 indicates primary base deficit (metabolic acidosis). *High* HCO_3 indicates base excess (metabolic alkalosis). HCO_3 fluctuates to compensate for Pco_2 imbalances.	Discuss: • Purpose of test. • Need for resting state 10–30 minutes before test. • The sample must be arterial, which causes discomfort. • Local anesthetic sometimes used. Encourage questions. Place specimen on ice and take to lab immediately. Apply firm pressure to site for 5–10 minutes and then apply firm dressing. Observe and report numbness, tingling, swelling at puncture site. Record amount of oxygen being administered and method used on lab request. Discuss implications of results.
Sputum Tests Analyze sputum for presence of pathogens or malignant cells. Common tests include: • Culture and sensitivity. • Gram stain. • Acid-fast bacillus (TB). • Fungal studies. • Cytologic studies (for cancer cells).	Sputum should be relatively free of microorganisms, but there will be some contamination by oral flora. Small numbers of alpha-hemolytic streptococci, staphylococci, diphtheroids may be present.	Pathogenic bacteria, fungi, parasites, cancer cells, viral inclusions.	Discuss: • Purpose of test. • Specimen must be sputum, not saliva; deep cough or suction required. • Discuss implications of results. Encourage questions. Use sterile specimen container. Send specimen to lab immediately. Refer to Procedures 30–1 and 30–2 for more information.

Data in this table were adapted in part from Treseler KM. Clinical Laboratory and Diagnostic Tests. *3rd ed. Norwalk, CT: Appleton & Lange; 1995; Kee JL.* Handbook of Laboratory and Diagnostic Tests With Nursing Implications. *2nd ed. Norwalk, CT: Appleton & Lange; 1994.*

TABLE 30-6. COMMON DIAGNOSTIC EXAMINATIONS TO ASSESS OXYGENATION

Examination/Description	Patient Preparation	Posttest Nursing Care
Chest x-ray Radiographic views of chest. Usually includes PA (back to front), AP (front to back), and lateral views. Can detect structural abnormalities, heart size, abnormal air accumulation, fluid in lung, atelectasis, tumors, abscesses.	Discuss: • Purpose of test. • Position of test: standing or lying down. • Need to remove clothing and jewelry above waist, wear hospital gown. • Need to take deep breaths during procedure. • Exposure to radiation is minimal. • X-ray results may reveal need for further tests. Encourage questions.	Assist as needed. Provide opportunities to discuss results of x-ray.
Pulmonary Function Tests A group of tests that measure various lung volumes and amount and rate of air movement. Used to diagnose and track progression of lung disease, discriminate between restrictive and obstructive disorders, determine the effects of medication.	Discuss: • Purpose of test. • Position for test: sitting or standing. • Breathing as directed through a mouthpiece is necessary; nose clip may be used. • Nonrestrictive clothing is advised. • Test may be repeated after bronchodilator spray used. • Need to avoid smoking 4–6 hours before test. • Need to avoid a heavy meal before test. Encourage practice of deep breathing, forced deep breathing, and rapid breathing techniques before test. Assess vital signs, note signs and symptoms of respiratory distress; delay test if distress present. Note patient use of bronchodilators and steroids on test request slip. Note patient age, height, and weight on request slip.	Assess for signs and symptoms of respiratory distress, report if present. Provide opportunities to discuss results of tests.
Bronchoscopy Direct visualization of airways with fiberoptic bronchoscope. May include fluoroscopy (direct projection of x-ray-type image on a screen). Can detect lesions, bleeding, secretions, mucus plugs. Suction, biopsy, or removal of foreign bodies may be done during procedure.	Discuss: • Purpose of test. • Position for test: sitting or lying down with neck hyperextended. • Bronchoscope is inserted through mouth or nose. It may create a feeling of being unable to breathe, but airway remains open. • Local anesthetic is sprayed on throat. • Sedation may be used. • Test takes about 1 hour. • Techniques and benefits of deep breathing and relaxation during procedure. • Keep npo 6–12 hours before test. • May have sore throat, hoarseness, and/or blood-tinged sputum after test. Encourage questions. Inquire if patient has loose or capped teeth; note on chart. Check/obtain informed consent. Request or assist with removal of dentures. Check for allergies to local anesthetic.	Assess vital signs until stable. Assess for respiratory difficulty, cardiac arrhythmias, laryngeal edema, bronchospasm, bleeding. Report frank bleeding, respiratory distress, or major changes in vital signs. Check gag reflex with tongue blade (may be obliterated by local anesthetic). Keep npo until gag reflex returns. If sedated, position on side for drainage of oral secretions. Encourage patient to avoid talking, smoking, coughing for 6–8 hours to reduce possibility of bleeding. Offer lozenges, ice bag for throat. Provide opportunities to discuss results of test.

TABLE 30-6. CONTINUED

Examination/Description	Patient Preparation	Posttest Nursing Care
Lung Scan (VQ-scan, PV) Provides a comparison of perfusion and ventilation. IV and inhaled radionuclides are used. Used to determine adequacy of blood flow to lungs and completeness of ventilation. Comparison of perfusion (Q) and ventilation (V) determines nature of pulmonary pathology. Can detect pulmonary embolism, distinguish between disease involving lung tissue versus vascular obstruction.	Discuss: • Purpose of test. • Position for test: lying down, sitting, several position changes necessary. • Q-scan takes 30 minutes; V-scan 10–15 minutes. • Minimal discomfort except for injection of IV radionuclide and nose clip. • Exposure to radiation less than with x-ray, no danger to patient or visitors; excreted in 6–24 hours. • Need to remove clothing and jewelry above waist, wear hospital gown. • For Q-scan, a scanning device will move over chest to detect presence of radionuclide in pulmonary circulation. Various position changes may be required. • For V-scan, patient will inhale oxygen with a small amount of radionuclide gas; need to take deep breath and hold briefly; scanner used during inspiration, holding, and exhalation to detect pattern of inflation. Encourage questions.	No specific test-related care. Provide opportunities to discuss results of test.
Electrocardiogram (ECG) Records electrical activity in heart; detects arrhythmias. Variations: stress test (ECG while patient walks on treadmill or over 24-hour period using portable Holter monitor device).	Discuss: • Purpose of test. • Position for test: supine unless treadmill or 24-hour test. • ECG is not painful or dangerous; no electricity is applied to body. • Need to remove clothing and jewelry above waist, remove nylon hosiery, wear hospital gown. • 12 electrodes (leads) are applied to the body using straps or suction device; conductive paste applied under electrode. • If exercise test is to be done, eat lightly (no coffee, tea, alcohol) 2 hours before test, wear loose comfortable clothing not made of nylon, rubber-soled shoes. Encourage questions.	Assist patient to wash off conductive paste if needed. Provide opportunities to discuss results of test.
Vectorcardiogram Records electrical impulses, like ECG, but produces three-dimensional picture of cardiac activity, useful in diagnosis of myocardial infarction (heart attack).	Same as ECG, above.	Same as for ECG, above.
Echocardiogram Noninvasive technique for examining heart size, position, movement of valves and chambers, and velocity of blood flow by means of reflected ultrasound.	Discuss: • Purpose of test. • Position for test—slight side-lying position. • Takes 30–45 minutes. • No pain or discomfort involved. • Electrocardiogram leads may be attached for simultaneous ECG reading during procedure.	Provide opportunities to discuss results of test.

Continued

TABLE 30-6. CONTINUED

Examination/Description	Patient Preparation	Posttest Nursing Care
Cardiac Catheterization Insertion of a long catheter into a vein or artery of the arm or leg and threading it to the chambers of the heart or coronary arteries. Contrast dye injected to visualize heart chambers, activity, or arteries. Can detect abnormal heart structure, size, valves; measure pressure in pulmonary circulation; detect coronary occlusions.	Discuss: • Purpose of test. • Position for test: supine on tilting table, ECG leads attached to chest. • Takes about 2 hours. • No food or fluids 6–8 hours before test. • IV will infuse during procedure; hot flushing sensation likely as dye injected; lasts 1–2 minutes. • Allergies to dye, seafood, iodine (if present, may use antihistamine night before test). • Possibility of palpitations as catheter is passed into heart. • Need to cough and deep breathe frequently during procedure. • Need to discontinue oral anticoagulants; IV heparin may be used, if needed. • Sedative given 30–60 minutes prior to procedure. • Need for bedrest 8–12 hours after test, cardiac monitoring may be used. Encourage questions. Check/obtain informed consent. Assess and record vital signs.	Monitor vital signs q 15 min for 1 hour, then q 30 min until stable. Assess for arrhythmias on monitor or apical pulse. Observe catheter-insertion site for bleeding. Change dressings as needed; report continued bleeding. Assess peripheral pulses distal to insertion site q 15 min for 1–2 hours, then q 1–2 h until stable. Assess for coolness, paleness, pain, numbness, tingling of catheter insertion site extremity; report signs of circulatory insufficiency. Assess and report chest pain. Administer pain medications as ordered for site pain. Encourage fluids unless contraindicated. Provide opportunities to discuss results of test.
Vascular Doppler Studies Evaluates blood flow in arteries and veins to arms, legs, neck, and abdomen using an ultrasound transducer placed over the skin. Can detect altered blood flow, arterial occlusion, deep vein thrombosis.	Discuss: • Purpose of test. • Position for test: supine. • Takes 10–30 minutes. • Test is not painful or uncomfortable. • Need to perform Valsalva maneuver at intervals during test. • Intermittent occlusion of extremity circulation manually or using blood pressure cuff. • External probe placement at several sites on affected extremities; opposite extremity also tested for comparison; conducting gel applied under probe. Encourage questions.	Assist patient to remove gel, if needed. Provide opportunities to discuss results of test.

Sources: Kee JL. Handbook of Laboratory and Diagnostic Tests. *2nd ed. Norwalk, CT: Appleton & Lange; 1994. Patrick ML, Woods SL, Craven RF, et al.* Medical-Surgical Nursing. *Philadelphia: Lippincott; 1991. Treseler KM.* Clinical Laboratory and Diagnostic Tests. *3rd ed. Norwalk, CT: Appleton & Lange; 1995.*

▲ NURSING DIAGNOSIS OF OXYGENATION STATUS

The data obtained in the oxygenation history and physical examination may indicate problems related to oxygenation status. The use of the taxonomy of nursing diagnoses can help beginning students identify relationships between the various data cues and associate these data with specific nursing diagnoses (Table 30–7). The diagnostic statement provides the basis for planning individualized care. For a nursing diagnosis to be most useful, it should include the cause or etiology, of the problem if known and the defining characteristics.

Several nursing diagnoses are directly related to oxygenation status. These include ineffective airway clearance, ineffective breathing pattern, and altered tissue perfusion. Other nursing diagnoses related to altered oxygenation status but not covered in detail here are listed at the end of Table 30–7. Although the nursing diagnoses are distinct, there is a great deal of overlap among them. This will be clarified as the diagnoses are discussed.

INEFFECTIVE AIRWAY CLEARANCE

Ineffective airway clearance is a state in which an individual is unable to clear secretions in the respiratory tract or to protect and maintain the patency (openness) of the airways. The extent to which this interferes with oxygenation varies with the degree of obstruction.

PROCEDURE 30–1. COLLECTING A SPUTUM SPECIMEN FROM A PATIENT ABLE TO COUGH

PURPOSE: To obtain a sample specimen of sputum for analysis for the presence of microorganisms or abnormal cells.
EQUIPMENT: Sterile specimen container with cover, nonsterile gloves, facial tissues, toothbrush and/or mouthwash, cup, and water, may require goggles and gown.

ACTION 1. Check medical orders for purpose of specimen and other specified conditions (amount of specimen, number of specimens, time of collection, purpose).

RATIONALE. Specifications may vary with test. Obtaining the smallest amount of sputum sufficient for test will minimize stress on patient.

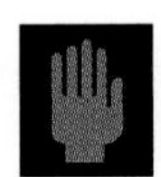

Bronchial secretions accumulate during sleep. It may be easier for patient to produce sputum in early morning. Another good time to collect sputum is just after a bronchodilator treatment or postural drainage and percussion.

ACTION 2. Discuss the procedure and its purpose with the patient.

RATIONALE. Active participation is more likely if the patient understands the desired behavior, its purpose, and anticipated benefits.

ACTION 3. Provide privacy by closing the door or bedside curtains.

RATIONALE. The procedure may be embarrassing to the patient or offensive to others.

ACTION 4. Ask patient to cleanse mouth with mouthwash or by brushing teeth and to thoroughly rinse mouth with water after cleansing.

RATIONALE. Cleansing the mouth reduces possible contamination by oral flora. Mouthwash may contaminate specimen or kill possible pathogens.

ACTION 5. Assess patient's ability to cough deeply and expectorate sputum. If patient has a nonproductive cough and/or severe chest or abdominal pain, suctioning may be necessary (see Procedure 30–2).

RATIONALE. A deep cough is essential to obtain mucus from the tracheobronchial tree. Simple clearing of the throat or spitting out saliva is inadequate.

ACTION 6. Assess patient's respiratory status: RR, depth, rhythm, skin color.

RATIONALE. Active coughing may alter status. Baseline data can help determine impact of coughing.

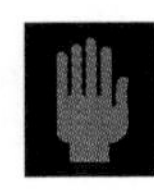

Do not attempt to obtain specimen from patient in respiratory distress.

ACTION 7. Request patient to assume upright position: high Fowler's, dangling, or standing. Assist to sit up if necessary. Patients who are able may prefer to take cup to bathroom after instruction on how to produce an acceptable specimen.

RATIONALE. Upright position facilitates lung expansion and cough effort.

ACTION 8. Instruct patient to hold sputum container without touching inside of container or cover. If patient is weak, or needs to splint an incision while coughing, don gloves and hold cup for patient.

RATIONALE. Normal flora from hands would contaminate inside of container, altering results of test.

If droplet spray is anticipated, don goggles and moisture impervious gown to protect uniform and eyes from potentially infectious secretions.

ACTION 9. Ask patient to cough deeply (Procedure 30–6) and expectorate into container, repeating as necessary until the necessary quantity of sputum is obtained.

RATIONALE. Deep cough is necessary to bring up sputum from lower respiratory tree. Lower respiratory tract specimen is necessary for accurate test.

ACTION 10. While wearing gloves, secure the cover on the container.

RATIONALE. Prevents contamination of specimen by environmental organisms, or transfer of organisms from specimen to environment.

ACTION 11. Offer patient facial tissues to wipe mouth or mouthwash or toothbrush as necessary. Assist patient to a comfortable position.

RATIONALE. Promotes patient comfort, reduces oral microorganisms.

Continued

Procedure 30–1. Collecting a Sputum Specimen from a Patient Able to Cough (continued)

ACTION 12. Reassess patient's respiratory status as above.

RATIONALE. The effort of coughing may cause oxygen deficit in patients with serious respiratory impairment.

ACTION 13. Label container and send to lab according to agency policy.

RATIONALE. Facilitates prompt analysis of specimen and receipt of results to assist in treatment plan.

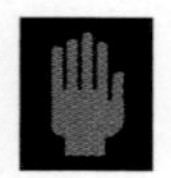

Specimen may require special bagging or refrigeration.

ACTION 14. When laboratory report is filed in patient's chart, share results with patient.

RATIONALE. Patient has a right to information about personal health status.

Recording:

Describe respiratory status before and after specimen obtained, method used to obtain specimen, quantity and character (viscosity, color, odor) of sputum, and disposition of specimen. When results are obtained, notify physician and place result in patient's record.

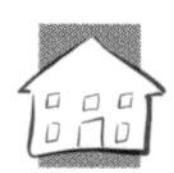

HOME HEALTH ADAPTATION: Place the specimen container in a plastic bag or pouch with the requisition in a separate compartment of pouch. Transport specimen to lab in an insulated container with artificial ice and labeled "Biohazard." Request lab to fax or phone results to the physician and Home Health Agency. Note time specimen is delivered to lab.

There are several potential causes of ineffective airway clearance. Accurate identification of the underlying cause of the problem is necessary, because the etiology often determines what type of nursing implementation is appropriate.

- *Etiology: decreased energy or fatigue.* Lack of energy may prevent coughing that is effective enough to clear the airways, even if a patient is motivated to learn effective coughing techniques. Strong contraction of the abdominal and respiratory muscles is required to build sufficient intrapulmonary pressure to expel secretions from airways. An effective cough requires pressures of 100 mm Hg or more, creating an explosive outflow of air at velocities up to 965 km (600 miles) per hour.[5]
- *Etiology: tracheobronchial infection, secretions, or obstruction.* Tracheobronchial infection often produces such copious secretions that coughing efforts cannot clear the airways. These secretions are often viscous and may form mucus plugs that obstruct airways and add to the difficulty in clearing them. If the underlying cause of increased secretions is an infection, treatment with antibiotic therapy may be required.

  Obstruction can also be the result of aspiration of small pieces of food or small objects. Irritants such as smog or general anesthesia are another possible cause of excessive secretions.
- *Etiology: trauma.* Injuries or incisions in the chest, shoulder, back, or abdomen make coughing painful, because they often involve the muscles used in coughing. Contraction or stretching of the damaged muscles causes pain, and so individuals often suppress or abort coughing despite the presence of secretions.
- *Etiology: perceptual or cognitive impairment.* Individuals whose cognitive processes have been impaired by injury or disease may have the physical ability to cough, but may have difficulty learning or remembering to cough effectively. In some cases, prompting can result in an effective cough.

INEFFECTIVE BREATHING PATTERN

Ineffective breathing pattern is a state in which a person's inhalation or exhalation does not bring about adequate inflation or emptying of the lungs. Examples include such respiratory patterns as hypoventilation, asymmetric breathing, and excessively rapid or shallow breathing. A patient who has chronic lung disease may panic easily when dyspnea occurs, causing an ineffective breathing pattern.

Several conditions, including ineffective airway clearance (discussed previously), can produce an ineffective breathing pattern. The discussion that follows addresses the etiologies listed in the taxonomy of nursing diagnoses.

- *Etiology: neuromuscular impairment.* Neuromuscular impairment implies that nervous control of the respiratory muscles is altered. Depending on the specific underlying problem, hyperventilation, hypoventilation, or asymmetric breathing may result. Some of the underlying problems cannot be treated by independent nursing implementation; nevertheless, nursing care frequently contributes to improvement.
- *Etiology: musculoskeletal impairment.* Examples of this etiology include bone fractures or changes in muscle functioning, such as weakness or contractures. Often, pain is a contributing factor. As in the previous etiology, nursing implementation alone may not always be sufficient to correct the underlying problem.
- *Etiology: pain.* Severe, acute pain frequently causes hyperventilation because the sympathetic nervous system response to pain causes increases in heart rate and oxygen

PROCEDURE 30–2. OBTAINING A SPUTUM SPECIMEN FROM A PATIENT UNABLE TO COUGH

PURPOSE: To obtain sample of sputum for analysis for presence of organisms (culture and sensitivity—C & S; or acid-fast bacilli—AFB) or abnormal cells (cytology).

EQUIPMENT: Suction device (wall or portable); sterile suction kit (includes catheter, glove, container for liquid), sterile water or saline; sterile sputum trap; towel or moisture-resistant pad; facial tissues; and mouthwash or toothettes, goggles and moisture impervious gown if droplet spray is likely.

ACTION 1. Refer to Procedure 30–1 for assessment and preparation of patient.

ACTION 2. Explain that suctioning should not cause great discomfort, but that it may stimulate gagging or coughing. This will diminish fear of the unknown and assist patient to participate rather than resist procedure. Remember that unconscious patients may retain hearing and comprehension abilities. Do not omit explanation.

ACTION 3. Request or assist conscious patient to assume semi-Fowler's position with head turned toward nurse to facilitate insertion of the catheter while diminishing feelings of helplessness of patient and minimizing risk of aspiration. Position unconscious patient in lateral position facing nurse to allow tongue to fall forward and facilitate drainage of secretions with decreased risk of aspiration.

ACTION 4. Attach suction tube to adapter on sputum trap to facilitate direct collection of sputum in container without risk of contamination of specimen or nurse.

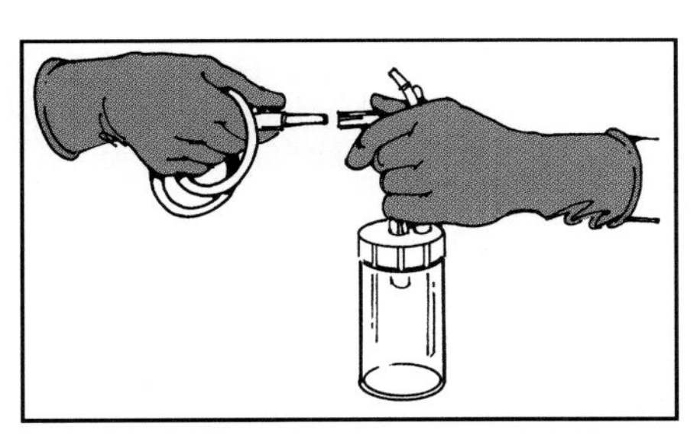

ACTION 5. Suction as described in Procedure 30–7. Repeat as necessary until sufficient amount of sputum is obtained.

ACTION 6. Provide for rest periods between catheter insertions to minimize stress.

ACTION 7. Detach suction tubing from sputum trap. Seal trap with attached rubber tubing to prevent contamination of specimen and transfer of microorganisms to environment.

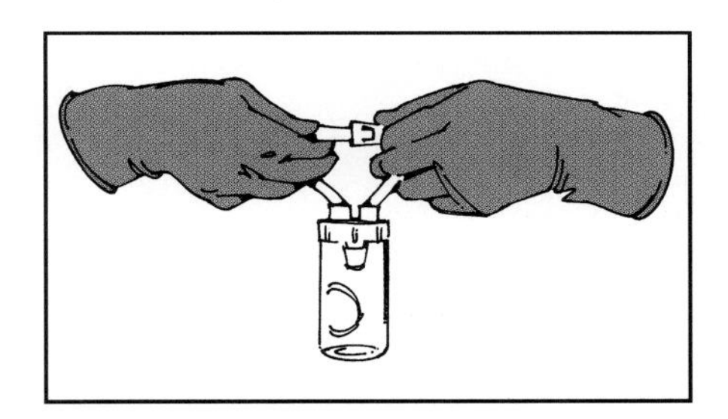

ACTION 8. Assist patient as needed and send specimen to laboratory as detailed in Procedure 30–1. When results are obtained, discuss with patient, notify MD, and place report in patient's record.

Recording:

Describe respiratory status before and after specimen is obtained, method used to obtain specimen, quantity and character of sputum, and disposition of specimen.

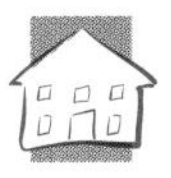

HOME HEALTH ADAPTATION: See Procedure 30–1 for specimen transport to lab.

TABLE 30-7. SAMPLE NURSING DIAGNOSES: OXYGENATION

Nursing Diagnosis	Defining Characteristics/Manifestations: *Subjective Data*	Defining Characteristics/Manifestations: *Objective Data*	Etiology
Ineffective airway clearance *1.5.1.2*	Reports inability to cough Reports fatigue	Gurgles, rumbles on chest auscultation. Decreased respiratory rate (RR). Weak, ineffective cough.	Physical: Decreased energy/fatigue.
	Severe dyspnea	Harsh or weak cough. Diminished breath sounds. Excessive mucus. Wheezing or inspiratory stridor. Rumbles. Shallow respirations. Use of accessory muscles.	Physical: Bronchial obstruction: mucus plug.
Ineffective breathing pattern: hypoventilation *1.5.1.3*	Reports incisional pain with deep inspiration	Decreased chest excursion. Shallow respirations. Diminished breath sounds. Hypercapnea Atelectatic crackles.	Physical: Acute pain: abdominal surgical incision.[b]
Ineffective breathing pattern: hyperventilation *1.5.1.3*	Reports feeling nervous, being "on edge" Reports feeling lightheaded, faint	Tachypnea. Nasal flaring. Hypocapnea. Shallow respirations. Tremors. Sweaty palms. Clenched fists, jaw. Random repetitive movements.	Emotional: Anxiety.
Altered peripheral tissue perfusion *1.4.1.1*	Reports coldness/numbness/tingling in extremity	Skin locally reddened or pale, cool to touch. 4 + edema in legs.	Physical: Exchange problems 2° edema[a]
	Reports tightness of treatment modality (eg, bandage) Reports coldness/numbness/tingling in extremity	Skin locally pale or bluish, cool, edematous. Peripheral pulse in affected extremity weaker than in other extremity.	Physical: Interruption of arterial flow by constricting cast, bandage, poorly fitted TED hose.[a]

OTHER NURSING DIAGNOSES RELATED TO OXYGENATION

PHYSICAL
Activity intolerance
Altered cardiac output: decreased
Pain
Altered fluid volume: excess or deficit
Fatigue
Risk for infection
Impaired gas exchange
Impaired home maintenance management
Risk for injury
Risk for aspiration
Impaired physical mobility
Altered nutrition: more or less than body calorie requirements
Self-care deficit
Impaired skin/tissue integrity
Sleep pattern disturbance
Altered tissue perfusion: cerebral, cardiopulmonary, renal, or gastrointestinal

COGNITIVE
Altered thought processes
Knowledge deficit
Impaired verbal communication

EMOTIONAL
Anxiety
Fear
Hopelessness

SELF-CONCEPTUAL
Ineffective individual coping
Powerlessness
Body image disturbance
Altered role performance
Self-esteem disturbance

SOCIOCULTURAL/LIFE-STRUCTURAL
Ineffective family coping
Altered family processes
Impaired social interaction
Social isolation
Ineffective individual coping

DEVELOPMENTAL
Diversional activity deficit

SEXUAL
Altered sexuality patterns
Sexual dysfunction

[a]Example only. Many other specific examples of altered functioning with this general etiology are relevant to nursing diagnosis. Defining characteristics, desired outcomes, and nursing implementation would differ for each specific etiology.

Sources: The nursing diagnoses and etiologies on this table and the definitions of nursing diagnoses in the body of the text not credited to other sources are from Nursing Diagnosis: Definitions and Classifications, 1997–1998. *Philadelphia: North American Nursing Diagnosis Association; 1996. Manifestation categories for etiologies and specifications of general etiologies on these tables are authors' original work.*

demand. Conversely, localized pain in the abdomen, chest, shoulders, or back may result in hypoventilation because of shallow breathing. As discussed above, stretching of injured muscles stimulates pain receptors; therefore, shallow breathing is a common response to pain.

- *Etiology: perceptual or cognitive impairment.* Perceptual or cognitive deficits play similar roles in ineffective breathing pattern as those discussed above under ineffective airway clearance.
- *Etiology: anxiety.* The role of anxiety in the development of ineffective breathing patterns relates to sympathetic nervous system response to stress as well as possible limbic system influence on the respiratory center. The most common anxiety-related alteration in breathing pattern is hyperventilation.
- *Etiology: decreased energy, fatigue.* The work of breathing can become burdensome to extremely debilitated individuals. Paradoxically, bed rest, the common treatment for individuals in this state, increases the amount of energy needed to expand the lungs. This is because in the recumbent position, abdominal organs impinge upon the thoracic cavity and must be displaced by the diaphragm to create space for full lung inflation.
- *Etiology: obesity.* Obesity creates the same impediment to full lung expansion as recumbency. Increased adipose tissue deposits on the chest and abdomen make full lung expansion more difficult. Hypoventilation is a common result.

ALTERED TISSUE PERFUSION

Altered tissue perfusion is the state in which an individual experiences a decrease in nutrition and oxygenation at the cellular level due to a deficit in capillary blood supply. The diagnostic statement should specify the location of the interference with perfusion: peripheral, gastrointestinal, renal, cerebral, or cardiopulmonary. This can be the result of inadequate pumping action by the heart, decreased circulating blood volume, gas exchange problems, or interference with arterial blood flow. The following discussion applies principally to altered peripheral perfusion.

- *Etiology: interruption in arterial flow.* Interruption in arterial flow is a major cause of impaired tissue perfusion. External pressure over bony prominences related to immobility is one cause of interrupted blood flow. Treatments such as casts, anti-embolism stockings, or improperly applied bandages on an extremity can interrupt arterial flow locally. Diseases that cause narrowing of arteries also impair perfusion.
- *Etiology: exchange problems.* Exchange problems refer to interference with the exchange of oxygen and carbon dioxide. Exchange problems can occur between alveoli and pulmonary capillaries (such as caused by secretions or fluid) or between peripheral capillaries and tissue cells, usually resulting from edema. Edema interferes with efficient diffusion of oxygen to the cells and carbon dioxide from the cells. In either case tissues receive insufficient oxygen.

STATING THE OXYGENATION DIAGNOSIS

A nursing diagnosis statement is most useful as a basis for planning patient care if it is individualized by specifying the problem statement, etiology, and defining characteristics as they are manifested by a particular patient. For example, a patient who remains in semi-Fowler's position for extended periods of time is noted to have a 2-inch-diameter reddened area over her sacrum; she states that "sometimes my tailbone feels a little numb." The redness is not relieved after lying on her side for 15 minutes. "Altered peripheral tissue perfusion related to interrupted arterial flow" is an appropriate nursing diagnosis, but the statement "Altered perfusion of tissue over sacrum related to interruption of arterial flow from prolonged periods in semi-Fowler's position as evidenced by erythema, 5-cm diameter over sacrum, and localized numbness" communicates the nature of the problem more clearly and gives stronger guidance for corrective action. Precisely stated nursing diagnoses based on the oxygenation assessment provide a foundation for collaborative management, discussed in Section 3.

SECTION 3

NURSE-PATIENT MANAGEMENT OF OXYGENATION

PLANNING FOR OPTIMAL OXYGENATION

An effective patient care plan clearly communicates measurable outcomes for patient care, related evaluation criteria, and nursing implementation to attain the outcomes. Desired outcome statements provide realistic goals for patient and nurse and guidelines for patient care; they are the basis for evaluation criteria.

Oxygenation outcomes, like other outcomes of care, are best determined through mutual goal setting. Nurse and patient work together to establish desired outcomes that both understand and accept. The desired outcomes for nursing care should also be compatible with the goals for medical treatment. Collaboration with the physician and other members of the interdisciplinary team is important if the nursing and medical goals are to be complementary and compatible. Setting outcomes can be difficult when a patient is in an extremely debilitated state with little or no awareness of the quality of life that may be possible if these problems are well managed. In this case, the family may collaborate with nurses and other caregivers if possible, or nurses and other members of the health care team may need to establish outcomes and plan care until the patient is well enough to participate in decision making.

Once desired outcomes are set, they should be stated clearly for mutual understanding. For example, an outcome for the sample nursing diagnosis in Section 2 might be: "improved tissue perfusion within 24 hours, as evidenced by progressive decrease in size of erythema and full return of sensation to area." Another sample oxygenation outcome might be "within 2 days, the patient will walk 50 feet while correctly using pursed-lip breathing techniques." Another might be "at the end of 3 days, the patient will correctly describe the structure and functions of normal lungs and how his or her own lungs differ from normal."

Sample nursing management of oxygenation, including appropriate outcomes, implementation, and evaluation criteria, is presented in Table 30–8, Nurse–Patient Management of Oxygenation Problems. This table provides guidelines for developing individualized nursing care plans in which outcomes are tailored to the strengths, needs, and lifestyle of a specific patient and family.

TABLE 30-8. NURSE-PATIENT MANAGEMENT OF OXYGENATION PROBLEMS

Nursing Diagnosis	Desired Outcome	Implementation	Evaluation Criteria
Ineffective airway clearance R/T decreased energy/fatigue *1.5.1.2*	1. Effective airway clearance	1a. Explain importance of effective coughing to reduce shortness of breath, DOE. 1b. Teach correct coughing technique (see Procedure 30–6). 1c. Encourage and positively reinforce effective coughing. 1d. Teach importance of refraining from smoking. 1e. Teach diaphragmatic breathing and pursed-lip breathing (Procedures 30–3, 4). 1f. Administer oxygen in collaboration with physician. 1g. Tracheobronchial suctioning PRN.	1. Airway clear, AEB: No gurgles, rumbles on chest auscultation RR and depth within expected range for age and health status.
	2. Decreased fatigue	2a. Reduce metabolic demands: space activities requiring exertion; no bathing, ambulating, eating, etc, during periods of acute distress. 2b. Plan regular rest periods, especially after coughing, meals, exercise. 2c. Collaborate with physician to treat cause of fatigue.	2. Progressive energy level improvement AEB increased participation in regular activities without reports of fatigue, DOE.
Ineffective airway clearance R/T bronchial obstruction: mucus plug[a] *1.5.1.2*	1. Clear airway with unlabored respiration	1a. Assist with effective coughing techniques (Procedure 30–6). 1b. Perform chest physiotherapy and postural drainage. 1c. Perform tracheobronchial suctioning if obstruction persists. 1d. Administer oxygen in collaboration with physician.	1a. RR and depth within expected range for age and health status. 1b. Stridor, adventitious breath sounds absent. 1c. Progressive decrease in cough, mucus. 1d. Patient reports decreased dyspnea.
Ineffective breathing pattern: hypoventilation R/T acute pain: abdominal surgical incision[a] *1.5.1.3*	1. Effective RR, rhythm, and depth	1a. Assess RR, rhythm, depth, lung fields at least q shift. 1b. Teach diaphragmatic pursed-lip breathing (Procedure 30–3).	1,2. Airway remains free of secretions AEB: No gurgles, rumbles, crackles, or diminished breath sounds on chest auscultation. RR and depth within expected range for age and health status.
	2. Lungs remain free of atelectasis and/or secretions	2a. Assist with coughing (Procedure 30–6) whenever secretions are present. 2b. Assist patient to use sustained maximal inspiration device (Procedure 30–5) qh. 2c. Encourage splinting of incision when performing deep breathing and coughing. 2d. Teach importance of not smoking.	
	3. Alleviation or elimination of pain	3. Provide pain-relief measures (see Chap. 32).	3. Patient states that pain is diminished or gone.
Ineffective breathing pattern: hyperventilation R/T anxiety[a] *1.5.1.2*	1. Effective RR, rhythm, and depth 2. Decreased anxiety	1. Teach diaphragmatic and pursed-lip breathing (Procedure 30–3). 2a. Teach breathing and relaxation techniques (see Clinical Guideline 25–2). 2b. Use active listening techniques to assist patient to resolve feelings of anxiety (see Chap. 15). 2c. Collaborate with other health care team members (social worker, counselor, psychiatrist) as needed.	1. RR and depth within expected range for age and health status. 2. Anxiety decreased AEB: Decreased tremors. No sweaty palms. Hands and jaw relaxed. Decreased random movements. Patient reports not feeling edgy, nervous.

TABLE 30-8. CONTINUED

Nursing Diagnosis	Desired Outcome	Implementation	Evaluation Criteria
Altered peripheral tissue perfusion R/T exchange problems: 2° edema[a] *1.4.1.1*	1. Peripheral tissue perfusion appropriate to patient's health status	1a. Teach importance of qh position changes. 1b. Assist with position changes if patient unable to perform independently (see Chap. 33). 1c. Elevate legs. 1d. Use protective devices as needed to decrease pressure (see Chap. 33).	1. Peripheral tissue adequately perfused AEB: Skin over all bony prominences appropriate color for patient. No lesions related to pressure.
Altered peripheral tissue perfusion R/T interruption of arterial flow by constricting cast, bandage, or poorly fitted TED hose[a] *1.4.1.1*	1. Peripheral tissue perfusion appropriate to patient's health status	1a. Assess extremity on which cast, bandage, or TED hose has been newly applied qh × 4, q4h × 12, then q shift for pallor, pulselessness, ischemic pain, paresthesia (abnormal sensation), poikilothermia (coolness), decreased capillary refill. 1b. When reapplying TED hose or bandages around an extremity, apply smoothly and snugly, but not tightly (see Procedure 30–15 and Table 27–10). 1b. Elevate extremity with cast, bandage, or TED hose.	1. Optimal peripheral perfusion AEB distal parts of extremity remain warm, appropriate color for patient, without abnormal sensation or pain, with strong peripheral pulse and immediate capillary refill.

[a]Example only. Many other specific examples of altered functioning with this general etiology are relevant to nursing management. Defining characteristics, desired outcomes, and nursing implementation would differ for each specific etiology.
Source: See Table 30–7.

Table 30–9, Partial Critical Pathway for Congestive Heart Failure: Oxygenation Function, and Table 30–10, Partial Critical Pathway for Total Hip Replacement: Oxygenation Function, show collaborative plans of care incorporating concepts from this chapter.

NURSING IMPLEMENTATION TO PROMOTE OPTIMAL OXYGENATION

Collaborative planning for oxygenation needs involves selecting nursing implementations to attain the desired outcomes. The appropriate level of care is suggested by the assessment data and the desired outcomes. Specific implementation is best derived collaboratively by nurse and patient. Nursing measures should allow patients to draw on their strengths and provide supportive care where needed.

PREVENTIVE CARE

Nurses have an important role in the management of oxygenation status in all levels of care. A nurse can do many things to assist a patient toward optimal oxygenation and to prevent oxygenation problems. Many oxygenation problems stem from lifestyle factors such as smoking, exposure to air pollution, failure to use masks during exposure to fumes and dusts, stress, improper diet, and lack of exercise. Preventive measures must begin early in life if long-term oxygenation problems are to be avoided. It is not enough to wait until symptoms occur and then change one's lifestyle. Nurses should be teachers and role models of how to keep healthy. Preventive care includes both screening and health education to facilitate lifestyle changes.

Screening

Nursing approaches to assist patients toward an optimal oxygenation status should include lifestyle analysis as a method of identifying problems or planning preventive strategies. Factors to be considered relative to patients' lifestyle are discussed under *General Health and Lifestyle* in Section 1.

Health Education

Health education is a major nursing responsibility. Nurses should not assume that patients are aware of the hazards of smoking, exposure to air pollution, stress, lack of exercise, or improper diet. In addition, many people are unaware of simple everyday activities that will help them stay healthy.

Discouraging Smoking. Smoking is the most important preventable cause of disease and disability in the United States.[14] According to the US Department of Health and Human Services, a sizable per-

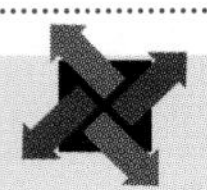

TABLE 30-9. PARTIAL CRITICAL PATHWAY FOR CONGESTIVE HEART FAILURE: OXYGENATION FUNCTION

Nursing Dx/Problem	Outcome Primary Care Visit	Outcome Home Care Week 1 (3 Visits)	Outcome Home Care Week 2 (3 Visits)	Outcome Home Care Weeks 3–4 (3 Visits)
Altered peripheral tissue perfusion R/T O_2–CO_2 exchange problems 2° pulmonary & peripheral edema		O_2 saturation > 90% c̄ O_2, room air > 85% Transfer to BSC prn s̄ SOB or chest pain	O_2 saturation > 94% c̄ O_2, room air > 90% Lungs CTA Ankle edema < 2+ Ambulates 10 feet s̄ SOB	O_2 saturation > 92% s̄ O_2 Lungs CTA Ankle edema < 1+ Ambulates s̄ SOB
Implementation	**Primary Care Visit**	**Home Care Visit Week 1**	**Home Care Visit Week 2**	**Home Care Visit Weeks 3–4**
Assessment	V/S, HR, BP, O_2 sat Breath sounds, edema, pain, dizziness, skin integrity, weight	Same Family ability/willingness to assist Response to meds Environmental limitations	Same Same Response/compliance to meds	Same Same Same Same
Tests/Consults	Refer to Home Health EKG, chest x-ray, electrolytes: Na, K, Cl, CO_2; BUN, creatinine Digoxin levels	Electrolytes		
Medications/Treatments	Diuretics, K supplements Digoxin, anticoagulants O_2 at 2 L/cannula Antithromboembolism stockings	Same O_2 continually Apply stockings	Same O_2 prn & @ night	Same O_2 prn
Psychosocial	Reflective listening	Explore adjustment to health status		
Teaching	Protect feet & legs Antithromboembolism stocking application O_2 use/precautions Medications: correct use, SE, precautions How to take BP, pulse S/Sx to report to MD, RN, 911	Skin care Reinforce as needed Elevate legs when up Reinforce as needed Disease process/care plan Food & fluid restriction	Energy conservation Reinforce as needed Reinforce as needed Reinforce as needed Reinforce as needed	Reinforce as needed Reinforce as needed Reinforce as needed Reinforce as needed Reinforce as needed
Activity/Safety/Self-care	Bedrest, HOB @ 30–45 degrees c̄ BSC or BRP Turn q2h Assist c̄ self-care	Chair c̄ legs elevated tid Remove obstacles to ambulation Bedside commode Assist c̄ ADLs	Progressive activity Self-care as tolerated	Same Independent ADLs
Nutrition	Low Na, fluid 1 L/d	Same	Fluid 1.5 L/d	Same
Transfer/Discharge Coord./Case Manager		Communicate status to MD	Communicate outcomes achieved to MD	Prepare for discharge

See inside back cover for abbreviations.

COLLABORATIVE STRATEGY

GENERAL HEALTH AND LIFESTYLE

Oxygen is fundamental to life. Collaboration with patients to help them understand the relationship of lifestyle factors to oxygenation, and to the quality and length of life, is one of the most significant contributions a nurse can make to a patient's care.

centage of smokers do not believe that smoking increases the risk of certain diseases or that quitting smoking decreases the risk.[15] Yet, in smokers who stop smoking when precancerous lesions are found, damaged lung tissue often returns to normal. Smokers who persist in smoking may form abnormal cell growth patterns that lead to cancer.[16]

Each year, 21 percent of all cardiovascular deaths, 30 percent of cancer deaths (including 87 percent of lung cancer deaths), and about 62,000 deaths from respiratory diseases are attributed to smoking.[17,18] In 1990, smoking caused about 419,000 deaths.[17] In addition, smoking shortens a person's projected life span by about 25 percent.[18] Lung cancer has long been the number one cancer killer of men. It is now the top cancer killer in women as well, because cigarette smoking is increasing among women in general, particularly young women.[14]

Smoking may also lead to emphysema, chronic bronchitis, heart and blood vessel diseases, bladder and pancreatic cancers, and worsening of existing cardiopulmonary conditions such as asthma. Chronic smokers and those who are exposed to large amounts of smoke have a high blood level of carbon monoxide and consequently a reduced level of oxygen in their blood. Statistically, there are changes in the airways after only 20 pack-years of smoking, though patients at this level of smoking usually are not yet symptomatic.[4] The fact that smoking leads to changes in both ventilation and perfusion becomes even more problematic in view of the fact that smoking elevates heart rate. The heart, therefore, needs more oxygen to support the extra work it is doing at the same time that less oxygen is available to it.

Smoking seems to have a synergistic effect with other risk factors for cardiopulmonary disease. For example, diabetes is a major risk factor for cardiovascular changes. The vascular changes are increased if the diabetic is also a smoker. Asbestos workers who smoke are 90 times more likely to die of lung cancer than people who neither smoke nor work with asbestos.[18] A woman who uses oral contraceptives and smokes increases her risk of heart attack and stroke many times compared with a woman who does neither.[2]

CRITICAL QUERY

Noting that current statistics point to heart disease as the number one cause of death in women, Hamel and Oberle[16] point out that health care professionals, who are unaware of this fact and are trained to think of heart disease as a man's illness may inadvertently project a less urgent attitude to women experiencing cardiac symptoms. What is the implication for nurses performing routine checkups on women without symptoms?

Those who share the smoker's environment are also at risk. Up to 85 percent of the smoke from a cigarette, pipe, or cigar may be sidestream smoke, or smoke that simply goes into the environment. This smoke contains a higher concentration of dangerous gases than the smoke that is exhaled by the smoker. An estimated 30,000 to 40,000 deaths from heart disease and 3000 from lung cancer each year are attributed to passive smoking.[18] In addition, 10 percent of infant deaths and 20 to 30 percent of low-birth-weight infants are attributable to tobacco use by family members.[19]

The best solution to the problem of smoking is never to start. Indeed, nicotine, the primary psychoactive agent in tobacco, has been shown to meet the criteria of a highly addictive drug.[18] Therefore, educational programs for adolescents in the schools and other community settings are important. Nurses who work with adolescents should discourage smoking in health teaching and patient care. Because adolescents are present-oriented, they are less likely to respond to discussions of long-term health risks than to emphasis on immediate negative effects, such as bad breath, stained fingers and teeth, and diminished performance in sports.

Education for those who already smoke is also important. A straightforward message advocating quitting and pointing out risks is most effective. Avoid scare tactics, guilt trips, or preaching.[20] Provide information about resources such as local offices of the American Lung Association, American Heart Association, and American Cancer Society, and about various smoking cessation methods, such as self-help strategies, nicotine replacement therapy,

INSIGHTS FROM NURSING LITERATURE

CARDIOVASCULAR RISK ASSESSMENT

Hamel L, Oberle K. Cardiovascular risk screening for women. Clin Nurs Specialist. *1996;10:275–279.*

Numerous factors, according to the authors, make cardiovascular risk assessment especially important in women. Cardiovascular disease is the leading cause of death in women in the United States and Canada. Further, prior emphasis on heart disease in men resulted in an inclination to minimize its existence and severity in women.

The author identifies several risk factors in women, many of which are shared with men: abnormal increases in low-density lipoprotein blood levels or decreases in high-density lipoprotein levels (more predictive in women); hypertension, particularly when paired with raised blood lipids; diabetes, which adversely affects lipid profiles and increases the risk threefold; smoking, associated with lower levels of high-density lipoproteins; obesity, particularly when distributed to the waist, abdomen, and upper body; sedentary lifestyle, which excludes the exercise needed to lower blood pressure, heart rate, and blood cholesterol and raise high-density lipoproteins; stress and multiple roles; and menopause, which is accompanied by estrogen deficiency. All these factors increase the risk of heart disease at any age among women. The incidence of coronary heart disease in women increases with age and reaches major proportions beyond age 55.

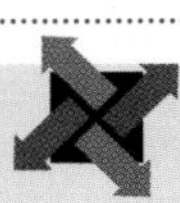

TABLE 30-10. PARTIAL CRITICAL PATHWAY FOR TOTAL HIP REPLACEMENT: OXYGENATION FUNCTION

Nursing Dx/Problem	Outcome DOS/Day 1	Outcome Days 2–3	Outcome SNF Days 4–6	Outcome Home Care 3 Weeks (6 Visits)
Risk for ineffective airway clearance, RF stasis of secretions, 2° anesthesia, immobility	Breath sounds clear to auscultation Achieves 50% of volume goals on incentive spirometer	Same Achieves 75% of volume goal on incentive spirometer	Same Achieves 100% of volume goal on incentive spirometer	Same Same
Implementation	**DOS/Day 1**	**Days 2–3**	**SNF Days 4–6**	**Home Care 3 Weeks**
Assessment	V/S, HR, BP breath sounds, O_2 sat q4h	Same qid	Same bid	Breath sounds V/S, HR, BP each visit
Tests/Consults	Respiratory therapy			
Medications/Treatments	DB q4h Incentive spirometer q1–2h Reposition q2h	Same qid Same Same	Same Same	
Psychosocial				
Teaching	Use of incentive spirometer DB techniques When coughing is needed, effective coughing techniques	Reinforce as needed Cough & DB c̄ position changes	Reinforce as needed	
Activity/Safety/Self-care		Encourage use of trapeze for self position change	Same Ambulate c̄ assistive devices as directed	Same Same
Nutrition			Encourage fluids by mouth to 2000 mL/day	Same
Transfer/Discharge Coord./Case Manager		Communicate outcomes achieved, problems/ interventions to SNF	Communicate outcomes achieved, problems/ interventions to Home Health	Communicate outcomes achieved, problems/ interventions to MD & prepare for discharge

See inside back cover for abbreviations.

hypnosis, acupuncture, and behavior modification. Group programs as well as individual approaches are available. Selecting a program is an individual decision based on individual needs and preferences; however, the *Stages of Change Model* provides a conceptual model for assessing smokers' readiness. According to this model, readiness can be described on a continuum with five stages: *precontemplation* (not at all ready to quit); *contemplation* (considering cessation at some future time); *preparation* (actively considering cessation soon and engaging in some quit-oriented behavior); *action* (having quit smoking within 6 months); *maintenance* (having quit for at least 6 months). Smoking cessation efforts should be matched to smokers' level of motivation for cessation.[18]

Nurses working with smokers who are trying to quit should remember that patience and support from those around the smoker are essential. Relapse is common. Many smokers try several times before quitting for good. Stress, being around other smokers, and weight gain are common causes of relapse. It is also important for individuals to know that when they stop smoking, their cough and sputum may remain for 3 to 6 months. Ex-smokers who do not understand this phenomenon may start smoking again to stop the cough. Actual tissue damage, such as emphysema, cannot be reversed by stopping smoking. However, the condition can be better treated and general health improved after quitting.

COLLABORATIVE STRATEGY

SMOKING

Nurses can make a significant contribution to patients' health by discouraging them from smoking, preferably before they start. When a patient is already a smoker, education is essential, and a straightforward message that advocates quitting and points out the risks is most effective. Chronic smokers usually know they should stop smoking, and frequently they have tried several times. Such individuals may already have symptoms related to smoking; nevertheless they may still benefit from the nurse's patience, support, and encouragement.

Air Pollution. Air pollution is a continuing problem in many areas of the United States and is a significant problem in almost every major city. It can be either an additive or potentiating risk factor with smoking for cardiopulmonary disease.[21] Air pollution may cause increased morbidity and mortality, exacerbate existing cardiopulmonary disease, and cause sensory, neurologic, and behavioral changes. Vulnerable individuals (such as those with cardiopulmonary disease) should stay indoors and quiet during times of air stagnation or severe pollution. Even people who are at low risk should not play or exercise outdoors during severe air pollution.

Occupational Hazards. Unlike most other body systems, the respiratory tract is in direct contact with the outside environment. It can, therefore, be injured directly by exposure to noxious materials. Occupational respiratory hazards include dusts, fumes, silica (glass, sandstone, other rocks), coal dusts, asbestos, beryllium, and chemicals such as formaldehyde and glutaraldehyde. Workers who are exposed to occupational hazards should always wear appropriate protective apparel. Occupational health nurses have a special mandate to be certain that workers understand safety regulations and adhere to them to prevent disability and disease.

Preventing Aspiration. Aspiration is what happens when foods, fluids, saliva, foreign objects, or other matter enters the nose, throat, or lower airways. The best way to deal with aspiration and the resulting asphyxiation or aspiration pneumonia is to prevent it.

Aspiration in young children frequently occurs because they put small objects, such as toys or coins, in their mouths. Small toys or toys with small removable parts should not be given to children under age 3. For example, children often pull or bite off the eyes or noses of some stuffed animals, so parents need to check these and other toys before allowing children to play with them.

Sometimes, aspiration or airway obstruction occurs when a person chokes on a piece of food during a meal. To some extent, such aspiration can be prevented. Children under 3 years old should not be given foods such as peanuts or pieces of chewy meats. Thorough chewing should be encouraged. In adults, aspiration of food may occur when the person has been drinking alcoholic beverages and the gag reflex and judgment are consequently impaired.

Heimlich Maneuver and CPR. The Heimlich maneuver is a technique for removing a foreign body that has lodged in the trachea or pharynx. It is effective and easy to learn. Teaching this maneuver to parents and others who care for individuals at risk for aspiration can prevent injury and save lives. CPR (cardiopulmonary resuscitation) is used when choking or another insult causes respiratory or cardiac arrest. Agencies such as the American Heart Association and the American Red Cross also provide classes for the general public on CPR and the Heimlich maneuver. These techniques are discussed later in this chapter. See Procedures 30–8 to 30–10.

Home Health Care

Home preventive care focuses on assessing patients and their environments to establish that the conditions for optimal oxygenation are present. As the section above on preventive care established, many oxygenation problems stem from lifestyle factors such as smoking, exposure to air pollution, failure to use masks during exposure to fumes and dusts, stress, improper diet, and lack of exercise. Home health nurses can assess the problems of patients and family members in their usual environment and counsel them about necessary adaptations according to their unique needs. Smokers are encouraged to reduce their smoking or give it up entirely, and all members are educated about healthful diet, stress reduction, and exercise. Family members are taught basic principles to prevent the spread of viral and other communicable illnesses. Further, home nurses routinely assess the adequacy of home ventilation systems and look for sources of allergens and pollutants that can bring on respiratory symptoms and distress. Families are encouraged, for example, to have their gas-burning space heaters periodically checked for the emission of poisonous carbon monoxide fumes, install filters in their air conditioners when members show a sensitivity to dust or other pollutants, or organize their homes to prevent any of a number of accidents such as drowning in home swimming pools. They may also be assisted to accommodate the needs of family members whose energy is limited by circulatory or respiratory alterations.

SUPPORTIVE CARE

Supportive care is aimed at supporting patients' physiologic and psychosocial adaptations so illness-related disruptions are minimal. As with preventive care, lifestyle modification and health education can often prevent mild health problems from becoming more serious. Additional approaches are discussed below.

Caring for Patients with Mild Upper Respiratory Infections

Patients often self-diagnose and self-treat upper respiratory infections such as colds, laryngitis, and mild influenza. Although these infections do not usually seriously compromise oxygenation, they do make breathing more difficult. Individuals having frequent colds can benefit from help in identifying contributing factors and ways to reduce discomfort.

Reducing Incidence. Colds are caused by viruses. The mode of transmission is via droplet nuclei, although direct transmission of a virus from hands to mucous membranes also occurs. Avoiding crowded places during the cold and flu season is one way to reduce one's incidence of colds. Individuals with respiratory allergies have heightened susceptibility to colds and should take preventive measures.

Advise individuals who have mild upper respiratory infections to avoid crowds and, in particular, contact with people with chronic respiratory disease because these individuals are particularly vulnerable to the negative effects of colds.[22] Covering the mouth and nose when coughing or sneezing, frequent handwashing, and appropriate disposal of facial tissues also help prevent transmission of the virus.

Smokers are at greater risk for upper respiratory infections than nonsmokers because of damage to the respiratory tract mucosa. Pointing this out to a smoker who has frequent colds may be an incentive to quit.

Managing Symptoms. The minor discomforts of colds are often greatly relieved by over-the-counter medications such as decongestants (phenylephrine, pseudoephedrine) and analgesics (aspirin, acetaminophen). Patients should be cautioned to read package inserts about side effects and necessary precautions. Generally, if symptoms persist despite self-medication, consultation with a health care provider is advised. Increasing fluid intake is important during a cold. Many patients find that gargling with salt water and using throat lozenges relieve sore throat and cough.

Patients should be advised that symptoms such as a fever over 100F, a very sore throat, rash, or thick copious secretions suggest the possibility of a bacterial infection that requires medical treatment. Individuals with heart or lung disease should seek care for even mild influenza, because they are at risk for extension of the infection to the lower respiratory tract and other more serious complications.

Assisting Patients with Respiratory Allergies

Many people have allergies that are manifested by respiratory symptoms. Most can lead normal lives with little change in lifestyle. Others need support from health care providers to make lifestyle changes that will enable them to remain healthy and active.

Allergic rhinitis is a reaction of the nasal mucosa to specific allergens. An allergen is a substance that can produce a hypersensitive (allergic) reaction in the body. These may include inhaled allergens (such as pollens), food allergens, or systemic allergens (such as drugs). The manifestations of allergic rhinitis include nasal drainage or obstruction and stuffiness; sneezing; headaches; itching of the nose, eyes, throat, or ears; mouth breathing; and redness of the eyes. These manifestations usually do not interfere with oxygenation, although breathing may be difficult if nasal and pharyngeal mucosa become swollen and congested. Asthma, which is characterized by airway inflammation, hypersecretion, and contraction of airway smooth muscles, occurs in response to exposure to allergens. This is a potentially serious condition and requires more intensive treatment.

In general, therapy for allergies includes use of mild antihistamines and identification of the offending allergens. If the allergens can be identified, it may be enough for the person simply to avoid the allergens as much as possible. In other cases, desensitization (allergy shots) may be recommended.

Nurses can be instrumental in helping patients identify possible allergens and eliminate them from their environment. Discussion should focus on timing and frequency of symptoms and possible exposure to common allergens at the time symptoms appear.

Some examples of substances that often stimulate allergic reactions include cigarette smoke, molds, perfume, fumes from certain household cleaners, propellants from common aerosol products, pollens, and animal dander (the dry scales that are shed from the fur of animals and the feathers of birds). A dusty environment entraps allergens and therefore tends to exacerbate allergies.

Preoperative Teaching

Nursing care given before surgery to prevent postoperative oxygenation problems is also supportive care. Postoperative patients are at risk of developing oxygenation problems because of general anesthesia, postoperative pain, pain medications, and immobility.

General anesthesia sometimes depresses respirations in the postoperative period, which may result in hypoventilation and atelectasis. Moreover, some inhalation anesthetics irritate the respiratory mucosa, causing increased production of mucus, which can obstruct airways and inhibit air exchange if it is not effectively cleared.

Postoperative pain, particularly from thoracic, abdominal, or flank incisions, promotes shallow respirations and suppression of coughing, as discussed earlier. The narcotic analgesics usually prescribed to treat postoperative pain may also depress respirations.

Many patients are reluctant to move and change positions because of postoperative pain. As discussed in Chap. 33, the venous stasis associated with immobility increases the risk of thrombophlebitis. Thrombophlebitis is the inflammation of a vein wall in conjunction with the formation of a clot. The clot adhering to the inflamed vein wall can compromise circulation locally.

Other factors related to surgery increase the risk of thrombophlebitis. Surgery stimulates the clotting mechanism because blood vessels are cut during the surgical procedure. Vein walls in the lower extremities are sometimes damaged during surgery, because of body positioning for optimal surgical access. Also, the extended immobility during the operation precipitates venous stasis.

Thrombophlebitis can lead to a more serious complication, pulmonary embolus. This occurs when a clot breaks free of the vein wall and becomes entrapped in the pulmonary artery, thereby interfering with lung perfusion. The management of pulmonary embolism is beyond the scope of this text.

People with preexisting oxygenation problems have a higher than normal risk of postoperative respiratory or circulatory complications. In the preoperative period, particular attention should be given to the patient's smoking history and to symptoms of cardiopulmonary problems such as dyspnea on exertion, wheezing, cough and sputum production, chest pain, or symptoms of right- or left-sided heart failure. Even if there is no evidence of long-term oxygenation problems, an acute respiratory disease as minor as the common cold can predispose to postoperative pulmonary problems. Other problems that may be associated in some measure with postoperative pulmonary or circulatory complications include advancing age, obesity, and varicose veins.

Some of the techniques to promote postoperative oxygenation are initiated in the immediate postanesthesia recovery period. Because patients' level of alertness is likely to be diminished at this time, preoperative teaching to orient patients to the techniques and equipment is beneficial. Nurses should consider the patients' level of anxiety regarding surgery when planning teaching sessions (see also Chaps. 21 and 25).

Techniques to promote optimal oxygenation after surgery include breathing exercises to maximize lung expansion, effective coughing to maintain airway patency, and leg exercises to enhance venous return.

Breathing Exercises. Exercises that enhance lung expansion and therefore prevent atelectasis and hypoventilation include diaphragmatic breathing (Procedure 30–3), pursed-lip breathing (Procedure 30–4), and use of an incentive spirometer (Procedure 30–5).

(continued on page 1039)

PROCEDURE 30–3. TEACHING DIAPHRAGMATIC BREATHING

PURPOSE: To increase ventilation in the lower lobes, strengthen the diaphragm, and promote relaxation. This exercise is not appropriate for patients with reduced lung capacity.
EQUIPMENT: None.

ACTION 1. Select a time and setting that is mutually acceptable to you and the patient.

RATIONALE. Learning is facilitated when attention, is focused. High anxiety levels interfere with learning; therefore, teaching should not be attempted when the patient is uncomfortable, stressed, or dyspneic.

ACTION 2. Discuss the procedure with the patient, including desired patient participation and anticipated benefits.

RATIONALE. Active participation is more likely if the patient understands the desired behaviors and the anticipated benefits.

ACTION 3. If patient has nasal congestion, suggest blowing the nose first.

RATIONALE. A clear airway is necessary for effective airflow.

ACTION 4. With patient in a low-Fowler's or sitting position, instruct the patient to place one hand lightly on the abdomen, just over the umbilicus; and the other hand at mid-chest. Knees should be flexed to relax the abdominal muscles.

RATIONALE. This hand placement enhances awareness of correct use of muscles during the exercises.

ACTION 5. Describe and demonstrate to the patient how to inhale slowly and deeply through the nose, while using the abdominal muscles to elevate the hand resting upon it. The patient should feel as if the abdomen is gradually filling with air during inhalation. The chest should move only a small amount during this exercise.

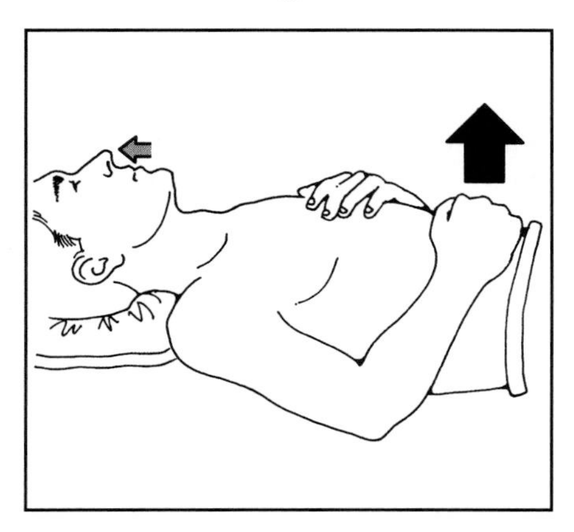

RATIONALE. Using multiple teaching modalities (in this case, auditory and visual) enhances learning. Use of the abdominal muscles facilitates relaxation and expands the chest cavity, inflating more alveoli.

ACTION 6. Describe and demonstrate slow and complete exhalation through pursed lips, while tightening the abdominal muscles. The abdomen should contract. Complete exhalation can also be facilitated by tightening the abdominal muscles and exerting light pressure with the hand on the abdomen.

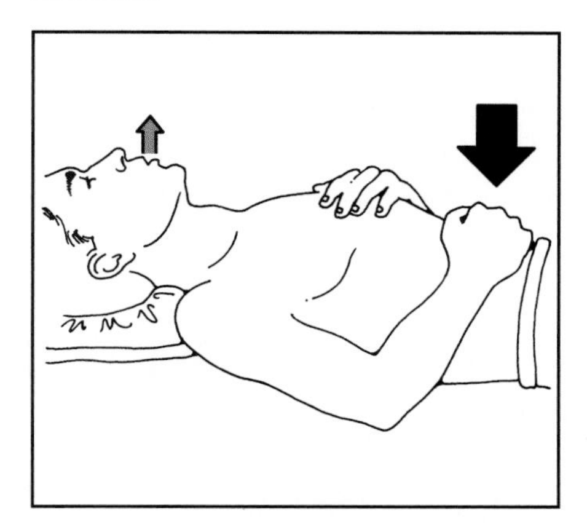

RATIONALE. See Action 5. Exhaling through pursed lips slows collapse of small airways by maintaining higher bronchiole pressure, allowing slower and more complete exhalation (see Procedure 30–4).

ACTION 7. Assess the patient's response during several repetitions of the exercise to determine the number of repetitions per session to suggest as a short-term goal.

RATIONALE. Patients with oxygenation problems fatigue easily. Several short exercise periods each day will promote maximum benefit with minimal fatigue.

ACTION 8. Give positive feedback for correct performance of the exercise.

RATIONALE. Positive reinforcement increases likelihood that the behavior will be repeated.

ACTION 9. Instruct the patient take three breaths in a row and then rest for 1 minute.

RATIONALE. Rest delays the onset of fatigue, allowing longer practice sessions.

Continued

ACTION 10. Instruct the patient to increase to about four 10-minute exercise sessions daily.

RATIONALE. Improved pulmonary function should result from regular exercise, so the patient will be able to tolerate longer exercise periods.

If dizziness or shortness of breath occurs during the exercise, the patient should rest and decrease the intensity or length of the exercise.

ACTION 11. As the patient gains competence in the technique, suggest performing the exercise in alternate positions, such as lying or standing, and during simple activities such as walking and stair climbing.

RATIONALE 11. Facilitates transfer of learning so the patient can use this technique to relieve respiratory distress if it occurs during regular daily activities.

Recording:

Note the specific exercise taught, the degree of proficiency demonstrated by the patient, the length of the exercise session, any problems noted, and mutual plans for continued practice. The exercise plan should be incorporated into the patient care plan and posted at the patient's bedside.

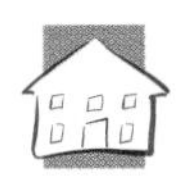

HOME HEALTH ADAPTATION: This is a beneficial technique to teach patients in the home setting.

PROCEDURE 30–4. TEACHING PURSED-LIP BREATHING

PURPOSE: To provide a means of controlling respirations during exercise, dyspnea, or panic situations; to increase tidal volume and prevent air trapping by maintaining patency of small airways; to reduce unintentional breath holding during activity. It is especially helpful for patients with chronic lung disease.

EQUIPMENT: None.

ACTION 1. Select a time that is mutually acceptable to you and patient.

RATIONALE. Learning is facilitated when attention is focused. Low stress levels facilitate concentration. High anxiety or panic interferes with learning; teaching should not be attempted when patient is uncomfortable, stressed, or dyspneic.

ACTION 2. Discuss the exercise and its purpose with the patient.

RATIONALE. Learning is facilitated when the individual sees the relevance of what is being learned to the personal situation.

ACTION 3. Request patient to assume a sitting position in bed or chair. After patient has mastered the technique, it can be performed in any position.

RATIONALE. Upright position reduces pressure of abdominal organs on the diaphragm, creating more space for lung expansion.

ACTION 4. Ask patient to inhale deeply through the nose while you count slowly to two. When the breathing technique has been learned, ask the patient to count with respirations.

RATIONALE. Learning is facilitated when the learner can focus on one behavior at a time.

ACTION 5. Ask patient to form pursed lips as if to whistle, then exhale evenly while you count to four. Tell the patient to listen for a soft whooshing sound as air is exhaled.

RATIONALE. It takes about twice as long to exhale a given volume as to inhale it because small airway collapse retards expiratory airflow. Whooshing sound indicates correct lip position.

ACTION 6. Ask the patient to repeat the exercise several times while you count. Give positive feedback for correct performance.

RATIONALE. Repetition enhances learning. Behavior that is positively reinforced is likely to be repeated.

ACTION 7. When patient can correctly perform the exercise as you count, ask him or her to breathe and count simultaneously, using the same rhythm as before. Reinforce correct performance.

RATIONALE. Patient must be able to perform the exercise independently for it to be useful in daily situations.

ACTION 8. Work with the patient to develop a regular practice schedule with increasing frequency of sessions per day until five sessions lasting 5 to 10 minutes a day are tolerated.

RATIONALE. Repetition is necessary for the acquisition of a motor skill. The patient is more likely to adhere to a schedule that he or she participates in developing. Short practice sessions are better tolerated by patients with respiratory dysfunction.

ACTION 9. Encourage use of the technique during exercise, and activities such as shaving, dressing, carrying light loads, climbing stairs, and doing housework, or when stressed. Sample instructions: Shave only while exhaling. Tie shoes by first inhaling, then bending to tie one shoe while exhaling. Use similar inhalation–exhalation rhythm while making beds, vacuuming, climbing stairs.

RATIONALE. Patients with respiratory dysfunction becomes short of breath after very short periods of breath holding. Breath holding is common during exercise, shaving, and other activities listed. Stress tends to cause tachypnea, which results in decreased oxygen intake and possible hypoxia.

Recording:
Document the specific exercise taught, the degree of proficiency demonstrated by the patient, length of the exercise session, any problems noted, and mutual plans for continued practice. The exercise plan should be incorporated into the patient care plan and posted at the patient's bedside.

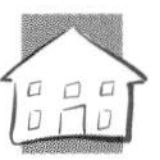

HOME HEALTH ADAPTATION: The procedure for teaching pursed-lip breathing is the same regardless of the patient's setting.

PROCEDURE 30–5. TEACHING USE OF THE INCENTIVE SPIROMETER

PURPOSE: To facilitate sustained maximal inhalation (SMI); and to prevent atelectasis, especially in patients who inhibit deep breathing because of postsurgical incisional pain or respiratory dysfunction.

EQUIPMENT: Incentive spirometer.

ACTION 1. Discuss volume goals for spirometry with physician or respiratory therapist. (If using Tri-flow or similar type spirometer, volume goals are not necessary.)

RATIONALE. Specific patient variables will determine appropriate volumes.

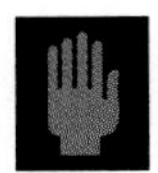

Postsurgical patients may simply be encouraged to take as deep a breath as possible; patients with respiratory dysfunction may need to increase volume goals gradually.

ACTION 2. Select a time and place that are mutually acceptable to you and the patient.

RATIONALE. Learning is facilitated when attention is focused. Pain, high anxiety, and distractions interfere with learning, so teaching should not be attempted when patient is anxious or during episodes of respiratory distress or pain.

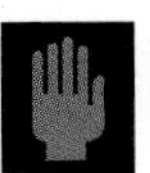

It may be appropriate to give analgesia ½ hour before exercise for postsurgical patients.

ACTION 3. Assess respiratory status: rate, depth, breath sounds, chest wall expansion, and symmetry.

RATIONALE. Provides a baseline for assessing treatment effectiveness.

Continued

ACTION 4. Discuss the procedure and its expected benefits with the patient.

RATIONALE. Active participation is more likely if the patient understands the desired behaviors and anticipated benefits.

ACTION 5. Instruct the patient to:

a. Hold the spirometer in an upright position (less critical in a flow-oriented spirometer).

RATIONALE. Less negative pressure is required to move the balls or discs in a flow-oriented spirometer.

b. Exhale normally.

c. Seal the lips tightly around the mouthpiece.

RATIONALE. If air leaks around the mouthpiece, less negative pressure will be generated inside the device. Feedback about performance will be inaccurate.

ACTION 6. Ask the patient to:

a. Take a slow, deep breath through mouth only, until the preset goal is reached; then hold the breath for 2 seconds, increasing to 6 seconds as tolerance increases.

RATIONALE. Greater lung expansion is achieved with slow inspiration. Holding one's breath after maximal inspiration facilitates lung expansion.

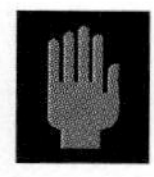

If incisional pain interferes with effective deep breathing, assist the patient to splint the incision (see Fig. 30–6). Patients should avoid rapid, shallow breaths; these do not inflate the alveoli effectively. If a patient has difficulty inhaling only through the mouth, a nose clip may be used.

b. Take the mouthpiece out of mouth and exhale normally.

RATIONALE. The spirometer is not designed to allow expiratory flow through the chambers.

c. Repeat the exercise five to ten times with a 15 to 30 second rest period between breaths as needed.

RATIONALE. Repetition increases inspiratory volume and improves alveolar ventilation.

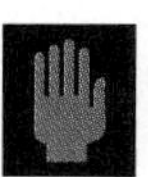

If the patient becomes dizzy or lightheaded, the exercise should be terminated and the number of repetitions decreased in subsequent sessions.

ACTION 7. If lung secretions are present, instruct the patient to cough with mouth covered at the completion of each series of deep inhalations (see Procedure 30–6).

RATIONALE. Deep breathing loosens secretions; coughing facilitates their removal, covering mouth prevents spray of secretions to environment and/or on nurse.

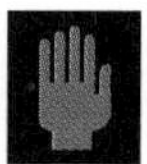

Patients with copious secretions may cough uncontrollably after deep breathing. In this situation, wearing a moisture impervious gown and goggles is advised.

ACTION 8. Reassess respiratory status to compare with baseline data.

ACTION 9. Instruct the patient to repeat the exercise hourly.

RATIONALE. Alveoli not being inflated tend to collapse within 1 hour.

Recording:

Note the type of spirometer, number of repetitions, the volume or flow achieved, presence of secretions, any problems noted. Some institutions use a flowsheet or checklist to document use of an incentive spirometer.

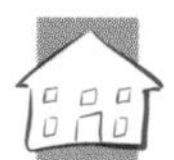

HOME HEALTH ADAPTATION: Many patients are sent home with an incentive spirometer. Plan with patients how to incorporate its use into their daily schedule.

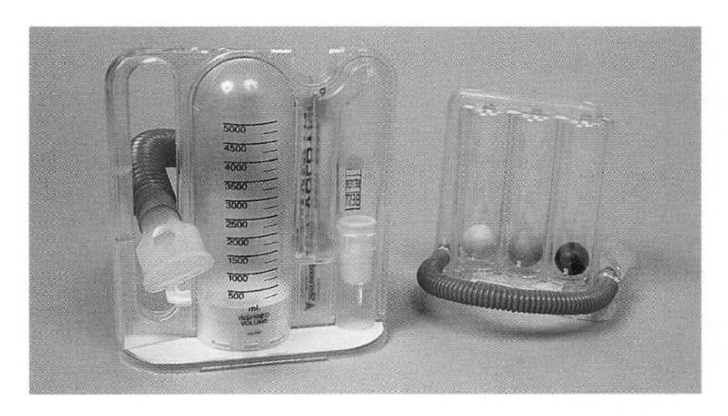

Figure 30–5. Incentive spirometers: volume type (left) and tri-flow (right).

Diaphragmatic and pursed lip breathing are also effective for relief of respiratory distress. An incentive spirometer encourages patients to breathe deeply and to hold the inspired breath briefly before exhaling. This is called **sustained maximal inspiration.** It is an effective way to prevent alveolar collapse. Different incentive spirometers are illustrated in Fig. 30–5.

Effective Coughing. Coughing is often necessary postoperatively to clear secretions and maintain airway patency. Postoperative patients are often reluctant to cough and therefore cough ineffectively, which causes pain but does not move secretions. Procedure 30–6 describes teaching effective coughing. Formerly, regular coughing concurrent with deep breathing was recommended as part of postoperative prevention of respiratory complications. However, current practice is to recommend postoperative coughing only when secretions are present. Routine coughing in the absence of secretions has been found to cause atelectasis and, because of associated pain, to decrease motivation for effective deep breathing. Splinting while coughing decreases the pain that postoperative coughing typically generates. **Splinting** is supporting the incision with interlaced hands and fingers and/or a pillow. As Fig. 30–6 illustrates, splinting can be done by patients themselves or by a nurse.

Leg Exercises. Several simple exercises that can be done in bed stimulate venous return and reduce the risk of thrombophlebitis (Fig. 30–7):

- Calf pumping: Alternate plantar flexion and dorsiflexion (Fig. 30–7A).
- Foot circles: Rotate the forefoot as if to draw a circle with the great toe (Fig. 30–7B).
- Hip rotation: Alternate inward and outward rotation of the hip (Fig. 30–7C).
- Leg spread: Alternate abduction and adduction of the hip (Fig. 30–7D).
- Knee flexion: Alternately flex and extend the leg at the knee (Fig. 30–7E).

The optimal frequency and number of repetitions of these exercises vary from patient to patient and are best decided postoperatively. The longer the period of postoperative bed rest, the more important it is to schedule these exercises several times a day. Patients should be cautioned to avoid holding their breath or using a Valsalva maneuver when doing these exercises.

Home Health Care

One aspect of supportive home health care is assisting patients with mild upper respiratory infections and respiratory allergies. Although such problems may not initiate home visits, they often are part of the care of families who have some other reason to need the assistance of a home health nurse. Assessing the nature of upper respiratory problems and particularly the need for a medical referral is part of the role of home health nurses.

Another service home nurses provide is to monitor vital signs and medications taken by patients with health problems that compromise oxygenation and to assure that medicines are appropriate, are used properly, and are not contraindicated by some other aspect of the patient's therapy (Fig. 30–8).

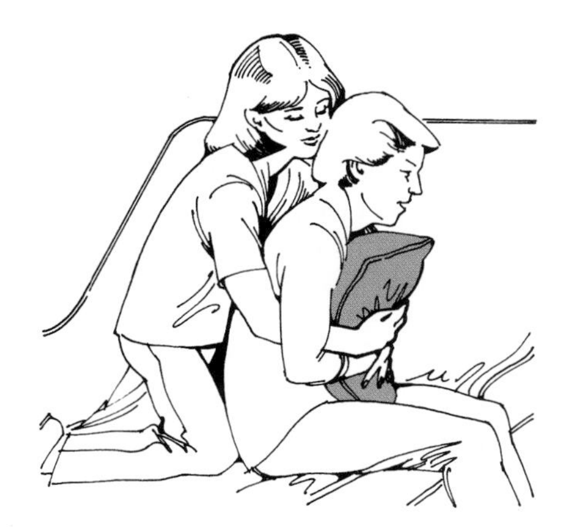

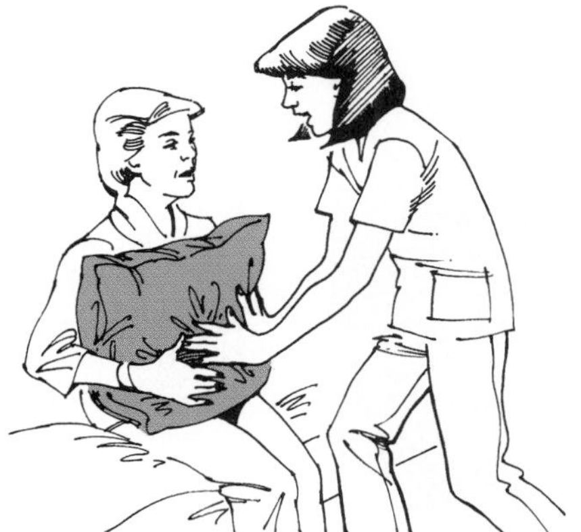

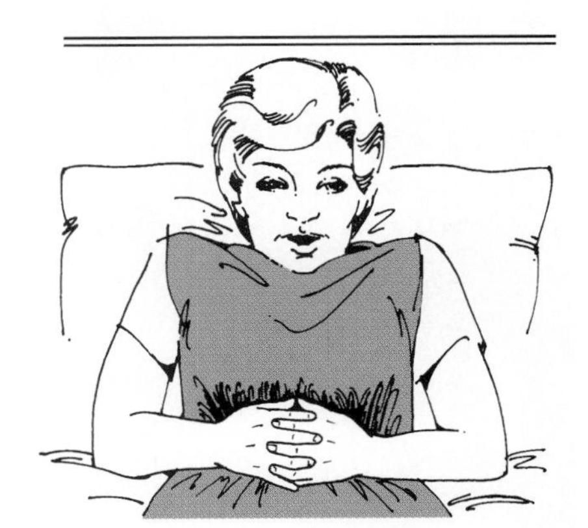

Figure 30–6. Splinting area of incision to alleviate pain when coughing.

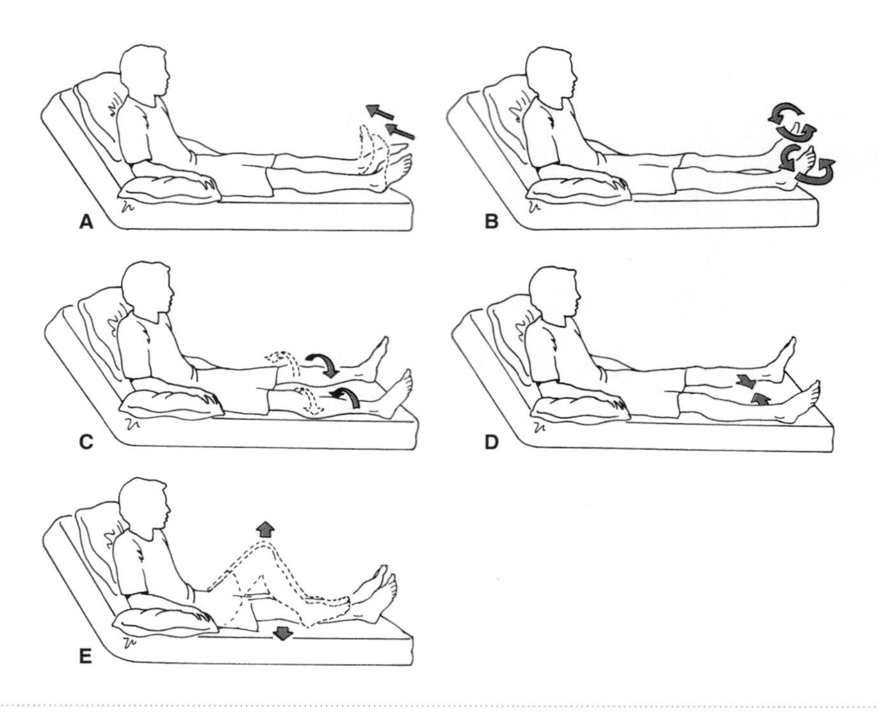

Figure 30–7. Leg exercises. **A.** Calf pumping. **B.** Ankle-foot rotation. **C.** Hip rotation. **D.** Hip abduction/adduction. **E.** Knee flexion/hyperextension.

RESTORATIVE CARE

Patients who experience major interferences with oxygenation or perfusion of body tissues need restorative care. This care may take the form of nursing implementation to reduce oxygen demands, mobilize secretions, maintain airway patency, administer ordered therapy, and promote circulation.

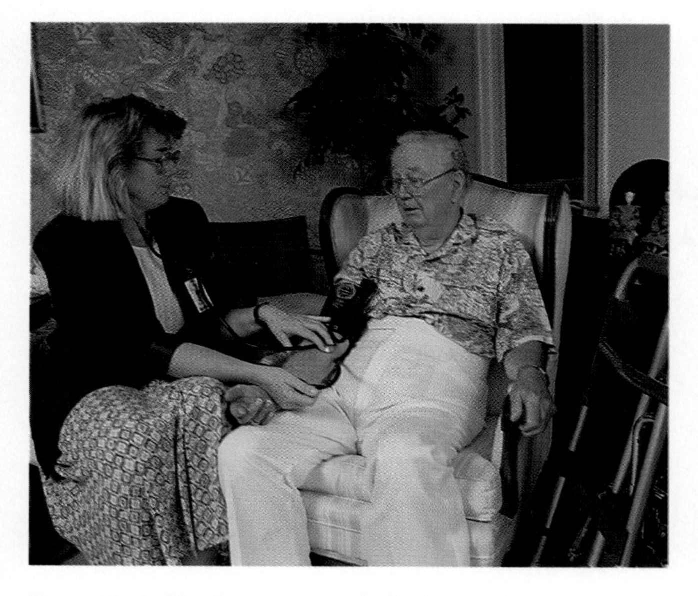

Figure 30–8. Blood pressure monitoring is a routine part of home health care for patients with oxygenation problems.

Reducing Oxygen Demands

One of the most important things a nurse can do for patients with oxygenation problems is to help them reduce demands for oxygen. Many activities increase metabolism and consequently increase the body's oxygen need. When a patient is in an oxygenation crisis, activities should be kept to a minimum so that energy is available for the life-sustaining activities of breathing and circulation.

Reducing Activity. Patients in respiratory distress should be encouraged to rest. Eating, entertaining visitors, ambulating, and bathing add to oxygen demands. Planning nursing care so that a patient has uninterrupted rest periods is an effective way to reduce oxygen demands. Because of the amount of care seriously ill patients require, they may not have a single hour of uninterrupted sleep for many days. Developing a schedule for essential care collaboratively with patients and other health care team members is necessary to support optimal oxygenation.

Digestion increases metabolic rate considerably. Therefore, many patients with oxygenation problems tolerate a light diet with frequent meals more readily than three large meals a day. Another reason for diet modification is that a full stomach presses upward on the diaphragm and tends to compromise its motion. This can lead to dyspnea or shortness of breath.

The patient who is acutely ill with oxygenation problems should be taught to avoid the Valsalva maneuver. The Valsalva maneuver increases intrathoracic pressure. This reduces or occludes the return of blood to the heart, which temporarily reduces cardiac output and may cause dizziness, lightheadedness, or fainting.

Reminding family members and other visitors of a patient's need for rest is also helpful. Making sure they are aware that the patient should not be awakened unnecessarily will help the patient

(continued on page 1042)

PROCEDURE 30–6. TEACHING CASCADE COUGHING

PURPOSE: To raise respiratory secretions from large and small airways, facilitating optimal oxygenation in patients at risk for airway occlusion (postoperative patients; patients with restrictive lung disease, laryngeal disease, central nervous system disease, neuromuscular disease; patients on prolonged bedrest; and patients being treated with restrictive binders/dressing or with artificial airways).

EQUIPMENT: None.

ACTION 1. Assess patient to determine respiratory status and need for scheduled and prn coughing.

RATIONALE. Regularly scheduled coughing (q 1–2 h) is necessary for immobile patients and those with diseases listed above, because secretion production interferes with oxygen exchange. Postoperative patients should cough prn (only when secretions are present) because coughing when there are no secretions present can cause alveolar collapse and causes unnecessary pain.

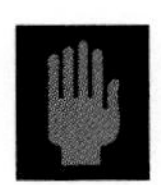

Pain associated with unnecessary coughing in postoperative patients may decrease motivation to cough correctly when coughing is needed.

ACTION 2. Discuss the procedure and its expected benefits with the patient.

RATIONALE. Active participation is more likely if a patient understands the desired behavior and its anticipated benefits.

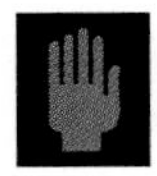

Discussing the technique and having a practice session preoperatively increases likelihood of postoperative participation.

ACTION 3. Assist or instruct patient to assume sitting position leaning slightly forward with feet on floor. Alternate positions for patient confined to bed: high or semi-Fowler's, or side-lying with legs flexed, HOB slightly elevated.

RATIONALE. Allows maximal lung expansion by diminishing pressure of abdominal organs on diaphragm and maximizes use of diaphragm and abdominal muscles to increase intrathoracic pressure by stabilizing torso.

ACTION 4. Verbalize and demonstrate each of the following:

RATIONALE. Use of multiple sensory modalities (visual and auditory) enhances learning.

a. Take a slow, deep breath (patients with severe airway disease may be able to take only somewhat shallow breaths).

RATIONALE. Slow, rather than quick, inhalation is less likely to pull secretions more deeply into the lungs.

b. Exhale, then repeat the deep inhalation. If first deep breath stimulates coughing, encourage the patient to go ahead and cough.

RATIONALE. Deep inhalations build up a volume of air behind the mucus, which will effectively propel it upward; inhaling deeply also stimulates the cough reflex.

c. Hold breath for 2 seconds; then exhale against closed glottis by contracting diaphragm. Telling the patient to try to exhale with the throat closed may be easier for some to understand.

RATIONALE. Builds up intrathoracic pressure. Combination of maximal air volume and pressure creates bolus of air, which moves secretions.

d. Open mouth, cover with hand, and cough repeatedly without inhaling until nearly out of breath. The object is several small coughs rather than a few large coughs.

RATIONALE. Cough with large lung volumes (immediately after inhalation) clears trachea and mainstem bronchi; later coughs at small volumes tend to milk mucus out of smaller airways.

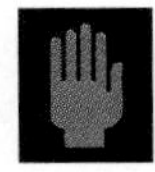

To assist patients with weak or paralyzed respiratory muscles, use quad coughing technique. If patient cannot accomplish cascade cough, try "huff" cough (see Clinical Guideline 30–5).

e. Pause, then inhale slowly.

RATIONALE. Pause prevents uncontrollable coughing, which may be stimulated by quick inhalation.

f. Rest, then repeat cough up to three times to clear airway.

RATIONALE. Excessive coughing can cause hypoxia, airway collapse, and discomfort.

Continued

Procedure 30–6. Teaching Cascade Coughing (continued)

ACTION 5. If paroxysmal coughing occurs, ask patient to attempt slow, regular respirations until the urge to cough passes. Offer sips of water. Pursed-lip breathing may assist some patients to suppress cough (see Procedure 30–4).

RATIONALE. Controlled breathing may suppress cough reflex. Water decreases mucusal irritation.

When assisting patients prone to paroxsmal coughing, wear moisture impervious gown and goggles to prevent droplet contamination of uniform or eyes.

ACTION 6. Assess secretions produced and respiratory status after coughing. Alert and oriented patients can be taught to self-evaluate secretions produced.

RATIONALE. Evaluates effectiveness of coughing.

ACTION 7. After completing coached cascade cough, ask patient to verbally describe the steps. Repeat instruction as necessary.

RATIONALE. Reinforces learning, allows nurse to evaluate understanding.

ACTION 8. Collaborate with patient to establish a coughing schedule if appropriate. Post schedule at patient's bedside and record it in the care plan.

RATIONALE. Patients are more likely to adhere to a schedule that is mutually developed. Posting a schedule will increase likelihood of adherence.

ACTION 9. Assist patient with coughing as scheduled. Intermittently observe patient who is coughing independently to reinforce correct technique and/or suggest improvements.

RATIONALE. Positive reinforcement increases likelihood that behavior will be repeated. Incorrect technique is ineffective and wastes energy.

Recording:

Initial note should describe what was taught, accuracy of patient performance, and plans for further teaching if needed. Describe patient's respiratory status before and after coughing, effectiveness of cough, and amount and character of secretions produced, if any, on initial and routing charting.

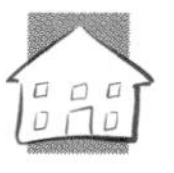

HOME HEALTH ADAPTATION: This is a beneficial technique to teach patients in the home setting.

---

conserve oxygen. Sometimes restricting visiting privileges to a few selected close family members is necessary.

Relieving Anxiety. Anxiety increases metabolism and therefore escalates bodily oxygen demands. A nurse can often reduce a patient's anxiety by honest explanations and answers to questions. Listening as patients vent feelings and fears can also decrease their anxiety. Sometimes, a nurse need only stay in the room with a patient to reduce anxiety. Encouraging a significant other to stay with the patient often has a calming effect. Relaxation techniques (Clinical Guideline 25–2) can also promote feelings of tranquility and reduce oxygen demand. Patients with chronic lung disease often panic when dyspnea occurs. Remind them that panic increases dyspnea and suggest using pursed-lip breathing to gain control and improve oxygen intake (see Procedure 30–4).

Alleviating Pain. Pain triggers a stress reaction that stimulates metabolism and increases the need for oxygen. Nursing measures aimed at both preventing and relieving pain are important. For example, preventing pain includes techniques such as teaching postoperative patients how to turn in bed and cough effectively without causing incisional pain. Chapter 33 details techniques for helping patients move in bed; coughing was discussed previously.

Pain relief can be accomplished in several ways, depending on the cause and nature of the pain. Changing positions in bed, massage, and other noninvasive techniques are often effective for mild pain. Severe acute pain usually requires analgesic medications prescribed by the physician. To be most effective, analgesics must be administered before pain reaches its peak intensity, so prompt response to complaints of pain are particularly important when oxygenation is compromised.

Pain medications and tranquilizers are ordered cautiously for patients who have pulmonary disease because these medications may reduce ventilatory drive. Patients with more severe pulmonary disease may suffer respiratory arrest because of this respiratory depression. Sometimes imagery, relaxation, or other noninvasive pain relief measures can relieve pain without compromising oxygenation.

Lowering Body Temperature. Each Fahrenheit degree of fever increases metabolism by about 7 percent. This increases the body's need for oxygen by a like amount. Patients with oxygenation problems may be unable to meet the extra oxygen and circulation demands caused by fever. Methods to reduce body temperature may be as simple as removing excess covers, improving room ventilation, or providing a sponge bath. Infection as a causative factor of fever must be ruled out or treated in collaboration with the physician. Antipyretic medications such as aspirin or acetaminophen may also be ordered.

Mobilizing Secretions

Excessive respiratory tract secretions are produced as a result of mucosal irritation associated with respiratory illnesses or immobilization (see Chap. 33). These secretions can interfere with ventilation and diffusion across the alveolar-capillary membrane. Facilitating movement of these secretions so that they can be easily removed by coughing promotes optimal oxygenation. Nursing measures to mobilize secretions include improving hydration, humidifying air, frequent turning, and chest physiotherapy.

Improving Hydration. Adequate hydration keeps sputum thin and easy to expectorate. If sputum is sticky and difficult to cough up, this is a good indication that a patient needs a higher fluid intake. In general, patients with chronic oxygenation problems need at least 64 ounces (1900 mL or 8 full glasses) of fluid daily (excluding milk, which may thicken secretions). More fluid is necessary if a patient has a respiratory infection. Strategies for assessing hydration status and increasing fluid intake are further discussed in Chap. 34.

Humidification. Even well-hydrated patients with copious secretions can benefit from breathing moist air rather than dry air. Dry air causes loss of moisture from mucosa by evaporation. Thick, tenacious secretions are created that are difficult for cilia to clear and for patients to expectorate. Bubbling air or oxygen through water enables it to carry more moisture, which in turn hydrates rather than dehydrates respiratory mucosa. Sometimes aerosolized (liquid transformed into a fine mist) water or saline is introduced into the respiratory tree to produce the same effect.

Frequent Turning. If a patient with copious respiratory secretions remains in the same position for several hours, the secretions pool in the dependent portion of the airway. This compromises the ability of the cilia to clear mucus. To prevent negative outcomes, nurses should encourage or assist patients to turn frequently from side to side and to the supine position. Patients should change positions at least every 2 hours; hourly is even better. Often deep-breathing and coughing exercises are done at the same time.

Chest Physiotherapy. Chest physiotherapy (CPT; also called postural drainage with percussion and vibration) may also be used to mobilize secretions. This method is performed by nurses, physical therapists, and respiratory therapists. Patients assume specific positions that use gravity to drain lung segments in which secretions have accumulated. Percussion and vibration are then applied to physically loosen and mobilize pooled secretions. **Percussion** is clapping the chest wall with cupped hands. **Vibration** is application of rapid oscillating pressure, either with the hands or with a mechanical vibrator. Patients are expected to cough in each position to remove secretions. If a patient is unable to cough effectively after CPT, tracheobronchial suctioning may be used. This is discussed in a later section.

Maintaining Airway Patency

Nursing implementation to maintain airway patency includes encouraging patients to perform the coughing and deep-breathing exercises discussed above, teaching patients positions that facilitate ventilation, administering medications to dilate bronchioles, performing pharyngeal and tracheal suctioning, and using artificial airways, the Heimlich maneuver, and CPR.

Breathing Exercises. Pursed-lip breathing, discussed under *Supportive Care* earlier in the chapter (see Procedure 30–4), is effective in maintaining the patency of small airways because the resistance created by pursing the lips during expiration preserves a low level of pressure throughout the respiratory tree. It is particularly effective when combined with exercise or with resting positions as described below. The incentive spirometer (see Procedure 30–5) also enhances airway patency, particularly if the sustained maximal inspiration technique is used.

Positioning. Generally, airways are most patent when a person is upright. Patients who have difficulty breathing therefore breathe most comfortably when sitting in a chair, with the head of the hospital bed raised, or when propped up on pillows in a regular bed. These positions also lower the abdominal contents and reduce pressure on the diaphragm. Patients in respiratory distress find that resting their arms on the overbed table or the arms of a chair (Fig. 30–9) or using the tripod position as discussed earlier (Fig. 30–4) enables them to breathe more effectively. In a standing position, leaning on a wall as shown in Fig. 30–10 works well. Using pursed-lip breathing in these positions adds to their effectiveness in maintaining airway patency.

Unconscious or partially conscious patients should never be positioned on their backs. In the supine position, the tongue tends to fall backwards, blocking the airway, and making aspiration of oral secretions more likely. For these reasons, anyone with a low level of consciousness or who has trouble swallowing oral secretions should be placed in a lateral position so that oral contents can drain out. Placing a towel or pad that can be changed frequently under the head will keep patients dry and comfortable. Often, oral suction is advisable to clear mouth of secretions. Frequent turning,

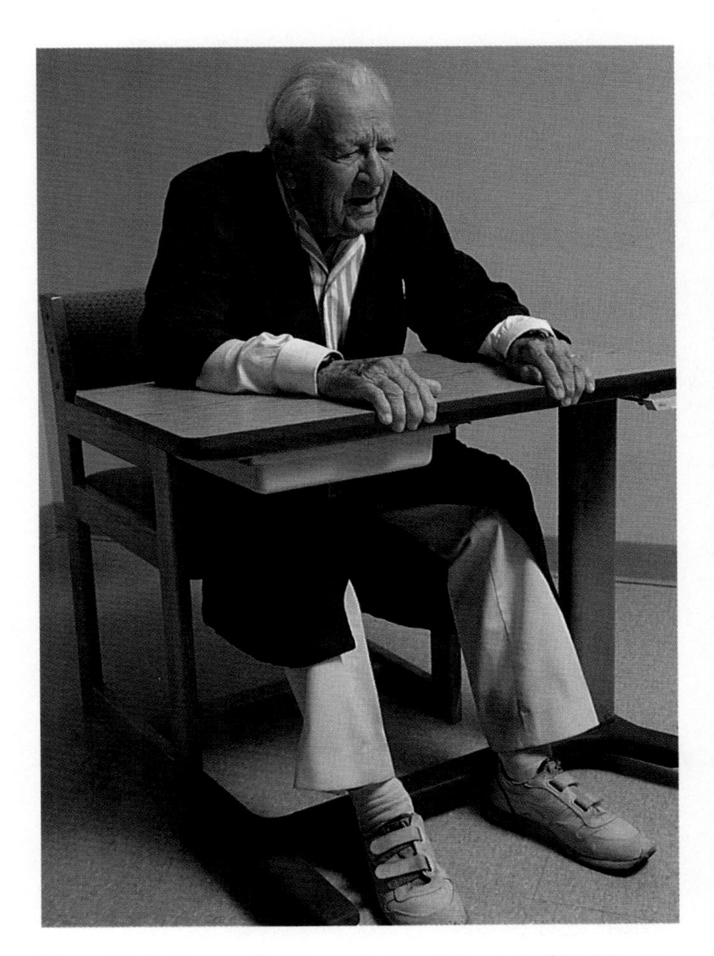

Figure 30–9. For a patient in respiratory distress, resting arms on a table will help breathing by increasing space for lung expansion.

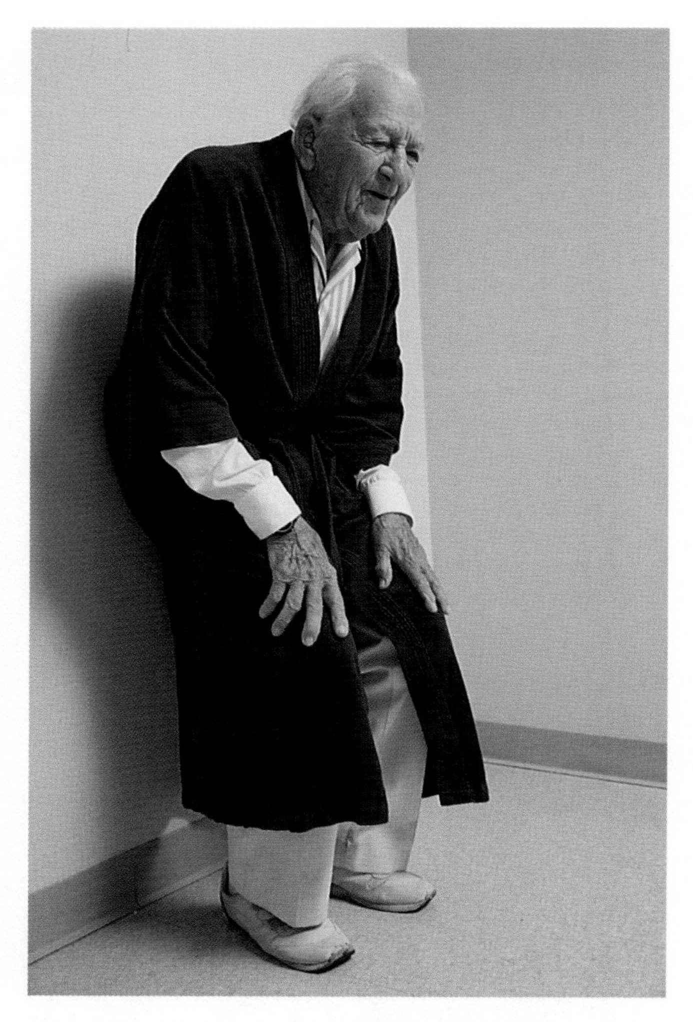

Figure 30–10. A patient may rest against a wall when respiration is difficult.

INSIGHTS FROM NURSING LITERATURE

BODY POSITIONING TO SUPPORT OXYGENATION

Swanlund SL. Body Positioning and the Elderly with Adult Respiratory Distress Syndrome: Implications for Nursing Care. J Gerontol Nurs. *1996;22:46–50.*

Age-related changes in the respiratory system may require that nurses use a different approach to meet the needs of elderly patients who have respiratory symptoms. Calcification of the costal cartilage, according to the author, reduces the compliance of the chest wall thus reducing respiratory excursions. Diminished elastic recoil results in premature airway closure and air trapping. This plus decreased strength of aging respiratory muscles leads to an increase of the residual volume and decreased forced vital capacity, a greater distribution of oxygen in the upper than in the lower airways, and suboptimal ventilation in the dependent areas of the lung—effects exaggerated by the presence of respiratory disease.

The author reviewed literature on body positioning for elderly patients who have respiratory disease. Studies comparing supine versus lateral positioning showed that oxygenation improved when patients with unilateral disease (disease in one lung only) were placed in a lateral position with the healthy lung down. This increased blood flow into the dependent healthy lung, enhancing oxygenation. Putting patients suffering from respiratory distress in the prone position also improved oxygenation, although the effect diminished after 120 minutes prone. A study comparing supine with semi-prone positions in patients with bilateral lung disease showed better oxygenation in the right semi-prone position. Noting that cases have to be evaluated individually, the author nevertheless concluded that therapeutic body positions can help maximize patients' oxygen supply and minimize energy demands. They recommended that nurses note patient position whenever arterial blood gases are drawn.

as discussed above, is particularly important for these patients, as their spontaneous movement is extremely limited.

Facilitating Effective Coughing. If secretions are present, a productive cough is the least traumatic way to clear airways. The cascade coughing technique shown in Procedure 30–6 generates optimal intrathoracic pressure to move secretions upward out of the respiratory tree. If patients are unable to cough effectively with this technique, try to determine the reason. Patients with pain from abdominal incisions or chest pain may need pain medication before they can cough effectively. Splinting the incision also helps, as discussed earlier. A patient with severe airway disease may cough more effectively at low inspiratory volumes. Follow the steps in Procedure 30–6, but suggest that the patient inhales less deeply before coughing. Alternative strategies to enhance coughing are presented in Clinical Guideline 30–5. Patients having no secretions should not be encouraged to cough, as it is painful, and serves no purpose.

? CRITICAL QUERY

Swanlund[23] reviewed the current research on therapeutic positioning, which showed that oxygenation improved when patients with respiratory problems were placed in therapeutic positions such as lateral, prone, and semi-prone, according to their condition. Given that these findings are based on studies using reliable methods and valid measures, how would a nurse evaluate their usefulness for individual patients?

Administering Bronchodilator Medications. Bronchodilators relax and open the airways. Using an inhaled bronchodilator before coughing can open the airways and enable the cough to clear the deeper, smaller airways more effectively. Bronchodilators may be delivered topically by hand-held cartridge inhalers (see Procedure 25–10); in nebulized form, in which patients breathe a mist of bronchodilator and air; or by intermittent positive pressure, in which the mist is delivered by a machine that blows air and mist in by positive pressure. Respiratory therapists usually administer bronchodilators by these routes.

CLINICAL GUIDELINE 30–5

ALTERNATIVE STRATEGIES FOR EFFECTIVE COUGHING

LOW INSPIRATORY VOLUME

- Use for patients with severe airway disease.
- Use techniques in Procedure 30–6, but inhale less deeply.

SPLINTING

- Use for patients with incisional or chest wall pain.
- Place a pillow, folded bath blanket, or interlaced fingers over the painful area. Apply even pressure over the painful area when the patient inhales prior to cough and during forced expiration. This technique can be done by a patient or nurse. (See Fig. 30–6.)

HUFF COUGHING TECHNIQUE

- Use to stimulate a cough reflex and raise secretions in patients who cannot perform the cascade cough. Progressive inhalations and exhalations in this technique gradually increase the lung volume and pressure to aid in producing a forceful cough.
- Ask patients to (1) hold their breath for 2 seconds, and then exhale in short puffs (with enough velocity for the air to be felt by a hand 2 inches from mouth); (2) again inhale slowly, hold the breath, and exhale in slightly more forceful puffs as if to blow out a candle; (3) repeat this process, this time saying "huff" on exhalation (the "huff" should have a breathy quality); and (4) repeat the process again, this time coughing once or twice on exhalation.

QUAD COUGHING TECHNIQUE

- Use for patients with muscle weakness or paralysis.
- Use a modified Heimlich maneuver (push upward at the base of the sternum) as the patient coughs or place heel of both hands at the base of the sternum (same hand position as for CPR, but lower). Or, teach patients to make a fist and lean over onto it if they have little arm strength or control. This makes the cough more forceful and improves clearance of secretions.

The use of inhaled bronchodilators is usually combined with the use of systemic bronchodilators. In patients who are in acute distress, these medications are given intravenously. Otherwise, they are given orally. Some patients will also need oral or intravenous steroids. All of these medications require a physician's prescription.

Suctioning. If bronchodilators, steroids, and coughing exercises are ineffective in clearing the airway, or if patients are unable to cough, oropharyngeal or nasopharyngeal suctioning may be necessary (Procedure 30–7). Nasotracheal suctioning, in which the suction catheter is passed from the nose down into the trachea and airways, is used in unconscious patients. This method is dangerous in the hands of an untrained person as it can cause laryngeospasm, closing the vocal cords and cutting off the air supply. Nasotracheal suctioning should be reserved for respiratory therapists and registered nurses who have been trained in its use. It is not described in this text, but is addressed in most textbooks of medical-surgical nursing.

Artificial Airways. If a patient needs assistance in keeping the airway open, an oral airway or a nasal airway may be used. These are most often used in postanesthesia recovery rooms or other situations in which the need for airway assistance is short term. Some practitioners use artificial airways when doing cardiopulmonary resuscitation to avoid contact with another person's oral secretions. (See Table 25–9, Infection Control Measures, and Procedure 30–9).

The oral airway helps to hold the tongue in place so it will not fall back and occlude the airway; however, conscious or partly conscious patients will gag and spit it out. These patients tolerate a nasal airway much better. This is a soft rubber airway that fits in the nose and extends into the pharynx so that even if the tongue falls back, there is an open airway.

A tracheostomy is an artificial opening into the trachea. It may be created to treat a respiratory emergency or for other therapeutic purposes, such as long-term mechanical ventilator use. A curved plastic tube is placed into the opening to maintain its patency. Tracheostomy care is an advanced clinical skill that is not addressed in this text.

Abdominal Thrusts (Heimlich Maneuver). If a person aspirates an object or piece of food that is large enough to obstruct the airway, he or she will immediately begin gasping for breath and coughing. The person with an obstructed airway will be unable to speak. Immediate intervention is imperative. A baby or young child is put over the lap in the head-down position and given several quick thumps on the back. This will often dislodge the object. Back thumps are not used for someone who is not in the head-down position, as they may drive the object further down into the airway. A person of any age, including a young child, can have the airway cleared by use of the Heimlich maneuver (Procedure 30–8). This maneuver is included as part of the American Red Cross and American Heart Association Cardiopulmonary Resuscitation (CPR) courses.

Cardiopulmonary Resuscitation. Cardiopulmonary resuscitation (CPR) is the act of giving mouth-to-mouth breathing and cardiac compressions (external pressure over the heart to circulate blood) to a person who has no pulse or respirations (cardiopulmonary arrest). Cardiac or respiratory arrest is a life-threatening problem that every member of the health care team must be prepared to handle at any time. Effective CPR must be initiated within 4 minutes of cessation of respiration, to prevent brain death. Techniques for maintaining an open airway and providing rescue breathing and external cardiac compressions are summarized in Procedures 30–9 and 30–10. People should not attempt to use these techniques unless they have completed a certification course. If the techniques are not used correctly, they will be ineffective and may cause harm, especially to infants and small children. Every nurse should complete a course in basic life support and recertify yearly. Nurses who work with critically ill and injured patients can also complete advanced cardiac life support (ACLS) courses.

An ambu-bag (hand-compressible breathing bag) may be used in the health care setting to aid in resuscitating a person who has suffered a cardiopulmonary arrest (Procedure 30–11).

Oxygen Therapy

Oxygen is commonly administered to people who are acutely or chronically ill with oxygenation problems. It improves cellular oxygenation while reducing cardiopulmonary workload. Oxygen therapy requires a physician's order. Orders for oxygen therapy should specify the type of delivery system or device and the rate of flow or oxygen concentration. Oxygen is *not* a "prn" (as needed) therapy. The patient should use the amount of oxygen that is prescribed and not adjust the oxygen flow rate up or down.

(continued on page 1066)

PROCEDURE 30–7. OROPHARYNGEAL AND NASOPHARYNGEAL SUCTIONING

PURPOSE: To relieve respiratory distress caused by upper airway secretions that patient is unable to expectorate.
EQUIPMENT: Wall suction setup cannister with filter, regulator, connecting tubing (portable suction machine may also be used); sterile suction kit containing catheter with thumb port, glove, water-soluble lubricant, and container for liquid; sterile water or normal saline; moisture-resistant bag; towel or disposable drape; nonsterile gloves, tongue blade, facial tissues; mouthwash; and toothbrush or toothettes; goggles and a moisture-resistant gown if secretions are copious.

ACTION 1. Determine need for suctioning by assessing respiratory rate, depth, quality, presence of gurgles or rumbles on auscultation or signs of acute distress: gasping, grasping throat, cyanosis. If secretions are present, encourage coughing.

RATIONALE. Presence of respiratory secretions interferes with optimum oxygenation. Patients who cannot cough effectively may need suctioning even if they are not in acute respiratory distress.

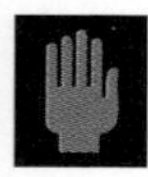

It is common practice to keep a suction setup ready for use and a supply of suction kits and appropriate-sized catheters in the room of a patient who may need assistance to clear the airway. The correct size catheter is about ½ the diameter of the patient's nostril: large enough to move secretions, but not so large as to block the airway. If patient is in acute distress, begin suctioning (see Action 7) without delay. If able to cough, he or she may still need assistance to completely clear the airway.

ACTION 2. Discuss the procedure and its expected benefits with the patient. Indicate that it may be uncomfortable, but is not painful, and that patient relaxation will decrease difficulty for patient and nurse. Let patient know that gagging or coughing may occur. If patient is expected or known to be uncooperative, have a second person available to restrain patient movement.

RATIONALE. Active participation is more likely if patient understands the desired behavior and anticipated benefits. Fear is diminished if honest explanation of what patient will experience is provided.

ACTION 3. Check cannister to see that connecting tubing attached to the vacuum port is clear, that it has a regulator and is securely attached to wall outlet.

RATIONALE. System must be intact to remove secretions effectively and safely. If cannister is full, it may overflow or automatic shutoff valve will make suctioning impossible. Regulator controls amount of negative pressure transmitted to patient.

ACTION 4. Close door or bedside curtains.

RATIONALE. Provides privacy. Procedure may be embarrassing to patient or offensive to others.

ACTION 5. Assist patient to semi-Fowler's position, with head turned toward you. Unconscious patients should be in lateral recumbent position, facing nurse, to minimize aspiration.

RATIONALE. Facilitates coughing to assist in removal of secretions without aspiration; aids insertion of catheter.

ACTION 6. Cover patient's pillow with towel or disposable drape. Don goggles and gown on first suctioning and thereafter if coughing is anticipated.

RATIONALE. Protects nurse and patient from possible contamination by sputum, as reflex coughing may transport secretions.

ACTION 7. Turn on and set regulator to appropriate setting:

Infant: 60–100 mm Hg
Child: 80–115 mm Hg
Adult: 80–120 mm Hg

Use lowest setting that will move secretions. Remove protective cap from tip of connecting tubing.

RATIONALE. Excessive amounts of negative pressure can damage respiratory mucosa by drawing it into the catheter.

ACTION 8. Prepare suction kit: open package; pour sterile liquid into container; squeeze lubricant onto sterile surface; open catheter package, if separately wrapped, maintaining catheter's sterility by preventing contact with unsterile objects. If unfamiliar with principles of asepsis, refer to Procedure 25–2 and Clinical Guideline 25–8.

RATIONALE. Aseptic technique is important because patients needing suctioning often have reduced pulmonary function and are more vulnerable to infection. If patient's resistance is low, it is recommended that each catheter be inserted only once.

ACTION 9. Oxygenate patient: instruct alert patient to take several deep breaths; use resuscitation bag with mask to hyperinflate lungs of unconscious patient. If patient is receiving nasal oxygen, it should be continued while suctioning.

RATIONALE. Suctioning removes oxygen from patient. Less distress occurs if patient is well oxygenated before suctioning.

ACTION 10. Don clean glove on nondominant hand, sterile glove on dominant hand. Some kits contain a pair, rather than a single glove, for nurse's convenience.

RATIONALE. The sterile gloved hand will be used to manipulate catheter, which is kept sterile to avoid introducing microorganisms into patient's respiratory tract. Clean glove protects nurse from contamination by sputum.

ACTION 11. Holding coiled catheter in dominant hand and connective tubing in the other, attach catheter to connective tubing. Catheter should not contact any other objects during connection.

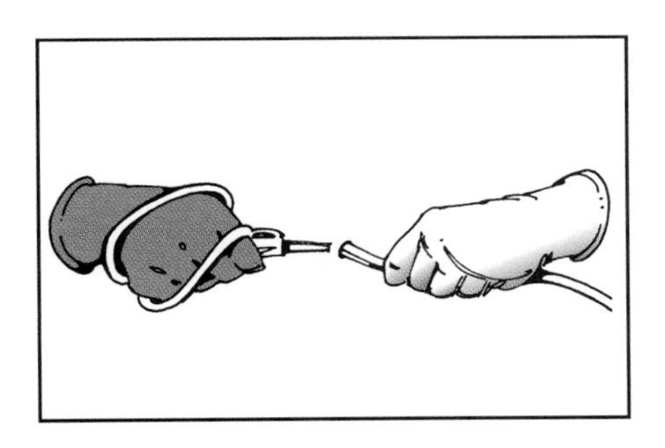

RATIONALE. Maintains sterility of catheter, provides pathway for secretions to travel to collection cannister.

ACTION 12. Place distal end of catheter into sterile liquid and cover thumb port; liquid should move into collection catheter. If liquid does not move through tube, check that all connections are secure and that regulator is set correctly.

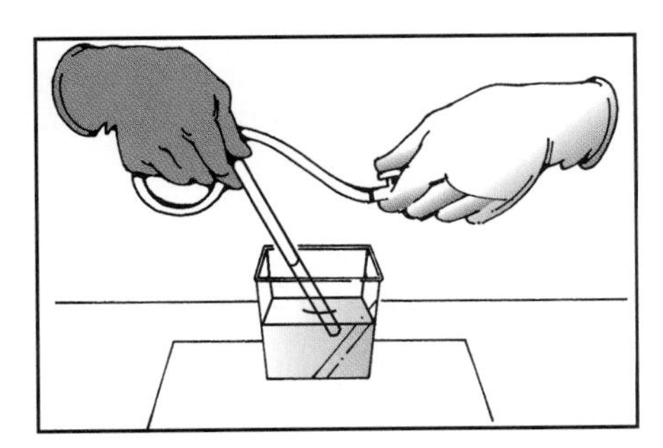

RATIONALE. Demonstrates if equipment is working; facilitates movement of secretions by lubricating lumen of catheter.

NASOPHARYNGEAL ROUTE

ACTION 13. Dip distal tip (6–8 cm or 3–4 in.) into sterile lubricant.

RATIONALE. Lubricant reduces friction between catheter and mucosa, preventing mucosal injury and irritation. Mucosal trauma increases infection risk.

ACTION 14. Note several markings on the catheter, which indicate average distances for insertion. Estimate the distance between the patient's nose and earlobe and note which marking most closely approximates this distance.

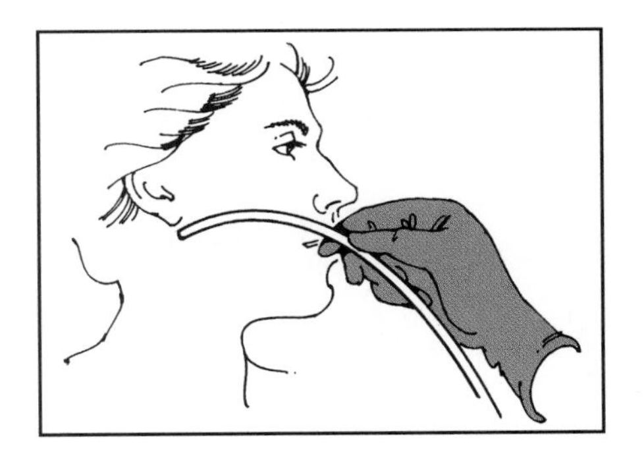

RATIONALE. The distance between nose and earlobe is similar to the distance from nostril to the distal pharynx. Advancing the catheter to this point will decrease the likelihood of inserting it too deeply, causing gagging or laryngeal spasm.

ACTION 15. Gently insert catheter into nares directing it along the floor of the nasal cavity, not upward. Thumb port should be open so no negative pressure is produced. Obtain patient preference for which nostril is to be used.

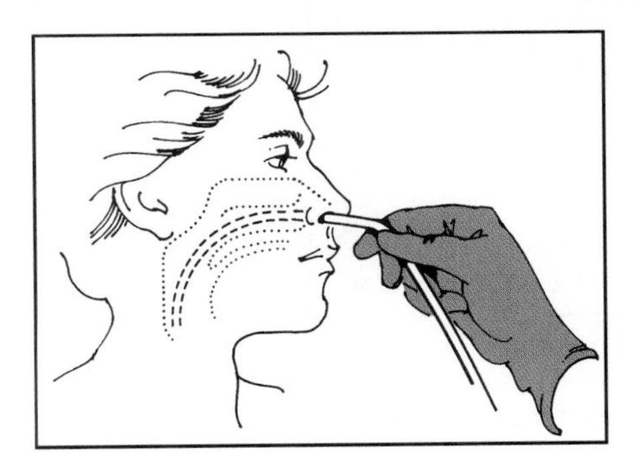

RATIONALE. Following the natural curve of the nasal floor reduces mucosal damage due to friction or pressure from the catheter tip. Lack of negative pressure during insertion minimizes oxygen depletion and prevents trauma from mucosa being drawn into catheter as it advances.

Continued

Procedure 30–7. Oropharyngeal and Nasopharyngeal Suctioning (continued)

ACTION 16. Advance the catheter smoothly and rapidly to the mark selected in Action 14.

RATIONALE. Airway should be cleared as rapidly as possible to optimize oxygenation and minimize discomfort.

Do not force catheter. If mucus plug is encountered, briefly cover thumb port to apply suction. Then advance catheter. If resistance is met, try opposite nostril.

ACTION 17. If patient coughs, pause, but do not remove catheter. Usually, it is not necessary to advance the catheter farther if effective cough occurs. If patient coughs uncontrollably, remove and reinsert catheter if needed to clear remaining secretions.

RATIONALE. Suction will remove coughed secretions. Removal and reinsertion increases mucosal trauma.

ACTION 18. If crowing noise (stridor) is heard, remove catheter quickly.

RATIONALE. Stridor indicates laryngeal spasm, which interferes with breathing.

ACTION 19. When catheter has been advanced to pharynx, cover thumb port intermittently while withdrawing the catheter with a twisting motion, in 10 seconds or less. (Count to 10 or hold your breath during suctioning to remind you to limit suctioning time.)

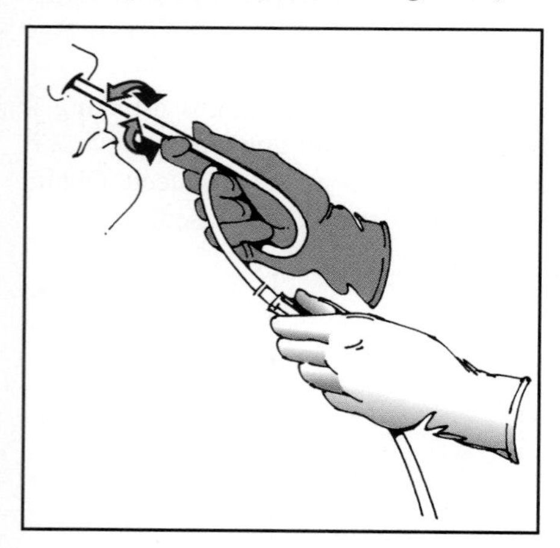

RATIONALE. Intermittent negative pressure reduces mucosal trauma; twisting rotates catheter tip, so all surfaces are cleared of mucus. Prolonged suctioning (greater than 10 seconds) can cause hypoxia.

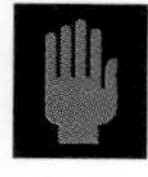

Do not move catheter up and down while suctioning, as this injures mucosa. Suction children for 5 seconds only.

ACTION 20. Rinse catheter in sterile liquid until all tubing is clear of secretions.

RATIONALE. Flushes secretions into collection cannister for disposal.

ACTION 21. Assess respiratory status to determine need for further suctioning. Repeat suctioning until pharynx is clear, allowing several minutes of rest and deep breathing between suction passes.

RATIONALE. Hypoxia is prevented by allowing patient time to take in oxygen between suction passes.

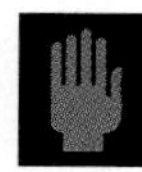

Hypoxia is more common with deep tracheal suction, but can occur if pharyngeal suctioning is repeated without rest periods.

ACTION 22. Check mouth for secretions; suction as above if needed. Most alert patients will be able to mobilize and expectorate oral secretions without assistance. Yankauer suction tip may be used to clear oral cavity, if desired.

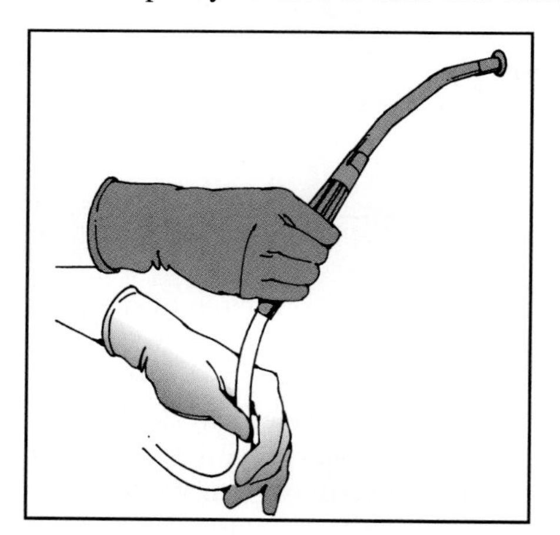

RATIONALE. Mouth should be suctioned last, as it has more organisms than nose. Yankauer tip is rigid and more easily directed to all parts of oral cavity.

ACTION 23. Assess secretions for color, amount, and odor. Complete procedure according to Actions 27–33.

RATIONALE. Assists in determining change in patient's condition.

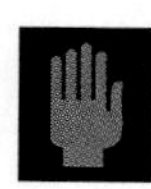

Bloody secretions suggest mucosal trauma; gray-green secretions, infection; thick, viscous secretions, dehydration.

OROPHARYNGEAL ROUTE

ACTION 24. Prepare suction kit as for nasal route, except for lubrication of catheter.

RATIONALE. Saliva provides sufficient lubricant for oral cavity.

ACTION 25. Ask patient to open mouth and stick out tongue; if patient is unconscious or weak, tongue blade may be used to hold tongue down.

RATIONALE. Allows visualization of pharynx and easy passage of catheter.

ACTION 26. Insert catheter over tongue to pharynx, then proceed with suctioning. (See Actions 17–23 above.)

RATIONALE. Pharynx should be cleared before mouth to optimize oxygen exchange.

ACTION 27. When airway is cleared, coil catheter in sterile gloved hand and remove glove so it turns inside out over catheter. Remove second glove in same fashion. Auscultate lungs to ascertain that airways are clear. Turn off suction device.

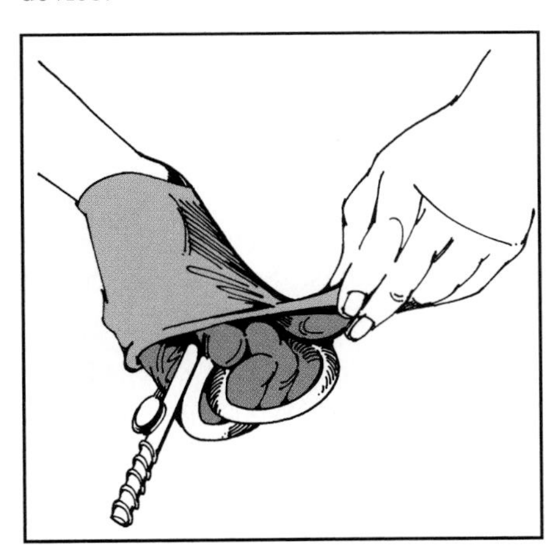

RATIONALE. Provides barrier to prevent transfer of microorganisms from catheter by direct contact with objects in environment.

ACTION 28. Dispose of goggles, gloves and gown according to agency policy.

RATIONALE. Secretions are considered contaminated; see rationale for Action 27 above.

ACTION 29. Provide mouth care if desired by patient.

RATIONALE. Promotes comfort and well-being.

ACTION 30. Discard remaining sterile liquid in sink, disposable equipment in trash, towel in laundry

RATIONALE. Promotes clean environment for patient.

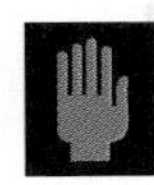

If patient is on isolation precautions, follow institutional guidelines for disposal of equipment.

ACTION 31. Reposition patient in correct alignment.

RATIONALE. Supports optimum oxygenation, motor function, and skin integrity.

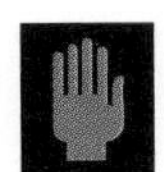

Many patients with oxygenation problems may be placed in semi-Fowler's position, but prolonged use of this position increases risk of pressure sores and contractures (see Chap. 33).

ACTION 32. Check cannister; if full, dispose of and replace. Cover end of connecting tubing with protective cap. Assure that ample supply of suction kits is readily available for future use.

RATIONALE. Prepares unit for prompt suctioning if respiratory distress occurs.

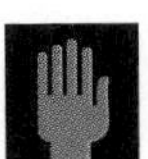

Some cannisters are completely disposable; others have disposable liners. Do not empty cannister in room or attempt to reuse a disposable cannister. Cannister and tubing must be changed every 24 hours.

ACTION 33. Collaborate with physician for revised treatment plan if sputum characteristics suggest change in condition.

RATIONALE. Suctioning treats symptom of airway occlusion, but not underlying cause.

Recording:
Describe patient status before and after suctioning, response to procedure, nature and amount of secretions, and additional nursing actions taken, if any.

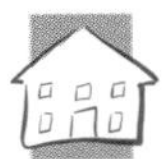

HOME HEALTH ADAPTATION: To contain costs, suction catheters and Yankauer tips are reused in the home, necessitating cleaning after each use. After suctioning, flush the catheter and/or tip and tubing with a vinegar solution made of equal parts of white vinegar and water, then rinse with cold water. Disconnect the catheter and wash the exterior of the catheter and tip in hot soapy water, then rinse. Prepare a basin of vinegar solution (1 to 1) and soak the catheter and tip for 30 minutes. Remove items from solution, rinse, then air dry on a clean paper towel. When dry store in a plastic zip-lock bag. It is recommended that at least two catheters or tips are available at all times. Instruct family caregivers how to suction, care for the equipment, observe for adverse signs and symptoms, and promptly report these to a health care professional.

PROCEDURE 30–8. CLEARING AN OBSTRUCTED AIRWAY: ADULT (HEIMLICH MANEUVER)

PURPOSE: To clear an obstructed airway.
EQUIPMENT: None.

CONSCIOUS VICTIM

ACTION 1. Upon observing a person who has apparently choked, but who is not coughing, ask, "Are you choking?" If patient speaks, take no action except encouraging coughing. The universal signal for choking is grasping the throat with one or both hands.

RATIONALE. Normal defenses of coughing are often more effective in clearing airway obstruction than external measures, which can actually interfere with a person's efforts to clear the airway.

ACTION 2. If person is unable to speak, explain that you will try to assist in removing the foreign body. Emphasize the importance of relaxation during the maneuver, then initiate abdominal thrusts (Heimlich maneuver).

RATIONALE. A person unable to breathe will be anxious and may tense the chest and abdominal muscles, which may reduce the effectiveness of the thrusts.

If patient is pregnant or obese, use chest thrusts (see below).

ACTION 3. Abdominal thrusts: Stand behind the victim. Make a fist; place it so thumb side is against victim's abdomen in the midline, just above the umbilicus.

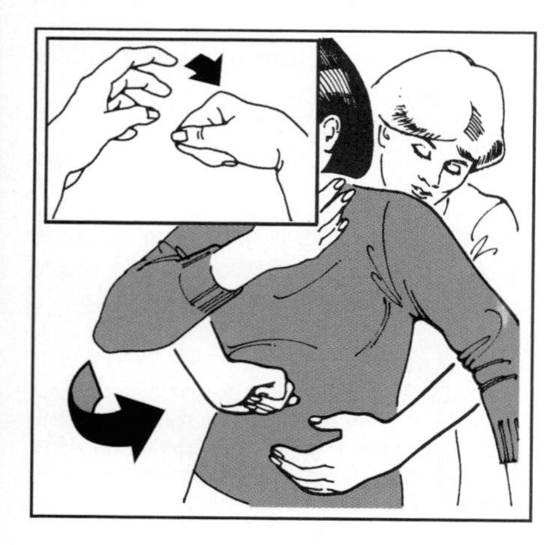

RATIONALE. Pressure will be exerted below the obstruction.

ACTION 4. Grasp your fist with your other hand, then thrust it upward vigorously, as if to push out the obstructing object. Repeat several times.

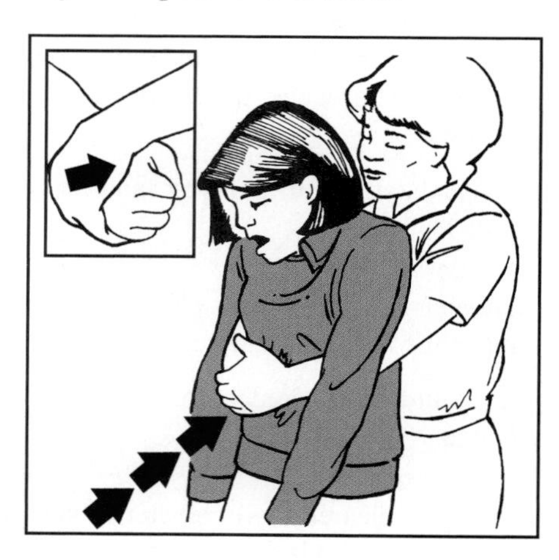

RATIONALE. Force of thrusts creates changes in air pressure producing a rush of air which will carry the obstructing object upward for expulsion.

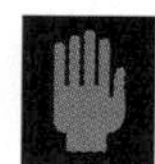

Do not squeeze rib cage with forearms or exert pressure on xyphoid process or ribs.

ACTION 5. Repeat until object is expelled or victim starts coughing or becomes unconscious. See next page for unconscious victim.

RATIONALE. Object may be too deep to be expelled with one to two thrusts. It must be removed to prevent brain damage due to anoxia. Coughing indicates patient is working to expel object.

CHEST THRUSTS

Used if conscious choking patient is pregnant or so obese that the rescuer cannot reach around the abdomen.

ACTION 1. Reach around patient from behind, make a fist, place thumb side against sternum at the level of the armpits, explaining your intentions as you position your arms.

RATIONALE. See Actions 2 and 3.

Procedure 30–8. (continued)

ACTION 2. Grasp your fist with your other hand and pull straight back sharply with a quick thrusting motion.

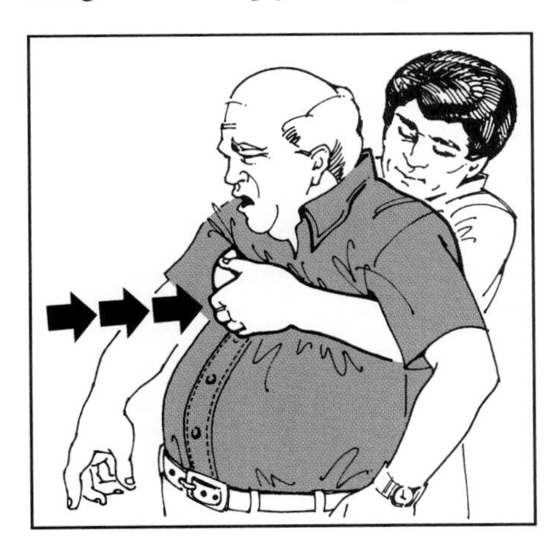

RATIONALE. See Action 4.

ACTION 3. Repeat until object is expelled or victim begins coughing or becomes unconscious.

RATIONALE. See Action 5.

UNCONSCIOUS VICTIM

ACTION 1. Activate Emergency Medical Service (EMS; call 911). If victim is in a healthcare facility, activate emergency call light.

RATIONALE. Assistance with CPR may be needed to prevent anoxia and brain damage.

ACTION 2. Place victim in supine position.

RATIONALE. Allows correct placement of hands for abdominal thrusts.

ACTION 3. Check for foreign body: Perform a finger sweep—place thumb in victim's mouth over tongue; grasp chin and pull lower jaw upwards. Slide index finger of other hand along inside of cheeks, deep into throat, using a hooking motion across base of tongue.

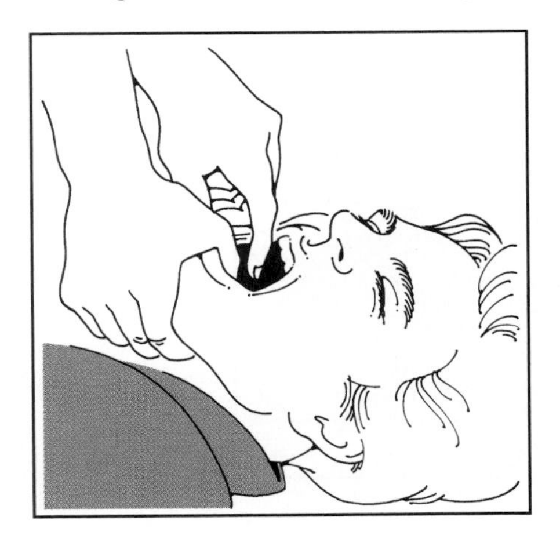

RATIONALE. Hooking finger sweep may dislodge an obstruction that is not deep in airway. Avoid straight poking motion of finger, which may push obstruction deeper.

ACTION 4. Attempt to ventilate victim (see Procedure 30–9). Make no further attempts to dislodge object if ventilation is possible.

RATIONALE. Relaxation of throat muscles due to anoxia may allow passage of air even though obstruction is not dislodged.

ACTION 5. If ventilation fails, initiate abdominal thrusts.

RATIONALE. Airway must be patent to deliver oxygen and prevent brain damage.

Continued

Procedure 30–8. Clearing an Obstructed Airway: Adult (Heimlich Maneuver) (continued)

a. Straddle victim. Place heel of one hand at the midline slightly above the umbilicus well below the xyphoid process; place the other hand on top of the first, pointing fingers of both hands upward, away from chest wall.

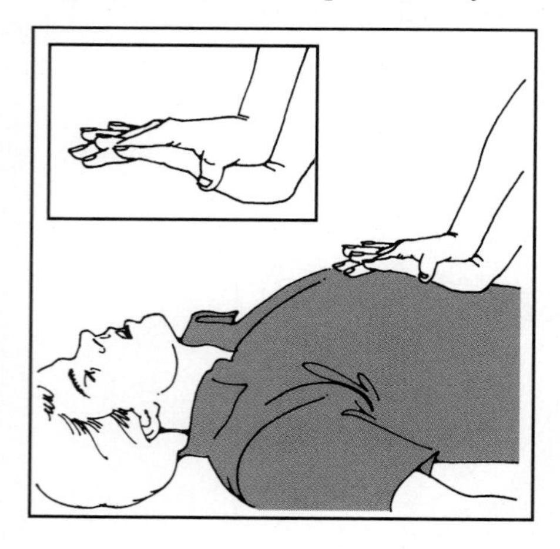

RATIONALE. Locates upward force below obstruction while avoiding injury to victim's ribs or lungs.

b. With elbows straight and your shoulders over victim's lower abdomen, press inward and upward quickly and sharply, six to ten times. Avoid thrusts on either side of midline to prevent injury to victim.

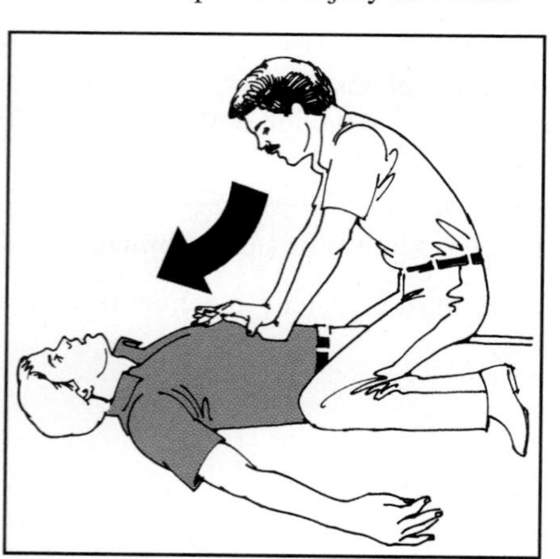

RATIONALE. Force of thrusts creates changes in air pressure, producing rushes of air, to carry the obstructing object upward for expulsion.

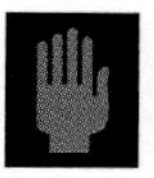

For pregnant or obese victims, place your hands on the lower one-third of the sternum, above the xyphoid process, and administer downward thrusts.

ACTION 6. If victim does not begin to breathe, repeat sequence of finger sweep, ventilation attempt, thrusts until airway is opened or EMS arrives.

RATIONALE. Relaxation of throat muscles after a period of anoxia may permit removal of object with subsequent attempts.

Recording:

If cessation of breathing occurs in a patient who is admitted to a health care facility, precise description of all events observed that could have contributed to cessation of respirations, or the state of the patient when first noted to have stopped breathing, as well as all actions taken and their results, should be noted on the patient's chart.

HOME HEALTH ADAPTATION: The technique for clearing airway obstruction is applicable to any setting.

PROCEDURE 30–9. CPR: ADULT

PURPOSE: To ventilate an unconscious person until spontaneous breathing resumes or an oxygen delivery system is available, and to circulate oxygenated blood to vital organs when heart is not beating.

EQUIPMENT: Oral airway or mask with one-way valve, emergency "crash cart" if available.

ONE RESCUER

ACTION 1. Assess whether victim is unconscious by grasping shoulder, gently shaking, and shouting, "Are you OK?"

RATIONALE. CPR contraindicated in a conscious victim.

ACTION 2. If victim is not responsive, call for help. Activate Emergency Medical Service (EMS; call 911) or Code Blue.

RATIONALE. Victim may also require external cardiac compressions and the assistance of specially trained resuscitation team.

ACTION 3. Place the victim in supine position and open **airway** by head-tilt, chin-lift:

RATIONALE. Loss of muscle tone due to unconsciousness causes tongue to fall backward, obstructing the pharynx. Head-tilt/chin-lift or jaw thrust move the jaw and attached tongue so pharynx is opened. Opening airway will restore spontaneous breathing and/or permit rescue breathing.

a. Place palm of one hand on victim's forehead.

b. Place fingers of opposite hand under victim's chin. Use care to avoid pressure on the soft tissue of the throat.

c. Simultaneously push down on forehead and lift upward on chin.

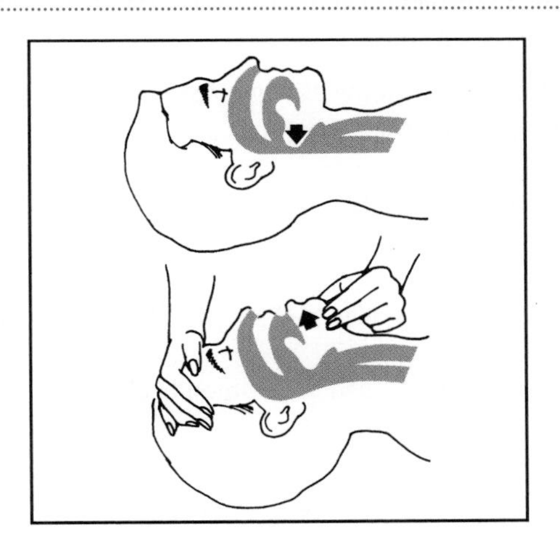

Or jaw thrust:
Pull upward on both mandibular angles (corner of jaw directly below ears) with tips of fingers; neck will hyperextend.

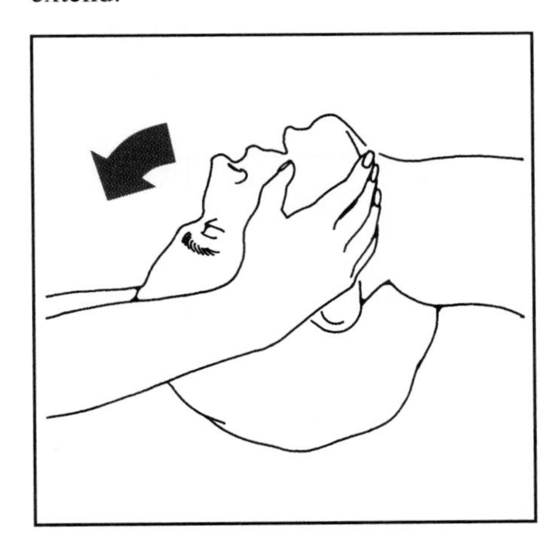

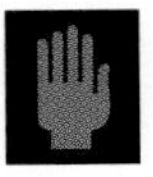

If there is evidence of injuries, support head and neck as you reposition victim. If neck injury is suspected, do not hyperextend neck. Instead put thumb into the mouth and grasp lower jaw and pull jaw upward. For infants, see Procedure 30–10.

Continued

ACTION 4. Assess for breathing:
Look for chest movement.
Listen for air movement.
Feel breath on your cheek.

RATIONALE. Rescue breathing is unnecessary if victim is able to breathe spontaneously.

ACTION 5. If victim is **not breathing:**

a. Pinch nostrils together.

RATIONALE. This prevents escape of air from nostrils.

b. Take a deep breath and place mouth over the victim's mouth, forming a tight seal.

RATIONALE. Deep breath to deliver sufficient oxygen to victim; seal to avoid loss of air.

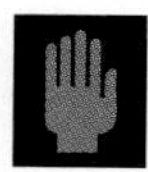

Oral airway or mask with one-way valve may be used if readily available. Do not delay ventilation to obtain one. If an airtight seal cannot be made with mouth-to-mouth or with airway, use mouth-to-nose resuscitation (Action 6).

c. Blow two full breaths, **1–1.5 seconds each,** pausing between breaths to allow passive deflation of lungs. Observe for chest expansion as ventilations are done.

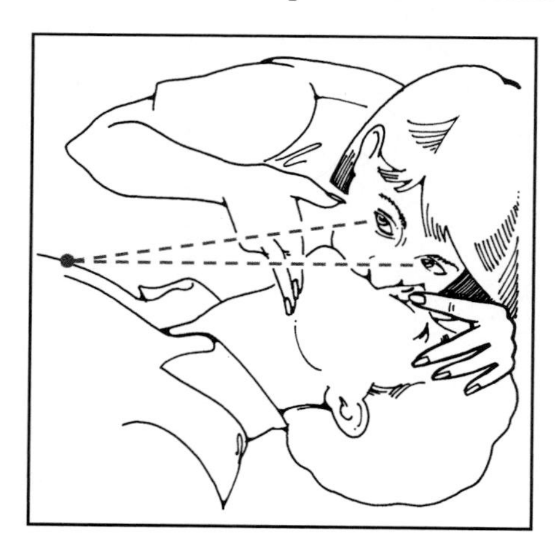

RATIONALE. Provides sufficient oxygen and reduces the possibility of gastric distension due to excessive rate or pressure. Filling of lungs will cause chest to rise if ventilation is adequate.

d. If chest does not rise, reposition head and ventilate again. If unsuccessful, repeat abdominal thrusts (see Procedure 30–8) and try again.

RATIONALE. Failure to ventilate may be due to obstructed airway, which must be corrected to oxygenate victim.

ACTION 6. **Mouth-to-nose resuscitation:**

a. Hold victim's mouth closed while maintaining hyperextension of neck.

RATIONALE. Prevents loss of air via mouth.

b. Place mouth over victim's nose, making a seal on cheeks, and place your cheek over victim's lips. Continue with Actions 5c–d.

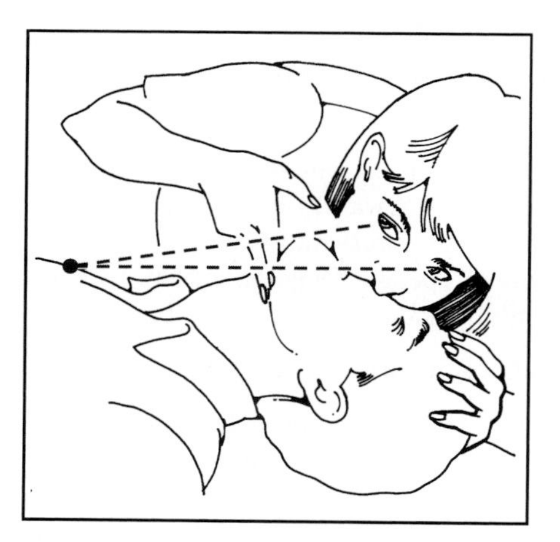

RATIONALE. Directs oxygen to victim's lungs.

ACTION 7. After administering two full breaths, check the carotid pulse for 5 to 10 seconds. The carotid pulse is just below the angle of the mandible (jawbone). Locate it by placing two or three fingers in the groove between the Adam's apple and the muscle.

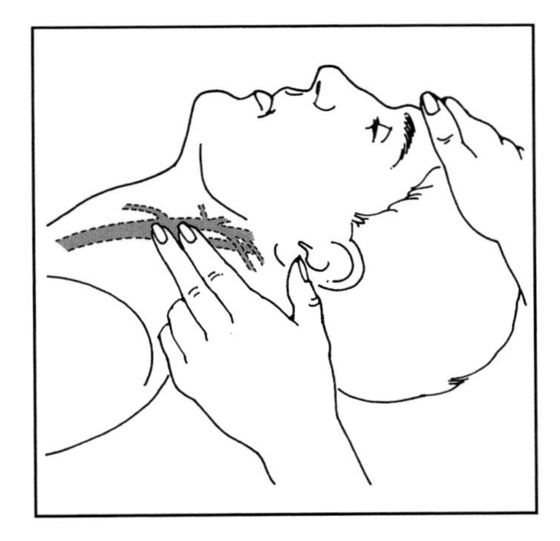

RATIONALE. Cause of cessation of breathing may be a cardiac arrest. The victim will then need chest compressions, as well. If the heart is beating, the carotid pulse is most likely to be palpable as it carries one fourth of the person's total blood volume.

ACTION 8. **If there is no pulse,** initiate cardiac compressions (go to Action 14).

RATIONALE. Lack of pulse signifies lack of circulation to vital organs.

ACTION 9. **If there is a pulse,** continue to ventilate victim at rate of **one breath every 5 seconds,** removing your mouth from victim's mouth (or nose) after each breath. Watch chest rise and fall and feel escape of air with your cheek.

RATIONALE. This rate and volume of air will provide sufficient oxygen to prevent damage to vital organs as long as heart is beating. Continued observation of chest movement verifies continued ventilation.

ACTION 10. Check pulse again after 2 minutes (24 breaths). Continue ventilation if pulse is present. Add compressions if pulse is absent (Action 14).

RATIONALE. Palpable pulse verifies continued cardiac function.

ACTION 11. If ventilations become impossible to administer, check the stomach for distension.

RATIONALE. Some of the air you are breathing into the victim may travel to the stomach via the esophagus. As the stomach fills with air, pressure increases and is transmitted to the mouth, causing resistance to incoming air.

Ventilation should not be interrupted. Remove gastric air only if pressure makes ventilation impossible.

ACTION 12. If distended stomach prevents ventilation, remove the air as follows:

a. Turn victim on side with back toward you.

RATIONALE. Air removal could cause vomiting. If supine, victim could aspirate emesis.

b. Place hand between victim's rib cage and waist and push on the stomach.

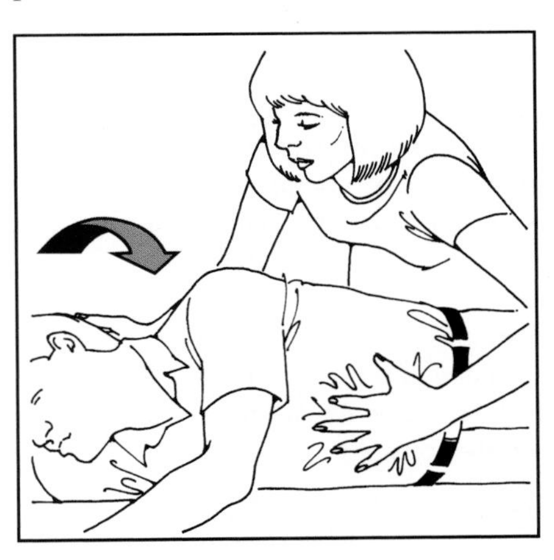

RATIONALE. Pressure should push air out via the path of least resistance, the esophagus.

c. Clear the mouth of emesis if vomiting occurs.

RATIONALE. Emesis could obstruct the airway or be pushed into the lungs with subsequent ventilations.

d. Return victim to supine position and continue ventilation, checking carotid pulse every few minutes, until spontaneous breathing begins or trained resuscitation team arrives, or victim is pronounced dead by physician.

RATIONALE. Efforts to maintain ventilation and perfusion should continue until known to be futile.

Continued

ACTION 13. If breathing resumes, observe carefully to verify continued spontaneous respiration. Maintain victim in a supine position with head and shoulders raised. Keep at a comfortable temperature until EMS (or Code Team in a healthcare facility) arrives and assesses victim.

RATIONALE. Airway may still be partially occluded and may easily become obstructed again. Position facilitates ease of respiration. Neutral temperature minimizes metabolic demands for oxygen. Complete assessment to determine and treat cause of respiratory arrest and any resulting complications is necessary to protect victim's health and well-being.

Do not raise head or shoulders of a potential spinal cord injured victim.

ACTION 14. **If no pulse,** begin compressions to support circulation. A person in bed must be moved to the floor, or a cardiac board or similar large, flat, firm object must be placed beneath the back. The head- or footboard of some hospital beds may be removed for use as a cardiac board.

RATIONALE. A firm surface facilitates the compression of the victim's heart between the sternum and spine. A soft surface absorbs the force of compressions so insufficient force is available to compress the heart. If head is higher than heart, the brain will not be perfused.

ACTION 15. Locate the position for compression by using the fingers of your hand nearest the victim's legs to follow the lower edge of the rib cage toward the sternocostal notch where the ribs join the sternum.

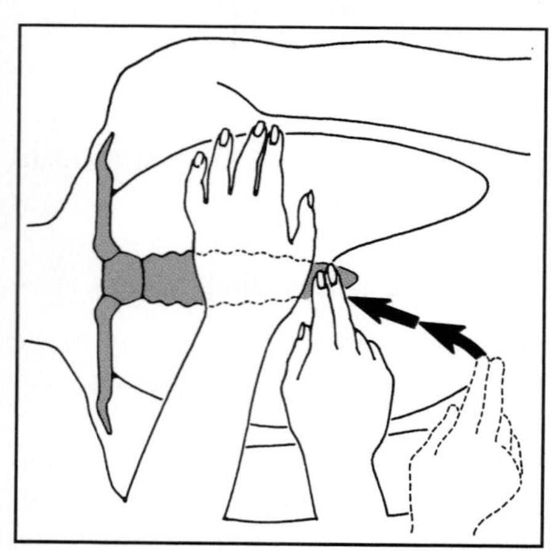

RATIONALE. Correct hand placement is critical to avoid injury. This method is a rapid and accurate way to avoid exerting pressure too low in the sternum. Liver lacerations may occur if compressions are administered too low.

ACTION 16. Place the heel of your other hand on the lower third of the sternum, two finger breadths above the notch, then place the heel of the opposite hand over it, interlacing and holding fingers off the chest. Fingers should be perpendicular to the sternum, heels of the hands directly over sternum.

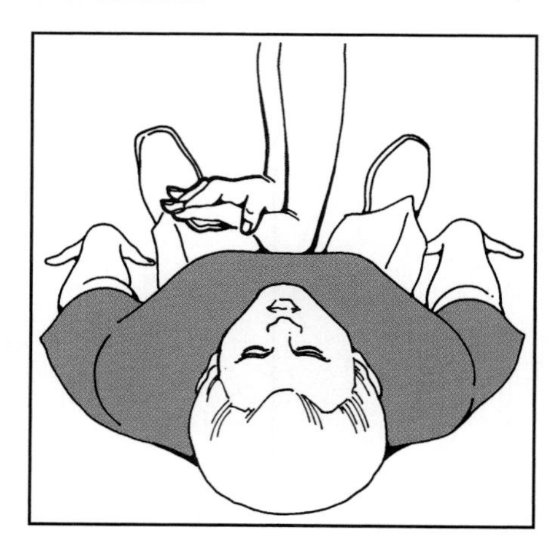

RATIONALE. This hand position will direct the force of compressions directly downward toward the heart without injuring the ribs. Pressing on the ribs or the edge of the sternum could fracture the ribs.

ACTION 17. Support your weight on your knees, then rock forward, bending at the hips, so shoulders are directly over victim's sternum, keeping arms straight and elbows locked.

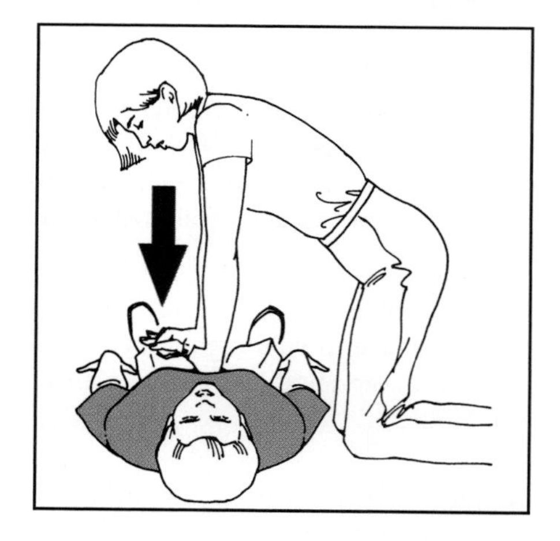

RATIONALE. This motion uses the rescuer's weight to compress the heart in a smooth, regular pattern, similar to the rhythmic action of a functioning heart. Locking the hips or flexing the elbows results in less forceful or uneven compressions.

ACTION 18. Press straight down on the sternum, compressing the chest 1½ to 2 inches.

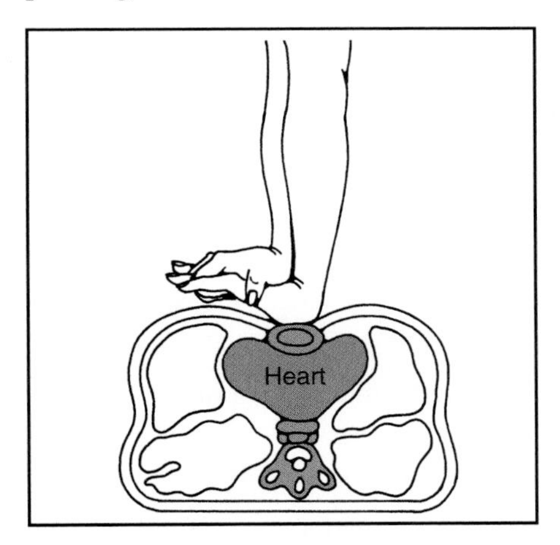

RATIONALE. The pressure squeezes the blood out of the heart.

ACTION 19. Rock back slightly, releasing pressure, but maintaining contact with body.

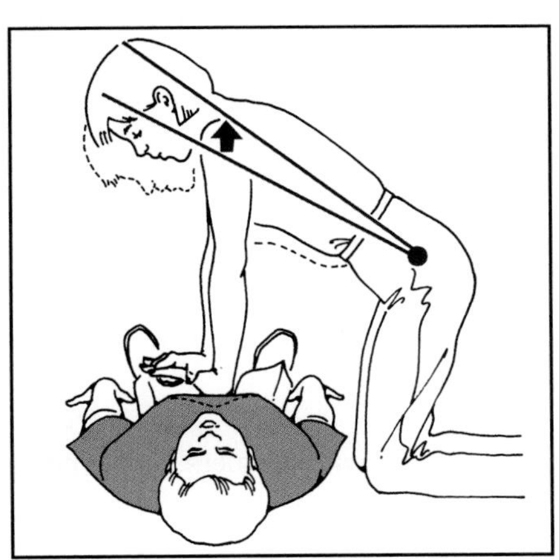

RATIONALE. Release of pressure allows heart to refill with blood. Maintaining contact prevents malpositioning of the hands and possible injury on subsequent compressions.

ACTION 20. Give compressions at rate of **80 to 100 per minute,** counting "one and two and," etc, up to 15.

RATIONALE. This rate will produce sufficient cardiac output to perfuse vital organs.

ACTION 21. After each group of **15 compressions,** give **two full ventilations.** Reposition hands correctly after ventilations as in Action 15.

RATIONALE. Blood must be oxygenated periodically.

ACTION 22. After the first minute of CPR (4 cycles) check carotid pulse and resume CPR if pulse is absent. Recheck pulse every few minutes, but do not interrupt CPR for more than 5 seconds to do so.

RATIONALE. Return of cardiac function signals that compressions may be discontinued.

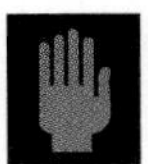

Pulse should also be checked if signs of recovery such as movement, swallowing, or returning facial color occur.

ACTION 23. If pulse if present, continue ventilations every 5 seconds without compressions if ventilations do not also resume.

RATIONALE. See Action 21.

ACTION 24. Continue CPR until heartbeat and breathing are restored, EMS team arrives, you are exhausted, or victim is pronounced dead by a physician.

RATIONALE. Efforts to maintain life must be maintained until a thorough assessment can be made by a qualified person.

ACTION 25. If heartbeat and breathing resume, continue to observe and arrange for transport of victim to health care facility.

RATIONALE. Determination and treatment of the cause of cardiac arrest are necessary for victim's well-being.

TWO RESCUERS

ACTION 1. When second rescuer arrives, ask that EMS be activated if you have not already done so.

RATIONALE. EMS team is equipped with drugs, oxygen, and transport vehicle so victim can receive definitive treatment.

ACTION 2. If second rescuer knows CPR, initiate two-person CPR.

RATIONALE. Two-person CPR is more effective because more breaths per minute can be delivered. It can usually be maintained for a longer period of time because it is less fatiguing.

ACTION 3. First rescuer should communicate to second whether to assume ventilations or compressions.

RATIONALE. Prevents confusion and possible lengthy interruption of CPR.

Continued

ACTION 4. If second rescuer ventilates:

a. First rescuer assesses for pulse and breathing while second takes a position near victim's head.

RATIONALE. Determines actual need for continued CPR.

b. First rescuer states: "No pulse, continue CPR" and gives five compressions while second reopens airway and prepares to ventilate after fifth compression.

RATIONALE. Maintains cardiac output of oxygenated blood and allows for assessment of effectiveness of compressions.

c. Second rescuer checks pulse during compressions.

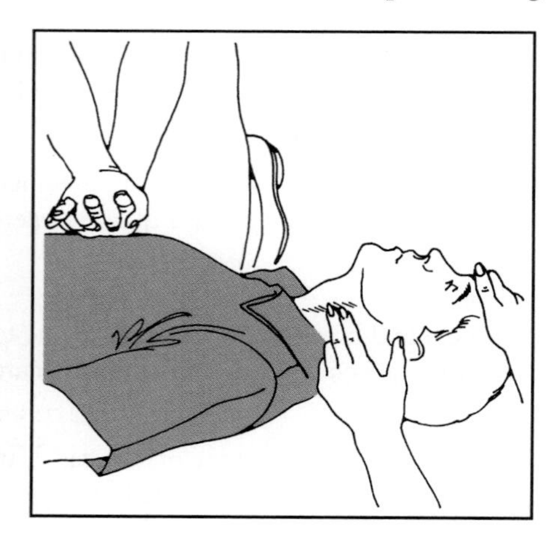

RATIONALE. Determines whether compressions are moving blood.

d. CPR continues at a ratio of **one ventilation** to **five compressions,** and a rate of **80 to 100 compressions/minute** with first rescuer counting aloud. A 1 to 1.5-second pause is allowed after the fifth compression to allow time for a full ventilation.

RATIONALE. Provides sufficient circulation to perfuse major organs while allowing enough time for full ventilation to oxygenate blood.

ACTION 5. If second rescuer does compressions:

a. First rescuer assesses pulse and breathing, second takes position near chest and locates xyphoid process (One Rescuer, Action 15).

b. First rescuer states "No pulse, continue CPR," and gives one ventilation.

c. Second rescuer begins compressions as above.

d. CPR is maintained as previously described.

ACTION 6. When either rescuer tires, a clear signal is given to change positions.

RATIONALE. Prevents lengthy interruption of CPR.

ACTION 7. Switch is done after a ventilation:

RATIONALE. Maintains oxygenation of blood during switch.

a. Ventilator moves to chest, locates xyphoid process, and awaits signal to begin.

b. Compressor simultaneously moves to head, then opens airway, assesses pulse and breathing, verbalizes whether pulse and breathing are present or absent, and gives one slow, full ventilation if needed. If pulse and/or breathing is noted on assessment, compression and/or ventilation are discontinued.

c. Compressor begins compressions at previous rate if told pulse is absent.

RATIONALE. Coordinated movement and rapid assessment facilitate continuous ventilation and perfusion of victim's vital organs.

d. CPR continues as above with rescuers switching as needed until EMS team arrives, victim is pronounced dead by a physician, or rescuers are exhausted.

RATIONALE. Efforts to maintain life must be maintained until a thorough assessment can be made by a qualified person.

Recording:

If victim is a patient in a health care facility, the following should be noted on the patient's record: events occurring before the arrest, if observed; condition of patient when found if arrest was not witnessed; all actions taken by health care providers; and patient's response to interventions.

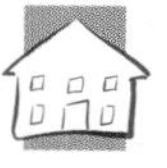

HOME HEALTH ADAPTATION: Adult CPR techniques are applicable in any setting if rescuer has had a current CPR course.

PROCEDURE 30–10. CLEARING AN OBSTRUCTED AIRWAY AND CPR: INFANTS AND CHILDREN

PURPOSE: To clear obstructed airway and circulate oxygenated blood to vital organs when cardiac function has been interrupted.
EQUIPMENT: None

A. OBSTRUCTED AIRWAY—Conscious Infant Less Than 1 Year Old

ACTION 1. Confirm airway obstruction: difficulty breathing, dusky color, or weak or absent cry. If obstruction is caused by swelling due to infection, rather than a foreign object, do not attempt to clear the airway. Rush the infant to the nearest advanced life support facility.

RATIONALE. Infants are unable to cough. If airway is completely occluded, color change is rapid. The techniques described here are of no benefit if the problem is caused by swelling; attempting them only delays effective treatment.

ACTION 2. Place infant face down with head lower than chest. Support head and neck with your hand, the trunk with your forearm, then rest your forearm on your thigh.

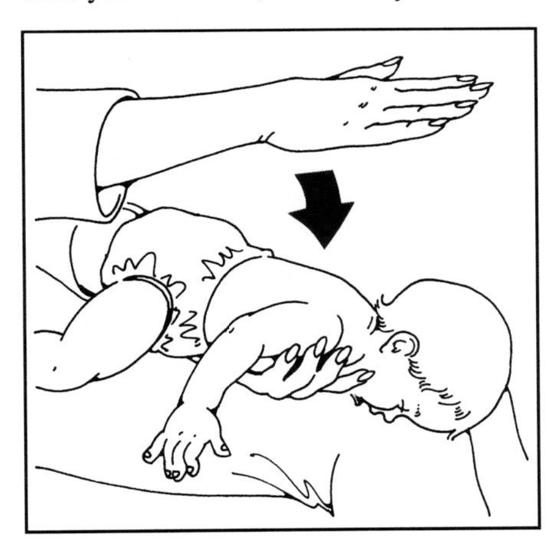

RATIONALE. Adds gravity to assist the movement of the obstruction while minimizing injury to infant.

ACTION 3. Deliver up to five sharp blows between the scapulae with the heel of the hand.

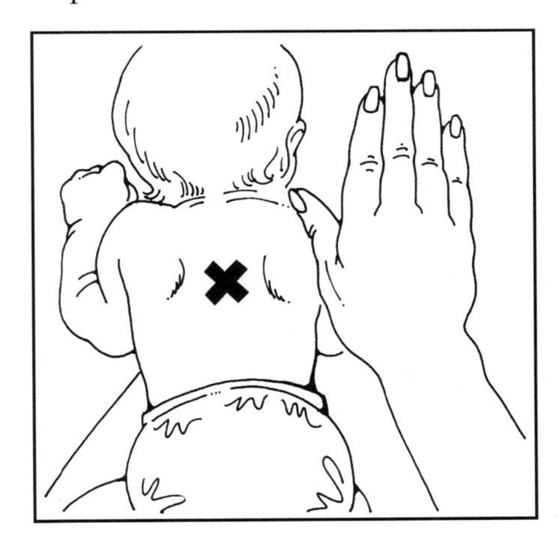

RATIONALE. Jarring of blows may dislodge object.

ACTION 4. Turn infant over for chest thrusts as follows: Place your free hand on the back of the infant's head, with your arm extending down the infant's back. With the infant sandwiched between your arms, turn your arms over so the infant is supine.

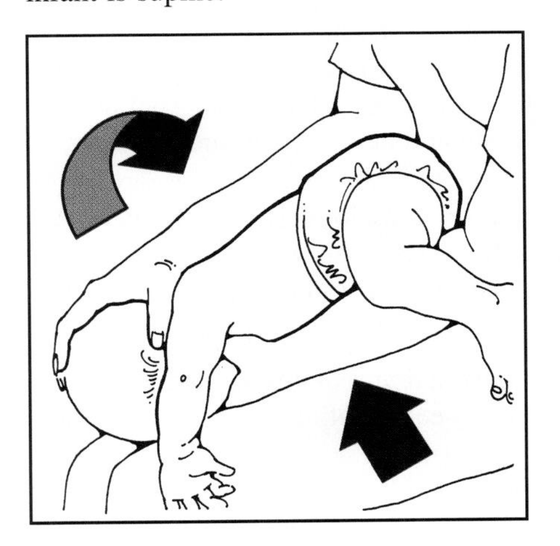

RATIONALE. The infant lacks muscle strength to support the head. Injury can occur if head is not supported when infant is turned.

Continued

ACTION 5. Support the infant so head is lower than trunk and deliver up to five sharp chest thrusts in the midsternal region with two fingers of one hand. Locate the correct position by placing three fingers in a vertical line on the sternum perpendicular to the nipple line, raising the finger on the nipple line and using the two remaining fingers to deliver thrusts.

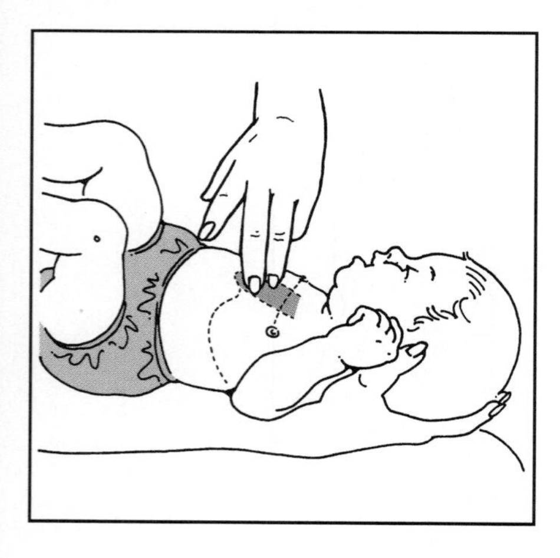

RATIONALE. Two fingers by an adult create enough force to dislodge the object.

ACTION 6. Alternate back blows and chest thrusts until spontaneous air exchange occurs or victim loses consciousness.

RATIONALE. Dislodging obstruction will permit air exchange. If object is not dislodged, hypoxemia will cause loss of consciousness. Life support must be continued to prevent damage to brain and other organs and death.

ACTION 7. If infant loses consciousness, call for help. Ask helper to activate EMS system (call 911). If in a healthcare facility, carry the infant quickly to the nearest wall suction unit.

RATIONALE. Deep obstruction requires suction equipment to dislodge. Infant may need additional advanced life support.

ACTION 8. With infant in supine position, inspect the mouth for obstructing object. Do not use fingersweep on infants unless object can be seen; place thumb over tongue and pull jaw upward while looking into mouth. Carefully remove visible object with fingers. Assess for breathing after fingersweep.

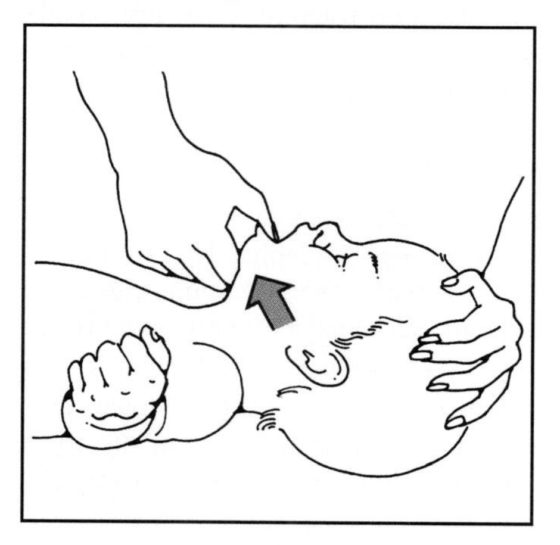

RATIONALE. Infant's mouth is so small that fingersweep is more likely to push object further down than to remove it.

ACTION 9. Open airway using head tilt-chin lift, but do not hyperextend neck as for adult victim.

RATIONALE. Infant has less muscle tone, so complete hyperextension of infant's neck may cause tracheal collapse or neck injury.

ACTION 10. Begin rescue breathing. Place mouth over infant's nose and mouth to form a seal.

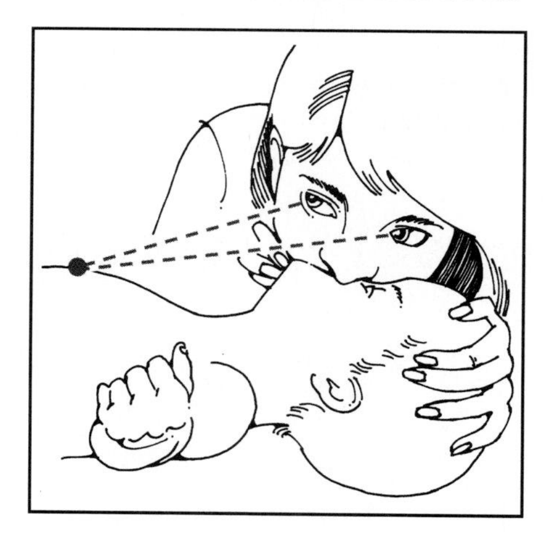

RATIONALE. The infant's face is too small to enable a tight mouth-to-mouth seal.

a. Gently blow **two breaths of 1 to 1.5 seconds each** into infant, pausing for passive deflation of lungs. Breaths should have just enough pressure to cause chest to rise.

RATIONALE. Inflates lungs at lowest possible pressure, avoiding gastric distension.

b. If chest does not rise, reposition infant's head and try again. If still unable to give breaths, repeat Actions 2 to 8 to clear airway until able to ventilate.

RATIONALE. See Actions 2 to 8.

ACTION 11. If you are alone and you are unable to restore breathing within 1 minute, activate Emergency Medical System (EMS) and then continue attempts to clear airway.

RATIONALE. See Action 7.

ACTION 12. If you are able to remove the obstruction, check for breathing: Place your ear above infant's mouth and
Look at the chest for rise and fall,
Listen for air movement,
Feel breaths on your ear, and check brachial pulse.

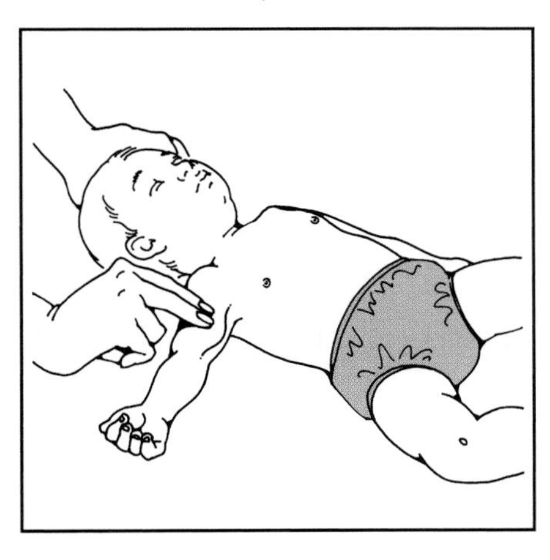

RATIONALE. The airway occlusion may have caused cardiac and respiratory arrest.

ACTION 13. If infant is breathing, position the infant on his or her side and continue to monitor breathing and pulse. If no breathing, give rescue **breaths at 20 per minute** (1 every 3 seconds) and monitor pulse.

RATIONALE. Side-lying position facilitates respiration with minimal effort and risk of aspiration; 20 rescue breaths per minute will provide sufficient oxygen until definitive treatment can be initiated. Continued monitoring indicates need for support.

ACTION 14. If no pulse, give 2 breaths and begin cardiac compression. See part C.

RATIONALE. If there is no pulse, compressions are necessary to circulate oxygenated blood.

B. UNCONSCIOUS INFANT—Less Than 1 Year Old

ACTION 1. Determine unresponsiveness by tapping or gently shaking shoulder. Shout for help.

RATIONALE. Rescuer's actions vary with conscious vs unconscious victim.

ACTION 2. Support the infant's head and position on his or her back. Open the airway using head tilt-chin lift. Do not hyperextend neck.

RATIONALE. See Action 9.

ACTION 3. Determine whether infant is breathing as in step 12 above.

RATIONALE. See Action 12.

ACTION 4. If infant is breathing, contact regular health care provider for advice. If infant is not breathing, initiate rescue breathing as in step 10a.

RATIONALE. See Action 10a.

ACTION 5. If unable to move air, reposition and try again. If second attempt also fails, activate EMS system or ask someone there to do so.

RATIONALE. Infant has not been breathing for an unknown period. Since immediate efforts to restore breathing have failed, definitive assistance is needed.

ACTION 6. Attempt to dislodge a possible foreign object by initiating back blows and chest thrusts as in Actions 2 to 5 in part A.

RATIONALE. See Actions 2 to 5 in part A.

ACTION 7. Continue rescue attempts using Actions 8 to 14, part A.

RATIONALE. See Actions 8 to 14, part A.

Continued

C. CHEST COMPRESSIONS:—Infant Less Than 1 Year Old

ACTION 1. Assess consciousness, breathing, and circulation, as described previously, initiate ventilations if infant is not breathing.

ACTION 2. If there is no brachial pulse, place the infant on a firm surface and begin chest compressions to restore circulation. Place the fingers of your other hand along the infant's sternum, one finger-breadth below nipple line.

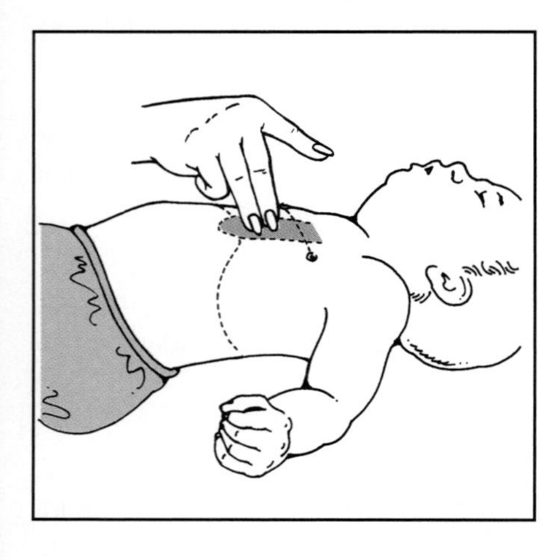

RATIONALE. Firm surface is needed to compress the heart. Hand position maintains head tilt for ventilation. Head must be at same level as or lower than heart to adequately perfuse the brain.

ACTION 3. Compress the chest ½ to 1 inch using two or three fingers at a rate of **100 compressions per minute.** Do not press on the xyphoid process.

RATIONALE. Greater pressure could cause injury; faster rate is nearer infant's normal heart rate.

ACTION 4. Continue to provide ventilations and compressions at a **ratio of one ventilation every five compressions,** pausing 1 to 1.5 seconds for ventilation as with adult victim.

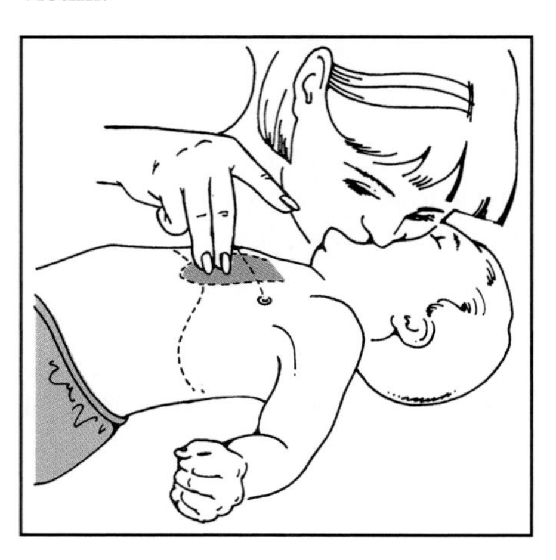

RATIONALE. Maintains adequate oxygenation and perfusion.

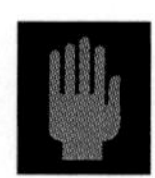

Keeping your face very close to the infant's during compressions facilitates giving ventilation quickly.

ACTION 5. After 20 cycles of compressions and rescue breaths, quickly activate EMS (call 911) or call for cardiac arrest team (Code Blue or Code Pink).

RATIONALE. Advanced life support is needed.

ACTION 6. Assess brachial pulse. If absent, resume compressions and ventilations. If present, check for breathing. If breathing is absent, continue ventilations at 20 per minute (1 every 3 seconds). If there is breathing, position infant on side and continue to monitor until help arrives.

RATIONALE. Life support must be continuous to prevent damage to brain and other organs and death.

ACTION 7. If CPR is resumed, reassess breathing and brachial pulse every few minutes.

RATIONALE. Verifies continued need for CPR.

ACTION 8. Continue CPR until EMS team arrives, infant is pronounced dead by a physician, or you are exhausted.

RATIONALE. Efforts to maintain life must be continued until a thorough assessment can be made by a qualified person.

Procedure 30–10. (continued)

D. CHILD VICTIM—1 to 8 Years Old

Performing CPR on young children is similar to adult CPR. The differences are as follows:

ACTION 1. If there is only one rescuer, give 20 cycles of CPR before activating EMS.

RATIONALE. EMS is activated before beginning basic life support for adults because in cardiac arrest (the common reason for needing CPR in adults) early advanced life support significantly improves survival rates. The cause of a respiratory arrest in children is not likely to be cardiac arrest, so prompt basic life support is the priority.

ACTION 2. Give compressions with heel of one hand, depressing chest only 1 to 1.5 inches.

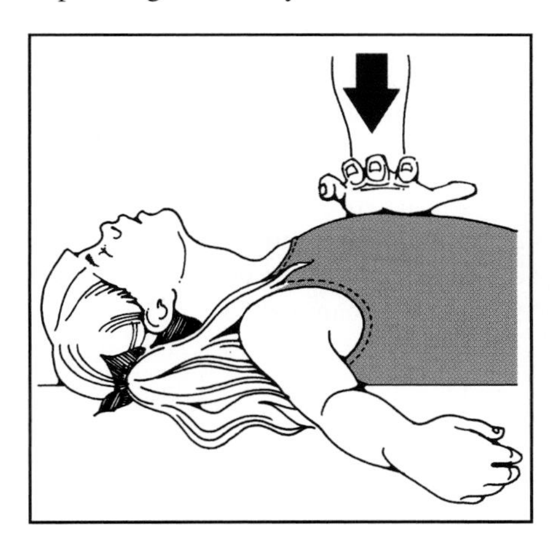

RATIONALE. Creates sufficient pressure to squeeze blood out of heart without injuring child.

ACTION 3. Provide compressions at a rate of **100 per minute** at a ratio of five compressions for each ventilation.

RATIONALE. Maintains adequate oxygenation and perfusion.

ACTION 4. Reassess breathing and carotid pulse as with adult victim. Continue CPR until EMS team arrives, child is pronounced dead by a physician, or you are exhausted.

RATIONALE. Verifies need for continued CPR. Efforts to maintain life must be continued until a thorough assessment can be made by a qualified person.

Recording:

If victim is a patient in a health care facility, the following should be noted on the patient's record: events occurring before the arrest, if observed; condition of patient when found if arrest was not witnessed; and all actions taken by health care providers, and patient's response to interventions.

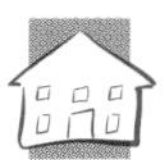

HOME HEALTH ADAPTATION: CPR techniques are applicable in any setting if rescuer has had a current CPR course.

PROCEDURE 30–11. USING A HAND-COMPRESSIBLE BREATHING BAG (AMBU BAG)

PURPOSE: To ventilate an unconscious person who is not breathing.
EQUIPMENT: Hand-compressible breathing bag with mask to fit patient. May be kept at bedside of patient experiencing frequent respiratory difficulty or be kept on the emergency "crash" cart.

ACTION 1. Assess consciousness and breathing as described in Procedure 30–9, Action 4. If patient is not breathing, open airway using one of the methods described in Procedure 30–9, Action 3.

ACTION 2. Apply mask securely over patient's nose and mouth, holding it in place and maintaining patient's head position with one hand to keep airway open.

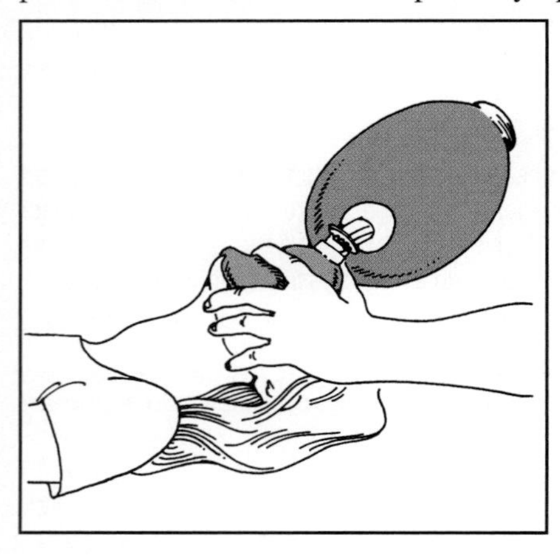

RATIONALE. If airway is closed by patient's head changing position, no oxygen will be delivered to lungs. If air escapes from sides of mask, less oxygen will be delivered.

ACTION 3. Compress bag forcefully with your free hand while observing chest for elevation. Allow bag to self-reinflate by relaxing hold on it.

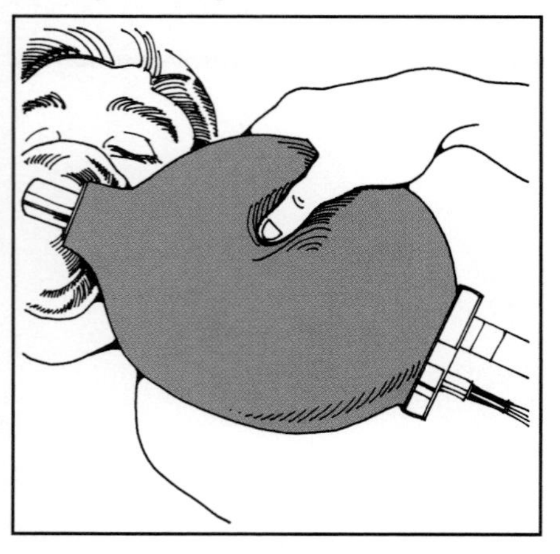

RATIONALE. Compression of bag should inflate lungs and cause chest to rise. Exhaled air will be released into room via an exhaust valve; bag will refill with room air.

ACTION 4. If no evidence of lung inflation is noted, reposition head and squeeze bag again. If still unable to verify lung inflation, attempt to remove possible foreign body obstruction using abdominal thrusts (Procedure 30–8). If tracheal suctioning equipment is available, suction to clear airway (Procedure 30–7).

RATIONALE. Rapid attempts to open airway and deliver oxygen are necessary to prevent brain damage and death.

ACTION 5. Assess for spontaneous breathing. If none, call for help. Give two full inflations, then assess carotid pulse for 5 seconds (Procedure 30–9, Action 7).

RATIONALE. Opening airway and ventilation may restore breathing. If cardiac and respiratory arrest has occurred, CPR must be initiated and code team called.

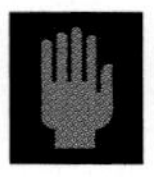

Many health care facilities have an emergency call button on wall to alert code team.

ACTION 6. **If there is a pulse,** continue to ventilate by squeezing bag at a rate of 12 breaths/minute (one per 5 seconds). If an oxygen source is available, connect it to the nipple at the top or bottom of the bag, set liter flow at 12 to 15 L/min, and ventilate at same rate.

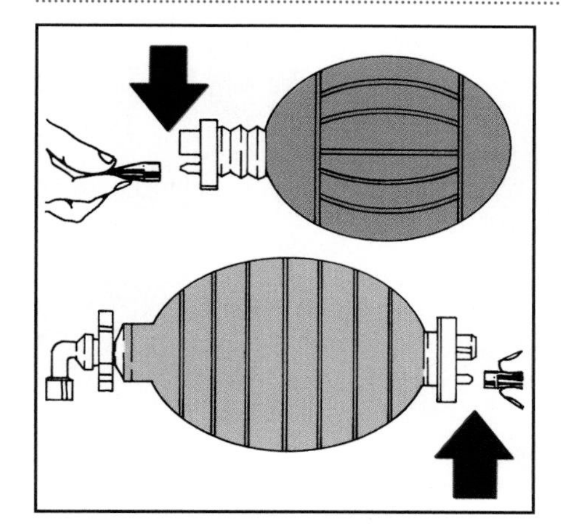

RATIONALE. Optimum perfusion is maintained by administering oxygen, as the apneic patient has an oxygen deficit. If oxygen source is not available, room air will provide adequate perfusion until code team arrives.

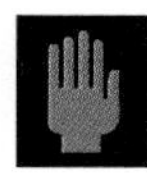

Do not increase rate of inflations; bag must refill and be firmly squeezed to sufficiently inflate lungs.

ACTION 7. **If there is no pulse,** initiate CPR (Procedure 30–9).

RATIONALE. Ventilation is ineffective without circulation.

ACTION 8. Be alert for vomiting, turning patient to one side immediately should it occur, and clearing mouth before continuing to ventilate.

RATIONALE. Ambu bag may deliver some air to stomach, causing distension and reflex vomiting. Side-lying position facilitates flow of emesis out of mouth. Emesis will cause pneumonia if aspirated or forced into lungs.

ACTION 9. Continue resuscitation until patient breathes spontaneously or until relieved by code team.

RATIONALE. Health care facility policy usually designates code team to be responsible for immediate definitive treatment of patient suffering cardiac and/or respiratory arrest. Nurse initiating ventilation may be asked to assist in this process.

ACTION 10. Notify patient's primary physician of respiratory arrest.

RATIONALE. Primary physician is responsible for ongoing medical treatment of patient.

Recording:

Note events precipitating arrest, if observed; condition of patient when found; action taken by all health care providers; and patient's response.

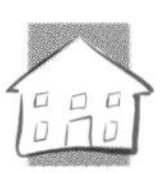

HOME HEALTH ADAPTATION: Ambu bags are not used in the home.

INSIGHTS FROM NURSING LITERATURE

PULSE OXIMETRY

Tallon RW. Oximetry: state-of-the-art. Nurs Manage. *1996; 27:43–44.*

Pulse oximeters are noninvasive devices that can be attached to a finger, ear lobe, nose, or forehead to analyze a patient's blood oxygen concentration. Pulse oximeters use light waves and internal algorithms to identify the differential absorption of red and ultraviolet wavelengths by oxygenated and deoxygenated hemoglobin in circulating arterial blood. Their use decreases the need to gather arterial blood samples for blood gas analysis. Further, through the use of defined "stop criteria," they enable oxygen therapy to be withdrawn sooner in postoperative and other clinical situations without, research indicates, adverse patient outcomes. These devices may also be useful for assessing wound healing and as a screening tool for sleep apnea.

The use of pulse oximetry may be limited in people with dark skin or decreased peripheral circulation; there is also a risk of pressure ulcer formation when probes are clipped to the same tissue site for prolonged periods of time. Care must be taken to remove probes before magnetic resonance imaging because of the potential risk of tissue burns.

Pulse oximeters are also limited in their use because they do not assess acid-base status or alveolar ventilation, critical factors in many situations.

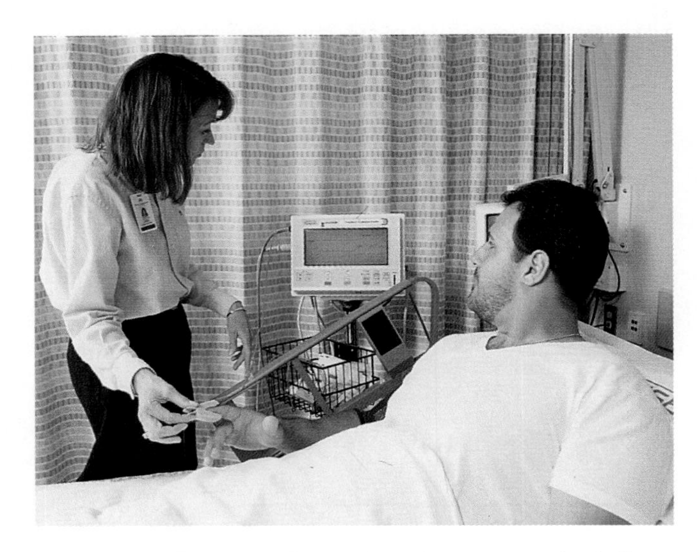

Figure 30–11. The nurse clips a pulse oximeter to a patient's finger and assesses the concentration of oxygen in the patient's blood.

A device for determining the amount of oxygen in the blood, called a *pulse oximeter,* is useful for assessing the effectiveness of oxygen therapy (Fig. 30–11).[24] The oximeter uses a noninvasive oxygen sensor that is clipped to a patient's earlobe or finger. Monitoring can be continuous or intermittent. The sensor determines the level of oxygen saturation with sufficient accuracy for monitoring most patients who are not critically ill. Some physicians order oxygen therapy with the flow rate dependent on pulse oximetry readings (for example, "Oxygen via nasal prongs, 2 to 4 L per minute, to keep oxygen saturation above 90 percent").

The safest way to administer oxygen is to give the lowest flow or concentration that will maintain acceptable arterial blood gases or oximeter readings. Forty percent is a safe concentration for most patients. Some patients require up to 60 percent. Very high oxygen concentrations should be given for as short a time as possible, because they may damage lung tissue.

In patients with chronic hypoxia, high concentrations of oxygen are particularly dangerous. As discussed earlier, some patients who retain carbon dioxide are insensitive to the normal respiratory stimulus of elevated CO_2. Instead, their stimulus to breathe is **hypoxemia,** a decrease in blood oxygen. Thus high concentrations of oxygen may eliminate such patients' stimulus for breathing and they may cease to breathe adequately. Such patients are usually treated with oxygen at low concentrations or flow rates.

Oxygen supports combustion, and so certain precautions are required when it is being used. Clinical Guideline 30–6 summarizes safety precautions related to oxygen administration.

CLINICAL GUIDELINE 30–6

SAFETY PRECAUTIONS DURING OXYGEN THERAPY

- Post "NO SMOKING, OXYGEN IN USE" signs on the door of any room in which oxygen is being used and near the bed of a patient who is receiving oxygen. Although smoking is not allowed at any time in patients' rooms, the sign will reinforce the need for caution.
- Explain to the patient and significant others why open flames, ungrounded electrical appliances, volatile materials, or any item capable of creating sparks may not be used in a room in which oxygen is in use.
- Show significant others the location and correct operation of the nearest fire extinguishers.
- Help the patient store personal effects that could support combustion in a secure but inaccessible place during oxygen therapy. These include:
  - Smoking materials such as lighter and matches.
  - Ungrounded electrical devices, such as radios, shavers, and hair dryers.
  - Items that can generate static electricity, such as blankets or clothing made of wool or synthetic fabrics.
  - Volatile toiletry products such as alcohol-based perfumes or colognes and nail polish remover.
- Make sure that all hospital electrical equipment—such as beds, monitors, infusion pumps, and portable suction machines—is properly grounded. Notify hospital engineering or maintenance departments of any faulty electrical equipment.
- Remove all volatile and petroleum-based hospital products from the room. Replace with water-soluble products when possible.

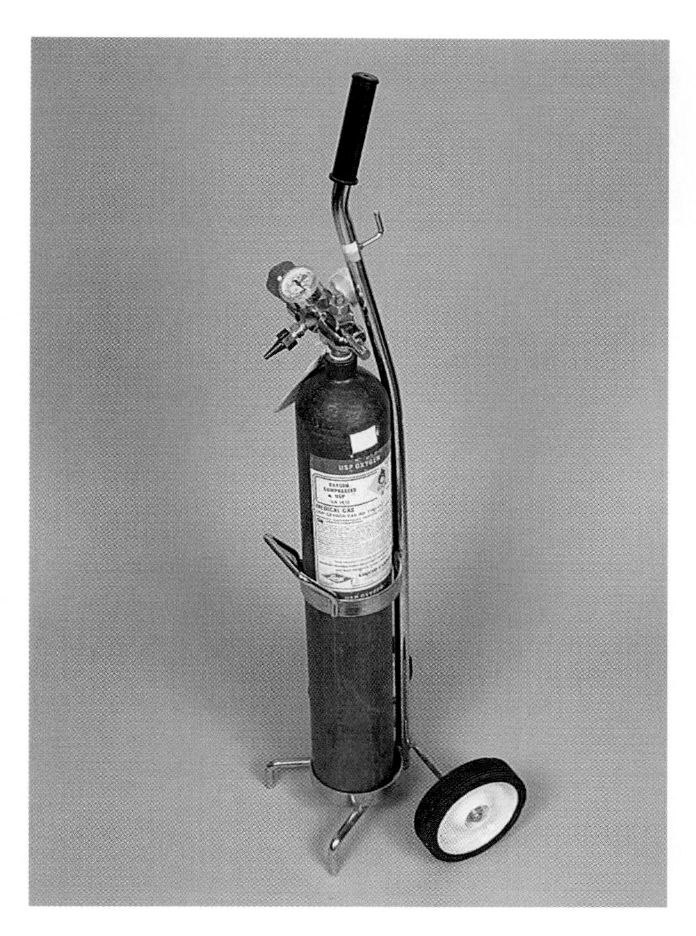

Figure 30–12. E cylinder of oxygen on a stand.

Oxygen Supply. Most health care agencies use oxygen piped to wall outlets from large, low-pressure storage reservoirs. When oxygen must be delivered in a setting that has no central oxygen supply system, such as in a patient's home, oxygen cylinders containing compressed oxygen are used. Both large and small cylinders are available. Small cylinders, called E cylinders or portable oxygen tanks, can be mounted on small wheeled carriers or on holders attached to wheelchairs or gurneys.

Because compressed oxygen is stored under very high pressure in cylinders, a pressure regulator must be used in conjunction with a flowmeter when using oxygen from a cylinder. The regulator has a pressure-reducing valve that limits the rate of release of oxygen from the cylinder. A gauge that indicates the amount of oxygen in the cylinder is part of the regulator. This gauge is calibrated in pounds per square inch (psi). Figure 30–12 illustrates an E cylinder on a stand with an attached regulator and pressure gauge. Procedure 30–12 summarizes nursing responsibilities when administering oxygen from an E cylinder.

Oxygen is also available in liquid form (when cooled to 460F below 0). Liquid oxygen is more concentrated than gaseous oxygen and, therefore, lasts longer (Fig. 30–13). An electrically driven device called a "concentrator" is also available. This device makes its own oxygen by removing the nitrogen from the air, thereby enhancing oxygen concentration.

Measuring Oxygen Delivery. Oxygen used for oxygen therapy is measured in liters per minute (L/min). This unit is the **flowrate,** that is, the rate at which oxygen is flowing to a patient. Flowrate is one way that oxygen therapy is prescribed. A device called a **flowmeter** is used to adjust and measure the flowrate. Two kinds of flowmeters are used: the Thorpe tube, which has a vertical flow indicator gauge; and the Bourdon gauge, which has a round flow indicator gauge (Fig. 30–14).

Oxygen dosage can also be ordered as a concentration, or percent of oxygen. Oxygen *concentration* is expressed as **FiO_2**, or **fraction of inspired oxygen.** All oxygen delivery devices mix supplemental oxygen from the supply source with room air (which is 21 percent oxygen). The FiO_2 indicates what fraction of the room air-oxygen mixture a patient is receiving as oxygen. FiO_2 is expressed as a percentage.

Oxygen delivery systems that can precisely control the FiO_2 delivered to the patient are called high-flow systems. If a specific oxygen concentration is critical for a given patient, the physician will order a high-flow delivery device and specify the FiO_2 at which the device should be set (for example, "O_2 per Venturi mask at 28 percent").

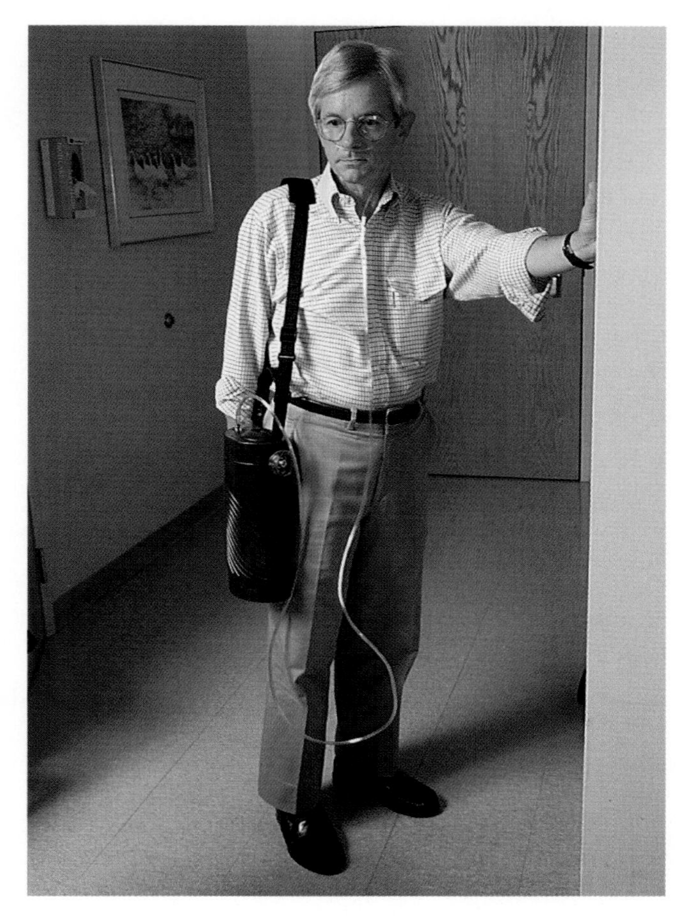

Figure 30–13. An individual needing full-time oxygen therapy can carry a liquid oxygen supply, enabling him to pursue daily activities.

PROCEDURE 30–12. ADMINISTERING OXYGEN FROM A PORTABLE OXYGEN TANK

PURPOSE: To supply oxygen continually while patient is ambulating or being transferred between departments (eg, treatments or tests).

EQUIPMENT: Portable oxygen tank (E cylinder), regulator with flowmeter, and patient's oxygen delivery device with humidifier and connecting tubing.

ACTION 1. Explain the procedure and its expected benefits to the patient. Obtain a portable tank.

ACTION 2. Check the gauge for the amount of oxygen (psi) in the tank. Compute the length of time this amount will last using the following formula:

$$\frac{\text{psi} \times 0.28}{\text{L/min ordered}} = \text{minutes of oxygen available}$$

Obtain a new tank if insufficient quantity remains for projected length of planned activity.

ACTION 3. For a new cylinder:

a. "Crack" the cylinder—turn the handwheel at the top slowly clockwise about one quarter turn, to clear the valve opening of any dust or particles, then close it quickly. Cracking the cylinder produces a loud hissing noise; this does not indicate malfunction.

b. Attach a regulator with flowmeter to the cylinder outlet. A wrench is attached to the tank for this purpose. Tank oxygen is stored under pressure. The regulator controls the *pressure* at which the oxygen exits the tank. A flowmeter is needed to regulate the *rate* of flow.

ACTION 4. To administer oxygen from an E cylinder, open the cylinder valve by slowly turning the handwheel until it is fully open to start the flow of oxygen, then turn it back one quarter turn.

ACTION 5. Set the flowmeter at the ordered rate.

ACTION 6. If the patient is receiving humidified oxygen, remove the humidifier with the connecting tubing from the wall source and attach it to the portable tank below the flowmeter to prevent drying of mucous membranes. (See Procedure 30–13.) Humidifiers should not be used by more than one patient. If left on tank from previous use, discard to prevent cross contamination.

ACTION 7. If no humidifier is in use, remove the connecting tubing from the wall source and attach it to the portable tank below the flowmeter. Turn the wall flowmeter to zero.

ACTION 8. Remind the patient not to be around smokers while using portable oxygen.

ACTION 9. After the patient has returned to the room, reconnect the delivery system to the wall source and reset the flowmeter to the ordered rate. Turn off the flow of oxygen from the portable tank by setting its flowmeter at zero and close the cylinder valve.

ACTION 10. Store the portable tank so that it cannot fall or be easily tipped over, which could damage the regulator, resulting in rapid escape of gas under pressure from the tank and making the tank a projectile.

Recording:
Document the use of portable oxygen, the specific activity, and the patient's response.

HOME HEALTH ADAPTATION: Teach patient and caregivers how to turn on E tank, attach a regulator, and adjust the flowmeter. Instruct the patient and family regarding no smoking precautions and safety factors, and to avoid petroleum as a lubricant. "Oxygen in Use" signs need to be posted in entryway.

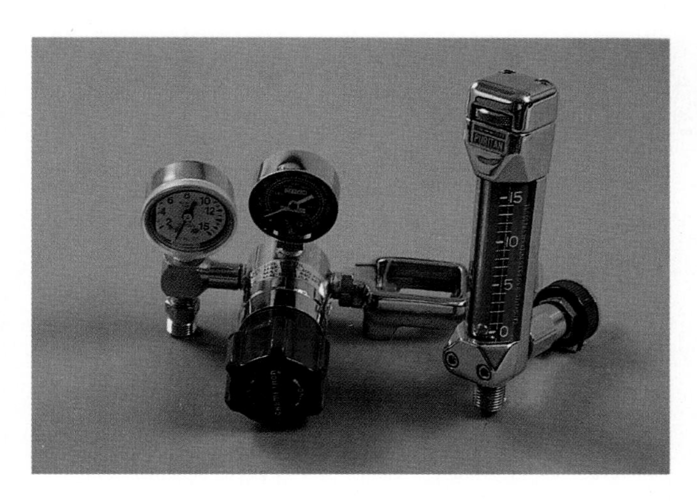

Figure 30–14. To administer oxygen, a flowmeter is used to determine the liters per minute of oxygen delivered. Bourden gauge (left), Thorpe gauge (right).

Most oxygen delivery systems cannot regulate the exact amount of oxygen a patient receives, because the device supplies only supplemental oxygen. The room air with which the oxygen is mixed enters the device as patients inhale. Therefore, a patient's rate and depth of respiration influence the amount of room air that mixes with the oxygen coming from the delivery system and affects the percentage of oxygen the patient takes in. These kinds of delivery systems are called low-flow systems. The approximate FiO_2 that low-flow devices supply can be predicted based on the oxygen flowrate being used (Table 30–11). Many patients who require oxygen therapy do not require precise concentrations of oxygen. In this situation, a physician orders a low-flow device, with a specified flowrate rather than a concentration (for example, "O_2 2 LPM via nasal prongs").

Humidifying Oxygen. Oxygen stored in cylinders or central reservoirs is dry. If given directly, oxygen can dry respiratory tract mucosa and thus compromise airway patency. Disposable or reusable humidifiers can be attached to oxygen delivery systems to prevent mucosal drying and irritation (see Procedure 30–13).

Oxygen Delivery Devices. Several kinds of oxygen delivery devices are available, each having advantages and disadvantages. Some, such as the oxygen hood and the croupette, or oxygen tent, are used only for pediatric patients.

OXYGEN HOOD. The rigid plastic hood, which covers only the head, is effective for neonates and premature infants who do not move independently.

BLOW-BY. A blow-by is a narrow oxygen catheter with small holes or large corrugated oxygen tubing place near a child's face. It is used when the child will not tolerate other delivery devices.

CROUPETTE. The croupette is a large clear plastic tent that is placed inside a crib, providing sufficient space for a young infant or small child to move around. The entire tent is flooded with humidified oxygen. The croupette is useful for a child who will not wear a mask, but it has several disadvantages. It is difficult to maintain oxygen levels because the tent must be opened to give care. Moreover, the child may feel isolated within the tent. The humidity creates a mist that interferes with visual monitoring of the child and makes the child's clothing and bed linen damp. Pediatric-sized masks or nasal cannulae are preferred delivery methods, if the child will tolerate them.

NASAL CANNULA. For older children and adults, the nasal cannula (also called nasal prongs) is the best tolerated form of oxygen therapy. It consists of two soft plastic prongs, curved to fit into the nostrils, attached to a plastic tube (see Fig. 30–15A and Procedure 30–14). The nasal cannula delivers oxygen effectively regardless of whether patients breathe through their nose or mouth. It does not interfere with eating and speaking nor does it cause a closed-in feeling, which is a common complaint with oxygen masks. Nasal prongs deliver 24 to 44 percent FiO_2, depending on flowrate and respirations. Flowrates of 1 to 6 L/min are recommended.

OXYGEN MASKS. If mist or a higher oxygen flow is desired, there are several types of masks available (Fig. 30–15B, D–F). Masks require flowrates of at least 5 L/min to flush exhaled CO_2 from the mask.

TABLE 30-11. APPROXIMATE FiO_2 DELIVERED BY VARIOUS DEVICES AT VARIOUS FLOWRATES

Device[a]	Flow	Flowrate (L/min)	FiO_2 (%)
Nasal cannula (prongs)	Low	1	24
		2	28
		3	32
		4	36
		5	40
		6	44
		(Higher flowrates not recommended)	
Simple mask	Low	Flowrates < 5 not recommended	
		5–6	40
		6–7	50
		7–8	60
Partial rebreather mask	Low	Flowrates < 6 not recommended	
		6	60
		7 and above	<60 (FiO_2 varies @ < 7 L/min)
Nonrebreather mask	Low	6	55–60
		8	60–80
		10–15	80–90
Face tent	Low	8–10	35–50
Venturi mask	High	4	24
		6	28
		8	35

[a] With low-flow devices, precise FiO_2 cannot be regulated. It is dependent upon respiratory rate and pattern. The figures here assume regular respiratory rate between 16 and 20 breaths per minute.

PROCEDURE 30–13. USING A HUMIDIFIER FOR OXYGEN THERAPY

PURPOSE: To prevent drying of respiratory mucosa with high-liter-flow oxygen delivery.
EQUIPMENT: Disposable or reusable humidifier, adapter to connect to oxygen source.

ACTION 1. Discuss the procedure and expected benefits with the patient. Assure patient that interruption in oxygen flow will be temporary.

ACTION 2. Attach the adapter to the top of the humidifier bottle to secure humidifier to oxygen flowmeter. Adapter is usually packaged with disposable humidifier.

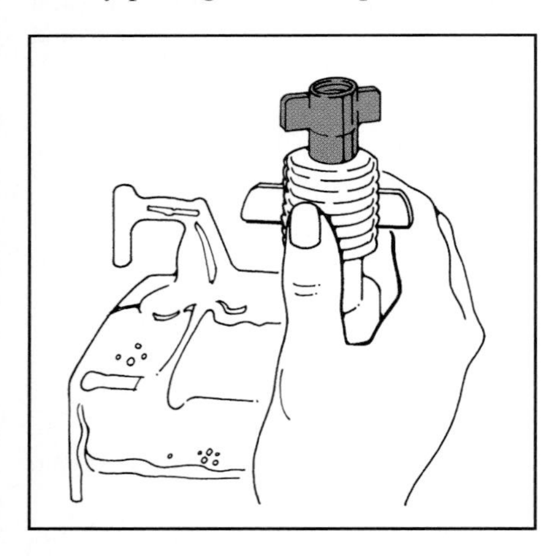

ACTION 3. Snap off seal from outlet port of prefilled disposable humidifier. Reusable units will be enclosed in sterile wrap, but must be filled before use.

ACTION 4. Attach humidifier to flowmeter by turning the adapter in a clockwise direction until it is tight. If not securely attached, oxygen could leak at connection and cause a fire hazard.

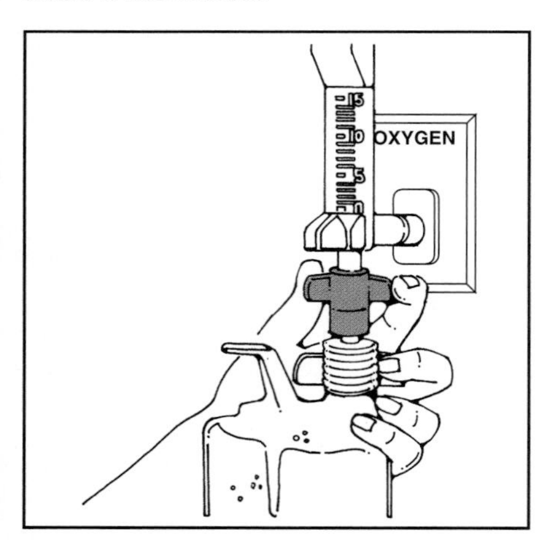

ACTION 5. Attach the small-bore oxygen tubing connected to the oxygen delivery device to the outlet port of the humidifier.

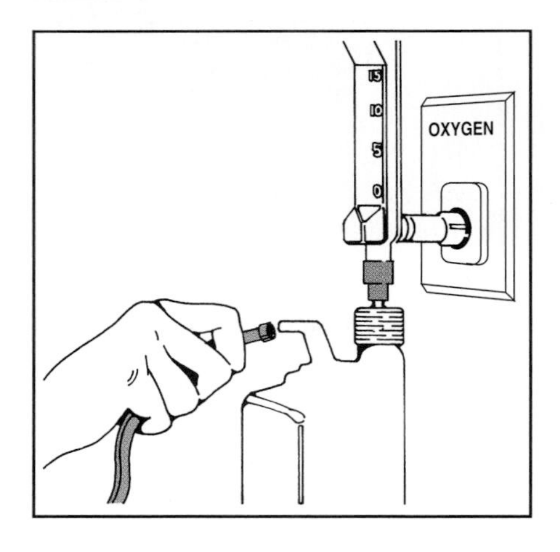

ACTION 6. Adjust the flowmeter to the ordered flowrate and observe for bubbles as oxygen flows through the water in the humidifier. If there are no bubbles, no oxygen is flowing. Obtain assistance from respiratory therapist if flow cannot be initiated.

ACTION 7. If delivery device is not already in place, apply to patient (Procedure 30–14) and complete assessment of patient's response to oxygen therapy.

Recording:

In most health care facilities, humidification is routinely included when oxygen is delivered at flowrates above 4 L/min, so no specific entry related to humidifier is needed. If humidifier was added to a system at low flowrate, document reason for addition in patient's progress notes. It may also be useful to post a sign for respiratory therapist that patient needs humidifier, despite usual policy, and note same in the Kardex.

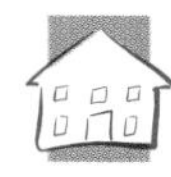

HOME HEALTH ADAPTATION: Oxygen concentrators are usually set up with humidifiers for home use.

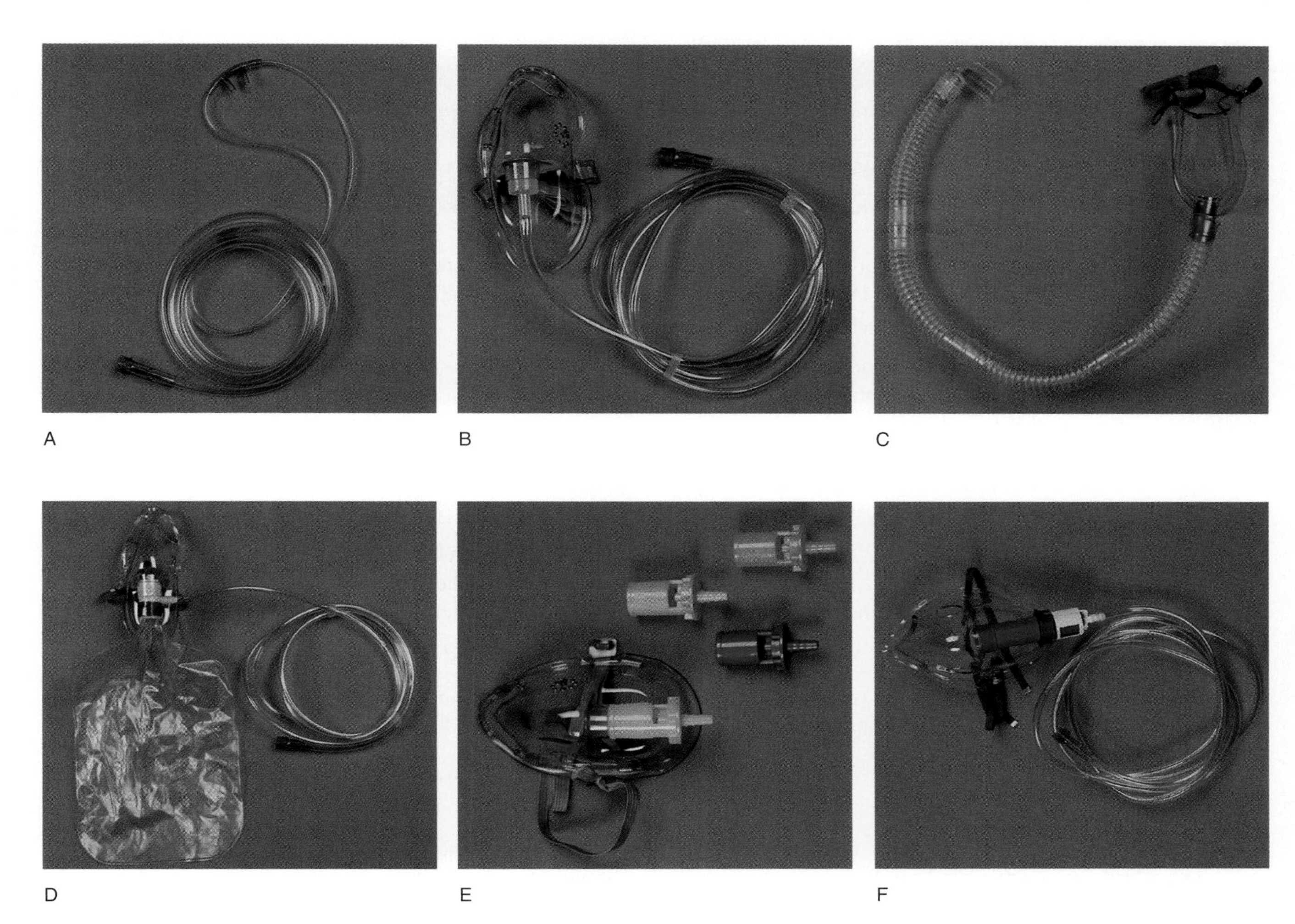

Figure 30–15. Oxygen therapy devices. **A.** Nasal prongs. **B.** Face mask which delivers moderately high flow of oxygen. **C.** Face tent. **D.** Partial rebreather mask. **E.** Venturi mask with adapters to regulate concentration of oxygen. **F.** Venturi mask with dial-in oxygen concentration control. *(From Smith S, Duell D.* Clinical Nursing Skills: Nursing Process Model; Basic to Advanced Skills. *4th ed. Norwalk, CT: Appleton & Lange; 1996:717.)*

The major disadvantage of masks is that patients find them uncomfortable and tend to remove them often. The masks must also be removed for eating, drinking, expectorating, and shaving. Oxygen should be supplied via nasal cannula during these activities. Disposable masks should be changed every 8 hours. Procedure 30–14 presents nursing considerations for each of the types of masks discussed below.

- *Simple mask.* The simple mask can deliver FiO_2s of 40 to 60 percent. Room air is mixed with oxygen and exhaled air expelled via small perforations on either side of the mask (Fig. 30–15B).
- *Partial rebreather mask.* The partial rebreather mask delivers 35 to 60 percent FiO_2. It has an attached reservoir bag at its base that collects the first one third of the patient's exhaled air. Because this air comes from the pharynx and trachea where no air is exchanged, its oxygen and CO_2 content approximate room air. Perforations on either side of the mask allow entry of room air and escape of the rest of the exhaled air (Fig. 30–15D).
- *Nonrebreather mask.* The nonrebreather mask has the same appearance as the partial rebreather, but a rubber one-way valve at the base of the mask prevents exhaled air from entering the reservoir bag and another on the side of the mask limits intake of room air. This mask can deliver FiO_2s of 60 to 90 percent if it fits snugly on the face.
- *Venturi mask.* The Venturi mask is the only mask that can deliver specific concentrations of oxygen. Adapters are attached to the base of the mask that cause a predictable amount of room air to mix with the incoming oxygen at a given flowrate (refer to Table 30–11). The mask has large ports on each side to allow exhaled air to escape. Venturi masks can deliver FiO_2s of 24 to 40 percent, or if used with a nebulizer and high flowrate, up to 100 percent (Fig. 30–15E and F).

FACE TENT. A face tent is a modified mask that is designed to deliver high-humidity oxygen. It does not fit closely against the face as oxygen masks do, and so it may be tolerated better than a mask. Because of its design, FiO_2 delivery is less predictable with the face tent than with other delivery devices (Fig. 30–15C).

(continued on page 1077)

PROCEDURE 30–14. ADMINISTERING OXYGEN VIA NASAL CANNULA, FACE TENT, OR VARIOUS MASKS

PURPOSE: To maintain optimal oxygenation status in patients unable to maintain sufficient oxygen concentration when breathing room air, thereby decreasing the work of respiration and improving oxygenation of body tissues.

EQUIPMENT: Oxygen source; flowmeter; humidifier; oxygen tubing to be used with the specified device; oxygen delivery device specified in medical order; and "No Smoking, Oxygen in Use" signs.

ACTION 1. Check the medical order for specific delivery device and oxygen flowrate or percent. Discuss the procedure and its expected benefits with the patient.

RATIONALE. Active participation is more likely if the patient understands the desired behaviors and anticipated benefits.

ACTION 2. Obtain baseline data regarding patient's oxygenation status: level of consciousness; vital signs (BP, P, R); respiratory pattern; O_2 saturation; airway patency; color; activity tolerance.

RATIONALE. Provides basis for evaluating effectiveness of oxygen therapy.

ACTION 3. Check to see that the control on the flowmeter is in the "off" position. Then push the flowmeter into the wall outlet, exerting very firm pressure.

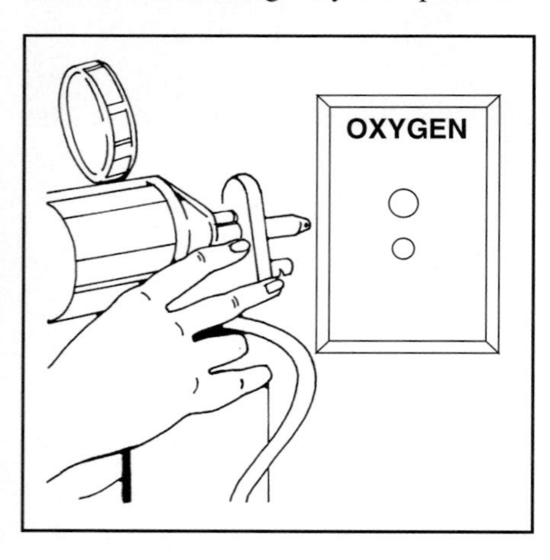

RATIONALE. If the flowmeter control is in the "on" position, oxygen will escape when the flowmeter is attached to the wall outlet. Firm pressure is needed to secure the flowmeter.

ACTION 4. Attach the humidifier to the flowmeter if this is institutional policy (see Procedure 30–13). Some institutions do not humidify oxygen at low flowrates.

RATIONALE. Unhumidified air often causes mucous membranes to dry out and sputum to become thick and tenacious.

ACTION 5. Securely attach one end of connecting tubing to nipple on humidifier, the other to the oxygen-delivery device.

RATIONALE. Provides a continuous leakfree system for oxygen delivery.

ACTION 6. Set flowmeter at ordered flowrate. Caution patient and others not to adjust the flowmeter under any circumstances.

RATIONALE. Oxygen is prescribed specific to patient condition. Rates higher or lower than ordered could result in danger to the patient.

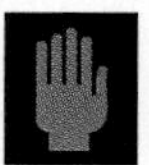

Decreasing oxygen flow will deliver insufficient oxygen to maintain desired blood oxygen concentration (Po_2). Increasing flowrate could cause respiratory arrest in patients with a hypoxemic breathing drive.

ACTION 7. Observe for bubbling in the humidifier as oxygen flows through the water.

RATIONALE. If no bubbles appear, no oxygen is flowing through the humidifier nor is it being supplied to the patient.

ACTION 8. Place the oxygen delivery device on the patient as follows:

A: NASAL PRONGS (CANNULA)

ACTION 1. Position the prongs so they curve toward the nares, then place tubing over patient's ears and under the chin. Adjust the tubing comfortably so oxygen is directed upward into nose, then pull up on slide until tubing is comfortably snug. Pad the tubing over the ears with gauze, if desired. Some models are secured by an elastic headband instead of a chinstrap.

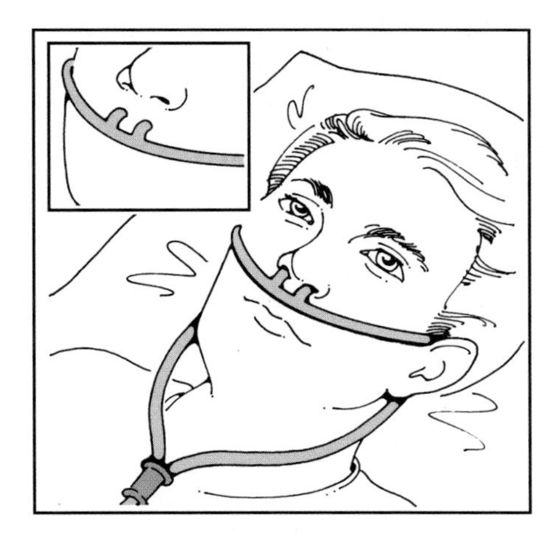

RATIONALE. If the prongs are not properly positioned, the oxygen flow may be blocked. If device is too snug, patient may remove it, or it may cause pressure sores on the face or ears.

ACTION 2. Instruct patient to breathe in the pattern that is most comfortable.

RATIONALE. Mouth breathing is acceptable and still produces adequate bodily oxygenation because oxygen is heavier than air and tends to go down into lungs along with air inhaled through the mouth.

ACTION 3. Check the prongs at least q shift for occlusion by mucus and irritation of nares. Clean prn with cotton applicators moistened with water. Check frequently for correct prong placement.

RATIONALE. Mucus will impede oxygen flow. Irritation from prongs may stimulate mucus production. The prongs tend to be displaced easily.

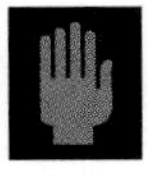

Water-soluble lubricant may be used to reduce irritation, but petroleum-based products are contraindicated because they support combustion.

B: SIMPLE, PARTIAL REBREATHER, OR NONREBREATHER MASK

ACTION 1. Place mask so it covers patient's nose and mouth. Adjust the elastic strap and the nose clip so mask fits snugly. Apply padding if strap irritates patient's ears.

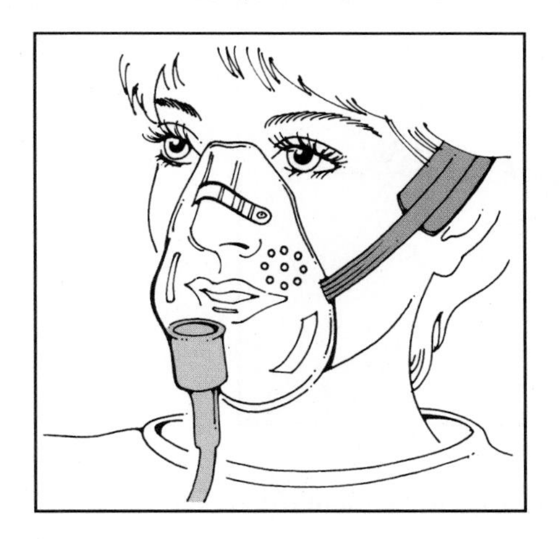

RATIONALE. To deliver maximum oxygen, the mask must be sufficiently snug so that oxygen cannot escape at edges of mask.

ACTION 2. Observe for correct functioning of partial rebreather and nonrebreather masks as follows:

a. *Partial rebreather:* Reservoir should fill on exhalation, and nearly collapse on inspiration.

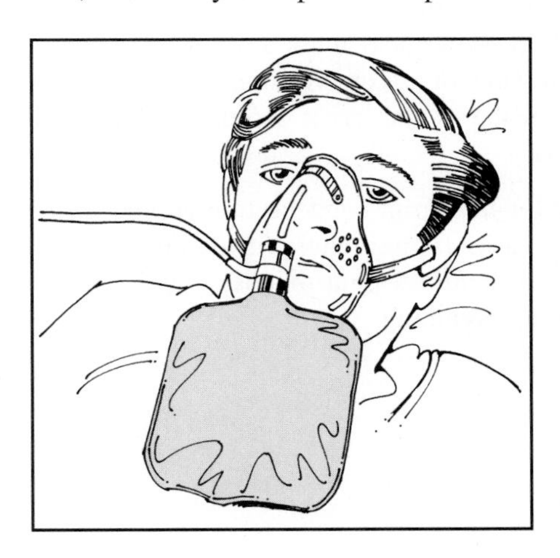

RATIONALE. If the reservoir on a partial rebreather mask does not fill on exhalation, air is escaping via another route and the rebreather function is not operating.

Continued

b. *Nonrebreather:* No change in reservoir on exhalation; slight deflation on inspiration.

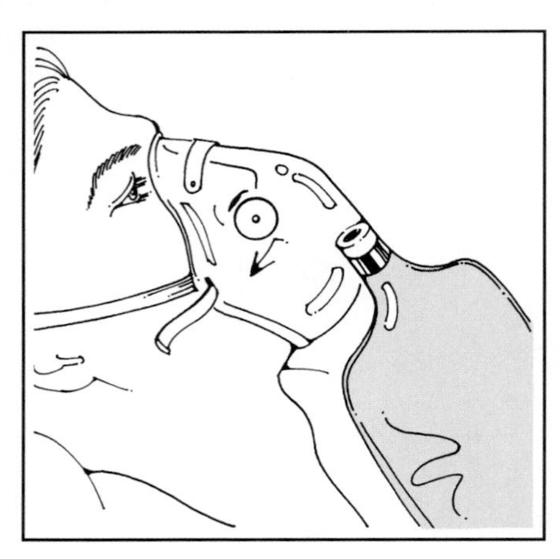

RATIONALE. No exhaled air should flow into the reservoir of a nonrebreather mask, so the bag inflation should not change on exhalation. If the reservoir on either mask collapses on inspiration, flowrate is too low. A collapsed reservoir indicates no oxygen is flowing into mask.

ACTION 3. Stay with patient until he or she adjusts to the sensation of breathing with mask on face.

RATIONALE. Some patients feel claustrophobic with mask on until hypoxia is relieved and even afterward.

ACTION 4. Check skin under mask several times per shift for signs of pressure or excessive moisture. Sputum may collect on the inside of the mask. Adjust, clean, and dry mask as necessary.

RATIONALE. Moisture from condensation and perspiration collects under mask. It may cause irritation and/or skin breakdown and discomfort. Oral mucosa may become dry if patient is mouth breathing.

C: VENTURI MASK

ACTION 1. Set dial on mask or select the jet adapter that delivers the percent of oxygen specified in the medical order. Connect it to the distal end of the wide-bore tubing attached to the mask.

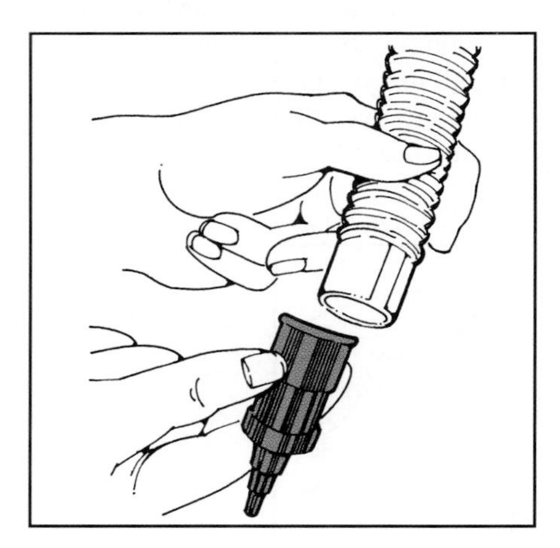

RATIONALE. The jet adapter restricts the flow of oxygen so it mixes with air to deliver precise concentration of oxygen. Respiratory rate does not change the flowrate. A Venturi mask is used when precise oxygen concentrations are necessary.

ACTION 2. Attach the humidity adapter (clear plastic sleeve) to the jet adapter to prevent blocking of the entrainment ports.

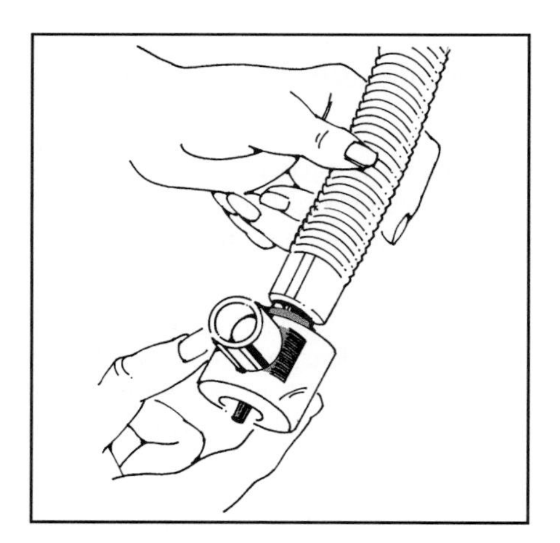

RATIONALE. If the mask's ports are blocked (eg, by bed linen), room air will not flow into the ports and higher concentrations of oxygen will be delivered.

Procedure 30–14. (continued)

ACTION 3. Attach the connecting tubing from the oxygen source to the jet adapter.

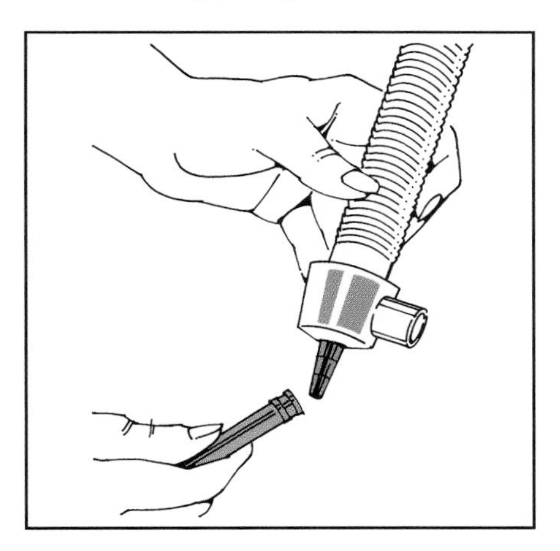

RATIONALE. Delivers oxygen at ordered concentration to the patient.

ACTION 4. Use wide-bore tubing to attach a humidifying device to this sleeve if oxygen concentration of 30 percent or greater is ordered.

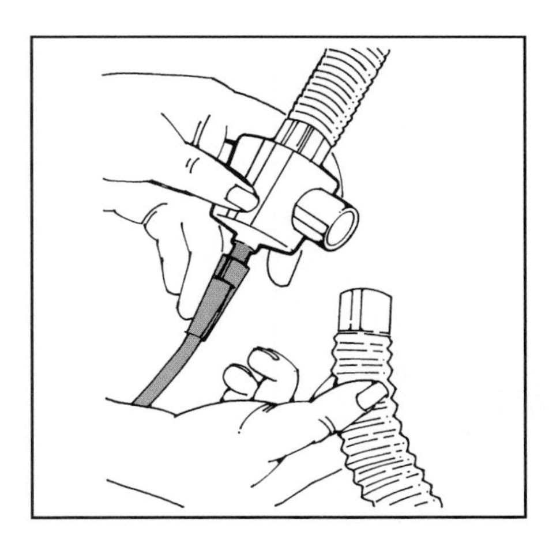

RATIONALE. At flowrates required for delivery of these oxygen concentrations, significant drying of mucosa occurs.

ACTION 5. Apply mask as described above. Continue with other steps as for other masks.

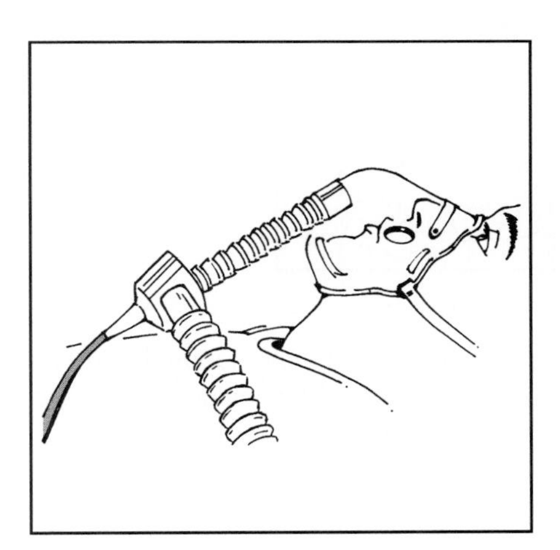

Continued

ACTION 6. Check wide-bore tubing for condensation several times per shift. If present, separate tubing from humidity adapter and drain liquid into a container for disposal. Take care to prevent backflow of the liquid into the humidifier reservoir.

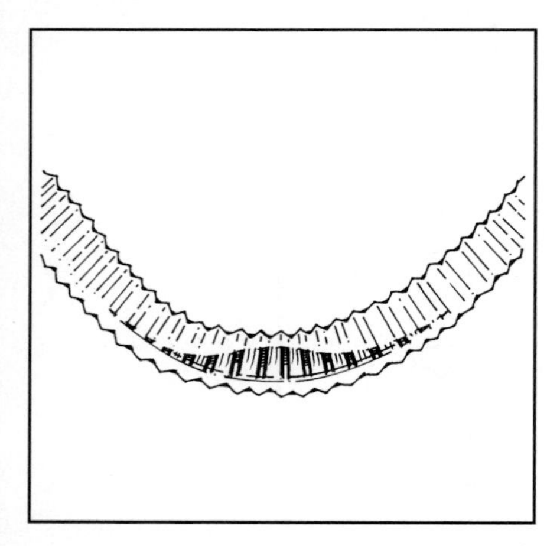

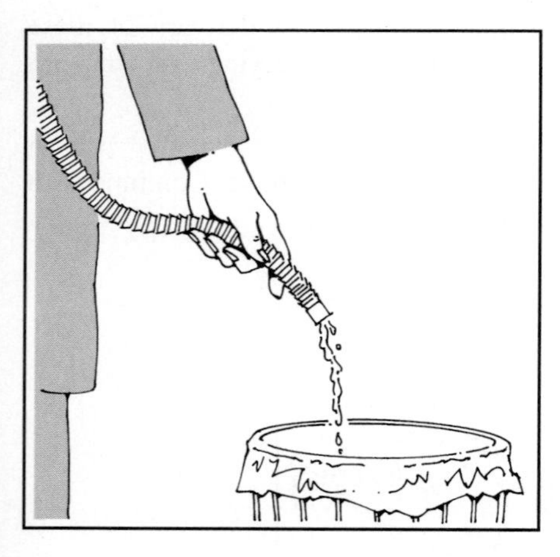

RATIONALE. Velocity of gas in wide-bore tubing is slower; hence moisture supplied by humidifier condenses. It is a potential source of contamination, so must be removed. If liquid is left in wide-bore tube, it impedes oxygen flow.

D: FACE TENT

ACTION 1. Apply the tent so it fits under chin and sweeps around face. Secure the strap behind head to keep the device in place. It does not fit snugly over nose and cheeks.

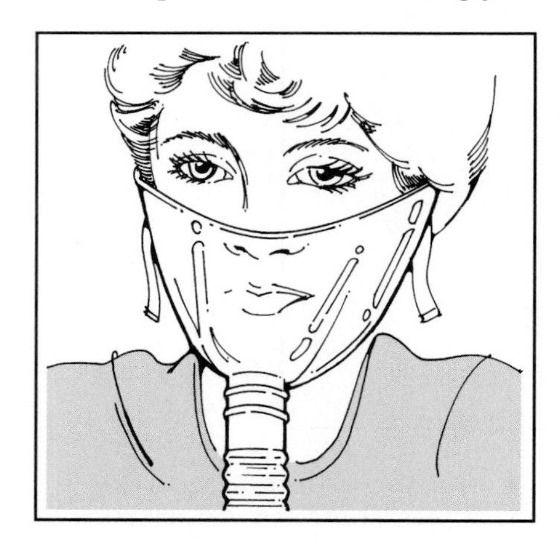

RATIONALE. A face tent is used to deliver aerosolized gas for treatment of thick secretions. It is also better tolerated by patients who find that conventional masks cause a feeling of claustrophobia.

ACTION 2. Use wide-bore tubing to connect face tent to humidifying device. An adapter may be needed.

RATIONALE. Wide-bore tubing transmits highly humidified gas more effectively.

ACTION 3. Check for presence of mist inside face tent.

RATIONALE. Mist indicates humidified gas is being delivered.

ACTION 4. Assess skin under tent, provide skin and mouth care, and clean mask as for conventional masks.

RATIONALE. Excess moisture could cause discomfort or skin irritation. Mucus from coughing could build up inside mask.

ACTION 5. Check wide-bore tubing for condensation, and dispose of as described for Venturi mask (C, Action 5).

RATIONALE. See C, Action 5, above.

Procedure 30–14. (continued)

FOR ALL DEVICES:

ACTION 1. Instruct patient to keep the delivery device in place at all times and to call for assistance if problems occur.

RATIONALE. Interruption of oxygen therapy may result in decreased Po_2, and deterioration of condition.

Patients receiving oxygen via mask or face tent should use nasal prongs while eating so no interruption of therapy occurs.

ACTION 2. Discuss safety precautions outlined in Clinical Guideline 30–6. Discuss with patient and significant others.

RATIONALE. Oxygen supports combustion so any situation that could create sparks must be prevented.

ACTION 3. Instruct patient to notify nurse if dyspnea, dizziness, or shortness of breath occurs.

RATIONALE. These symptoms suggest insufficient oxygen.

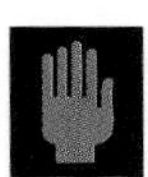

Physician should be notified if respiratory problems occur so oxygen therapy prescription can be reevaluated.

ACTION 4. If patient is ambulatory, be sure connecting tubing is long enough to allow movement about the room without disconnecting oxygen. Proximal end of oxygen tubing can be secured to the patient's clothing with a rubber band and safety pin to reduce pulling on prongs or mask when patient moves.

RATIONALE. If movement is restricted by tubing that is too short, patient may remove device while walking to bathroom or moving about the room.

ACTION 5. Ask ambulatory patient to obtain assistance to ambulate outside the room.

RATIONALE. A portable oxygen source must be used for ambulation outside the room (Procedure 30–12).

ACTION 6. Post signs indicating that oxygen is in use on door to patient's room and at bedside.

RATIONALE. Alerts visitors of necessary precautions.

ACTION 7. Assess patient's oxygenation status as described in Action 2 at least q8h.

RATIONALE. Determines effectiveness of oxygen therapy. Frequency of assessment is determined by patient condition.

Recording:

Note assessment findings, mode of oxygen delivery, flowrate, patient's response to therapy, any adverse effects noted, and corresponding nursing action. These data should be recorded when oxygen therapy is initiated, and at least every shift thereafter.

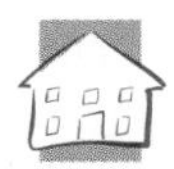

HOME HEALTH ADAPTATION: Oxygen concentrators and cannulas are the most common route of oxygen delivery in the home. E tanks for portability and/or H tanks for backup for power outages should also be present. Instruct family and caregivers regarding no smoking precautions, safety from falls when using very long connecting tubing, and avoidance of petroleum as a lubricant. "Oxygen in Use" signs need to be posted on entryway.

Chest Tubes

When air has entered a patient's pleural space (pneumothorax) or body fluids have accumulated in the pleural space (pleural effusion), the lung may be completely or partially collapsed. As a result, oxygenation status is severely compromised. The air is removed from the pleural space by placing one or more chest tubes through the skin and into the pleural space, allowing the lung to reexpand. The distal ends of chest tubes are connected to a water-sealed drainage system to prevent air from reentering the pleural cavity. Patients who need chest tubes are usually seriously ill and require advanced nursing care that is beyond the scope of this text.

Supporting Circulation

Restorative care for oxygenation problems may also involve support of circulation. Examples include anti-embolism stockings, venous compression stockings, foot pumps, and special exercises to promote circulation, positioning, and external cardiac compressions. These techniques result in improved oxygenation to various tissues of the body.

Anti-embolism Stockings. Anti-embolism stockings are used to enhance venous return, which improves peripheral circulation, reduces orthostatic hypotension, and reduces the risk of clot formation in the legs. There are two types of anti-embolism stockings. The elastic type is much like support hose. Procedure 30–15 describes their application. These stockings are supplied in knee-high and thigh-high styles. It is important to measure patients' legs carefully and apply the right size stocking.

Another type of anti-embolism stocking is the *pulsatile anti-embolism stocking* (PAS) or *venous compression device*. These devices have an inflatable sleeve that fits into a pocket running along the length of the stocking or a series of inflatable cuffs that wrap around the leg (Fig. 30–16). They are rhythmically inflated and deflated by a pneumatic pump, creating pulsations that enhance fibrinolytic activity, stimulate leg circulation and improve venous return. As with the elastic stockings, it is important to apply the right size stockings and to assess circulation in the legs carefully before application and periodically during use. The stockings may be deflated during ambulation. They should be removed for 15 minutes each shift to provide skin care and assess skin and circulation.

A variation of venous compression stockings called foot pumps operates similarly but is applied only to the foot. The patient's foot is placed on the rigid sole, and the soft side flaps are secured snugly over the top of the foot with Velcro straps.

Buerger-Allen Exercises. These exercises were developed for patients with compromised arterial circulation to the feet and legs. They can also be used to promote peripheral circulation in patients whose activity is limited because of illness or its treatment. The exercises shown in Fig. 30–7 can also be used in conjunction with Buerger-Allen exercises for patients who are gradually increasing their activity level. Both can be continued into the rehabilitation phase of care, in combination with walking. Patients who use the exercises for severe peripheral vascular disease should follow the advice of the physician.

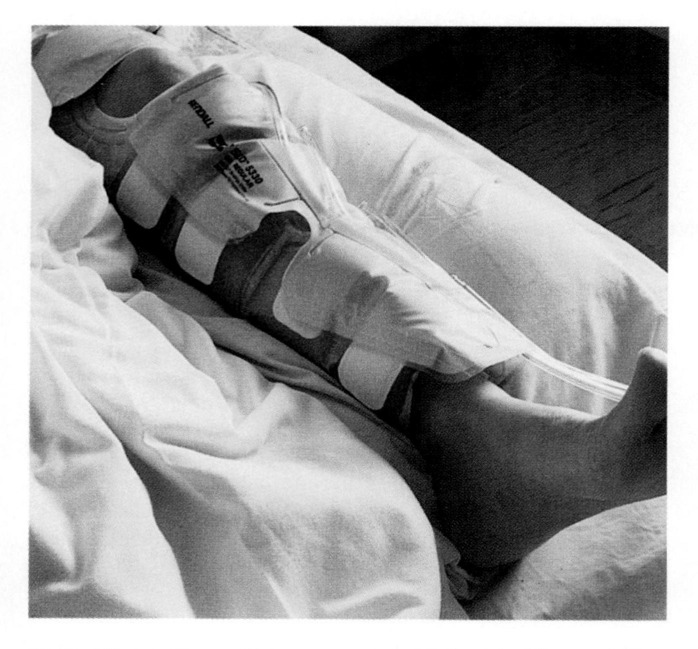

Figure 30–16. Sequential venous compression stockings enhance venous return. They are available in knee-high or above the knee length.

To perform Buerger-Allen exercises, patients should:

1. Lie flat on their back and elevate both legs and feet on a padded surface for 1 to 3 minutes. A large cushion or a chair tipped so its back creates an incline works well. The purpose of this step is to drain stagnant blood from the feet and lower legs, so feet should remain elevated until blanching occurs.
2. Sit in a chair or on the edge of the bed and repeat alternating flexion and extension of the feet, first with the feet in a normal position, then with the feet everted, and finally with the feet inverted. Each position should be held for 30 seconds. By this time the feet should be very pink, indicating that circulation has improved.
3. Conclude the exercise by lying flat in a supine position for 3 to 5 minutes. The entire set may then be repeated three to six times.

If at any time during the exercises the legs or feet become blue and painful, patients should lie down immediately with the feet elevated as in step 1 for as long as necessary to reverse the symptoms. These exercises usually are done three to four times a day.

Positioning. Positioning to promote circulation and avoid pressure on bony prominences is important for all patients whose mobility is limited. It is particularly important for patients with oxygenation problems.

When the patient is lying in the lateral position in bed, support the nondependent leg on pillows so that it does not put pressure on the dependent leg and compromise circulation in both legs. Frequent repositioning will also help combat venous stasis. If spontaneous arm movement is limited, patients' hands should be supported so that they are at or above heart level. When a person with compromised circulation lies in bed for a prolonged period with hands even slightly dependent, they can swell significantly. Placing their hands on pillows can prevent this. Refer to Chap. 33 for more information about positioning patients.

External Cardiac Compression. External cardiac compression, discussed above, is an emergency method to support circulation when cardiac function has ceased. The steps of basic life support (CPR) as outlined in Procedures 30–9 and 30–10 should be closely followed, including verification that CPR is necessary.

Monitoring

Monitoring patients for adequacy and changes in oxygenation is part of restorative care. Several methods are used to monitor oxygenation status. These include vital signs, pulse oximetry, and special measurements such as arterial blood gases, central venous pressure (CVP), and pulmonary artery monitoring.

Vital Signs. Vital signs, specifically pulse and blood pressure, are important indicators of both circulatory status and the effectiveness of the pumping action of the heart. Respiratory rate and quality is an indicator of oxygen exchange. These measurements are discussed in detail in Chap. 17. Pulse oximetry, a measure of blood oxygenation, is discussed on page 1066.

Special Measurements. The measurement of arterial blood gases (ABGs) can be an essential part of assessing of oxygenation status. The tests that are included in ABGs are: pH, Po_2, Pco_2, and HCO_3 (bicarbonate level). Sometimes base excess (a measurement of buffers in the bloodstream), oxygen saturation (how much oxygen

(continued on page 1081)

PROCEDURE 30–15. USING ANTI-EMBOLISM STOCKINGS (THROMBOEMBOLI DETERRENT OR TED HOSE)

PURPOSE: To enhance venous return, thereby improving peripheral circulation, minimizing orthostatic hypotension, and reducing the risk of clot formation. Indicated for postoperative patients or patients who are immobilized.

EQUIPMENT: Stockings, tape measure.

ACTION 1. Be sure there is a valid medical order for hose.

RATIONALE. Anti-embolism stockings require a physician's order

ACTION 2. Discuss the procedure and its expected benefits with the patient.

RATIONALE. Active participation is more likely if the patient understands the desired behaviors and anticipated benefits.

ACTION 3. Assess the circulation in the patient's legs by:

a. Palpating posterior tibial and dorsalis pedis pulse, rhythm, and volume.

b. Noting signs of arterial insufficiency (skin cool, shiny, taut, pale), or venous insufficiency (ankle pigmentation, thickened skin, pitting edema).

c. Observing for positive Homans' sign (calf pain on ankle dorsiflexion).

d. Noting varicosities (distended leg veins when supine).

RATIONALE. This assessment establishes a baseline against which to compare assessment data on circulation status obtained in periodic checks when stockings are in use.

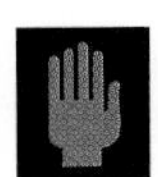

If previously unreported circulatory deficits or new skin lesions are detected, consult patient's physician before applying hose.

ACTION 4. Measure the patient's legs. Compare measurements to size chart to select correct size; order two pairs. *For knee-high hose:* Midcalf circumference, heel to popliteal space.

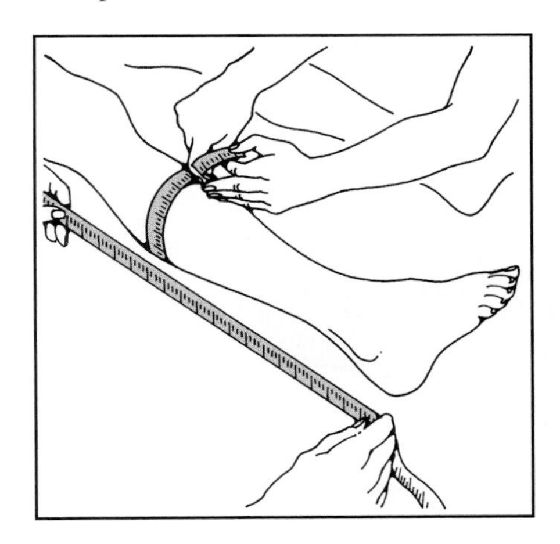

For thigh-high hose: Midcalf and midthigh circumferences, heel to gluteal fold.

RATIONALE. Stockings must fit properly to achieve therapeutic effect. If they are too large, they will not provide adequate support. If they are too small, circulation may be impeded.

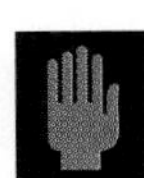

The best time to measure and apply hose is in the morning before patient arises or after at least 1 hour of bedrest, to prevent dependent edema.

Continued

Procedure 30–15. Using Anti-embolism Stockings (Thromboemboli Deterrent or TED Hose) (continued)

ACTION 5. Apply stockings:

a. Turn leg portion of the stocking inside out over the foot portion by placing one hand into the stocking and holding the toe while inverting the stocking to its heel over your arm. The leg of the stocking should extend past the foot, rather than being bunched or rolled. Patient's leg should be dry. Talcum powder may be applied sparingly to reduce irritation.

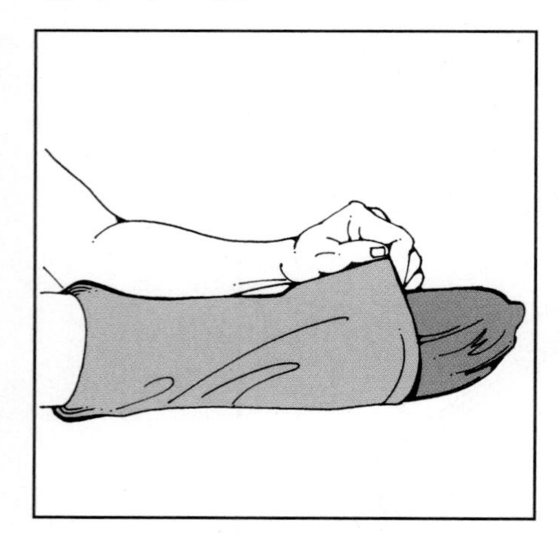

RATIONALE. Inverting rather than rolling or bunching the stocking prevents constrictions in the stocking, which would make its application difficult or even painful to the patient.

b. Grasp each side of the stocking and slip it smoothly over the patient's foot. Be sure the heel of the stocking is centered correctly over patient's heel.

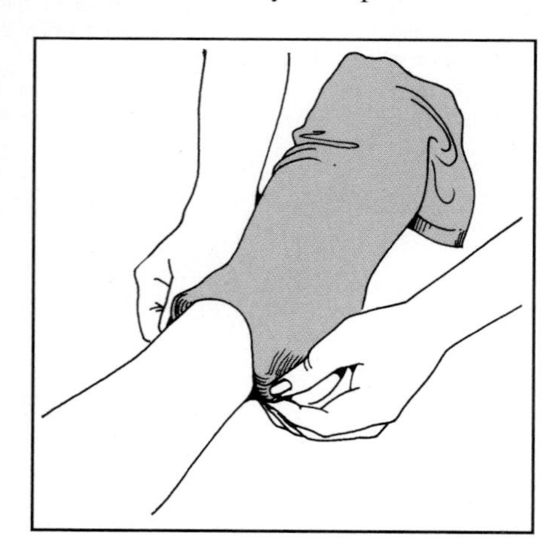

RATIONALE. Wrinkles or ripples could create a tourniquet effect, impeding circulation.

c. Slide the remainder of the stocking bit by bit up the patient's leg, smoothing ripples if they develop. The stocking should fit snugly without wrinkles or bunching.

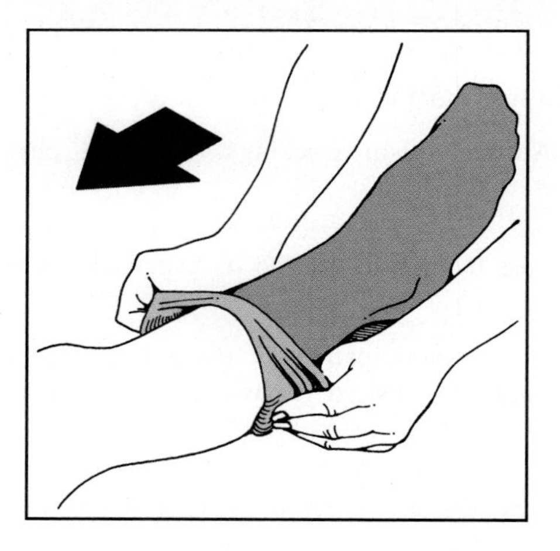

RATIONALE. See part b.

d. Check to see that the patient's toes are covered, not extending out of the open area of the stocking, and that the stocking is correctly aligned for its entire length.

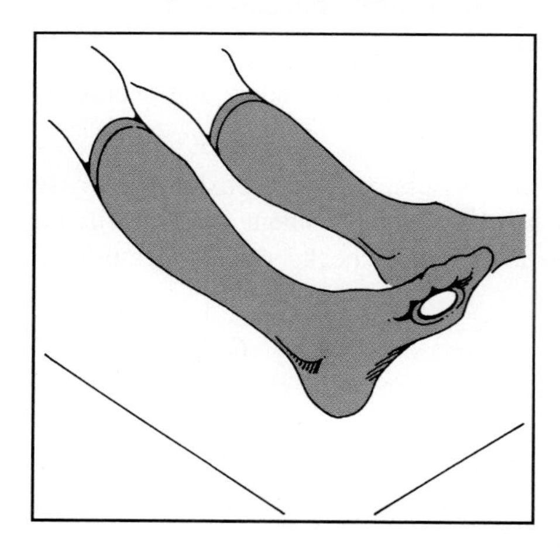

RATIONALE. If the toes extend out of the opening, circulation may become constricted. The opening is provided for periodic assessment of the toes. (See Action 7.)

ACTION 6. Repeat for second leg.

Procedure 30–15. (continued)

ACTION 7. Discuss with the patient how to assess for proper application, and ask patient to notify the nurse to correct problems. Dangers of rolling stockings should be emphasized. Inspect the legs periodically to see that the stockings remain properly applied, that the legs above the stockings are not swollen, and that the toes remain warm and pink with good capillary refill.

RATIONALE. Stockings may roll or twist as the patient moves, with resulting circulatory constriction.

ACTION 8. Remove the stockings for 30 minutes each shift, assess circulation, and provide skin care as needed.

RATIONALE. Provides patient comfort and opportunity for complete circulation assessment.

ACTION 9. To remove stockings, grasp the top of the stocking on each side and pull it off. The stocking will be inside out. Avoid rolling to remove stocking.

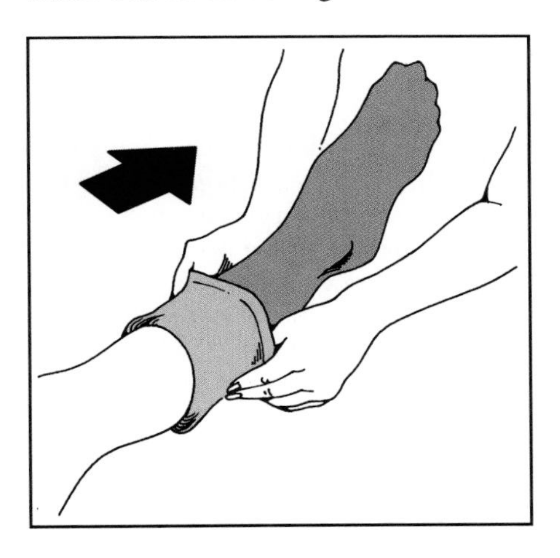

RATIONALE. Rolling or bunching even for a short time will cause constriction with resulting discomfort and temporary impairment of circulation.

ACTION 10. Launder hose about every 1 to 2 days in mild soap and water. Dry flat and away from direct heat. Use spare pair of hose during drying.

RATIONALE. This care will prolong the life of the hose.

ACTION 11. If signs of venous or arterial insufficiency or thrombophlebitis are noted, notify the patient's primary nurse or physician.

RATIONALE. These are complications that may require additional treatment.

Recording:

Record the data and time of application of hose, the circulatory status, and the condition of the skin before application. When hose are removed, record skin and circulatory status and length of time hose remain off.

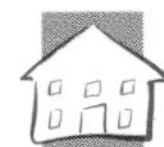

HOME HEALTH ADAPTATION: Observe patient or family member apply hose to be sure they can do it correctly. Emphasize the importance of correct technique and the risks associated with bunching, rolling, or twisting the stocking. Instruct patient and family caregiver to observe for adverse signs and symptoms and report them promptly to the health care professional. When stockings are used for dependent edema, the patient may be more comfortable if they are removed at night and reapplied before getting out of bed in the morning.

the hemoglobin is carrying), and $CaPo_2$ (Pao_2 plus hemoglobin, which reflects total plasma oxygen concentration) are included. ABGs can help health care providers determine if there are disturbances of acid-base balance related to respiratory or metabolic function. (For further discussion of acid-base balance, refer to Chap. 34).

If ABGs are to be drawn, patients must be stabilized beforehand. They should rest in bed without stimulation for about 30 minutes so that their metabolism will be at its lowest level before the gases are drawn. This is to allow comparison among successive readings. Once the metabolism is stabilized, a specially trained health care provider draws a blood sample via an arterial puncture, then applies firm pressure to the puncture site for 5 to 10 minutes to prevent a hematoma. Pressure is applied directly with the hand, not simply by placing a dressing on the site. An adhesive bandage or similar dressing is applied after the 5- to 10-minute period of manual pressure.

Hemodynamic monitoring such as central venous pressure (CVP) and pulmonary artery pressure assessment also provide data about oxygenation. CVP reflects the pressure in the circula-

INSIGHTS FROM NURSING LITERATURE

OXYGENATION AND FUNCTIONAL PERFORMANCE

Leidy NK. Functional performance in people with chronic obstructive pulmonary disease. Image. *1995;27:23–34.*

Functional performance, the extent to which people with chronic illness execute certain activities as they resume their normal activities of daily living, is not well understood in respiratory illness. Consequently, the author reviewed relevant studies to identify new directions for practice and research. Her focus was chronic bronchitis and emphysema, with or without an asthmatic component. This cluster of related diseases causes airflow obstruction, air trapping, lung hyperinflation, impaired gas exchange, and a syndrome of shortness of breath, cough, sputum production, wheezing, poor exercise tolerance, easy fatigability, dyspnea, and related problems such as sadness, depression, a sense of impending doom, anger, anxiety, and social isolation.

The literature showed that disease severity (as measured by forced expiratory volume, a pulmonary function test) did not directly affect performance, but played an indirect role through its effect on symptoms (dyspnea, fatigue). Anxiety and depression were significant predictors of decreased performance in several studies; however, some patients were not anxious or depressed, suggesting that other factors such as strong resources facilitating mastery, well-being, and physiologic stabilization may promote higher levels of performance.

tory system as the blood is returned to the right atrium. One cause of a high CVP is ineffective pumping of the blood to the peripheral circulation, causing blood to back up into the right side of the heart. A low CVP may be caused by low blood volume. Either situation can compromise perfusion.

CVP can be assessed using a glass manometer attached to an intravenous catheter, which goes from the subclavian vein to the right atrium. A catheter placed in this location is called a central line. For an accurate reading the manometer must be held at heart level when a reading is taken. CVP is measured in centimeters of water (cm H_2O). The usual range is 5 to 10 cm H_2O. Some intravenous infusion controllers and pumps can also measure CVP when connected to a central line. The central line insertion site requires a sterile occlusive dressing. Meticulous aseptic technique is required when the dressing is changed, because of the risk of introducing organisms into the subclavian vein and subsequently to the heart (see Chap. 34).

More sophisticated indicators of cardiac function and fluid load, such as *pulmonary artery pressure* (PAP) and *pulmonary artery wedge pressure* (PAWP), are often necessary for critically ill patients. These measurements directly reflect the functioning of the left side of the heart. They are done only in intensive care units and are addressed in advanced nursing courses.

Home Health Care

Restorative home health care focuses primarily on the needs of patients who have chronic respiratory conditions such as severe chronic bronchitis, asthsma, or emphysema. Such patients require increasing levels of direct care once their conditions enter a phase of progressive deterioration. Implementations of home health nurses include teaching effective coughing and pursed-lip breathing to patients, as well as educating caregivers in the techniques of chest physiotherapy, delivering aerosol medications, using intermittent positive pressure breathing machines and nasotracheal suctioning for patients unable to independently rid themselves of respiratory secretions.

Patients with chronic respiratory disease often require home oxygen therapy and may rely on oxygen concentrators, liquid oxygen canisters, or high-pressure oxygen cylinders as sources of oxygen-concentrated air. Thus, training in the operation, maintenance, and cleaning of oxygen systems, begun in the hospital prior to discharge, is a regular part of the home health nurse's family education plan. Home oxygen delivery systems vary in their components but commonly incorporate nasal cannulas or Venturi masks.

Home health restorative care also focuses on preventing respiratory and circulatory complications in all home patients who are bedridden. Turning and positioning patients to prevent pooling of secretions and pneumonia is as important in the home as in the hospital. Thus, a role of home health nurses is to teach caregivers the principles of managing the care of their bedridden relative. Occasionally venous compression stockings are part of the therapy, but more often standard elastic anti-embolism stockings are used to prevent vascular thrombosis and pulmonary embolism during long periods of inactivity.

REHABILITATIVE CARE

Fourth-level patient care focuses on rehabilitation. Patients with chronic lung disease can improve their quality of life and their well-being with an effective rehabilitation program; however, rehabilitation programs and standard therapy for chronic lung disease do not statistically prolong life.

Patient Education

Patient education plays a significant role in rehabilitative care (see also Chap 21). The rehabilitation program for a patient with a chronic oxygenation problem involves teaching about the problem and how to manage it.

? CRITICAL QUERY

Leidy[25] makes the point that studies assessing the functional performance of patients are difficult to evaluate because "functioning" is culturally and economically based, and not well understood. For example, autonomy of aging parents and their offspring is highly valued in some cultures, whereas familial interdependence is the norm in others. What is the implication for nurses who assess the functional performance of individual patients with oxygenation problems?

COLLABORATIVE STRATEGY

EDUCATION FOR SELF-CARE

To assume self-responsibility, patients with long-term oxygenation problems need to learn to be alert to changes in their own physical status. Exchanges between nurse and patient that focus on common subjective and objective manifestations of altered oxygenation can help prepare patients to take responsibility for health care decisions. Patients may ignore worsening symptoms that signal a deterioration in their condition. Nurses can make a significant contribution by reviewing before discharge the critical factors for patients to monitor, once they return to their home setting.

Pathophysiologic Process. A good place to begin is to describe normal physiology of the heart and lungs. Then, provide information about the pathophysiology of the patient's condition; that is, how the patient's lung or heart function is altered.

Medications. Many patients with chronic oxygenation dysfunction must take medications; teaching about prescribed medications is therefore essential. Patients should be taught the expected therapeutic effects, side effects, toxic effects, and pertinent information about medication administration. They should also know whether medications are to be taken with food or on an empty stomach. For example, bronchodilators can cause gastric irritation if they are taken on an empty stomach, so they should be taken with food. Patients must also be made aware of any specific combinations of food and drugs to be avoided. Patients using a cartridge inhaler for medications, should know how to use and clean it. Patients should be instructed not to use over-the-counter medications without consulting their physicians first.

Patients who are using oxygen at home must know why they are using it, when to use it, how much to use, and how to clean and care for the equipment. They must learn how to recognize when the oxygen supply is low. They must be encouraged to keep up usual activities while using oxygen and may also learn how to travel with oxygen. They should also learn breathing techniques and exercises, as previously described.

Signs and Symptoms. Patients who have oxygenation problems should learn to be alert to changes in physical status so that they can contact their physician when such changes occur. Individuals with chronic conditions often ignore signs of increasing illness or are unaware of which symptoms to report. Pulmonary patients should be advised to notify their physician if the cough is worse, sputum is thicker and more difficult to cough up or a different color, or they are dyspneic or orthopneic. Both cardiac and pulmonary patients should monitor their weight at least three times a week and report any sudden weight gain, which may signal heart failure with fluid retention.

Changes in Daily Routines. Nurses should also discuss changes in self-care or daily routines that may prevent further complications. For example, the importance of hydration must be emphasized to patients with pulmonary problems. Most patients need to drink at lease 2000 mL of fluids per day.

Measures to promote circulation can also be made part of daily routine for patients with chronically compromised circulation. Anti-embolic stockings, as discussed under *Restorative Care,* are often continued into the rehabilitation phase of care. If patients are at risk for thrombophlebitis, their legs should be inspected and the calves measured to see that they are of equal size (assuming that they were equal to begin with). Ask patients to report any change in size, redness, heat, or discomfort to their physician. A positive *Homans' sign* (pain in the calf when dorsiflexing the foot) may be a sign of thrombophlebitis and should also be reported.

There are several cautions that patients with compromised circulation can use when sitting or standing. People with vascular compromise should not sit with their legs crossed at the knees or stand in one position for long periods of time. Sitting with legs crossed at the ankles is acceptable. Sitting with the legs elevated on a footstool is better than allowing the legs to be dependent. Whenever extended periods of sitting are necessary, walking around for about 5 minutes each hour will help combat venous stasis.

Assisting With Lifestyle Modification

Patients need information about modifiable risk factors. They need assistance and encouragement in modifying these risk factors as well as education about dietary and other lifestyle changes.

Quitting Smoking. If a patient still smokes, teaching should focus on risks associated with smoking and provide encouragement and support to stop smoking. See also *Discouraging Smoking* in the *Preventive Care* section earlier in the chapter.

Graded Aerobic Exercise Programs. Individually tailored exercise programs are important for people who have oxygenation problems. Graded aerobic exercise improves circulation and reduces the oxygen need per unit of work that a muscle does. A person with oxygenation problems who exercises appropriately will be able to accomplish more activities and have a better quality of life than one who does not exercise. Often, in the early stages of rehabilitation, patients are asked to exercise in a setting where their activity can be closely observed and heart function and blood oxygen levels can be monitored (Fig. 30–17). Patients with obstructive lung disease should use pursed-lip breathing while exercising and should use oxygen if it has been prescribed. Patients should be taught how to decide if they need to rest during exercise and given helpful tips for resting positions.

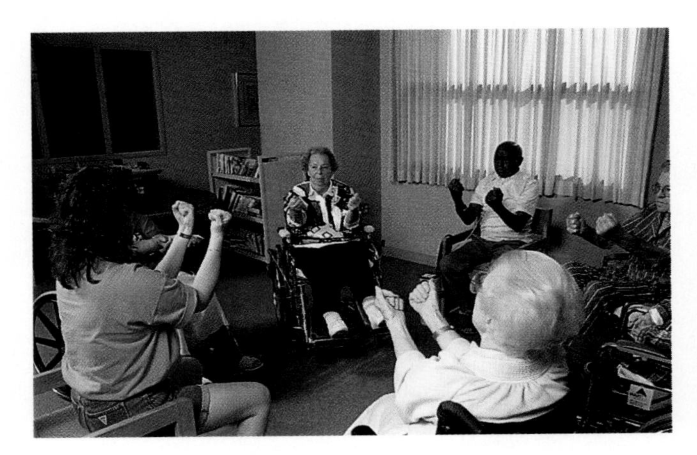

Figure 30–17. Exercise, important in rehabilitative care, encourages blood flow, thereby oxygenation.

Isometric exercises should generally be avoided by those with oxygenation problems. These exercises—which include activities like weight lifting and using many of the machines at traditional exercise studios—increase cardiac workload, promote the Valsalva maneuver, and cause reflex hypertension. Even performing mild isometrics such as quadriceps setting, requires prior consultation with a physician, as most patients hold their breath during such exercises and they tend to increase blood pressure.

Energy Conservation Techniques. Energy conservation techniques can be helpful for persons with compromised oxygenation. Patients should do as many tasks as possible while sitting down. For example, they can assemble all items needed for food preparation and then sit to prepare the food. At the grocery store, patients should ask that groceries be divided into several lightweight bags. The use of a long-handled dustpan will enable patients to sweep floors without bending over. Long-handled tongs can be used to retrieve items from hard-to-reach shelves (Fig. 30–18). Men can sit rather than stand while shaving. Many men habitually hold their breath while shaving with a razor. Using pursed-lip breathing techniques during shaving will eliminate the shortness of breath problems related to this. Patients can sit during a shower using a shower chair (see Chap. 32). Nurses and patients can collaborate to discover many safe and effective methods to minimize the patient's energy expenditures.

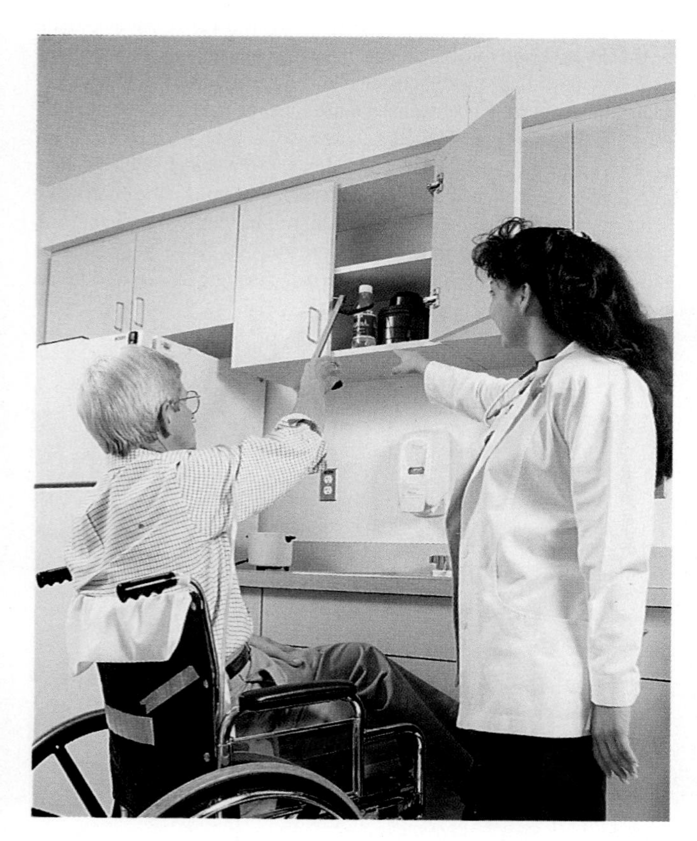

Figure 30–18. Long-handled tongs help an individual unable to stand to perform some activities of daily living.

? CRITICAL QUERY

Leidy[25] points out that recognizing declines in functional performance, that is, patients' independence in carrying out activities of daily living, enables nurses caring for patients with oxygenation problems to identify factors contributing to poor adaptation, facilitate anticipatory intervention, and improve the quality and sensitivity of outcome indicators. Should patients' functional performance be used as a measure of nurses' success in caregiving? Why or why not?

Counseling and Emotional Support

The lifestyle changes required to maintain adequate oxygenation may be difficult for patients to make. Often, they involve restrictions on recreational activities and activities of daily living. Sometimes occupational changes are also required. Often patients' independence is compromised.

Adaptation to these changes may be stressful and may cause economic hardship. Health care providers may inadvertently add to patients' stress by implying that modifications are easy to accomplish. In fact, the effects of the oxygenation problem itself and the reorganization in lifestyle that it demands are usually quite complex. Patients need empathy and support from health care providers and significant others. Many patients benefit from professional counseling to help them explore the implications of the oxygenation problem and associated lifestyle modifications. Counseling can help patients accept their condition, decide which lifestyle changes are possible, and make a commitment to accomplish them.

▲ EVALUATION

When nurses and patients have stated precise, measurable outcomes or specific evaluation criteria in the planning phase of care, both ongoing and terminal evaluation are straightforward. To evaluate accomplishment of outcomes, nurse and patient look for evidence that the criteria identified were attained. An example of a specific measurable outcome for a patient who has altered ventilation due to a postoperative atelectasis might be that within 3 days, the patient's lungs will be free of secretions, as evidenced by absence of adventitious breath sounds and regular, unlabored respirations at about 20 per minute. To evaluate, the nurse would auscultate the patient's lungs and assess respirations regularly, informing the patient if the lung sounds seemed to be improving. Thus, ongoing evaluations can be an incentive for the patient to participate in activities that will promote progress toward the agreed-upon outcomes.

Evaluation is essential if nurse and patient are to know what outcomes have been achieved and whether modifications are necessary. As these examples indicate, the nursing process is circular. Once evaluation is done, the decision about whether to continue implementations or to change them can be made.

▲ SUMMARY

Working collaboratively, nurses and patients can greatly improve patients' quality of life. An understanding of the physiology of healthy oxygenation, including functioning of the heart, lungs, and blood vessels, is required to ensure competent and knowledgeable nursing care of patients with oxygenation problems. Ventilation, diffusion, perfusion, and cellular respiration mechanisms in oxygenation are essential for optimal health.

Oxygenation is affected by an individual's developmental stage, general health and lifestyle, and environment. Alterations in oxygenation may involve ventilation, diffusion, perfusion, or cellular respiration and may result in hypoxemia, hypoxia, hypercapnia, hypocapnia, and tissue necrosis.

Oxygenation is assessed by examining the functioning of various body systems. The oxygenation history and physical assessment includes examining the integument, chest and cardiovascular systems, abdomen, and mental status as they relate to oxygenation. Selected diagnostic and laboratory testing is also done. Nursing diagnoses for patients with oxygenation problems include ineffective airway clearance, ineffective breathing pattern, and altered tissue perfusion.

Nurse–patient management of oxygenation problems—including planning, nursing implementation, and evaluation—assists patients to maintain or regain optimal functioning. Nursing implementation addresses four levels of care: preventive, supportive, restorative, and rehabilitative. When oxygenation is compromised, many other functional dimensions are threatened as well. Optimal oxygenation contributes significantly to a patient's well-being.

LEARNING OUTCOMES

Upon completing this chapter, the student should be able to:

1. Discuss the major organs involved in each of the following processes: ventilation, diffusion, perfusion, and cellular respiration.
2. Define and describe the processes of ventilation, diffusion, perfusion, and cellular respiration.
3. Discuss the impact of general health, development, and the environment on oxygenation.
4. Discuss at least two factors that cause altered ventilation, diffusion, perfusion, and cellular respiration.
5. Discuss how these factors can cause hypoventilation, hyperventilation, or tissue necrosis.
6. List data that are important in an oxygenation history.
7. Describe essential elements of an oxygenation examination.
8. List at least five laboratory tests or diagnostic examinations relevant to oxygenation.
9. Define three nursing diagnoses describing altered oxygenation and identify and explain at least two etiologies for each nursing diagnosis.
10. Describe at least two examples of nursing implementation for preventive, supportive, restorative, and rehabilitative oxygenation care.
11. Discuss nurses' responsibilities associated with oxygen administration.
12. Identify strategies to evaluate effectiveness of nursing implementation to support oxygenation.
13. Write a patient care plan to promote optimum oxygenation for a specific patient.

REVIEW OF KEY TERMS

anatomic dead space
atelectasis
diastole
diffusion
dyspnea
expiration
Fi_{O_2} (fraction of inspired oxygen)
flowmeter
flowrate
hematocrit
hemoglobin
hyperpnea
hyperventilation
hypoventilation
hypoxemia
hypoxia
hypoxic respiratory drive
inspiration
oxygenation
percussion
perfusion
pulmonary edema
retractions
splinting
surfactant
sustained maximal inspiration
systole
tachypnea
tidal volume
total lung capacity
ventilation
vibration
vital capacity

Having Read the Chapter, consider again the opening scenario, page 999, and the following responses to the questions concerning Mrs. Jacobson's care following her heart attack.

Georgette Jacobson is receiving low-flow oxygen by nasal cannula to improve her cellular oxygenation and reduce her cardiopulmonary workload as she awaits surgery. The nasal cannula, a common oxygen delivery device, is the best tolerated form of oxygen therapy for adults and children. To evaluate the effects of the therapy, Mrs. Jacobson's blood oxygen saturation is to be monitored by a device called a pulse oximeter. The pulse oximeter requires no blood sample be drawn. Instead it uses a probe attached to the skin, and thus is noninvasive, painless, and generally well tolerated by patients of all ages. Oxygen therapy prescriptions commonly specify a flowrate to achieve a level of oxygen saturation as measured by pulse oximetry ("Oxygen by nasal prongs, 2 to 4 LPM, to keep oxygen saturation at 92 percent").

Mrs. Jacobson is having major surgery to correct the pathology that caused her heart attack. In the postoperative period, she will be at risk for the oxygenation problems accompanying general anesthesia, postoperative pain, pain medication, and immobility, all of which depress respiration and may result in hypoventilation and atelectasis. To prevent complications, Mrs. Jacobson should be taught that she will be asked to participate in certain postoperative procedures such as breathing exercises and use of an incentive spirometer to enhance pulmonary ventilation, leg exercises to prevent thrombophlebitis, and periodic coughing to maintain airway patency if lung secretions accumulate. She needs to know that even if she suffers from incisional pain, such measures are necessary to prevent serious postoperative complications.

To prevent a recurrence of her disease, Mrs. Jacobson will need to undergo a complete assessment of her cardiovasculary risk factors (smoking, diet, blood pressure, blood lipid levels, stress-reducing habits) as part of a comprehensive rehabilitation program. To prevent recurrence, it will benefit Mrs. Jacobson to make changes in her habit patterns. For example, smoking is likely to cause a recurrence of her heart problem. Other habits, such as trail hiking, are contraindicated during the immediate postoperative period, but may be resumed as a form of regular exercise after she fully recovers from surgery.

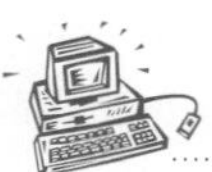

INTERNET RESOURCES

Web Site

American Heart Association:
http://www.amhrt.org

American Cancer Society:
http://www.cancer.org

REFERENCES

1. American Lung Association. *Statistical Update on Lung Disease—March 1997.* New York: American Lung Association; 1997.
2. American Heart Association. *1997 Heart and Stroke Statistical Update.* Dallas, TX: American Heart Association; 1996.
3. Bullock BL, Rosendahl PP. *Pathophysiology: Adaptations and Alterations in Function.* 4th ed. Boston: Scott, Foresman; 1995.
4. West JB. *Pulmonary Pathophysiology: The Essentials.* 4th ed. Baltimore: Williams & Wilkins; 1992.
5. Ganong WF. *Review of Medical Physiology.* 17th ed. Norwalk, CT: Appleton & Lange; 1995.
6. Guyton AC, Hall JE. *The Textbook of Medical Physiology.* 9th ed. Philadelphia: Saunders; 1996.
7. Des Jardins TR. *Cardiopulmonary Anatomy and Physiology: Essentials for Respiratory Care.* 3rd ed. Albany: Delmar; 1997.
8. Williams SR. *Essentials of Nutrition and Diet Therapy.* 6th ed. St. Louis: Mosby; 1996.
9. McKenry LM, Salerno E. *Mosby's Pharmacology in Nursing.* 19th ed. St. Louis: Mosby; 1995.
10. Sherwen LN, Scoloveno MA, Weingarten CT. *Nursing Care of the Childbearing Family.* 2nd ed. Norwalk, CT: Appleton & Lange; 1995.
11. Avery ME, First L, eds. *Pediatric Medicine.* 2nd ed. Baltimore: Williams & Wilkins; 1994.
12. Betz CL, Hunsberger MM, Wright S. *Family-centered Nursing Care of Children.* 2nd ed. Philadelphia: Saunders; 1994.
13. Carroll P. Spotting the differences in respiratory care. *RN.* 1996;59:26–29.
14. American Cancer Society. *Cancer Facts & Figures—1997.* Atlanta, GA: American Cancer Society; 1997.
15. US Department of Health and Human Services. Public Health Service, Centers for Disease Control, Center for Chronic Disease and Health Promotion, Office of Smoking and Health. *The Health Benefits of Smoking Cessation.* DHHS pub no. 90–8416; 1990.
16. Hamel L, Oberle K. Cardiovascular risk screening for women. *Clin Nurs Specialist.* 1996;10:275–279.
17. Centers for Disease Control. Cigarette-attributable mortality and years of potential life lost—United States, 1990. *MMWR.* 1993;42:645–649.
18. American Thoracic Society. Cigarette smoking and health. *Am J Respir Crit Care Med.* 1996;153:861–865.
19. McGinnis JM, Foege WH. Actual causes of death in the United States. *JAMA.* 1993;270:2207–2212.
20. Osterud H. *Dealing with the Nicotine Addiction.* Portland: Oregon Health Sciences University; 1989.
21. American Lung Association. *Breath in Danger.* New York: American Lung Association; 1989.
22. Berkow R. *The Merck Manual.* 16th ed. Rahway, NJ: Merck & Co; 1992.
23. Swanlund SL. Body positioning and the elderly with Adult Respiratory Distress Syndrome. *J Gerontol Nurs.* 1996;22:46–50.
24. Carroll P. Pulse oximetry at your fingertips. *RN.* 1997;60:22–26.
25. Leidy NK. Functional performance in people with chronic obstructive pulmonary disease. *Image.* 1995;27:23–34.

31

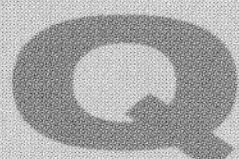

Recently, 72-year-old Ms. Richards has had repeated episodes of shortness of breath, violent coughing spells with occasional bloody sputum, and some pain associated with respiration. After a complete physical examination, including a chest x-ray and lung biopsy, Ms. Richards is diagnosed with lung cancer. Today, she is being admitted to the hospital for surgery and chemotherapy. During her initial admission assessment, Ms. Richards mentions that she has been a "nervous wreck about all of this for weeks" and she is "very tired." Ms. Richards also states that she is very anxious about the treatment she is about to receive, sad about her future, and worried about her family's response to her illness.

What symptoms does Ms. Richards exhibit that may interfere with her sleep?

What factors may interfere with her sleep during hospitalization?

What purpose do REM and NREM sleep serve?

What interventions could her nurse implement to encourage satisfactory sleep for Ms. Richards during her hospitalization?

How can Ms. Richards and her family be involved in the plan to encourage satisfactory sleep?

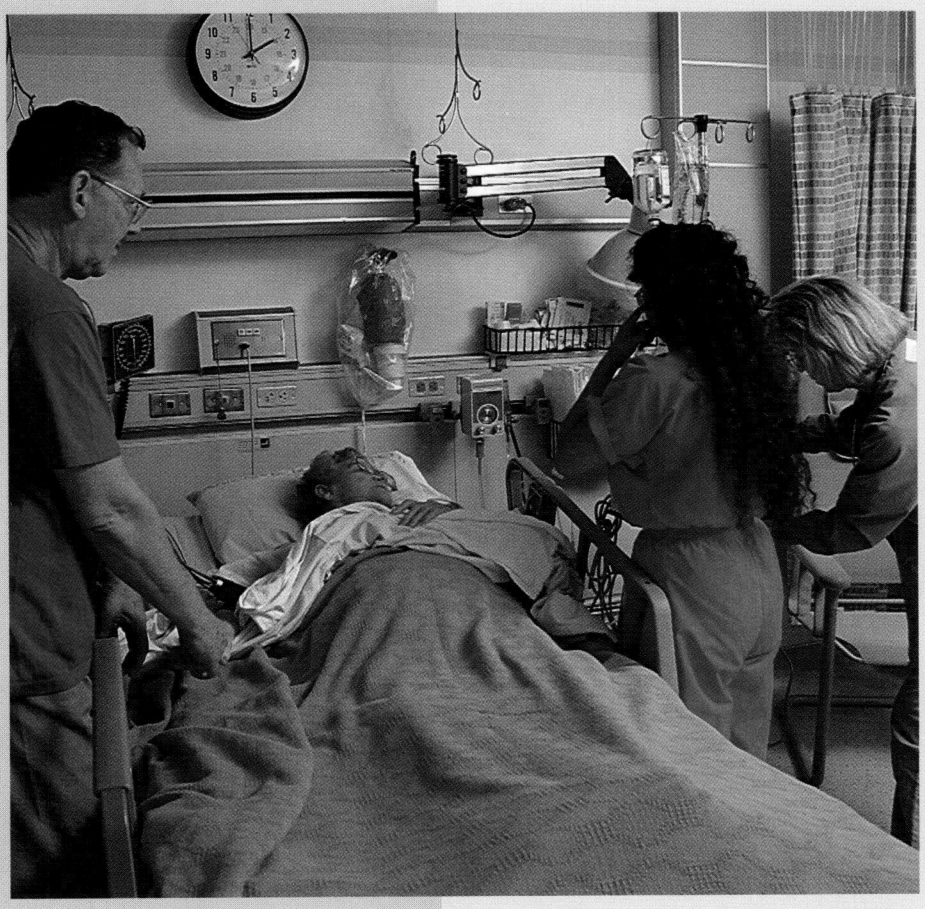

Sleep–Rest Patterns

Julie E. Johnson

CHAPTER OUTLINE

About one-third of our lives is spent sleeping. Experts know that sleep is a normal and complex physiologic rhythm that permits periods of nonresponding to the environment.[1] Although the individual appears to be idle during sleep, activity increases in certain parts of the brain: the hypothalamus, thalamus, and basal forebrain. In addition, sleep is closely associated with biochemical and neuroanatomic processes, nerve cell activity, bodily movement, and changes in heart rate, blood pressure, and temperature.[2]

The purpose of sleep is a mystery; however, it is necessary to health and a sense of well-being.[1] Loss of sleep results in daytime sleepiness, alteration in mood, and inability to concentrate.[3] Sleep loss of greater than 48 hours results in altered hormone production, decreased psychomotor ability, and diminished perceptual ability. Hallucinations, nervousness, and irritability occur with continued sleep loss.[4]

Sleep is an individual experience.[1] Different people sleep for varying lengths of time. Some sleep better at certain times of the day or night than others. Consequently, people have varying degrees of satisfaction with their sleep experience. Difficulty sleeping is a common reason why individuals seek care from health professionals.

Nurses play a key role in maintaining a patient's sleep–rest pattern and assessing and managing sleep problems. Through a collaborative approach, the nurse and patient share information about the patient's sleep patterns and problems, and ways that healthful sleep can be maintained or sleep problems handled. This chapter discusses healthful sleep patterns and factors affecting them, alterations in sleep–rest patterns, sleep–rest assessment, nursing diagnoses related to sleep–rest status, and nursing interventions to promote sleep and rest.

SECTION 1
UNDERSTANDING SLEEP AND REST

OPTIMAL SLEEP AND REST

Rest and sleep, both basic human needs, are not the same. **Rest** is a period of inactivity that is dependent on the simultaneous relaxation of the body and mind (Fig. 31–1).[5] A person who lies quietly in bed cannot rest if stress and worry cause muscular tension. Resting prepares the individual for sleep.

Sleep is often defined as a period of time during which bodily functions are partially suspended and consciousness is partially or completely interrupted.[2] Temperature, pulse, blood pressure, and respirations decrease; kidneys are less productive; and digestive secretions diminish.[6] As muscles relax, the basal metabolic rate declines and most reflexes disappear or weaken, except for the cough reflex. Sleep renews the body's energy.

REGULATION OF SLEEP–WAKEFULNESS

Circadian Rhythms

Circadian rhythms refer to those events that occur at approximately 24-hour intervals.[6] These rhythms include the sleep–wake cycle, core body temperature changes, and fluctuations in hor-

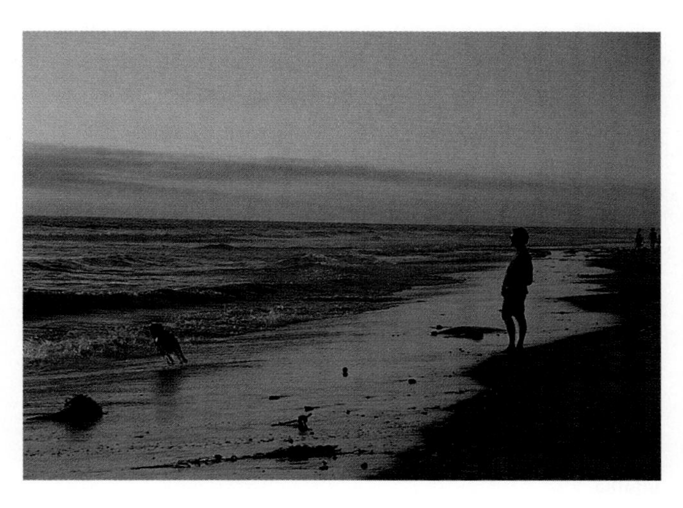

Figure 31–1. By giving oneself time to think and relax, a person achieves rest for mind and body.

monal secretions. They are interrelated and coincide with given external events, such as day and night and light and dark. For example, a person's body temperature is highest while awake and is at its lowest while asleep. A change in the timing of the circadian rhythms may be precipitated by a change in the environment. For example, people who fly across several time zones must adjust to sleeping at a different time than they do at home. Their inherent circadian rhythms must change to accommodate the new environment. This process may require several days, and some people never adjust.

Neuroendocrine activity—release of growth hormone, adrenocorticotropic hormone (ACTH), adrenocortical hormones, and antidiuretic hormone—has been linked to the 24-hour sleep–wake cycle.[2,6] A disruption in the individual's inherent sleep–wake cycle alters the secretion and release of these hormones. As a result, many target organs and body systems are affected by the changing levels of these hormones.

Circadian rhythms are subject to individual variation. People differ in when they function best and when they prefer to go to bed. Hospitals often overlook these differences, and staff organize routines around work flow rather than patient sleep needs.[7]

Neurologic Regulation of Sleep–Wakefulness

The **ascending reticular activating system** (RAS) is responsible for awareness, consciousness, wakefulness, and arousal. Increased activity in this part of the brain results in wakefulness; decreased, or inadequate, activity causes sleep. Irreversible coma may occur when the reticular activating system is destroyed.[6]

CRITICAL QUERY

Kirkwood and Sood[8] point out that the neuronal complexes regulating sleep–wakefulness are located in the basal forebrain, brainstem, and hypothalamus. What role does the reticular activating system (RAS) play in sleep–wakefulness? How can nurses apply understanding of RAS activity to help patients with sleep problems?

To regulate wakefulness, the RAS must be stimulated from external sources. Pain impulses, visual and auditory signals, visceral sensations, and proprioceptive signals from the muscles will cause arousal. Once arousal occurs, RAS excitation is maintained through three feedback systems:

- The RAS increases activity in the cerebral cortex. In turn, the cerebral cortex enhances RAS activity.
- Increased RAS activity enhances muscular activity throughout the body, which promotes greater RAS response.
- The RAS stimulates the release of epinephrine from the adrenal medulla, which increases RAS activity.

After a period of wakefulness, RAS cells become less excitable and activity of the feedback systems decreases. As a result, the reticular activating system is further depressed and sleep occurs. After a period of inactivity or sleep, RAS excitability is reestablished, and wakefulness occurs and is maintained for a period of time.

Chemical Regulation of Sleep–Wakefulness

Chemicals that influence sleep–wakefulness including epinephrine, high concentrations of norepinephrine, dopamine, serotonin, indoleamine, and catecholamines are found in the brainstem.[6] Dopamine and norepinephrine are associated with wakefulness and rapid eye movement (REM) sleep; serotonin is linked to nonrapid eye movement (NREM) sleep. However, the exact mechanism by which these chemicals influence sleep is unclear.

HEALTHFUL SLEEP PATTERNS

Healthful sleep patterns are composed of nonrapid eye movement sleep and rapid eye movement sleep.[1] These patterns change throughout the life cycle, amounts of sleep decreasing with age. **Nonrapid eye movement (NREM) sleep,** is that period of sleep during which no eye movements can be observed and the eyelids are still. There are four stages of NREM sleep. They are discussed in the following section. NREM sleep is a time of energy conservation and tissue repair.[5]

Rapid eye movement (REM) sleep is that period of sleep when eye movements occur and the eyelids twitch.[1,6] REM sleep serves the following functions: it restores one mentally; is important for memory, learning, and psychological adaptation; provides a review of the day's events; and allows information to be categorized and assimilated into the brain's storage system. The need for REM sleep increases when one is faced with new experiences and psychological stress.[2] The consequences of REM sleep deprivation include irritability, apathy, increased sensitivity to pain, and a lack of alertness. A repeated loss of REM sleep results in increased anxiety, decreased coping abilities, confusion, and disorientation.[2,3]

The basic physiologic mechanisms underlying the stages of sleep are complex and much is unknown about them. It is believed that a minimum of three major neurotransmitters are associated with the sleep stages: serotonin, acetylcholine, and norepinephrine.[2,6]

Because serotonin is responsible for sleep onset and sleep maintenance, it initiates the physiologic mechanisms involved in stages I, II, III, and IV (NREM) sleep.[2,6] Little is known about the causes of serotonin activation.

The neurotransmitter acetylcholine is responsible for maintaining REM sleep. Norepinephrine may be involved in maintaining wakefulness.

NREM SLEEP STAGES

Stage I

Stage I of NREM sleep lasts only a few minutes and is the lightest of the sleep levels.[1,3] It is characterized by decreases in temperature and in respiratory, pulse, and metabolic rates. A slight decrease in blood pressure occurs and the muscles relax. The individual is easily aroused in this stage.

Stage II

During stage II, the individual becomes more relaxed, but continues to be easily awakened. This stage lasts approximately 5 to 10 minutes.[3]

Stages III and IV

Stages III and IV are the deepest levels of sleep and last from 15 to 30 minutes.[2,3] The sleeper is not disturbed by sensory stimuli and seldom moves. In stage III, there is loss of muscle tone (the muscles are most relaxed), reflexes diminish, and snoring may occur. The person may be aroused by touch only. Stage IV sleep rests, relaxes, and physically restores the body.

REM SLEEP

Following approximately 90 minutes of sleep, the individual returns from stage IV up through the lighter stages of sleep to stage I.[3,6] Rather than entering stage I or awakening, one enters REM sleep. This stage is characterized by frequent bursts of rapid eye movements, dreams, muscular twitching, and profound muscle relaxation. Erections may occur in men. The sleeper is most difficult to awaken during this stage.

Following the period of REM sleep, the sleeper again descends through stages II to IV.[2] Everyone averages 4 to 5 of these sleep cycles per night, each lasting approximately 90 to 100 minutes. With each cycle, stage IV sleep decreases and REM sleep increases. Thus, the major portion of stage IV sleep occurs early in the night, the majority of REM sleep takes place in the last several hours before awakening. When awakened during any stage of this cycle, one must resume sleep at stage I and progress through the stages to REM sleep.

FACTORS AFFECTING SLEEP AND REST

Age, environment, and physical and psychological factors affect the quantity and quality of sleep.[3] The effect of these factors varies among individuals.

AGE

Sleep changes from one developmental stage to another.[3]

Infants

Infants sleep about 14 to 18 hours a day. Sleep episodes last from 20 minutes to 6 hours, and are evenly distributed over 24 hours.[2,3]

By the age of 6 months, infants experience 3 to 4 sleep periods during 24 hours.[2] This pattern occurs as a long period of nighttime sleep, with shorter afternoon and morning naps. By the age of 6 months, 80 percent of infants sleep through the night.

Infants with food allergies or colic are irritable and uncomfortable and experience delayed sleep onset.[2] Parents who are accustomed to providing comfort for such an infant may have difficulty limiting their attention when distress is no longer present. They should be encouraged to intervene only when a problem, such as a wet diaper, exists.

Toddlers

By 2 years of age, most toddlers sleep 12 to 14 hours in a 24-hour period, and no longer nap in the morning.[2] Most children stop napping completely by the age of 3. Efforts to continue the child's napping beyond the child's need, excessive nighttime fluid intake, illness, medication, and fear of the dark may result in sleep problems. Establishing a regular daytime schedule and bedtime routine, and offering comfort measures (for example, a doll or blanket) may help establish sleep patterns.

Children and Adolescents

Total sleep time decreases very slowly to 8 hours a day between the ages of 4 years and adolescence.[2] Difficulty falling asleep is less prevalent; however, sleepwalking, sleeptalking, confusional arousals, and enuresis (bedwetting) may occur. Such episodes are usually caused by stress or anxiety.

Young Adults

Normal young adults usually sleep from 7 to 8 hours per night. In the United States, this age group participates in a variety of nighttime activities. Except in cultures where a siesta is the norm, young adults usually do not nap.

Middle-aged and Older Adults

The middle-aged adult begins to experience an increased time to sleep onset, an increased number of nighttime awakenings, and less total sleep time.[1] These trends continue with advanced age, and are more pronounced in women than men.[9] Older adults also return to napping, with men napping more than women. Common disorders of initiating and maintaining sleep and excessive somno-

> **INSIGHTS FROM NURSING LITERATURE**
> **MEETING PATIENTS' SLEEP NEEDS**
>
> *Southwell MT, Wistow G. Sleep in hospitals at night: are patients' needs met?* J Adv Nurs. *1995;21:1101–1109.*
>
> Noting that sleep deprivation is common among hospitalized patients, and that noise, light, treatments, pain, and other discomforts are the causes, the researchers studied the hospital inpatient night. Their findings showed that sleepless patients complain about uncomfortable beds and pillows, of being too warm or too worried to sleep, or of other patients' noise or telephones ringing. Although patients and nurses both perceived that patients did not get as much sleep as they needed, the study also found that nurses were not always aware of the sleeplessness of their patients—pointing to the importance of systematically asking patients about their sleep experiences.

lence in this age group are discussed in the *Alterations in Sleep–Rest Patterns* section later in the chapter.

ENVIRONMENT

Loud or unfamiliar noise, uncomfortable room temperature, lighting, type and size of bed, mattress firmness, and the loss or addition of a bed partner may influence one's ability to fall asleep and remain asleep.[4] Soft music may help.

PHYSICAL FACTORS

Regular physical exercise early in the day promotes sleep.[10] Excessive exercise done late in the day or a change in the usual exercise pattern may interfere with sleep.

Prolonged use of certain medications, such as sedatives, antidepressants, barbiturates, or anxiolytics, alter the sleep–wake cycle.[8] For example, a sedative used for 3 days will enhance sleep. One used for 2 months, however, may cause difficulty falling asleep due to drug tolerance. Prescription and nonprescription drugs used to treat other health problems, such as hypertension, may also interfere with sleep due to their secondary effects.[8]

The amino acid L-tryptophan enhances one's ability to fall asleep,[5] and is found in such foods as dairy products, meat, peanuts, green leafy vegetables, and beans. Sleeplessness, on the other hand, is caused by caffeine in coffee, tea, chocolate, and cola drinks.[3] Alcoholic beverages induce sleep; however, excessive alcohol causes nighttime wakenings and difficulty returning to sleep.[8]

Physical discomfort, such as the pain from arthritis or an uncomfortable position, interfere with sleep. Potentially, any illness can disrupt sleep.[3] Individuals with cardiac, pulmonary, renal, gastrointestinal, or urologic disorders may be particularly vulnerable to sleep disturbance.

PSYCHOLOGICAL FACTORS

Grief, anxiety, worry, depression, and stress lead to sleep loss in some individuals and to excessive sleep in others.[1,4] Alterations in one's daily routine, working various shifts, or participation in late-night social activities also change sleep patterns.

INSIGHTS FROM NURSING LITERATURE
SLEEP PROBLEMS IN WOMEN

Clark AJ, Flowers J, Boots L. Shettar S. Sleep disturbance in mid-life women. J Adv Nurs. *1995;22:562–568.*

The researchers used a sleep-disturbance questionnaire, an anxiety measurement scale, and blood hormone analysis to explore the relationship between sleep disturbance and the psychological and physiologic status of middle-aged women. They found no statistically significant relationship between sleep disturbance and menopausal state, anxiety, or depression. As the authors note, their findings challenge the widely held opinion that sleep disturbance in midlife women is caused by hot flashes or depression.

COLLABORATIVE STRATEGY
FACTORS AFFECTING SLEEP AND REST

Although the body's physiologic processes normally support optimal cycles of sleep and rest, many factors alter the internal mechanisms that regulate those cycles. To minimize the factors that interfere with sleep, nurses exchange information with the patient valuable to promoting an optimal sleep pattern.

ALTERED SLEEP–REST PATTERNS

Each alteration in sleep patterns has its own set of symptoms. The most common and severe alterations in adult sleep are described here. Age variations are noted when applicable.

INSOMNIA

Insomnia is the subjective complaint of having difficulty falling asleep, remaining asleep, and/or wakening too early in the morning.[11] About 50 percent of the population experiences insomnia at some time during their life.[8] It is more prevalent in middle-aged and older adults, and its incidence increases dramatically in those older than 65 years.[5] The common causes of insomnia are environmental, physical, and psychological factors previously described. Insomnia may be transient (2 to 3 nights), short term (1 to 3 weeks), or chronic (more than 3 weeks or recurring over the individual's life).[5,8]

SLEEP APNEA

Sleep apnea is the repeated, temporary loss of breathing for at least 20 seconds while asleep.[2,8] There are three types of sleep apnea: central, obstructive, and mixed. Central apnea is caused by the central nervous system's failure to control respiration, and is characterized by the absence of diaphragmatic movement and airflow. Obstructive apnea is caused by an obstruction of the upper airway, and is characterized by diaphragmatic movement and the absence of airflow. Mixed apnea is a combination of central and obstructive apnea. Individuals with sleep apnea experience loud snoring, gasping for air, and daytime drowsiness. Sleep apnea is prevalent in infants born before 34 weeks of gestation or in those weighing less than 1500 grams,[12] overweight middle-aged men,[2] and those older than 60 years.[5]

PERIODIC LIMB MOVEMENT SYNDROME

Periodic limb movement syndrome (PLMS) is characterized by twitching of the legs that occurs at 20 to 60-second intervals while asleep.[1] Twitching causes a brief awakening, which alternates with periods of quiet sleep. PLMS may occur in children and adolescents, but is most prevalent in adults older than 50 years. Individuals with PLMS report insomnia, daytime drowsiness, and cold or hot feet. Its cause is unknown.

NARCOLEPSY

Narcolepsy is a chronic condition characterized by repeated, uncontrollable episodes of sleep and drowsiness from which the individual may be easily awakened.[8] Onset is usually in the second decade of life, and peaks at 14 years of age.[2] Narcolepsy occurs in men and women equally, and tends to run in families. Daytime sleepiness, hallucinations, and loss of muscle control are common manifestations.

SECTION 2

ASSESSMENT OF SLEEP–REST PATTERNS

SLEEP–REST DATA COLLECTION

In carrying out the nursing process to help patients meet their sleep-rest needs, nurses use the knowledge they have of sleep patterns and alterations in sleep. For example, a 55-year-old overweight man tells the nurse that his wife complains about his snoring and he is drowsy during the day. The nurse knows that these complaints are common in obstructive sleep apnea. The nurse assesses the patient to determine the severity and frequency of these symptoms. Data reveal that symptoms occur nightly and that the patient's wife has noticed he seems to stop breathing while asleep. The nurse uses this information to collaborate with the patient and his wife and refers them to a sleep disorders clinic.

An assessment of a patient's sleep status is necessary in order to plan individualized, comprehensive nursing care. Assessment entails gathering information related to the patient's sleep–rest history and performing a sleep–rest examination.

Collaboration with the patient, family, and health care team members is essential to ensure accurate assessment. Ideas and information are exchanged freely about sleep patterns and sleep problems. The collaboration facilitates establishing a trusting, productive, and ongoing relationship between the patient and nurse as they develop the plan of care to manage sleep problems.

A complete history, physical examination, and review of pertinent laboratory reports are essential to assess sleep–rest patterns. The nurse may gather information from the patient, family, physician's report of the medical examination, and medical history.

SLEEP–REST HISTORY

Primary Concern

The patient's primary concern may be directly or indirectly related to sleep. Some complaints directly related to sleep are excessive daytime fatigue and loss of appetite as well as narcolepsy, sleep apnea, insomnia, bedwetting, and sleepwalking. Concerns indirectly related to sleep are discussed in the next sections.

Current Understanding

The patient may perceive that a current health problem interferes with obtaining satisfactory sleep. For example, a respiratory or cardiovascular problem (such as pneumonia or congestive heart failure) may be the patient's primary concern. Shortness of breath associated with the problem may inhibit sleep. Similarly, a sudden onset of acute chest pain may cause difficulty falling asleep or remaining asleep. The same is true for someone experiencing chronic pain such as from arthritis. The treatment of the problem may also interfere with the patient's usual sleep patterns, as when diuretics given for congestive heart failure increase the need to void at night. Therefore, it is important that the nurse ask about the patient's current understanding of the health problem and treatment in relation to any possible impact on the patient's sleep. For example, the nurse should discuss any recent changes in sleep patterns with the patient. It is important to assess when these changes occurred, what precipitated the changes, and how significant the changes are to the patient. The nurse should also ascertain the onset, duration, and exacerbating and relieving conditions of the current health problem. In assessing the impact of the health problem on the patient's sleep, it is also appropriate and necessary for the nurse to discuss any alterations in sleep patterns with the patient's sleep partner. The partner can often identify disturbances that the patient is not aware of, such as snoring, muscle twitching, and restlessness.

Past Health Problems/Experiences

The patient's past health problems/experiences may disclose chronic problems or treatments related to sleep. Ask if the patient has had previous problems with sleep or with illnesses or injuries that have affected sleep. If so, determine when, and the severity, treatment, and any residual effects of the illness or treatment. The current use of prescription or over-the-counter medication that could affect sleep should be noted (ie, those that act on the neurologic, endocrine, respiratory, cardiovascular, or gastrointestinal systems). It is important to ask if any drugs are used to induce or maintain sleep, how long they have been taken, how often they are used, and whether any changes in usual sleep patterns have been noted since taking the medication. The following example illustrates the importance of past health problems/experiences.

> A nursing student is visiting the home of 3-year-old Karen and her mother to complete a developmental screening for class. As part of the screening, the student must obtain Karen's past history. Upon questioning Karen's mother, the student learns that Karen has had frequent upper respiratory infections followed by otitis media. Karen's pediatrician has recommended that her mother administer antihistamines to Karen at the onset of an upper respiratory infection in an attempt to prevent the otitis. Karen's mother states that she gave the antihistamines several times, but after several days Karen woke up screaming at night. The mother also states she becomes frightened because she doesn't know what is wrong with Karen. Because the nursing student knows that antihistamines may cause restlessness and interfere with children's usual sleep patterns, she decides to educate Karen's mother about the medication. She also recommends that the mother ask the pediatrician to change Karen's medication in an attempt to alleviate her sleep problems.

Personal, Family, and Social History

The patient's personal, family, and social history can provide information for making nursing diagnoses about sleep status. Table 31–1 lists suggested questions for obtaining this information. Anything that the individual does each night to prepare for sleep should be considered a bedtime routine. For example, many people have a snack, watch television, listen to the radio, bathe, brush their teeth, pray, or read before bedtime. The nurse should also inquire about the importance of these activities to the patient and what happens to the sleep pattern if they are omitted from bedtime preparation. When feasible, routines should be incorporated in the

TABLE 31-1. SLEEP-REST HISTORY: PERSONAL, FAMILY, AND SOCIAL HISTORY QUESTIONS

A. Vocational
1. What type of work do you do?
2. What hours do you usually work?
3. Does your work involve physical activity?
4. Have you noticed drowsiness or inability to concentrate while you work?

B. Home and Family
1. Are you married?
2. Any difficulties with a relationship that disturbs your sleep? How?
3. Do you have children? Ages? How do they sleep at night?
4. Do you have other family members living with you? Who? Ages?
5. What type of care, if any, do they require? How do they sleep at night?
6. Describe a typical day.

C. Social and Leisure
1. What are your favorite leisure activities?
2. Do drowsiness or feelings of tiredness ever interfere with these activities?
3. Have you given up any of these activities due to tiredness or lack of energy?

D. Sexual
1. Has your sexual relationship been satisfactory?
2. Have you noticed changes related to your current illness? If so, what?
3. Does tiredness interfere with this relationship?
4. Do you have sexual concerns that disturb your sleep? How?

E. Habits

Exercise
1. Do you exercise regularly? How often?
2. What time of day do you exercise?
3. Have you given up exercising due to tiredness or feeling sleepy?
4. Do you notice any changes in your sleep when your exercise pattern changes?

Sleep
1. Describe a typical night's sleep.
2. How many hours do you sleep at night?
3. Do you feel rested in the morning?
4. Do you nap? How often? How long?
5. Do you feel rested after napping?
6. Have you ever been told that you snore? That you're a restless sleeper?
7. How often do you awaken at night?
8. Do you have difficulty returning to sleep?
9. Do you have a bedtime routine? If so, what is it?
10. Do you need assistance with bedtime routines?
11. Have you had difficulty sleeping since becoming ill?
12. Has this illness altered your sleep patterns?
13. If so, how? Do you think you sleep too much? Too little?
14. Describe factors in the environment that interfere with your sleep (noise, room temperature, being awakened for treatments or medication, roommate).

Diet
1. How many meals do you eat per day?
2. Do you snack? When?
3. Do you ever have trouble sleeping due to indigestion?

Beverages
1. Do you use alcohol?
2. What do you usually drink?
3. How much do you drink in a typical week?
4. Have you ever noticed any difficulty sleeping after using alcohol?
5. Do you use caffeine? Tea? Coffee? Soft drinks?
6. How much of each per day?
7. What time do you have your last cup of coffee? Tea? Soft drink?
8. Do you notice sleep changes when you use caffeine at night?

Other Substances
1. Do you use sleeping pills? How often?
2. What other medications do you take?
3. Do you use diet pills? Marijuana? Tobacco? Water pills? How often?

F. Psychological/Coping
1. Do you feel "blue" or downhearted? How often?
2. Do you feel like crying? How often?
3. Do you feel restless? Nervous? Irritable? How often?
4. Do you have problems making decisions?
5. Do you still enjoy things you used to?
6. Do you get upset easily? How often?
7. What do you usually do when you are "blue" (substitute "nervous," "irritable," "restless," "upset" as needed) to feel better?
8. Are you able to talk with anyone when you are "blue" (nervous, irritable, restless, upset)?
9. How do you sleep when you are "blue" (nervous, irritable, restless, upset)?

patient's plan of care. Nurses also need to gather information about the patient's family. What changes in the family relationships could adversely influence sleep? For example, a newborn baby, confused elderly adult, fearful child, or unsatisfactory marital relationship may alter sleep patterns. The following example illustrates the use of this information.

Mr. Warren is admitted to the medical floor for treatment of a gastric ulcer. While gathering his personal, family, and social history, the nurse notes that Mr. Warren follows a very specific bedtime routine. He brushes his teeth, takes a warm bath, listens to the radio, and likes to use two pillows. He states that this routine is extremely important to him. He also indicates that he usually retires at 10:30 PM and awakens at 6:30 AM. The nurse uses this information to plan with the health care team to maintain Mr. Warren's bedtime routine during his hospital stay. The nurse also consults with his physician regarding the ordering of medication that has a long duration of action and so does not need to be administered during the nighttime hours.

Subjective Manifestations

A review of subjective manifestations furnishes a complete picture of the symptoms the patient perceives as related to sleep problems. Chapter 17 provides sample questions for subjective manifestations.

SLEEP–REST EXAMINATION

Assessments of the integument, head, neck, eyes, chest, abdomen, musculoskeletal system, and neurologic system are major components of the sleep–rest examination. Abnormalities could precipitate sleep disturbances or complicate existing sleep problems. Many clues regarding sleep status can be obtained from general observation of the patient. These observations may indicate other areas needing more detailed assessment.

Objective Manifestations

General Observations. General observation of the patient's overall appearance indicates status of rest and alertness. Note the patient's posture. Is it slumped forward? Is the body properly aligned? Guarding or a stiff posture suggests pain that can interfere with sleep. Poor posture can indicate tiredness caused by poor sleep. Correct posture can indicate feeling rested and alert.

The patient's gait and motor activity should also be noted. Patients who move with vigor and perform tasks with enthusiasm are indicating that they have energy provided by adequate sleep and rest. Loss of sleep may cause uncoordinated movements even when performing simple tasks.

During this general observation period, the nurse should also assess the patient's facial features. Eyes that appear dull or puffy, have darkened areas under or around them, accompanied by a masklike facial expression, may indicate a lack of sleep.

Patients' general physical condition; psychological state, orientation to time, place, and person; anxiety level; and general mood should be noted. Prolonged loss of sleep often leads to disorientation, nervousness, and mood swings. A distinct personality change in someone who is sleep-deprived may be noted. For example, a usually cheerful person may look unhappy and cry without provocation. Upon questioning, this individual may admit to feeling anxious, a sense of not being "real," or feeling as if the head is going to explode. Individuals who are not sleeping well often have vague complaints of not feeling well in general. Mental status is usually assessed throughout the sleep examination. If the patient is inattentive to the nurse, disoriented, anxious, uncooperative, or has vague physical complaints, further examination is warranted. Methods for further assessment are discussed in the section on the neurologic examination later in the chapter.

Personal observation during sleep provides another objective means of examining the patient. It is also important for the nurse to observe whether the patient appears rested after sleeping.

Integument. During the sleep examination the integument should be observed for color, texture, and integrity. Healthy-appearing skin indicates adequate rest. Cyanotic skin may indicate a cardiac or pulmonary problem, such as bronchitis, that may interfere with sleep. Impaired skin integrity (such as painful sores or pruritic rashes) may interfere with the ability to obtain adequate sleep due to discomfort.

HEENT. In addition to the assessment of facial features discussed, a head, eyes, ears, nose, and throat (HEENT) examination should be completed. The nurse should determine whether the patient experiences any difficulty breathing through the nose when lying down. Obstruction of the nasal passages can be disruptive to sleep. Any neck vein distension should be noted, as it may indicate congestive heart failure (CHF). Patients with CHF typically have difficulty sleeping in a flat position. The patient should also be assessed for distorted vision. Prolonged sleep loss causes the individual to see halos around lights or a webbing effect on the floor.

Chest. Chest inspection may disclose conditions that could interfere with sleep; for example, the "barrel-shaped chest" of chronic obstructive pulmonary disease (COPD) or the arrhythmia of a cardiac abnormality. The respiratory rate, depth, rhythm, and quality should also be inspected. Shallow breathing, labored breathing, coughing, or rapid breathing may disrupt sleep.

Chest auscultation will detect heart rate, rhythm, and any abnormal closure of the valves. Disturbances in any of these areas may interrupt sleep either through physical symptoms or from psychological distress due to fear or anxiety over one's cardiac status.

Abnormal breath sounds, such as crackles or wheezes caused by secretions or obstructions, may also be detected upon auscultation. If they are present, it is necessary to assess whether these respiratory problems interfere with the patient's rest or sleep. Refer to Chap. 17 for a detailed discussion of the chest assessment.

Abdomen. In addition to the questions asked about gastrointestinal function, the nurse should auscultate the abdomen for the presence of hyperactive or hypoactive bowel sounds. Such sounds may indicate abnormalities that interfere with sleep, such as diarrhea or

COLLABORATIVE STRATEGY
DATA COLLECTION

Collaboration on sleep problems involves the exchange of information concerning sleep. In the hospital setting, the nurse and patient need to discuss the patient's usual activity and bedtime routines to determine how an optimal sleep–rest pattern can be maintained. In other settings, the nurse and patient may also need to identify new approaches for solving rest and sleep problems.

CRITICAL QUERY

In a study conducted by Southwell and Wistow,[7] hospitalized patients reported that numerous factors prevented them from receiving sufficient sleep. What parameters should nurses assess to determine if their hospitalized patients are receiving adequate sleep?

constipation. Percussion and palpation of the abdomen may reveal an enlarged liver, spleen, or areas of flatus in the intestines. If either is present, inquire about symptoms that may affect sleep, such as pain, tenderness, generalized itching, or the need to pass flatus at night. Chapter 17 provides more detail about the abdominal examination.

Musculoskeletal System. For the sleep examination, the musculoskeletal system should be assessed for joint mobility and muscle tone and strength (see Chap. 33). The results of this assessment indicate how much activity the patient can tolerate. Also ask how much physical activity is engaged in on a weekly basis. Moderate amounts of exercise several hours before bedtime enhances sleep.

Neurologic System. If information gathered during the general observation period of the patient's mental status indicates a problem, further neurologic assessment is necessary. Additional assessment of mental status is part of the neurologic examination and involves determining the patient's state of awareness, reaction time in performing motor activities, and the capacity for recall of recent and remote memories. The nurse also needs to assess the patient's attention span, ability to understand what is being said, and degree of cooperation during the examination. With progressive loss of sleep, the patient's state of awareness and attention span decrease while reaction time increases. The individual may exhibit difficulty in recalling the timing of recent events as one day blends into the next. Remote memory remains intact. The patient also has difficulty understanding what is being said and may become less cooperative in the plan of care. The individual with severe sleep deprivation may even be unable to understand and carry out simple commands, such as "Please be seated" or "Take a deep breath."

Other neurologic symptoms may develop with sleep loss. The patient should be assessed for skeletal muscle strength, evidence of muscle tremor, and degree of coordination while performing motor tasks (see Chaps. 32 and 33). Lack of sleep results in loss of muscle strength, tremor, and uncoordination.

DIAGNOSTIC TESTS

Objective methods for examining the patient with a sleep dysfunction include the administration of a **nocturnal polysomnogram.** This test involves measuring the sleeping patient's brain waves through an electroencephalogram (EEG), eye movements through an electrooculogram (EOG), and muscle movements through an electromyogram (EMG). As part of the examination, the patient's respiratory rate, oxygen saturation, and leg movements while asleep are also measured.

The nocturnal polysomnogram reveals how long it takes the patient to fall asleep, shows the night's progress through the stages of NREM and REM sleep, and indicates the soundness of sleep. Although the test is performed by someone other than a nurse, the results are used as assessment data.

▲ NURSING DIAGNOSIS OF SLEEP–REST STATUS

Analyzing the data obtained in the sleep–rest history and examination indicates whether a patient is experiencing a sleep problem that could be corrected by nursing treatment: a sleep pattern disturbance. This nursing diagnosis and associated etiologies are discussed in the next section and in Table 31–2. Assessment data may also suggest other nursing diagnoses that may result from disturbed sleep–rest patterns or be caused by sleep disruptions.

SLEEP PATTERN DISTURBANCE

A sleep pattern disturbance is a condition in which an individual is at risk for or experiencing changes in sleep patterns that cause discomfort or interfere with the desired lifestyle. The quality or quantity of sleep is altered for a prolonged time period, not only 1 or 2 days. Often the reason for the disturbed sleep is an emotional or physical illness. The prolonged loss of sleep may interfere with the individual's emotional, physical, or daytime functioning.

STATING THE SLEEP–REST DIAGNOSIS

Data analysis to determine the exact nature of the sleep problem and its etiology should result in a precise statement regarding the patient's sleep status. The assessment data provides clues that may be used to refine broad statements from the taxonomy (such as "sleep pattern disturbance related to impaired bowel function") into concise statements with defining characteristics. For example, a more precise statement of this broad diagnosis would be "sleep pattern disturbance related to diarrhea as evidenced by eight liquid stools from 1 to 3 AM, complaints of the continued need to use the bathroom during the night, and complaints of not feeling rested."

Complete assessment of a patient's sleep patterns is an important aspect of comprehensive care. After arriving at an accurate diagnosis, nurses collaborate with patients, family, and other health care professionals to manage the identified sleep disturbance.

SECTION 3

NURSE-PATIENT MANAGEMENT OF SLEEP-REST PATTERNS

Management of sleep problems involves collaborative nurse–patient planning to meet the patient's sleep needs. Appropriate nursing implementation to enhance, promote, or reestablish sleep patterns is determined by the patient's level of care and the cause of disrupted sleep.

▲ PLANNING FOR OPTIMAL SLEEP AND REST

An effective patient care plan communicates the desired outcomes for care and the methods for achieving those outcomes. The statements of desired outcomes should specifically describe the changes in sleep or rest anticipated as a result of nursing care. These statements provide a guide to specific implementation that can be used, and criteria by which the effectiveness of these implementations can be evaluated.

Sleep outcomes are best determined by mutual goal setting. From the assessment data, the nurse formulates perceptions about disruptions in the patient's sleep and what can realistically be done to alleviate the problem. The nurse then shares these perceptions with the patient and asks for input. In this way, the patient

TABLE 31-2. NURSING DIAGNOSES: SLEEP-REST PATTERNS

Nursing Diagnosis	Defining Characteristics: *Subjective Data*	Defining Characteristics: *Objective Data*	Etiology
Sleep pattern disturbance *6.2.1*	States pain causes difficulty falling asleep. States awakens frequently during night because of pain. Reports not feeling rested.	Frequent yawning Increasing irritability Restlessness Lethargy Listlessness Expressionless face Slight hand tremor Drooping eyelids Dark circles under eyes	*Physical:* Illness: Pain/discomfort
Sleep pattern disturbance *6.2.1*	Reports not feeling rested. States newborn baby interfering with sleep—awakened early AM and throughout night.	Frequent yawning Increased irritability Listlessness Dark circles under eyes	*Developmental:* Social cues: Awakening to feed newborn
Sleep pattern disturbance *6.2.1*	Reports not feeling rested. Reports difficulty falling asleep. States awakens earlier than desired. States has used a sleeping pill every night for 2 months so should be sleeping without problems.	Restlessness Lethargy Expressionless face Drooping eyelids Dark circles under eyes Thick speech with mispronunciation and incorrect words	*Cognitive:* Knowledge deficit: Inappropriate use of sleeping medication
Sleep pattern disturbance *6.2.1*	Reports not feeling rested. States has difficulty falling asleep—"too much on my mind," "on edge." States hard to get back to sleep if awakened—"feel tense." Reports unfamiliar noises and roommate's need for frequent care cause frequent awakening.	Frequent yawning Increasing irritability Listlessness Dark circles under eyes Halls are noisy Roommate requires 24-hour care Observed awake 4 or 5 times at night	*Environmental:* Environmental changes: Recent hospitalization

OTHER NURSING DIAGNOSES RELATED TO SLEEP-REST PATTERNS

PHYSICAL
- Activity intolerance
- Diarrhea
- Decreased cardiac output
- Fluid volume deficit
- Hypothermia
- Hyperthermia
- Impaired physical mobility
- Altered nutrition: less than body requirements
- Ineffective airway clearance
- Ineffective breathing pattern
- Impaired gas exchange
- Impaired skin integrity
- Altered tissue perfusion
- Altered urinary elimination patterns
- Potential for injury

COGNITIVE
- Pain
- Sensory perceptual alteration

EMOTIONAL
- Anxiety
- Ineffective individual coping
- Fear
- Grieving

SELF-CONCEPTUAL
- Disturbance in self-esteem
- Powerlessness
- Hopelessness

SOCIOCULTURAL/LIFE STRUCTURAL
- Ineffective coping
- Diversional activity deficit
- Altered family processes
- Social isolation
- Impaired home maintenance management
- Spiritual distress

SEXUAL
- Altered sexuality patterns
- Sexual dysfunction
- Rape-trauma syndrome

Sources: The nursing diagnoses and etiologies on this table and the definitions of nursing diagnoses in the body of the text not credited to other sources are from Nursing Diagnosis: Definitions and Classification, 1997–1998. *Philadelphia: North American Nursing Diagnosis Association; 1996. Manifestation categories for etiologies and specifications of general etiologies on these tables are authors' original work.*

COLLABORATIVE STRATEGY

PLANNING TO MEET SLEEP NEEDS

Planning for a patient's individual sleep needs means determining the desired outcome related to sleep and rest. Collaborative planning ensures that goals and approaches will be compatible with the patient's needs.

can contribute to setting goals that are acceptable and important to individual care. The nurse may also need to consult with other health care professionals involved in the patient's care (eg, the physician, physical therapist, and respiratory therapist) in order to establish realistic desired outcomes.

For example, Mr. Torcello and the nurse note that his sleep is interrupted every 4 hours during the night for medication. Mr. Torcello states that physical therapy interrupts his morning nap and he feels "exhausted." After consulting with the physician, the nurse determines that Mr. Torcello's medication schedule cannot be changed. The physical therapist, however, agrees to change his session to early afternoon, which enables Mr. Torcello to nap for 3 hours in the morning.

When planning to reach a long-term outcome, it may be necessary to first set short-term outcomes. In the example of Mr. Torcello, the long-term outcome would be: "The patient will receive 8 hours of uninterrupted nocturnal sleep within 2 weeks." A short-term outcome would be: "The patient will receive 2 hours of uninterrupted morning nap time every 24 hours." As the patient's medication schedule changes, it will be possible to meet the long-term outcome with appropriate planning. In the meantime, it is possible to attain the short-term outcome. It is important to remember that the individualized outcome statement describes specific patient behavior and establishes a time period within which the outcome should be attained. Thus, it is possible to measure and document progress toward outcome achievement.

The next part of planning for a patient's sleep needs is determining what nursing measures should be used to achieve the desired outcomes. The assessment data and outcomes suggest the appropriate patient care. Again, collaborative or mutual planning among nurse, patient, and other health care professionals provides the most realistic and workable approaches to care.

A complete sleep care plan addresses all of the problems stated in the nursing diagnoses and the implementation to be used to attain each outcome. The nursing treatment is then carried out, and its effectiveness is evaluated in terms of what progress the patient is making in achieving the desired outcomes. If this ongoing or day-to-day evaluation reveals that progress is slow or nonexistent, it is necessary to reassess the desired outcome and the treatments for their appropriateness to the patient's needs. Revisions in the plan of care are made as needed.

Specific nursing approaches to assist patients with sleep needs involve a variety of nursing skills and depend on the etiology of the sleep pattern disturbance and the related nursing diagnoses. These are described in Table 31–3. Age-appropriate implementation for each level of care is shown in Table 31–4. Table 31–5, Partial Critical Pathway for Total Hip Replacement: Sleep–Rest Function, and Table 31–6, Partial Critical Pathway for Congestive Heart Failure: Sleep–Rest Function, are interdisciplinary plans that incorporate concepts from this chapter.

NURSING IMPLEMENTATION TO PROMOTE OPTIMAL SLEEP AND REST

PREVENTIVE CARE

Preventive care focuses on the individual who is at risk for developing sleep pattern disturbances. Nursing implementation is formulated to prevent the development of these problems with the knowledge that patients are responsible for their care. Preventive care for sleep may occur in the hospital, but is more common in the home.

Screening and Risk Assessment

For the healthy individual at risk for developing disturbed sleep, screening and risk assessment are appropriate nursing actions. Nurses should explore any variables in the patient's lifestyle that may disrupt sleep. Factors that place an individual at risk for developing sleep-pattern disturbance were described earlier in this chapter.

Health Education

Health education is an important part of preventive care. Patients at risk should be taught the importance of maintaining a bedtime routine, remaining active during the day, and reducing or eliminating environmental distractions at bedtime. Many people find that quiet activity such as reading or listening to soft music promotes relaxation and facilitates sleep.

The nurse can also teach patients the importance of certain comfort measures to induce sleep, for example, using an additional pillow or blanket or making the bed with fresh linen. Some patients may find a warm bath relaxing. Progressive relaxation (a combination of rhythmic, slow breathing and progressive relaxation of the body's muscle groups) may reduce anxiety and tension that delays sleep onset and/or interferes with sleep maintenance. (See Clinical Guideline 25–2 for further discussion of the use of progressive relaxation.)

Many people who experience occasional sleep problems view over-the-counter (OTC) sleep medications as a quick, easy solution. Teaching about the dangers associated with these preparations is another focus for health education. Inform patients that these drugs alter normal sleep cycles, especially REM sleep, and that prolonged use can result in dependency. Rebound insomnia and vivid dreams, even nightmares, often occur when OTC sleep medications are discontinued after regular use. Patients who are aware of the risks associated with inappropriate use of OTC preparations to induce sleep are more likely to select other approaches to enhance sleep and to use any medication for sleep with caution.

Home Health Care

Home health nurses assess a patient's home environment to identify whether it is conducive to optimal rest. They ask patients about their sleep routines and habits, and assess all of the factors mentioned earlier in the chapter, including age, physical condition,

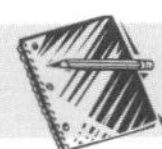

TABLE 31-3. NURSE-PATIENT MANAGEMENT OF SLEEP-REST PROBLEMS

Nursing Diagnosis	Desired Outcomes	Implementation	Evaluation
Sleep pattern disturbance R/T pain, discomfort *6.2.1*	1. Progressive decrease in time between going to bed and sleep onset.	1a. Assist patient into comfortable sleeping position. 1b. Teach patient progressive relaxation (Clinical Guideline 25–2). 1c. Offer a back massage. 1d. Reduce environmental distractions. 1e. Suggest bedtime snack containing tryptophane and carbohydrates, such as milk with fruit or cookie. 1f. Maintain patient's usual bedtime routine. 1g. Suggest warm bath before bedtime.	1. Patient reports falls asleep within 15 min after going to bed.
	2. Progressive increase in amount of uninterrupted sleep each night to 8 h.	2. Consult with physician regarding an analgesic to be given before bedtime.	2. Patient reports sleeps 6–8 hours each night without interruption.
	3. Progressive improvement in quality of rest each night.	3. Patient reports sleeps 6–8 h each night without interruption.	3a. Patient reports feels rested in AM; is less irritable. 3b. No dark circles under eyes. 3c. No yawning noted.
Sleep pattern disturbance R/T social cues: awakening to feed newborn *6.2.1*	1. Increase in total sleep time per 24-h period to total of at least 8 hours sleep per 24 h.	1a. Suggest patient feed and change infant immediately before retiring at night. 1b. Suggest patient nap when infant naps during day. 1c. Teach progressive relaxation, suggest warm bath before bedtime.	1. Patient reports receiving two 4-hour periods of uninterrupted nighttime sleep and napping 2 hours a day.
Sleep pattern disturbance R/T knowledge deficit; inappropriate use of sleeping medication *6.2.1*	1. Patient aware of risks of long-term use of sleeping medications.	1a. Teach the adverse effects on sleep of routine use of medication. 1b. Collaborate with physician and patient to schedule gradual decrease in drug dosage until discontinued.	1. Patient correctly states risks associated with use of sleeping medications.
	2. Progressive decrease in time between going to bed and sleep onset.	2a. Teach progressive relaxation (Clinical Guideline 25–2). 2b. Reduce environmental distractions. 2c. Suggest bedtime snack containing tryptophane and carbohydrates, such as milk with fruit or cookies. 2d. Maintain patient's usual bedtime routine. 2e. Suggest warm bath before bedtime.	2. Patient reports falls asleep within 15 min after going to bed.
	3. Progressive increase in amount of uninterrupted sleep each night to 8 h. 4. Progressive improvement in quality of rest each night.	3,4a. Discuss value of regular exercise in promoting healthy sleep patterns. 3,4b. Suggest limiting evening fluid intake, especially of alcoholic beverages and beverages containing caffeine.	3,4a. Patient reports receiving 6–8 h of restful sleep 10 days after discontinuing sleeping medication. 4b. Dark circles under eyes/drooping eyelids absent. 4c. Speech clear. 4d. Facial expression animated.
Sleep pattern disturbance R/T recent hospitalization *6.2.1*	1. Progressive decrease in time between going to bed and sleep onset.	1a. Teach progressive relaxation (Clinical Guideline 25–2). 1b. Offer a back massage. 1c. Suggest warm bath before bedtime. 1d. Assess patient's usual bedtime routine and incorporate into care.	1. Patient reports falls asleep within 15 min after going to bed.
	2. Uninterrupted nighttime sleep.	2a. Reduce environmental distractions (close door to room, reassign to another room, reduce lighting). 2b. Give treatments, medications at same time when possible and time other than when patient usually sleeps.	2a. Patient reports sleeps 6–8 h each night without interruption. 2b. Noted to be asleep when checked by night shift nurses.

Source: See Table 31–2.

TABLE 31-4. AGE-APPROPRIATE NURSING IMPLEMENTATION FOR SLEEP PATTERN DISTURBANCE

Developmental Stage	Level of Care			
	Preventive	*Supportive*	*Restorative*	*Rehabilitative*
Infant/toddler	Screening and risk assessment with parents. Health education with parents regarding usual sleep patterns of developmental stage; reduction of environmental distractions and use of bedtime routines and comfort measures to induce sleep. Encourage outdoor play using large muscles at least one time per day (toddlers)	See preventive care. Initiate a daily schedule to incorporate sleep opportunities. Quiet activities only after evening meal. Teach parents importance of consistent response to toddlers' attempts to delay sleep.	See preventive and supportive care. Use of any ordered medications and treatments for underlying illness interfering with sleep. Comfort measures, such as rocking, singing; soft music and/or bedtime story; appropriate room temperature, clothing, and bed covers.	See preventive and supportive care. Referrals to other health care professionals to reestablish healthful sleep patterns. Health teaching on ways to induce and maintain sleep.
Preschooler	Screening and risk assessment with parents. Health education with parents regarding usual sleep patterns of developmental stage; reduction of environmental distractions and use of bedtime routines and comfort measures to induce sleep.	See preventive care. Initiate a daily schedule to incorporate sleep opportunities. Have parents keep a sleep log of child's sleep patterns. Have parents complete assessment tool of child's sleep patterns.	See preventive and supportive care. Use of any ordered medications and treatment for underlying illness interfering with sleep. Comfort measures, such as rocking, singing; appropriate room temperature, clothing, and bed covers, reading a bedtime story; offering a bedtime snack; warm bath.	See preventive and supportive care. Referrals to other health care professionals to reestablish healthful sleep patterns. Health teaching on ways to induce and maintain sleep.
Child	Screening and risk assessment with parents. Health education with parents regarding usual sleep patterns of developmental stage; reduction of environmental distractions and use of bedtime routines and comfort measures to induce sleep. Routinely scheduled exercise to promote sleep.	See preventive care. Initiate a daily schedule to incorporate sleep opportunities. Have parents keep a sleep log of child's sleep patterns. Have parents complete assessment tool of child's sleep patterns. Initiate an exercise program.	See preventive and supportive care. Use of any ordered medications and treatments for underlying illness interfering with sleep. Comfort measures, such as appropriate room temperature, clothing, and bed covers; reading a bedtime story; offering a bedtime snack; warm bath, back rub; allowing older children to read, listen to soft music.	See preventive and supportive care. Referrals to other health care professionals to reestablish healthful sleep patterns. Health teaching on ways to induce and maintain sleep.
Adolescent/young adult through older adult	Screening and risk assessment related to lifestyle and stressors that interfere with sleep. Health education on reduction of environmental distractions and use of bedtime routines and comfort measures to induce sleep, and routinely scheduled exercise to promote sleep, as well as relaxation techniques.	See preventive care. Initiate a daily schedule to incorporate sleep opportunities. Initiate an exercise program. Have patient complete a sleep log. Have patient complete a self-assessment tool.	See preventive and supportive care. Use of any ordered medications and treatments for underlying illness interfering with sleep. Comfort measures such as appropriate room temperature, clothing, and bed covers; bedtime snack; warm bath, back rub; listening to music; reading; positioning. Limited use of sedatives. Use of noninvasive pain relief, such as imagery, distraction.	See preventive and restorative care. Referrals to other health care professionals to reestablish healthful sleep patterns. Health teaching on ways to induce and maintain sleep.

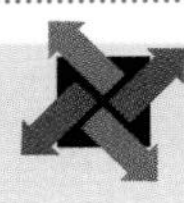

TABLE 31-5. PARTIAL CRITICAL PATHWAY FOR TOTAL HIP REPLACEMENT: SLEEP-REST FUNCTION

Nursing Dx/Problem	Outcome DOS/Day 1	Outcome Days 2–3	Outcome SNF Days 4–6	Outcome Home Care 3 Weeks (6 Visits)
Sleep pattern disturbance R/T hospital environment	Obtains 2 hr uninterrupted sleep × 3	Obtains 2 hr uninterrupted sleep × 4	Obtains 4 hr uninterrupted sleep × 2	Increase in uninterrupted sleep each night to 8 hr or sufficient sleep to feel rested
Implementation	**DOS/Day 1**	**Days 2–3**	**SNF Days 4–6**	**Home Care 3 Weeks**
Assessment	Pain-comfort level: 1–5 scale # hr of uninterrupted sleep	Same Fatigue, tiredness	Same Same	Same Same
Tests/Consults		Physical therapy for safe exercise program		
Medications/ Treatments	Pain relief/comfort measures Arrange care to allow uninterrupted sleep	Same Same	Same Same	Same Same
Psychosocial				
Teaching	Relaxation techniques	Reinforce relaxation techniques	Same	
Activity/Safety/ Self-care			Large muscle exercise per PT	Progressive increase in daily large muscle exercise per PT.
Nutrition		Eliminate caffeinated beverages late in day	Same	Same
Transfer/Discharge Coord./Case Manager		Communicate outcomes achieved, problems/ interventions to SNF	Communicate outcomes achieved, problems/ interventions to Home Health	Communicate outcomes achieved, problems/interventions to MD & prepare for discharge

See inside back cover for abbreviations.

and mental and emotional status. Diet, for example, and the patient's ingestion of foods or drinks that may foster or hinder sleep, are part of the preventative home health sleep assessment, as is the daily exercise pattern and medication regimen.

Teaching is an important part of home preventive care. A simple but effective intervention is to teach patients about comfort measures that promote sleep, so that patients and their families are equipped to deal with sleep problems as they arise. Some patients may not have thought about approaches that nurses take for granted, such as soft music or a warm milk drink before bedtime to induce rest.

Finally, one of the common causes of sleep deprivation is interruption of an individual's sleep. In home health care, nurses have the flexibility to schedule their visits to meet the patient's needs. Thus, part of the preventive role is not to interfere with the patient's sleep time.

SUPPORTIVE CARE

Supportive care for sleep focuses on patients who are experiencing mild problems with sleep, such as a frequent traveler with jet lag or new parents experiencing sleep disruptions due to an infant's sleep–wakefulness cycle. This care usually occurs in a nonhospital setting, such as a community-health agency, physician's office, or the patient's home; however, supportive implementation may also be appropriate for use with hospitalized patients. The primary goal is to prevent further disruption of sleep patterns. Nurse and patient should collaborate to determine the cause of the sleep problems and make a daily schedule that incorporates adequate opportunities for sleep.

Sleep Log

The use of a sleep log in which patients record sleep periods can be used to identify sleep patterns. To keep a sleep log, patients can take a blank piece of paper and write down each time they sleep in a 24-hour period. They should include the approximate time they fall asleep and awaken for each sleep period. Finally, they total the number of hours slept for the past 24 hours. The sleep log should be kept for at least 7 days.

Self-assessment Tool

A self-assessment tool to be completed by patients is useful in identifying risk factors that can be altered to promote sleep. Such

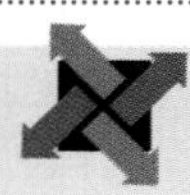

TABLE 31-6. PARTIAL CRITICAL PATHWAY FOR CONGESTIVE HEART FAILURE: SLEEP-REST FUNCTION

Nursing Dx/Problem	Outcome Primary Care Visit	Outcome Home Care Week 1 (3 Visits)	Outcome Home Care Week 2 (3 Visits)	Outcome Home Care Weeks 3–4 (3 Visits)
Sleep pattern disturbance R/T anxiety response to altered health status		Verbalizes less anxious p̄ included in discussion of plan of care Sleeps 2 hr during day	Sleeps 6 hr each night c̄ 2 interruptions	Progressive increase in sleep to 8 hr per night
Implementation	**Primary Care Visit**	**Home Care Visit Week 1**	**Home Care Visit Week 2**	**Home Care Visit Weeks 3–4**
Assessment	Fatigue, weakness	Same # hrs of sleep each night, physical, emotional, & cognitive symptoms of anxiety Level of knowledge & experience c̄ relaxation techniques	Same Same Same Use of relaxation techniques	Same Same Same Same
Tests/Consults	Refer to Home Health			
Medications/ Treatments			Relaxation techniques	Reinforce as needed
Psychosocial	Reflective listening	Explore adjustment to health status	Same Involve family in problem solving Explore realistic solutions	Reinforce role adaptations
Teaching	Introduce relaxation techniques S/Sx to report to MD, RN, 911	Review, reinforce as needed Plan of care, chest pain scale Disease process/Care plan	Review, reinforce as needed Review, reinforce as needed Review, reinforce as needed	Effect of exercise on sleep Same
Activity/Safety/ Self-care	Bedrest, HOB 30–45 degrees c̄ BSC or BRP	Progressive ADLs & activity as tolerated Regular rest periods Reading/soft music ā bed	Same Same Same	Same
Nutrition	Eliminate caffeine	Same Bedtime tryptophane & carbohydrate snack	Same Same	Same Same
Transfer/Discharge Coord./Case Manager		Communicate outcomes achieved to MD	Same	Same Prepare for discharge

See inside back cover for abbreviations.

risk factors have been discussed previously in this chapter. Most self-assessment tools ask patients to record the time they go to bed, how calm they feel at bedtime, how tired they feel at bedtime, and to estimate the time they fall asleep. Patients indicate their bedtime routines; illnesses; exercise routines; and use of medications, alcohol, and caffeine-containing products, including the times these substances are ingested. In the morning, patients record the number of nighttime awakenings they experienced, their perceived movement during sleep, the time they awakened in the morning, and how satisfied they feel with the previous night's sleep. Sleep assessment tools should be used for at least 3 to 4 nights so that any patterns can be noted.

Supportive approaches to promote sleep include reestablishing the patient's usual bedtime routines, exercising vigorously 6 to 8 hours before bedtime, reducing or eliminating environmental distractions, providing comfort measures, and teaching a relaxation technique (see Clinical Guideline 25–2). Progressive relaxation is also appropriate supportive care.

Home Health Care

Home health nurses may intervene effectively to help patients who show mild sleep disturbances. Home health nurses assess the nature of the patients' sleep loss and document the symptoms that result from sleep deprivation. Part of that assessment is to consider whether a patient requires referral for further workup or diagnostic appraisal.

One of the nurse's most important actions is to assist patients and their families to modify the home environment to support their needs for rest. Controlling noise and overall activity levels may be important, particularly in families where there are children. Banging doors and ringing telephones do little to foster rest. The home health nurse may need to review the activity of the entire family to help its members find solutions.

Teaching family members how to help their sleep-deprived member is also important. For example, home health nurses often demonstrate how to give a back rub or may work with patients to help them learn sleep-inducing techniques, such as progressive relaxation, music therapy, or guided imagery.

Supportive home care also considers the family caregiver. One of the most important contributions the nurse makes is to assess the sleep–rest needs of those who are caring for ill family members. Not infrequently caregivers go without rest themselves to care for their loved one. It is sometimes necessary to structure time for them to rest, and to assist them to identify others who can care for the ill family member while they rest. For example, it may be necessary to bring in volunteers on a regular schedule to make rest possible for the home caregiver.

INSIGHTS FROM NURSING LITERATURE

UNDERSTANDING SLEEP

Davidhizar RE, Poole VL. What nurses need to know about sleep. J Nurs Sci. *1995;1:61–67.*

The authors of this article focused on sleep deprivation, a problem with decreased amount, quality, and consistency of sleep, as distinguised from sleep disorders such as insomnia, sleep apnea, narcolepsy, sleepwalking, bedwetting, and tooth grinding.

They noted that sleep is linked with the circadian rhythms of the human biological clock. When these rhythms are disrupted, as happens in sleep deprivation, a person's mood, cognition, judgment, sensory integration, vital signs, and vulnerability to pain may be affected. They advised that a detailed sleep history be done whenever a sleep problem is suspected—one that inventories the patient's normal sleep pattern, usual bedtime rituals and environment, emotional, mental, and physical status, and the symptoms of sleep deprivation the patient is experiencing. Further, they recommended strategies for sleep promotion such as promoting bedtime rituals, using relaxation techniques and comfort measures, promoting relief from anxiety, pain, and discomfort, and controlling factors in the environment, including health procedures that may serve to disrupt sleep.

RESTORATIVE CARE

Restorative care for sleep focuses on acute sleep pattern disturbances. Here, lack of sleep has become so pronounced that the patient's physical and psychological well-being is threatened.

Noninvasive Measures

Nursing implementation for acute sleep disturbance includes treating the underlying cause of the sleep problem. In some cases, the cause of the patient's sleep disturbance may be treatable by nurses using noninvasive pain relief measures (see Chap. 32) or assisting with positioning for comfort (see Chap. 33). *Evening care,* including a back rub, is a planned part of patient care and can assist in promoting sleep. Procedure 31–1 presents the routine evening or PM care that should be given by a nurse. Procedure 31–2 outlines the correct procedures for a back rub. For patients at home, the procedure can be taught to a spouse or other significant individual.

Administering Medications

Sometimes correcting the cause of the sleep problem involves collaborating with other health care providers, such as administering medications and treatments ordered by the physician. When the underlying illness is resolved, healthier sleep patterns return. The use of preventive and supportive implementation to promote comfort and reduce environmental stimuli is also appropriate during the acute phase of most illnesses if sleep is disturbed.

Nurses may also administer sedative–hypnotic or tranquilizer drugs to hospitalized patients that have been ordered by the physician to induce sleep directly. In the home, patients or significant others administer medications. These medications should be used only on a short-term basis while normal sleep patterns are being restored. Prolonged use of these medications (over 2 weeks) may cause *rebound sleep pattern disturbance,* restlessness, depression, and drug dependency. Table 31–7 compares the various medications for sleep.

Reassessment of sleep during drug therapy is an important nursing function. If medication has been used every night for 10 to 14 nights, the nurse should discuss with the physician discontinuing it. The patient also needs information about a drug's actions and side effects so that the medication will not be used on a routine basis.

In addition to monitoring the patient's use of sleep medication, the nurse should also assess the drug's effectiveness in treating the sleep problem. If sleep is improved, the drug is serving its purpose. The patient also needs to be assessed for side effects of

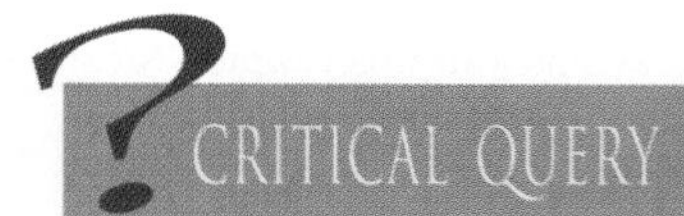

Foreman and Wykle[9] state that sedatives should be considered the intervention of last choice for older hospitalized patients with sleep pattern disturbance. What nursing interventions should be implemented for those patients who must receive these medications?

PROCEDURE 31–1. PROVIDING EVENING (PM) CARE

PURPOSE: To assist the patient in preparing for bed and to promote sleep.
EQUIPMENT: Basin of warm water; washcloth; towels; dental care items; cup; emesis basin; skin lotion or powder; deodorant; urinal, bedpan, bedside commode, toilet paper.

ACTION 1. Gather equipment.

ACTION 2. Discuss the purpose of evening care with the patient.

ACTION 3. Provide privacy.

ACTION 4. Wash hands.

ACTION 5. Adjust bed to a comfortable working position, with siderail farthest from nurse in up position.

ACTION 6. To reduce possibility of interrupted sleep, if patient is unable to walk to the bathroom, assist with bedpan, urinal, or bedside commode (see Procedure 29–4).

ACTION 7. Provide basin with warm water and soap to wash face and hands. Assist as needed.

ACTION 8. To promote comfort and relaxation, assist with dental/mouth care (see Procedure 27–1), and hair care as needed.

ACTION 9. If needed or requested by patient, assist with bath (see Procedure 27–10).

ACTION 10. Clean and store reusable equipment; discard disposables according to agency policy.

ACTION 11. Replace any soiled linens. Straighten unsoiled linen and fluff pillow.

ACTION 12. Provide sleep medication if ordered.

ACTION 13. To promote muscle relaxation and minimize RAS activation, provide back rub (see Procedure 31–2).

ACTION 14. Assist patient into comfortable position for sleep.

ACTION 15. Straighten top covers. Provide additional covers as needed.

ACTION 16. To promote safety, place bed in low position. Place call light within reach. For some patients, raise siderails.

ACTION 17. Wash hands.

ACTION 18. Turn off or dim lights to decrease RAS stimulation.

Recording:
Note specific care provided and patient response. Many agencies use a checklist for procedures such as evening care.

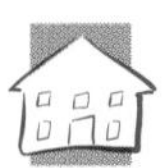

HOME HEALTH ADAPTATION: For a patient needing additional rest, this procedure can be initiated at any time to promote relaxation and sleep. It can easily be implemented in the home by caregivers and family.

the particular sleep medication being used. If any are present, the physician should be notified and the sleep medication discontinued or changed. Safety factors, such as keeping the bed in a low position and using siderails, must also be observed while sleep medication is in use.

Other nursing measures for acute sleep disturbances depend on the patient's age and developmental stage. Many times, these measures are similar to those for rehabilitative care.

Home Health Care

Restorative care for a home patient with a sleep problem requires not only that nurses do the preventive and supportive implementations described, but also that they take additional measures. The progression of actions begins with the noninvasive, comfort measures already mentioned, and progresses to pharmaceutical measures, which may require collaboration with other health care providers to adequately assess the patient's problem and need. Nurses working in the home setting are always careful to conduct a full assessment of all of the drugs a patient is taking, including those given for problems other than disturbed sleep. It is important to know whether anything the patient is ingesting is contributing to the sleep problem.

Patients with serious illnesses often have related sleep problems that may not respond to comfort measures alone. Whenever sleep-inducing medications are given, it is vital that the nurse work with the family to ensure that the home environment is safe for the patient. The effects of sleep medications often render patients more vulnerable to accidents. Thus, barriers such as furniture, which may impede a patient's route to the bathroom or other living areas, should be identified and removed. It is also important that the family is alerted to the need to assess their elderly relatives for signs of excessive dosage. Older individuals may not adequately metabolize or eliminate ingested medications.

REHABILITATIVE CARE

Rehabilitative care is focused on reestablishing the patient's usual sleep patterns or on establishing new habits because of health

(continued on page 1107)

PROCEDURE 31–2. GIVING A BACK RUB

PURPOSE: To promote relaxation and induce sleep.
EQUIPMENT: Skin care lotion; bath towel optional.

ACTION 1. Discuss the purpose and expected benefits of the back rub and ask the patient if one is desired.

RATIONALE. Patient is more likely to agree to the activity if its purpose is clearly explained, and if the opportunity to provide consent is given.

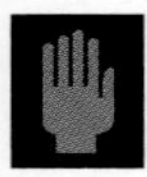

Use language that is easily understood. Some patients may view the back rub as an invasion of privacy or place it in a sexual context. A clear explanation of benefits of back rub can prevent misinterpretation.

ACTION 2. Provide privacy. Use low lighting.

RATIONALE. Personal care is considered a private activity in most cultures; patient relaxation is facilitated if need for privacy is respected. Low light reduces RAS activation.

ACTION 3. Wash hands.

RATIONALE. Removes transient microorganisms from nurse's hands, preventing transfer to patient.

ACTION 4. Adjust bed to a comfortable working position.

RATIONALE. Prevents nurse's backstrain.

ACTION 5. Assist or request that patient assume prone or semiprone position. Pillow under head is optional. Pregnant patients, and those with recent abdominal surgery, may be unable to assume these positions. Use sidelying position instead.

RATIONALE. These positions provide greatest exposure of back and buttocks.

ACTION 6. Arrange bed covers and gown or clothing so that skin of back, shoulders, and upper buttocks is exposed, but legs are covered.

RATIONALE. Provides warmth, minimizes feelings of exposure, while permitting access to skin.

ACTION 7. Pour a moderate amount of lotion onto the palm of your hand. Rub your hands together to warm lotion. Lotion may also be warmed by placing bottle in a basin of warm water during preceding care activities.

RATIONALE. Lotion reduces friction between nurse's hands and patient's skin. Cold lotion is uncomfortable and may cause chilling.

ACTION 8. Tell patient you are ready to begin. Warn that lotion may feel a bit cool at first.

RATIONALE. Avoids startling patient.

ACTION 9. Using firm, steady pressure, move your hands slowly up either side of the spine from the buttocks to the base of neck, across the shoulders, and down the lateral aspects of the back, returning to the buttocks. Repeat 3 to 5 times.

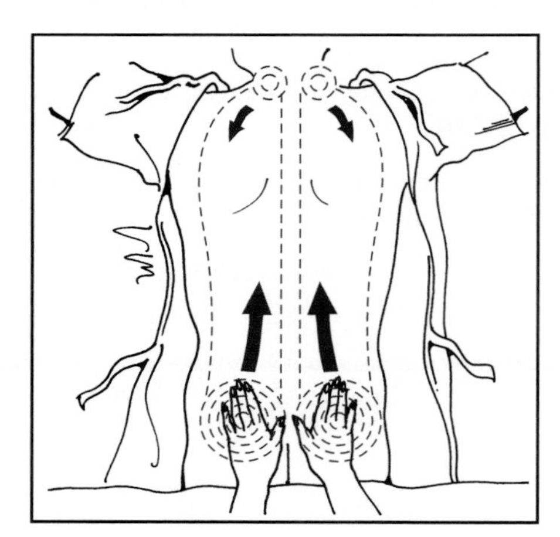

RATIONALE. Firm pressure is relaxing and reassuring. Light pressure may be perceived as a tickling sensation. Rapid movements are stimulating rather than relaxing.

Procedure 31–2. (continued)

ACTION 10. Next, using a kneading motion, rub your hands over the scapulae and upper shoulders. Work down to the sacrum and posterior illiac spines. Kneading should be done gently to avoid pinching the patient. Obtain more lotion as needed.

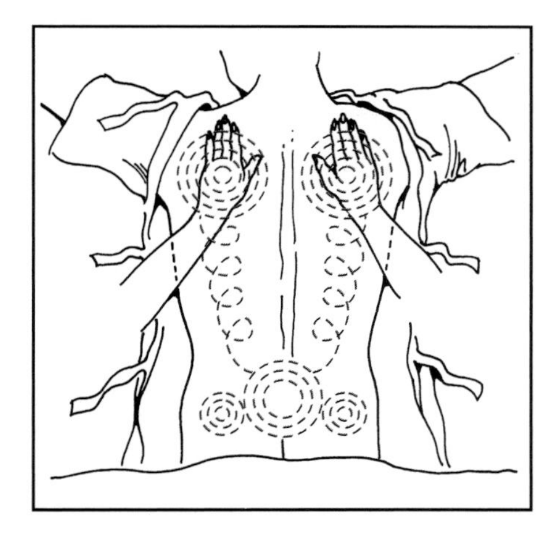

ACTION 11. Using a figure-8 motion, massage from the sacrum over each buttock. Repeat 3 times.

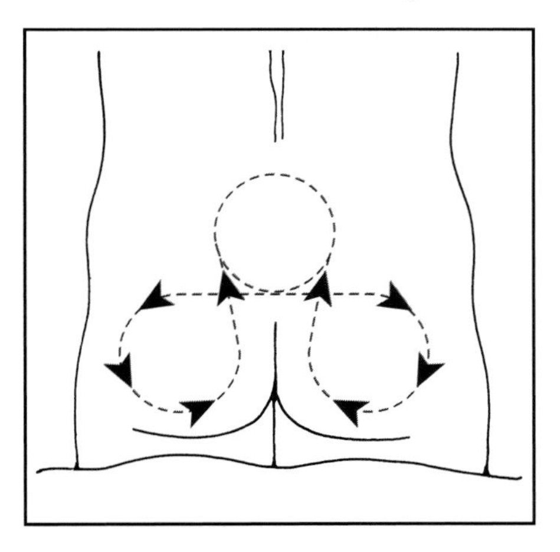

ACTION 12. Rub up and down the back with a long, stroking motion. Repeat 3 times.

RATIONALE. These movements promote muscle relaxation in all major muscle groups of posterior trunk, many of which may become tense and/or sore from bedrest. Tense or sore muscles may cause RAS activation, promoting wakefulness. Circulation over boney prominences (scapulae, sacrum, posterior illiac spines) is also stimulated, thereby reducing the risk of pressure ulcers (see Chap. 33).

ACTION 13. Repeat Actions 9 to 12 for 5 to 10 minutes.

RATIONALE. Time required to achieve relaxed state is variable.

ACTION 14. Wipe excess lotion off the patient's back with the bath towel.

RATIONALE. Excess lotion may cause skin, gown, or sheets to feel damp or sticky, interfering with relaxation.

ACTION 15. Close gown, assist patient into desired position and adjust bed covers. Place bed in low position and call light within reach.

RATIONALE. Promotes comfort and safety, which reduces cortical activity, thereby minimizing RAS activation.

ACTION 16. Wash hands.

RATIONALE. Removes transient microorganisms, preventing transfer to other patients.

Recording:
Note procedure, condition of skin, degree of relaxation reported by patient, and any complaints of discomfort. If skin lesions noted, record associated action taken.

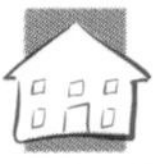

HOME HEALTH ADAPTATION: Use good body mechanics to avoid back strain when working with low stationary beds. Instruct family caregivers to rub the patient's back with each position change to maintain skin integrity and promote relaxation.

TABLE 31-7. MEDICATIONS USED FOR SLEEP

Medication	Mode of Action	Duration of Action	Side Effects	Nursing Implementation
Barbiturates Pentobarbital (Nembutal) Secobarbital (Seconal)	Produce all levels of CNS depression.	PO = 1–4 hr IM = 1–4 hr IV = 15 min Rectal = 1–4 hr	*CNS:* Drowsiness, lethargy, hangover, depression, delirium, excitation, restlessness. *Dermatologic:* Urticaria, rashes. *GI:* Nausea, vomiting. *Misc.:* Hypersensitivity reactions, psychological dependence, tolerance to increasing doses, physical dependence at high doses.	• Assess sleep patterns before and during drug therapy. • Caution patient of possibility of increased dreaming upon discontinuing therapy. REM sleep is suppressed by barbiturates. • Limit amount of drug available to patient, especially if suicidal, depressed, or has history of addiction. • Caution patient to avoid daytime activities requiring alertness until effect of medication is known. • Advise against concurrent use of alcohol or CNS depressants. • Use siderails and place call light within reach after drug administration. • Assist with ambulation after administration. • Monitor respirations, pulse, and blood pressure during IV administration.
Benzodiazepines Sedative–hypnotics Flurazepam (Dalmane) Temazepam (Restoril) Triazolam (Halcion) Estazolam (ProSom) Quazepam (Doral)	Act on CNS to produce general depression.	Flurazepam: 7–8 hr Temazepam: 10–20 hr Triazolam: 2–5 hr Estazolam: 12–18 hr Quazepam: 2–4 days	*CNS:* Dizziness, drowsiness, lethargy, hangover, confusion, mental depression, headache, paradoxical excitation. *Dermatologic:* Rashes. *GI:* Nausea, vomiting, diarrhea, heartburn. *Misc.:* Psychological dependence, physical dependence, tolerance.	• Assess sleep patterns before and during drug therapy. • Limit amount of drug available to patient, especially if suicidal, depressed, or has history of addiction. • Caution patient to avoid daytime activities requiring alertness until effect of medication is known. • Advise against concurrent use of alcohol or CNS depressants. • Use side rails and place call light within reach after drug administration. • Assist with ambulation after administration • For triazolam and temazepam, do not administer within 1 h of antacids, as they impair absorption. May administer with food to prevent gastric irritation.
Tranquilizers Alprazolam (Xanax) Chlordiazepoxide HCl (Librax) Diazepam (Valium) Lorazepam (Ativan) Oxazepam (Serax) Trazodone (Desyrel)	Produce CNS depression and skeletal muscle relaxation. Have antianxiety properties.	Alprazolam: up to 24 hr Chlordiazepoxide HCl: 4–8 hr Diazepam: up to 24 hr Lorazepam: up to 48 hr Oxazepam: 6–12 hr Trazodone: 6–12 hr	*CNS:* Dizziness, drowsiness, lethargy, hangover, confusion, mental depression, headache, paradoxical excitation. *Dermatologic:* Rashes. *GI:* Nausea, vomiting, diarrhea, heartburn. *Respiratory:* Respiratory depression. *Misc.:* Psychological dependence, physical dependence, tolerance.	• Assess sleep patterns before and during drug therapy. • Limit amount of drug available to patient, especially if suicidal, depressed, or has history of addiction. • Caution patient to avoid daytime activities requiring alertness until effect of medication is known. • Advise against concurrent use of alcohol or CNS depressants. • Use siderails and place call light within reach after drug administration. • Assist with ambulation after administration. • Assess degree of anxiety before and during therapy. • Caution that abrupt withdrawal of medication may cause insomnia, nervousness, irritability. • May administer with milk to reduce gastric irritation.
Chloral Hydrate Aquachloral, Noctec, Oradrate	Generalized CNS depression.	4–8 hr	*CNS:* Excess sedation, hangover, disorientation. *Dermatologic:* Rashes. *GI:* Nausea, vomiting, diarrhea, flatulence. *Respiratory:* Respiratory depression. *Misc:* Tolerance, psychological dependence, physical dependence.	• Assess sleep patterns before and during drug therapy. • Caution patient to avoid daytime activities requiring alertness until effect of medication is known. • Use siderails and place call light within reach after drug administration. • Assist with ambulation after administration. • Advise that concurrent use of alcohol may cause vasodilation, flushing, tachycardia, hypotension, headache. • Caution that abrupt withdrawal may result in anxiety, CNS excitement, tremor, hallucination, delirium. • Advise patient to swallow capsules whole with a full glass of water to avoid gastric irritation.

Sources of information: DiPiro JT. Pharmacotherapy: A Pathophysiologic Approach. *3rd ed. Stamford, CT: Appleton & Lange; 1996. Ebersole P, Hess P.* Toward Healthy Aging: Human Needs and Nursing Responses. *St. Louis: Mosby; 1994.*

COLLABORATIVE STRATEGY
EVALUATION

Evaluation of sleep and rest is a collaborative process to gain a patient's subjective appraisal of how rested he or she feels. This requires that nurse and patient communicate directly about the amount of sleep or rest the patient has had, the quality of the rest, and the energy level that the patient experiences as a result. The nurse should also observe how well the patient appeared to rest. Based on this mutual assessment, care plan approaches are revised.

alterations or their treatment. Appropriate health teaching and referrals comprise the key implementation in this stage. Nurses should acquaint patients with the type and amount of sleep appropriate for their ages, assist in reducing stress that interferes with sleep, explain the causes of sleep pattern disturbances and ways to avoid them, and explain measures that can be used to relieve symptoms of disturbed sleep, such as physical exercise 6–8 hours before bed, relaxation exercises, and a glass of warm milk before retiring. Once again, the use of preventive and supportive implementations is appropriate in this stage and may be discussed with the patient. Rehabilitative care may occur in the hospital or home.

EVALUATION

In evaluating the effectiveness of patient care plan, nurse and patient consider progress toward the desired outcomes and the influence of current sleep patterns on physical and psychological well-being. If the evaluation reveals that satisfactory sleep has not been achieved, reassessment and replanning must be undertaken in collaboration with the patient in another attempt to reach that outcome.

When the desired outcome has been achieved, a notation should be made in the chart. If it has not been achieved by the time indicated in the outcome statement, a notation of reassessment findings and alternative plans should be given.

SUMMARY

Sleep and rest are basic human needs essential to all individuals' physical and psychological well-being. Promoting adequate rest and sleep is a primary nursing responsibility. Collaboration with the patient, family, and health care team is essential to the success of this function. Appropriate nursing interventions are based on the patient's age and level of care. Evaluation to determine whether the desired outcome is achieved—adequate restful sleep—is essential to this process.

LEARNING OUTCOMES

Upon completing this chapter, the student should be able to:

1. Differentiate between the functions and characteristics of REM and NREM sleep.
2. List the consequences of REM sleep deprivation.
3. List the factors affecting sleep.
4. Summarize how sleep–rest patterns differ in each of the following age groups: infants, toddlers, children, adolescents, young adults, middle-aged adults, and older adults.
5. Describe five disorders of initiating and maintaining sleep.
6. Describe two causes of excessive somnolence.
7. Describe three causes of disorders of arousal in individuals under 20 years of age.
8. State four causes of sleep problems in the elderly.
9. List data to be obtained in a sleep–rest history.
10. List several nursing diagnoses related to the diagnosis of sleep–rest patterns.
11. List five nursing implementations for the promotion of sleep and rest.
12. Discuss the importance of collaboration in the management of sleep–rest problems.

REVIEW OF KEY TERMS

ascending reticular activating system
insomnia
narcolepsy
nocturnal polysomnogram
nonrapid eye movement (NREM) sleep
periodic limb movement syndrome
rapid eye movement (REM) sleep
rest
sleep
sleep apnea

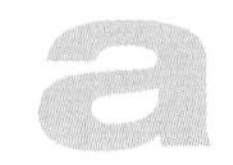

Having Read the Chapter, consider again the opening scenario, page 1087, and the following responses to the questions concerning Ms. Richards's sleeping difficulties.

Symptoms that Ms. Richards might exhibit that would interfere with her sleep are shortness of breath, cough, pain, anxiety, grief, and worry. Other disturbing factors during hospitalization would be chemotherapy, unfamiliar sounds and noises, a different bed, and the hospitalization itself.

REM and NREM sleep serve several purposes. During NREM sleep, body temperature, pulse, respirations, and metabolic rate all decrease, and the blood pressure drops slightly. There is a loss of muscle tone as the body relaxes. These changes are conducive to rest, and thus NREM sleep provides the body with time for energy conservation and tissue repair. REM sleep, which is a deeper sleep, is important for mental rest and is important for memory, learning, and physical adaptation.

Interventions that her nurse might implement to encourage satisfactory sleep for Ms. Richards during her hospitalization include short-term use of a sedative ordered by the physician; reducing the noise around Ms. Richards' room; adjusting the room temperature and lighting to the patient's preference; encouraging Ms. Richards to pursue her usual bedtime routine (if she has one); having the patient do progressive relaxation; and giving a back massage at bedtime.

To include Ms. Richards and her family in a plan to encourage satisfactory sleep, the nurse should ask them about activities that have encouraged sleep for Ms. Richards in the past; ask for suggestions that might be helpful during hospitalization; implement activities at a time when Ms. Richards feels they will be effective; and ask Ms. Richards to evaluate the effectiveness of efforts that are made.

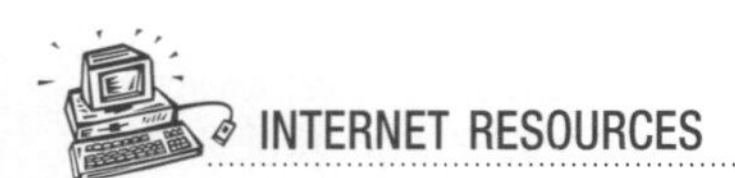

INTERNET RESOURCES

Web Site

Sleep disorder information:
http://www.asda.org

REFERENCES

1. Ancoli-Israel S. *All I Want Is a Good Night's Sleep*. St. Louis: Mosby; 1996.
2. Robinson C. Impaired sleep. In: Carrieri-Kohlman VK, Lindsey AM, West CM, eds. *Pathophysiological Phenomena in Nursing: Human Responses to Illness*. 2nd ed. Philadelphia: Saunders; 1993.
3. Carskadon MA, Dement WC. Normal human sleep. In: Kryger MH, Roth T, Dement WC, eds. *Principles and Practice of Sleep Medicine*. 2nd ed. Philadelphia: Saunders; 1994.
4. Davidhizar RE, Poole VL, Giger JN. What nurses need to know about sleep. *J Nurs Sci*. 1996;1:61–67.
5. Ebersole P, Hess P. *Toward Healthy Aging: Human Needs and Nursing Response*. St. Louis: Mosby-Yearbook; 1994.
6. Guyton AC, Hall JE. *Textbook of Medical Physiology*. 9th ed. Philadelphia: Saunders; 1996.
7. Southwell MT, Wistow G. Sleep in hospitals at night: are patients' needs being met? *J Adv Nurs*. 1995;21:1101–1109.
8. Kirkwood CK, Sood RK. Sleep disorders. In: DiPiro JT, ed. *Pharmacotherapy: A Pathophysiologic Approach*. 3rd ed. Stamford: Appleton & Lange; 1996.
9. Foreman MD, Wykle M. Nursing standard-of-practice protocol: sleep disturbances in elderly patients. *Geriatr Nurs*. 1995;16:238–243.
10. Taylor SR, Driver HS. Is sleep affected by physical exercise and fitness? *Crit Rev Phys Rehabil Med*. 1995;7:131–145.
11. American Psychiatric Association. Sleep disorders. In: *Diagnostic and Statistical Manual of Mental Disorders*. 4th ed. Washington, DC: American Psychiatric Press; 1994.
12. Dullock HL. Apnea. In: Carrieri-Kohlman VK, Lindsey AM, West CM, eds. *Pathophysiological Phenomena in Nursing: Human Responses to Illness*. 2nd ed. Philadelphia: Saunders; 1993.

32

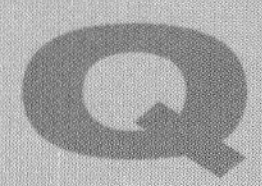

Mr. Martin Bergstrom, a 68-year-old retired textile worker, was found unconscious at his home by his family having apparently fallen and injured his head. Upon arrival at the hospital, the intensive care interdisciplinary team assessed his overall health status, including his neurosensory functions. His past health problems included high blood pressure and diabetes. Diagnostic measures (CT scan and laboratory tests) showed a cerebral vascular accident (stroke) involving the middle cerebral artery of the left hemisphere of his brain.

Mr. Bergstrom's current findings include a continued loss of consciousness and no movement of extremities (flaccidity). He has no response to verbal stimuli nor does he speak. His respirations are shallow and irregular.

Mr. Bergstrom's family lives in the same town and has helped him maintain his independent living situation. They are concerned about his plan of care and want to be involved in decisions about his treatment.

What are the priority nursing assessments and implementations to include in Mr. Bergstrom's plan of care?

At what point should the family be included in the discussions about their father?

How might Mr. Bergstrom's nurse support the family during this difficult time?

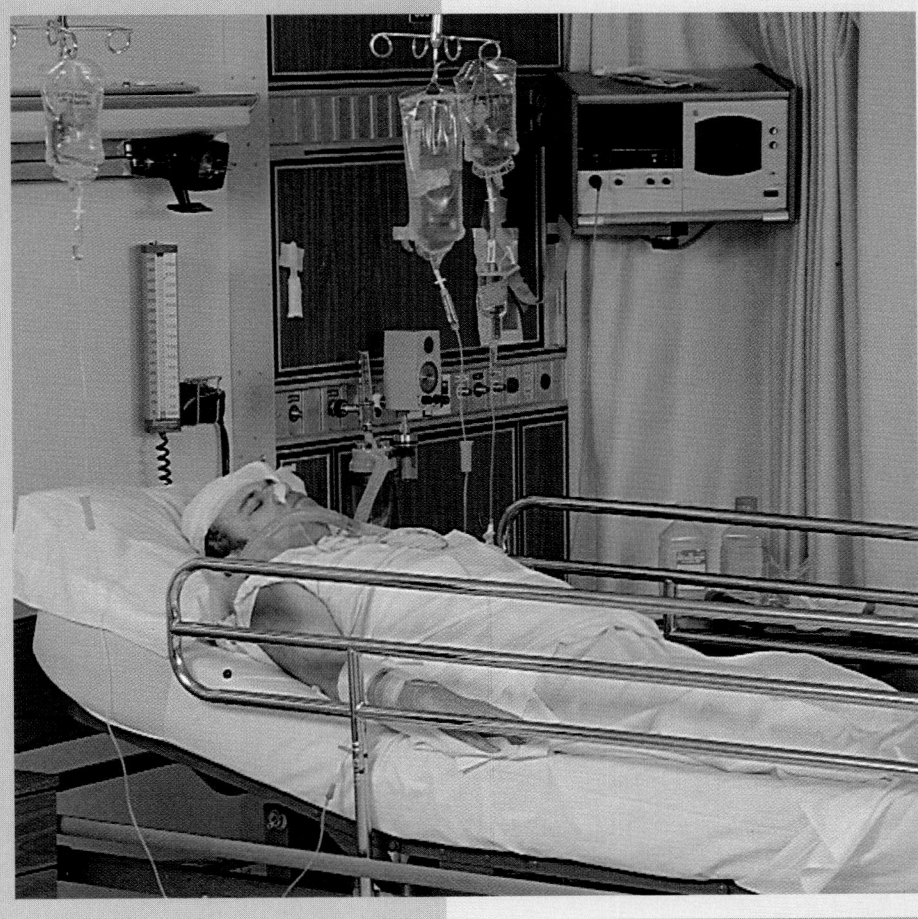

Neurosensory Integration

Janet A. McNelly and Barbara St. Marie

CHAPTER OUTLINE

The neurosensory system is a complex entity incorporating the central nervous system (CNS—the brain and spinal cord), and the peripheral nervous system, (the nerves that connect the CNS to other parts of the body).

The nerve tissue of the brain and spinal cord is made up of masses of nerve cells known as **neurons.** The millions of neurons in the neurosensory network serve as pathways for impulse conduction. Different types of neurons carry different messages. *Afferent* neurons transmit sensory stimuli from the periphery to the spinal cord and brain. *Efferent* neurons transmit impulses from the CNS to the peripheral nerves, which results in a motor response from muscles or glands.

The CNS and the peripheral nervous systems perform three general functions: a sensory function, a conscious or integrative function, and a motor function. The sensory function gathers data from sensory receptors located at the ends of the peripheral nerves. These receptors convey information regarding environmental changes in and around the body, including temperature, noise, light, and oxygen concentration in the blood.

All information gathered by the sensory receptors is converted into nerve impulses that are transmitted to the brain via the peripheral nerves. These impulses are then brought together—or integrated—creating sensations, perceptions and memories, which aid the formation of thoughts. The integrative function of the brain produces conscious and subconscious thoughts and decisions, enabling a person to see, hear, respond, eat, think, move, and act. Neurosensory integration occurs as a result of the networks and circuits of the neurosensory system, which blends information from all other systems into a unified whole so that individuals can function and think.

The motor function of the nervous system occurs as a result of CNS activity. The peripheral nerves carry impulses from the brain to responsive nerve endings located in muscles and glands known as effectors. Effectors cause muscles to contract and glands to produce hormones or secretions when stimulated by nerve impulses.

Neurosensory integration is fundamental, not only to individuality, but to one's responses to illness. Neurosensory integration enables patients to cope and therefore influences their requirements for nursing care. Coping is particularly important in illness because it affects the capacity to interact with others. Successful coping can support the healing process. Collaboration between the patient and health care providers can be a crucial part of recovery. Without a significant level of neurosensory integration, a patient's capacity to engage in a collaborative relationship may be seriously impaired, or the patient may only be able to function in a limited capacity. Nursing assessment of the neurosensory system is thus essential to determine to what extent patients will be able to participate in care.

Important nursing management decisions are derived from the nurse's impressions about the patient's level of neurosensory function and ability to engage in a collaborative nurse–patient relationship.

SECTION 1

UNDERSTANDING NEUROSENSORY INTEGRATION

The neurosensory network is an intricate collection of communication circuits that transmits sensory information, in the form of electrical and chemical energy, to central control centers in the brain. The circuits of the neurosensory network reach out to the sense organs and muscles, extend up and down the spinal cord, and bind the very different parts of the brain into an interlocking, coordinated control unit. The information processed produces perception, channels attention, creates thought and emotion, and initiates motor responses involved in carrying out effective action. All of the aspects of the network work together to coordinate behavior.

OPTIMAL NEUROSENSORY INTEGRATION

NEUROSENSORY FUNCTIONS

The functions served by neurosensory integration are consciousness; perception; memory; thought; speech, language and communication; and movement. Although the following discussion deals with each neurosensory function separately, these functions in actuality are closely interrelated, each function serving and supporting the others.

Consciousness

Consciousness (awareness) is the state of being aware of one's self and one's surroundings. It is the ability to interpret sensory information, to react critically with thoughts and movements, to take appropriate action, to permit the accumulation of memory traces, and to develop an intellect.

Consciousness has two components, arousal and content.[1] **Arousal** corresponds to wakefulness. It is a state in which an individual attends to people, things, and events in the environment and is ready for activity. Wakefulness is not a constant state, but fluctuates normally with the state of sleep. Changes in consciousness, from sleep to wakefulness and back again, are the most visible manifestations of the body's circadian (daily) rhythms and, in fact, are accompanied by changes in several physiologic processes. For example, a sharp reduction in the formation of urine occurs during sleep, the basal metabolic rate is decreased, heart rate slows, pulse and blood pressure decrease, and body temperature decreases.

Content, the second component of consciousness, is also controlled by and involves broad areas of the brain. **Content** is what is contained in the consciousness; the ideas, feelings, and sensations of which the individual is aware. Content is the sum of cognitive and affective (emotional) processes—the result of awareness, judgment, and emotional reaction. The generation of mental content is a particularly complex aspect of neurosensory integration.

Neurosensory Basis. Arousal level is controlled by the reticular formation of the brain stem, which enables the body to shift from states of alertness to states of lethargy and sleep. The reticular formation consists of neurons distributed in the medulla oblongata, pons, mesencephalon, and portions of the diencephalon. Responding to sensory information, the reticular formation screens messages to the brain, activating consciousness and responsiveness or protecting a restful state as appropriate to normal daily patterns and needs.

Relationship to Other Neurosensory Functions. Consciousness depends on the interaction between the intact cerebral cortex and the upper brain stem. The cerebral cortex is responsible for consciousness and higher mental processes such as speech, language, memory, abstract reasoning, and learned responses to stimuli. It is comprised of two hemispheres joined by the corpus callosum. One hemisphere is dominant.[2] The brain stem is involved in arousal and vital body functions such as breathing. Consciousness is required for voluntary activities such as interacting with others, walking, and playing tennis, but not for autonomic processes such as breathing.

Implications for Collaboration. Without consciousness, the ability to think and to communicate are drastically diminished. Collaboration with patients is dependent on the patient's state of consciousness. Altered states of consciousness place the patient in a dependent condition. When a patient's consciousness is diminished, it may become necessary for nurses to shift the focus of collaboration from the patient to others in the patient's family.

Perception

Perception is the ability of the mind to interpret and analyze input from the senses in order to understand the internal and external environment. Perception requires experience. Multiple stimuli must be evaluated, organized, and integrated to provide meaning. Human life, in fact, depends on successful and accurate relaying and interpretation of body signals and cues from the environment.

Sensory Input. Perception depends on sensory input received by sensory organs—eyes, ears, nose, tongue, and skin—and by spatial sensors—muscles, tendons, joints, and visceral organs. These sensors send a barrage of internal and external stimuli to support consciousness and arousal. Cutaneous stimuli assist in maintaining consciousness while visual, acoustic, and psychic stimuli influence arousal, attention, and perception. Because the brain cannot react completely to a barrage of incoming stimuli, the incoming messages are sorted and screened.[3] Thus, a person will generally only react to meaningful stimuli.

SIGHT. Sight is the most important of the human senses. People receive 90 percent of their information about the world using the sense of sight. Through vision, color can be appreciated, and spatial and object discrimination allow the detection of shapes and the movement of objects. Both central and peripheral vision are important.

Central vision is sight that results from images falling on the macula of the retina and is used when focusing on an object. **Peripheral vision** is the ability to see objects that reflect light waves falling on areas of the retina other than the macula and is used to see out of the corners of the eyes. It contributes to depth perception and assists in detecting objects and sensing movement.

CRITICAL QUERY

Leukenotte[5] has stated that a majority of institutionalized elders have hearing problems. For which nursing actions would this be problematic? How can the nurse assist patients who have decreased hearing?

The complex functions of the sense of vision enable people to perceive objects and events surrounding them in the context of their environment, assigning meaning to the events.

The visual sense develops from birth as newborn infants begin to see light and recognize familiar objects, such as the mother's face, shapes, colors, and toys. Learning, whether cognitive, affective, or psychomotor, is dependent on sight. Approximately 13 percent of people over 65 years old have some form of visual impairment.[4]

HEARING. Hearing is important for protection, survival, and communication. Accuracy of perceptions, communication, and quality of life are also affected by one's sense of hearing. The acoustic nerve (CN VIII), the temporal lobes, and a portion of the frontal lobes of the cerebrum are involved with sound perception and interpretation. The sense of hearing is developed in utero and is used throughout the life span. It is estimated that 50 percent of people over 65 and 90 percent of institutionalized elders have a hearing problem.[5]

SMELL. The sense of smell is the least developed of the human senses. The limbic system of the brain is closely associated with the area perceiving smell and may have developed from it. Because the limbic system serves the functions of memory, emotion, and learning, smell can awaken strong memories that can be perceived as good or bad. Smell is also a component in heightened sexual awareness. All of these effects of smell greatly enhance the depth of perception of stimuli.

TASTE. Taste is an unrefined sense that detects only four qualities: sweet, sour, salty, and bitter. Chemical receptors, located separately on the tongue, enable individuals to taste foods. Taste is a major factor in selection of foods, leading people to form opinions of foods and thus influencing nutritional habits. The sense of taste is also protective. People are less likely to ingest harmful substances if they have a foul taste. Enjoyment of the flavors of food is not a function of taste, but rather of the smells associated with food. The facial nerve (CN VII) and glossopharyngeal nerve (CN IX) also link with temporal and frontal lobes of the cerebrum to interpret the taste.

TOUCH, OTHER BODY AWARENESS SENSES, AND TEMPERATURE. Touch and related sensory modalities, temperature and pain, are the last senses to vanish in unconsciousness, and the first to reawaken.

The sense of touch is comprised of several sensory modalities. Special receptors send stimuli to relay stations in the brain via special nerve tracts. These modalities include vibration, pressure, and touch; stereognosis (identifying objects by touch alone, through texture, size, and shape); and kinesthetic proprioception (ability to perceive movement of muscles and joints to control and refine movements, posture, and equilibrium).

The sense of temperature transmits information about hot and cold. The ability of the brain to interpret this information, identifying extremes of temperature, protects individuals from injury.

BALANCE. The last of the special senses is balance or equilibrium. Equilibrium provides sensory information about gravity and rotation of the body. Receptors are located in the vestibular apparatus of the acoustic nerve (CN VIII) in the ear. Several higher brain centers and the sensory association areas make interpretations about the body's upright position and execute careful reflex adjustments to maintain balance. People are unaware of the operation of these reflexes when standing, sitting, and walking.

Sensory Interpretation. The senses provide the input that is the basis of perception. However, perception also depends on the ability of the brain to integrate and interpret this input.

Cognition, the act or process of knowing, plays an important role in perception. Integration and interpretation are cognitive activities. Through cognition, various stimulus sensations are coordinated and united into a whole for complete awareness. For example, when one sees and smells a pizza, the brain interprets this and responds by causing salivation and stomach rumbling. Sensory integration refers to the assembly of this sensory input in a perceptual unit.

Sensory interpretation involves comparison of a current event to previous experience. This interpretive capacity also enables the brain to recognize and differentiate incoming sensations. An example of multisensory interpretation is using vision, touch, hearing, and shape to correctly identify a set of car keys.

Variables affecting sensory interpretation include many parts of personality such as emotions, motivations, past life experiences, and coping styles. Sensory interpretation allows for the significance of an event to be shaped through mental activities of comparison and analysis unique to each personality. No two people have the same life experiences; thus, no two people perceive events in the same way. Hospitalization may mean confinement to some persons, danger and a threat to life for others, and a source of comfort and healing for still others.

Relationship to Other Neurosensory Functions

EMOTION. Emotions play an important role in sensory interpretation. **Emotion** is an affective state of consciousness in which joy, fear, anger, rage, and pleasure are experienced. Strong emotions are usually accompanied by physiologic changes (such as increased heart rate) in the body. An example of a strong emotional response is the fight-or-flight response. Mild emotions, such as appreciation, affection, or irritation, may not manifest such apparent bodily changes.

COLLABORATIVE STRATEGY

NEUROSENSORY FUNCTIONS

Collaboration as an interpersonal process is impossible without the support of the neurosensory functions: consciousness, perception, memory, thought, and communication. These functions of the nervous system comprise the anatomic and physiologic foundation of humanness and social interaction. When any one of these functions is altered or impaired, collaborative exchanges become difficult. In essence, neurosensory integration is the necessary condition for collaboration.

Emotions seem to be linked to and inform the brain of an undefined sense of disruption or upset. Upsets can be pleasant, such as getting an A grade in a course, or unpleasant, such as hearing footsteps from behind while walking alone in a dark alley. Emotions influence the ability to respond to stress, to take corrective action, and to restore equilibrium.

Emotion has subjective and objective aspects. The subjective aspect is the feeling state of an individual, described in terms of feeling, mood, affect, or tone. **Feeling** refers to the cognitive awareness of emotions such as happiness, fear, pleasure, anger, and irritability. When feeling is prolonged, a mood occurs. **Mood** refers to one's subjective description of feelings. In contrast, **affect** is the outward appearance of an emotional state to others. **Tone** describes the character or style in which a person communicates. Tone is influenced by affect and feelings (eg, "she spoke with a friendly tone in her voice").

The limbic system plays an essential role in processing the sensory input that produces emotions and accompanying physiologic expressions. The deep cerebral structures of the limbic system form a loop or circuit around vital structures in the center of the brain, linking these structures and drawing on resources of the brain (eg, perceptions, memory, and cognition) to interpret or analyze stimuli and, subsequently, to produce an emotional expression. Emotional expression is also mediated by information stored in memory about past events.

As sensory input flows through this loop or circuit, brain chemicals known as neurotransmitters are released. Neurotransmitters influence emotional behavior and may have tranquilizing and mood-elevating properties.

Implications for Collaboration. Because no two individuals perceive any event in the same way, it is essential in the collaborative process for nurses to assess a patient's perception of an event when the event is related to the patient's health. For example, a nurse who admits two women for labor and delivery may find that they interpret their situations differently despite the fact that both are undergoing the birthing process. Understanding the unique perceptions of each patient enhances their care.

Pain

Pain is a warning that alerts the individual to the presence of injury or illness. Sternbach describes pain as an "abstract concept that refers to (1) a personal, private sensation of hurt; (2) a harmful stimulus which signals current or impending tissue damage; (3) a pattern of responses which operate to protect the organism from pain."[6] This is a theoretical definition. A more useful definition for nurses has been developed by McCaffery, who defines pain as "whatever a person says it is, existing whenever the person says it does."[7]

Pain is a common symptom and a universal human experience. It is the most common reason that people seek health care. Pain is a warning that something is wrong. It serves as an adaptive mechanism that alerts individuals of a potentially harmful situation. The capacity to perceive pain is a normal function. The absence of pain response is abnormal.

The Pain Response. The pain response has three components: reception, perception, and response.

RECEPTION. Reception is the neurologic component of the pain response. Special receptors receive the painful stimulus and transmit it along afferent fibers in the peripheral nerves to the spinal cord. There, the simplest neurologic response—reflex—occurs; a contraction of the muscle leads to a protective withdrawal from the source of the pain. Pain impulses travel quickly to the brain, where the stimulus is processed.

PERCEPTION. Perception involves the interpretation of the painful stimulus. It begins when the individual first becomes aware of the pain. Both physiologic and psychological factors contribute to an individual's pain perception.

Pain impulses travel up the spinothalamic tract, activating the reticular formation, before proceeding to the higher brain centers in the cerebral cortex. The interpretation of data from all of these neurologic centers provides perceptual information on the location, severity, and probable cause of the painful stimulus.

For pain to be perceived, the individual must have an intact neurologic system. Factors that alter alertness lower pain perception; for example, anesthetics, pain medication, spinal cord trauma, or brain dysfunction. On the other hand, factors that heighten awareness to stimuli, such as stress and fatigue, will increase pain perception.

Psychological factors also affect how people perceive pain. Individuals do not perceive pain in the same way. Interpretation of pain is influenced by past experiences. If a person in the past had severe pain without relief, present pain may be viewed with anxiety and fear. On the other hand, if past experiences in coping with pain have been successful, the person may be better prepared to deal with another pain event.

Anxiety increases a person's perception of pain. Someone who has used a great deal of psychological energy in coping may not be able to deal well with pain. Other emotions also heighten pain perception, for example, loneliness, depression, boredom, fear, hopelessness, and anger.

Cultural background regarding the meaning and significance of pain is an important aspect of pain perception. Cultural background influences how people think about pain, how they show pain, and decisions they make about pain. People of one culture may take pride in not recognizing pain, while others may view pain as something to endure. Values about pain include the perception that pain is punishment for past deeds.

Age also influences pain perception. Young children and the elderly may experience more pain than others. Because they are often unable to communicate their needs, these patients may not receive adequate pain relief measures.

RESPONSE. Response to pain has physiologic and behavioral components. They may appear to conflict. For example, although the objective data may indicate the presence of pain (eg, elevated pulse, blood pressure, a gaping wound), a patient may demonstrate behaviors indicating that pain does not exist.

As the pain stimulus ascends the spinal cord, the autonomic nervous system is alerted as a part of the stress response. Acute pain evokes the sympathetic fight-or-flight response. Unrelenting visceral pain, on the other hand, causes the parasympathetic nervous system to act. Therefore, patients with severe sustained pain may reach a state of equilibrium where they do not show acute signs of pain.

Of the many behavioral responses to pain, most are observable. Patients may grind their teeth, clench their hands, rock side to side, pace, hug themselves, cry or moan, hold the painful area, or tense groups of muscles.

Pain Nerve Fibers. Specialized nerve endings in the skin and viscera send messages of noxious stimuli (such as mechanical, chemical, or thermal stimuli) to the brain. These specialized nerve endings, or receptors, send impulses along specific fiber types, all of which are part of peripheral nerves. These fiber types, identified as A beta, A delta, and C fibers, differ in their rate of impulse conduction, diameter, and the types of stimuli to which they respond. *A beta fibers,* large-diameter myelinated fibers, conduct impulses rapidly, are located near the surface of the skin, and respond to thermal and mechanical pain stimuli. They cause a sensory pain that responds best to nonsteroidal anti-inflammatory drugs (NSAIDS). *A delta fibers,* also myelinated, are smaller in diameter, and conduct impulses more slowly than A beta. Along with the unmyelinated, slow-transmitting *C fibers,* they are located in the skin, the cornea, and the joints and viscera. A delta and C fibers respond to chemical as well as persistent mechanical and thermal irritants, and the intense pain stimuli produced when tissue is damaged or inflammed. Because of this dual innervation system, a sudden pain stimulus often produces a dual pain sensation—a sharp pain transmitted fast by the myelinated fibers which apprises the person rapidly of danger and the need to withdraw from the stimulus. This is followed a second or two later by slow, dull pain, the kind of pain that intensifies over time, produces suffering, and often requires narcotic medication for its alleviation.[6]

Gate-control Theory of Pain. The gate-control theory of pain, proposed by Melzak and Wall, describes how neurons in the dorsal horn of the spinal cord act as gates that regulate the transmission of pain impulses to the brain.[8] It is the most commonly accepted pain theory today.

Gate-control theory speculates that an area in the dorsal horn of the spinal cord known as the substantia gelatinosa acts as a gate that can increase or decrease the number of nerve impulses from the peripheral nerves to the brain. The gate is opened or closed depending on the input from small and large nerve fibers. Increased activity in the small fibers opens the gate, allowing the pain sensation to enter the brain. Conversely, increased activity in the large fibers closes the gate so that pain stimuli do not get through to the brain. Pain is perceived when the stimuli reaching the brain surpass a certain threshold limit.

Melzak and Wall also describe a cognitive influence on pain perception. Age, anxiety, previous experiences, attention, expectation, sex, cultural background, and socioeconomic status all play a role in perception of pain. The overall pain recognition in the brain is modulated by input received from the spinothalamic tract, reticular formation, limbic system, and certain cerebral areas that control memory retrieval of past pain experiences. Thus, pain is determined by a combination of sensory input and impulses from the higher brain centers.

Endorphins and Other Endogenous Opioids. The brain produces chemical regulators called *endogenous opioids* that modify pain. It is thought that they bind with opiate receptor sites throughout the body and, in particular, in the dorsal horn of the spinal cord. The release of these endogenous opioids closes the gate by decreasing the number of pain impulses that are transmitted to the brain. To date three types of endogenous opioids have been discovered: endorphins, dynorphins, and enkephalins.

Endorphins probably modulate pain by binding with opiate receptor sites throughout the nervous system, inhibiting release of neurotransmitters. It is thought that endorphins are made and stored in the pituitary gland. The abundance of opiate receptor sites in the limbic system supports the assumption that opiates relieve pain by altering, rather than preventing, pain perception. Several subgroups of endorphins have been identified, including beta-endorphin, which is found in high concentration in the hypothalamus.

Dynorphins, 50 times as potent as beta-endorphin, are found in the hypothalamus, pituitary gland, and spinal cord.

Enkephalin, a small polypeptide, binds to opiate receptor sites in the dorsal horn of the spinal cord and inhibits the release of a neurotransmitter referred to as substance P. Substance P acts to enhance pain transmission across synapses. By reducing pain transmission, enkephalins serve as an analgesic. Outside the spinal cord enkephalins are found in the brain stem, limbic system, hypothalamus, adrenal glands, and gastrointestinal tract. Subgroups of this endogenous opioid include levenkephalin and metenkephalin.

Classification of Pain. The International Association for the Study of Pain has established three different categories of pain: acute, chronic, and cancer. *Acute pain* is a protective mechanism and historically has been measured in time (pain lasting less than 6 months). Acute pain may be reflected physiologically with an increase in heart rate, respiratory rate, blood pressure, peripheral blood flow, muscle tension, palmar sweating, and pupil size. It is caused, for example, by traumatic injury, a surgical procedure, or a medical disorder. Acute pain gets better over time.

Chronic pain does not subside and is disabling and persistent. It is usually defined as pain lasting longer than 6 months. However, the idea has been forwarded that chronic pain can exhibit itself before the 6-month point.[9] An individual who has chronic pain may show the same clinical picture as the person suffering from acute pain, or his or her body may condition all signs of pain with normal heart rate, normal blood pressure, and no facial grimacing. Persons with chronic pain frequently exhibit signs of psychological depression.

Approximately 30 to 40 percent of cancer patients in the intermediate stages of cancer, and 55 to 90 percent of terminal cancer patients, have pain. Sixty percent of these patients report their pain as moderate to great severity.[9] Cancer pain is related to malignancy or the treatment of the malignancy.

Implications for Collaboration. Patients experiencing pain are a challenge to nurses. To collaborate effectively with patients who have pain, nurses must examine their personal attitudes about pain in general and an individual patient's pain. Nurses often underestimate patients' pain, and consequently give insufficient medication. To collaborate effectively with patients to control pain, nurses must be aware of these subjective judgments and objectively assess the nature of pain and its meaning for the patient.

Memory

Memory is the mental capacity of receiving, registering, encoding, consolidating, storing, and retrieving information, impressions, or experiences. Without memory, people would only be able to experience stimuli, sensations, and events of the moment. Information would only be stored for seconds. The information would not be

COLLABORATIVE STRATEGY
MEMORY

Memory is a neurosensory function that many people take for granted; yet it underlies even the most basic human activity or social exchange. Chronic illnesses often have a harmful effect on memory by their primary and secondary effects on the central nervous system and by the severe stress they cause. Current population dynamics suggest that more and more older people with chronic illnesses will need health care in the future. Skill in assisting people with memory difficulties will determine whether or not nurse-patient collaboration is successful. Supportive implementation that is constantly focused on bridging the cognitive gap created by a memory deficit will be a prominent feature of the care of many patients.

INSIGHTS FROM NURSING LITERATURE
SUPPORTING MEMORY

Green PM, Gildemeister JE. Memory aging research and memory support in the elderly. J Neurosci Nurs. *1994;25:241–244.*

The authors reviewed research on memory and aging that showed little relationship between older persons' perceived memory problems and their performance scores on standard memory tests. The recognition memory of older adults proved as efficient as that of younger adults. However, older people sometimes had difficulty remembering conversations, a function connected with their ability for self-care. The authors emphasize that memory problems can be readily identified during history-taking. Older patients with memory problems frequently prove to be poor historians. The author suggests strategies in health care settings which focus on reducing the need to remember by such techniques as labeling the call button and bathroom door, and by positioning important items so they are not forgotten. Cuing devices such as the use of alarm clocks or kitchen timers to remind the patient to do something may also be helpful, as can systems for storing information externally, such as notebooks, diaries, and tape recorders.

registered, and thus could not be retrieved or used for future comparative interpretation.

Types of Memory. Memories are distinguished by their duration and purpose.

IMMEDIATE MEMORY. **Immediate memory,** which occurs in the sensory registers, refers to activity at the site of sensory registration. Information enters the system through the senses and is held briefly in the sensory form in which it was received (eg, a sound such as a fan turning is heard in auditory form). There is a sensory register for each of the senses in which information stays only briefly. While the information is in the sensory register, it undergoes pattern recognition, which results when a group of pieces or elements is associated with previously acquired knowledge. It is a way of encoding the stimulus in a combined form; for example, a friend's face is stored as a face, not just a nose, eyes, and mouth. Once encoded, the stimuli can be moved to short-term memory.[10]

SHORT-TERM MEMORY. **Short-term memory** (STM), or working memory, is the site of ongoing cognitive activities such as word meaning and symbol manipulation as is used in mental arithmetic, and reasoning. These processes are carried out with the immediate awareness of the individual.

The STM stores information in a processed form that can be called up at the individual's discretion. STM is capable of holding five to nine pieces of information for a short amount of time, generally for minutes to hours. It can be held indefinitely by using a process called rehearsal.

Rehearsal is an overt or covert practicing or repetition of information, such as in reciting a grocery list or phone number. For example, STM will hold a telephone number long enough to enable the person to dial the number. Then the number is forgotten. Or if that telephone number is significant and the individual needs to remember it, or if the number is dialed many times (rehearsed), the memory trace becomes permanent and is transferred to long-term memory.

LONG-TERM MEMORY. **Long-term memory** (LTM) is the storage of information that lasts for hours to a lifetime. Without long-term memory, learning could not occur, and the brain would not have past experience with which to compare current events.

As memories move from short- to long-term memory, sensory associations are made that become a part of the memory trace. For example, words and ideas or visual memories of past similar stimuli are mechanisms by which information is categorized before it is sent to LTM. These associations influence retrieval.

Once information is transferred to long-term memory, it is there forever. Memory is a complex and active process. Information is not stored in isolation; it is related to previous memory stores, put in a certain framework or file of knowledge, and these frameworks are organized. Knowledge and information are always changing and always being reexamined and reformulated as new facts and other data are gathered, processed, and stored. Retrieval of information then becomes the challenge.

Process of Memory. Retrieval of information depends on attention and how memories are stored. People remember by concentrating, by relating information in elaborate ways such as mnemonics, by noting similarities and differences, or by noting a relationship of the information to something already known. People recall information when they are given a stimulus or a cue to retrieve stored information. Although no study has pinpointed an exact location, several areas of the cerebral cortex and related brain structures contribute to recall, revival, and recognition of information.

Scientists have long pondered and investigated the neurologic basis of memory. It is believed that the sensory system stimulates neurons in such a way that a pattern is fired over millions of neurons, producing an imprint or memory trace, which eventually becomes the memory. One neuron can be a part of several memory traces; thus memory is represented in many neural networks and can be evoked or reached through several inputs. It is also believed that memories are not static, but constantly restructured in the neural networks as the brain receives new information and as learning occurs.

RETRIEVAL OF MEMORIES. Sensory input is involved in evoking memories. The sense of smell, in particular, is known to evoke strong memories. Consider how the smell of cinnamon rolls baking reminds one of a grandmother baking. Not only is a scent pattern recalled, but scents can be remembered as well. As a stimulus causes a few neurons to fire in long-term memory to evoke memories of an event or fact, those neurons fire other neurons and the recall becomes greater.

Emotions may well underlie memory imprinting, especially in long-term memory. Emotions associated with significant events evoke memories of those events; they become part of the neuronal circuit.

Memory and Learning. Learning and memory are interrelated. The simplest kind of learning implies that something has been remembered. Learning has been defined in many ways. Psychologists view learning as a relatively permanent change in behavior as a result of experience, practice, or training. Physiologists define learning as the ability of the nervous system to store memories for future retrieval.[11]

IMPORTANCE OF LEARNING. Learning helps human beings know and recognize their environment and surroundings. It is important for the development of thought, knowledge, physical skills, and fine-tuned motor responses. Thus, learning is essential for actualization of the growth potential of human beings.

People who cannot remember cannot learn and lack the ability to store or recall items of information. Without learning, there could be no change in an individual's responses, behaviors, or thoughts; life would be a moment-to-moment existence, lacking meaningfulness and connections to the past or future. An example might be the patient who has a stroke damaging half of the brain. As a result, learning is impaired. The patient forgets how to dress himself. Because the patient cannot learn, directions from others will not help him learn to dress himself again. The act of instruction occurs as a single-moment experience for the patient and lacks meaning.[11]

TYPES OF LEARNING. People learn by simple and complex means. Chapter 21 discusses theories on human learning. The reader is referred to that chapter for additional information.

The three kinds of simple learning are (1) habituation, (2) sensitization, and (3) classical or Pavlovian conditioning.

Habituation is a form of learning that occurs when a stimulus that originally produced a response is presented so often that the individual stops responding to it.[12] Nurses observe learning by habituation in patients who must learn to give themselves injections. The individual gradually comes to view the pain from injections as nonthreatening and insignificantly painful, and thus through habituation learns to deal with the pain.

Sensitization, a form of nonassociative learning, occurs when a person attends to a previously neutral stimulus. Sensitization has the opposite effect of habituation. It arouses human interest and helps to determine dangerous stimuli. Persons who experience shortness of breath with exercise, for example, may consider this a normal response to exercise. However, if a healthy individual develops a chest cold, with shortness of breath, he or she may become sensitized, viewing it as abnormal or potentially threatening.

Classical conditioning (Pavlovian conditioning) is a form of learning in which an individual learns to link two separate stimulus elements. This occurs when a primary stimulus (a stimulus that naturally yields a certain reaction) is paired with another neutral stimulus and ultimately becomes conditioned. Eventually when the neutral stimulus is presented, it elicits the reaction formerly elicited only by the primary stimulus. The classic example is that of Pavlov's dogs, which became conditioned to salivate (a normal reaction to the primary stimulus of food) in reaction to the presence of white-coated attendants (neutral stimulus) who brought the food.

Humans learn by conditioning. Infants and children who experience pain in a visit to the clinic may be conditioned to view physicians and nurses with fear. Health care professionals (neutral stimulus), associated with injections or other procedures (primary stimulus), evoke fear (response) in the child, even when the primary stimulus is absent.

Complex learning is voluntary and requires the use of cognitive (thinking) skills involving learning facts and rules, classifying objects, making associations to previously learned material, analyzing data, and evaluating. It is associated with the ability to transfer information from short-term memory to long-term memory.

The variables that affect how information is stored are many. Age determines how much an individual can learn. For example, a small child will learn differently than an adolescent or adult. Attention to material will enhance the transfer into long-term memory. Rewards for learning and punishments for not learning contribute to learning. A person's verbal level may affect the way the information is transferred to memory. Cognitive skills relate to the ways in which individuals regulate their own internal process such as attention, learning, remembering, and thinking.[4] These strategies allow people to solve new problems, perform mathematical calculations, and carry out self-management behaviors.

Implications for Collaboration. Memory problems present a challenge to a nurse who wishes to establish a collaborative nurse–patient relationship. Memory loss refers to the inability to recall or store memories. Patients who lack memory have trouble learning and may have difficulty remembering explanations or instructions. They therefore may be unable to carry out tasks independently. Such patients are often confused and disoriented and may require nursing interventions directed at safety and self-care. Of necessity, patients with memory problems often assume a more dependent role, shifting the focus of the collaborative nurse–patient relationship to the family.

Thought

Thought is the mental process that assigns meaning to and designs actions in response to the integration and interpretation of sensory input. It is the process whereby the brain sorts and integrates every relevant piece of information gathered throughout each day. The term "thought" is applied to that which is intellectual—having to do with logic and reason and is distinguished by the capacity of reasoning. Mere perceiving, feeling, or willing are mental activities that do not require reasoning.

Thought comprises several mental functions. They are comprehension, reasoning, judgment, problem-solving, and conception (Table 32–1). The combination of these structured mental activities is also referred to as the cognitive capacities or the ability to think.

Importance of Thought. Humans have the ability to construct ideas, memories, and concepts in sequential fashion, to have insight into

TABLE 32-1. FUNCTIONAL CAPACITY OF THOUGHT

Function	Definition
Comprehension	Understanding.
Reasoning	Drawing inferences or conclusions using the power of comprehension.
Judgment	The capacity of the brain to form an opinion of an idea or event.
Problem-solving	The mind's ability to determine an action or solution based on judgment of a particular internal or external event.
Conception	The capacity, or function, of forming concepts or understanding ideas or abstractions; reflective thinking.

situations, to make appropriate decisions, to solve problems, to demonstrate reality-based thoughts, and to produce appropriate behaviors. Thought allows individuals to make careful adjustments in order to adapt to their environment and work toward the goal of health and to generate long-range goals and take action in light of those goals. A blending of sensory impressions and input from memory stores allows people to assign meaning to these specific events or goals and determine subsequent behaviors or thoughts.

Process of Thought. Thought is a complex, integrative mental activity involving many areas of the brain. For example, the frontal lobe of the cerebral cortex is responsible for emotions, intellect, learning, concentration, focusing attention, problem-solving, and the ability to follow instructions. All of these functions are requisites of thought.

It is difficult to pinpoint where thought occurs. Neuroscientists have found that for any task requiring thought, specific neural pathways perform that task.[13] Moreover, the pathways may differ depending on the nature of the thoughts. It is known that certain parts of the thought process occur in a somewhat sequential fashion.

- *Phase I.* Perception, or attending to sensory stimuli, produces a conscious awareness of a particular stimulus. For example, when one experiences soft rubbing sensations on the skin, the sensory system sends information that produces a general and nonspecific awareness. To discern what is causing the sensation, an intact sensory system, an appropriate attention span, and the ability to recognize and interpret the incoming stimuli are necessary.
- *Phase II.* The integration of stimuli results in interpreting and pinpointing the event. It is interpreted in terms of words, concepts, and relationships. Symbols, particularly linguistic symbols, are assigned to a given perception. This step is dependent on language. The fuzzy creature might be a cat or a bear.
- *Phase III.* An expressive thought or execution of motor activity, or change in mood and action, occurs based on the symbols attached to the perception. One pets the cat, talks to it, and feels pleasure; or one sees the bear, runs away, and feels intense fear.

Relationship to Other Neurosensory Functions. Thought is an integrative neurosensory function that is related to, dependent upon, and necessary for other functions. Perception and consciousness are necessary initially in the process of thought. Memory and memory retrieval and the ability to learn contribute to the store of neurosensory resources the brain uses during the analysis phase of thought. Finally, thought is necessary for speech, language, communication, and movement. The brain is highly dependent on language to process conscious brain events.

The networks of neurons that produce thought are vast, complex, and highly ordered. This network lies on the outer surface of the brain and is dependent on input from neural pathways. Thought is produced at a speed much faster than a person's consciousness can keep pace with.

Implications for Collaboration. A collaborative nurse–patient relationship requires that a patient have organized thinking, an intact neurosensory network, and the higher cognitive functions of comprehension, reasoning, judgment, problem-solving, and conception. When altered thought processes occur, they become apparent in almost every aspect of an individual's behavior. In many cases, the patient will be dependent on the nurse for guidance, safety, instruction, and interpretation to accomplish activities of daily living and achieve a satisfactory and safe level of independence.

Speech, Language, and Communication

Speech, language, and communication are intertwined. **Communication** is the act of sending and receiving messages by the use of verbal and nonverbal language. **Language** is a formal system of signs and symbols used for communication. **Speech** uses language to articulate or express thoughts and ideas using language.

Neurosensory Basis. Communication is a complex neurosensory process involving the entire brain. Language function is widely distributed throughout the dominant side of the brain. It relies on information stored in the front of the brain, as well as the touch, auditory, and visual interpretative areas that contribute comprehension of concepts, people, and thoughts.

NEUROSENSORY PROCESSES OF COMMUNICATION. The neurosensory processes involved in communication and the understanding of messages are complex. They involve reception, perception, conceptualization, formulation, and expression of verbal and written speech.

In *reception,* spoken words are converted into neural signals in the cochlea of the ears with ongoing passage of these signals to an area of the brain where perception takes place. Visual information is also telegraphed to the brain. *Perception* is the awareness of the stimuli. Then the message or idea is reconstructed through language into symbols or thought in areas of the brain. This is known as *conceptualization.* Knowledge, past experience, feelings, attitudes, and emotions are a frame of reference influencing the perception and conceptualization of a message. Thought *formulation* is the detailed, coordinated plan for vocalization. It results from the neural signal sent to the brain area telling the facial muscles, lips, and tongue to move in a specific motor pattern and sound sequence so that a particular sound is expressed. *Expression* is the articulatory and mechanistic vocalization known as speech. In order for articulation or speech to occur, the neurosensory network for communication must be intact.

SENSORY AND MOTOR ASPECTS OF COMMUNICATION. Communication involves both sensory and motor aspects. The sensory aspect includes the use of ears, eyes, and touch for reception and the ability to understand both the written and spoken word. The motor aspect involves the muscles used in vocalization and its control as well as the ability to produce speech and to write words.

PROCESS OF SPEECH. Speech sounds and their meaning arise in the dominant hemisphere of the brain and travel to an area of motor cells in the frontal lobes. The neural impulse evokes a detailed and coordinated program for vocalization that is then transmitted to adjacent motor cells that control the facial muscles. When words are read, the back of the brain where vision cells are located is activated, and the brain must work to match the visual input with the sounds those words have when spoken.

Relationship to Social Interaction. Communication is an individual's way of expressing himself or herself and relating his or her needs. Relationships, whether casual or intimate, are established through communication. Communication is necessary for intellectual, spiritual, and physical growth, and occurs throughout the lifespan.

Language and speech are prerequisites to communication. They allow humans to express knowledge that is learned; to describe events and happenings never before experienced; to share emotions, needs, and desires; and to influence role behaviors, lifestyles, and social interaction.

The social impact of problems of communication, language, and speech can have dramatic consequences for patients and their significant others. Language and communication are inextricably bound with the culture of the patient. Poor communication can cause feelings of fear, frustration, anger, anxiety, hostility, depression, confusion, and isolation.

Relationship to Other Neurosensory Functions. Communication is related to all of the other functions of the neurosensory system, both supporting them and depending on them. In order to use language, one must be conscious; in turn, language provides much of the content of conscious awareness. Language is dependent on information retention, recall, and the integration of symbols, and is necessary for thought. As a consequence, it is intimately involved in the capacity to interpret the sensory stimuli that comprise perceptions.

?

CRITICAL QUERY

Ebersole and Hess[10] state that language and communication are bound to one's culture. What are important factors or issues for the nurse to consider when addressing a patient from a different culture? What observations might the nurse make to differentiate communication problems arising from the fact that the patient speaks a different language from those caused by hearing loss, for example?

Much of the content of memory and learning is structured around language. The capacity to use language in thought and speech is also dependent on memory and learning. Moreover, language has the capacity to evoke emotions that become associated with ideas embedded in the memory.

Speech depends on the interpretation of auditory and visual images that reach the higher intellectual centers during differing states of consciousness. To use speech, one must initially formulate the thought to be expressed, choose appropriate words, and then control the motor activity of the muscles of speech.

Implications for Collaboration. Communication is vital to the development of a collaborative nurse–patient relationship. Communication is the tool by which nurses validate their inferences and judgments with patients to develop nursing diagnoses and outcomes that clearly reflect patient needs. Nursing care is most effective when patients can communicate their needs and desires. When communication is insufficient or patient input lacking, the nurse–patient relationship is one in which the nurse must anticipate the needs of the patient. Eye contact, voice intonation, and facial expression are a few of the ways in which nurses demonstrate caring and increase effectiveness of communication with patients experiencing impaired communication.

Movement

Movement can be defined as a change of place, position, or posture of any portion of the body. Movement may appear to be a simple maneuver, but in actuality it is a highly complex neurosensory function. Controlled, purposeful movement as a result of neurosensory integration brings great fulfillment and joy to people's lives. To be effective, movement must be purposeful, controlled, balanced, upright, fluid, and smooth.

Types of Movement. Movement occurs through the use of over 600 muscles in the human body to perform a large number of actions, ranging from walking to blinking to swallowing. Movement can be classified as voluntary or involuntary. **Voluntary movement** is carried out consciously and intentionally under a person's will or volition. Brushing the teeth, piano playing, and driving a car are conscious movements. **Involuntary movement** is performed unconsciously, without the person's will, or unintentionally. The quick release of the hand from a hot stove, and excursion of the chest during respiration, occur spontaneously, quickly, and usually without conscious control.

Neurosensory Basis. The motor system controls movement. In contrast to the sensory system, which relays signals from the periphery (skin, visual field) upward to specific brain sites, the motor system originates in specialized brain cells, that make up the motor cortex, and passes stimulation through the spinal cord, ending at the periphery in the movement of muscles. The motor cortex is like a map, with regions (brain cells) specialized to move each muscle of the body by controlling and coordinating the push and pull forces of opposing muscle groups. Without this input, movement would be awkward and erratic.

Relationship to Other Neurosensory Functions. It is not known exactly how the brain comes to a decision to perform a particular action or in what area of the brain the decision originates. It is apparent, however, that movement is interrelated with other functions of the neurosensory system.

- *Movement and perception.* Movement and perception might seem to be very separate systems, yet very few of the sensory signals sent to the brain end without initiating and modifying muscle action in some way. The pleasant smell of fresh flowers often stimulates the sensory system in such a way that one is drawn toward the smell and to find the flowers.
- *Movement and thought.* Interrelationships are necessary in order for purposeful movement to occur. The brain operates in lightning-like fashion in response to stimuli. Because people have the ability to analyze and judge, they also have the capacity to control movement.
- *Movement and learning.* Movement and learning are linked in the achievement of skilled activities, such as handwriting. Dexterity, coordination, and sequencing of movements are part of skilled activities. Their efficiency increases and skill improves with learning.
- *Movement and emotion.* Emotion and movement are linked through the activation of the autonomic nervous system. The fight-or-flight response initiates a cascade of autonomic physiologic responses.
- *Movement and communication.* Communication is so closely associated with movement that if one cannot communicate either verbally or in written word, the outer world becomes shut out.

Importance of Movement. One of the benefits of movement is the capacity for independence which is highly prized by human beings. Parents thrill with their baby's first steps. Exercise, through activities such as walking, running, and bicycling, diminishes tension and promotes mental rejuvenation. Society values both independence and movement. Individuals who can move are able to take care of their own self-care needs and thus preserve independence.

The integration of thought and movement is also linked to social functioning through purposeful, controlled actions. Smiling, shaking hands, and laughter control are some examples of "thoughtful" action.

Movement also allows expression of the self. Each person has certain movements that accompany various emotions. A happy smile, drooped shoulders, or raised eyebrows characterize differences in emotions. Sexuality is influenced by movement. To touch, kiss, and express and receive love are integral to human behavior and growth.

Overall health is affected tremendously by movement. Exercise strengthens the heart, brings oxygen to the tissues, and relieves mental tension. Skin and bone breakdown, decreased mental stimulation, and increased dependence on others are examples of the negative health effects of immobility.

Implications for Collaboration. One effect of not being able to move one or more parts of the body is dependence. Patients become dependent on nurses to assist them in activities of daily living. The collaborative nature of the nurse–patient relationship is shifted to focus on safety and protection under these conditions, and the patient becomes temporarily dependent on nurses for mobility and interpretation of the surrounding environment. The nurse's roles in the collaborative relationship will be those of supporter and promoter of independence. Including the family and monitoring the patient's needs is of prime importance.

FACTORS AFFECTING NEUROSENSORY INTEGRATION

GENETIC HERITAGE

Genetic heritage is important in neurosensory integration. Through the genes, genetic information is conveyed that shapes both the characteristics of the neurosensory apparatus common to humans and the unique features that are characteristic of the individual. Genetic information may also cause malformation of the neurosensory apparatus. Features of the neurosensory apparatus that in health protect neurosensory functions include the following.

- *Skull.* The skull is a bony structure composed of several bones that fuse after birth to form a rigid vault. This vault absorbs trauma to the head, protecting the brain.
- *Vertebral (spinal) column.* The vertebrae form a protective covering for the spinal cord and a support for the cranium and trunk. Each vertebra is cushioned from the next by a structure called the intervertebral disc, which has a high water content. With age, this water content decreases, which potentiates a loss of protective function. When the core of the disc herniates through the outer layer, the disc will again lose its protective function. Further movement of the damaged disc can actually cause injury by compressing the spinal cord or spinal nerves.
- *Meninges.* The meninges are protective membranes covering the brain and spinal cord. Meningeal layers also provide blood supply and act as a cushion to the brain. There are three layers: the dura mater, arachnoid, and pia mater.
- *Cerebrospinal fluid.* The cerebrospinal fluid (CSF) provides a cushion to prevent damage to the brain, helps regulate intracranial pressure, and provides a mechanism for nutrient supply and waste removal. The CSF is produced by the filtration that occurs between the circulatory system and the choroid plexus. It filters out and coats the brain and spinal cord as it travels through the subarachnoid space. About 800 mL of CSF is secreted every day, although only approximately 150 mL is present at any one time in an adult. Reabsorption of CSF occurs through the arachnoid mater. CSF and molecules such as protein, glucose, and certain waste products are released back into the circulatory system. If the arachnoid villi are blocked, CSF cannot be reabsorbed and may result in injury.
- *Blood–brain barrier.* The blood–brain barrier is a protective structure of capillaries that supplies blood to the brain. The capillaries form a continuous wall that prevents many substances from entering the brain. Water, oxygen, carbon dioxide, glucose, and selected electrolytes easily pass through this barrier. Extra nutrients and waste products of cell metabolism are filtered out. If this barrier is injured, molecules that are normally excluded may enter the brain, disrupting its fluid and electrolyte balance.
- *Cerebral circulation.* The cerebral circulation transports elements that are vital for the central nervous system, including oxygen and glucose, which the brain is unable to store. When arterial circulation ceases, the brain is depleted of oxygen in 4 to 6 minutes and is depleted of glucose in less than 1 minute. Arterial blood enters the CNS by two internal carotid arteries and two vertebral arteries.

AGE

Children

Young children have immature neurosensory systems. As they grow and learn, neurosensory functioning matures. Perception also changes with age. Infants and children need stimulation and parental affection to develop. Too little stimulation can lead to the inability to conceptualize in later years. Too little affection can develop into failure to thrive in infants.

Many childhood diseases can affect the sensory organs. For example, measles can affect sight, resulting in blindness. Chronic ear infections, mumps, measles, or rubella can cause impaired hearing.

Older Adults

Cortical size and blood flow to the brain diminish with aging. The decrease in blood flow may result in a decrease of the oxygen supply, thereby compromising neurosensory function.

The senses also diminish with aging. Most elderly people develop some sight loss, hearing loss, loss of taste and smell, and loss of sensation. Balance may be affected as well, as the muscles become weaker or the neurosensory system degenerates.

Emotional changes may result from these neurosensory changes. The elderly may become depressed because of these changes. Sleep deprivation may cause delirium. Deprivation of NREM sleep (see Chap. 31) results in a reduction of hormones and produces lethargy and depression. Sensory deprivation may occur from the loss of sensory function.

Memory can be altered with the aging process. Decreased blood flow to the brain, atherosclerosis, and Alzheimer's disease are a few examples of aging changes contributing to altered memory. In addition, ability to learn may be altered and the speed of central processing is slowed.

Gait changes such as the slowing of step, widening of the base of support, and shuffling are related to a decrease in muscle mass and loss of large motor nerve fibers regulating nerve function.

GENERAL HEALTH STATUS

Certain alterations in health can affect neurosensory functioning. Diseases or conditions that reduce blood circulation to the brain result in decreasing awareness and slowed responses. Diseases that alter brain tissue, such as Alzheimer's disease, result in a decreasing awareness. Diseases of the central nervous system can produce varying degrees of paralysis and sensory loss.

Physical alterations in other body systems can have an impact on neurosensory functioning. Decreased respiratory or cardiac function can lead to confusion, as can an imbalance in fluids and electrolytes. Renal alterations can result in a buildup of body toxins that can lead to an altered level of consciousness, as can liver dysfunction. An alteration in almost any body system can have an impact on neurosensory function.

CULTURAL FACTORS

Neurosensory integration and cultural diversity are interrelated, especially in the interpretation of a person's pain. Stating that one has pain can be viewed as a weakness by people in one culture or as an expected occurrence by people in another culture. Every culture also interprets its distinctive beliefs into how its members learn and collaborate with members of the health care team. For example, folk healers may be viewed as essential to healing in some cultures.[5,14]

DIET

Deficiencies in certain nutrients can influence sensory functioning. For example, semineural deafness is thought to be related to dietary deficiencies in vitamin D and calcium, which may affect the action potentials generated by the cochlea. Thiamin C is essential for neurosensory integration (Chap. 28). Electrolytes (chiefly sodium and potassium) are essential for nerve conduction and cellular integrity (Chap. 34).

ENVIRONMENT

Stimuli

The environment is a major factor influencing conditions such as sensory deprivation or sensory overload. Too few meaningful stimuli can result in altered neurosensory integration, as can too many stimuli.

Excessive noise in the environment can lead to diminished hearing. Teenagers are at risk for hearing loss because of very loud music.

Toxins

The word "toxin" means poison. Many substances in the home, workplace, and environment are toxic agents and act like poison in the body, particularly on neurosensory integration. Toxic agents are commonly found in solvents, paints, pesticides, and chemicals used in industry. In the hospital workplace, there is added risk of accidental exposure to mercury, a heavy metal, or to chemotherapy agents.

Bacteria are another source of toxins that affect neurosensory integration. Tetanus and diphtheria are diseases produced by bacterial toxins. Both can be prevented with proper immunization. Another disease, botulism, is produced by a toxin that is potentially present in unrefrigerated foods, such as mayonnaise or salad dressings, and in meats, particularly chicken or pork, that are improperly cleaned or cooked. Simple prevention through proper preparation of food and refrigeration eliminates the potential harm from botulism toxin.

Toxins interfere with the transmission of impulses over the neurosensory network. A primary mechanism by which toxins exert their harmful effects is by interfering with the production, transfer, or release of neurotransmitters that relay signals from one neuron to another. The effects can be slight to overwhelming in nature. The functions of consciousness, memory, perception, speech, and movement may be affected.

The effects of toxic agents or chemicals on neurosensory integration can result in reversible or irreversible loss of function. Treatment is aimed at removal of the toxic agent and initiation of supportive and rehabilitative interventions. The extent of reversibility is evaluated as functions return.

PSYCHOSOCIAL FACTORS

Changes in mental health can result in neurosensory alterations. Depression or withdrawal, for example, leads to sensory deprivation. Stress also affects behavior and thought. An individual's reaction to a stressful event will depend on the amount of stimulus presented by that stressful event and the number of other stresses simultaneously occurring. Failure to cope with stress in itself perpetuates stress. Eventually the stress may become overwhelming, and the individual may become disoriented or confused.[13]

MEDICATIONS AND OTHER SUBSTANCES

Many medications can affect neurosensory function. Sedations and tranquilizers may reduce alertness or lead to lethargy, drowsiness, or confusion. Antibiotics, such as streptomycin, neomycin, and gentamicin, can cause injury to the auditory nerve.

Alcohol and drugs can also result in toxicity to the neurosensory system. Ingestion of large amounts of alcohol and drugs is like ingesting a poison. Although each drug interferes with the neural cell in its own way, the effect is the same: neurosensory dysfunction. Altered consciousness, perception, movement, thought, or memory can occur with alcohol and drug toxicity.

ALTERED NEUROSENSORY FUNCTIONING

OVERVIEW

Altered neurosensory functioning may require supportive, restorative, and rehabilitative health care. Serious long-term disability can interfere with the patient's quality of life and capacity to cope with the problems of life and living.

The preceding discussion of factors affecting neurosensory integration suggests some of the etiologies involved in altered functioning. For example, genetic factors may cause illnesses that directly or indirectly affect neurosensory function. Genetic anomalies of the brain and spinal cord alter the structure and electrochemical processes of the central nervous system.

Deterioration of general health from nongenetic causes also can have pathophysiologic consequences for neurosensory functions. Chronic kidney and liver disease, for example, can produce derangements in body chemistry that affect the whole body, including the nervous system. Wide fluctuations in the body's internal environment can disrupt the metabolism of cells in the neurosensory network, which interferes with neurosensory functions.

Altered neurosensory functions may also result from advancing age, poor nutrition, or environmental hazards. Ventricular accidents and other trauma are common causes of altered functioning that may result in disability.

Moreover, a number of diseases can attack virtually any aspect of the central or peripheral nervous systems. Depending on their location and severity, they can alter an individual's consciousness, perception, memory, thought, communication, or movement. These processes include tumors, infection, toxicity, vascular lesions that disrupt circulation to the brain or spinal cord, and impaired neurosensory transmission.

ALTERED CONSCIOUSNESS

Alterations in consciousness result in decreased wakefulness (arousal) or decreased orientation or awareness of the environment (content). Causes can be physical damage to the brain tissue or abnormalities that interfere with the metabolism of the nerve cells.

Unconsciousness is a state in which people become unresponsive to external stimuli (noise, voices, pain). The unconscious state may be characterized by varying reductions in degree of arousal. Ambiguous terms, such as "disorientation," "semiconsciousness," and "coma," are often used to describe altered levels of consciousness. It is more important to describe the patient's response to verbal or painful stimuli than to label the change in consciousness (Table 32–2). Use of the Glasgow Coma Scale (see Fig. 32–3, page 1135) allows for clearer objective descriptions.

ALTERED PERCEPTION

Any sensory modality can be impaired with damage to the brain tissue or cells in the sensory pathway.

Altered Vision

Patients experiencing visual impairments or sight loss are disabled. Loss of vision may create a threat to safety, incomplete perceptions of events, and potential limitations in education, occupation, and mobility. The nurse's role will involve assisting patients to adapt in various ways to their environment and sense of perception.

Visual alterations occur when there is external damage to the structure of the eye and its muscles, or internal damage to the optic nerve and nerve pathway. The result is decreased or absent visual capacity that manifests as refractive errors, dystopia, or blindness.

Refractive errors include such conditions as myopia, hyperopia, and presbyopia. *Myopia* (nearsightedness) occurs from elongation of the eyeball and causes objects that are distant to be out of focus. Glasses with concave lenses correct this problem. *Hyperopia* (farsightedness) is having difficulty focusing on close objects while seeing distant objects clearly. Glasses with convex lenses correct this problem. *Presbyopia* occurs with aging, usually around age 40. It occurs when the lens of the eye loses elasticity and persons cannot focus on close objects. Bifocals, trifocals, or reading glasses may be prescribed to correct the problem.

Diplopia is double vision or seeing two images of a single object. It can result from dysfunction of cranial nerves III, IV, and VI, which can cause muscle weakness and uncoordinated eye movements, and the resulting diplopia.

Cataracts, common in older persons, are opacities of the lens of the eye that decrease the light reaching the retina. Diminished vision results because the opaque area is impervious to light.

Glaucoma is a condition of increased intraocular pressure that can lead to blindness. Increased pressure from accumulating aqueous humor damages the eye, producing visual field defects. This results in a person seeing only what is straight ahead, a situation that is referred to as tunnel vision. If untreated, total loss of vision can result.

A *detached retina* occurs when the sensory layer of the retina separates from the pigment layer, depriving the sensory layer of a blood supply. Patients may complain of flashes of light, blurred or sooty vision, blank spots of vision, or complete loss of vision.

Alterations in color vision happen as a result of a defect in the visual color receptors of the retinal cones. The inability to distinguish certain colors is referred to as color blindness and is most

TABLE 32-2. TERMS DESCRIBING ALTERATIONS IN CONSCIOUSNESS (IN DESCENDING ORDER)

Alert
- Fully arouseable and conscious.
- Fully oriented to person, place, and time.
- Responses: Appropriate acknowledgment of people in environment with turning of head and/or body in person's direction (unless impaired motor function present). Ability to focus attention on the environment.

Confused
- Needs encouragement to focus on person or things in environment.
- Has difficulty correctly interpreting and attending to stimuli and is easily distracted.
- Responses: Disoriented first to time, then to place, and then to person. Has difficulty following commands and remembering.

Delirious
- May be loud or physically abusive. Therefore, arranging for safety of self and all near him or her is necessary.
- Responses: Restless, incoherent, agitated, and may have altered thought processes such as delusions, illusions, or hallucinations.

Obtunded
- May be sleepy or drowsy but arouses easily.
- Responses: Speech may be appropriate or inappropriate, and may be limited to two or three-word sentences.

Stuporous
- Lethargy, slow to arouse, and drowsy.
- Painful stimuli required for arousal and often repetition is needed.
- Responses: Withdrawal from painful stimuli occurs.

Semiconsciousness (Semicoma)
- Unresponsive. Does not spontaneously move unless noxious superficial stimuli are applied.
- Responses: Moaning or groaning with brief responses to this stimulation.

Coma
- Unarouseable except by deep noxious stimuli.
- Responses: Lack of withdrawal to stimuli. Slight muscle movement may be seen. Reflexes (corneal, pupillary, and gag) are present.

Deep Coma
- Complete unresponsiveness.
- Responses: No response to deep noxious stimuli. Lacks reflexes (corneal, pupillary, gag, tendon, and plantar).

commonly manifested as the inability to distinguish between red and green.

Blindness is the loss of sight and occurs as a result of congenital malformation or from detachment of the retina, the visual reception area of the eye. *Partial blindness* is a loss in limited areas of the visual field. Hemianopia is a form of partial blindness that occurs as a result of damage to the optic nerve behind the optic chiasm. A patient with *hemianopia* experiences blindness in one half of the visual field of one or both eyes. A patient who has had a stroke may have hemianopia.

Complete blindness is the total loss of vision from both eyes. Not all blind persons have a total loss of vision. The term "legal blindness" is used to describe severe, but incomplete, blindness. Legal blindness is defined as central visual acuity of 20/200 or less in the better eye, even when corrective lenses are worn.

Altered Hearing

Accurate assessment of the hearing loss, its meaning to a patient, and adaptations for communicating with the patient (hearing aid, sign language), influence the ability of nurse and patient to collaborate effectively. Changes in the structure and function of the ear can impair an individual's ability to hear. Almost every type of hearing loss can be classified into one of three areas: conductive hearing loss, sensorineural (perceptive) hearing loss, or mixed hearing loss.[13]

Conductive hearing loss can result from obstruction of the external canal by cerumen or a foreign body, damaged eardrum (tympanic membrane), or immobility of the tympanic membrane or ossicles.[15,16] When sound vibrations are not adequately transmitted to the inner ear, partial hearing loss results. If the basic cause cannot be corrected, the patient can use hearing aids to enhance hearing.

Sensorineural hearing loss, or perceptive hearing loss, occurs when there is a disorder of the inner ear (for example, as a result of certain drugs), damage to the hair cells of the cochlea, or pathology in the acoustic nerve (cranial nerve VIII) or the brain. In this type of hearing loss, vibrations are transmitted to the inner ear, but the nervous impulses from the cochlea to the brain are weakened. This type of hearing loss may be helped with hearing aids. Recently, devices known as cochlear implants have been designed to assist individuals with this type of hearing loss. The implants are inserted directly into the ear and compensate for damage to the sound-producing hair cells by sending out electrical signals to the hearing center in the brain.

Mixed hearing loss is a combination of conductive and sensorineural loss in the same ear. Mixed losses reduce both hearing sensitivity and discrimination, but because part of the loss is conductive, the ability to discriminate among sounds is reduced less than in sensorineural loss. Overall, hearing losses may also result in speech deterioration, irritability and fatigue, social withdrawal, insecurity, indecision, suspiciousness, paranoia, and anger.

Altered Smell and Taste

Alterations in the ability to smell can be caused by the common cold, strokes, head trauma, brain tumor, specific viral infections,

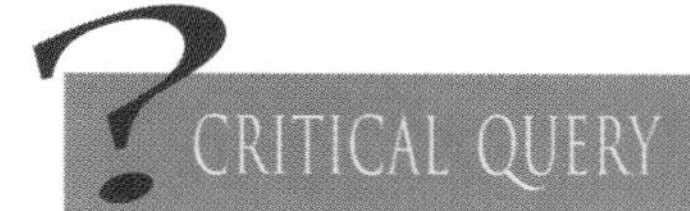

Souder and Yoder[17] describe olfactory disorders as affecting 5 to 10 percent of individuals with head injuries and occurring with increasing frequency in those over age 40. How would knowing these facts change the care nurses provide to patients?

cancer, nasal polyps, or heavy smoking, and frequently occur as a result of damage to cranial nerves II or V.

Patients sometimes experience impaired smell or a distorted sense of smell from congestion. The complete absence of smell can be an important symptom of a brain tumor.

Damage to cranial nerves V or IX, which innervate the tongue, can result in alterations in taste. The effects of certain drugs also cause taste alterations.

Loss of smell may be a barrier to occupational choices, and pleasure or a major health concern.[17] For instance, a person who cannot smell will have difficulty detecting smoke or fire. Individuals employed in the preparation of foods, such as cooks and bakers, may not be able to pursue their occupations without their sense of smell.

Altered Touch

Alterations in tactile sensation or touch can result from damage to the peripheral sensory pathway, to the brain cells, or to pathways associated with sensation. The sensations perceived with altered touch—paresthesia, hyperesthesia, and anesthesia—are perceived as pain or lack of sensation and are discussed later under *Altered Pain Perception.*

Loss of position sense is referred to as *altered proprioception.* Sensory nerve endings in muscles, tendons, and the labyrinth of the ear give individuals this sense of position. Proprioception includes the sense of movement, the sense of vibration, deep pressure, and touch. With loss of proprioception, patients are susceptible to falls and injury, and may experience dizziness.

A patient's inability to detect or accurately gauge temperature sensations cutaneously results in altered thermoreception and can make the patient vulnerable to accidental freezing or burning of the skin and subcutaneous tissue. The nose, ears, fingers, and toes are the first areas to freeze with exposure to cold. Prolonged exposure to cold results in frostbite, with sequelae of painful inflammation, blistering, ischemia, and gangrene.

Altered Sensory Input

Perceptual alterations occur as the result of the inability to interpret and integrate incoming sensory stimuli and messages into a meaningful whole. They frequently occur as a result of brain injury or stroke, especially with damage to the right cerebral hemisphere. It is concerned with perception, spatial proportion, distance and rate, ability to recognize faces and familiar objects, perception of time, and ability to follow visual instructions. When perceptual deficits are compounded by other neurologic deficits, interpreting the environment can become very difficult.

Perceptual alterations include alterations in body awareness and visual–spatial relationships, apraxias, agnosias, sensory deprivation, and sensory overload.

One-sided neglect is an alteration in body awareness in which patients are not able to integrate and use perceptions from the affected side of the body and/or from the environment on the affected side. It often occurs in patients with right brain damage. One-sided neglect is manifested when people simply deny the existence of one side of the body and pay no attention to the environment on the affected side. It may accompany one-sided blindness and interferes with self-care and safety.

Alterations in visual–spatial relationships involve difficulties in perceiving the position of two or more objects in relation to one's self and in relation to one another. Depth and distance perception may be affected, and patients may have difficulty differentiating in–out, front–behind, or up–down. Patients may bump into objects, hit doorways with their wheelchairs, knock objects over on a table, have balance problems, and demonstrate confusion.

Inability to conceptualize, plan, and execute skilled or nonhabitual motor activity despite adequate muscle power, sensation, and coordination is called *apraxia.*[18] This is a complex problem, a result of left or right cerebral hemisphere damage. A patient with apraxia is able to understand the voluntary act required, but is either unable to carry out the act or does so incorrectly or inconsistently.

Inability to recognize objects or faces through the senses is called *agnosia.* The different types of agnosia are usually labeled according to the sensory function that is impaired (Table 32–3).

TABLE 32-3. TERMS RELATED TO AGNOSIA

Term	Definition
Visual agnosia	The inability to name or recognize common objects by sight; damage is usually present in the visual cortex.
Auditory agnosia	The inability to name or recognize the meaning of environmental sounds. Patients can hear the sounds but not put meaning to them. Lesions of the temporal lobe are associated with auditory agnosia.
Tactile agnosia	The inability to recognize common objects through the sense of touch. Inability to recognize car keys, pencils, or combs with the eyes closed is a result of parietal lobe lesions.
Autotopagnosia	The inability to identify body parts and/or their relationships. This is a result of posterior–inferior parietal lobe damage.
Prosopagnosia	The inability to recognize familiar faces.
Unilateral asomatognosia	The inability to recognize or unawareness of one side of the body and its visual space (usually left asomatognosia due to right hemisphere damage).

Perceptual alterations include two other phenomena, sensory deprivation and sensory overload. **Sensory deprivation** occurs when input from the senses is lacking. A person's sense of reality may be altered and result in irritability, restlessness, confusion, boredom, sleepiness, decreased attention span, false sense of reality (hallucination), or false beliefs (delusions). Manifestations of sensory deprivation vary with an individual's adaptation ability and vary at different times for any individual.

Sensory deprivation may occur when sensory input is interrupted. Blindness, deafness, or paralysis can result in sensory deprivation. Lack of environmental stimulation may precipitate sensory deprivation when a person is confined to a hospital room or is on bedrest. Socialization and conversation stimulate thought and emotions. When social input is lacking, whether from mobility restrictions, communication problems, or confinement from hospitalization, sensory deprivation may occur.

Darkness may also contribute to sensory deprivation. The lack of light and lack of visual stimulation from a lighted room can decrease sensory input and alter perceptions. This situation is common in older persons. They may be fully oriented during daytime hours, but with the onset of night and darkness, confusion, hallucinations, and irritability may set in. This condition is sometimes referred to as "sundowners' syndrome."

Sensory overload occurs when too much sensory input impinges on the sensory network and brain, which alters a person's sense of reality and results in slowed thinking, distractibility, impaired memory, confusion, irritability, difficulty sleeping, inability to concentrate, fear, anxiety, hallucinations, and delusions. The symptoms or results of sensory overload are very similar to those of sensory deprivation. Again, a person's ability to adapt and the timing of events influence that person's reaction to sensory overload.

Factors contributing to sensory overload are altered sleep patterns, pain, hospital or health care facility routines, an unfamiliar environment, and a different culture or language barrier. Any combination of one or more of these factors predisposes patients to sensory overload.

Sensory overload, which can be viewed as sensory bombardment, originates in the external environment. For hospitalized people, sensory overload usually occurs in the intensive care unit. There, patients are subjected to a vast array of noises coming from beeping machines and alarms. Frequent nurse checks and physician rounds interrupt rest and sleep schedules. Consequently, sleep patterns are altered and/or shortened, producing irritability and anxiety.

Altered Pain Perception

Pain is a naturally occurring phenomenon that protects the body from serious injury and alerts an individual to an alteration in health. If individuals did not experience pain when exposed to painful stimuli, they would not instinctively withdraw or be able to identify pain, allowing for more cellular damage to occur. Absence of the sense of touch or absence of pain sensation is known as **anesthesia.** Reduced pain sensation can also result in injury or tissue damage. This condition is known as **hypoesthesia.**

Abnormal or strange sensations are called **paresthesias.** These sensations may include burning, itching, tingling, or the feeling of an electrical shock.

Hyperesthesia is a heightened sense of touch or pain. A sheet covering a person who experiences hyperesthesia can produce severe pain.

ALTERED MEMORY AND LEARNING

Memory and learning are integrally related, thus manifestations of their dysfunction are related. Brain injury, sensory overload or sensory deprivation, impaired neural transmission, and altered perception states interfere with the input of sensory stimuli and/or their reconstruction into meaningful patterns.

Alterations in memory involve difficulty retaining or storing thoughts, information, and learned experiences. The loss of memory is termed *amnesia.* With a loss of recent memory, new information or events cannot be stored and the patient may demonstrate difficulty learning. Sometimes with a concussion or mild head injury a person loses consciousness momentarily and, upon awakening, cannot remember the events following or surrounding the head injury.

Loss of remote memory—difficulty remembering long-term memories of events and experiences of several years past—is referred to as retrograde amnesia. The person who sustains a head injury and has problems with remote memory would be unable to remember his or her birth date, names of family members, or the schools attended.

Forgetfulness involves disrupted retrieval, rather than storage, of information or experiences. It is usually seen as an inability to recall people's names or an item on a mental list. Forgetfulness is a functional problem rather than brain tissue damage as with amnesia.[18] In the process of retrieving information, single items of information are lost. A person with forgetfulness can be prompted to remember an item of information. Etiologies associated with forgetfulness include depression, disorientation, the aging process, and certain organic brain disorders.

ALTERED THOUGHT

Thought is closely related to memory and learning. Impaired thinking involves the inability to carry out activities of logic, reasoning, insight, calculations, judgments and decision-making, dealing with reality, and abstract thought. External traumatic events as well as altered in internal neurologic structure or process may disrupt this complex process. Alterations in thought present problems in orientation, memory, and perception, and may also manifest in agnosias and apraxias (Table 32–4). Emotional disturbances can also result in disturbances in thought processes and neurosensory integration.

ALTERED SPEECH, LANGUAGE, AND COMMUNICATION

People with motor communication alterations experience mechanical difficulties in articulation of thought. For example, the lips, throat, or facial muscles may be paralyzed or damaged in some way. Inability to express needs and desires is impaired, the consequence of which is feelings of frustration and anger.

Whether communication problems are the result of unclear messages or of problems with reception and expression, patients experience interference in interpersonal relationships and satisfaction of human needs. Alterations in language and speech produc-

TABLE 32-4. TYPES OF ALTERED THOUGHT

Alteration	Definition
Impaired thought content	The inability to interpret internal and external stimuli accurately and meaningfully in one's environment. May be manifested as doubting and indecision, feelings of unreality and control by others, and compulsive phenomena, such as obsessions, phobias, or repetitive thinking about issues.
Illusions	A false interpretation of external, usually visual or auditory, sensory stimuli. For example, a patient who is restrained in bed may falsely interpret the external environment as a department store in which she is tied to a playpen, with many people around whom she does not recognize.
Delusions	Fixed, irrational beliefs not consistent with cultural mores. May be persecutory, grandiose, nihilistic, or somatic. For example, a patient receiving medication might have delusions that he is part of a drug ring and is being forced to take drugs.
Hallucinations	False sensory perceptions occurring without any external stimuli. Patients can see, feel, hear, smell, or taste things not apparent to others. For example, an alcoholic patient experiencing drug withdrawal may see insects crawling on the wall; a confused elderly person may see deceased relatives in a familiar setting unrelated to the patient's current environment.
Impaired attention span	The inability to attend to incoming stimuli. The patient is distracted, unable to engage in a conversation or to concentrate on activities, and requires assistance in nursing activities. Etiologies contributing to impaired attention span include confusion, depression, sensory overload, and sensory deprivation.
Loss of abstract thinking	Patient retains only the ability to deal with the concrete. Patients can manipulate objects correctly and deal with the here-and-now, but unfamiliar events and concepts pose problems. Problem-solving ability is decreased because abstract representations cannot be used for making decisions. Implications are in the arena of social relations. A limited, dependent lifestyle will result with loss of interpretative abilities, sense of humor, and limited conversational abilities.
Confusion	A state in which a person's thoughts are disorganized and incongruent with reality. Although found in many metabolic and psychological disorders, it is very characteristic of brain damage. It is manifested by misinterpretation of stimuli, paranoia, illusions, delusions, hallucinations, and confabulation.
Confabulation	Occurs when people make up stories or explanations to correctly explain surrounding events or situations.
Emotional lability	Rapid transition from one emotional state to another. Emotional outbursts may occur in response to ordinary activities, such as receiving a glass of water.

tion are thus related to alterations in thought and are manifested as aphasias and dysarthrias.

Aphasia is an impairment of language in which there is loss of ability to communicate. *Expressive aphasia,* also known as Broca's aphasia or motor aphasia, is the inability to transfer words into articulation. Damage to Broca's area (the speech motor association cortex in the dominant cerebral hemisphere) results in slowness of speech, difficulty in forming words for speech, and use of simple phrases. Patients with expressive aphasia understand written and spoken words and know what they want to say but cannot utter the words to express themselves. Patients may resort to using only main ideas to convey wants and needs.

Receptive aphasia or sensory aphasia involves difficulty in comprehension of incoming messages. Damage occurs in Wernicke's area, the area of the cortex that involves interpretation of the spoken and written word. Incoming messages make no sense, but the patient is able to speak easily and to formulate words without difficulty. After a time, listeners become aware that even though speech is fluent, coherence and logic are missing. Patients may also have difficulty naming objects correctly.

Global aphasia is the combination of both expressive and receptive aphasia whereby all systems for communication are damaged. This has the poorest prognosis and causes the greatest problems for patients. Patients cannot understand what they see or hear, nor can they convey thought in speech or writing.

Dysarthria is a language disorder in which there is defective articulation caused by motor deficit of the tongue or speech muscles (cranial nerves V, VII, IX, X). Patients have slurred speech and difficulty pronouncing the letters m, b, p, t, d, and the number one. However, the content of speech is intact. All forms of communication, language, and speech alterations pose a concern for the nurse, a member of the modern health care team,[19,20] and especially for the speech pathologist.

ALTERED MOVEMENT

Alterations in body movement may occur as a result of injury to the neurons and pathways in the central nervous system or as a result of injuries to the peripheral nervous system. The reader is referred to Chap. 33 for a discussion of alterations in movement related to loss of strength, mobility, and flexibility.

Mobility can be altered in a variety of ways. **Paralysis** is the loss of voluntary muscle movement. Hemiplegia, paraplegia, and quadriplegia are types of paralysis. *Hemiplegia* refers to loss of motor function in one half of the body; *paraplegia* involves loss of motor function to the lower extremities; *quadriplegia,* loss of lower extremity function plus varying amounts of loss of upper extremity function, depending on the spinal cord level involved.

Ataxia, the incoordination of voluntary muscle action (especially the walking muscles), is the result of impaired balance and cerebellar function. With an ataxic gait, the feet are lifted high and then hit the floor heavily. There may also be a lurching walk. Another problem of balance and coordination is the inability to maintain normal or desired body posture.

Change in muscle tone, such as *spasticity* or hypertonic muscle tone, is the result of damage to neural pathways or cells in the central nervous system, and results in undue resistance of the muscle to passive lengthening (the muscle is tight and resists stretching). *Flaccidity* or hypotonic muscle tone is caused by neuron damage in the peripheral nervous system, and results in muscle that is soft, floppy, and without tone. Rigidity involves a constant state of resistance and is seen with dysfunction of the extrapyramidal system, as in Parkinson's disease.

Tremors are involuntary muscle movements of the body or limbs resulting from contraction of opposing muscles. Resting tremors are tremors that occur when the person is at rest and are diminished by purposeful activity. *Intention tremors* are tremors that are increased or precipitated by purposeful activity. These involuntary, abnormal movements interfere with patients' coordinated movement.

Tics are involuntary, compulsive stereotyped movements. Some tics are viewed as "nervous habits"; others are hereditary conditions.

Seizures are sudden, brief, jerky contractions of a muscle, muscle group, or the whole body. They occur because of uncontrolled and excessive electrical impulses in the brain cells; some are localized to the motor strip. A seizure is a phenomenon or symptom of a health alteration, not a disease. Seizures may be seen in patients of any age (Table 32–5).

Seizures are classified as generalized and partial. *Generalized seizures* involve both hemispheres of the brain. *Partial seizures* occur when the electrical discharge involves only a part of the brain. Partial seizures may occur with a wide variety of symptoms, depending on which section of the cerebral cortex is involved. With seizures, there is altered movement as well as alterations in consciousness, perception, thought, and communication.

CAUSES OF ALTERED NEUROSENSORY FUNCTIONING

Trauma

The major types of trauma that affect neurosensory integration include head trauma, spinal cord trauma, and peripheral nerve injury. Major alterations in neurosensory integration are associated with traumatic injuries. Mobility, independence, health maintenance, skin integrity, bowel and bladder elimination, respiratory functions, thermoregulation, and self-care abilities can all be affected. These effects can be overwhelming to patients and their significant others. Interpersonal relationships, sexuality, and self-concept can become strained by overwhelming dependence for activities of daily living. The social impact of these changes disrupts every aspect of the injured person's life. For some individuals, the injury may mean the end of a career. Lifestyle may be drastically altered.

The potential for recovery for patients experiencing various types of nervous system trauma is dependent on the location, extent, and severity of damage to the brain, spinal cord, and peripheral nerves and muscles. Although some injuries may be permanent, such as paralysis from a spinal cord injury, others result in full recovery. A minor head injury may have only temporary consequences but should not be overlooked as a potential cause of neurosensory integration difficulties.

Tumors

Tumors are a spontaneous new growth of tissue, resulting in an abnormal mass that interferes with the function of normal tissue. Tumors can develop in any area of the neurosensory system, particularly in the brain and, occasionally, the spinal cord. Although many neurosensory tumors are malignant with a poor prognosis, others are benign and can be treated effectively.

The impact of a tumor is similar to that of head and spinal trauma and may include (1) destruction of nerve cells by infiltration or compression, resulting in interrupted transmission of neural signals; (2) pressure on nerve tracts in the spinal cord or brain, interrupting transmission of neural signals; (3) irritation or destruction of specific brain tissues or structures, causing functional alterations (for example, thought and intellectual impairment); and (4) increased intracranial pressure as the tumor swells, grows, and enlarges. Any of the effects can be devastating to neurosensory function and can result in altered consciousness, perception/sensation/vision, emotions, speech/language/communication, memory, thought, and movement, depending on what areas of the brain or spinal cord are involved.

Infection

Infections can alter neurosensory function. Commonly, infections of the nervous system result when some other area of the body has become infected and the infection spreads. Infections of the ear, sinuses, and tonsils are the most common initial sites for infections that spread to the neurosensory system. The brain or its parts, the meninges, the spinal cord, spinal nerves, and peripheral nerves, are all susceptible to infection.

The impact of infection on neurosensory integration depends on the location of the infection in brain tissue and the function of the affected brain tissues. A localized infection may produce very specific altered neurosensory functions, such as speech impairment, or weakness or paralysis of an extremity. If the infection is widespread, the result may be generalized manifestations, such as loss of consciousness and alteration in vital functions.

Infections of the nervous system are dangerous because even when they are temporary, they can cause serious interference with functions of the nervous system and with other systems of the

TABLE 32-5. ALTERED MOVEMENT: SEIZURE ACTIVITY

Type	Description
I. Generalized Seizures	
1. Tonic–clonic (grand mal)	Major motor activity with loss of consciousness. Four phases with routine duration. a. Preictal (aura). b. Tonic: 15–60 seconds. Rigid muscles, loss of consciousness, no respirations, pupils dilate. c. Clonic: 2–5 minutes. Rapid breathing. Rapid, violent, bilateral jerking. Incontinence and sweating. d. Postictal. Muscle flaccidity. Drowsiness, confusion, headaches, and muscle fatigue. Can occur in all age ranges.
2. Absence (petit mal)	Loss of awareness, lasting 10–30 seconds, but no loss of consciousness. Appears to stare but does not lose muscle tone. No aura or postictal phase. Usually begins between ages 4 and 8 years. May resolve in adolescence. May continue or may convert to tonic/clonic seizures into adulthood.
3. Tonic	Sudden rigidity of muscles with loss of consciousness, flushing, increased heart rate, and pupil changes. No clonic jerks seen. Rare.
4. Clonic	Brief generalized spasm followed by asymmetric bilateral jerks, no tonic phase. Lasts several minutes. Seen in children between the ages of 4 and 8 years.
5. Myoclonic	Brief, sudden muscle contraction in arms and legs or trunk. Little or no loss of consciousness. Associated with fevers, spinal cord lesions, or biochemical alterations.
6. Atonic and akinetic	Loss of body tone resulting in falling. May catch themselves before hitting the ground. Does not lose consciousness.
II. Partial Seizures	
1. Elementary partial	May demonstrate motor, sensory, or autonomic symptoms. Loses control of affected area for 5–15 second time span.
2. Complex partial (temporal lobe or psychomotor)	Generally present with aura. Demonstrates fear, paranoia, and inappropriate activities, such as smacking lips or picking at clothing.

body, and because they can lead to permanent loss of function. Infections are more prevalent among the very old, the very young, patients with nutritional deficiencies, and those whose immune defenses are impaired by illness or medication.

Vascular Lesions

In the United States, vascular lesions of the brain strike more than half a million people each year and remain in third place (after heart disease and cancer) as a cause of death. These lesions represent an interruption to the blood supply to brain tissue (ischemia). They result in lack of oxygen and glucose to the neurons and the accumulation of end products from metabolism. These ischemic events are commonly referred to as a *stroke* or *cerebral vascular accident (CVA)*.

Vascular lesions include blood clots or rupture of a blood vessel (hemorrhage). Blood clots occur when blood cells collect in the wall of a cerebral artery (thrombosis) or when a clot or foreign material dislodged from another site (embolism) travels to a brain vessel and lodges in the vessel, causing a blockage. Rupture of a blood vessel, on the other hand, causes blood to surround brain tissue and cells, and disrupts the blood supply and available oxygen to the surrounding brain tissue. This may occur when the patient has high blood pressure, when disease weakens the walls of a cerebral artery, or when a congenitally malformed vessel finally breaks open. Vascular lesions can adversely affect consciousness, perception, sensation, memory, thought, learning, language/speech/communication, emotions, and movement.

Impaired Neurosensory Transmission

Alterations in neurosensory functions can also result from impaired nerve impulse transmission. This can accompany trauma, clots, lack of oxygen, or a host of degenerative conditions (Parkinson's disease, multiple sclerosis, muscular dystrophy, and amyotrophic lateral sclerosis), which result in progressive loss of muscle movement.

The functions affected by neurosensory transmission disorders can include perception, memory, thought, emotion, language/speech/communication, and movement. Because the impact on movement and thought functions is so devastating, patients suffer severe economic and social costs. The economic costs of home care and rehabilitation can be overwhelming. The social costs include the consequences of restricted mobility, and the decreased socialization and recreational opportunities for patients. Families also suffer in having to deal with the changed personality and altered, deteriorating physical condition of a loved one.

Because of the resulting impaired mobility, mental incapacitation, and dependency on others, the collaborative relationship between nurse and patient is often affected by illnesses of the neurosensory system. Patients with unimpaired perceptual and cognitive function can collaborate with nurses in determining care. In cases of perceptual and cognitive impairment, or disorders of consciousness, however, nurses assume greater direction in the nature of the patient–nurse relationship.

INSIGHTS FROM NURSING LITERATURE
UNDERSTANDING NEUROSENSORY DEBILITATION

McGuinness S. Learned helplessness in the multiple sclerosis population. J Neurosci Nurs. *1996;28:163–169.*

Multiple sclerosis, a progressive degenerative disease of the motor and sensory nerves, is probably initiated by a virus that triggers an autoimmune response in genetically predisposed individuals and follows an unpredictable course. Affected patients have symptoms that advance unexpectedly. These include increasing motor incoordination and weakness progressing to paralysis, sensory impairment, cognitive changes, and bowel, bladder, and sexual dysfunction. According to the researchers, patients sometimes adapt to the uncertainty of multiple sclerosis with a pattern of learned helplessness—a pattern in which they come to view their own actions as insufficient to control events. The researcher studied 72 patients using scales to measure social and functional capacities and learned helplessness. She found helplessness higher among patients with greater disability, and recommended that nurses focus nursing care on realistic achievable goals. This reinforces the patients' sense of ability to affect outcomes, and discourages patients from generalizing helplessness derived from one area of disability to other areas of ability.

SECTION 2
ASSESSMENT OF NEUROSENSORY INTEGRATION

NEUROSENSORY DATA COLLECTION

Assessment of neurosensory integration enables a nurse, with patient or family collaboration, to gather data on a patient's condition and functional ability. Specifically, nurses perform a neurosensory assessment to gain data about altered neurosensory function such as level of consciousness, altered memory and learning, altered perception, altered thought, altered communication, and/or altered movement; altered functions of body systems other than the neurosensory system that may lead to or result from loss of neurosensory integration; and pain.

Sharing information between nurse and patient is essential to the assessment process. Neurosensory assessment incorporates a patient history, patient examination, and review of relevant diagnostic tests. Important nursing questions such as the following can be answered as the result of a neurosensory assessment:

- Can the patient see and hear adequately?
- Will sensory losses impede the patient's ability for self-care?
- Does the patient have the balance necessary for safe ambulation?
- Is the patient's judgment adequate for safe performance of activities of daily living?
- Can the patient communicate sufficiently to make needs known?
- Does the patient have the coordination needed for bathing and eating?
- Is the patient alert enough to perceive dangers in the environment?
- Is the patient aware of limitations?
- Does the patient have appropriate memory capabilities to give adequate information?

Neurosensory assessment is extremely important to planning patient care and to identifying the type of nursing assistance patients may want and need.

Neurosensory assessment need not always be a formal process. In a sense, every time a nurse interacts with a patient, a neurosensory assessment is being performed. In the course of a conversation with a patient, for instance, a nurse will make observations about how alert the patient appears, the clarity of the patient's speech, the coherence of the ideas the patient is expressing, or the coordination of the patient's gestures or movements. For the most part, neurosensory assessment does not require taking the patient to an examination room but occurs during the course of other activities, such as the bed bath.

The formal neurosensory assessment is presented here in its entirety. Once all aspects of the assessment are mastered and clinical uses are understood, a nurse may elect to carry out a full neurosensory history and examination or select aspects according to the demands of a particular clinical situation. A thorough assessment is especially important when initially establishing the patient care plan. Thereafter, specific observations may be sufficient to evaluate progress.

NEUROSENSORY HISTORY

The neurosensory history provides vital information about losses in neurosensory integration that may interfere with a patient's adaptation and ability to perform activities of daily living. It may be necessary to include family members in this process, particularly when memory and thought are impaired. The level of neurosensory deficit can vary markedly and may affect patients' ability to complete a history, particularly if family members or significant others are not present. History-taking is also an opportunity for nurses to begin a working relationship with patient and family.

Primary Concern

The primary concern is that aspect of a patient's problem for which he or she seeks health care. For example, a woman with weakness in her right arm may be most concerned not about an underlying disease state that the weakness may represent, but rather about her ability to work to earn money to support her family. By gathering this type of data, nurses are able to identify areas of patient needs and validate them with patients. Moreover, nurses can use this information to make clinical appraisals not only of patient concerns, but also of neurosensory functions. The integrity of the following neurosensory functions may become apparent as a patient responds to a nurse's questions.

- *Consciousness:* Is the patient alert enough to identify the primary concern?
- *Perception:* Does the patient's concern relate to the problems the nurse sees?
- *Emotion:* Does the patient express the concern with appropriate emotion?
- *Memory:* Does the patient remember what the concern is?
- *Thought:* Does the patient's statement of concern indicate difficulty in evaluating the seriousness of the condition?
- *Communication:* Does the patient have problems with speech or understanding speech?

The following example illustrates a primary concern related to neurosensory functioning.

> Erin, a 13-year-old girl, has injured her right arm while swimming butterfly during swim practice. She is unable to fully raise her arm. The nurse who is interviewing Erin in the emergency department confirms that Erin's primary concern is being unable to swim in an upcoming swim event. Erin is not aware that there may be underlying damage to the neurosensory system, although the nurse recognizes this possibility. This data is used to establish initial nursing diagnoses that will be used in developing a plan of care for Erin.

Current Understanding

The current understanding relates to the patient's interpretation of the health problem and understanding of the causes and consequences of the problem. A nurse obtains this information by establishing the patient's own understanding of the causes and effects of his or her health problem. The nurse may also help define the onset, sequence, and duration of the problem.

Pain History. Pain history is an essential component of the patient's current understanding. Problems often arise in taking a pain history because of the subjectivity of the pain experience. Patients should be encouraged to describe pain in their own words. A pain history should be modified to fit the patient's need; for example, questions asked a postoperative patient would differ from those asked a patient in chronic pain. Several factors that are relevant to pain include location, intensity, onset, duration, quality, what makes it worse or better, and associating factors.

LOCATION. Pain may be generalized or quite focused. Asking a patient to accurately identify or trace location may require repeated questioning to obtain the necessary level of specificity. The description should include the extent and spread of the pain, as well as identification of pain-free areas. The patient may be entirely focused on the pain, or may be unable to adequately describe it because of neurosensory involvement. Anatomic diagrams may be useful if patients cannot adequately locate their pain or if there are multiple areas of pain interspersed with pain-free areas.

Terms that describe pain location include *localized*—confined to the area of focus; *radiating*—extending beyond the focus of the pain; *projected*—transmitted along nerve pathways; and *referred*—occurring in an area other than the source. When gathering data on pain location, the nurse should determine if the pain is superficial or deep, and if the pain location remains constant or if it moves. If location changes, ask the patient to identify related factors. For example, does the location of the pain change when the patient sits up?

INTENSITY. Intensity is probably the most subjective characteristic of pain. Certain types of pain are more severe (eg, chest pain) or more annoying (eg, low back pain) than others. Pain intensity can reflect the intensity of the stimulus, the extent of tissue damage, the amount of psychological distress, or any combination of these factors. Patients can be asked to rate their pain intensity on a scale of 0 to 10, with 0 representing no pain and 10 representing the most severe pain. This provides a rough measure of the patient's subjective experience of pain.

It is difficult to gather objective data on pain intensity. Descriptive scales have also been created to assist in this effort. Patients are asked to point to the place on the scale where they perceive their pain intensity is.

ONSET. Information about onset of pain includes when it started, mode of onset, pattern of pain, and history of pain. Was onset sudden or gradual? What was the patient doing at the time? Is the pain steady or intermittent? If intermittent, does it follow a pattern? How frequently does pain occur? Has this type of pain occurred before? If so, was a cause determined?

DURATION. Duration pertains to the length of time the pain is felt. How long does the pain last with each occurrence? When did the patient last experience the pain? How frequently does it recur? In addition, it is important to ask patients what they have found that alleviates pain and what they do that aggravates it. These questions will further assist nurses in their evaluation of pain and gives an opportunity to listen for the values patients place on self-care methods.

Inquiring about the associated factors aids in determining other events accompanying the pain, which is the only stimulus. Perhaps nausea is interfering with the patient's quality of life. Physical pain is rarely isolated from other physical conditions that create a problem for the patient. Psychosocial issues are also important to investigate.[19]

Patients's name: ______ Diagnosis: ______
Pain medication(s): Date: ______ Time: ______ a.m./p.m.
______ Dosage: ______ Time given: ______ a.m./p.m.
______ Dosage: ______ Time given: ______ a.m./p.m.

PRI: S ______ (groups 1-10) A ______ (groups 11-15) E ______ (group 16) M ______ (groups 17-20)

NWC: ______ Comments: ______

PPI: ______

PRI

SENSORY (S)

1. 1. FLICKERING 2. QUIVERING 3. PULSING 4. THROBBING 5. BEATING 6. POUNDING

2. 1. JUMPING 2. FLASHING 3. SHOOTING

3. 1. PRICKING 2. BORING 3. DRILLING 4. STABBING

4. 1. SHARP 2. CUTTING 3. LACERATING

5. 1. PINCHING 2. PRESSING 3. GNAWING 4. CRAMPING 5. CRUSHING

6. 1. TUGGING 2. PULLING 3. WRENCHING

7. 1. HOT 2. BURNING 3. SCALDING 4. SEARING

8. 1. TINGLING 2. ITCHY 3. SMARTING 4. STINGING

9. 1. DULL 2. SORE 3. HURTING 4. ACHING 5. HEAVY

10. 1. TENDER 2. TAUT 3. RASPING 4. SPLITTING

TOTAL

AFFECTIVE (A)

11. 1. TIRING 2. EXHAUSTING

12. 1. SICKENING 2. SUFFOCATING

13. 1. FEARFUL 2. FRIGHTFUL 3. TERRIFYING

14. 1. PUNISHING 2. GRUELLING 3. CRUEL 4. VICIOUS 5. KILLING

15. 1. WRETCHED 2. BLINDING

TOTAL

EVALUATIVE (E)

16. 1. ANNOYING 2. TROUBLESOME 3. MISERABLE 4. INTENSE 5. UNBEARABLE

MISCELLANEOUS (M)

17. 1. SPREADING 2. RADIATING 3. PENETRATING 4. PIERCING

18. 1. TIGHT 2. NUMB 3. DRAWING 4. SQUEEZING 5. TEARING

19. 1. COOL 2. COLD 3. FREEZING

20. 1. NAGGING 2. NAUSEATING 3. AGONIZING 4. DREADFUL 5. TORTURING

TOTAL

PPI

1. MILD 2. DISCOMFORTING 3. DISTRESSING 4. HORRIBLE 5. EXCRUCIATING

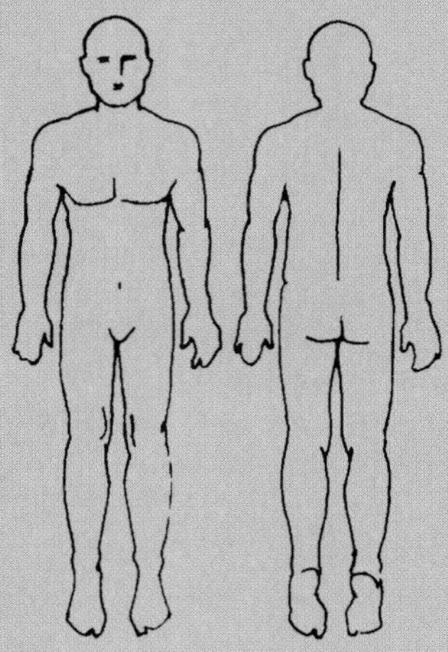

CONSTANT
PERIODIC
BRIEF

Mark E if pain is external; I if internal; if pain is both external and internal, mark EI.

ACCOMPANYING SYMPTOMS
NAUSEA — COMMENTS
HEADACHE
DIZZINESS
DROWINESS
CONSTIPATION
DIARRHEA

SLEEP
GOOD — COMMENTS
FITFUL
CAN'T SLEEP

FOOD INTAKE
GOOD — COMMENTS
SOME
LITTLE
NONE

ACTIVITY
GOOD — COMMENTS
SOME
LITTLE
NONE

Figure 32–1. McGill–Melzack pain questionnaire. *(Courtesy of R. Melzack. Copyright 1970, R. Melzack.)*

QUALITY. Assessing pain quality may require extensive questioning, as many patients experience difficulty in articulating their pain experience. Nurses can begin by asking, "How does your pain feel?" After giving the patient enough time to think and respond, the nurse may suggest such words as stabbing, burning, aching, throbbing, and the like. The McGill–Melzak Pain Questionnaire was designed to assist health care providers to assess the dimensions of pain (Fig. 32–1). The questionnaire has five basic sections:

- *Pain rating index.* This consists of 20 word groups used to determine pain quality. The groups are divided into subgroups: 1–10, sensory (S); 11–15, affective (A); 16, evaluative (E); 17–20, miscellaneous (M). Words in these categories aid patients in choosing a verbal description of their pain.
- *Present pain intensity.* A 5-point pain scale. The patient points to the pain location on the scale.
- *Number of words chosen.* The total of pain rating index words chosen by the patient.

- *Line drawing of the body.* The patient points to areas of pain and describes whether pain is superficial or deep.
- *List of symptoms.* The patient indicates associated symptoms.

Although this assessment tool was developed to be used in conjunction with pain medication administration, it is useful in general pain assessment as well.

Past Health Problems/Experiences

Past health problems may directly relate to the patient's present problem or may alert the nurse to begin assessment of other pertinent areas. For instance, a patient may reveal having had a traumatic injury to one of the peripheral nerves in the left lower extremity. This information would indicate to the nurse that careful assessment of neurosensory integration of that extremity and mobility is necessary.

Questions about prior drug therapy may contribute additional assessment data. For example, when a patient who is admitted for a foot ulceration reveals he is diabetic and requires insulin injections, the nurse would assess the patient's compliance with his diabetic management and would ask the patient about the sensory perception from his feet, which can be reduced in diabetes contributing to ulcer-causing foot injuries.

Prior hospitalizations and prior interactions with the health care system can also affect patients' expectations and attitudes. Positive experiences lend a positive trustful attitude, while a previous negative experience may make a patient wary and make it more difficult to establish a trusting relationship.

The past health history provides a wealth of valuable data to use in patient assessment, as illustrated by the following example.

> Paul Williams is a 39-year-old factory worker who is admitted to a neurology floor from the emergency room for diagnostic tests to determine the cause of low back pain incurred at work. He reports bending over to lift a large, heavy box and feeling his "back go out." Mr. Williams states that this has never happened to him before. He relates that he once had a kidney stone and when he passed it, the pain was horrible. He states that he hopes the current pain that he is experiencing can soon be relieved because he can't stand it. He also reports he has had a past health problem with hypertension, controlled with an antihypertensive medication.
>
> The nurse understands that Mr. Williams' current health problem, involving the neurosensory network, may enhance his stress and aggravate his hypertension. In addition, Mr. Williams has experienced severe pain in the past and is apprehensive about the present pain. The nurse decides to collaborate with Mr. William's physician to assure that Mr. Williams' hypertensive medication is ordered and to monitor his blood pressure. Keeping Mr. Williams free of pain should reduce some of his anxiety.

Personal, Family, and Social History

Obtaining the personal, family, and social history is very important for patients experiencing a neurosensory alteration, as any alteration in function will affect all of these aspects of patients' lives. Alterations in neurosensory function can cause changes in the patient's ability to perform self-care and can also strain family and social relationships.

The personal, family, and social history also provides pertinent data about lifestyle patterns that may have contributed to the client's neurosensory function. For example, if a patient has injured the spinal cord in a motor vehicle accident and is unable to work, the nurse would assess the patient's personal, family, and social history to determine whether the patient has support systems, coping mechanisms, and necessary personal habits to aid in recovery. If the patient's history indicates he or she does not have sufficient resources, the nurse would determine to collaborate with other health professionals to address long-term needs.

Table 32–6 provides sample personal, family, and social history questions related to neurosensory assessment.

Subjective Manifestations

The neurosensory history includes subjective manifestations (symptoms the patient reports). Chapter 17 outlines a systematic approach for collection of this data.

NEUROSENSORY EXAMINATION

Nurses conduct a neurosensory examination to gain data about clinical manifestations of loss of neurosensory or neurosensory-related functions. It is by identifying these alterations that nurse and patient are able to determine mutual goals of care to assist the patient to attain a higher or a stable health state.

Measurements

Temperature, pulse, blood pressure, and respiration are a necessary part of a neurosensory assessment. Measurements of height and weight may also be made (refer to Chap. 17).

Temperature. Temperature is regulated by the hypothalamus and brainstem. A patient with an injury or lesion to these areas may lose the ability to regulate body temperature. An increase in temperature may also indicate infection.

Temperature may also affect the CNS. Body temperature below 97F (hypothermia) results in decreased metabolic rate, causing a decrease in cerebral blood flow and oxygen concentration. Body temperature above 101F (hyperthermia) increases the metabolic rate and cerebral metabolism, thereby placing an additional demand for oxygen and glucose on the body. Furthermore, CNS function is impaired when body temperature varies 9F either above or below the normal range.

Pulse and Blood Pressure. Changes in vital signs are usually a late sign of increasing intracranial pressure. More than transitory changes in pulse and blood pressure represent neurologic deterioration. The rise in pulse and blood pressure is a compensatory mechanism. As edema, hemorrhage, blockage of cerebrospinal fluid, or lesion growth increase, pressure is exerted on the blood vessels that supply the brain. This causes ischemia of the brain tissue. Blood is pumped to the brain under increased pressure so that the ischemic tissue can receive both blood and glucose, resulting in an increase in blood pressure. At the same time, a slowing of the pulse occurs because of stimulation of the vagal nerve.

Respirations. Assessment of respiratory patterns assists the nurse to determine the patient's level of brain functioning. CNS respiratory failure results when neurons of the medulla become damaged. Severe bilateral hemisphere dysfunction may result in Cheyne-Stokes respirations (rapid, deep respirations alternating with periods of apnea). Involvement of the posterior hypothalamus and midbrain produces rapid respirations. Damage at or below the pons is manifested by irregular breathing patterns. Lesions in this area produce various patterns such as cluster breathing, gasping,

TABLE 32-6. NEUROSENSORY HISTORY: PERSONAL, FAMILY, AND SOCIAL HISTORY QUESTIONS

A. Vocational
1. What type of work do you do?
2. Does your work require mental concentration or coordinated physical activities?
3. Have you noticed any problems doing your work lately? If so, what? How long?
4. How do you usually get around? Drive? Ride the bus? Walk?

B. Home and Family
1. Are you married? Single? Involved in a relationship?
2. How long have you been in that relationship?
3. Do you have children? Ages?
4. If older children or other family members, do they live with you? Or near by?
5. How will they assist you in this situation?
6. Tell me about where you live. Stairs?
7. Describe a usual day.

C. Social and Leisure
1. What are your favorite leisure activities?
2. With whom do you do these?
3. Have these changed in the past because of a change in your health? If so, how?
4. Has your home life changed because of your health? If so, how?

D. Sexual
1. Has your sexual relationship been satisfactory?
2. Any changes related to this illness? What changes have occurred?

E. Habits

Exercise
1. How often do you exercise? Weekly? More or less often?
2. What types of exercise/activity do you enjoy?
3. Has your exercise pattern changed because of a change in health status? If so, how?
4. Is regular exercise an important part of staying healthy for you?

Sleep
1. How much sleep do you get? At night? From naps?
2. Do you feel rested?
3. Do you have sleep problems? How long? How have you dealt with them?
4. Describe a typical night's sleep.
5. Has this health concern affected your sleep? How?

Diet
1. How many meals do you eat every day? Are weekends different? Snacks?
2. Describe your appetite. Has it changed? If so, how?
3. What is a healthy diet? Is it important to you?
4. Has this health problem changed your eating habits?

Beverages
1. How much alcohol do you usually drink each week? What types?
2. Has this amount changed recently? Why?
3. Do you drink coffee, tea, or cola? How much?
4. Has your alcohol or other beverage intake changed recently because of your health status? How?

Drugs
1. Do you use any medications, such as aspirin, sleeping pills, diet pills, nerve pills? What are their names? How many do you take?
2. What other drugs do you use? Do you use marijuana, cocaine, or other drugs of this type? If so, what types and how often?
3. Do you find a difference in your health after you take these drugs? How so?
4. Has your use of these drugs changed since your health concerns became evident? How so?

F. Psychological/Coping
1. Have you noticed a change in how you feel about yourself?
2. Does this worry or concern you?
3. How have you dealt with this?
4. Has it been effective?
5. Do you feel your health has had something to do with this? How?
6. How do you feel about your health change? Are you coping? How so?
7. Do your past experiences with health changes help you cope?
8. What assistance do you think you will need during your hospital stay? At home?

or ataxic breathing. Extensive damage to the medullary reticular formation usually destroys central control of respiration, leading to apnea and death.

Objective Manifestations

General Observations. General observations of the patient's overall appearance are really an informal neurosensory assessment, and can be made quickly as the patient enters a room or interacts with the nurse. A more detailed assessment can then be completed as a part of the complete neurologic examination; however, general observations continue throughout the examination. In some instances, the initial impression may set the focus of the interview and examination.

The general health status, sex, race, and apparent age are noted. Much initial information can be gathered regarding the patient's neurosensory function. Do the eyes track? Limited movement may indicate a problem with the cranial nerves that innervate the eyes. Does the patient look alert? Do the patient's facial muscles move appropriately? Paralysis of the facial nerve will produce altered facial movement. Note the patient's facial expression. Is the patient dressed appropriately? Are the clothes clean? What is the patient's level of hygiene? Inappropriate dress can indicate mental disorders or confusion. Soiled clothing and poor hygiene may indicate the inability to perform self-care as a result of neurosensory dysfunction such as Alzheimer's disease, paralysis, pain, or weakness.

General assessment of mental status includes the apparent level of consciousness and orientation, both of which are discussed in detail below. Orientation provides data regarding the patient's perception of who or where he or she is, and what time it is. Memory and thought content are also assessed by the nurse in this process. Station, posture, body movement, and gait, also discussed in Chap. 17, are assessed. Changes in these characteristics may indicate conditions such as Parkinson's disease, tremors, or seizure activity.

Gait patterns affect patient mobility and are regulated by the neurosensory network. Is the patient's gait fluid and coordinated? Deficits in gait are manifested by short steps, wide-based gait, loss of arm movement, or dragging of feet. Neurosensory deficits such as stroke or peripheral nerve injury often result in problems with gait.

Both sides of the body are observed for symmetry. Usually the dominant side is slightly larger because it is used more. However, a marked asymmetry may indicate cranial or peripheral nerve dysfunction.

Handedness indicates cerebral dominance. Assess whether the patient is left- or right-handed. In states of neurosensory dysfunction, the patient may lose the ability to use only one side of the body. If the dominant side is involved, the patient will have difficulty in performing activities of daily living.

Energy level reflects the patient's ability to function in a consistent manner appropriate to the situation. Fatigue may accompany neurosensory problems, such as multiple sclerosis, head injury, or infection. Odors from a patient's breath may also indicate that a health problem is present. Scents such as acetone, alcohol, or ammonia may be signs of a disease process or personal or social habits causing a change in neurosensory status.

Does the patient appear to be in pain? Pain can indicate a wide variety of neurosensory alterations, such as lesions, pinched nerves, tumors, or pressure ulcers. Pain may be apparent as the nurse observes the patient. Although pain is a subjective manifestation, the patient may demonstrate observable signs. Pain behavior encompasses changes in facial expression, mental status, posture, gait, and energy level—virtually every aspect of general observation. When patients are in severe pain, their mental status may change. In chronic pain, patients may appear older than their chronologic age. Posture, movement, and gait may be altered. Energy level may also be diminished. Patients in pain demonstrate diffuse general observation alterations.

Integument

Skin is observed for skin integrity or defects such as areas of breakdown, discoloration, or lesions. Intact skin, free of bruises, cuts, and burns, therefore generally indicates that individuals can feel pain and have intact pain reflexes.

HEENT

Head. The head is assessed for facial nerve function (CN VII). This nerve has both motor and sensory function. Motor functions include maintenance of facial symmetry at rest and facial expressions such as smiling, frowning, or raising the eyebrows. Spasms, tremors, weakness, or atrophy are unusual findings that should be noted. The sensory function of this nerve involves the sense of taste on the anterior two-thirds of the tongue. The tastes of sweet, salty, sour, and bitter should be tested on each side of the protruded tongue with water given between each side and each taste. Loss of taste can lead to a loss of appetite.

The trigeminal nerve (CN V) has both motor and sensory components. The nurse observes motor strength during mastication (chewing). The jaw reflex is elicited by tapping the jaw with a reflex hammer while the jaw is slightly open. The normal response, although weak, is closure of the mouth. The sensory component of this nerve is responsible for sensation on the skin of the face. The nurse asks the patient to close the eyes and assesses both sides of the face for the sensations of temperature, light touch, and light pain.

Eyes. The eyes provide sensory data for the brain to process. Patients who experience a loss of vision often demonstrate alterations in balance, gait, and ability to perform self-care, in addition to losing one of the main senses of the body.

The *visual fields* of the patient are tested as a part of the neurosensory assessment. This is done by using confrontation, an advanced technique learned later in the nursing curriculum. Blind spots may be due to loss of a portion of the visual field from strokes, carotid artery pathology, optic nerve interruptions, or tumors pressing on the optic pathways. Blurred vision may be caused by disturbances in the optic pathways in the brain. Diplopia (double vision) may result from cranial surgery or multiple sclerosis. Visual changes may result from past head injuries, altered sleep patterns, or abnormal ocular physiology. Loss of peripheral vision may result in injury as the patient is unable to see out of the "corner" or outer portion of the eye.

The *ophthalmoscopic examination* is performed to view the inside of the eye by shining a light into the eye. This is another advanced technique, learned later in the nursing curriculum. The normal disc is round with a clear distinct margin. A swollen optic disc (papilledema) is indicative of increased intracranial pressure.

Pupil size and reactivity are essential indicators of neurosensory integration. Pupil size is determined by the balance of activity between the sympathetic and parasympathetic nervous systems. Checking the pupils involves first observing the size of one pupil and then observing its size in relation to the other pupil. Pupils should be equal in size and are measured in terms of millimeters (Fig. 32–2).

The pupils are also assessed for response to light. Response should be brisk; sluggish response or no response should be noted, as this can indicate a serious alteration in function of the third cranial nerve or the brainstem. The other pupil should also respond

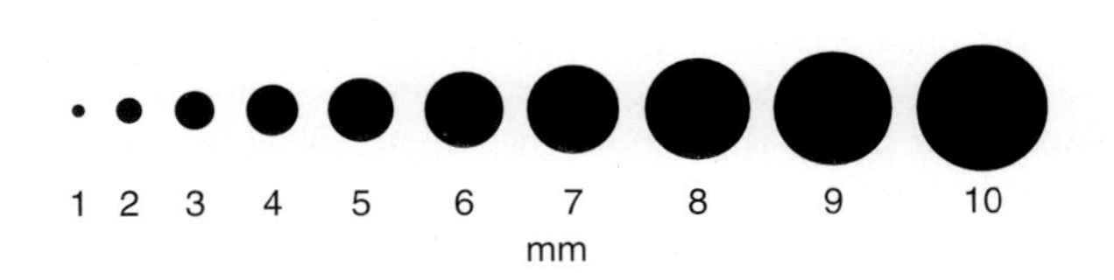

Figure 32–2. Pupil diameter is measured in millimeters.

when the light is shined into one eye, but to a lesser degree. This is called the *consensual response*. Pupils should be round and equal in size. Unequal pupils may indicate brain damage.

The unconscious person may be assessed for the oculocophalic reflex, also called the doll's eyes phenomenon. In this procedure the head is rotated briskly from side to side while the examiner watches for movement of the eyes relative to head movement. The normal finding is for the eyes to move in the direction opposite that of the head; hence the name "doll's eyes." Eyes that do not move, but merely follow the motion of the head, may indicate brainstem injury.

Ears. The acoustic nerve (CN VIII) is involved with the sensory functions of hearing and equilibrium. The cochlear nerve branch is responsible for hearing. Damage to these nerves causes diminished hearing and balance changes.

The ear canal may be examined with an otoscope to determine if structural abnormalities exist. Hearing tests are routinely performed and include the watch ticking test, the *lateralization test* (Rinne test), and the *bone-air conduction test* (Weber test) as in Chap. 17.

The nurse should assess for pain in the ear caused by otitis media, which may cause inner ear damage. Altered hearing has many causes, including use of certain medications. Difficulty in hearing may be due to the aging process, obstruction of the ear canal by cerumen (ear wax), or congenital anomaly.

Nose. The sense of smell (CN I) is assessed. Damage to this nerve results in diminished smell and generally a loss of appetite as well.

Mouth and Throat. The glossopharyngeal and the vagal nerves (CN IX and X) are tested together because of their similar functions. Nurses perform a motor examination of these nerves by assessing the muscles of the pharynx and larynx for symmetry of movement, while watching how effectively the patient swallows, and listening to the patient speak (phonation). Dysarthria occurs as a result of altered speech due to a motor deficit of the tongue and other speech muscles. Dysphonia is due to a disruption of the larynx that manifests as vocal hoarseness. Aphonia is also due to injury to the larynx or its innervation and results in whispering. Abnormality of these nerves may limit the patient's ability to communicate and make his or her needs known.

The pharyngeal (gag) reflex is assessed by touching each side of the posterior soft palate with a tongue depressor. Loss of the gag reflex places patients at risk to aspirate foods and fluids. The palatal reflex is tested by stroking each side of the mucous membrane of the uvula. The uvula should rise and deviate to the side stimulated. The sensory component of these nerves involves the interpretation of pain, touch, and temperature in the pharynx, larynx, trachea, lungs, and esophagus. Taste on the posterior one-third of the tongue is also regulated by these cranial nerves. The autonomic functions include slowing of heart and bronchial constrictions.

The nurse should note tongue movement and strength (CN XII). Fibrillations, indicating muscle atrophy, should be noted. Weakness or paralysis of the tongue will not allow the patient to swallow correctly or speak.

Nurses also assess the spinal accessory nerve (CN XI), which innervates two large muscle groups, the sternocleidomastoid and the trapezius muscles. Its effect on those muscles is purely motor. The nurse assesses the first muscle group by asking the client to turn the head sideways. The trapezius muscle is assessed by placing resistive pressure down with the hands when the patient shrugs the shoulders. Both of these muscles should be inspected and palpated for symmetry of muscle mass, equality of strength, and any wasting or spasm. Nerve damage in this area may result in limited movement of the head.

Chest and Cardiovascular System

Alterations in neurosensory function are generally associated with changes in pulse, blood pressure, and respiration (see *Measurements* section).

Abdomen

The abdomen should be auscultated, for quantity and quality of bowel sounds to detect the presence of fecal retention, and palpated for extreme firmness or tenderness. Normal bowel sounds occur every 3 to 5 seconds. The patient may experience fecal retention as a result of spinal cord injury, a degenerative disease, or the aging process.

Also nurses observe for signs and symptoms of fecal incontinence. Skin integrity, especially in the perianal area, may be disrupted if fecal incontinence is chronic.

Genitourinary Tract

The patient who has a neurosensory deficit may demonstrate urinary retention or incontinence. Nurses should ask when the patient last voided. If the patient cannot provide this information, palpate the bladder and percuss for normal position, slightly above the symphysis pubis bone. If the bladder is palpated much above this level, urinary retention may be present. The skin of the perineal region should also be assessed for redness and possible breakdown, which may indicate problems with urinary incontinence.

Musculoskeletal System

The musculoskeletal examination is discussed in Chap. 33. Refer to that chapter for discussion of musculoskeletal findings.

Neurologic System

The first portion of a neurologic assessment is the mental status examination, part of the general observation portion of the examination. Other areas that are assessed include level of consciousness, orientation, mood and behavior, knowledge and vocabulary, judgment and abstraction, memory, language and speech, sensory and motor function, and reflexes.

Level of Consciousness. Level of consciousness is the key indicator of brain function. Altered states of consciousness indicate some level of brain failure.

The nurse first checks for response to auditory commands. Depending on the level of functioning, the patient may respond appropriately, may answer with only a simple response, may appear unsure of what to do, or may not respond.

This initial level of consciousness is important because it gives baseline data for comparison if changes occur in the patient. A simple, consistent, and well-accepted guide for grading level of consciousness is the Glasgow Coma Scale (Fig. 32–3).

In an unconscious patient, painful stimuli such as compression of the nail beds, pressure on the trapezius muscle, sternal rubbing, or pressure on the Achilles tendon of the lower leg may be

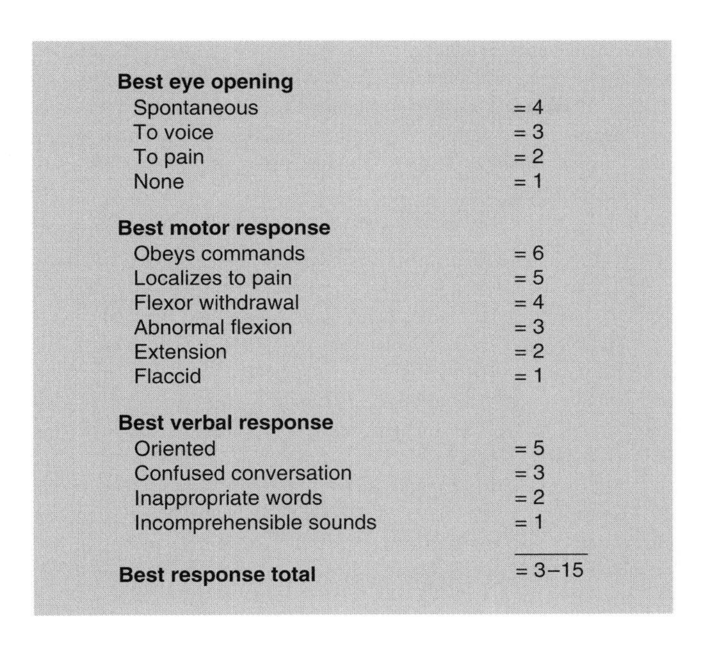

Best eye opening	
Spontaneous	= 4
To voice	= 3
To pain	= 2
None	= 1
Best motor response	
Obeys commands	= 6
Localizes to pain	= 5
Flexor withdrawal	= 4
Abnormal flexion	= 3
Extension	= 2
Flaccid	= 1
Best verbal response	
Oriented	= 5
Confused conversation	= 3
Inappropriate words	= 2
Incomprehensible sounds	= 1
Best response total	= 3–15

Figure 32–3. Glasgow Coma Scale.

required to elicit a response. Responses may include purposeful actions (grimacing and pushing the examiner away), nonpurposeful actions (withdrawal from source of pain or inappropriate flexion or extension of arms), or no reaction to stimuli.

The Glasgow Coma Scale focuses on cognitive behaviors. However, individuals with significant brain injury may demonstrate behavioral, cognitive, and long-term memory deficits beyond the scope of the scale.[4] Any decrease in the level of consciousness of these patients must be compared to baseline data. Decrease in level of consciousness is a serious sign and must be reported to the physician immediately.

Orientation. Orientation is the awareness of person, place, and time. Orientation to person means the patient knows his or her own name, family names, or names of health care professionals. Place is awareness of present location and address of home. Time consists of knowledge of hour, date, day of week, month, year, and noteworthy events, such as current season or recent holidays. Confusion may indicate brain deterioration. Confused patients will need to be reoriented consistently.

Mood and Behavior. Mood and behavior are states that can indicate a patient is attentive to the examiner without being hostile, agitated, hypoactive, or bizarre. Delusions, illusions, or hallucinations indicate psychological dysfunctions. It is very difficult to establish a good nurse–patient relationship with patients who are suffering from delusions, illusions, or hallucinations. Mood and behavior are assessed throughout the neurologic assessment and should be continually assessed and compared for changes.

Knowledge and Vocabulary. Overall knowledge and vocabulary may be affected by cerebral hemorrhages, brain tumors, psychiatric disorders, or mental retardation. The nurse assesses the patient for common knowledge, taking into account cultural or age differences.

Judgment and Abstraction. Judgment and abstraction are tested to determine the integrity of higher cerebral functions. (Refer to Chap. 17, *Neurologic System*, for details.)

Memory. Memory tests evaluate immediate recall, recent memory, and remote memory.

Immediate recall should occur within 3 to 5 minutes of initial information presentation. Note if a related question is answered correctly, indicating intact immediate memory, or incorrectly, indicating some memory deficit. Patients with impaired memory can be difficult to teach. They cannot remember information about medications and their health requirements. Family members should be taught significant facts regarding care.

Recent memory is assessed by evaluating recall of events that happened hours to several days ago. Loss of recent memory can be very frustrating for patients and can lead to anxiety. Good communication technique is essential, as is frequent reinforcement of who the patient is, how the patient got to the hospital, and topics addressed in health teaching.

Remote memory is memory of things long passed. The nurse questions the patient about place of birth or names of family members, and then verifies this information with family members.

Language and Speech. Language and speech assessment provides necessary information regarding how a patient is processing and relating to the environment.

Nurses should continually note the patient's speech. Is it fluent, well-articulated, and appropriate to age? Dysarthria and aphasia are commonly associated with neurosensory dysfunctions. To assess speech formally the patient is asked to repeat the days of the week or months of the year (automatic speech), and then to repeat sounds and words of increasing difficulty (speech motor qualities). Nurses should listen to the quantity and quality of speech occurring. The amount and the pace of the speech may indicate abnormalities. Little speech, paced very slowly or with many silences, may indicate anxiety, depression, or organic brain disorders. The quality of speech includes how clear it is, how loud it is, and the inflections used. A very loud speech pattern, poor enunciation, or inappropriate inflection warrant further assessment.

Noting organization and coherence of speech assists nurses to determine the level of consciousness and orientation. Patients who change words in midsentence or speak in a confused manner need further assessment. There may be other reasons, however, for altered language and speech besides a neurosensory problem.

Sensory and Motor Function. Assessment of special cortical functions includes the patient's ability to recognize common objects by using the senses of sight, hearing, and touch. Nurses may point to an object, ask the patient to listen to a familiar sound or ask the patient to touch a familiar object with eyes closed; then ask the patient to identify the sound or the object. An incorrect response to visual stimuli reflects occipital lobe alterations. Inability to interpret sounds indicates a temporal lobe deficit. Inability to identify items by touch suggests alterations in the parietal lobe. If patients are unable to perform a skilled act, such as writing their names or buttoning a shirt, in the absence of paralysis, the deficit may be caused by injury to several areas in the dominant hemisphere.

Cerebellar function is determined by assessing balance and coordination. Balance can be assessed by performing Romberg's test and by evaluating gait (see Chap. 33). Gait is one of the first observations a nurse makes when meeting a patient and should be assessed while the patient is walking independently back and forth in the room. Posture, movement of body parts, stance of feet, and the types of steps taken should be noted. (See Chap. 33 for further details on normal gait.) Coordination can be assessed through a series of activities, which are described in Table 32–7. Abnormalities include lack of coordination between muscle groups, overexaggeration of movements, incomplete or weak movement, uncoordinated rapid alternating movements, or incoordination of large muscle groups.

Motor function involves an assessment of the muscles and their movement. Muscles are examined for size, symmetry, and tone. Refer to Chaps. 17 and 33 for more details. Nurses should palpate the muscles and joints of each extremity at rest. Abnormal muscle tone findings include spasticity, manifested by undue resistance of the muscles to passive lengthening; rigidity, a constant state of resistance; and flaccidity, extreme fixing of muscles. Muscle strength is tested by placing the joints through passive range of motion, against gravity, and with active resistance from the nurse.

Spontaneous muscle movements should be observed. Abnormal muscle movements indicate an abnormality of nerve impulse transmission to or from the motor cortex. The nurse should note whether abnormal movements occur at rest or with motion, where they are located, what causes them, and whether they cease.

The *primary* sensory stimulation tests are superficial touch, temperature, position, vibration, superficial pain, and deep pressure pain. Refer to Chap. 17 for assessment technique. These assessments are performed when there are symptoms of numbness, tingling or loss of sensation, loss of motor function, areas of tissue breakdown, or muscle atrophy. Loss of sensation may indicate lesions in the posterior column of the spinal cord or the sensory cortex. Bilateral sensory loss in both lower extremities is indicative of peripheral neuropathy.

Reflexes. Assessment of deep tendon reflexes provides information regarding the function of the reflex area and spinal cord segments. Five common deep tendon reflexes are the biceps, triceps, brachioradialis, patellar, and achilles reflexes (see Chap. 17).

Reflexes may be altered in physiologic changes involving the sensory pathways from the muscles and tendons or the motor components (upper motor neurons), or the anterior horn cells or their axons (lower motor neurons). Deep tendon reflexes are graded in Table 17–44.

Abnormal (pathologic) reflexes generally denote deficits in the pyramidal tract, which assists with control of gross motor movements. The main pathologic reflex, *Babinski's reflex,* is assessed by stroking the lateral side of the sole of the foot and underneath the toes. Do *not* stroke the center of the foot. A normal (negative) response is flexion of the toes. An abnormal (positive) response is dorsiflexion of the big toe with fanning of the other toes.

TABLE 32-7. COORDINATION SKILLS TEST

Component	Action
1. Finger to nose	1. With outstretched arms, patient touches nose with index finger. Speed is increased with each successive attempt. Eyes are open at first, then are closed.
2. Finger to finger	2. Patient is asked to touch examiner's index finger with own index finger. The examiner moves the finger several times. Repeat with patient's opposite index finger.
3. Hand tapping	3. While sitting, the patient is asked to supinate and pronate the left hand on the left knee and the right hand on the right knee.
4. Heel to shin	4. In a sitting or lying position, the patient is asked to run the heel of one foot down the opposite leg. Repeat procedure for other foot.
5. Figure 8	5. While sitting, the patient is asked to use the foot to draw a figure 8 in the air. Repeat procedure for opposite foot.
6. Tandem walking	6. With the patient standing, arms at side, and eyes open, ask patient to walk heel-to-toe across the room.

DIAGNOSTIC TESTS

A review of the findings of diagnostic tests of the neurologic system aids in understanding the underlying cause of a patient's loss of neurosensory function.

Nurses play a vital role in preparing patients for diagnostic tests by providing necessary information in a professional way with appropriate depth. Many patients desire to know what the test is, why it is being done, what they will experience, and when they may be obtaining results. Teaching is individualized to meet patients' needs. Too much or too little information may cause anxiety about the procedure. Listening to patient's concerns and answering questions are priorities.

Clinical Guidelines 32–1 and 32–2 outline nursing implementation for neurosensory testing.

Lumbar Puncture

The lumbar puncture is performed for a variety of therapeutic and diagnostic purposes. Therapeutically, it is administered to give medications and anesthesia, and to remove blood, pus, and cerebrospinal fluid (CSF). Diagnostically, it allows for removal of CSF for inspection, measurement, and laboratory evaluation. A physician performs this test with nurse assisting.

Complications of lumbar puncture include leakage of CSF, infection, damage to the spinal cord, damage to the vertebrae, respiratory failure, postpuncture headache, difficulty in voiding, backache, numbness, and tingling or pain radiating to the legs. Contraindications include local tissue infection, increased intracranial pressure, broken vertebrae, neck trauma, and anticoagulation therapy.

Nurses should explain to patients that there may be slight pain but it may feel more like pressure. The physician will administer a local anesthetic to reduce discomfort. The needle is inserted below the level of the spinal cord, so there is little danger of the needle entering the spinal cord. Aseptic technique is essential throughout the procedure to prevent contamination of the punc-

CLINICAL GUIDELINE 32–1

ASSISTING PATIENTS BEFORE, DURING, AND AFTER NEUROSENSORY TESTS

BEFORE PROCEDURE

1. Discuss procedure with patient.
2. Invite questions.
3. Attempt to reduce anxiety and fear.
4. Instruct the patient to lie very still and maintain position.
5. Monitor vital signs.
6. Assess neurological status.
7. Ascertain drug allergies, particularly those related to local anesthetics and skin preparation.
8. Premedicate as needed, as per physician order.

IMMEDIATELY BEFORE PROCEDURE

1. Instruct patient to empty bladder.
2. Administer muscle relaxants or sedatives, as per physician order, to decrease anxiety and reduce movement.
3. Assemble required equipment or obtain disposable tray.

DURING PROCEDURE

1. Assist the patient to maintain position.
2. Assess respiratory function.
3. Provide comfort as needed.
4. Assist the physician as needed.

FOLLOWING PROCEDURE

1. Assist patient with positioning if needed.
2. Obtain vital signs and compare to preprocedure vital signs.
3. Monitor neurosensory status.
4. Monitor for complications.
5. Document procedure as to date, time, patient response, physician, any measurements made (eg, opening and closing pressures during lumbar puncture), appearance of samples taken, medications administered, and so forth.

ture site. Infection is a serious complication of the procedure in the normally sterile subarachnoid space.

The procedure is performed with the patient lying on the side in a knee-to-chest position (Fig. 32–4) to allow easy passage of the needle into the subarachnoid space in the lumbar region. In adults, the needle is inserted into the lower lumbar vertebrae (L3 or L4) below the level of the spinal cord. In children, the spinal cord may end in the sacral area, necessitating an even lower needle insertion. Placing the back close to the edge of the bed facilitates needle insertion.

After the procedure, nurses instruct patients to remain supine and monitors patient position. Often patients are restricted to bedrest for 4 to 8 hours with the head of the bed flat or slightly elevated to prevent a "spinal" headache. Headaches can result from CSF loss or leakage or from meningeal irritation. Analgesics can be given for these headaches. The insertion site is monitored for edema or hemorrhage. Fluids should be encouraged to replenish CSF.

CLINICAL GUIDELINE 32–2

TEACHING PATIENTS ABOUT NEUROSENSORY TESTS

Review the procedure with the patient, even if patient is semiconscious or unconscious. Review the following areas. Additional information may be added if needed.

PURPOSE

Provide information that is relevant to specific indication for this test.

PROCEDURAL INFORMATION

1. *Position:* Describe position required for the test and position changes if any. Emphasize the need to remain still until requested to move.
2. *Specific information:* Time of procedure; location where procedure will occur; health professionals in attendance during procedure; length of time for completion.

AFTERCARE INFORMATION

1. *Positioning:* Advise patient that some tests require lying flat for specified amount of time to lessen chances of a headache.
2. *Reporting:* Advise patient to report anything unusual (dizziness, difficulty breathing, abnormal sensations, headache, numbness, tingling, or pain).

Cerebral Angiography

Cerebral angiography assesses the status of cerebral vessels—their size, position, and integrity. The procedure involves the injection of radiopaque dye into a carotid or vertebral artery while radiographic exposures are taken of the blood vessels of the brain. Indications for this procedure include visualization of cerebral arteries and veins and detection of intracranial lesions (abscesses, aneurysms, hematomas); however, the introduction of computerized axial tomography, magnetic resonance imaging, and magnetic resonance angiography has changed the use of this procedure.

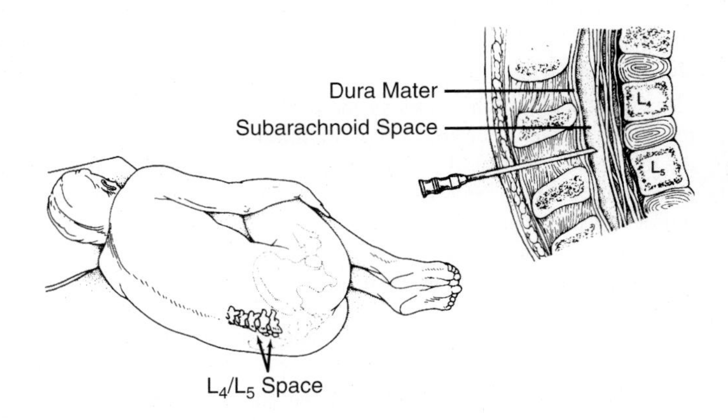

Figure 32–4. For a lumbar puncture, having patient in Sims' position facilitates insertion of needle into subarachnoid space. *(From Smith S, Duell D.* Clinical Nursing Skills: Nursing Process Model; Basic to Advanced Skills. *4th ed. Norwalk, CT: Appleton & Lange; 1996:516.)*

Computerized Axial Tomography

Computerized axial tomographic (CAT or CT) scans combine radiographic imaging with detailed analysis of tissue density by a computer. Radiographs of thin cross-sections of the brain are analyzed by computer to discern tissue density differences that cannot be visualized by conventional x-ray films. After assessing for sensitivity to contrast dye, it may be used to highlight small differences in tissue densities, as in diagnosis of intracranial lesions.

Before the procedure, patients require little physical preparation. The CT scan does not produce pain and is noninvasive. Patients should be informed of the appearance of the CT scanner and that it will make humming sounds. In addition, patients must remain still for 15 to 30 minutes until the test is finished. This may seem like a long time to some patients, who become anxious and fearful. Results may show the areas of change that have caused neurosensory alterations.

During the procedure, the patient is placed on a table with the head strapped into a rigid support. During the CT scan, the head is exposed 180 times to a narrow x-ray beam that penetrates through the various types of brain tissue. If a radiopaque dye is injected, the patient may sense a warm feeling or a metallic taste in the mouth. The patient should be monitored for anaphylactic or allergic reactions to the dye.

After the procedure, nurses continue to monitor for adverse reactions to the contrast medium and to evaluate fluid status, as the hypertonic medium may increase blood volume and cause eventual diuresis.

Magnetic Resonance Imaging

Magnetic resonance imaging (MRI) uses magnetic polarity fields instead of x-rays, as the CT scan does. A computer is used to differentiate tissue densities to detect lesions and analyze central nervous system structures. Foreign metal objects in the body, such as cardiac valves or orthopedic devices, may be disturbed because of the electromagnetic force fields applied during the procedure and serve as contraindications to the procedure.

No specific preprocedure preparation is needed, but patients should be told that they will be placed in a chamber similar to that used for CT scans with a sound like mild hammering. All metal must be removed and the patient wears a hospital gown. After the procedure, the patient may resume normal preprocedure activities.

Electroencephalography

Electroencephalography assesses the brain's electrical activity by recording activity from the surface of the brain. The purposes of the test are assessment of overall brain activity, detection of abnormal brain activity, and determination of extent of abnormal impulses. The electroencephalogram (EEG) provides a visible record in the form of brain wave patterns of the electrical potentials generated by the brain. Because the test is noninvasive, contraindications are rare.

Patient preparation involves discontinuing all anticoagulants, tranquilizers, and stimulants (alcohol or caffeine) for 24 to 48 hours before the test. Patients may be fearful that the electrode placement will hurt, and that they might receive an electric shock, but can be reassured that these fears are unfounded. The need for scalp electrodes should be explained. No meals should be missed, as hypoglycemia can alter brain wave patterns. The hair should be clean and dry and without oils, sprays, or lotions. It is best if the patient goes to sleep late and arises early because this may increase the likelihood of abnormalities being recorded.

The procedure may be performed in an EEG laboratory or at the bedside. Adhesive surface scalp electrodes or subdermal needle electrodes may be used to detect the brain's electrical output. A baseline EEG will be documented in a dim, quiet environment. Three maneuvers may be performed. In the first, the patient is asked to hyperventilate after the initial EEG is performed. This allows the blood pH to become alkalotic (pH > 7.45), which increases excitability of the nerves and the patient's potential of seizure activity. The patient may feel faint or experience tingling, but this will cease as soon as hyperventilation is stopped. The second maneuver involves exposure to a flickering light with the eyes closed. This helps to identify abnormal brain wave patterns that may indicate seizures. The third maneuver is performed when the patient is drowsy or sleeping.

After the procedure, the hair may need cleansing. Necessary medications are resumed and vital and neurosensory assessments are completed. Results of the test aid in evaluating patients who have seizure disorders and in localizing brain tumors. Conditions such as meningitis, encephalitis, infection, and drug overdose produce irregular EEGs.

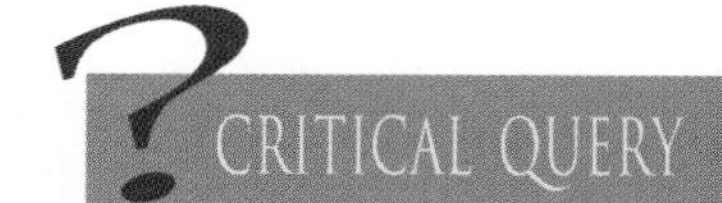

Foreman and Zane[20] found that acute confusion in the elderly can jeopardize recovery. What are the key assessments and implementations a nurse can apply to either identify or resolve this state that affects neurosensory integration?

NURSING DIAGNOSIS OF NEUROSENSORY INTEGRATION

The neurosensory assessment provides nurses with data that leads to development of nursing diagnoses. These diagnoses then form the basis for collaborative planning with patients to promote optimum neurosensory functioning. The following discussion focuses on nursing diagnoses representative of neurosensory dysfunction and their respective etiologies. These diagnoses have been approved by the North American Nursing Diagnosis Association (NANDA). Examples of subjective and objective data, defining characteristics, and etiologies for these diagnoses are presented in Table 32–8. Other nursing diagnoses related to neurosensory alterations are also listed at the end of Table 32–8.

ALTERED THOUGHT PROCESSES

The diagnosis of altered thought processes describes a state in which a person experiences a disruption in mental activities and cognitive processes. Defining characteristics include inaccurate interpretation of the environment, distractibility, difficulty remembering, focus on the self (egocentricity), disorientation to person, place, or time, delusions (fixed false beliefs), and hallucinations. Patients who have difficulty conceptualizing, who think slowly,

TABLE 32-8. SAMPLE NURSING DIAGNOSES: NEUROSENSORY INTEGRATION

Nursing Diagnoses	Defining Characteristics/Manifestations: *Subjective Data*	Defining Characteristics/Manifestations: *Objective Data*	Etiology
Altered thought processes *8.3*	Reports inability to remember events, people prior to car accident.	Retains new information in short-term memory for 3–4 minutes. Oriented to person only; disoriented to place and time. Unable to carry out directions unless cued verbally with each step. Inappropriate answers to questions.	*Physical:* Head trauma.
Impaired verbal communication *2.1.1.1*	No subjective data. Patient is unable to speak.	Indicates understanding and written communication. Unable to speak. Grunts, attempts to vocalize. Able to communicate by pointing to pictures, diagrams. Gestures to indicate requests.	*Physical:* Decrease in circulation to the brain.
Pain *9.1.1*	Reports fell off ladder 30 minutes ago, twisting knee. Sharp, piercing, shooting pain in knee. States pain is constant, and worsened by movement.	Left knee bruised; diameter slightly greater than right knee. Holds and leans over knee, rocks back and forth. Intermittent crying, moaning. Contorted facial expression.	*Physical:* Traumatic injury to left leg.
Sensory–perceptual alteration: auditory *7.2*	Reports inability to hear voices. Requests other people to speak louder. Reports humming or ringing in the ears.	Does not respond to people speaking in a normal conversational tone when they cannot be seen. Increases volume of radio and TV beyond normal hearing levels. Ticking clock and tuning fork tests indicate hearing loss.	*Physical:* Altered auditory reception, transmission.
Syndrome of impaired environmental interpretation *8.2.2*	Reports inability to understand what is occurring in current environment.	Unable to follow simple directions or instructions. Unable to reason. Responds slowly to questions.	*Physical:* Dementia.
Acute confusion *8.2.2*	Reports perceiving sounds and objects when no observable stimuli are present.	Intermittently disoriented to place and time. Fluctuates in sleep/wake cycle. Agitation/restlessness	*Physical:* Alcohol abuse.
Chronic confusion *8.2.3*	Reports nonvalid information.	Unable to retain information in short-term or long-term memory. Unable to socialize.	*Physical:* Head injury.
Impaired memory *8.3.1*	Reports forgetting recent events.	Not able to remember how to perform newly learned task. Forgets to dress self in morning.	*Physical:* Head injury.

OTHER NURSING DIAGNOSES RELATED TO NEUROSENSORY ALTERATION

PHYSICAL
Altered nutrition
Altered oral mucous membranes
Altered tissue perfusion (cerebral)
Bowel incontinence
Constipation
Dysreflexia
High risk for aspiration
Risk for infection
Impaired physical mobility
Impaired skin integrity
Impaired swallowing
Ineffective airway clearance
Ineffective breathing pattern
Ineffective thermoregulation
Self-care deficit
Sleep pattern disturbance
Total urinary incontinence
Urinary retention

COGNITIVE
Altered thought processes
Knowledge deficit
Impaired verbal communication

EMOTIONAL
Anxiety
Ineffective denial
Ineffective individual coping
Grieving
Pain
Powerlessness
Social isolation
Spiritual distress
Posttrauma response

SELF-CONCEPTUAL
Altered role performance
Body image disturbance
Hopelessness
Personal identity disturbance
Self-esteem disturbance

SOCIOCULTURAL/LIFE STRUCTURAL
Altered family processes
Altered role performance
Diversional activity deficit
Impaired adjustment
Impaired social interaction
Ineffective family coping
Social isolation
Caregiver role strain

DEVELOPMENTAL
Altered growth and development

SEXUAL
Altered sexuality patterns
Sexual dysfunction

ENVIRONMENTAL
High risk for injury
Impaired home maintenance management

Sources: The nursing diagnoses and etiologies on this table and the definitions of nursing diagnoses in the body of the text not credited to other sources are from Nursing Diagnosis: Definitions and Classification, 1997–1998. *Philadelphia: North American Nursing Diagnosis Association; 1996. Manifestation categories for etiologies and specifications of general etiologies on these tables are authors' original work.*

misinterpret events, or are confused reflect the diagnosis of altered thought processes.

- *Etiology: physical changes.* Many physical conditions can cause an alteration in thought processes. Injury to the brain, brain tumors, or increased intracranial pressure can produce an altered level of consciousness or damage to the brain cells needed to think and respond. Other factors such as decreased cardiac output result in hypoxia to the brain. Dehydration can cause brain cells to shrink, whereas alteration in electrolytes can result in disruption of the sodium–potassium pump. All of these conditions can result in altered thinking.
- *Etiology: psychological stress.* Psychological stress such as anxiety, fear, depression, or acute grief may produce temporary changes in a patient's thought processes. Some patients become so overwhelmed with the changes in their lives that they become disoriented.[20]
- *Etiology: environmental changes.* Individuals who are admitted to a hospital may experience sensory overload or sensory deprivation. This results in upsetting the balance of the reticular activating system. Multiple simultaneous stimuli, such as the sounds generated by monitoring equipment, alarms that signal malfunction of IV pumps or similar machines, or the rumble of carts delivering supplies can produce sensory overload. Conversely, other patients, when alone in a stark clinical room, experience sensory deprivation.
- *Etiology: medications, drugs, or alcohol.* Many medications can cause confusion, including excess or deficiency in insulin, digitalis toxicity, narcotics, sedatives, and tranquilizers. Use of illegal drugs may lead to altered awareness, as can alcohol abuse.

ACUTE PAIN

Acute pain describes temporary encounters with pain and is limited by time. Acute pain may last from a moment up to 6 months. McCaffery describes acute pain as pain that subsides as healing takes place or pain that has a predictable end.[7] Acute pain is associated with a specific event, including: (1) fractures of bones, muscle spasms associated with injuries or accidents; (2) migraine headaches, gout, sickle cell crisis, or myocardial infarction; and (3) health treatments such as biopsies, surgery, diagnostic procedures, or dental procedures.

- *Etiology: injuring agents.* Agents causing pain are categorized as biologic, chemical, physical, or psychological. Biologic agents, such as bacterial or viral agents, can disrupt tissue integrity resulting in pain. Chemical agents are toxins within the environment, such as pesticides, ingested chemicals or drugs, that can disrupt neurosensory integration. For example, they can cause burn injuries, tissue breakdown, damage the respiratory tract if inhaled, or destroy the esophagus if swallowed.

  Physical agents exacerbating an episode of acute pain are broadly categorized under trauma. Whether trauma occurs as an assault by another person, or an injury sustained from a moving object, such as a baseball bat, or from collision with an immovable object, such as the ground, acute pain is likely to develop.

  Psychological factors may aggravate episodes of acute pain and arise within or outside the person. Fears regarding the nature and intensity of anticipated pain, and external psychological factors, such as suggestions from health care workers about the nature of a diagnostic procedure, may alert the patient to the potential for pain, causing fear and anxiety, which may then interact with actual pain to enhance the pain response.

CHRONIC PAIN

Prolonged pain that occurs continuously, pain that has active and inactive states over a lifetime, or pain that is acute for a lengthy, time-limited period are variations of pain that characterize the diagnosis of chronic pain. There is controversy regarding how long pain must occur before being termed chronic; however, pain existing longer than 6 months is considered chronic.

Chronic pain can be limited, intermittent, or persistent. Individuals with chronic pain may have adapted so that physical manifestations may not be obvious, such as grimacing or guarding of a painful area. Behaviors like depression, anger, withdrawal, or manipulation may characterize individuals who suffer with long-term pain. These behaviors can be frustrating for family, patients, and health care personnel.

- *Etiology: chronic physical or psychosocial disability.* Chronic pain may be a result of persistent diseases, such as low back pain, rheumatoid arthritis, or degenerative diseases of the joints; progressive diseases, such as cancer; or other physiological processes that are not clearly understood.

  After an injury, pain receptors may become sensitized and continue to fire even after the injury has healed. Pain messages continue to be sent to the brain. It appears that the cellular damage as a result of degeneration or injury causes changes in the central processing system of the brain, resulting in the self-sustaining neural activity. It is also hypothesized that chronic pain results from a series of biochemical changes that cause depletion of serotonin. Serotonin affects sleep, mood, and perception of pain. Still other theories suggest that chronic pain may be a result of abnormal functioning of the endogenous opiate system.

  Persons who experience chronic pain often become overwhelmed with the pain. As a result of loss of locus of control anxiety and depression result.

IMPAIRED VERBAL COMMUNICATION

Impaired verbal communication reflects an individual's inability or decreased ability to send and/or receive messages. Effected individuals have difficulty relating thoughts, needs, and desires. Behavioral characteristics of this diagnosis include inappropriate or absent speech response, confusion, weak or absent voice, and stuttering or slurring. Individuals may have difficulty finding the correct word when speaking, or have decreased hearing comprehension or deafness.

- *Etiology: impaired circulation to the brain.* Impaired circulation to the brain can result from occlusion of blood vessels, brain tumors, and blood clots leading to tissue damage and cell death. If the impairment involves the brain areas responsible for speech or for motor control of speech organs, loss of ability for verbal expression results, as discussed earlier. The local inflammatory reaction often exaggerates the loss of function immediately after the injury; partial return of function in many patients is therefore possible after inflammation resolves.

- *Etiology: cultural differences.* Impaired verbal communication can be a result of not being able to speak the language of the dominant culture. Although such a person is able to express thoughts and needs verbally, caregivers are usually not able to understand.
- *Etiology: physical barriers, tracheostomies, intubation, or laryngectomy.* Some patients require a tracheostomy to allow them to breathe. Because air cannot pass the vocal cords, the patient cannot speak without plugging the tracheostomy. Tracheal intubation has the same effect. Laryngectomy (removal of the vocal cords) presents an irreversible loss of capacity for normal speech, but artificial aids and speech therapy make verbal communication possible.

SENSORY–PERCEPTUAL ALTERATIONS

Sensory–perceptual alterations refer to altered visual, auditory, kinesthetic, gustatory, tactile, or olfactory modes of perception. It is defined as the change in the amount or patterning of incoming stimuli and subsequent diminished, exaggerated, distorted, or impaired response to stimuli.

Defining characteristics of this diagnosis include disturbed sense of time, place, or person; a change in usual response to stimuli; change in behavior patterns; report of or measured change in sensory acuity; and change in ability to problem-solve and communicate. Restlessness, irritability, fear, anxiety, apathy, and auditory, visual, or other perceptual hallucinations are examples of behavioral characteristics of this diagnosis.

- *Etiology: altered environmental stimuli.* Excessive stimuli from the hospital environment might include such things as beeps and noises from machines (eg, suction machines and IV pumps), various monitors, many health care personnel assisting one patient, and sleep interruptions. The extremely ill, the critically ill, and the elderly are most likely to experience sensory overload or sensory deprivation. For patients who have diminished perceptual input, normal amounts of environmental stimuli may be too much. Astute nursing assessment and discussion with patients can result in diagnosis statements that accurately reflect nurse–patient collaboration in problem identification.

  Insufficient environmental stimuli implies diminished sensory perceptual input, darkness, or simply lack of naturally occurring stimulating activities. The resulting understimulation of the reticular-activating system caused altered perception. Sensory deprivation is characterized by auditory or visual hallucination, restlessness, and anxiety. Nurses who collaboratively assess and plan for patients' needs for sensory stimulation achieve optimal interventions.
- *Etiology: altered sensory reception, transmission, and integration.* Whether the dysfunction involves reception, transmission, or integration, the end result is lost communication between the sensory input and the brain. When the sensory receptors or their respective pathways to the brain become damaged, altered sensory reception occurs. This altered sensory reception can happen as a result of a traumatic event, of some internal degenerative process to the sensory organ, or of lack of neurotransmittors, necessary for neural communication.

  Altered sensory integration is disorganized or ineffective processing of sensory input. It is characterized by decreased cognitive abilities and by memory alterations. Causes include traumatic events, intracranial tumors, lack of neurosensory neurotransmitters, and abnormal firing of neural impulses from highly active neurons. The cells or structures necessary for integrative function are not properly functioning, whether from the results of direct pressure, cell death, or anoxia, and as a result do not process input into meaningful ideas or thoughts. Nurses can assist patients by providing sensory input for the unaffected senses, providing reality orientation, protecting patients from injury, and providing emotional support.
- *Etiology: chemical alterations.* Chemical alterations can be endogenous or exogenous alterations. Endogenous chemical alterations are changes within a cell or organism that are harmful to neurosensory integration. Examples of cellular changes are impaired oxygen transport and electrolyte disturbance within the cells, which may cause the accumulation of hydrogen ions resulting in confusion or brain death.

  Exogenous chemical alterations are changes introduced to the neurosensory network or cells that cause damage and impair sensory–perceptual function. Ingestion of drugs, toxins, and growth of bacteria in the neurosensory network can produce such chemical alterations.
- *Etiology: psychological stress.* In this state, a person experiences a changed perception of events; that is, certain stimuli are viewed as stressful and may be accompanied by altered coping mechanisms. Psychological stress causing altered sensory–perceptual function can be experienced as actual or perceived threats to self, anticipation of pain, or misinterpretation of persons or situations in the environment.

IMPAIRED ENVIRONMENTAL INTERPRETATION SYNDROME

Impairment of environmental interpretation suggests that the patient demonstrates a lack of orientation to person, place, time, or other circumstances for longer than 3 to 6 months.

- *Etiology: chronic confusional states.* Patients with chronic conditions, such as Alzeheimer's disease, AIDS, depression, or alcoholism, experience the inability to relate, perceive, understand, and interpret the environment. Nurses, with the family and other members of the care team, must identify safety concerns for the patient and modify the activities in the environment to provide for safety. These interventions include adequate assessment of patient history and condition progression, environmental restructuring to remove unsafe hazards, and behavioral interventions such as reorientation techniques with clear, simple communication and distraction techniques when the patient becomes agitated. Resources that will be available to the patient after discharge must be identified.

ACUTE CONFUSION

Patients with acute confusion demonstrate an abrupt onset of global, yet transient, changes in their attention, thought processes, psychomotor activity level of consciousness, and/or the sleep–wake cycle. The nurse's role is to assess causative factors, including degree of impairment; maximize the patient's level of function; and prevent further deterioration. Conditions such as dementia, alcohol abuse, medication reaction, severe pain, and sleep deprivation alter the patient's view of internal and external stimuli.

- *Etiology: severe pain.* A patient with severe pain perceives and inaccurately interprets messages from internal and external sources, adding to the acute confusional state. Nurse assess the patient for adequacy of pain control measures and alter the plan of care accordingly. Patients might also deveslop acute confusion from medication administered to alleviate their discomfort. Careful evaluation of patients' response to medication will minimize acute confusion.
- *Etiology: medication reaction.* Some medications affect patients' level of orientation and may cause confusional states. Nurse should determine the most appropriate schedule of medications based on potential drug interactions. Common medications when combined with each other sometimes cause acute confusion (cimetidine with an antacid, or digoxin with a diuretic, for example).
- *Etiology: sleep deprivation.* Consistent and prolonged sleep deprivation, particularly REM sleep, produces confusion and disorientation which resolve when a normal sleep pattern is resumed.
- *Etiology: chronic disease exacerbation.* Flare–ups of many chronic conditions produce confusion. A completely oriented person with congestive heart failure, for example, may experience acute confusion when the disease worsens. The patient with obstructive lung disease will become acutely confused when the pulmonary lung status deteriorates due to a respiratory infection.

CHRONIC CONFUSION

With chronic confusion, a patient has an irreversible, long-standing, and/or progressive deterioration of personality and intellect. The person has a decreased interpretation of environmental stimuli and a decreased capacity for intellectual thought processes with disturbances of memory, orientation, and behavior. Examples of conditions associated with this nursing diagnosis are Alzheimer's disease, cerebral vascular accidents, and head injuries.

- *Etiology: altered brain circulation (CVA or head injury).* A continuous supply of oxygen and glucose is essential for effective brain function. When trauma or other insult permanantly interrupts brain blood flow, neurosensory function deteriorates, evidenced by confusion.

IMPAIRED MEMORY

A person with impaired memory is unable to remember information and relate it to purposeful behavior. Impaired memory can be connected with specific disease states or situational causes that are either temporary or permanent. Defining characteristics include forgetfulness, inability to recall recent or past events, inability to retain or learn new behaviors, and forgetting to perform a behavior at a scheduled time.

- *Etiology: alteration in circulating blood components/fluid/electrolyte status.* The patient who has inadequate levels of circulating blood volume, oxygen, or fluid and electrolytes will not be able to support the higher level of functioning consistent with neurosensory integration, including memory.
- *Etiology: change in structure of brain mass related to aging or disease states.* Loss of brain mass, for example as a result of a tumor, disrupts the neural networks that permit information storage and retrieval.

STATING THE NEUROSENSORY DIAGNOSIS

Once the assessment is completed, meaningful clustering of data and analysis regarding the patient's neurosensory functioning culminates in the formulation of nursing diagnoses.

Nursing diagnoses are most meaningful and relevant to the care of a particular person when they include specific descriptions of how the person exemplifies the diagnosis. Likewise, defining characteristics can be made more descriptive to assist in identifying appropriate evaluation criteria and recognizing the absence of symptoms that originally validated that the diagnosis applied. "Moaning and restlessness" as defining characteristics of pain more clearly explains the patient's situation than "distraction behaviors." Individualization of etiologies and defining characteristics is appropriate for all neurosensory integration diagnoses.

SECTION 3

NURSE–PATIENT MANAGEMENT OF NEUROSENSORY INTEGRATION

Once the nursing diagnosis of a neurosensory deficit has been made, the management phase begins. It involves collaboration with other health care providers, and with the patient and the patient's family. Appropriate implementation is instituted to prevent further alteration, or to promote, support, or restore optimal functioning.

PLANNING FOR OPTIMAL NEUROSENSORY INTEGRATION

Planning includes formulating desired outcomes that determine priorities of effective care. Mutual goal setting is the ideal approach in determining neurosensory outcomes. Patients who share their perceptions are more likely to participate and progress toward achieving the mutually determined goals.

When patients experience alterations of neurosensory function with impaired cognition and thought, it may be difficult to engage in mutual goal setting. The nurse should then include close family members or significant others. At other times, particularly when the patient is unconscious, nurses may be required to assume full responsibility for decisions on goals and approaches.

In addition to family members, nurses may need to consult other members of the health care team: physicians, physical therapists, occupational therapists, speech pathologists, respiratory therapists, clinical nurse specialists, and others. The care of the patient with a neurosensory problem can be complex and frequently necessitates professional interdisciplinary collaboration. The plan of care for the patient addresses all of the identified nursing diagnoses.

Table 32–9, Nurse–Patient Management of Neurosensory Integration Problems, summarizes appropriate outcomes, approaches, and evaluation criteria for neurosensory problems. Table 32–10, Partial Critical Pathway for Congestive Heart Failure:

(continued on page 1145)

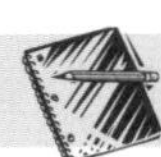

TABLE 32-9. NURSE-PATIENT MANAGEMENT OF NEUROSENSORY INTEGRATION PROBLEMS

Nursing Diagnosis	Desired Outcomes	Implementation	Evaluation
Altered thought process R/T head trauma *8.3*	1. Improved orientation (within limitations of physical condition).	1a. Give stimuli to achieve/maintain orientation: • Call patient by preferred name. • Remind patient of location. • Keep clock and calendar in patient's view. • Encourage family involvement in care and stimulating activities. • Encourage family to bring photos and personal items from home. 1b. Speak slowly and clearly; allow ample response time. 1c. Establish/maintain a routine for personal care and other activities. 1d. Encourage patient choice-making and participation in care.	1a. Patient able to: state name, location, and time; identify family members and regular caregivers; remember recent events.
	2. Freedom from injuries.	2a. Maintain adequate lighting. 2b. Keep bed in low position; use siderails if necessary, but avoid restraints, if possible. 2c. Assist with ambulation.	2. Patient remains free of injury.
	3. Improved ability to respond to environment (within limitations of physical condition).	3a. Involve patient in conversations about surroundings and daily events. 3b. Provide opportunities for interactions outside patient's room.	3a. Responds appropriately to questions, events. 3b. Performs activities of daily living with assistance relative to physical condition.
Impaired verbal communication R/T decrease in circulation to the brain secondary to CVA (stroke) *2.1.1.1*	1. Needs communicated by alternate means.	1a. Speak to patient in a normal conversational tone. 1b. When communicating, position yourself so patient can readily see you; maintain eye contact. 1c. Provide alternate means of communication for patient to use to express needs: magic slate, pictures or flashcards of common objects, pad/pencil, magnetic board with alphabet. 1d. Encourage use of gestures, nods, eye blinks to respond to questions. 1e. Provide time for patient to express needs; meet needs promptly. 1f. Verbalize empathy and acceptance of anger, frustration. 1g. Explain the cause of speech loss to patient; share prognosis for recovery, if known. 1h. Encourage and positively reinforce attempts to speak. 1i. Encourage family to engage in frequent communication with patient.	1a. Patient consistently uses alternative method of choice to communicate needs. 1b. Patient indicates needs are met.
	2. Improved ability to communicate verbally commensurate with medical diagnosis.	2. Consult with speech therapist for collaborative plan to maximize speaking ability.	2. Comprehensible verbal communication at level permitted by medical condition.
Pain R/T traumatic injury to left leg *9.1.1*	1. Pain remains at tolerable level until definitive treatment of injury commences.	1a. Speak to patient in soothing monotone voice. 1b. Position in good alignment; support and elevate left leg so it is above heart level. 1c. Apply ice bag to knee. 1d. Suggest and assist patient with noninvasive pain relief measures: deep breathing/relaxation, guided imagery.	1a. States pain is tolerable. 1b. Cessation of crying, moaning. 1c. Facial and torso muscles relaxed.
Sensory–perceptual alteration: auditory R/T altered auditory reception/ transmission *7.2*	1. Communication with others via measures to support/augment hearing to aid independent functioning.	1a. Collaborate with patient to select preferred hearing support strategies: lip reading, hearing aid. 1b. If patient has hearing aid, encourage its use; teach and assist as necessary with care, cleaning (see Procedure 32–2). 1c. Speak slowly and clearly with voice slightly louder than normal conversational level; keep messages short and concise. 1d. Use tactile and visual stimuli to compensate for auditory sensory loss. 1e. Make sure other caregivers are aware of hearing loss: post sign with preferred communication methods on patient's bed. 1f. Teach patient and family safety measures to compensate for hearing loss; increased visual vigilance; amplifier on telephone. 1g. Refer to community resources (eg, Teletype for Hearing Impaired, American Organization for the Education of the Hearing Impaired).	1a. Uses hearing aid and/or lip reading to help receive messages. 1b. Responds appropriately when others communicate with him or her.

Source: See Table 32–8.

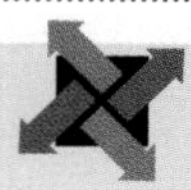

TABLE 32-10. PARTIAL CRITICAL PATHWAY FOR CONGESTIVE HEART FAILURE: NEUROSENSORY FUNCTION

Nursing Dx/Problem	Outcome Primary Care Visit	Outcome Home Care Week 1 (3 Visits)	Outcome Home Care Week 2 (3 Visits)	Outcome Home Care Weeks 3–4 (3 Visits)
Risk for altered thought processes RF decreased cardiac output (compromised cerebral perfusion)		Oriented × 2	Oriented × 3 Correctly subtracts 9 from 100 Correct interpretation of truism	Same Same Same

Implementation	Primary Care Visit	Home Care Visit Week 1	Home Care Visit Week 2	Home Care Visit Weeks 3–4
Assessment	Orientation/mentation Restlessness/anxiety Jugular venous distension V/S, arrhythmia, O_2 saturation Breath sounds, edema Chest pain, dizziness, dyspnea, ā & p̄ activity	Same Same Same Same Same Same Safe environment	Same Same Same Same Same Same Same	Same Same
Tests/Consults	Refer to Home Health			
Medications/Treatments	ECG, chest x-ray, electrolytes: Na, K, Cl, CO_2, BUN, creatinine Digoxin levels O_2 at 2 L/cannula Diuretics, K supplements Digoxin, anticoagulants Antithromboembolism stockings	Stimulate cognitive function Assist family with appropriate responses to patient	Same Encourage socialization	
Teaching	Teach family O_2 use and precautions, how to take pulse & BP, applying antithromboembolism stocking application, medications: correct use, SE, precautions S/Sx to report to MD, RN, 911	Reinforce as needed Importance of uninterrupted rest periods Injury prevention Reinforce as needed	Same Reinforce as needed Reinforce as needed Same	
Activity/Safety/Self-care	Bedrest, HOB 30–45 degrees c̄ BSC or BRP	Assist c̄ ADLs Chair c̄ legs elevated tid Restraint device if needed Position change precautions	Progressive activity as tolerated Same	Same
Nutrition				
Transfer/Discharge Coord./Case Manager		Communicate to MD outcomes achieved	Same	Same Prepare for discharge

See inside back cover for abbreviations.

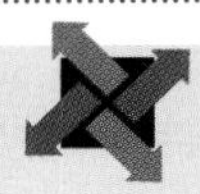

TABLE 32-11. PARTIAL CRITICAL PATHWAY FOR TOTAL HIP REPLACEMENT: NEUROSENSORY FUNCTION

Nursing Dx/Problem	Outcome DOS/Day 1	Outcome Days 2–3	Outcome SNF Days 4–6	Outcome Home Care 3 Weeks (6 Visits)
Pain R/T surgery: hip replacement	Pain rated at 4 or less	Pain rated at 3 or less	Pain rated at 2 or less	Same
Implementation	**Outcome DOS/Day 1**	**Outcome Days 2–3**	**Outcome SNF Days 4–6**	**Outcome Home Care 3 Weeks (6 Visits)**
Assessment	Rate pain 1–5 scale Effectiveness of pain control measures Overt & covert signs of pain	Same Same Same	Same Same	Same Same
Tests/Consults				
Medications/Treatments	Pain control meds (PCA, epidural, or IV analgesia) & comfort measures	Same Relaxation & guided imagery techniques	Same Same	Same
Psychsocial				
Teaching	Side effects & effective use of ordered pain meds Relaxation & guided imagery techniques	Reinforce as needed Reinforce as needed	Same Same	
Activity/Safety/Self-care	Pain medication before activities	Same	Same	
Nutrition				
Transfer/Discharge Coord./Case Manager		Communicate outcomes achieved, problems/interventions to SNF	Communicate outcomes achieved, problems/interventions to Home Health	Communicate outcomes achieved, problems/interventions to MD & prepare for discharge

See inside back cover for abbreviations.

Neurosensory Function, and Table 32–11, Partial Critical Pathway for Total Hip Replacement: Neurosensory Function, illustrate concepts from this chapter. Such interdisciplinary plans are valuable because they improve provider efficiency and may shorten the hospital stay.[21]

NURSING IMPLEMENTATION TO PROMOTE NEUROSENSORY INTEGRATION

Nurse–patient management involves implementation of planned goals. Measures to alleviate patient problems should focus on the patient's strengths, as well as needs, and provide support where needed.

PREVENTIVE CARE

Preventive care includes health education and health promotion and maintenance. Health education focuses on safety and accident prevention, whereas health maintenance involves encouraging patients to participate in or schedule hearing and vision checks, blood pressure monitoring and control, and exercise programs.

Health Education

Health education for neurosensory health focuses on accident prevention and safety issues such as risks associated with automobiles and motorcycles. Nurses explain the importance of wearing seat belts when driving or riding in cars, driving without consumption of alcohol or drugs, turning on lights at twilight, avoid-

COLLABORATIVE STRATEGY
HEALTH EDUCATION

Many permanent neurosensory alterations are caused by accidents and subsequent trauma to the nervous system that could have been prevented or avoided. Motor vehicle, motorcycle, and bicycle accidents are frequently causes of severe head and spinal cord injury. Drug overdose is another way that individuals impair their neurosensory functions. Nurses are in a good position to educate the public on the tragic and costly consequences of preventable accidents, and can help individual patients by routinely asking them about their activities and their safety practices such as wearing helmets and seat belts.

ing driving if experiencing night blindness, and wearing an approved helmet when using a bicycle or motorcycle. Young adults and teenagers are at increased risk for motor vehicle accidents because of inexperience and risk taking, making them prime candidates for teaching about vehicular safety.

Motorcycle accidents are a common cause of spinal cord and head injuries. Although some motorcycle enthusiasts resist wearing helmets, the incidence of serious brain injury is lower when helmets are worn.

Diving accidents are another cause of cervical spine injury, and result from diving into shallow water. Teenage males are frequent victims, along with people under the influence of alcohol.

Health Maintenance

Screening for health problems is another preventive nursing activity. Vision screening should be done on a yearly basis or as prescribed by an ophthalmologist or optometrist. Teaching individuals to protect and preserve their eyesight is an important nursing role (for example, to wear goggles when using power tools). Individuals with eye disorders should be taught about their condition and about how to prevent further alterations.

Hearing screening helps detect hearing loss. Preschools and secondary schools schedule periodic hearing checks to detect abnormalities in children. Environmental precautions should be taken to reduce noise levels that might injure hearing.

Blood pressure screening is important for detecting high blood pressure and hypertension. Hypertension can precipitate cerebrovascular accidents (strokes) if prolonged and if blood pressure is very high (eg, 200/100).

Home Health Care

All of the information conveyed in the *Preventive Care* section may be used as a foundation for health promotion and disease prevention by home health nurses. The prevention of motor vehicle accidents and related injuries is a major way to reduce neurosensory health problems. Reinforcing principles of safe driving, such as obeying speed limits, not drinking alcoholic beverages if driving, and using seat belts and headlights, is part of the nurse's role in the home. In addition, educating patients about the causes and prevention of sports accidents is important, particularly when there are children in the home. Home nurses also identify factors in the home that contribute to accidents and injury. They identify potential home hazards and assess the safety practices of family members; for example, in a swimming pool. Home health nurses also screen their patients for vision, hearing, and memory loss, and for mental confusion, which may result from accidents. Furthermore, alcohol and drug use is another part of the patient database accumulated by nurses working in the home.

SUPPORTIVE CARE

Supportive care focuses on care for patients who experience mild to moderate interruption in neurosensory integration and who require some assistance with self-care. The primary goals of care are to alleviate the neurosensory dysfunction and to prevent further loss of neurosensory integration.

Supporting Patients with Impaired Vision

Supporting patients whose vision is impaired enhances their optimal vision; promotes comfort, hygiene, and body image; and prevents infection (see Chap. 27 for eye hygiene).

Approaches to Help Patients with Impaired Visual Acuity. Supporting impaired or reduced vision in patients entails proper knowledge and use of vision supports and care of eyeglasses, contact lenses, and glass eyes.

VISION SUPPORTS. Vision supports are devices or environmental modifications that enhance vision, such as proper lighting for reading and adequate night lights for comfort and safety. Large-print reading materials and magnifying glasses may assist patients in reading and are especially helpful for those with myopia or prosbyopia, who are without glasses. In planning care, daily routines or medication schedules, bedside marker boards can facilitate patients' visual access to necessary information.

EYEGLASSES. Clean eyeglasses enhance vision. Eyeglasses require daily cleansing and special care when handling to prevent damage and scratching of lenses. If patients request that nurses not clean their eyeglasses, ask them if they plan to do so, and explain the need.

Eyeglasses with glass lenses should be cleaned with soap and warm water, and dried with a tissue or cloth that will not scratch the lenses. Plastic lenses scratch easily and require specific cleaning solutions and drying tissues. Fingernails or sharp objects must not be used to remove debris.

If patients need help removing eyeglasses, gently grasp each side of the frame in front of the ears and raise the bow up from the ears. Avoid grasping only one side. Reverse the process when placing eyeglasses on a patient.

Eyeglasses and cases should be labeled with the patient's name. Store hospitalized patients' eyeglasses in bedside units when not in use. Decide with the patient where in the unit the eyeglasses will be kept.

CONTACT LENSES. Contact lenses are thin, curved plastic discs that fit on the cornea of the eye directly over the iris and pupil. Lenses float on the thin layer of fluid that bathes the eyes. Hard, nonpermeable lenses can be worn up to 18 hours; some gas-permeable lenses for 1 to 3 days; soft contact lenses from 1 to 30 days, depending on the manufacturer.

Contact lenses are relatively easy for patients to insert and remove, although it is difficult for someone to insert lenses in someone else's eye. The lenses are usually inserted and removed by the patient. Soft lenses in particular are easily torn if handled improperly, and incorrect manipulation can injure the eye. Most contact lense wearers have eyeglasses for situations in which they are temporarily unable to wear contact lenses.

Nurses may be asked to help care for a patient's contact lenses. Several cleaning and care systems are available for both hard and soft lenses. Each time the lenses are removed they should be cleaned and/or disinfected with a solution the patient chooses. Collaborating with the patient will provide the nurse with necessary information. Cleaning lenses over a towel is a good idea to prevent loss or damage if they are dropped during cleaning.

Assisting Patients Who Are Blind. Lack of vision produces anxiety, particularly for a person who recently became blind. When a blind person is in an unfamiliar environment, usual coping methods and adaptations for performing daily activities may no longer be successful. Blind persons depend on routine placement of objects. Asking for help and otherwise being dependent is difficult for blind persons who are striving for independence.

Lack of social support hinders adjustment. Blind individuals can be helped to adjust to loss of vision by being with other visually impaired persons. A trusting nurse–patient relationship can be established by spending time with the patient and encouraging expression of apprehension and fears.

When speaking with patients who are visually impaired, face toward them. Describe events and situations that are occurring around them. When talking with someone who is blind and in a group of people, address the person directly, stating his or her name first.

Clinical Guideline 32–3 outlines nursing implementations for supporting patients who are blind.

Most blind persons have a keen sense of hearing and touch and are sensitive to spatial perception. These senses become more developed and assist blind persons in adapting to their condition. Nurses can orient patients who are blind to unfamiliar sounds in the environment, such as noises at the nurses' desk, the beeps on certain machines, and other unfamiliar noises.

Walking canes provide patients who are blind with a sense of spatial perception; alert them to steps, curbs, and obstacles; and complement their increased acuity in hearing. Seeing eye dogs and canes are supports for the blind person. Blind persons who cannot have their seeing eye dogs with them feel helpless, lonely, and less organized. The nurse can explore with the patient alternative methods for promoting independence.

Many blind people are sensitive to breezes. This use of spatial–perceptual abilities gives them information about location of doors and windows. When voices, music, and sounds reverberate against walls or other objects, there is an effect of an echo to note solid walls, fences, or other high objects.

Safety is of great importance for hospitalized patients who are blind. Precautions include keeping one siderail up, assisting patients when ambulating, removing hospital instruments from the bedside, and arranging bedside items according to patient preference to facilitate locating them.

The newly blind patient requires sensitivity and understanding on the part of caregivers. Loss of vision can be a traumatic loss; nurses can facilitate the grieving process by supporting patients' expressions of emotion—be it anger, sadness, or grief (see Chap. 26 for discussion of patients who are grieving a loss). The assistance of other occupational therapists, physical therapists, social workers, psychiatrists, or pastoral care can facilitate adjustment and rehabilitation of the newly blind patient.

CLINICAL GUIDELINE 32–3

SUPPORTING PATIENTS WHO ARE BLIND

1. Introduce yourself to patients each time you enter the room.
2. Speak to the patients before touching them or performing a procedure. Prepare them for what is going to happen next.
3. Introduce patients to their surroundings. Provide opportunities for blind persons to touch objects in the environment.
4. Always make sure call lights are secured to the bed or siderail in patient's preferred location.
5. Encourage independent activities of daily living: grooming, hygiene, eating, dressing.
6. Keep personal items and other important objects (eg, water pitcher, cup) in the same place or notify and describe to patients any changes made in the placement of items in the environment.
7. Inform patients when you are leaving the room.
8. When in a group of people, call the patient out by name when speaking specifically to him or her.
9. When walking with a patient, do not grasp the patient's elbow, but rather suggest that the patient hold onto your forearm as you stay one-half step ahead when moving. Describe stairs, doorways, obstacles, and other key elements in the environment. Move slowly and smoothly. Do not hurry with blind patients.
10. Gently inform patients of any facial grimaces or postures that call unnecessary attention to them.
11. Place food on meal trays in a similar location for each meal, or inform patients of the specific location and layout of foods and items on the meal tray.
12. Keep doors wide open or completely shut to protect patients from bumping into doors.
13. Be alert to objects on floor and notify patients as to location of temporary objects, such as cleaning equipment.
14. Provide sensory stimulation for the other senses.
15. Orient patients to time of day and date.

Supporting Patients with Impaired Hearing

Many people over 65 years of age experience some degree of hearing loss. People experiencing hearing loss demonstrate inattentiveness to sounds and voices, and may respond inappropriately in conversations because of "unheard" phrases or misinterpretation of words. Inappropriate shouting occurs when people lose the ability to hear their own voices.

Compensatory measures that supplement hearing acuity or offset the loss of hearing include lip reading, sign language, gestures, and hearing aids.

Ear Hygiene. Ear hygiene, performed daily, aids in preventing debris build-up and infection. Simple cleansing of the ear is carried out using a washcloth folded over the tip of an index finger and carefully wiping out the ear canal. Cerumen, or ear wax, also may be removed in this manner. Build-up of cerumen is a common cause of diminished hearing. Cotton swabs and hairpins should never be used to clean ears or remove cerumen. In some cases, ear irrigations with warm tap water may be done to cleanse the ear canal. Ear drops for cerumen removal (Debrox) can be inserted into the ear canal to help dissolve large accumulations of cerumen. Procedure 32–1 describes irrigation of the ear.

Lip Reading. Lip reading involves understanding speech by carefully observing lip movements, facial gestures, and body movements. Lip reading may be used by patients in combination with hearing aids. It is therefore very important to face directly persons who lip read and to maintain good eye contact during conversations. Lip reading requires a great deal of skill and concentration. Patients experiencing a great deal of pain, stress, or fatigue may therefore have difficulty using lip reading.

Sign Language. Sign language, although most commonly used by the deaf, may be used by hearing-impaired patients to supplement their communication. Sign language is communication by hand signals that represent the letters of the alphabet, certain phrases, and words.

Hearing Aids. Hearing aids are battery-operated mechanical devices that improve hearing by amplifying or intensifying the level of sound reaching the ear. Over 700 types of hearing aids are currently available, enabling a hearing aid to be tailored to a particular patient's need. For example, a patient with a conductive hearing loss may benefit from amplification alone if it can overcome the blockage or damage that prevents sound from reaching the inner ear. Someone with a sensorineural hearing loss may need to have low tones depressed and high tones enhanced, rather than needing to have all sound amplified.

Collaboration with an otologist and/or audiologist will determine type of loss and assist in choosing the most appropriate hearing aid.

Before getting a hearing aid, patients should be told that using a hearing aid does not guarantee perfect hearing, and that not every person is a candidate for a hearing aid. Persons with middle ear problems benefit the most from hearing aids. Hearing aids are most useful when hearing loss is conductive rather than sensorineural in origin. Their effectiveness depends on the degree of loss of ability to hear high frequencies, personal tolerance for loud noises, and cognitive ability to understand speech. Hearing aids amplify background noise as well as conversation, and some people find this distracting and annoying. In addition, as sound becomes louder, it does not necessarily become clearer. Individuals may require auditory training in addition to the hearing aid.

The amount and type of hearing loss determines the types of hearing aids that a patient may choose. Smaller, less visible hearing aids tend to be most desired. Unfortunately their small size and the proximity of the hearing aid and the receiver limit the amount of amplification that can be achieved. Therefore, individuals with severe hearing loss cannot use them.

BEHIND-THE-EAR HEARING AID. The behind-the-ear (BTE) hearing aid is the most common. It fits behind the ear and is connected to an ear mold inside the ear. This device is comfortable and has cosmetic appeal. It is useful for hearing loss in the range of 20 to 80 decibels (dB).[5]

IN-THE-EAR HEARING AID. The in-the-ear (ITE) hearing aid is also popular with its small, one-piece design. All components—hearing aid, receiver, and battery—fit directly into the ear. Because of its small size, it has aesthetic appeal, but it cannot be used by individuals with severe hearing loss. This device is useful with hearing losses in the 25 to 55 dB range.[5]

EYEGLASSES HEARING AID. The eyeglasses hearing aid is similar to the BTE unit. A limitation of this type of hearing aid is that the eyeglass style is somewhat bulky to disguise the hearing aid equipment. This type of hearing aid is used for hearing loss in the 20 to 70 dB range.[5]

BODY AID. The body aid is a device used for individuals with severe hearing loss. It consists of a fitted ear mold connected to a round receiver that attaches to a transmitter the size of a cigarette case that can be concealed in clothes. The body aid is used for hearing losses in the 40 to 110 dB range.[5]

COCHLEAR IMPLANT. The cochlear implant is a device that is surgically implanted into the ear and is known as the "artificial ear." The cochlear implant is intended for people with sensorineural deafness in which the hair cells of the cochlea are impaired. The implant bypasses the damaged hair cells to stimulate the intact nerve fibers, which then send auditory impulses to the brain.

CARING FOR HEARING AIDS. Hearing aids require delicate care and protection from moisture, heat, and breakage. Procedure 32–2 outlines the correct insertion, removal, and cleaning of hearing aids.

Volume control and tone can be individually adjusted for patients. Patients may require practice and many trials before an optimal setting is achieved. When hearing aids are turned on too loud, a high-pitched noise will come from the unit. Do not assume that patients whose hearing aids are in place have correct volume settings or properly functioning hearing aids.

Communicating with Hearing-impaired Patients. Hearing impaired persons benefit from sensitivity on the part of nurses and others to the consequences of hearing loss. A first and most vital consequence is the lost ability to communicate with others and to detect environmental sounds. Persons may find themselves treated as incompetent or receiving undeserving irritation from others who cannot understand them. The loss or impairment of hearing leaves people socially and environmentally deprived and at risk for injury.

Communication with patients who are hearing impaired involves approaches that reduce social and environmental sensory deprivation and enhance effective communication. The following approaches are helpful.

- Make sure your presence is known by moving into the patient's visual field as soon as possible .
- When speaking, position yourself in front of the patient so that he or she can lip read, or near the patient's good ear or hearing aid.
- Assure proper lighting so the patient can see you.
- Speak normally or in a slightly raised voice; do *not* shout.
- Speak slowly, distinctly, and evenly so your voice does not trail off at the end of sentences.
- Use longer sentences or repeat themes so the patient may understand the gist of the conversation; elements important to understanding may be missed in short phrases or may not be heard or understood.
- Listen intently and focus on the patient.
- Turn off television or radio, fan or other machinery (if possible).

PROCEDURE 32–1. EAR IRRIGATION

PURPOSE: To remove excess cerumen or foreign body.
EQUIPMENT: Ordered solution (usually 500 mL is needed), 50-mL syringe or rubber bulb syringe (some agencies use a mechanical irrigation device such as that used to clean teeth), curved (enemsis) basin, waterproof pad, towel.

ACTION 1. Review the medical order. Wash your hands. Discuss the procedure with the patient, including the usual sensations, and desired participation.

ACTION 2. Warm the ordered solution to body temperature to prevent vertigo or discomfort from cold solution stimulating the vestibular apparatus. Tap water, normal saline, or 50 percent hydrogen peroxide solution are commonly used irrigants.

ACTION 3. Request or assist the patient to a sitting position with the head tilted away from the affected ear. Protect the patient's clothing with a towel and waterproof pad. Inspect the external auditory canal with an otoscope to assess the location and amount of cerumen or foreign body and to assure that the typanic membrane is intact. Note the condition of the outer ear.

ACTION 4. Place the basin with the concave side facing the patient's cheek, directly below the ear. If the patient holds the basin tightly against the cheek, more of the return will be collected in the basin.

ACTION 5. Fill the syringe (or turn on the mechanical irrigation device). Straighten the ear canal to facilitate cleansing the entire canal: for adults, pull the pinna upward and backward; for young children, pull the pinna slightly downward.

ACTION 6. Carefully position the syringe so that the tip is directed toward the top or side of the auditory canal to prevent solution from flowing directly onto the tympanic membrane. Administer solution until foreign body is removed or until returned solution is clear. Stop if patient complains of dizziness or a sudden pain in the ear. To prevent dizziness, warm solution slightly and administer slowly. Pain suggests rupture of the tympanic membrane. Assess immediately with the otoscope. If rupture is confirmed, report this to the physician; if membrane is intact, continue with irrigation, using care to avoid irritating the membrane.

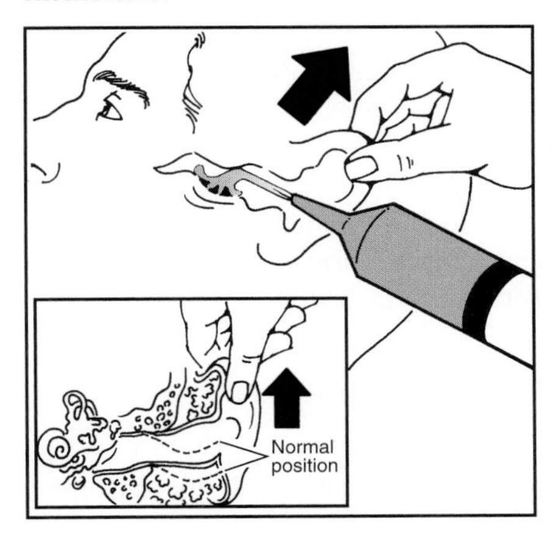

ACTION 7. Reassess external auditory canal to assure that it is clear. Dry ear, cheek, and neck. Dispose of or clean equipment according to agency policy.

Recording:
Note type and amount of solution, character of return, condition of external auditory canal and external ear before and after procedure, and patient's response to irrigation.

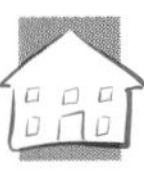

HOME HEALTH ADAPTATION: Ear irrigation adapts well to the home setting.

- Supplement conversations with nonverbal gestures, cues, and pictures.
- Write out portions of conversations, if necessary.
- Communicate with the patient by talking about the major topic first, then ask for details: "Bath time—do you want a shower or to wash up in your room?"
- Repeat phrases, when necessary, using a calm reassuring manner.
- Use different words to communicate the same idea if patient does not seem to understand.

PROCEDURE 32–2. INSERTING, REMOVING, AND CLEANING A HEARING AID

PURPOSE: To improve hearing and maintain optimal functioning of hearing aid.
EQUIPMENT: Hearing aid, soap and water, hearing aid case, towel or drying cloth, basin.

ACTION 1. Wash hands.

ACTION 2. Insertion:

a. Check the hearing aid batteries: remove hearing aid, turn volume to maximum. A continuous whistling indicates the battery is working. To replace a dead battery, place a towel over the working area. Open battery unit, replace battery, and be sure (+) and (–) signs of battery match the hearing aid.

b. Turn the volume down and the hearing aid off to prevent sudden, high-pitched sounds directed in the ear during insertion.

c. Check with the patient for proper ear location and position of hearing aid.

d. Place earmold in the external ear and gently press and rotate hearing aid into place. For behind-the-ear device, bring the connecting tubing and battery device up-over-and behind the ear; for body device, attach housing for microphone and battery pack to patient's gown.

e. Turn the hearing aid on and adjust the tone and volume to patient preference.

ACTION 3. Trouble-shooting if hearing aid does not function properly:

a. Adjust volume.

b. Check earmold for debris buildup.

c. Assess ear canal for buildup of cerumen.

d. Recheck the battery.

e. If the patient reports hearing a whistling sound, turn down the volume and check earmold placement.

ACTION 4. Removal:

a. Turn the hearing aid off and decrease the volume to prevent sudden, high-pitched sounds directed in the ear during removal.

b. Turn the earmold slightly forward and pull outward.

c. Remove batteries if hearing aid is not to be used for several days, as battery may corrode the hearing aid if left in the unit.

d. Store the hearing aid in its case to protect it from damage due to moisture, heat, or cold.

ACTION 5. Cleaning:

a. Remove the earmold from the receiver if detachable. (An earmold secured by a small metal ring or glued cannot be detached.)

b. Soak detachable earmolds in soap and water, wipe nondetachable earmold with a damp, soft cloth.

c. Wash and dry earmold.

d. Check the earmold for patency and cerumen buildup. Blow through the tube or remove wax with a pipe cleaner.

e. Do not use alcohol. It can dry and crack the plastic.

Recording:
Describe assistance and care, any difficulties experienced, corrective measures taken, and patient response.

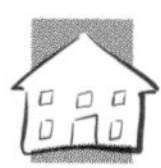

HOME HEALTH ADAPTATION: Assisting a patient with a hearing aid is the same regardless of the patient's setting.

Supporting Patients with Loss of Smell or Taste

Taste and smell promote an individual's desire to eat. To some persons foods may taste flat as a result of a loss of smell. They may subsequently lose their appetites. People with a dysfunctional sense of smell or taste are at risk of eating spoiled foods or of being malnourished.

The focus of collaboration is to assist patients in making meaningful adjustments to compensate for a temporary or permanent loss of smell. Specific approaches include the following.

- Monitor the diet to be sure patients are getting enough trace minerals, such as zinc, and adequate vitamins.
- Encourage the labeling of all foods with the type and date, as patients will be unable to smell spoiled food.
- Encourage thorough cooking of all foods.
- Emphasize having a smoke detector with active batteries for patients who have a smell alteration.

Supporting Patients with Loss of Sensation

Loss of sensation can be rapid or slow and insidious depending on its cause. Loss of sensation may result from disease of one or more peripheral nerves (peripheral neuropathy). Common causes of peripheral neuropathy include decreased circulation, deficiency of B vitamins, alcoholism, and diabetes mellitus or renal failure. Loss of all sensation occurs below the area of a severely damaged spinal cord.

Peripheral nerve degeneration begins with temporary episodes of pain, tingling, burning, prickling, or numbness in the lower extremity. Varying degrees of sensory, motor, and reflex loss typically occur in the feet before the hands and arms. As the degenerative process continues, muscle weakness, wasting, and diminished sensation occur, characterized by an ataxic (unsteady), wide-based gait. Patients may also develop foot drop and paraplegia.

Patients who experience peripheral neuropathies and loss of sensation are at risk for injury. These injuries include falls, cuts, bruises, and burns. Patients at risk should be taught to carefully bathe their feet, dry between each toe, and use talcum powder and lotions. Never use alcohol since it tends to dry skin and may result in breakdown. They should be encouraged to wear cotton socks and well-fitting shoes. A method to reduce the risk of burns is to have the patient use a bath thermometer to measure the temperature of the bath, shower, or foot tub water.

Patients should be encouraged to seek a podiatrist for removal of corns and calluses and trimming the toenails. Further, patients should be told not to perform these procedures themselves because they may cut themselves and may develop an infection.

Supporting Patients with Altered Body Image

Loss of body parts or functions or a change in body image activates a period of grief and mourning for the lost part or body image. Chapter 26 discusses nursing approaches for people who experience an alteration in body image.

Supporting Patients' Memory, Learning, and Thought

Many patients with memory loss and impaired learning and thought have problems evaluating reality. Inability to concentrate, distractibility, disordered thinking, and poor judgment are problems for these patients.

Effective communication is required in a therapeutic relationship. Nursing strategies include approaching patients in a calm manner, being an attentive listener, and recognizing one's own body position, facial gestures, and tone of voice.[20,22] Nurses should talk directly to patients and explain expectations required of them. They should *not* talk about patients in front of family members or health care personnel.

Reality orientation is essential to aid people who have memory loss or misconceptions about reality. Asking patients to state where and who they are and to identify the date and time gives information about their orientation. Patients with head injuries who are recovering from memory loss, or others experiencing memory loss from brain damage, may require reality orientation many times in one day. Cues such as family albums and favorite toys, books, clothing, and music can also provide stimuli to enhance memory. Patients may be instructed as to day and date (Fig. 32–5). This should be done in a patient, reassuring manner.

Focusing on the present is important for any patient experiencing thought alterations, such as hallucinations. Nurses should also validate meanings of conversations with patients who experience disordered or altered thinking.

Breaking tasks into small steps often aids people who experience distractibility and shortened attention span. Accomplishing small steps increases self-esteem and feelings of success along with achievement of goals.

Measures to promote safety are necessary for patients who exhibit poor judgment or an inability to reason correctly. Patients may need careful supervision to prevent accidents. Patient conversation may need to be monitored to ensure that patients are not bothering others.

Teaching must be validated. Patients should be asked to repeat material, using examples and their own words. Reading materials can be supplied to reinforce learning. It is also important to reduce pain and stress prior to teaching, as they are barriers to learning.

Supporting Patients' Speech, Language, and Communication

To work effectively with individuals experiencing impaired communication, it is important to assume a calm, reassuring, and supportive manner that conveys a sense of caring and acceptance. Adequate time must be given for patients to communicate and respond.

Supporting Patients with Expressive Aphasia. In caring for patients experiencing expressive aphasia, nurses should encourage conversation and ask open-ended questions. Allow time for patients to find the right word, disregard incorrect word choices, and encourage pointing and pantomime for self-expression. Provide pictures of common activities or objects to stimulate conversation or choice of words. Acknowledging patients' frustration lets them know their feelings are recognized. If appropriate, reassure patients that their speech will improve over time and that speech skills can be relearned.

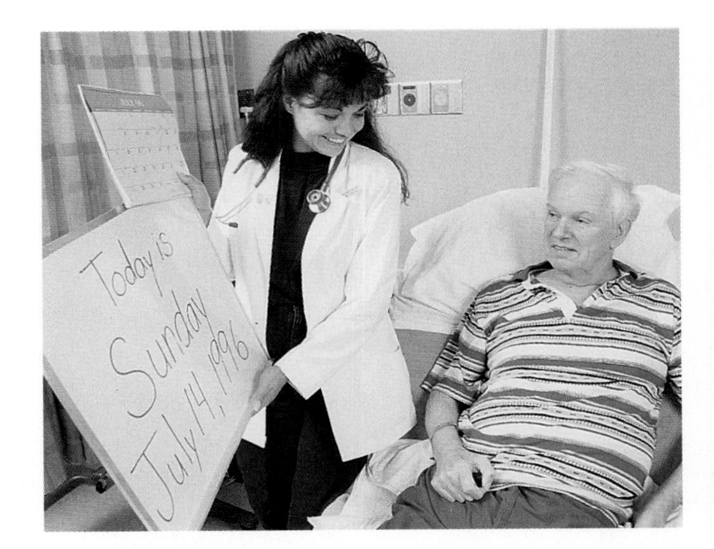

Figure 32–5. Reality orientation is essential for patients who have a memory loss, for example, following a stroke.

For patients with expressive aphasia who cannot speak at all, it is helpful to ask closed, yes-no questions. Instead of asking "How was your visit with your family?" one could ask several yes-no questions, such as "Did your family visit last night?" and "Did you enjoy seeing your family?" Yes-no questions can thus enable patients to communicate. If patients' writing ability and vision are not impaired, be sure to provide paper and pen to facilitate written communication. Pictures can also be used to convey basic requests and needs. For example, patients can point to a picture of a glass of water to indicate that they are thirsty. Another method to facilitate effective communication is through use of an alphabet board (Fig. 32–6).

Supporting Patients with Receptive Aphasia. Receptive aphasia necessitates nursing approaches that address patient comprehension problems. Patients may be unaware of a speaker's facial expressions, body position, or tone of voice. They may understand only fragments of conversation, and consequently answer inappropriately or incorrectly.

Comprehension can be facilitated by reducing environmental noise; for example, by turning off radio, television, and vibrating machines. Excessive environmental stimulation should also be eliminated. Too much clutter may be distracting to patients.

Approaching the patient slowly and speaking distinctly in short phrases facilitates comprehension. Do not shout. Use gestures, touch, and lip movements as cues in speaking. The patient's understanding of speech can be augmented by repeating and rephrasing statements calmly and without signs of irritation. To facilitate accomplishing tasks, it is essential to divide each task into small units. The patient's level of understanding and comprehension is best suited for achieving small steps.

Supporting Patients with Dysarthria. For individuals with dysarthria, the speech difficulty is motor weakness. Patients usually have unimpaired thought processes. Although therapy may not help the patient's speech, facial exercises such as pursing lips, smiling, whistling, sticking out the tongue, and grimacing can assist patients to maintain remaining muscles of speech. Reading aloud several times a day exercises muscles and encourages breath control.

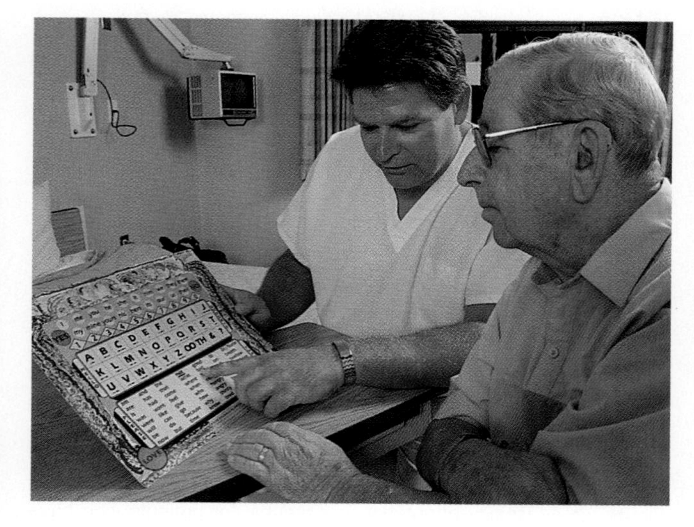

Figure 32–6. Aphasic patients may be helped to communicate by learning to use an alphabet board.

Articulation can be improved by having patients speak more slowly and exaggerate each spoken word. Encouraging patients to rephrase and shorten messages can facilitate articulation and improve communication. Use of gestures and written messages increases the likelihood that patients' communications will be understood by others. An alphabet or picture board can also facilitate communication. Patients point to letters on the board to spell a word, or point to pictures that communicate their needs.

Supporting Patients' Movement

Chapter 33 discusses specific approaches for increasing mobility with range of motion, proper positioning and body alignment, procedures for transfers, and assisting ambulation. The reader is referred to that chapter for discussion of those topics.

For many people experiencing an inability to move, the impact is devastating. Suddenly, people become dependent on others. For example, people who suffer brain damage due to a stroke may become paralyzed on one side of the body and experience an impaired ability to communicate. This translates into dependence on others. They will need help with self-care activities (brushing teeth, dressing), moving from bed to wheelchair to car, attending social activities, and exercise. The impaired ability to communicate complicates expression of needs and desires and may precipitate depression, anger, hostility, and loneliness. Rehabilitation strategies are designed to help such individuals gain independence, but this requires much effort and energy.

Special appliances or modified devices assist patients with impaired movement to carry out activities of daily living (Figs. 32–7 to 32–9). The purpose of assistive devices is to maintain or increase independent self-care and activities of daily living.

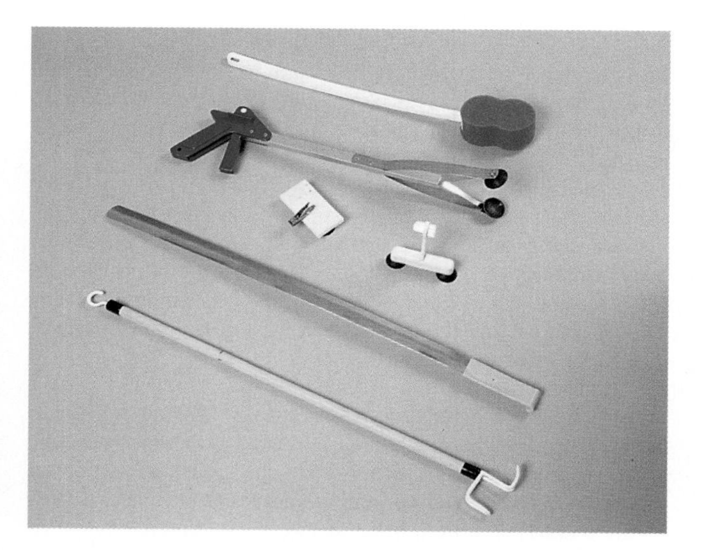

Figure 32–7. Many instruments have been devised to help disabled patients perform activities of daily living (ADLs). The assistive devices shown (beginning at the top) are a long-handled sponge, pick-up tongs, (left) stationary nail clipper, (right), stationary denture brush, long-handled shoe horn, and multipurpose dressing device that assists in pulling on pants and socks or pulling a zipper.

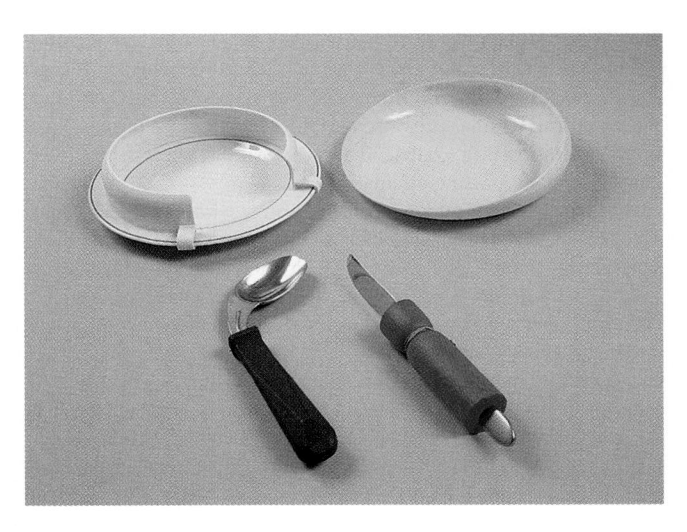

Figure 32–8. Appliances assist patients who have a neurologic/neuromuscular disorder causing weakness or a coordination deficit. These plates are constructed to make scooping food easier. Curved spoon and knife have built-up handles to help a patient grip better.

For patients with impaired hand functioning, either from a stroke (brain damage), spinal cord injury or peripheral nerve injury, the following assistive devices and measures may be helpful.

- Velcro closures can be substituted for buttons and zippers to make clothing easier to put on.
- Button hook and zipper pulls can be used for closing buttons and zippers.
- Plate guards, or metal half-circles, can be attached to plates to aid patients with impaired hand functioning. The patient uses the guard to provide an edge with which to push food onto the fork.
- Hand utensils can be built up with foam to improve the grip for persons with limited hand grasp.
- Hand straps or molds with clasps can be used to secure utensils or toothbrushes for those lacking hand grasp.
- Knives with curved blades that rock back and forth can be used to cut meat.
- Long-handled brushes or sponges are useful in washing hard-to-get body areas.
- Sophisticated equipment is continually being developed to promote independent living and occupational work for patients with neurosensory alterations. Such devices as mouth-operated wheelchairs, electric wheelchairs, and computers with laser beam pointers and correctable displays and printers offer new opportunities to enhance living.

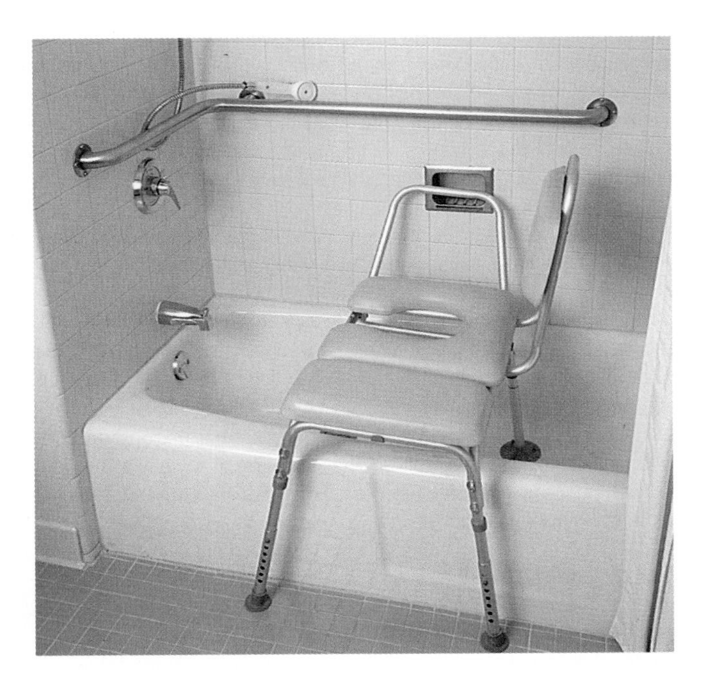

Figure 32–9. Safety bars and shower chair helps a disabled individual to bathe safely.

Activities of daily living (ADLs) become complicated for patients with mobility problems. With various modifications, nurses can assist patients to perform activities independently.

To assist with brushing teeth, a person with only one strong hand can stabilize the toothbrush on a flat surface with the affected hand while squeezing out the toothpaste with the strong hand. Independent hair combing and brushing is a straightforward procedure if the hairstyle is simple. Other hairstyles may require assistance from the nurse or significant others. Electric razors are safe for shaving and can be used by persons with only one strong hand.

A patient with only one strong hand and leg needs help dressing. When putting on a shirt, the patient should sit on the edge of the bed and spread the shirt out on the lap. Insert the weak arm into the correct armhole, pull up the sleeve and throw the garment over the back. Use the strong arm to get into the remaining sleeve. The patient should pull the pants leg over the weak foot first. The other pants leg should then be put on the strong leg as far as possible. In the standing or lying position, the pants can be pulled up over the hips and fastened.

Assistance with feeding may be required for people with weak or paralyzed upper limbs or with severe tremors.

Collaboration with occupational and physical therapists is often a component of rehabilitation of patients with impaired mobility. Nurses can facilitate rehabilitation by understanding the goals and approaches in ADL training, dressing, hygiene, and exercises offered by physical and occupational therapists.

Home Health Care

A patient's neurosensory health may be assessed in the home using indicators not present in other settings, and may be used to identify a need for supportive care. Orientation to time, for example, is easily observed in the home, reflected in whether a patient is able to keep appointments, pay bills on time, and prepare and eat meals and take medications on a regular schedule. Similarly, orientation to place is reflected in patients' ability to move purposefully from room to room in the home, while memory and recall are reflected in the ability to attend to, and perform safely, the activities of daily living. Thus, in merely observing behavior in the home, the home health nurse accumulates information helpful to assessing mental status and capacity for self-care.

To promote safety for patients with neurosensory deficits, home nurses check the patient's living area for adequate lighting and night lights. They assess the patient's need for magnifying glasses and other implements to support activities requiring close vision. They monitor and fill the patient's medication cassette—a tray with compartments for scheduled medications—to ensure the prescribed medicines are taken correctly. To prevent accidents, nurses may help patients rearrange furniture and rugs, reduce general clutter, and place personal items conveniently. Hearing loss is also common. Home nurses inspect patients' ears for ear wax, and encourage patients to use hearing aids to prevent the social isolation that may accompany hearing loss.

Cognition and memory are central to patients' capacity for independent living. Many elderly patients take numerous drugs, sometimes prescribed by more than one physician. Some drugs, particularly when taken in incompatible combinations, cause or contribute to mental confusion. Home health nurses must be careful to review the patient's entire prescription list. The objective is to determine whether all of the drugs are indicated by the patient's current condition, or whether some could be eliminated with a physician's order.

Home nurses are particularly interested in elderly patients' cognitive capacity. Patients unable to remember that something is cooking on the stove, for example, are at risk for serious accidents. It is not surprising, then, that confusion and loss of memory are common reasons why elderly patients are institutionalized, particularly after an acute illness that temporarily impairs their mental status. Professionals caring for such patients in the hospital may underestimate their capacity for recovery and independent living. Home nurses who see patients before they become acutely ill have an advantage in making an accurate assessment, and can assist members of the interdisciplinary team to appropriately evaluate the patient's need for long-term institutionalization.

RESTORATIVE CARE

Restorative care focuses on several acute disturbances in neurosensory dysfunction that are most often related to consciousness, movement, and pain. Patients who require nursing approaches that focus on physiologic restoration are comatose patients, patients experiencing seizures, patients with sensory overload or sensory deprivation, and patients with severe pain.

Caring for Comatose Patients

Care of comatose patients is a challenge because they are completely dependent on nurses for all of their care. Prioritization of patient needs is essential, and the first priority is oxygenation.

The brain is highly dependent on oxygen. Proper oxygenation is important to cerebral function, prevention of increased intracranial pressure, and tissue healing. Assuring that the patient's airway is clear is essential. Proper use of oxygen support devices, whether nasal cannulas, masks, or ventilators, assists in meeting the oxygen requirements. Suctioning may be necessary to clear obstructed airways of sputum and other secretions and allow proper oxygenated air flow. Maintaining proper head position is important so that airways do not become obstructed. Turning patients from side-to-side allows for lung expansion and for settled lung secretions to be dislodged (see Chap. 30 for more on supporting and restoring the oxygenation function).

Perfusion must be monitored through measurement of vital signs or blood gases per physician's order. Patients may be attached to a cardiac (ECG) monitor to monitor cardiac rhythm.

Fluid status must be carefully managed in comatose patients, who may require supplemental IV fluids and electrolytes. Nurses must carefully infuse IV fluids per physician's order to prevent increased intracranial pressure and at the same time provide adequate hydration (see Chaps. 30 and 34 for more on restoring fluid balance and supporting circulation).

Monitoring of comatose patients is essential, as their status can change quickly. Assessment of vital signs and neurochecks may range from every 15 minutes, if the patient is unstable, to every 2 to 4 hours, for a stabilized (noncritical) patient. Refer to Section 2 of this chapter for additional information on vital signs and neurochecks.

Nutrition for comatose patients is one of the greatest challenges for health care providers. A nasogastric or feeding tube may be inserted in order to give liquid supplemental feedings (see Chap. 28). Adequate nutrition is essential for recovery of any patient. Supplemental liquid feedings provide the nutrition and calories necessary for patient needs. If not contraindicated, a high-vitamin, high-protein feeding with 2300 to 3100 calories is recommended for an adult. Patients with severe head trauma can require 4000 to 5000 calories per day. For patients receiving liquid feeding, it is important to note the character and consistency of stools. Diarrhea is a frequent problem, and may indicate a need for a change in the formula of liquid nutrition used. Patients receiving supplemental tube feedings may also require supplemental water feedings to assure proper hydration. Nutritionists should be consulted for assessment of nutritional needs and problems associated with feedings. The reader is referred to Chap. 28 for discussion of nutrition.

Activities of daily living need to be performed for the patient. Nurses should discuss with the family the patient's pre-illness schedule and preferences. This information can be adapted for inclusion in the patient care plan, if feasible.

Hygiene measures include daily bathing and hair washing as appropriate. Mouth care is needed at least every 4 hours. This includes applying petroleum jelly to the lips to avoid drying and cracking. Hair should be combed every shift, if possible, and at least daily. Long hair can be braided. Range-of-motion can be performed conveniently during the bath.

Skin and tissue care is an important part of the hygiene routine and should be performed every 2 to 4 hours (Chap. 27) with vital sign checks.

Bowel and bladder regimens need to be initiated and maintained to promote adequate functioning and prevent complications. Most comatose patients have a Foley catheter in place. Proper cleansing around the meatus aids in prevention of infection (see Chap. 29). Urine output and the nature and color of urine should be monitored, and any cloudiness, blood, or infectious material reported.

To maintain bowel evacuation, patients may require daily or every-other-day suppositories. It is important to assess for and prevent stool impactions. Chapter 29 provides additional information on bowel and bladder management.

Safety. Comatose patients must be protected against injury. If a patient has seizures, the siderails should be padded and kept up at all times. Immobility and its complications, such as contractures, skin breakdown, and decubitus ulcers, require attention. Contractures, such as wrist drop and foot drop, can be prevented with range-of-motion exercises, proper positioning, and appropriate use of splints (refer to Chap. 33 for additional information).

Stimulation. Communication is an area of special need. While patients are comatose, it is important to talk to them while performing care. Many times these patients are aware of their surroundings and can hear but not respond. Nurses, physicians, and other health care personnel should refrain from talking at the bedside. Touching and stroking patients during care, and encouraging family members to do so as well, promotes communication and provides stimulation for the patient.

During the day, appropriate stimulation, such as tuning the radio to the patient's favorite station, or setting the television to a favorite program, are ways to provide stimulation. Family members can relate the day's events, tell the patient about friends and family members, and read stories.

At night, nurses should dim lights and coordinate nursing activities to promote a somewhat normal daily body rhythm, and to promote sleep.

Environmental Considerations. Many patients with altered consciousness are placed in an intensive care unit. Equipment is noisy and can fill the patient's immediate environment with meaningless stimuli that can contribute to sensory overload or deprivation.

The patient's dignity and humanity should be maintained by providing privacy when giving care, administering medications, and performing invasive techniques. If patients recover from the comatose state, it will become very important to reorient them to person, place, and time, and to help them understand what has happened.

Caring for Patients with Seizures

Patients who are comatose, who have brain injury or brain tumors, or who have internal excitability of brain cells may develop seizures. Seizures are the sudden discharge of electrical activity in brain cells (see Table 32–5). Those that last several minutes can be potentially life-threatening; however, most seizures last a few seconds up to a few minutes. Memory function is affected by seizures.

Nursing management of patients experiencing seizures is an advanced skill and is directed toward accurate data gathering based on observation, protecting the patient from injury during a seizure, and employing seizure precautions. Key points of observation and management during a seizure are included in Clinical Guideline 32–4. Seizure precautions are as follows:

- Padded siderails are kept in the up position to protect patient from injury.
- An artificial airway is available at the head of bed, however, it is never inserted if the jaw is clenched.
- Suction is available at the bedside in the event patient chokes or airway becomes blocked.
- Beds are kept in low position for patient safety.
- Patients may be required to wear protective headgear or helmets for uncontrolled seizures.
- Supervised ambulation may be required to prevent falls.

Priorities during a seizure include ensuring a patent airway, staying with the patient, calling for help, protecting the patient's head and arms and providing safety, and careful observation.

CLINICAL GUIDELINE 32–4

NURSING OBSERVATIONS AND MANAGEMENT DURING SEIZURE

OBSERVATIONS

1. Determine whether there were any warning signs or an aura.
2. Assess where the seizure began and how it proceeded.
3. Note the type of body movements and what parts of the body were involved.
4. Note any changes in the size of pupils.
5. Assess for urinary and bowel incontinence.
6. Determine the duration of the seizure and phases, if any.
7. Assess patient consciousness level throughout the seizure.
8. Describe the behavior of the patient after the seizure.
9. Note any weakness or paralysis of extremities after the seizure.
10. Note lethargy and amount of sleep required after the seizure.

MANAGEMENT

1. If the patient is in a chair at the onset of a seizure, ease to the floor.
2. Provide for privacy by pulling curtains or closing doors. Encourage onlookers to leave if there are no privacy measures.
3. Maintain a patent airway to ensure adequate ventilation. Constrictive clothing around the neck should be loosened.
4. Guide the patient's movements so that the head or extremities do not bang against hard surfaces.
5. Always stay with the patient during a seizure. Observation and prevention of injury cannot occur if the nurse is looking for help.
6. Turn the patient on one side to allow for drainage of secretions.
7. Offer the patient the option to sleep after a seizure.

It is important to obtain any history of seizures during the neurosensory assessment. Patients who suffer head trauma may not have a seizure at the time of injury. Years later, however, seizures can develop spontaneously. Being alert to past traumatic events to the head and to the presenting diagnosis of patients, and carefully assessing for seizures when taking the patient's history will identify those at risk for seizures.

Caring for Patients with Sensory Deprivation or Sensory Overload

Sensory deprivation may occur in patients with brain damage or conditions that decrease input through the senses (blindness, deafness), in patients with spinal cord injury (loss of touch), and in aphasic patients who experience altered reception or expression of language and, occasionally, decreased sensation and movement in one half of the body. Patients who suffer from severe pain may be vulnerable to sensory overload. It is also common in patients in an intensive care unit, and in patients who cannot process incoming stimuli at their previous speed. An unfamiliar environment with many machines and other stimuli enhances sensory overload. Informing patients and significant others of the deprivation or overload state can facilitate their interaction with others and generate other ideas for stimulation.[7]

COLLABORATIVE STRATEGY

SENSORY OVERLOAD AND SENSORY DEPRIVATION

Sensory input is necessary for healthy functioning of neurosensory mechanisms. However, both excessive sensory input (sensory overload) and deficit sensory input (sensory deficit) contribute to altered neurosensory functioning and stress. Individuals vary in their capacity to handle sensory input. What may be stressful to some may be pleasant to others. Nurse–patient collaboration is necessary to determine the optimal amount of sensory input—visual, auditory, tactile, olfactory, and gustatory—for individual well-being.

Nursing Approaches for Patients with Sensory Deprivation. Use visual stimuli such as pictures, calendars, or posters and auditory stimuli such as talking with the patient and playing music, radio, or television. Tactile stimulation is important, and may include the use of touch, back rubs or hand-holding. Social stimulation—encouraging visitors, sitting with patients, or encouraging group activities—is also beneficial.[23] Environmental stimulation includes providing proper lighting for reading or opening or closing of drapes.

Nursing Approaches for Patients with Sensory Overload. Reducing stimuli to eliminate overload involves shutting off nonessential lights, alarms and other equipment, using earplugs, avoiding loud noises, and encouraging personnel to hold conversations away from the patient's room. Promoting movement (turning, chair activity, and ambulation) and providing reorientation also reduces sensory overload.

Planning rest periods and providing privacy reduce excess stimuli. Excessive activities should be eliminated.[24] Grouping procedures and care activities reduces the continuous incoming pattern stimuli or interruptions. Orientation to daily activities and schedules of care or treatment assists patients in realistic expectations of their daily routine.

Caring for Patients with Pain

The Pain Continuum. The continuum of pain refers to the pain experience which begins with a mild sensation of acute discomfort in response to an irritating stimulus. Mild pain may progress to moderate or severe acute pain depending on the cause. If nothing is done to alleviate acute pain, chronic pain may ensue. Chronic pain, unlike acute pain which acts as a protective mechanism for the body, serves no protective purpose. Cancer pain may have elements of acute and chronic pain.

Types of Pain. Physiologically, pain is classified as fast or slow, according to the speed with which the pain fibers stimulated conduct pain impulses.[25] Fast pain, conducted by the A fibers, is felt 0.1 second after a pain stimulus is applied, and is usually described as a sharp, prickling, or electric sensation. It originates superficially in the skin, is felt when a knife cuts the skin or when the skin is burned or subjected to an electric shock. Slow pain, conducted by the C fibers, begins more than a second after the application of a stimulus, and increases over several seconds or minutes. Slow pain is often described as burning, aching, throbbing, or nauseous pain and may be chronic. The reader is referred to a textbook of physiology for a detailed discussion of the nerve pathways for pain reception.

Pain Stimuli. Pain, as previously indicated, is elicited by many types of stimuli: mechanical, chemical, and thermal. Mechanical and thermal stimuli usually elicit fast pain, but can also elicit slow pain in some situations. Chemical stimuli are especially important in causing the pain that accompanies deep tissue injury. Deep tissue pain may be caused by a loss of blood flow, referred to as tissue ischemia. Such pain results from an accumulation of lactic acid and other pain-causing substances in the tissue. It may also be caused by muscle spasm. In muscle spasm, the contracting muscles directly activate pain receptors and may also compress blood vessels in the tissue, leading to tissue ischemia.[25]

Monitoring Pain. The nursing assessments for acute and chronic pain are somewhat different. Individuals with mild to moderate acute pain will generally manifest their discomfort by withdrawing from the pain stimulus and may show a facial expression and body posture that express distress. Patients may also report the presence of pain but show few other signs. Severe acute pain, on the other hand, is manifested by grimacing, muscle tension, reduced activity, or movement patterns. Patients often protect the painful area by assuming a fixed posture. This is known as splinting.

Severe acute pain is a stressful experience that alters the body's homeostatic balance. As mentioned previously, it is associated with the activation of the sympathetic branch of the autonomic nervous system. Thus, the patient may show an increased heart and respiratory rate, breathing may be shallow, and blood pressure may be elevated; the patient may have dilated pupils, become pale, sweat profusely, and sometimes vomit. When the pain is alleviated, there is a return to baseline vital sign measurements as sympathetic activity decreases.

Pain and emotion are closely linked. Thus, patients in pain may cry out, moan, or communicate frustration, and may sometimes lash out in an angry manner. Furthermore, patients in severe acute pain are understandably anxious about the cause of their pain and what can be done to alleviate it.

Individuals with chronic pain, on the other hand, may show a similar clinical picture but more often become conditioned to pain. A return of parasympathetic tone allows them to maintain their usual heart rate and blood pressure. Chronic severe pain, often demoralizing, is manifested by habit changes made to accommodate pain, by loss of appetite and weight loss, and by mental depression and an apathy apparent in patients' loss of interest in their usual activities.

When assessing pain initially or monitoring its progress after pain treatment is begun, it is important to take a thorough history of the current pain episode as described earlier. Changes in pain pattern or new pain should not be attributed to previous causes and should trigger a thorough evaluation. To reiterate, the nurse should question patients about the location, quality, severity, and duration of their pain, about other related symptoms, and about what they have done to alleviate the pain. Nurses should ask patients with pain about how changes in their activity or habits affected their pain. Such questions provide the data needed to evaluate the cause and severity of the patient's pain. It is also important to ask patients to describe their pain and to document the words they use. Does the patient indicate the pain is "sharp,"

INSIGHTS FROM NURSING LITERATURE

PAIN IN OLDER ADULTS

Forrest J. Assessment of acute and chronic pain in older adults. J Gerontol Nurs. *1995;21:15–19.*

The author's review of the literature showed pain, which is two times more likely among people 60 years of age and older, is not a normal part of the aging process. Furthermore, numerous factors make pain in elders difficult to assess. For example, some elders believe pain is a natural aspect of aging, and fail to report it. Furthermore, visual, hearing, speech, or cognitive difficulty may also impair elders' ability to report pain. The author notes that undetected, poorly relieved pain is linked to depression, diminished quality of life, and family distress. Acute pain behavior includes verbal complaints, grimacing, moans, pupillary changes, diaphoresis, and posturing; however, chronic pain may not be accompanied by these signs. Other behavior changes—such as when the cognitively impaired elder becomes more withdrawn or combative—may signal pain. In addition, the elder with chronic pain may be less active, sleep more, appear stoic, or act confused.

"stabbing," "dull," "aching," "burning," "prickling," or "tingling"? Documenting these words helps other members of the interdisciplinary team better understand the nature of the patient's pain.

Planning Pain Implementations. Nurses caring for patients with mild to moderate pain usually have a variety of pain relief modalities from which to choose. Making an appropriate selection involves identifying the cause of the patient's pain and, if possible, removing it. For example, superficial skin pain may be caused simply by lying too long in a fixed position and may be alleviated by turning the patient in bed. Pain aggravated by environmental stressors may be alleviated by removing those stressors.

Identifying the cause of the patient's pain demands patient involvement. Patient collaboration is therefore an important first step in planning for pain alleviation. The nurse's primary objective is to provide comfort. To do that the nurse must understand what comfort means to the patient. Inviting the patient's participation in the planning process increases the likelihood that the approaches selected will be successful and helps patients to feel more in control of the situation. Approaches for helping patients with mild to moderate pain are discussed below.

In contrast to moderate pain, which may be simply resolved, planning to alleviate severe pain is often a complex matter and involves an interdisciplinary process. Input comes not only from nurse, physician, and patient, as is typical when pain is mild or moderate in intensity, but may also involve pharmacist, physical and occupational therapists, social worker, and the chaplain.

Management techniques for mild, moderate, and severe pain include support and comfort measures and noninvasive pain alleviation approaches such as massage, relaxation therapy, heat and cold therapy, music therapy, and medication.

Choosing the Method. In choosing techniques, nurses consider many factors, most importantly, the patient's pain intensity, the measures that have proved to alleviate the patient's pain in the past, and the patient's preferences. In general, nurses aim to provide pain relief that

- alleviates the patient's discomfort and distress
- protects the patient's lifestyle and enhances the patient's quality of life as he or she defines it
- does not sedate the patient unnecessarily
- produces a level of comfort sufficient to promote willingness to ambulate at the earliest possible point in his or her recovery from illness, trauma, or surgery, thus enhancing respiratory function and preventing complications of bedrest
- improves the patient's functional capacity

Assisting Patients with Mild to Moderate Pain. Several methods may be used to alleviate moderate pain. These include supportive approaches, noninvasive pain-relief measures, and medications, which may also be employed in conjunction with other measures.

SUPPORTIVE APPROACHES. Sociocultural beliefs, childhood experiences, and misconceptions may influence the meaning individuals place on pain. It is important for nurses to determine factors influencing the pain experience. Those that may augment or worsen the pain experience for a patient include the disbelief of others, fatigue, fear, knowledge of the event, misconceptions, and monotony.

- *Others' disbelief.* Individuals in pain may be frustrated or angered when others fail to acknowledge their pain. It is important, therefore, for nurses and others to acknowledge, with the patient, the presence of pain, and to be responsive to a patient's descriptions of pain. Family members or significant others may question the patient's pain. While it is important to listen to the family's concerns, it is most important to support the patient. The following approaches may be helpful in alleviating the factor of disbelief and help patients understand that nurses are interested and concerned about their pain.
  - Acknowledge the pain to the patient. Effective approaches are, "Tell me about your pain." "You mentioned you had a headache. Could you specifically describe it for me?" "How are you handling this pain you have just described?"
  - Listen responsively to patient statements about pain.
  - Respond to patient's other needs. Provide a quiet environment for rest or offer distractions, such as television, games, and books.

  Approaches that may be useful with family members or significant others include the following.
  - Relate to the family that pain is a subjective, individual experience of human beings.
  - Provide opportunities for family members to share their concerns privately.
- *Fatigue.* Fatigue influences patients' perceptions of pain. Individuals who are overly tired focus on the self. Consequently, patients focus on the pain experience. Providing adequate rest, assessing sleep patterns for adequate intervals of sleep, and evaluating with patient and physician the need for nocturnal sleep medications are important approaches. It is important for patients to understand that pain itself can cause fatigue. Fatigue, in turn, may heighten the perception of pain.

- *Fear.* Suffering may influence the amount of pain perceived. Fear increases apprehension and physical tension, thereby increasing pain and anxiety, which further increases fear. A vicious cycle thus becomes established.

  Fear, as experienced by the patient, needs to be explored. Fear of addiction to pain medication, fear of constant pain, and fear of revealing one's anxieties to others are examples of different kinds of fears that may contribute to a patient's pain experience.

  In providing care, the nurse should observe the following guidelines.
  - Discuss the pain experience and what it means for the patient.
  - Share with the patient the various methods for handling pain.
  - Reassure the patient that everything possible will be done to alleviate or reduce the pain.
  - Educate the patient about addiction to drugs.
  - Tell the patient to request pain medication before the pain becomes too intense.
  - Protect the patient from other discomfort. Therapy should not cause more distress than the pain itself.
- *Pain understanding.* The patient's knowledge of the painful event will contribute to how he or she responds to pain. Nursing approaches to address this factor include the following.
  - Inform the patient about the source of the pain.
  - Teach the patient about pain medication.
  - Use measures the patient believes are effective.
  - Invite the patient to participate in pain relief planning.
  - Use pain relief measures appropriate to the patient's pain intensity.
  - If therapy is ineffective at first, encourage the patient to try it again before abandoning the therapy.
- *Misconceptions.* Misconceptions about pain and its cause may intensify the pain experience, for example, as when patients incorrectly relate their pain to other events. To avoid misconceptions, nurses should carefully explain that pain is a very individual experience. Exploring with the patient why pain intensifies or occurs at certain times of the day can help nurses identify the patient's misconceptions about pain. For example, a patient whose pain intensifies upon returning home from work may attribute the pain to the car ride home when, in fact, the pain intensifies as a result of fatigue.
- *Monotony.* Monotony intensifies the pain experience because the individual's focus of attention is on the pain. Therefore, distractions, which draw attention to an alternative focus, are often effective in minimizing pain.

NONINVASIVE PAIN–ALLEVIATING APPROACHES. Noninvasive approaches are often helpful in preventing mild to moderate pain from becoming severe.

- *Transcutaneous Electric Nerve Stimulation.* Transcutaneous electric nerve stimulation (TENS) is used during and after painful procedures, such as dressing changes and to control post-operative pain. Research shows that TENS works nicely as an adjunct with other forms of analgesia, but is only 20 percent effective in providing analgesia when used alone. The TENS unit is a battery-powered device that transmits a low-voltage electrical impulse to the body through electrodes attached to the skin. The exact mechanism of pain relief is not known, but it is hypothesized that electrical stimulation of large nerve fibers serves to "close the gate" to painful stimuli. Another theory is that nerve stimulation triggers the release of endorphins, causing the transmission of noxious stimuli to be inhibited. Elderly patients are good candidates for TENS. Individuals who are not candidates include those who have a cardiac pacemaker, especially the demand type, because the electrical impulse for the TENS unit may interfere with pacing. In addition, TENS should not be used for pregnant women during the first trimester. The primary adverse effect of TENS is skin irritation. The TENS unit impulses should begin low and be adjusted to slowly increase.[26]

  Vibration is effective in relieving headache pain, muscle aches or spasms, itch, rheumatoid arthritis pain, phantom limb pain, or as a substitute for TENS.
- *Heat.* Heat therapy is a form of cutaneous stimulation. Heat has been employed historically to relieve aches and pains. Heat has many physiologic effects, such as vasodilation and increased metabolic activity in tissue and cells. Heat therapy can improve oxygen transport and blood flow to tissues. This also allows for metabolic end products to be transported away from injured tissue, accelerating the inflammatory response. Heat relieves pain by raising the pain threshold and promotes joint mobility by decreasing stiffness.

  Heat therapy must be used judiciously, because extremes of temperature can cause burns and expose patients to risk of tissue injury. Dry or moist heat may be used. Both require careful monitoring. Heat applications increase circulation to a local area, decrease pain, increase warmth, and aid removal of infectious material.

  Aquathermic pads are a source of dry heat and, when used with warm, moist compresses, the aquathermic pad and moist compress together provide moist heat. Procedure 32–3 discusses the application of an aquathermic pad (see Chap. 27 for guidelines on the application of moist heat compresses).

  Another form of heat therapy is the sitz bath, commonly used for persons with hemorrhoids and for women following pelvic surgery or vaginal deliveries. This method promotes healing, pain relief and comfort, relaxation, and hygiene.
- *Cold.* Cold therapy also produces cutaneous stimulation. Cold therapy is used to reduce inflammation and swelling and effectively alleviates pain. Types of cold application include ice massage, aerosol sprays, cold soaks or compresses, ice bag or collar, ice glove, cold pack, (Fig. 32-10) cooling sponge bath, and hypothermia blankets. Procedure 32–4 provides guidelines for application of ice packs.

  Cold therapy is effective because of its vasoconstrictive effect. Vasoconstriction reduces blood flow to an injured or painful area. Decreased blood flow reduces inflammation and swelling, a local anesthetic effect. As cold therapy decreases tissue temperature, cell metabolism and need for oxygen and nutrients is reduced as well.

  When applying cold therapy, it is important to remember three points.
  1. Skin temperatures fall quickly. Subcutaneous tissue and muscle cool more slowly, depending on the amount of fatty subcutaneous tissue. Direct application of cold applications for 2 to 3 minutes causes frostbite of the skin, although underlying cutaneous layers are not yet cooled. Thus, direct cold therapy must be applied for a period of 15–30 minutes,

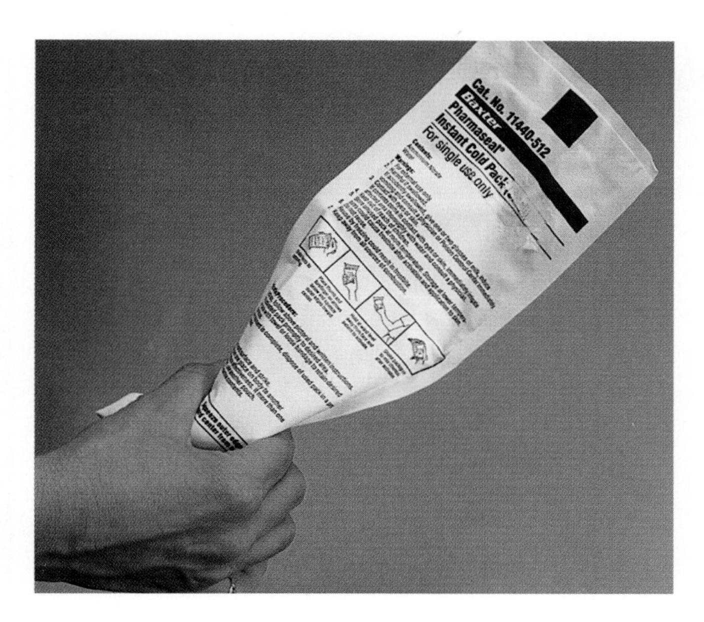

Figure 32-10. A commercially packaged, single-use ice pack. Directions for use of commercially prepared products are outlined on package and should be followed closely. *(From Smith S, Duell D. Clinical Nursing Skills: Nursing Process Model; Basic to Advanced Skills. 4th ed. Norwalk, CT: Appleton & Lange; 1996:649.)*

removed, and reapplied to produce effective results without danger of frostbite. (Frostbitten skin appears white, pale, blue, and mottled, is pulseless, and feels firm to the touch.)

2. When applying cold therapy to the skin, using a towel or flannel cloth provides an insulating layer between the skin and the source of cold. The insulating layer absorbs moisture and slows the effects of frostbite, enabling the cold to penetrate more deeply into the tissue.
3. Knowledge of the stages of sensation experienced with cold therapy is necessary to properly evaluate patient responses. Nurses should explain the effects of the different stages of cold therapy to patients before initiating treatment and assure them that the period of discomfort is short. The initial stage occurs within 1 to 3 minutes of application; cold may feel uncomfortable. Stage 2 occurs within 2 to 5 minutes following application; a sense of burning and aching occurs. Stage 3 occurs 5 to 12 minutes following application; local numbness occurs with decreased pain. Stage 4 occurs 12 to 15 minutes following application; changes occur in deep tissue, including alternating vasodilation and increased metabolism.

- *External analgesic medication.* External analgesic medications are topically applied substances containing menthol, which acts as a counterirritant. Their mechanism of action is to create a sensation of coolness or warmth on the skin, which serves to relieve the pain or draw attention away from the pain.

  Menthol preparations are nonprescription, over-the-counter gels or lotions used for muscle, joint, and tendon aches, sports injuries, and neck and shoulder pain. Menthol products provide continuous stimulation to the site of application but are contraindicated for use on open wounds, mucous membranes, and painful or uncomfortable skin areas. If menthol increases pain, it should be discontinued.
- *Relaxation.* Relaxation is another category of noninvasive pain relief. Relaxation can be defined as the state in which an individual has reduced anxiety and skeletal muscle tension, thereby interrupting the spiral of pain, anxiety, and muscle tension. The body responds physiologically by decreasing blood pressure; respiratory rate, and heart rate; decreasing muscle tension; and decreasing oxygen consumption of the tissues.

  Relaxation techniques stimulate the body's natural pain suppression system, consisting of the endogenous opiates that protect the body against the harmful effects of painful stress. Two endogenous opiates—the enkephalins and the endorphins—are involved. The enkephalins, the endogenous opiates released in the spinal cord, and the endorphins, the endogenous opiates released in the brain and central nervous system, are enhanced by relaxation techniques and massage.

  Relaxation techniques include meditation, progressive relaxation, biofeedback, yoga, and hypnosis. Most relaxation strategies necessitate a quiet environment, a comfortable position, a passive attitude, and a mental device or focus of concentration. The reader is referred to Clinical Guideline 25–2 for details on methods of relaxation.
- *Distraction.* Another category of noninvasive pain relief is distraction. Distraction can be simply defined as focusing on a source of attention other than pain. Although distraction cannot make the pain go away, it takes the patient's attention away from the pain. Benefits include (1) increased pain tolerance, making pain more bearable; (2) offering patients a "sense of control" over pain; (3) improved affect or mood; (4) decreased intensity or quality of pain; and (5) enhancing rest.

  Music therapy is one method of distraction. The purpose of music therapy is to reduce anxiety thereby reducing the patient's perception of pain. Any portable player for tape cassettes or CDs that is equipped with earphones can be used for music therapy. (Fig. 32–11) Tapes may contain soothing music or the patient's favorite music.

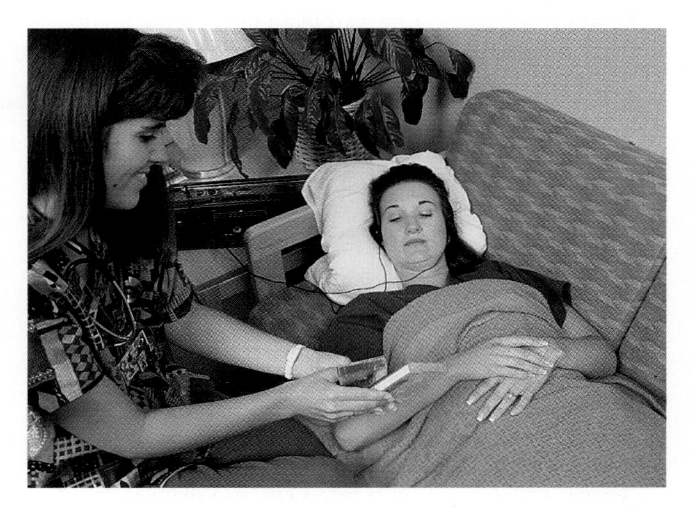

Figure 32–11. Music is a pleasant distraction for patients in the hospital or at home.

PROCEDURE 32–3. AQUATHERMIC PAD APPLICATION

PURPOSE: Application of dry or moist heat to reduce muscle spasm, provide comfort to painful tissue, and reduce or eliminate localized areas of inflammation and swelling.

EQUIPMENT: Aquathermic pad (also called Aqua K-Pad) and control unit, moisture barrier—waterproof disposable pad, plastic (Saran wrap), tape, Kerlex, gauze, petroleum jelly (for moist heat), normal saline, bath thermometer.

ACTION 1. Check physician's order for type of application, area to be treated, and length of time of treatment.

ACTION 2. Assess condition of the skin over which pad is to be applied (aquathermic pads are rarely applied to open wounds); level of discomfort of area receiving aquathermic pad treatment; and sensitivity to temperature, pain, and light touch.

ACTION 3. Prepare equipment and supplies:

a. Check the control unit. Temperature setting should be between 40.5° and 43°C (105° and 115°F).

b. Check the reservoir to see that it is two thirds full of water. Use only distilled water to refill.

c. Connect the waterproof plastic pad with (attached) two hoses to the control unit.

ACTION 4. Discuss the procedure and goals for treatment with the patient, including nurse's action and behavior desired of patient. Explain anticipated sensations and those to be reported.

ACTION 5. Application:

a. Provide privacy and position patient comfortably.

b. For dry heat, cover the plastic pad with a pillowcase or soft covering, then apply to the body part and secure with tape, gauze, or ties. (Do not use pins.)

c. For moist heat:

- Apply a thin layer of petroleum jelly on the body part to protect the skin.
- Moisten gauze, washcloth, or towel, wring out, and apply to affected area.
- Cover with Saran wrap, then apply and secure.

d. Monitor:

- Temperature of aquathermic pad.
- Skin condition.
- Time elapsed in treatment.

e. Discuss importance of calling nurse if pad becomes too warm, cools off, or creates other discomfort, rather than removing pad.

ACTION 6. Evaluation:

a. Evaluate color, temperature, and intactness of skin exposed to aquathermic pad treatment.

b. Assess pain relief or level of discomfort.

Recording:
Identify site of application. Describe temperature setting; duration of therapy; patient's responses; skin condition; evaluation of relief provided; problems, if any, and action taken.

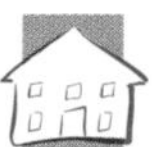

Home Health Adaptation: Inform patients, especially the elderly or those with neurologic deficits, and family members, of safety precautions needed to avoid burns when using a aquathermic pad independently.

Although it may provide some distraction, placing a radio beside a patient's bed is not music therapy. Nurses must assess the type and kind of music to be used, its particular effects, when to use it, and for how long.

To be effective, the distraction technique should have the following characteristics.

- Is interesting to the patient.
- Is consistent with patient's energy level and ability to concentrate.
- Uses and emphasizes rhythm; for example, keeping time to music.
- Stimulates the major sensory modalities: hearing, vision, touch, and movement.
- Provides a change in stimuli when the pain changes; for example, stimulus can be increased when pain increases.

- *Guided imagery.* Guided imagery is a specific distraction technique. It involves the structured use of the imagination and mental images to reduce pain. As persons engage in pleasant mental images, the images are stimuli to the autonomic nervous system and replace painful stimuli. Pleasant mental imagery activates calming responses of the autonomic nervous system. A well-chosen image supersedes the effects of painful stimula-

PROCEDURE 32–4. COLD APPLICATION

PURPOSE: To decrease pain, reduce inflammation and edema.
EQUIPMENT: Ice, ice bag, ice collar, disposable glove, or chemical cold generation pack; disposable waterproof underpad; bath towels or washcloth.

ACTION 1. Check physician's order for type and length of treatment. If not specified, cold treatments are applied for 20–30 minutes. If used to treat an injury, cold is effective for the first 24–36 hours postinjury.

ACTION 2. Assess:

- Condition of the skin at site of application.
- Level of discomfort at site of application.
- Sensitivity to temperature, pain, and light touch. To avoid frostbite injury, do not apply cold to an area of diminished sensitivity.

ACTION 3. Discuss procedure with the patient, including expected sensations, desired patient participation, and sensations to be reported to nurse.

ACTION 4. Prepare and apply ice:

- Fill ice bag, collar, or glove two thirds full of chipped ice.
- Remove excess air to promote bag comforming to body contours and reduce interference to conduction of cold.
- Ask or assist patient to assume a comfortable position.
- Apply a layer of cloth (towel or washcloth) over site of application to reduce risk of skin injury.
- Apply ice, shaping for close contact with affected part.
- For chemical cold generation pack, squeeze to activate; then apply as above.
- Hold ice application in place with towels or pillowcase; tape as needed.
- Place waterproof disposable underpad under part being treated.

ACTION 5. Monitor affected part in 10 minutes for color, temperature, and sensation. Skin should be cool and slightly pale with reduced sensitivity to touch. Redness indicates reflex vasodilation; lack of sensation and whiteness indicate frostbite. If no negative effects noted, leave ice in place 20–30 minutes. May be reapplied 30 minutes later.

ACTION 6. Evaluate effectiveness of therapy: assess comfort, swelling, and skin condition.

Recording:
Identify site of application. Describe site condition before and after treatment; patient response; degree of relief obtained; problems, if any, and action taken.

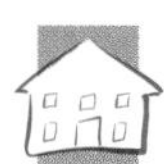

HOME HEALTH ADAPTATION: Teach patient and family members frequency, duration, and safety precautions of cold application therapy.

tions, which cause increased heart rate, increased blood pressure, increased respiratory rate and cool skin. Guided imagery techniques are presented in Clinical Guideline 25–2.

MEDICATION FOR MILD AND MODERATE PAIN. Relief of mild to moderate pain, using drugs, focuses on nonnarcotic analgesics. Nonnarcotic analgesics include over-the-counter (OTC) drugs referred to as nonsteroidal antiinflammatory drugs (NSAIDs). The three main characteristics of nonnarcotic analgesics are antiinflammatory, analgesic, and antipyretic properties. An antiinflammatory drug is one that counteracts or reduces inflammation; an analgesic is a drug that reduces pain perception; and an antipyretic is one that reduces fever. Aspirin (ASA) and salicylic derivatives such as acetaminophen (Tylenol) and ibuprofen (Advil, Nuprin) are OTC drugs used in treatment of mild to moderate pain. Their effectiveness is enhanced when they are administered before pain becomes severe.

When an individual has a cut through the skin, the chemical prostaglandin is released. Prostaglandin is the precursor to the painful impulse; it sends the message of pain to the spinal cord, where a neurotransmitter, substance P, transmits the message on to the brain. NSAIDs inhibit the synthesis of prostaglandins, thereby breaking the pain pathway at the peripheral nerve site. Patients describe the pain that best responds to NSAIDs as "sharp, stabbing." The pain is usually localized and the patient can point to where it hurts. NSAIDs play an important part in breaking the pain cycle and should be considered in planning pain intervention.

Indications for the use of NSAIDs include pain of peripheral origin such as low back pain, ordinary headaches, muscle strains; inflammatory conditions such as rheumatoid arthritis; trauma; surgery; cancer; bone metastasis; dysmenorrhea; or when patients desire to avoid narcotics and request to be alert and in control. Contraindications to the use of NSAIDs include intolerance or allergy to the drug. Stomach ulcers or bleeding disorders may limit the use of some NSAIDs.

The oral (po) route medications in the form of capsules or tablets are preferred (see Chap. 25 for considerations in medication administration). If patients are unable to ingest pills or capsules because of decreased consciousness or difficulty swallowing pills, crush the pills and give them with applesauce or yogurt, check to see if the drug is available as a liquid, or seek a physician's order for a rectal form of the drug, if available. These drugs generally need to be taken every 4 hours.

Individuals may respond more favorably to one drug than to another. Thus, it may require some experimentation to determine the most effective drug for a particular patient.

Side effects of NSAIDs include decreased clotting time (bleeding), impaired liver and kidney function with chronic use, gastrointestinal irritation and gastric ulcers, fluid retention, and decreased growth of new bone. Aspirin may cause gastric irritation, tinnitus, and decreased clotting time, whereas acetaminophen in large doses impairs kidney function. Laboratory values and patients' physical status need to be monitored to observe for any changes indicating these side effects.

GUIDELINES FOR PLANNING IMPLEMENTATION. Nursing implementation for a person in pain involves more than giving a medication. Careful assessment of the nature of the pain, how it is experienced, factors influencing pain, and the patient's sociocultural, personal, and past experiences with pain is needed to develop an appropriate management approach. Other considerations include the following.

- Nurses should examine their own feelings about pain and their reactions to the patient's pain. This will make them more understanding of the patient's pain.
- Careful listening is essential in communicating with patients in pain. An accurate pain assessment aids in directing the pain management strategy.
- Patients who report pain are having pain; the challenge is to help them identify the source of the pain and manage it effectively.
- Once the source of a patient's pain has been identified, consider simple comfort measures that might relieve the pain; for example, a back rub or other noninvasive approaches, either in conjunction with pain medication or alone.
- Know the action, purpose, and side effects of all pain medications. Plan for potential side effects; for example, monitor laboratory values, or offer fluids if constipation is a side effect.
- Identify and manage factors that influence pain: disbelief, fatigue, fear, knowledge, misconceptions, and monotony.
- Collaborate with patients in management of their pain. Nurses can offer alternatives and, when patients try new relief measures with a nurse's guidance, pain alleviation can be accomplished.

Caring for Patients with Severe Pain. Patients who experience severe pain are generally those who have had recent surgery, sustained some form of trauma, or are experiencing some acute, disruption in the neurosensory network. Care of patients in severe pain requires skill and sensitivity. At first, inexperienced nurses may find the behavior of patients in severe pain intimidating or frightening. In time, however, nurses become expert at assessing and responding to the psychological and physiologic needs of the patient as they recognize the behaviors associated with severe pain and master a variety of approaches that relieve pain.

Pain is a very stressful experience for patients. It can be fatiguing and can make individuals irritable and tense. Thus prevention of pain is of primary importance for patient comfort. Using a variety of pain-relief methods is useful. Incorporating the patient's beliefs about pain and pain relief enables the patient to collaborate in pain relief. Medications used in conjunction with alternate measures of pain relief may be required.

MODALITIES FOR SEVERE PAIN. Acupuncture is a method of pain relief which involves the placing of slender needles at specific points around the body. These points are associated with areas where nerves enter muscles (over 800 motor points) or where nerves lie close to the surface of the skin. Although it has been used extensively in Asia with good effect, it is less common in Western medicine.

Comfort measures are also helpful in reducing severe pain. These include positioning patients to relieve pressure and promote comfort; keeping bed linens free of wrinkles; eliminating as many environmental stressors as possible; keeping noise to a minimum; and employing other measures such as relaxation and music therapy.

Patient teaching includes informing patients to ask for medication before they are in severe pain. Once pain is severe, it may take from 20 minutes to several hours after an implementation to obtain pain relief. If patients take medication prior to experiencing severe pain, they obtain pain relief much faster.

Many patients have personal methods of pain relief or methods for comforting themselves. These include sitting in a certain position, pacing, drinking warm beverages, self-hypnosis, or taking hot baths or showers. Nurses should always ask patients about any personal pain relief methods and incorporate them in the pain-relief protocol.

MEDICATION FOR SEVERE PAIN: NARCOTICS. Narcotics are drugs that bind to multiple opioid receptor sites in the neurosensory network. When bound to receptor sites, they provide pain relief or analgesia, and euphoria, which alters pain perception. Narcotics are controlled substances and are prescribed by a physician. Refer to Chap. 25 for procedures and legal aspects of narcotics administration.

- *Types of narcotics.* There are three main groups of narcotics. Narcotic agonists are drugs such as morphine, codeine, methadone, dilaudid, and meperidine. The receptor site they occupy, called the "mu" receptor, which is the most powerful receptor, causes cognitive effects such as euphoria, analgesia, respiratory depression, physical dependence, tolerance for the drug, and constipation. These drugs bind tightly to receptor sites and stop or block activity at that site. A second group, narcotic agonist–antagonists, occupy a weaker receptor called the "kappa" receptor, but, in addition, antagonize the effects of the narcotic agonist drugs, such as respiratory depression and physical dependence. The effects of these drugs are analgesia and sedation. Drugs in this category are sometimes referred to as "mixed agonists." They are called "mixed" because, if given alone, they provide analgesia, but if given with a mu agonist drug, they reverse the analgesia provided by the mu agonist. Butorphanol (Stadol), nalbuphine (Nubain), and pentazocine (Talwin) are mixed agonist narcotics. A third group of drugs occupy the "sigma" receptors, which are very weak receptors. Drugs occupying these sites do not produce quality analgesia and may cause side effects such as hallucinations, anxiety, restlessness, or psychosis. See Table 32–12.
- *Administration of narcotics.* Narcotics are available in pure or synthetic form. They can be administered by oral, intramuscular

TABLE 32-12. ACTION OF OPIATE RECEPTORS WITH SPECIFIC DRUGS

Opiate Receptor	Agonist	Antagonist
Mu	Morphine Meperidine Fentanyl Sufentanil Alfentanil Hydromorphone Codeine, oxycodone Hydrocodone Methadone Levorphanal	Naloxone (Narcan) Pentazocine (Talwin) Nalbuphine (Nubain)
Kappa	Pentazocine Nalbuphine hydrochloride (Nubain) Butophanol tartrate (Stadol) Buprenorphine (Buprenex)	Naloxone (?)
Sigma	Pentazocine Ketamine	Naloxone

(IM), or intravenous (IV) routes. IV narcotics are recommended postoperatively to manage severe pain because (1) smaller doses can be given and (2) severe pain is managed quickly and effectively. IM narcotics provide 3 to 4 hours of pain relief for most postoperative pain and are often given prn (as needed) upon the patient's request. Nurses must thus be watchful to ensure that gaps in analgesia do not occur. Nurses must understand the action of the drugs to accurately assess side effects and need for readministration. The oral route for narcotics administration is convenient and inexpensive. It is used commonly after surgery done in outpatient settings as soon as a patient is able to tolerate oral intake.

Sublingual, subcutaneous, and rectal routes can also be used for administering narcotics. The sublingual and buccal mucosa of the mouth have a generous supply of veins and lymphatic drainage for rapid absorption, avoiding a "first pass" through the liver. Absorption, however, is variable and depends on the amount of drug dilution by the saliva. It is also easy for the patient to swallow the sublingual medications before maximal benefit is gained. The subcutaneous route may be preferred if the patient is unable to take oral, rectal, or sublingual pain medications, or if IM or IV administration is not an option. This route is less invasive and less expensive, and analgesia is comparable to that obtained by the intravenous route.[27,28] Rectal administration of narcotics may be offensive to some patients and is not usually selected unless other routes are not appropriate for the patient's situation. The absorption of narcotic suppositories is slower and depends on the suppository base, the presence or absence of feces, and the total volume content within the rectum.[29]

The intraspinal (epidural and intrathecal) route of narcotic administration provides effective pain relief, but is usually managed by specially trained nurses. The intraspinal spaces surround the spinal cord, and the intrathecal space, next to the spinal cord, contains cerebrospinal fluid. A spinal headache may thus result from the leakage of cerebrospinal fluid when this route is used. The delivery of postoperative narcotics intraspinally includes continuous epidural infusions, intermittent epidural injections, and single-shot epidural or intrathecal narcotics. Numerous studies show that postoperative epidural analgesia improves the patient's pulmonary function, expedites early ambulation, and provides continuous quality analgesia.[30,31]

Narcotics in combination with nonnarcotics can be helpful in relieving severe pain. Narcotics are given with nonnarcotics because each contributes to the effect of the other in pain relief. The combination results in an additive effect and reduces the narcotic dose needed for pain relief, thereby decreasing narcotic side effects. Common narcotic–nonnarcotic combinations are meperidine with promethazine or hydroxyzine given IV or IM and oral preparations such as Empirin #3, Tylenol #3, and Percodan.

Patient-controlled analgesia (PCA) is a method of pain management commonly used postoperatively or for patients with cancer pain. PCA is self-administered by the patient and operates with a pump and a timing device hooked up to an intravenous line. The patient presses a button on the PCA unit whenever experiencing pain. The PCA unit controls the total dosage and delivers a preset amount of analgesic. PCA can be used to deliver boluses of medication with or without continuous maintenance dosage infusion. Overdosage is prevented because of an inactivation period on the PCA unit. The major advantage of this system is that is puts patients in control of pain and pain relief and eliminates the wait for a pain medication.[32]

- *Side effects of narcotics.* Common side effects of narcotics are sedation, constipation, nausea and vomiting, dry mouth, and respiratory depression.
  - *Sedation* is common for most narcotics. Inform patients that the drowsiness may subside after 2 or 3 days. If sedation seems excessive, consult the physician regarding the need for an adjustment of the dosage.
  - *Respiratory depression,* which follows sedation, is always a concern with narcotic pain relief, but particularly so with large doses of morphine. Monitoring respiratory status while patients are resting is important. Be sure to count the respiratory rate for a full minute. Encouraging coughing and deep breathing while patients are awake stimulates breathing and encourages good lung ventilation. Report respiratory depression to the physician immediately.
  - *Constipation,* another common narcotic side effect,[29] occurs as a result of decreased peristalsis caused by narcotic medications. The stool becomes hard as water is absorbed from the fecal matter in the intestinal tract. Encourage patients to increase roughage (fruits, vegetables) in their diet, and increase water intake. A physician may need to write an order for a stool softener. Encourage exercise if patients are mobile.
  - *Nausea and vomiting* may occur as a result of pain or from the narcotic itself. An antiemetic may be given intramuscularly or

rectally to relieve nausea. It may be necessary to change the narcotic given if nausea and vomiting persist. Reduce unpleasant odors and sights that might stimulate vomiting.
  - *Dry mouth* occurs because narcotics reduce saliva production. Instruct patients to rinse the mouth frequently, suck on sugarless candies, eat pineapple or watermelon, and drink plenty of fluids to enhance moisture in the mouth. Good oral hygiene and dental care are essential.
- *Care of patients receiving narcotics.* Many nurses, and many patients alike, fear addiction as a side effect of narcotics administration. However, research shows that when individuals take a narcotic for pain relief, addiction is extremely unlikely.[33] Thus, nurses should be more concerned about providing pain relief than about preventing addiction. Appropriate use of narcotics does not result in addiction. Indeed, "addiction" is an outdated term and in fact has been removed from the taxonomy of many societies of pain experts. Terms in current usage include "tolerance," "physical dependence," and "drug-seeking behavior."

Tolerance occurs when patients require an increasing dose of medication to control the same amount of pain. However, research now challenges the assumptions on which the concept of tolerance rests, and it is important to note that as disease progresses, pain often increases. Thus, it is important to explain to patients that it is appropriate to take whatever amount is needed to control pain. Tolerance can be handled as it arises.

Physical dependence or withdrawal symptoms from discontinuing narcotic drugs is another fear. However, because most acute pain gradually subsides and along with it dosage and frequency of narcotic analgesics, physical dependence rarely occurs. Physical dependence is evident when a patient on long-term narcotics is abruptly taken off of narcotics and withdrawal symptoms develop. Symptoms are usually prevented, however, if a patient is slowly withdrawn from the narcotic. Drug-seeking behavior, the consumption of narcotics in the absence of pain, requires a chemical dependency program for resolution. Examples of behaviors that may suggest a drug-seeking tendency include eliciting sympathy or guilt, threatening physical, social, or financial harm, or offering bribes to obtain narcotics, or being uncooperative in care. If this behavior is suspected, objective observation must be documented and communicated to the physician.

Respiratory depression is always a concern. Indeed, no narcotic dose is automatically safe or fatal. The only safe way to administer a narcotic is to watch the first dose given to an individual. Indeed, safe administration requires that nurses titrate the narcotic effect. That means administering a certain dose according to prescription and watching a patient's response to the drug. Repeated doses are then administered, as outlined by the physician or hospital protocol, until the patient's pain is controlled, sedation occurs, or the maximum dosage has been given. This is called "titration to effect" and is an advanced nursing skill requiring special training. Once analgesia is obtained, patient-controlled analgesia is begun using the dosage information obtained from this procedure. Subsequent doses tend to be safe unless the drug accumulates or the patient's condition changes.

The nurse's responsibility in administering narcotic analgesics is an active one. Important choices to be made by nurses include (1) choosing the appropriate analgesic or narcotic, as prescribed by the physician; (2) deciding whether to give a narcotic, based on accurate pain assessment; (4) evaluating effectiveness of the narcotic; (3) determining if a change in pain medication is needed; (5) monitoring for side effects of medications; and (6) educating patients about drugs, dosage, side effects, and an effective schedule for taking the drug, and addressing fears or misconceptions.

OTHER MEDICATIONS FOR SEVERE PAIN. Tricyclic antidepressants are excellent analgesic agents for individuals with neuropathic pain. Patients describe the pain that best responds to tricyclic antidepressants as "burning," "prickling," or "tingling." Tricyclic antidepressants work at the descending tract of the spinal cord and prevent the reuptake of serotonin and norepinephrine at the spinal cord.[34]

SUMMARY OF SEVERE PAIN MANAGEMENT. Key points in the management of acute pain are as follows.

- Patients should be medicated before significant pain occurs, or before pain increases; prn (or as needed) pain medications should be given before pain worsens. This facilitates management of pain so that pain does not become unnecessarily severe. When pain becomes severe, it takes longer for pain medication to be effective.
- General comfort measures should always be considered in conjunction with administration of narcotics. Supportive approaches include keeping patients comfortable, dry, and warm (or cool, if preferred). Provide back rubs and massages as requested by patients. Repositioning patients can greatly affect comfort levels, or remove a source of pain.
- Rest periods are essential to combat fatigue, which can worsen pain. Rest can also enhance the effectiveness of pain medications as they begin to work in the body.
- Coordinate care and pain-producing activities with the schedule for pain medications. Providing medication to patients in time to act before transferring to a chair or turning enhances the ease of such activities.
- Immobilization and elevation of painful extremities will reduce swelling and pressure, and facilitate removal of waste products, which can cause pain and discomfort.

Approaches to Patients with Chronic Pain. For some patients, approaches used for acute pain management prove unsuccessful and pain becomes chronic. Chronic pain, as previously defined, is pain that lasts 3 to 6 months or longer. Approaches to assist patients with chronic pain include use of analgesics, medical and surgical treatment measures, and noninvasive approaches to pain control.

ANALGESICS. Analgesics may be helpful for chronic pain and should be administered orally, if at all possible. It is essential to give high enough doses to provide sufficient pain relief. Often, however, oral and other common routes of administration are ineffective and analgesics must be delivered by other routes, such as spinal or epidural catheter.[26] Administration by these routes requires advanced technical skill. Collaborating with patients in the adjustment of narcotics doses can facilitate the effectiveness of the drug therapy during acute flare-ups. Trust on the part of the patient will be enhanced if he or she understands the pain relief plan.

MEDICAL TREATMENT MEASURES. Medical treatment measures include electrical stimulation and nerve blocks. Such measures require patient education and understanding of the potential benefits and disadvantages associated with the treatment that is being considered.

Neuroaugmentation, the use of electrical stimulation of areas of the brain and spinal cord, is used to assist those with cancer pain and chronic pain[26] to manage severe, chronic pain when other methods have failed. Implanted electrodes connected to an external transmitter, which uses a battery device, may be employed to block pain impulses to the spinal cord. Such methods may prove effective where other methods have failed.

Nerve blocks are another approach for treating chronic pain. In this procedure, specially trained anesthesiologists inject solutions into the nervous structure, such as nerve trunks, nerve roots, sympathetic ganglion, or the spinal cord. The procedure destroys or anesthetizes nerves that carry the pain messages to the brain. This procedure carries the risk of neurologic injury and systemic side effects. Nerve blocks can be temporary or permanent.

SURGICAL MEASURES. Surgical approaches are also used. One approach is cutting sensory nerves to eliminate pain. A cordotomy is a more extensive surgical procedure designed to alleviate pain. It involves resecting the thoracic or cervical spinal cord at various levels. This procedure is used to relieve unrelenting or intractable pain. The higher the focus of the pain, the higher the site for the cordotomy. The procedure is not curative since the stimulus for the pain remains, but the stimulus does not reach the higher cerebral structures to be identified as pain. The patient will have permanent loss of both pain and temperature sensation in the areas in which the resected nerves lie. Patients do, however, retain sense of touch and position. Patients should be cautioned to measure temperature of bath water and any warming devices (such as hot water bottles) to avoid burns to those areas.

A posterior rhizotomy, another surgical procedure, entails the resection of the dorsal roots of a spinal nerve. This type of surgery is effective for relieving localized acute pain in the area supplied by the nerve root and deep visceral pain. As with a cordotomy, this procedure is not curative but only provides pain relief.

Home Health Care

Patients with many conditions for which hospital care was once routine—conditions such as coma—are now cared for in the home following the acute phase of illness. Teaching home caregivers to care for a comatose family member, for example, is a role of home health nurses. Instruction may include airway suctioning, vital signs measurement, fluid status monitoring, feeding a patient through a nasogastric tube, caring for a Foley catheter, turning and positioning to prevent skin breakdown and limb contractures, and carrying out the full range of hygiene procedures. Often home caregivers are assisted by home health aids to maintain the rigorous care required by a comatose patient.

The terminally ill also often require home care. Indeed, hospice care for the dying now extends into the home, and provides an interdisciplinary team and trained volunteers to assist with the patient's care. Hospice patients often experience severe pain, and may be candidates for PCA, which the home health nurse monitors and supervises. An important role of home health nurses is to ensure that patients receive adequate support and pain relief to keep them as comfortable as possible.

Chronic conditions impairing neurosensory integration also provide a challenge to home nurses. Arthritis is common among the homebound elderly, and many arthritis patients experience mild to moderate pain for which they take analgesics, particularly NSAIDs. Such medicines have serious side effects if not taken properly. Home nurses not only monitor the intake of pain medication but teach patients that aspirin and ibuprofen, for example, must be taken after eating to prevent gastrointestinal complications.

Stroke, or cerebrovascular accident, are also common in the later years of life. Stroke may cause temporary or permanent loss of speech and language comprehension and the ability to move one side of the body. Therefore, supporting such patients' communication and movement, particularly the abilities that affect patients' capacity for self-care, is essential. The role of the home nurse, however, is to assess the patient's needs and teach the family caregiver to provide the needed care. Caring for a patient totally dependent on others requires a great deal of caregivers. Thus, the home nurse is cognizant of caregivers' needs for relief. Day care for stroke patients is now available in many areas of the country, and is an option that may enable home caregivers to restore and maintain their own strength and energy.

REHABILITATIVE CARE

Rehabilitative care focuses on reestablishing patient lifestyle to adapt to or incorporate neurosensory alterations, if present. The optimal outcome is achieving the highest level of independence possible.[35] For some patients, major lifestyle changes may occur.

Lifestyle Changes

Lifestyle changes may require adjustment in patients' level of independence. Services such as home health care, day-care clinics, or volunteers or attendants in the home can provide much-needed relief for families or significant others from the day-to-day responsibility of patient care.

Occupational changes may be necessary for paralyzed patients or those with impaired communication, memory, or thought. Vocational retraining may provide assistance in some cases. Social workers can serve as resources in planning home and occupational referrals. Local and state agencies can be consulted to inform patients and their families of services they provide for special needs.

Environmental Adaptation

Special appliances may be required as patients adjust to different levels of independence. Use of special appliances should be encouraged. Some will view adaptive devices negatively. Encourage expression of such emotions, but gently remind patients that special appliances can enhance independence, which enhances self-esteem.

Modified telephones with large printed numbers are effective for people with visual acuity changes, as are telephones that have prerecorded numbers that can be automatically "speed-dialed."

Environmental adaptations in the home can be made as rehabilitation in hospitals or other facilities is completed. Ramps and modified doorways for wheelchairs and flat door handles for people with rheumatoid arthritis, are examples of modifications that provide adaptation in homes for patients with permanent neurosensory deficits. Bathroom fixtures with flat control bars and shower stalls with seats are other adjustments that can be made.

EVALUATION

Evaluation of care is the final component of nurse–patient management of neurosensory integration. Specific neurosensory outcomes identified in the care plan provide the framework for monitoring progress. Evaluation of the care in terms of how well the care was given is inadequate.[36] If the desired outcomes have been met and the problems are resolved, a notation is made in the patient's chart. If the desired outcomes have not been achieved, reassessment and replanning are necessary.

SUMMARY

Neurosensory integration represents the coordinated and unified functions that are essential to wholeness and individuality. Consciousness, perception, memory, learning, thought, communication, and movement—functions that form the basis of human personality—are only possible through neurosensory integration and are dependent upon the complex, interconnected circuitry of the nervous system for their elaboration. Together these functions make it possible for individuals to sense their environments, respond to stimuli in appropriate ways, and address the problems that people face in everyday life.

Each of the major neurosensory functions contributes to individual coping, self-care, and capacity for collaborative interaction. *Consciousness* is the state of being aware of one's self and one's surroundings and perception is the ability of the mind to interpret and analyze input from the senses. Without these functions individuals become dependent on others to assist them in problem-solving. *Pain,* a natural phenomenon related to perception, serves a protective function, alerting the individual to the possibility of injury or illness. Research is addressing the neurologic basis of pain, such as pain receptors, pain pathways, and endogenous opiates. *Memory,* the mental capacity for receiving, registering, encoding, consolidating, storing, and retrieving information, is essential to virtually every aspect of mental functioning and is closely associated with learning, which is a permanent change in behavior related to memory. Memory is vital to the accomplishment of even the simplest of human tasks. *Thought* is a complex set of mental processes that assigns meaning to sensory input and designs actions in response to interpretations of sensory input. *Communication,* closely related to thought, is the act of sending and receiving messages through the use of speech. *Speech,* in turn, is the vocal articulation of thoughts using language, a formal system of signs and symbols for communication. *Movement* is a change in place, position, or posture of any portion of the body, and is vital for engaging in activities of daily living. All of these functions, alone or in combination, are essential for a person's independence and for individuals to meet the demands of their environments.

The variables of neurosensory integration include genetic heritage, age, health, nutrition, environment, psychosocial factors, and medication. Alterations in neurosensory integration disrupt neurosensory functions. Certain deficits and disabilities, correspond to changes in consciousness, perception, memory and learning, thought, communication, and movement. Deficits interfere with self-care, independence, and collaboration. Trauma, tumors, infection, vascular lesions, and impaired neurosensory transmission are common causes of altered neurosensory integration.

Nurses assess patients' neurosensory functions by conducting a thorough health history and health examination focusing on the subjective and objective manifestations of the neurosensory system and on the health of other body systems that contribute to maintaining neurosensory integration. Data collected clinically is correlated with the results of neurosensory diagnostic tests, and nursing diagnoses of neurosensory status are derived.

Frequently, nurses find that patients manifest some disturbance to neurosensory integration that requires management. Depending on the nature of the problem, these patients will need preventive neurosensory care and will benefit from related health education and health screening. Many patients will also require supportive care to assist them with sensory perception, including vision and hearing, mild to moderate pain, or communication difficulties.

Restorative and ongoing care are necessary for many patients who have problems with neurosensory integration. Individuals who have experienced coma or seizures, or who have chronic pain, are examples. Ongoing medical treatment and altering patients' life activities are frequently required to cope with chronic problems. Rehabilitative care mediates chronic problems through adjustments in lifestyle and rehabilitative therapy. Nurse–patient collaboration may be limited by disruption in neurosensory function, but nevertheless is important not only in assessment but also in further implementation to enhance health.

LEARNING OUTCOMES

Upon completing this chapter, the student should be able to:

1. Describe functions served by neurosensory integration.
2. Identify and describe the anatomic components and pathways and the physiologic mechanisms involved in pain.
3. Discuss the importance of neurosensory integration for the collaborative nurse–patient relationship.
4. Identify factors affecting neurosensory integration.
5. Identify protective structures and processes involved in neurosensory functioning.
6. List and describe the basic causes of neurosensory alterations.
7. List and describe alterations in neurosensory functioning.
8. Identify essential components of a neurosensory history and examination.
9. List elements of the pain history.
10. Explain the purpose of selected neurologic diagnostic tests.
11. State nursing diagnoses for patients experiencing altered neurosensory integration.
12. Identify appropriate nursing implementations for preventive, supportive, restorative, and rehabilitative levels of care for patients experiencing alterations in neurosensory integration.
13. Describe the nursing implementations appropriate to mild, moderate, and severe pain.

REVIEW OF KEY TERMS

affect
anesthesia
aphasia
arousal
central vision
classical conditioning
cognition
communication
consciousness
content
emotion
feeling
habituation
hyperesthesia
hypoesthesia
immediate memory
involuntary movement
language
long–term memory
memory
mood
movement
neurons
pain
paralysis
paresthesia
perception
peripheral vision
sensitization
sensory deprivation
sensory overload
short-term memory
speech
thought
tone
voluntary movement

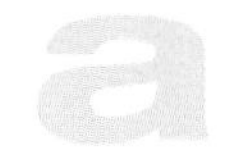

Having Read the Chapter, consider again the opening scenario, page 1109, and the following responses to the questions posed about the plan of care for Mr. Bergstrom after his stroke.

Unconscious patients are dependent on nurses for all of their needs. Although Mr. Bergstrom's plan of care should include careful, ongoing assessment of all body functions, the monitoring of his neurosensory status is a top priority. In particular, it should include careful evaluation of his level of consciousness as evidenced by his motor and reflex activity, his responsiveness to verbal and other environmental stimuli, and reaction to pain. As Mr. Bergstrom awakens from coma and grows in awareness, his orientation to person, place, time, and situation will be important to document, and his caregivers will want to assess his progress by noting, among other important signs, his memory of recent and past events, the quality of his speech and ability to communicate, and his capacity for abstract thought and judgment.

Because Mr. Bergstrom is unable to meet his own physiological needs, his caregivers will undertake nursing implementations to support his oxygenation function and fluid and electrolyte balance. These implementations are essential to Mr. Bergstrom's recovery and their success will be monitored by careful observations of the respiratory, circulatory, and hydration status. Mr. Bergstrom's nurses will assess his vital signs on a frequent basis, looking for changes in respiratory and pulse rate and blood pressure. While he is comatose, they will also frequently check his pupillary size and reactivity to light, an important indicator of brain oxygenation. Mr. Bergstrom will also require turning and repositioning at least every two hours and nutritional support via a feeding tube to keep him in nitrogen balance while he remains unable to eat.

Mr. Bergstrom's nurses should at all points incude his family members in his plan of care, and help them to interpret the information shared with them about his care. It can be anticipated that grief and anxiety will affect their ability to communicate. They will need information on the purpose of the nurses' activities, and can participate by conveying their observations of the patient's behavior to the nurses which will help in the evaluation of Mr. Bergstrom's neurological status.

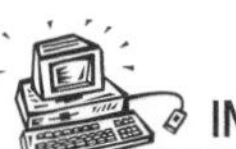

INTERNET RESOURCES

Web Sites

Management of Cancer Pain, Clinical Practice Guideline:
http://www.AHCPR.gov/guide/

Headache:
http://www.ayurvedic.org

Listserv

Pediatric Pain—Subscribe at: mailserv;caac.dal.ca (message: Subscribe Pediatric_Pain Yourfirstname Yourlastname)

REFERENCES

1. Temple C. *The Brain.* New York: Penguin; 1993.
2. Springer S, Duetsch G. *Left Brain, Right Brain.* New York: W.H. Freeman; 1993.
3. Nolte J, Angevine J. *The Human Brain.* St. Louis: Mosby; 1995.
4. Hickey J. *Neurological and Neurosurgical Nursing.* Philadelphia: Lippincott; 1992:61, 115, 117, 391.
5. Lueckenotte A. *Gerontologic Nursing.* St. Louis: Mosby; 1996: 827.
6. Sternbach R. *Pain: A Psychophysiological Analysis.* New York: Academic Press; 1963:12.
7. McCaffery M, Beebe A. *A Pain Manual for Nursing Practice.* St. Louis: Mosby; 1989.
8. Melzack R, Wall PB. Pain mechanisms: A new theory. *Science.* 1986;150:197.
9. Bonica J. *The Management of Pain.* 2nd ed. Philadelphia: Lea & Febiger; 1990;1:28–35.
10. Ebersole P, Hess P. *Toward Healthy Aging.* St. Louis: Mosby; 1994:381, 693, 391.

11. Rose S. *The Making of Memory: From Molecules to Mind.* New York: Doubleday; 1992:115, 171–173.
12. Desimore R. The physiology of memory: Recordings of things past. *Science.* 1992;258:245–246.
13. Beare P, Myers J, eds. *Adult Health Nursing.* 2nd ed. St. Louis: Mosby; 1994:1178.
14. Leininger M. *Transcultural Nursing: Concepts, Theories and Practice.* 2nd ed. New York: McGraw-Hill: 1995.
15. Seidel, HM, Ball, JW, Dains, JE, Benedict, GW. *Mosby's Guide to Physical Examination,* 3rd ed. St. Louis, MO: Mosby Year Book; 1994.
16. Meador J. Cerumen impaction in the elderly. *J Gerontol Nurs.* 1195;21:15–20.
17. Souder E, Yoder L. Olfaction: The neglected sense. *J Neurosci Nurs.* 1992;24:274.
18. Evans MJ. *Neurologic–Neurosurgical Nursing.* Springhouse, PA: Springhouse; 1995:46.
19. Terry J, Baranowski L, Lonsway R, Hedrick C. *Intravenous Therapy: Clinical Principles and Practice.* Philadelphia: Saunders; 1995:294.
20. Foreman M, Zane D. Nursing strategies for acute confusion in elders. *Am J Nurs.* 1996;96:44–52.
21. Gregor C, Pope S, Werry D, Dodeck P. Reduced length of stay and improved appropriateness of care with a clinical path for total knee and hip arthroplasty. *J Qual Improve.* 1996;22: 617–627.
22. Greene P, Gildemeister J. Memory aging research and memory support in the elderly. *J Neurosci Nurs.* 1994;26:242.
23. Danner C, et al. Cognitively impaired elderly: using research findings to improve nursing care. *J Gerontol Nurs.* 1993;48: 157–171.
24. Janeson D, Cimprich B. Attentional impairment in persons with multiple sclerosis. *J Neurosci Nurs.* 1994;26:95–102.
25. Guyton AC, Hall JE. *Textbook of Medical Physiology,* 9th ed. Philadelphia: Saunders; 1996.
26. Agency of Health Care Policy and Research. *Clinical Practice Guideline. Acute Pain Management: Operative or Medical Procedures and Trauma.* Rockville, MD: U.S. Department of Health and Human Services; 1994.
27. Bruera E. Palliative care rounds: The use of subcutaneous patient-controlled analgesia. *J Pain Symptom Manage.* 1982;72: 285.
28. Bull P, et al. Subcutaneous opiods: The painless approach. *Anaesthesia.* 1992;47:276.
29. DeBoer AG, et al. Rectal drug administration: Clinical pharmacokinetic considerations. *Clinical Pharmacokinetics.* 1982;7: 285.
30. Cuscheri R. Postoperative pain and pulmonary complications: Comparison of three analgesic regimens. *Br J Surg.* 1985;72: 495–498.
31. St. Marie B. Narcotic infusions: A changing scene. *J Intraven Nurs.* 1991;14:334–344.
32. Jackson D. A study of pain management: Patient-controlled analgesia versus intramuscular analgesia. *J Intraven Nurs.* 1989;12:42–51.
33. Porter J, Jicks H. Addiction is rare in patients treated with narcotics. *N Engl J Med.* 1980;302:123.
34. Patt R. *Cancer Pain.* Philadelphia: Lippincott; 1993:214, 228, 572.
35. Hoeman S. *Rehabilitative Nursing.* St. Louis: Mosby; 1994.
36. McMahon R, Pearson A, eds. *Nursing as Therapy.* New York: Chapman & Hall; 1991:68.

33

Mobility

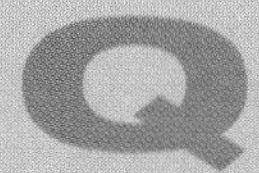

Mr. Adam Dodd, age 76, lives with his wife in a one story condominium in a quiet, grassy complex. He has had residual weakness (strength: grade 3) in his left leg since suffering a stroke 2 years ago. Although he is able to take several steps independently, he uses a walker for most ambulation. He is able to carry out ADLs independently. He had safety bars installed in the tub/shower and beside the toilet after his stroke. He likes to sit outside on his patio when the weather is nice. He watches TV, and he enjoys occasional visits from grandchildren. He takes an antihypertensive medication daily. A home health nurse visits every other week to evaluate Mr. Dodd's blood pressure.

What other assessments are appropriate for his nurse to make on her regular visits?

What are Mr. Dodd's mobility risks?

What recommendations would be appropriate for his nurse to make to reduce these risks and maintain optimum mobility?

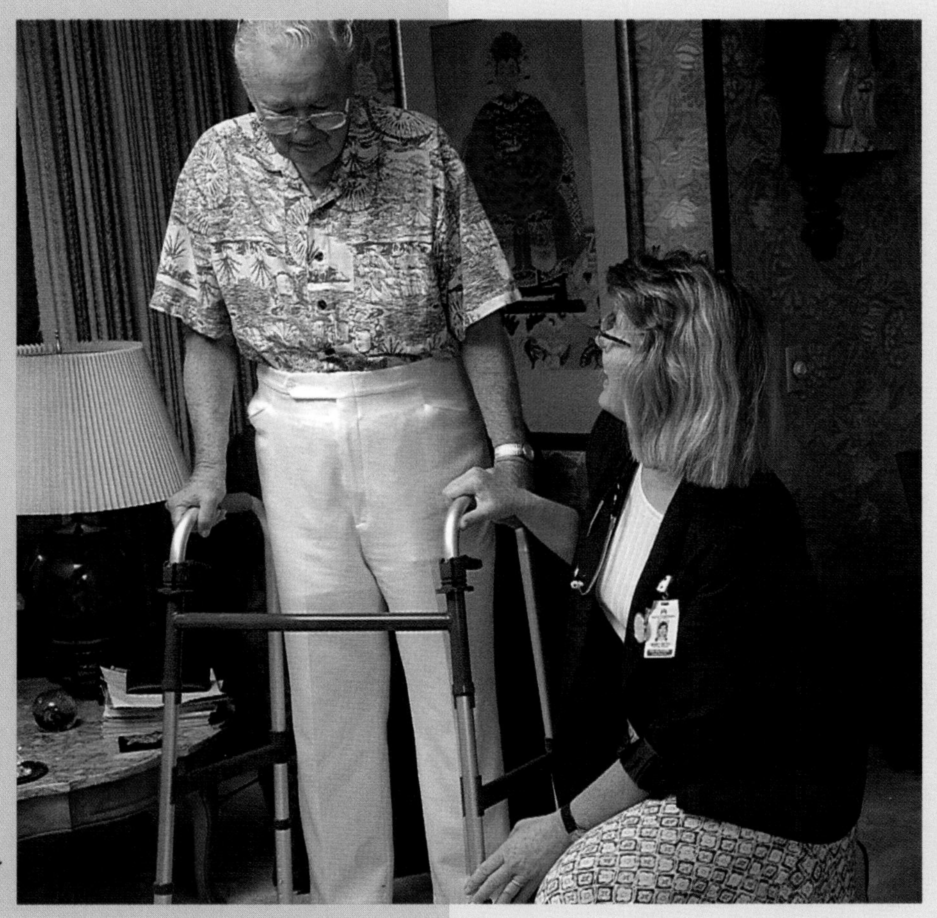

CHAPTER OUTLINE

Human **mobility** is the movement of the body as a whole and the movement of body parts in relation to one another. That humans have an innate need to move seems confirmed by the number of forms of movement that we pursue as recreation. Hiking, jogging, skating, skiing, swimming, tennis, golf, and bowling are a few of the popular activities enjoyed by hundreds of thousands of individuals. All are forms of movement and rely on the basic human capacity for mobility. They are pursued because people feel good doing them; people need to move!

The relationship of movement to wellness is complex. Scientific research documenting the importance of movement to physical health is vast and continues to grow. In addition, a balance between movement and psychological integrity is related to one's level of self-esteem. Psychologically, we relate mobility to a sense of independence and power. To move one's body through space is liberating. To be unable to move, on the other hand, is profoundly frustrating and discouraging.

When the capacity for movement is lost or diminished through illness, as it frequently is, discouragement is often evident and can be severe. When the loss is permanent, the adaptation requires a change in self-concept, which can make extremely expensive demands on psychological energy. Grieving for the lost function—and the lost part of self—is not uncommon.

Considering that mobility is so important to human wellness and the quality of human life, and recognizing that disease is a common factor in mobility dysfunction, it is not surprising that nurses have a significant role in assisting patients with mobility problems. This chapter addresses optimum mobility, including physiologic integration of mobility and fitness; factors that alter mobility and the effects of diminished mobility on other body functions; and nurse–patient assessment and management of mobility.

SECTION 1
UNDERSTANDING MOBILITY

OPTIMAL MOBILITY

Optimum mobility refers to the ability to willfully execute all of the many movements of which humans are capable. The concept suggests maintaining peak physiologic functioning, for all body systems support mobility and are in one way or another affected by mobility or the lack of it. An understanding of the physiologic integration of mobility and an awareness of how to attain and maintain fitness are basic to recognizing and supporting optimum mobility.

PHYSIOLOGIC INTEGRATION OF MOBILITY

Musculoskeletal, neurosensory, cardiorespiratory, and metabolic functioning underlie the physiologic integration of mobility. Each has a distinctive role, yet all are interdependent.

Musculoskeletal Functioning

The skeleton provides a rigid framework for the body and protection for the major body organs. Bones articulate in six types of joints (Table 33–1), which facilitate a wide range of possible movements:

- *Flexion,* bending, reducing the angle at a joint.
- *Extension,* straightening, increasing the angle at a joint.
- *Hyperextension,* movement beyond the normal extended position in the opposite direction from flexion.
- *Abduction,* movement away from the midline (midsaggital plane).
- *Adduction,* movement toward the midline.
- *Rotation,* turning in a medial or lateral direction, pivoting on an axis.
- *Circumduction,* moving the distal portion of an extremity in a circle.
- *Specialized movements.* These include *supination,* turning the palm of the hand forward or upward; *pronation,* turning the palm of the hand downward or backward; *inversion,* turning the sole of the foot inward; and *eversion,* turning the sole of the foot outward.

Characteristically, joints are surrounded by ligaments, which provide stability and enclose the joint capsule.

The muscles directly responsible for movement are the skeletal or striated muscles. Each is composed of many contractile fibers bound together by connective tissue called fascia. The fascia attaches the muscle to bone by forming a tendon that fuses to the bone. Tendons are relatively inelastic tissue with high tensile strength, which makes them resistant to injury.

When a muscle is stimulated by impulses from the nervous system, calcium is released from muscle cells and the contraction process is initiated. The splitting of high-energy adenosine triphosphate (ATP) bonds in muscle cells releases energy for muscle contraction.

When a muscle contracts, it shortens in length. One end, called the origin, remains relatively stable during the contraction, while the other end, the insertion, moves toward the origin. The shortening of the muscle results from structural rearrangement of the muscle proteins, actin and myosin in the myofibrils, the fine elements making up the muscle fiber.

During the recovery phase, the high-energy bonds are resynthesized. Without adequate oxygen for the recovery phase, ATP cannot be resynthesized and fatigue ensues. Normally, the energy to sustain muscular contraction comes from the oxidation of glycogen stored in the muscle. When muscular work is prolonged, liver glycogen and, ultimately, fat are metabolized for fuel.

Movement is the result of coordinated muscle activity. When two or more muscles interact together to accomplish a given movement, they are called **synergists.** The muscles that flex the elbow

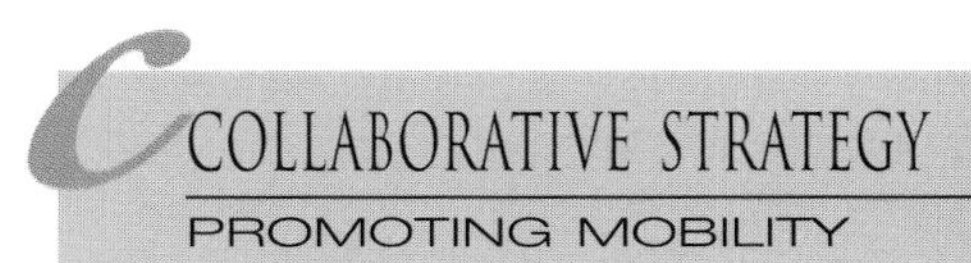

The capacity to move has always been important to human survival and adaptation. Humans seem to have an innate need to move just for the sheer joy of it. Mobility is related to wellness and physical fitness, but just as importantly, to self-actualization. Working in partnership with patients to reach mobility outcomes addresses more than the function itself: it also promotes self-esteem and affirms patients' personal identity.

TABLE 33-1. TYPES OF JOINTS

Joint	Description	Movement
Ball and socket *Example:* Shoulder	Ball-shaped head fitting into a concave socket formed by another bone or bones	360 degrees: Flexion–extension, adduction–abduction, circumduction, hyperextension
Hinge *Example:* Knee	One convex surface articulating with the concave surface of another bone or bones	180 degrees: Flexion–extension in one plane only
Pivot *Example:* Atlas, axis joint of spine	Ring-shaped bony structure rotates on the rounded surface of another bone	Rotation only
Condyloid *Example:* Carpo/metacarpal	Ovoid bony projection fits into elliptical cavity	All movements except axial rotation
Saddle *Example:* Carpo/metacarpal at thumb	Convex–concave surface of one bone fits into concave–convex surface of another	Flexion, extension, circumduction, hyperextension, abduction–adduction
Gliding *Example:* Wrist	Two flat/slightly curved bony surfaces articulate	Flexion–extension, hyperextension, rotation, adduction–abduction, circumduction

are among many synergistic muscles in the body. Another type of coordination is required between muscles whose contraction results in opposite movements of the same body part. These muscle pairs are called **antagonists.** One must contract and the other relax for movement to be accomplished.

The complexity of function is controlled by the central nervous system, which plays a significant role in all movement.

Neuromuscular Integration

Many complex cerebral mechanisms underlie voluntary movement. Automatic responses (reflexes) are controlled by the reflex arc involving spinal neurons. Complete mobility depends upon CNS integration of both reflex and voluntary movement.

Reflexes are essential for normal mobility. No cortical interpretation or integration occurs in reflex movement. Because the response is automatic, it is predictable. A stimulus that excites a particular type of receptor will result in an invariable response. A familiar example is someone withdrawing a body part from a painful stimulus. Relexes are also responsible for maintaining positive muscle tone and posture. Reflexes undergo developmental changes; some disappear with growth, and others emerge. Pathologic conditions that affect the nerves or muscles alter reflexes, causing sluggish responses, brisk responses, or a return of infantile reflexes. For this reason, testing reflexes is part of the nursing and medical assessments of motor functioning.

Voluntary, or purposeful, movement is initiated in the cerebrum. Sensory information comes to the cerebral cortex from visual stimulation and from proprioceptors (receptors that respond to stimuli originating within the body, such as stretch or position). They are located in the semicircular canals of the inner ear and in muscle spindles, tendons, and joints. Afferent (sensory) fibers carry the impulses to the cerebrum where the input is interpreted to facilitate intentional, coordinated movement.

The cerebellum also has an important role in this process. It receives some proprioceptive signals and influences the amount of neural activity in the motor cortex. When the afferent signals have been interpreted by the cerebellum and the premotor cortex of the cerebrum, efferent impulses from the motor cortex are initiated. They travel down to the brainstem, cross to the opposite side, and then synapse with lower motor neurons in the ventral horn of the spinal cord. Each motor neuron sends an axon to the skeletal muscle. There it divides to innervate signal muscle fibers. When the electrical impulse crosses the motor endplate at the myoneural junction, contraction results. Separate motor fibers carry inhibitory impulses that result in relaxation. This complex integration of brain, nerve, and muscle activity is necessary for all intentional movement.

Cardiovascular and Respiratory Functioning

Increased blood circulation is essential for sustained muscle activity. Working muscles demand more oxygen and metabolic fuel. They produce more waste products—carbon dioxide and lactic acid—which must be removed in order for muscle work to continue. The heat produced as muscles work must be dissipated. Each of these demands is met by enhanced blood circulation.

The cardiopulmonary system must be able to accomplish a series of actions to meet increased demands for oxygen in the muscles. First, a sufficient amount of environmental air must be inspired and mixed with lung gases in the alveoli. This occurs with the contraction of the respiratory muscles and a corresponding elevation in rate and depth of respiration. If depth of breathing approaches a person's vital capacity, there is a sensation of being out of breath, or winded. Next, oxygen enters capillary blood and carbon dioxide is retrieved. This diffusion of oxygen and carbon dioxide requires competent pulmonary circulation, adequate lung surface to which the blood can be exposed, and sufficient hemoglobin to carry the oxygen.

Next, the supply of oxygen-rich blood to exercising muscles is enhanced. This is brought about by vasodilation in muscles, corresponding vasconstriction in other organs, and a rise in cardiac output. The elevation in cardiac output is accomplished by accelerated heart rate and greater stroke volume. Sympathetic stimulation causes stronger ventricular contraction, and therefore more blood is ejected from the heart with each beat. The stronger contraction of working muscles enhances venous return. These changes result in increased systolic blood pressure. If arteries have diminished elasticity secondary to arteriosclerosis, or if exercise is excessively vigorous, diastolic pressure also may rise.

When oxygenated blood reaches muscle tissue, effective exchange of oxygen and carbon dioxide must occur in the muscle cells. Finally, the muscle must use the oxygen it has received. The proper functioning of the complex enzyme systems discussed above which bring about the breaking and reforming of the high-energy bonds in the muscle cells, is essential for efficient use of oxygen by muscles. It is only when all of these physiologic processes are carried out effectively that an individual can exercise at high levels of energy expenditure for a significant length of time.

Metabolism

Physical activity requires energy, which is usually derived from oxidation of foods. The amount and quality of food ingested affects performance. Effective digestion, absorption, and excretion of wastes is critical for maintaining sufficient energy stores (glycogen and fat) to support optimal mobility.

At the onset of activity, glycogen stores in the muscles supply energy for muscle activity. The stress of muscular work causes an increase in the production of adrenocortical hormones. These hormones stimulate the release of liver glycogen for use as metabolic fuel. The resulting rise in blood sugar levels is sustained until glycogen stores are exhausted. When blood sugar falls as a result of depletion of liver glycogen, symptoms of fatigue result. If continuing demands on the body are made, fat is oxidized to supply fuel for muscular work. These processes normally are aerobic and require a continuous supply of oxygen.

If the supply of oxygen is inadequate to allow oxidation of available glycogen, **anaerobic glycolysis** occurs. Although anaerobic breakdown of glycogen is a relatively quick source of energy, its end-product is lactic acid. Accumulation of lactic acid in muscles produces fatigue. The aerobic process is considerably more efficient. It produces almost 20 times more ATP than a comparable amount of anaerobic metabolism. It can use carbohydrate, fat, or protein as energy sources and it avoids the fatiguing byproducts. To use aerobic metabolic pathways for intense and prolonged activity, cardiorespiratory function must be optimal.

The heat produced by muscular work is dissipated by vasodilation in the skin and the production of perspiration. Considerable amounts of water and sodium can be lost in this way.

These metabolic changes affect kidney function, and for two reasons, less urine is produced. First, tubular reabsorption of water increases to compensate for losses through perspiration. Second, the glomerular filtration rate is decreased because of decreased renal blood flow. The kidney is one of the organs from which blood is shunted to increase circulation to the muscles. If anaerobic metabolism occurs, urine produced during exercise is more acidic due to higher lactic acid levels. Glucose may be present because the blood glucose concentration may increase faster than the tubules can reabsorb it. Sodium and chloride levels decrease, which partly compensates for increased losses via the skin.

The rate of all metabolic processes is increased by exercise. More activity requires more energy. When overall exercise is increased without a corresponding increase in intake of nutrients, the additional energy required is obtained from body stores of adipose tissue. This state, in which energy expenditure exceeds energy (caloric) intake, is referred to as negative energy balance. It is a desirable state for a person who is overweight. Ideally, total caloric expenditure matches caloric intake. This is energy balance. Positive energy balance occurs when more calories are ingested than are expended through activity. In this case, excess energy is stored as fat. Chapter 28 includes a more detailed discussion of energy balance and metabolism.

FITNESS

Fitness is the ability to sustain vigorous physical exertion without overtaxing cardiopulmonary or muscular capacity. It implies optimal functioning of all body systems. The following criteria define the type and intensity of exercise needed for fitness.[1]

- Use large muscles in rhythmic, repetitive movements.
- Maintain 60 to 90 percent of maximal heart rate.
- Exercise three to five times per week.
- Maintain continuous activity for 20 to 60 minutes.

Examples of appropriate large muscle exercise include swimming, walking, running, cycling, and rowing. Accurately determining one's maximal heart rate (HR_{max}) requires graded exercise testing. A person can estimate HR_{max} by subtracting his or her age from 220. It is best to start an exercise program at 60 percent of HR_{max}, then gradually increase the target heart rate.

In 1990, the US Department of Health and Human Services sought to make Americans more aware of the benefits of physical fitness and exercise. A DHHS publication, *Healthy People 2000*, set high goals for the numbers of Americans who would participate in regular vigorous exercise. Moderate exercise was also encouraged. As we move through the 1990s, it is clear that most of the goals set forth in *Healthy People 2000* are not being met. The 1996 *Surgeon General's Report on Physical Activity and Health*[2] stated that more than 60 percent of adults did not exercise regularly and 25 percent did not exercise at all. Other studies report that only 20 percent of Americans are active.[3,4]

According to many experts, at least part of the reason for such low levels of participation in exercise is the public perception that exercise must be strenuous to have beneficial effects. Because evidence is mounting that light to moderate exercise also confers health benefits, the thrust of the new Surgeon General's report is to emphasize the benefit of any physical activity. The report stresses that more exercise is better, but indicates that physical activity that uses 150 calories per day (15 minutes of running or 30 minutes of brisk walking) significantly reduces risk factors associated with a sedentary lifestyle.[2] Encouraging physicians and other health care providers to inquire about patient's exercise habits and provide

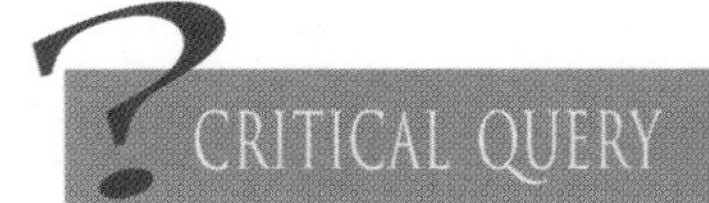

The 1996 Surgeon General's Report on Physical Activity and Health[2] and other research indicates that the majority of Americans do not exercise. However, there is ample evidence that physical activity has a positive effect on health status and general well-being. How can individuals be influenced to change their sedentary habits? Who should be involved in efforts to bring about this change?

information about the benefits of physical activity is one of the goals stated in the report.

Nurses have many opportunities to educate patients about fitness and physical activity. Information about the components of fitness, the benefits of various levels of exercise, and types of exercise programs can be part of health teaching in many types of health care and community settings. Many people assume that fitness programs are unpleasant, strenuous, even boring. Emphasis on the variety of fitness programs and on social and recreational aspects of fitness can help to change these perceptions and attitudes.

Components of Fitness

Fitness has four components: body composition, strength, flexibility, and endurance. Different sorts of activity promote each component.

Body Composition. Body composition refers to maintaining a healthy body weight. It is impossible to be really fit if one is grossly overweight or underweight. Individuals who are physically fit have a lower percentage of body fat and greater lean body mass (body weight minus fat content) than individuals who are not. Height–weight tables are available that describe a healthy weight range for persons of both sexes of varying age and body build (see Table 12–2).

The concept of energy balance, discussed previously, is relevant here. People who maintain this state will remain at a stable weight. Overweight individuals should strive for a negative energy balance, one in which energy expenditure exceeds energy (caloric) intake. Underweight individuals should aim for the converse. A balanced diet is critical to achieving a healthy energy balance. Refer to Chap. 28 for more information about diet and nutrition.

Strength. **Strength** refers to force exerted against resistance by a muscle or group of muscles. Isotonic, isometric, and isokinetic exercises are effective for building strength. **Isotonic exercises,** such as lifting free weights, are exercises in which the tension within a muscle remains constant as its length changes to move the resistance (weight). **Isokinetic exercise** requires movement through a joint's full range of motion while maintaining consistent tension on muscles. Computerized exercise equipment is necessary for isokinetic exercise. **Isometric exercise** involves near-maximal contraction against a fixed object. The length of the muscle does not change, because there is no joint movement during the contraction. Strength training results in hypertrophy of individual muscle fibers, increases the number of active muscle fibers, and decreases the amount of fat within a muscle.

Flexibility. Developing flexibility requires joint movement. The amount of movement possible at a given joint defines **flexibility.**

Stretching, yoga, and calisthenics increase joint range of motion. Isokinetic and isotonic exercise can increase flexibility as well as strength.

Endurance. **Endurance** refers to a person's ability to persist in the performance of an activity without becoming fatigued. Endurance incorporates cardiorespiratory efficiency and muscular efficiency. It requires whole-body **aerobic exercise.** Exercise is considered aerobic when it increases the body's oxygen consumption for a sustained period of time (at least 5 minutes). Aerobic exercise produces a sustained increase in heart rate and stroke volume. Activities that provide continuous cardiorespiratory demand, such as jogging, swimming, or basketball, contribute to endurance. Sprinting, which immediately depletes the cardiorespiratory reserve, is not aerobic. Aerobic activities lead to improved oxygen use by muscles, increased vascularity in cardiac and striated muscle, increased oxidation of fat for energy, and more effective aerobic metabolism of ATP.

Benefits of Regular Exercise

A consistent exercise program results in beneficial adaptations that contribute to overall well-being. Recent recommendations shift the emphasis from intensity of exercise to frequency. The Centers for Disease Control and Prevention (CDC) encourage accumulating 30 minutes or more of physical activity on 5 or more consecutive days of the week to achieve at least some of the benefits listed here.[5] Exercise of sufficient intensity, frequency, and duration to achieve and maintain fitness confers greater gains in all of the functions listed.

- *Greater cardiac efficiency:* increased stroke volume and overall cardiac output, lower resting heart rate and blood pressure, smaller increase in heart rate with moderate activity, greater tolerance for near-maximum heart rate, and faster return to baseline after exercise.
- *Improved pulmonary functioning:* expanded vital capacity, diminished dead space, maximal oxygen intake during exercise, smaller increase in respiratory rate and depth during exercise.
- *Improved circulation:* development of new capillaries in muscles, increased production of red blood cells and hemoglobin, decreased peripheral resistance, lower incidence of pathologic clotting, decreased tendency toward plaque deposits, better delivery of oxygen and nutrients to tissues and elimination of wastes, more efficient dissipation of heat.
- *Better neuromuscular coordination:* elimination of unnecessary movements, simpler more automatic motions, reduced energy to perform a skill.
- *Improved muscle functioning:* increased tone and strength; more rapid contractions; capacity for longer sustained activity; faster oxygen uptake; more efficient use of oxygen; greater storage of ATP and phosphocreatine; more efficient use of fatty acids during exercise, sparing glycogen.
- *Increased bone density and strength:* bone hypertrophy due to weight bearing against gravity, increased mineral content; of particular benefit to females to prevent postmenopausal osteoporosis.[6]
- *Improved digestion and metabolism:* more efficient use of carbohydrates, altered fat metabolism resulting in lower serum triglycerides and increased HDL (high-density lipoprotein) level, improved gastrointestinal motility.
- *Enhanced elimination of wastes:* increased lung and skin excretion, better elimination via intestine because of enhanced motility, improved urinary excretion because of less shunting away from kidneys during exercise when fit.
- *Achieving and maintaining appropriate body weight:* reduced total body fat, increased lean body mass, correction of obesity when fat intake is also reduced.
- *Enhanced psychological well-being:* reduced stress related to emotional release and lower catecholamine levels, euphoria related to endorphin release, improved body image and self-concept, decreased anxiety and depressive symptoms.
- *Improved cognitive functioning:* improved academic performance in children and improved performance on cognitive tests in adults.
- *Protection against disease:* protection against heart disease, high blood pressure, atherosclerosis, osteoporosis, arthritis, lipid disorders, colon cancer, and diabetes.[2,4,6,7]

Individuals can achieve these all-encompassing benefits by a commitment to a lifetime habit of regular physical activity. Nurses have a responsibility to teach patients the benefits of regular, prudent exercise. Our credibility as teachers will be greater if we demonstrate at least a moderate level of fitness ourselves.

Risks Associated with Exercise

Despite all of the advantages and benefits associated with a lifestyle that includes regular exercise, physical activity is not without risk. This is true for those participating at a recreational level as well as for elite athletes. Most exercise-related risks are associated with incorrect performance or inappropriate intensity of exercise for an individual's level of fitness. These injuries, although temporarily disabling, are not usually serious or life-threatening. The potential effects of exercise on those at risk for cardiovascular or other diseases is of greater concern, however.

Complications of Preexisting Disease. Apparently healthy active exercise participants under the age of 35, competitive athletes, children, and adolescents are considered to have no major risk factors that would prevent exercise participation. With appropriate training techniques, they are able to avoid significant injury. Sedentary individuals or recreational exercisers over 45 years old, and those of any age with symptoms of or known risk factors for liver, thyroid, or renal disease or diabetes, risk complications associated with exercise. They should undergo health assessment prior to beginning an exercise program. Those at highest risk include individuals with a known pulmonary, metabolic, or cardiovascular disease. They not only require pre-exercise screening, but should undergo periodic assessments as well. This latter group, in particular those with cardiovascular disease, is at the highest risk for sudden cardiac death related to exercise. Despite substantial evidence that exercise training is beneficial for individuals with coronary artery disease and is likely to extend their life expectancy, careful screening and lower-intensity exercise is strongly suggested.

Musculoskeletal Injuries. There are two basic types of exercise-related musculoskeletal injuries: acute injuries and overuse injuries. Both should be distinguished from stiffness after exercise or transient ischemic pain during exercise. These discomforts are common when extending the limits of workouts to improve performance, but don't indicate actual tissue damage.

Strains and sprains are the most common types of acute injuries related to exercise. They occur most commonly among "weekend" athletes who most often exercise in bursts without the benefit of warming up. *Strains* or "pulls" are injuries to muscles or tendon attachments. They occur when a muscle is vigorously overstretched, such as when forcefully throwing a ball, stroking a tennis racket, or lifting a heavy object. Depending on the number of muscle fibers involved, the injury may be mild to severe. *Sprains* involve ligaments and joint capsules. They most often occur with rapid changes of direction or sudden starts and stops. Sprains are usually more severe than strains. Bone fractures can also occur as a result of exercise, but are less common.

Overuse injuries develop gradually from a repetitive activity. They are typical when a person regularly performs the same types of exercise, such as running. Often overuse injuries have no obvious cause. They are the result of gradual microscopic injuries due to pushing beyond the body's ability to absorb the force of exercise. If exercise is continued despite the injury, the damage is extended and an acute injury at the site of the weakness is likely. Tendinitis (inflammation of a tendon) and stress fractures are examples of overuse injuries.

Negative Psychological Consequences. Some people who participate in regular, frequent exercise experience *exercise addiction*, characterized by feelings of irritability, restlessness, and fatigue when unable to exercise.[8] *Tolerance*, the need to constantly increase the amount one exercises in order to feel good about oneself, is another characteristic of this condition. Experts are divided on whether the symptoms are principally related to other psychological events in one's life so that exercise becomes an escape; are a result of obsessive traits that drive other behaviors as well as exercise behaviors; or have other origins. Research has identified no risk factors for this condition. Individuals experiencing any of the symptoms suggestive of exercise addiction generally benefit from counseling to identify potential stressors and assist in modifying responses. It is worth noting that the concept of positive addiction has also been applied to exercise. In this concept the enhanced well-being that regular exercisers derive provides continued motivation to participate in exercise, but does not generate symptoms of tolerance and withdrawal described above.

Trauma Related to Extremes of Temperature. Because exercise generates heat, efficient heat dissipation is necessary to maintain normal body temperature during strenuous exercise. Exercise in hot, humid weather makes efficient cooling more difficult, even for well-conditioned individuals. It is especially stressful for those who are less fit. Profuse perspiration leading to dehydration is likely. More serious heat effects such as heat exhaustion and heat stroke occur if exercise continues.

Hypothermia and frostbite can be a consequence of exercise in cold environments. They are more likely if protective clothing becomes wet and when wearing insufficient protective clothing. Prolonged exercise with little fluid intake leads to dehydration and increases the risk of hypothermia, even at relatively mild temperatures. Hypothermia is discussed further in Chap. 17.

FACTORS AFFECTING MOBILITY

Because mobility is to a large degree under voluntary control, a person's level of mobility is influenced by personal choices. Although physiologic limitations and psychological attributes influence mobility, they can often be overcome or altered if one is highly motivated. Physiologic factors that may limit mobility include age, disability, and health status. Self-concept, emotions, motivations, values and beliefs, lifestyle, and personal definition of health can have a positive or negative impact on mobility.

AGE

Mobility develops rapidly during the infant and toddler periods. It is refined and expanded throughout childhood and adolescence. Strength, endurance, and coordination continue to increase throughout adolescence and into young adulthood. Individuals who desire to can continue to increase their level of fitness into middle adulthood and maintain fitness into late adulthood. However, age-related changes ultimately create a constraining influence.[9] There is gradual loss of strength related to a decrease in size of muscle fibers and altered hormonal and metabolic function. Neurologic alterations including slowed conduction velocity and diminished amounts of neurotransmitter substances contribute as well. Joint changes interfere with mobility as individuals age. Cartilage thickens and its surface roughens due to the stress of long-term use. This causes joint irritation and risk for osteoarthritis. Bones lose density and strength and develop bone spurs, which increases the tendency for joint irritation.

Aging also affects cardiovascular and respiratory fitness. The resting stroke volume falls gradually from ages 25 to 85. The maximum attainable heart rate falls and resting and exercise blood pressure rise due to loss of elasticity in major blood vessels. Lung vital capacity decreases, and the length of time necessary for heart rate, blood pressure, and oxygen consumption to return to baseline after exercise is longer.

The timing of all of these changes is highly variable. An active lifestyle and good general health can delay both their onset and progression, as well as reverse some age-related changes.[6,9,10] In fact some researchers believe that it is difficult to separate the effects of factors such as heredity and lifestyle from those generally associated with aging.[11]

DISABILITY

Disability refers to impaired ability to perform usual activities expected for a given age. Congenital abnormalities, trauma, or disease may cause disability. Neurologic, musculoskeletal, and cardiorespiratory problems are most likely to interfere with mobility.

HEALTH STATUS

Acute and chronic illnesses can affect mobility. Most individuals curtail activity as a consequence of diminished well-being associated with illness. Some illnesses interfere with mobility by causing weakness, impaired oxygenation, or pain. Sometimes activity limitations are imposed as part of therapy. As detailed later in the discussion of altered mobility, there are often as many risks associated with therapeutic rest as there are benefits.

SELF-CONCEPT AND EMOTIONS

Mobility has a reciprocal relationship to self-concept. Developing a healthy self-image requires mastery of a variety of skills and tasks, many of which require coordinated movement (see Chap. 12). Participation in childhood games and sports develops muscle coordination and promotes a sense of accomplishment, both of which enhance a positive self-concept.[12] In adolescence, the importance of mobility to healthy self-concept continues to be evident. Not only is there renewed emphasis on athletic performance, but popular adolescent social activities such as dancing also require coordinated movements. Children or adolescents unable to match the performance of peers may retain a persistent image of themselves as clumsy and inadequate. This negative self-concept can actually limit mobility by causing these individuals to avoid participating in sports and exercise during adulthood, compromising physical, social, and emotional health.[13] If individuals with a poor self-concept begin to increase their activity level and become regular exercisers, their self-concept often improves considerably.[14]

Emotional status also affects ability to move about freely. One of the symptoms of depression is a low energy level with minimal or very slow movement. Another example of the relationship between emotions and mobility occurs with stress. Stress is often localized in the muscles. Setting of the jaw and tension in the neck muscles are characteristics of emotional strain. Alexander Lowen[15] has postulated that chronic muscular tension or "muscular armoring" results from continuing emotional conflict. This armoring can cause abnormal body posture and interfere with fluid movement.

The role of motivation and personality in determining the amount or type of mobility or exercise in which an individual engages deserves mention. C. L. Hull[16] believed that along with such commonly recognized drives as hunger and thirst, there also exists an activity drive. This drive is expressed in a variety of ways, from exploration of one's environment to participation in organized physical activity such as sports and games. Not all theorists accept the concept of an innate drive for activity, but most recognize the influence of motivation. The motivation to engage in activity may be complex and related to other anticipated benefits such as health, social experiences, or a shapely body rather than purely for the sake of activity itself.

VALUES AND BELIEFS

Values and beliefs influence motivation and behavior. An individual's definition of health and the value placed on health strongly influence choices related to activity and mobility.[17,18] For some, exercise is synonymous with health. They consider regular exercise essential to well-being and would not define themselves as healthy if unable to exercise. This definition of health and the high value placed on feeling fit would demand and enhance a significant level of mobility. Others place less emphasis on activity as a measure of health. They may place greater value on pursuits congruent with a sedentary lifestyle and feel no particular motivation to be physically active as well. They would be likely to be content with a lower level of mobility, requiring only that sufficient for basic activities of daily living to consider themselves healthy. Many individuals value balance among physical and other types of pursuits and strive for excellence or at least participation in many different life activities. The influence of health beliefs and one's concepts about personal efficacy and locus of control on health and health-related choices are discussed in greater detail in Chaps. 7, 13, and 25.

LIFESTYLE

Health status, values, beliefs, motivation, and self-concept, among other factors, influence lifestyle (see Chap. 26). Lifestyle influences mobility. Pender[19] considers lifestyle an expression of health, and activity one of the dimensions through which it is expressed. She defines activity as encompassing meaningful work, meaningful play, and positive life patterns such as eating well, exercising regularly, resting adequately, and managing stress. To the extent that individuals share these ideas, their lifestyle will be an active one, in which choices for leisure, social, and avocational endeavors will involve mobility. Their choice of an active lifestyle will even be evident in small ways, such as their walking or cycling on errands rather than driving, or using stairs rather than elevators. Likewise, lifestyle choices may be sedentary, reflecting other values and beliefs and not enhancing or emphasizing mobility.

ALTERED FUNCTION ASSOCIATED WITH LIMITED MOBILITY

Altered mobility occurs at many levels and for diverse reasons. Whatever the reason for diminished activity, predictable detrimental effects occur. These effects, called **disuse phenomena** or the **disuse syndrome,** occur at all levels of inactivity. The greater the activity limitation and/or health impairment at the onset of restricted activity, the more serious the disuse effects. For example, a healthy, active man of 23 who remains in bed for 5 days because of influenza, would be at lesser risk for disuse phenomena than a 60-year-old man already weakened by a chronic disease who became ill with influenza. If the 23-year-old were to remain on bed rest for several weeks because of a more serious health problem, his risk for disuse problems would increase.

Section 2 of this chapter, *Assessment of Mobility,* provides a framework for identifying mobility problems and, predicting risk for developing immobility-related problems.

ACTIVITY AND MOBILITY PROBLEMS

Inactivity limits options for activity. Greatly restricted exercise results in bone, muscle, and joint changes that inhibit normal mobility. Because the drive for motor activity is diminished after deconditioning, restoring functional mobility can be challenging. Even well-conditioned individuals who experience a short-term period of diminished activity may find returning to their former exercise routine requires considerable mental discipline. However, they will probably not experience the serious musculoskeletal problems associated with more extensive limitation of activity, discussed next.

Bone Changes

Bone integrity is normally maintained by complimentary functioning of osteoblasts and osteoclasts. In a state of wellness, weight bearing and large muscle activities stimulate osteoblasts to generate new bone matrix. This new tissue replaces that destroyed by osteoclasts, keeping living bone in a state of dynamic equilibrium. When bedrest or diminished muscle activity is prolonged, bone building ceases while destruction of bone continues. This releases calcium and phosphorus into the bloodstream. The demineralization results in *osteoporosis*—literally, porous bone. The rate of loss of bone density because of immobility is most rapid in weight-bearing bones. Although osteoporosis also occurs as a normal aspect of aging, lack of exercise hastens the process.

Immobility-induced osteoporosis takes place in several stages. The initial stage occurs in the first 12 weeks of immobility. It is the most rapid, but is also readily reversible with return to weight bearing. If immobility continues, bone loss continues at a slower pace. Ultimately, people whose immobility is very long term or permanent may lose more than half of their bone volume. Bone loss associated with long-term immobility is irreversible. Bones weakened as a result of osteoporosis are easily deformed and fracture readily. A significant percent of fractures among the elderly are a result of osteoporosis.

Muscle Changes

Like bones, muscles depend on activity to function efficiently. The demands of exercise cause an increase in the size and strength of muscles, as discussed earlier. The opposite occurs when activity is reduced. Muscles **atrophy,** that is, decrease in size. Circulation to muscles is reduced and muscle protein is lost. This results in shortened muscle fibers as well as diminished tone and strength. Endurance declines and muscles become stiff. The flabby appearance of inactive middle-aged adults represents a less severe form of this phenomenon.

Severe muscle wasting is associated with prolonged bedrest. The lower leg muscles that are ordinarily used to resist gravity are the first muscles to weaken and atrophy when recumbent. Muscles also lose oxidative efficiency when they are inactive. This means that when exercise is attempted, oxygen debt occurs sooner and lactic acid builds up more rapidly.

Joint Changes

Flexibility is diminished with inactivity. Shortened muscle fibers contribute to this. Also, healthy sedentary people experience relatively minor muscle shortening, connective tissue changes involving ligaments, tendons, and the joint capsule. These changes are more severe with bedrest. When confined to bed, individuals frequently assume flexed positions, favoring shortening of the flexor muscles. The position of comfort assumed by many patients fosters flexion contractures of the knees and hips and plantar flexion (foot drop). As the muscles become increasingly resistant to stretching, the range of motion (ROM) of the joints is diminished. This compromises walking and self-care. Contractures may eventually become so severe as to require surgical intervention.

REST AND SLEEP PROBLEMS

Rest implies a sense of tranquility or relaxation. Sleeping is a necessary form of rest. The prescription to curtail activity or to remain in bed is usually based on the assumption that increased rest will be the result. This is not always the case.

Regular physical exercise promotes restful sleep. Increased amounts of stage 3 and 4 sleep occur after exercise. Individuals deprived of regular exercise may find restful sleep difficult to attain. Sedentary people sometimes experience a chronic diminution of the deeper stages of sleep. A sleep period with less time in deep sleep is less restorative. One may awaken unrefreshed, with a lingering sense of fatigue.

A prescribed activity restriction is often emotionally stressful and can compound the physiologic stress associated with illness or injury. This state of tension may make relaxation and sleep difficult. If the treatment requires being in a hospital, the stress may be greater, for many people have problems sleeping in an unfamiliar environment. Also, the usual sleep–wakefulness rhythm is disturbed by inactivity. Daytime napping is common, but naps may actually diminish the quality of nighttime sleep by decreasing the amount of deep (stages 3 and 4) sleep. Sleep and rest are the subject of Chap. 31.

INSIGHTS FROM NURSING LITERATURE

REVERSING THE EFFECTS OF BEDREST

St. Pierre BA, Flaskerud JH. Clinical nursing implications for the recovery of atrophied skeletal muscle following bedrest. Rehabil Nurs. *1995;20:314–317, 354.*

The authors reviewed several studies done on animal models that simulated the effects of bedrest on skeletal muscles. These studies showed that several physiologic changes occur in muscle disuse, including muscle fiber damage, death, and regeneration. The recovery process involves inflammation and a shift of white blood cells (macrophages) to the damaged tissue.

Noting that similar changes may occur in the muscles of patients after a period of bedrest, the authors review nursing measures to support recovery. They recommend that nurses (1) monitor patients who are resuming activity for symptoms of decreased strength and/or fatigue; (2) encourage sufficient protein intake to ensure muscle repair; and (3) avoid the use of immunosuppressive therapy, if possible, to ensure adequate macrophage function during the muscle recovery process.

OXYGENATION PROBLEMS

Oxygenation involves taking oxygen into the body (ventilation), moving it from the lungs into the bloodstream (diffusion), transporting it to the tissues (perfusion), and moving it into the tissues from the bloodstream. All of these processes are less efficient in sedentary individuals. They are compromised when well-conditioned individuals are inactive for a period of time.

Decreased metabolic demands associated with limited activity cause reduction in depth of respiration. Shallow respirations promote alveolar collapse, reducing the functional lung surface area. This effect is enhanced when recumbent. Abdominal organs then exert pressure on the diaphragm and constrict the size of the chest cavity. Weakening of the accessory muscles used in respiration also contributes to decreased oxygen and carbon dioxide exchange.

Another factor interfering with ventilation and diffusion when individuals are confined to bed is pooling of mucus. Mucus is normally distributed evenly around the lumen of the bronchi. The action of gravity in the supine position favors collection of secretions in the dependent portion of the tubes, and drying of the upper portion. The pooling and drying interfere with the functioning of the cilia, resulting in still more pooling.

Generalized weakness related to the primary disease process or to bedrest and the supine position decrease the effectiveness of coughing. The static secretions become obstructive and are an excellent medium for the growth of microorganisms. A resulting complication is pneumonia.

A period of bedrest as short as 3 to 5 days leads to cardiovascular deconditioning, which compromises perfusion. The initial cardiovascular effect of bedrest is increased cardiac workload. This occurs as a result of a greater circulating blood volume because of less capillary pooling when legs are not dependent.[20] After this initial increase, cardiac output and stroke volume progressively decrease and oxygen uptake diminishes. The loss of cardiopulmonary efficiency is manifested by a higher resting pulse and considerably reduced stamina and endurance.

Patients confined to bed often use the Valsalva maneuver when using the trunk and arm muscles to change positions. The **Valsalva maneuver** is attempting a forced expiration with the glottis closed. No movement of air occurs, but intrathoracic pressure increases, thereby decreasing blood flow in the major thoracic and coronary blood vessels. When the breath is suddenly released, the thoracic pressure falls and a surge of blood flows into the heart. The myocardium stretches more to accommodate the larger blood volume and contracts more forcefully to eject it. This may strain cardiac capacity in debilitated patients, causing arrhythmias and temporarily compromised perfusion.

Orthostatic (postural) hypotension, a precipitous drop in blood pressure associated with standing, is another bedrest-related phenomenon that interferes with perfusion. When active individuals rise from a recumbent position, reflex vasoconstriction of peripheral arterioles maintains blood pressure and blood supply to the brain. This reflex is dulled with bedrest. Therefore, vessels remain dilated, blood pools in the legs upon standing, and central blood pressure falls. Patients feel dizzy and light-headed and may faint because less blood is delivered to the brain.

Perfusion may also be altered when on bedrest by **DVT (deep vein thrombosis).** The formation of clots (thrombi) is enhanced by increased coagulability, venous stasis, and damage to the intima of the vein walls. Bedrest induces two of these three factors and often plays a role in the third. Increased coagulability occurs because bedrest lowers plasma volume. This raises blood viscosity, which enhances the potential for clotting.[21] If patients are not well hydrated, the increase in blood viscosity and the possibility of DVT is further magnified. Venous stasis occurs during bedrest because of the lack of pumping action of the calf muscles. There is often additional interference with blood return because of improper positioning. For example, many patients favor a semi-Fowler's (sitting) position when on bedrest. They often adjust the bed so their knees are bent to prevent slipping toward the foot of the bed. This creates pressure on the veins behind the knee and interference with venous return. A similar problem occurs when side-lying with the superior leg resting on the dependent leg. Moreover, pressure on vessels in each of these situations may irritate or damage the inside of the blood vessels, therefore establishing the third contributing factor to thrombus formation. Clots compromise local circulation or may become dislodged and move through the circulatory system. This is called an *embolism*. *Pulmonary embolism,* a clot that lodges in the pulmonary artery or one of its branches, is a life-threatening complication of DVT.

Another serious result of decreased perfusion is pressure ulcers. When patients are improperly positioned or remain in one position for more than 1 hour, external capillary pressure at bony prominences may increase as much as tenfold, making the exchange of oxygen, nutrients, and wastes impossible. This ischemia brings about *necrosis* (tissue death) of skin and underlying tissues, a pressure ulcer or pressure sore (see discussion in Chap. 27). Figure 33–1 shows the pressure points at which pressure ulcers are most likely to develop in common positions. Patients at high risk for developing pressure ulcers include the following:

- *Patients with limited mobility* whose activity is restricted to bed or chair, who have limited limb mobility, or who are unconscious, paralyzed, and/or heavily sedated.
- *Obese patients,* whose weight and dense subcutaneous tissue create greater external pressure on capillaries over bony prominences.
- *Patients with edema.* Edematous tissue is more vulnerable to circulatory interference because the edema fluid creates a barrier to exchange of oxygen, nutrients, and wastes.
- *Poorly nourished patients.* Meager amounts of subcutaneous tissue and weakened collagen and elastin diminish tissue capacity to absorb and tolerate pressure. Diminished tissue perfusion secondary to nutritional anemia further compromises resistance to pressure.
- *Patients who are incontinent.* Urine and feces are irritating to skin, and dampness causes tissue maceration. Inflamed and macerated tissue is more vulnerable to breakdown.
- *Patients favoring Fowler's position.* Sitting upright against the raised mattress exposes the skin over the sacrum and heels to shearing force. Shearing force results from the simultaneous downward and forward pressures created as people slide gradually toward the foot of the bed. It tears the skin surfaces and damages capillaries and deeper tissues.

These risks are highlighted in Clinical Guideline 33–1.

NUTRITIONAL PROBLEMS

A healthy energy balance is difficult for inactive individuals to attain. More frequently, they remain in positive energy balance, which leads to weight gain. Sedentary individuals are frequently overweight.

Patients whose activity and environment are restricted by bedrest frequently have a poor appetite (anorexia). This may seem to be a beneficial effect, because caloric needs are diminished when activity is decreased. When bedrest is prescribed, however, it is usually to facilitate tissue repair. In this case, the body's demand for certain nutrients is greatly increased (see Chap. 28).

The anorexia is compounded by altered metabolism associated with decreased activity. When on bedrest, anabolic processes are slowed, while catabolic processes accelerate. Weight is lost, primarily lean body mass rather than fat. Inactive individuals on bedrest develop carbohydrate intolerance. Inactivity seems to increase resistance to endogenous insulin (insulin produced within the body), so that even though serum levels are at or above normal, carbohydrate metabolism is not optimum.

Protein metabolism is also altered. Protein synthesis is reduced and protein breakdown is increased. The increase in nitrogenous wastes resulting from the breakdown of protein pre-

CLINICAL GUIDELINE 33–1

RISK FACTORS FOR DEVELOPING PRESSURE ULCERS

- Limited mobility
- Obesity
- Edema
- Poor nutritional state
- Incontinence
- Prolonged use of Fowler's position

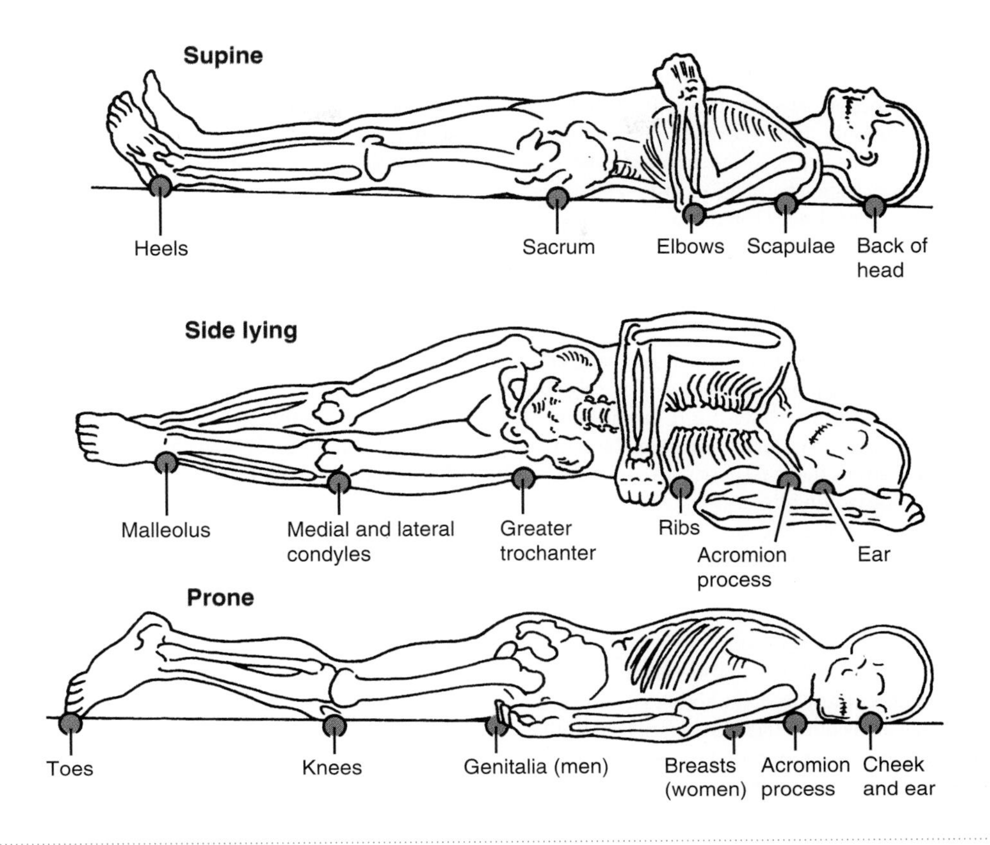

Figure 33–1. Pressure points in common positions.

cipitates a state of negative nitrogen balance: excretion of nitrogenous products (from protein catabolism) exceeding their ingestion. Negative nitrogen balance causes diminished interest in food. If the lack of desire for food results in reduced intake and/or a nutritionally unbalanced diet, increasingly greater needs for nutrients in the face of a paradoxical decrease in appetite will prolong the recovery period.

Anorexia may also cause decreased fluid intake. Several changes in fluid metabolism discussed in the next section actually increase patients' fluid needs when on bedrest. As in the case of nutrients, the greater need accompanied by reduced desire often results in complications.

FLUID AND ELIMINATION PROBLEMS

All of the body's processes for elimination of waste products are altered by inactivity. The effect on carbon dioxide excretion via the lungs was discussed earlier.

Skin

Being sedentary produces no appreciable change in excretion of wastes by the skin. Although there is less obvious perspiration when one in not actively exercising, insensible losses continue. When one is confined to bed, there is increased loss of water, sodium, potassium, and chloride via the skin. Dilation of blood vessels occurs, which raises the skin temperature and therefore promotes perspiration, especially in areas where skin surfaces touch. Sheets and blankets prevent heat loss by irradiation and conduction, which also stimulates sweating. This profuse perspiration, called diaphoresis, contributes to skin breakdown and general discomfort.

Kidney

Bedrest creates demands on kidney function. As a result of the catabolic processes previously discussed, serum levels of calcium, phosphorous, and nitrogenous wastes increase significantly. This intensifies the filtration load in the glomeruli. Expanded circulating blood volume due to recumbency gives rise to *diuresis* (increased urine output) and subsequent loss of plasma volume. This is because antidiuretic hormone (ADH) is suppressed when central blood volume increases, and because the glomerular filtration rate (GFR) is greater when renal blood flow is increased. Unless fluid intake is augmented, the effect of a lower plasma volume and higher levels of wastes is a rise in urine specific gravity. High urine specific gravity is related to another problem, renal calculi, discussed later in this section.

The increased production of urine creates a need for more frequent voiding. Some patients confined to bed, however, have difficulty with voluntary relaxation of the external sphincter. Using the bedpan or urinal may be embarrassing or uncomfortably awkward. Thus, patients may suppress the urge to void, causing urinary stasis. Gradually, the detrusor muscle becomes stretched and less sensitive. Bladder distension without the accompanying urge to void increases the intravesicular pressure. This can be transmitted to the kidney via the ureters, damaging the nephron or result in overflow incontinence.

Urinary stasis predisposes patients to two further problems, *urinary tract infection* and *renal calculi* (stones). Ordinarily, the bladder is rather resistant to infection. Despite frequent exposure to microorganisms, most commonly from normal gastrointestinal flora, infection rarely occurs. This is due to the inherent antimicrobial properties of the bladder mucosa, phagocytosis, and to the mechanical flushing action of voiding. Distension of the bladder reduces mucosal blood flow, however. Ischemic tissue is less resistant to invasion by microorganisms. Additionally, the urine of a person on bed rest becomes alkaline, favoring the growth of certain bacteria.

Static urine and the presence of bacteria enhance calculus formation. High levels of serum calcium, discussed earlier, promote precipitation of crystals in the urine, which form the nucleus of stones. *Lithiasis* (stone) formation can occur anywhere in the urinary tract, but in the recumbent position, the renal pelvis is a common site. These stones become quite large, giving rise to a characteristic severe colicky pain. The presence of stones and damage to the mucosa caused by movement of the stones increases the risk of infection, creating a cycle of stone formation and bacterial proliferation.

Bowel

Bowel elimination requires motility of intestinal smooth muscle and voluntary contraction of skeletal muscles of the abdomen and pelvic floor. Inactivity can interfere with both of these aspects of bowel elimination. Constipation is a common complication of bedrest and, not infrequently, a problem of sedentary individuals. Active exercise stimulates peristalsis and strengthens abdominal muscles. Conversely, intestinal motility is diminished with inactivity, and the loss of muscle tone associated with bedrest weakens the abdominal muscles. If using a bedpan is necessary, defecation is even more difficult, for the physiologic squatting position cannot be used.

Dietary changes due to illness or lack of appetite and changes in daily schedules or routines interfere with usual bowel habits, compounding the risk for constipation. Lack of privacy also contributes to constipation in hospitalized patients. Patients confined to bed may ignore the urge to defecate due to embarrassment associated with minimal screening and the unavoidable proximity of others. Repeated suppression of defecation diminishes sensitivity to rectal distension and produces a harder, drier stool that is more difficult to eliminate. A more serious complication, *fecal impaction*, may then result (see also Chap. 29).

SEXUAL PROBLEMS

There is no consistent relationship between sexual dysfunction and a physically inactive lifestyle. However, mobility restrictions because of illness, injury, or their treatment are potentially disruptive to meeting sexual needs. Being ill or depressed because of loss of independence may consume physical and emotional energy to such an extent that libido is diminished. This situation may be more stressful for the sexual partner than for the individual who is ill. Although illness does not always cause disinterest in sexual activity, some types of illness or injuries make usual sexual relations physically impossible on a temporary or permanent basis. In these situations, counseling assistance should be considered.

If immobility is imposed in an inpatient setting, achieving sexual satisfaction is directly inhibited. Any sexual expressions involving a partner are impossible. Rarely is there adequate privacy even for masturbation, which is a natural substitute under these circumstances. The resulting sexual frustration can add to the overall stress of being ill.

Self-concept alterations related to loss of mobility (see next section) can also have a significant impact on sexuality and sexual expression. Feelings of inadequacy or dependency, or believing that one is no longer attractive lead to fears of rejection by one's partner. These fears may diminish sex drive and even cause impotence. As a result, patients often withdraw from their partners. This can cause conflict and sexual tension between partners.

PSYCHOLOGICAL PROBLEMS

As discussed above, being physically active and physically fit contributes to a positive self-image and increased self-esteem. It is also true that many people who choose a sedentary lifestyle have a tendency to be overweight. Many have less self-esteem and are less satisfied with their bodies than physically active people. These feelings sometimes produce social withdrawal, particularly from group activities that involve sports or exertion. Those who must restrict their activity because of a diminished level of wellness often experience a similar loss of social options; however, prolonged restriction of mobility has even more far reaching psychological effects.

Immobility alters identity. Some of the complex components comprising who we are—self-concept, body image, relationships, perceptions, emotions, drives, roles, and choices—are modified when the ability to move about is partially or entirely curtailed. Moreover, physical mobility enhances psychological mobility. Moving through one's environment facilitates emotional contact with people and objects within it. Restricted physical mobility limits individuals' control over their interactions with others. This loss of control is most dramatic for those confined to bed. Rather than seeking out or initiating exchanges with others, they must wait for others to initiate. There is a significant limitation of personal space when immobilized. This, too, is a potential stressor.

The American culture ascribes great significance to productivity and participation. Involuntary limitation of involvement in desired activities is a major stressor. Valued roles are threatened in the family, workplace, and social contexts. When the ability to move about is critical for job performance, or being physically fit is central to self-concept, restricted movement may dramatically affect emotional status. This may occur even if the restriction is recognized as temporary.

Exercise is also a healthy way to dissipate stress. When illness or injury interferes with opportunities to engage in exercise, the result is often more intense feelings of stress and an increase in stress-related behaviors. The restrictions and changes produce role conflict, altered body image, and disturbed self-concept. These alterations may cause immobilized individuals to experience a greatly diminished sense of worth.

Withdrawal and apathy, which delay recovery and compound the reduction in self-esteem, are potential manifestations. Conversely, anger, hostility, frustration, or even guilt may be responses to the loss of power to make choices. Mood changes are common. Many people become preoccupied with themselves and with bodily functions. When the disability is prolonged or permanent, these reactions are typically more intense. The behaviors characteristic of the grieving process—denial, anger, and bargaining—are common.

Immobility also affects perception. A reduction in environmental stimuli (sensory deprivation), which occurs when a person is confined to a small space such as a bed, impairs the ability to interpret pattern, form, time, pressure, and temperature. Sensory deprivation compromises both motivation and capacity to learn cognitive and motor skills. The learning and perceptual deficits restrict problem solving ability, further threatening independence and self-esteem.

The far-reaching effects of immobility on all body systems and on all human needs underline the need for patient–nurse collaboration to identify creative, holistic approaches to care. Nurses must be alert to clues indicating immobility-related problems in patients with all levels of mobility curtailment, from inactivity to complete bedrest. Individual differences result in a wide range of reactions, not necessarily directly related to the degree of limitation. The following sections provide guides for nursing assessment and management of problems related to alterations in mobility.

COLLABORATIVE STRATEGY

THE PROBLEMS OF IMMOBILITY

Having one's mobility curtailed can be stressful, physically and mentally. Diligent care is needed to prevent the many complications of immobility. Collaborating with patients in assessing for manifestations of complications is essential until mobility is reestablished. Ongoing monitoring, the assessment that occurs during implementation, is a central aspect of any plan of prevention for immobility complications.

SECTION 2

ASSESSMENT OF MOBILITY

MOBILITY DATA COLLECTION

MOBILITY HISTORY

The mobility history includes information about a patient's current level of mobility, usual exercise patterns, attitudes about mobility, and level of knowledge about related subjects such as rest and nutrition. It provides important subjective data about a patient's strengths and deficits relating to movement and activity. Sharing the purpose of the history with the patient encourages full participation.

If mobility has recently changed as a result of illness or injury, it is also important to determine how patients feel about their current situation. What are their expectations for recovery? Level of understanding about the type of mobility or exercise that is appropriate during the acute, convalescent, and rehabilitation stages is also important to assess. For example, a patient may resist attempts to increase activity after surgery because of erroneous fears that disruption of the incision could be caused by movement. A patient who has suffered a stroke may not be aware that rehabilitating currently nonfunctioning limbs can be facilitated by passive exercise in the period immediately following the stroke. Someone being treated for cardiac problems may not realize the preventive and rehabilitative effects of prudent aerobic exercise.

Information about family or other support persons is a necessary element in the mobility database. Not only can these people contribute significantly to a patient's recovery, they can also provide additional insights into a patient's needs. The family is a primary source of data when a patient is unable or unwilling to communicate.

The following sections present a description of each part of the mobility history, using a modification of the standard health history format. This model yields data useful to nurses in planning patient care and also assists in collaborative planning with other members of the health care team.

Primary Concern

Loss of mobility is alarming to most individuals. Because many types of health problems threaten mobility, distress about real or anticipated mobility impairment is a frequent primary concern. Respiratory, circulatory, cardiac, neurologic, and musculoskeletal problems interfere directly with ease or capacity of movement. Pain related to dysfunction anywhere in the body is a common cause of mobility limitations.

For some patients, the results of altered mobility—such as time away from work or school, limited social and recreational activities, or the inability to carry out usual role functions in the home—are the primary concern. In all of these cases, a detailed mobility history is appropriate. The following example illustrates the implications a patient's primary concern can have for nursing assessment and care.

> During a routine health checkup, Mrs. Kung expresses distress that she in no longer able to manage her home tasks as she desires. The nurse questions her further and learns that she "runs out of energy" and sometimes feels dizzy. Also Mrs. Kung says, "I take a lot of pills every day for my heart and my arthritis." The nurse realizes that medications, arthritis, and cardiac problems could contribute to Mrs. Kung's primary concern and makes a note to follow up on these topics later in the history.

Current Understanding

A patient's ideas about the causes, seriousness, and possible effects of the current problem are an important aspect of the mobility history. Explore the course of the problem and consequences that have been troubling. Determine what remedies patients have tried and whether relief was obtained. The following example illustrates the importance of a patient's current understanding in identifying appropriate patient care.

> When discussing the reason for seeking care, Mr. Nelson states that he has been having acute epigastric pain that has been diagnosed as an ulcer. He is now scheduled for surgery after several months of taking medications without improvement in symptoms. During the hospital admission, Mr. Nelson expresses frustration about the interference his illness has caused in his usual physical fitness regimen, stating how much better he will feel after resuming regular jogging and weight lifting after his discharge from the hospital. The nurse makes a note of these apparently unrealistic expectations for activity immediately after surgery for later health teaching.

Past Health Problems/Experiences

Chronic conditions and their treatment, and past experiences with health care, are often relevant to current mobility status and related nursing care. Ask patients if they have ever had other illnesses, injuries, or operations that have affected mobility. Determine the date, severity, treatment, and residual effects, if any, of these. Note medications currently used that could affect mobility status, such as those acting on the cardiac, respiratory, circulatory, musculoskeletal, or neurologic systems. The following example illustrates the relevance of past health problems and their treatment to mobility.

> Ms. Shapiro is being evaluated for apparently minor head injuries sustained when she fell at home as a result of having "blacked out." When questioned about medications used on a regular basis, Ms. Shapiro indicates that she has recently begun taking a new medication for high blood pressure (hypertension). The nurse is aware that this medication often causes transient dizziness, especially when rising quickly from supine to standing. He decides that the care plan for Ms. Shapiro should include education about side effects of her medications and safety measures such as sitting briefly before rising from a lying to a standing position.

Personal, Family, and Social History

Personal, family, and social history provides significant data needed to make nursing diagnoses related to mobility status. Lifestyle choices, particularly diet and exercise habits, contribute to many of the health problems that cause limited mobility. Exploring daily routines and activities provides insights important to mobility care. Conversely, altered mobility can affect many facets of a person's life and often imposes lifestyle changes. If possible, it is a good idea to observe patients in their home environments to more clearly understand their routines and lifestyle. This will also provide an opportunity to assess the environment for hazards or barriers to mobility, note habits or actions that create risks to mobility, and suggest modifications to promote mobility and safety. Clinical Guideline 33–2 lists important observations in a home assessment for mobility hazards.

Clues about resources and limitations affecting ability to adapt to necessary changes come from the personal, family, and social history. The following example shows the relevance of this part of the history to mobility care. Table 33–2 lists sample questions to elicit appropriate information.

> Mr. Rothenberg is admitted to the surgical floor for a minor surgical procedure. The nurse notes that he appears to be overweight. When questioning him about his habits, she learns that he and his wife enjoy cooking together. Their usual diet includes foods high in calories for both meals and snacks. Mr. Rothenberg also reveals that he does not exercise regularly, preferring to watch television in his leisure time. The nurse decides that Mr. and Mrs. Rothenberg could benefit from health teaching about exercise and nutrition to help them to make informed decisions about their overall health status. She plans to consult with the physician and dietitian to develop a collaborative education plan for the Rothenbergs.

Subjective Manifestations

A review of subjective manifestations provides an overall picture of symptoms a patient is experiencing, categorized according to body systems. The questions in Table 33–3 focus on symptoms that may interfere with mobility. Information about symptoms experienced helps determine the nursing assistance needed for movement and daily care activities. The example on page 1184 illustrates the use of subjective manifestations data.

CLINICAL GUIDELINE 33–2

HOME ASSESSMENT FOR BARRIERS TO MOBILITY

GENERAL

- Are walks, driveways, floors and floorcoverings free of obstacles and in good repair?
- Is the yard level and free of obstacles?
- Do all balconies or porches have sturdy railings in good repair?
- Are carpeting and stair treads securely anchored?
- Do throw rugs, if used, lie flat and have nonslip backing?
- Are nonslip floor waxes or pollishes used on hardwood or linoleum/tile floors?
- Does arrangement of furniture permit a relatively straight traffic pattern?
- Is furniture adjacent to traffic paths sturdy enough to provide support?
- Is the home (including garage and attic) generally free of clutter on the floor?
- If an attic is used for storage, is flooring adequate?
- Are frequently used tools and appliances stored where easily accessable?
- Is a sturdy stepstool or ladder available to reach high objects?

STAIRS

- Are treads/carpeting or stair edges in good repair?
- Are handrails present (preferably on both sides of stairwell) and in good repair?
- Are stairs free of clutter?

LIGHTING

- Are adequate lights available in garage, entryways, porches? Motion-sensistive lights are very practical in these areas.
- Are all traffic areas, especially hallways and stairs, well lighted?
- Is floor-level lighting available wherever there is low furniture or plants?
- Are there switches at the top and bottom of all stairs?
- Are nightlights available in bedrooms, bathrooms, and connecting hallways?

BATHROOMS

- Are sturdy hold bars present in showers and tubs? (For some patients, bars beside toilets are advisable.)
- Do showers and tubs have nonslip mats or adhesive decals on stepping surfaces?
- Is toilet seat raised for patients who are weak or elderly?

HABITS

- Do shoes, slippers fit well, have nonslip soles, laces securely tied?
- Are pants, skirts, robes short enough so patient won't trip on them?
- Are spills on floors cleaned up promptly and effectively?
- Does patient use appropriate body mechanics for lifting, doing housework, and other tasks?
- Are items usually put away after use rather than left where they could cause accidents?
- Are ladders or stepstools used rather than chairs or other furniture to access items out of reach?
- Are ladders in good repair and used correctly? (Stepladders: do not stand on top two rungs, lock spreader braces before using; straight ladder: angle so its base is 1 foot away fom support wall for every 4 feet of ladder's height.)
- Are pets kept from lying in traffic areas?
- Are ambulation aids (canes, walkers) appropriately fitted to patient and do they have intact rubber tips?

TABLE 33-2. MOBILITY HISTORY: PERSONAL, FAMILY, AND SOCIAL HISTORY QUESTIONS

A. Vocational

1. What type of work do you do?
2. Does you current work involve physical exertion? Please describe activities.
3. Have you noticed any problems doing your work lately? How long has this been a problem?
4. What other job skills or interests do you have?
5. How do you usually get around—for example, to work, to shop? Do you drive? Ride the bus? Walk?
6. Have driving or walking become more difficult lately?

B. Home and Family

1. Are you married? In a relationship? How long?
2. Is the relationship satisfactory?
3. Do you have children? How many? Ages? Any with special care needs? Do you provide care?
4. What other family members live with you? Nearby? Where do nearest family members live?
5. How do you see family members as helping you as you deal with current health problem?
6. Do you perform many home maintenance tasks—cooking, cleaning, repairs?
7. Tell me about a typical day at home (tasks, activities).
8. Is there anything about your home—for example stairs, lighting, appliances—or your garage or yard that makes it more difficult to accomplish these activities or tasks?
9. Do you have adequate storage spaces for the appliances or tools you need to do these tasks?
10. Have you had to arrange for help for any of the tasks you were used to doing or allow them to go undone because of your health problem?

C. Social, Leisure, Spiritual, and Cultural

1. What are your favorite leisure-time activities? With whom do you usually do these?
2. Are there other pastimes you enjoy or have enjoyed in the past?
3. Do you belong to any clubs or groups?
4. Has your health problem affected your choice of leisure activities? How?
5. Has your social or family life been affected by the recent change in your health status? Please tell me about it.

D. Sexual

1. Has your sexual relationship been satisfactory?
2. Any changes related to current health problem?
3. What changes have occurred?

E. Habits

Exercise

1. Do you exercise regularly? Weekly? More often?
2. What type of exercise/activity do you enjoy most—games, individual sports, fitness activities?
3. Do you feel that regular exercise is an important part of staying healthy?
4. Has this health problem affected your pattern of exercise? How?

Sleep

1. How many hours do you usually sleep each night?
2. Is this enough for you to feel rested?
3. Do you have any sleep problems? How have you dealt with these?
4. Do you notice any change in your sleep patterns when you increase or decrease your exercise? How does sleep change?
5. Has this health problem affected your sleep? How?

Nutrition

1. How many meals do you usually eat daily? Any difference on weekends? Snacks?
2. What foods you do you eat most every day?
3. What kind of diet do you feel is necessary to stay healthy?
4. Describe your appetite.
5. Has this health problem affected your eating habits? How?

Beverages

1. Do you drink coffee? Tea? Soft drinks? Water? How much of each per day?
2. Do you drink alcoholic beverages? What do you usually drink? Beer, wine, liquor?
3. How much alcohol do you drink in an average week?
4. Does your alcohol intake affect your activity? How?
5. Do you notice a change in your ability or motivation to exercise when you are drinking more?
6. Does alcohol intake affect your overall mobility? How?
7. Have you ever injured yourself as a result of your alcohol intake?
8. Has your alcohol intake changed since you became ill?

Tobacco

1. Do you smoke? Cigarettes, pipe, cigar?
2. How long have you been smoking?
3. How much do you smoke?
4. Have you ever quit? For how long?
5. Does smoking affect your activity? How?
6. Do you note a change in your ability to exercise when you are smoking more?

Drugs

1. Are there any drugs you use regularly, such as aspirin, sleeping pills, diet pills, nerve pills?
2. How frequently do you take these? For what reason?
3. Do any of these affect your ability or motivation to exercise as usual?
4. Do they affect your overall mobility? How?
5. Have you ever injured yourself as a result of taking these drugs? What was the injury?
6. Has your use of any of these drugs changed recently? How?

Other Substances

1. Do you ever use marijuana? Cocaine? Crystal? Other drugs?
2. Do any of them influence your level of activity? Your motivation to exercise? Carry out usual home or work responsibilities?

F. Psychological

Coping

1. Has (current health problem) caused any worries for you? For example, about your overall health? Possibility of improvement? Relationships with spouse, family? Money?
2. How have you dealt with these concerns?
3. Has this been effective?

Self-image

1. Do you think the change in your mobility has changed the way you feel about yourself (for example, about the way you look, do your job, carry out your home responsibilities, parent, or relate to your spouse)?
2. How would you describe the change?

TABLE 33-3. SUBJECTIVE MANIFESTATIONS QUESTIONS

A. General

1. Describe your overall state of health.
2. Has there been a recent change?
3. Do you require any help to move about, cook, shop, care for yourself or your children?
4. Has there been a recent change in these abilities?
5. How much activity do you feel up to now? Sitting up? Walking to the door? In the hall? More strenuous activity?
6. Do you ever experience difficulty walking due to problems with your eyesight? When does this happen?
7. How about difficulty with transportation due to eyesight?
8. Can you drive?
9. Have you ever had difficulty orienting yourself because of hearing problems? When does this occur?

B. Respiratory

1. Do you ever experience difficulty breathing (dyspnea)? Coughing? Sneezing? Wheezing? Congestion?
2. What precedes or aggravates these?
3. Do you experience any of them or do they get worse when you are active?
4. What kind of activity causes these symptoms—for example, walking, running, housework, stair climbing?
5. How much can you do before these symptoms appear?
6. Do you notice improvement when you rest?
7. How much rest is necessary to relieve the symptoms?

C. Chest, Cardiovascular

1. Do you ever experience a pounding sensation in the chest (palpitations)? A very rapid heart rate (tachycardia)? Sharp shooting pains in your legs (claudication)? Dizziness? Passing out (syncope)?
2. Do any of these occur or become worse with activity? What kind?
3. How much of this activity can you do before these occur?
4. Are they improved with rest?
5. How long do you have to rest before they are better?

D. Musculoskeletal

1. Do you ever experience muscle weakness? Cramps? Muscle aches and pains? Joint stiffness? Back pain or stiffness? Back pain that radiates to the legs (radicular pain)?
2. What precedes or aggravates these?
3. Are any of them caused or worsened by activity? What kind?
4. How much activity before they appear?
5. Do they get better with rest? How much rest?
6. Do these symptoms keep you from being able to care for yourself?
7. Have you ever experienced a fracture? Dislocation?
8. Was it related to exercise? How did it happen?

E. Neurologic

1. Do you ever have headaches? Problems with vision? A sense of confusion/disorientation? Loss of balance? Loss of coordination? Tingling in the arms, legs, fingers, toes? Numbness? Other changes in sensation or touch, such as "pins and needles" (paresthesia)?
2. Are any of these related to activity? What kind of activity?
3. Does rest or stopping the activity improve them?
4. How long do you have to rest before they improve or disappear?
5. Have you ever had convulsions? Are they associated with exercise or with a specific activity?
6. Have you ever been injured as a result of a convulsion?

F. Psychological

1. Do you notice mood swings associated with activity/exercise? When you don't exercise?
2. How do these mood changes affect your interaction with others? Your job? Your interest in usual leisure activities?

Mrs. Johnson, an elderly patient being admitted to the hospital, tells her nurse that she has been experiencing joint stiffness in her back and legs, which is most severe when she first gets up in the morning. It has sometimes been severe enough to make walking difficult, but improves if she goes about household activities at a slow pace. Mrs. Johnson has been bothered by this stiffness for about 5 years and occasionally takes aspirin for relief. The nurse realizes that lying in bed during the period of hospitalization will probably aggravate the stiffness and resolves to include ROM and other in-bed exercises in Mrs. Johnson's care plan to prevent the stiffness from becoming more severe.

The mobility history should be initiated when a patient is admitted to a hospital or seeks care for a concern related to mobility. It is important, however, for nurses to be sensitive to patients' ability to respond. Anxiety, fatigue, or pain may necessitate obtaining baseline data in several short interviews. Nurses must also review patients' medical records. Frequently, data gathered by other health care team members, such as the physician or dietitian, are useful in planning nursing care. Collaborative data gathering is efficient, conserving energy of patients and health care professionals.

MOBILITY EXAMINATION

The mobility examination provides critical information about mobility status. The examination comprises measurements, inspection, palpation, and auscultation.

Measurements

Measure patients' height and weight and compare to normative charts. Is the patient underweight? Overweight? Excess weight hints at a sedentary lifestyle. Lack of exercise and obesity can lead to a variety of health problems affecting mobility. Overweight people may have a significantly lower exercise tolerance than would be predicted for their age. Many have hypertension, cardiac problems, or respiratory difficulties that make activities of daily living or strenuous exercise difficult. When confined to bed, they have increased risk for such problems as pressure ulcers, hypostatic pneumonia, and thrombophlebitis.[22]

Conversely, underweight individuals may suffer from nutritional deficiencies and musculoskeletal weakness, both of which could affect endurance. They would have minimal energy reserve to withstand the stress of illness or injury and may require a prolonged period of convalescence. This could lead to many of the disuse phenomena discussed in Section 1.

Measure vital signs as discussed in Chap. 17. Resting pulse predicts activity tolerance and implies general activity level. Individuals who are physically active usually have a lower than expected resting pulse for their age. Pulse irregularities, respiratory difficulties, or hypertension suggest limitations in activity tolerance.

Objective Manifestations

Integument, eye and ear, chest, cardiovascular, musculoskeletal, and neurologic examinations contribute to nursing diagnosis of mobility status.

General Observations. General observations at the beginning of the examination signal areas needing more detailed assessment later in the examination.

MENTAL STATUS. Information about mental status and sensory capacity is necessary to determine whether independent mobility is safe for a patient. Responses to questions during the history and patient participation during measurements are general indicators of mental status. Patients who are confused or apparently unaware of their surroundings could injure themselves if they attempt activity without assistance. Patients who have trouble hearing questions during the history and examination, or difficulty seeing where they are going, are at risk for injury during many activities. Consideration for assistance in the home, community, or health care facility should be given.

BODY PROPORTIONS AND ENERGY LEVEL. Body proportions and energy level also suggest potential strengths and deficits pertaining to mobility. Note the general body build. Is the patient slender? muscular? Do the muscles appear well toned? Overdeveloped? Flabby? Does the patient seem fatigued? Lethargic? Energetic? Poor muscle tone implies a sedentary lifestyle. Fatigue or lethargy may point to nutritional deficits, oxygenation problems, or emotional problems, all of which can hinder mobility. Optimum tone, well-developed muscles, and a dynamic energy level suggest regular exercise habits. Individuals who exercise regularly usually have the capacity for optimum mobility, but often have difficulty adapting to restricted mobility during convalescence from illness, surgery, or injury.

SKIN COLOR. Noting overall skin color is also part of general observations. A person who is unusually pale may be anemic (have an abnormally low concentration of circulating red blood cells). Not only would this patient have a low energy level, but tissue perfusion, especially during increased activity, would be diminished.

POSTURE, GAIT, AND BODY MOVEMENT. Posture, gait, and body movement are also important mobility indicators. Ideal standing posture consists of an erect position, with weight evenly distributed over both feet. The head is erect, shoulders level. The shoulders are aligned directly above the hips, which are centered over the knees and ankles. The knees should be slightly flexed, not locked, and the pelvis level. Figure 33–2 contrasts ideal and incorrect posture.

Slumped posture or guarding of body parts could indicate pain or structural problems interfering with mobility. These can be more thoroughly investigated during the musculoskeletal and neurologic assessments.

INSIGHTS FROM NURSING LITERATURE

BACK PAIN AND IMMOBILITY

Galindo-Ciocon D, Ciocon JO, Galindo D. Functional impairment among elderly women with osteoporotic vertebral fractures. Rehabil Nurs. *1995;20:79–83, 130.*

Galindo-Ciocon and associates studied a group of elderly women who had sustained vertebral bone fractures due to a loss of bone density, and a comparable group of elderly women who had sustained no such fractures. Using a scale to assess their capacity to complete activities of daily living, the researchers found the patients with the fractures—all of whom suffered from a loss of bone density and back pain—were significantly more dependent on others for help with bathing, toileting, dressing, and transferring than were subjects without fractures. Such patients, therefore, are likely to require more nursing time and assistance than those without fractures.

Gait can also provide clues about mobility status. Walking should be fluid and coordinated, with even weight bearing on each foot. The feet should be parallel. As a step is taken, the heel should strike the ground before the toe and the opposite arm should swing forward slightly. Shuffling, limping, or uncoordinated gait require further investigation later in the examination.

Gait assessment includes taking note of a patient's need for a prosthesis (artificial replacement for a body part) or assistive device

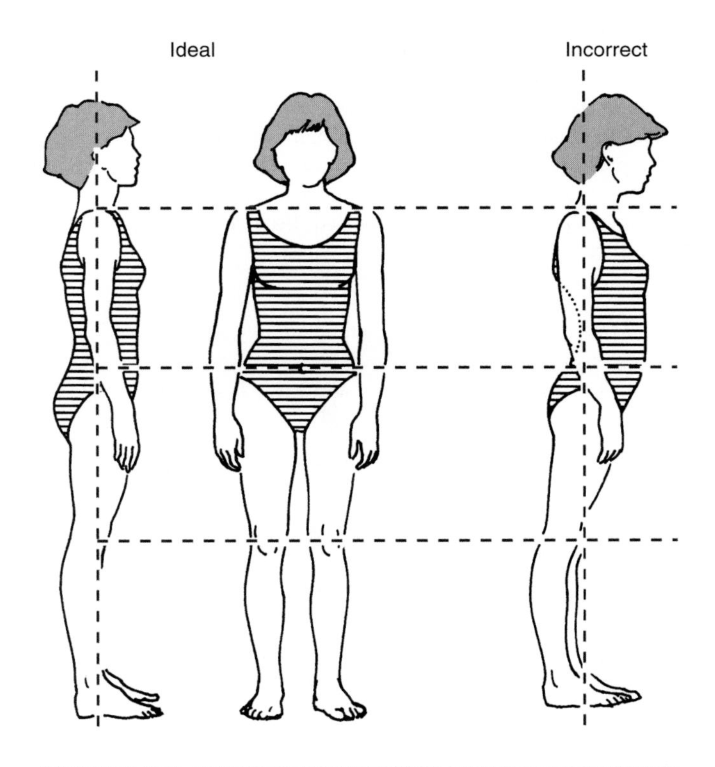

Figure 33–2. Ideal and incorrect postures.

such as a cane or walker to walk. If possible, also assess walking without the assistive device and compare the assisted and unassisted gaits.

Observe patients' mode of sitting, lying, and rising from a sitting or lying position. Difficulty with these position changes may indicate a need for strengthening exercises or other nursing assistance with activity. Assess spontaneous body movements for coordination, speed, and symmetry. Uncoordinated, jerky movements; very slow, guarded movements; or marked differences between movements on one side of the body and the other may signal pain, injury, or a disease process that will interfere with mobility. Be aware, also, of apparently involuntary movements such as tics or tremors. Note whether the latter occur during movement or when a patient is at rest. This information may be useful for later diagnosis.

If a patient is not ambulatory, note the posture usually assumed in bed or chair. Consistent use of one position, constant flexion of the extremities, or infrequent spontaneous movement increase the likelihood that problems related to disuse will develop.

Integument. Skin should be inspected for signs of vulnerability to pressure ulcers, as well as for actual skin breakdown. Skin changes indicating risk for pressure ulcers include edema, circulatory stasis, and poor hydration. Edema fluid increases the distance between cells and the capillaries that supply them with nutrients and carry off wastes. Edematous tissue is thus more susceptible to perfusion problems caused by external pressure. Skin that appears thin and shiny is indicative of poor circulation. Skin that appears dry and cracked with poor turgor is poorly hydrated (see Chap. 34). When dehydrated, skin loses elasticity and is more vulnerable to damage from pressure and shearing.

To assess for pressure ulcers, apply finger pressure to reddened skin over bony prominences to temporarily occlude blood flow. If the skin does not blanch (become pale) with digital pressure, inspect that area again when there has been no position-related pressure there for a time period half as long as the person was in the prior position. Redness (erythema) of intact skin that does not blanch, and that remains half to three-fourths as long as the pressure caused by the prior position, is considered a stage 1 ulcer.[23] Superficial or partial-thickness skin loss is a stage 2 ulcer.[23] Chapter 27 presents a more detailed discussion of assessment for pressure ulcers and their characteristics.

HEENT (Head, Eyes, Ears, Nose, and Throat). If general observation indicates a possible hearing or vision deficit that could interfere with safe mobility, test for visual and auditory acuity. Techniques for these examinations are discussed in Chap. 17. Recent research indicates that poor vision in an important predictor of hip fractures in elderly women because of its relationship to falls.[24]

Chest and Cardiovascular System. Signs of limited capacity for activity can be detected by inspection of the chest. Is breathing labored at rest? With activity? Is the chest symmetric? Rapid shallow breathing (tachypnea), rapid deep breathing (hyperpnea), or difficult breathing (dyspnea) at rest or with moderate exertion imply limitations.

Abnormalities such as barrel chest or funnel chest, discussed in Chap. 30, are caused by pathologic processes that limit air exchange. Abnormal spinal curves, discussed in the next section, can decrease the size of the thoracic cavity, compromising respiratory function, which would also decrease activity tolerance.

Chest auscultation (see Chap. 17) may reveal abnormal breath sounds that are caused by secretions in the respiratory tract. Absence of breath sounds, which may be caused by pneumonia, atelectasis, or pneumothorax, is also significant. All of these conditions could be expected to limit mobility. Cardiac rate and rhythm can also be determined by auscultation of the chest. Additional data about cardiac function are provided by assessing peripheral pulses (see Chap. 17). A later section, Exercise Tolerance, elaborates on assessing cardiorespiratory function to determine mobility status. Chapters 17 and 30 give a more detailed discussion of the chest and cardiovascular assessments.

Musculoskeletal

BODY ALIGNMENT. Inspect and palpate spinal curves. Normal spinal curvature is shown in Fig. 33–3. The thorax is convex and the lumbar region concave. Compare the normal curvature to the examples of abnormal curvature shown in the same figure. Lateral curvature (scoliosis) is more easily observed when a patient bends at the waist when the prominent scapulae (winging) associated with scoliosis is more evident.

JOINT MOBILITY. Inspection and palpation are also used to assess joint mobility (range of motion, or ROM). All joints should also be observed for swelling, tenderness, or deformity. Note whether the temperature in one or more joints is elevated compared with that

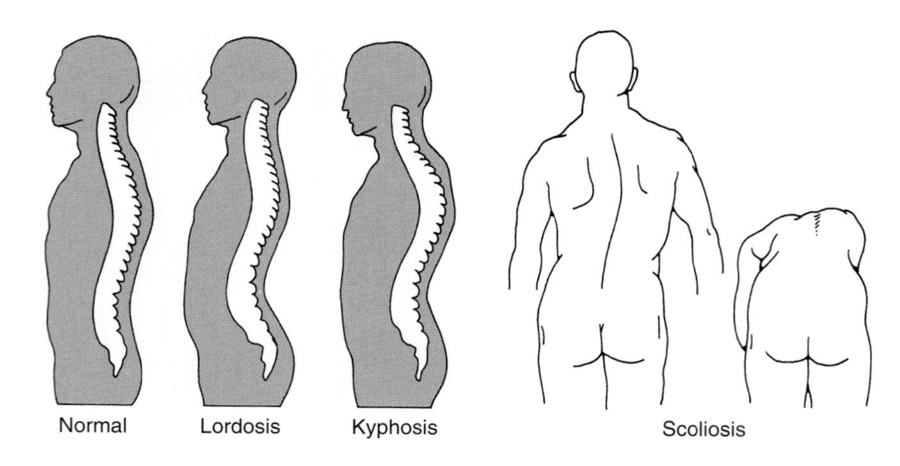

Figure 33–3. Normal and abnormal spinal curves.

CLINICAL GUIDELINE 33–3

JOINT RANGE OF MOTION

1. Discuss the procedure and the purpose with the patient, including the nurse's actions and patient participation desired, using language the patient can understand. Even apparently unconscious individuals may be able to hear and benefit from verbal communication.
2. Active ROM
   - Describe and demonstrate the desired movements for each joint (see Table 33–5 for details).
   - Repeat demonstration/instruction as needed. Relate movements to usual activities of daily living—walking, sitting, eating, hygiene—to show how these contribute to mobility.
   - Ask patient to perform each exercise while you watch. Give immediate feedback.
   - Provide positive reinforcement for correct performance. Give suggestions for change in technique, if exercise is performed incorrectly.
   - If ROM is done for therapy rather than assessment, ask patients to perform ROM three times every day and to repeat each movement smoothly at least three to five times. Point out that pacing is important to prevent fatigue. Emphasize the importance of stopping the exercise if pain occurs and to report it immediately. Work with patients to develop a schedule for ROM based on their usual daily pastimes to increase the likelihood that they will do the exercises regularly.
3. Passive ROM
   - Support each extremity to prevent stress on all joints due to torsion or hyperextension. (See Table 33–5).
   - Move each joint through all possible movements smoothly and rhythmically.
   - Move each joint as far as it will go without forcing it, then hold at the point of maximum stretch for 15 to 30 seconds to stimulate Golgi tendon organs. This inhibits reflex muscle contractions in response to extension and therefore reduces soft tissue resistance to stretching.
   - Repeat each movement three to five times. Opposing movements can be done together: flexion, extension; abduction, adduction.
   - Provide ROM at least every 8 hours.
4. Assess the degree of mobility possible for each joint according to the frequency specified in the patient care plan.
5. Recording: Note which joint or extremities were exercised; the number of repetitions for each; whether exercise was active, passive, or active with assistance; and whether pain or resistance was felt. Describe specific movement (in degrees) possible for each joint and compare to evaluation criteria.

in other parts of the body. An elevation could indicate inflammation in the joints. Ask patients to move all joints through normal ROM. See Clinical Guidelines 33–3, Joint Range of Motion. Normally, a person should be able to move all joints smoothly and without pain through the full range of motion. Inability to do so could be related to weakness, pain, contractures, or other pathology. If a patient is unable to move joint through the ROM independently, you should attempt to move that joint. Observe the approximate ROM active and/or passive, for each joint and compare it to the norms listed in Table 33–4. Do not attempt to force the joint if resistance or pain is noted. Table 33–5 illustrates the techniques for active and passive ROM that may be used as an assessment or a therapeutic measure. If a patient is hospitalized, ROM is often done while assisting with hygiene.

TABLE 33-4. NORMAL RANGE OF MOTION

Part/Movement	Adduction	Abduction	Rotation	Flexion	Extension	Hyperextension	Other
Neck (head)	0	0	70°	45°	0	35°	Lateral flexion 45°
Spine (trunk)	0	0	35°	90°	0	30°	Lateral flexion 35°
Shoulder	45°	135°	Internal 90°	180°	0	60°	Elevation 30°
			External 90°		0	50°	Depression 20°
Elbow	0	0	0		0	0	Supination
				160°			Pronation
Wrist	45°[a]	20°[b]	0	90°	0	70°	
Thumb	45°	45°	0	90°	0	5°	Opposition
Finger	15°	15°	0	90°	0	45°	
Hip	30°	45°	Internal 45°	120°	0	35°	
			External 45°				
Knee		0	0	130°	0	10°	
Ankle	0	0	0	Dorsi 20°	0		Inversion 35°
	0			Plantor 50°		0	Eversion 20°
Toes	10°	10°	0	45°	0	70°	

[a] Ulnar deviation.
[b] Radial deviation.

TABLE 33-5. ASSESSING OR ASSISTING WITH RANGE OF MOTION

Movement	Active: Illustration	Active: Instructions for Patient	Passive: Illustration	Passive: Description of Nurse's Action
Head		Tell patient to:		
Rotation	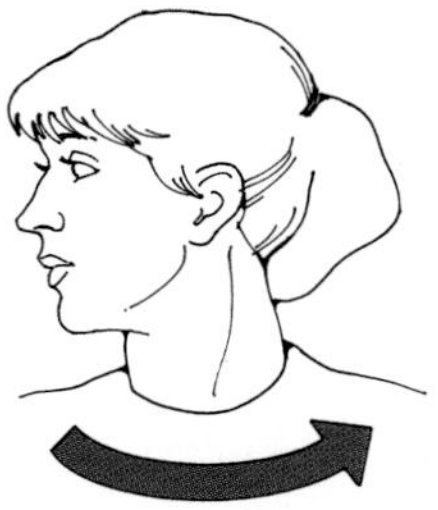	Turn head as far as possible to the left, then to the right.	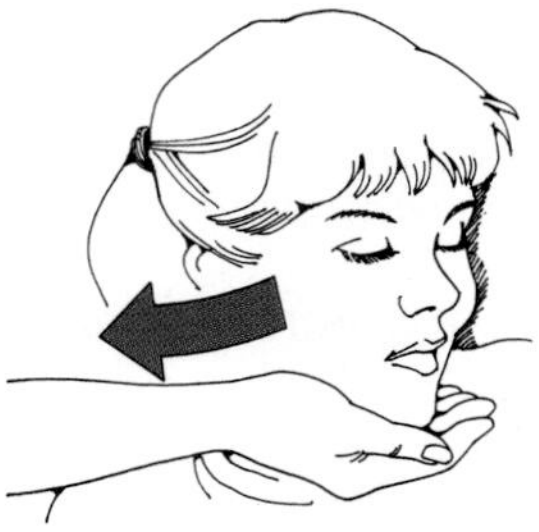	Cup the palm of your hand under the patient's chin. Pull or push chin in an arc toward each shoulder and return. (Note: no pillow)
Forward Flexion	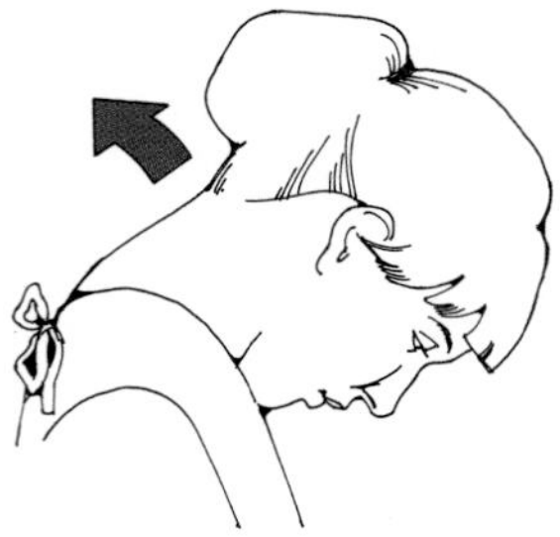	Move head as if to look at feet, then return to resting position.	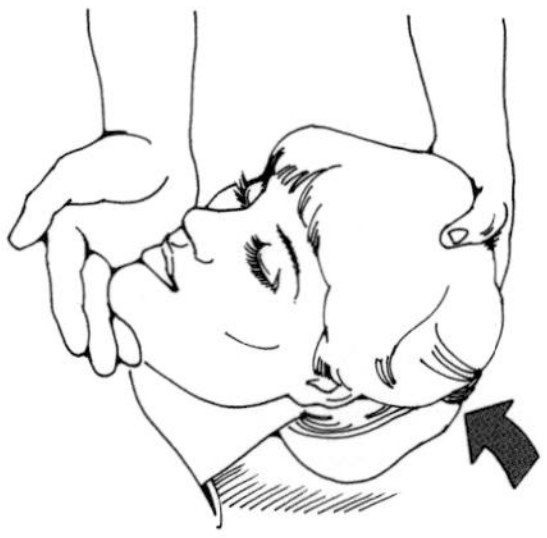	Cup hands behind patient's head, pulling head upward toward chest.
Lateral Flexion	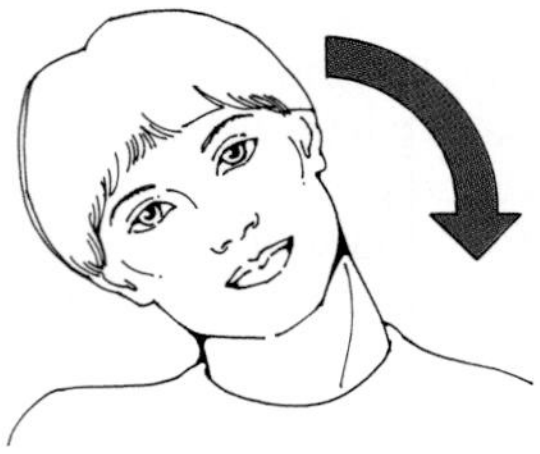	Tilt head so that left ear moves toward left shoulder. Repeat for right.	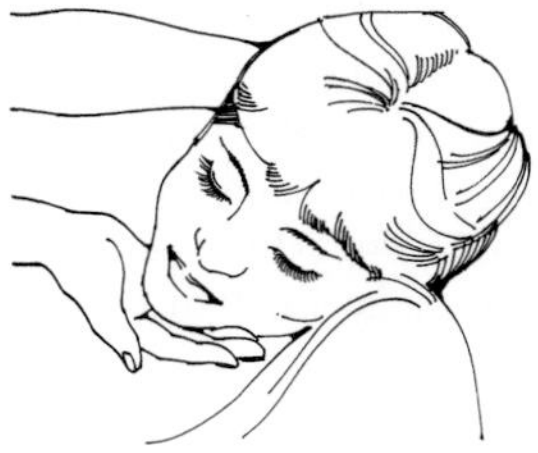	Supporting the head as above, tilt the head so that left ear moves toward the left shoulder. Repeat for right.
Hyperextension	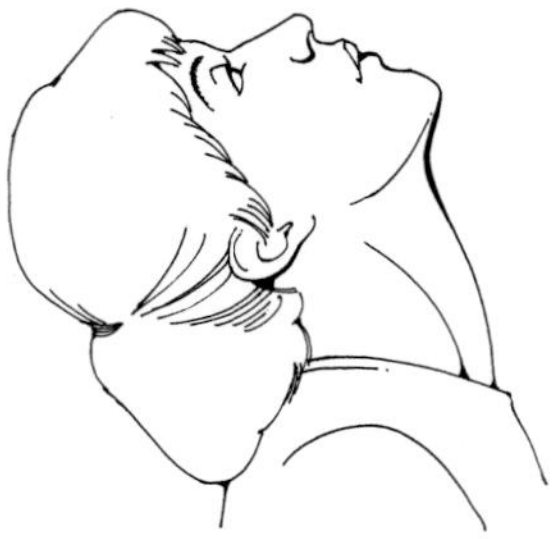	Tip head back as if looking up.	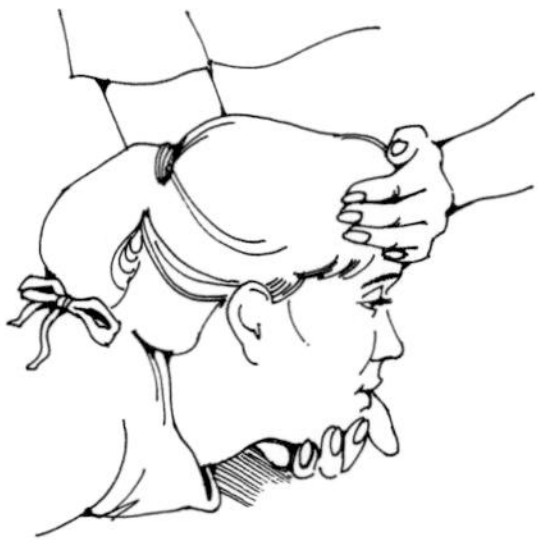	Seated or side-lying—done after all supine exercises. Place one hand on the patient's forehead, the other under chin. Move the head in an arc toward the back. *Note:* Contraindicated in some patients. Check with physician or physical therapist.
Circumduction	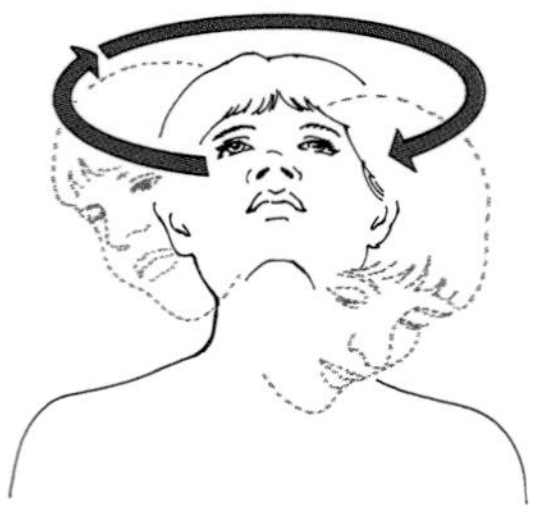	Roll head as if drawing a large circle with the top of the head, left to right, then right to left.	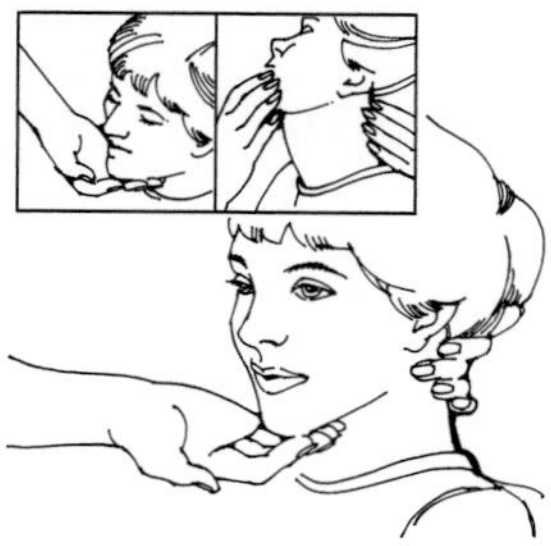	Support chin and occiput with palms of hands when patient is sitting up. Rotate head in circular motion to right, then to left.

TABLE 33-5. CONTINUED

Movement	Active: Illustration	Active: Instructions for Patient	Passive: Illustration	Passive: Description of Nurse's Action
Shoulder				
Flexion	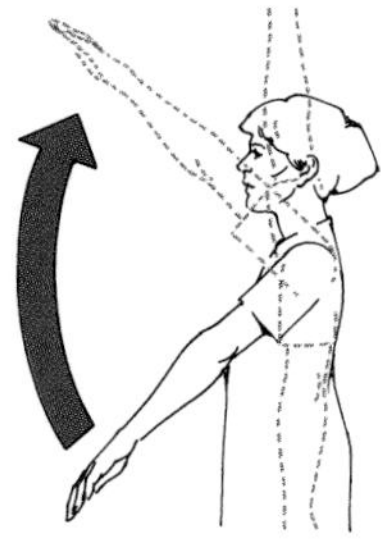	Start with arm at side or flexed so that forearm is across chest. Move arm above head in a smooth arc. (Hand or elbow will make a half-circle in movement.)	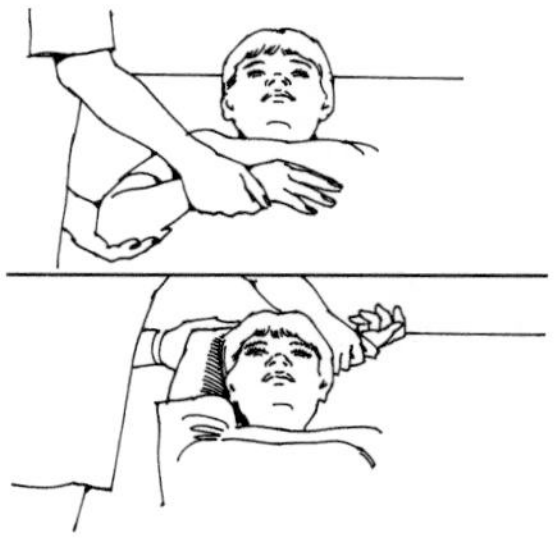	Flex patient's arm across chest. Cup elbow in one hand, grasp wrist joint to support wrist and hand. Move arm above patient's head so elbow describes 180° arc. Return to starting position.
Adduction	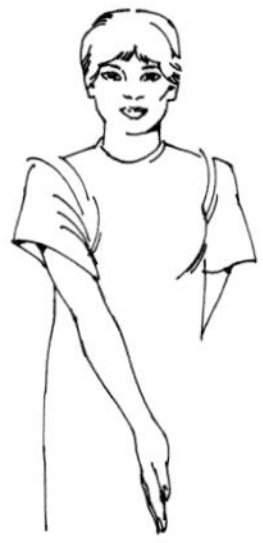	Bring arm across chest, moving elbow as close to middle of body as possible.	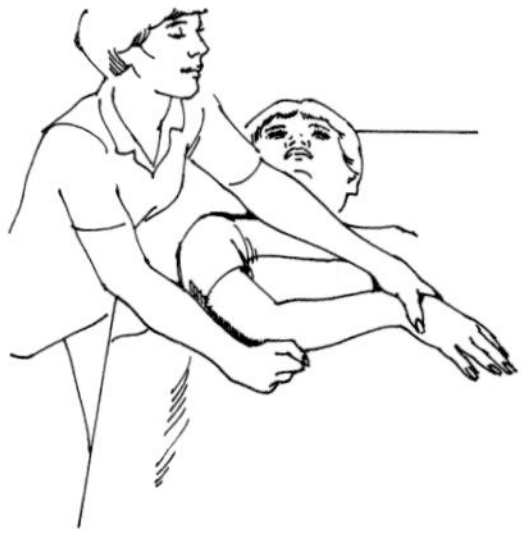	*Bracketed movements are performed together:* Grasping elbow and wrist joint as above, move elbow across chest toward midline.
Abduction	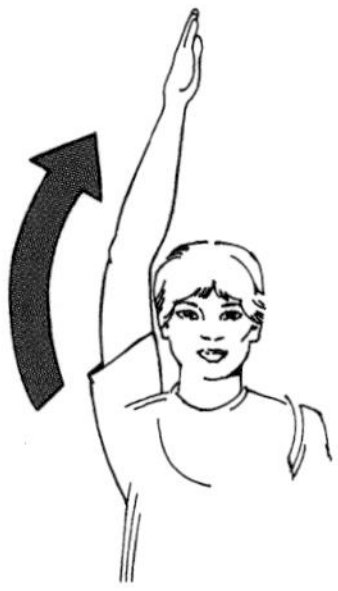	After the above, move arm outward, away from the body, then up over head.	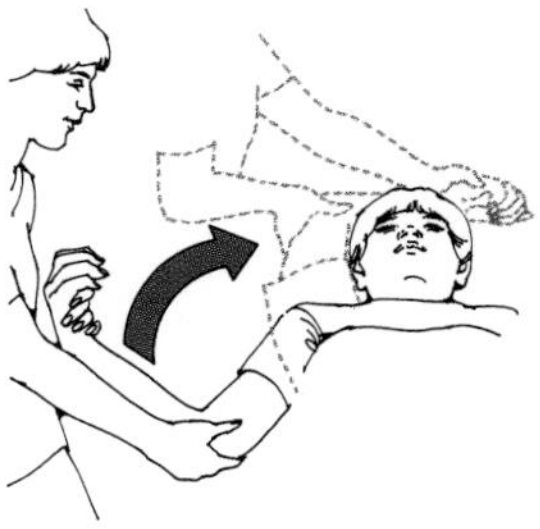	Starting in adduction and keeping arm flexed and supported as above, move arm away from the body, then over the head.
Internal Rotation	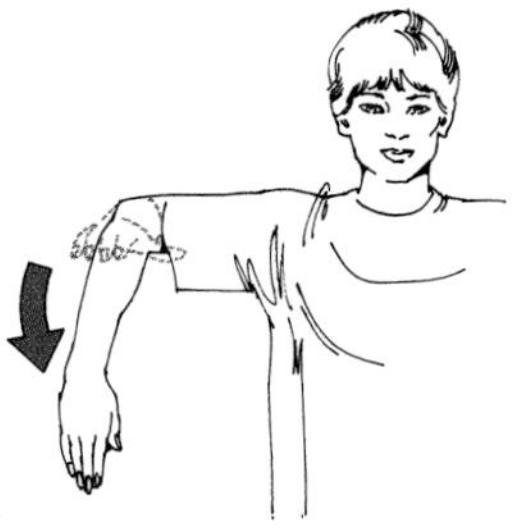	Start with arm straight out to the side from shoulder with palm facing floor and elbow bent in 90° angle. Move hand downward so fingers point to floor. If lying down, rest upper arm on bed with fingers pointing up. Move hand forward so it touches bed next to hip.	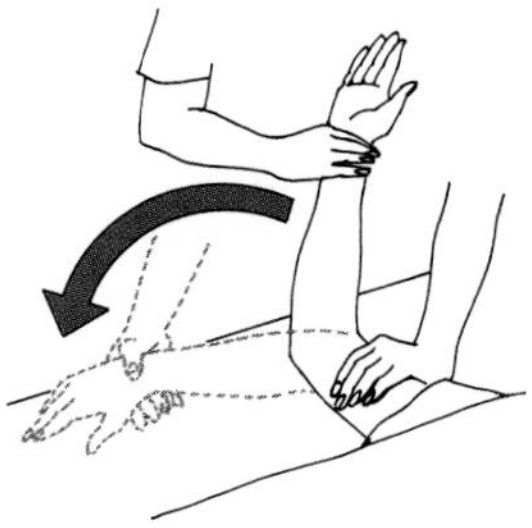	Move arm straight out from shoulder; flex elbow so hand is raised. Support wrist joint as above and stabilize upper arm. With elbow as fulcrum, move the hand downward so hand describes an arc, touching bed next to patient's hip if possible.
External Rotation	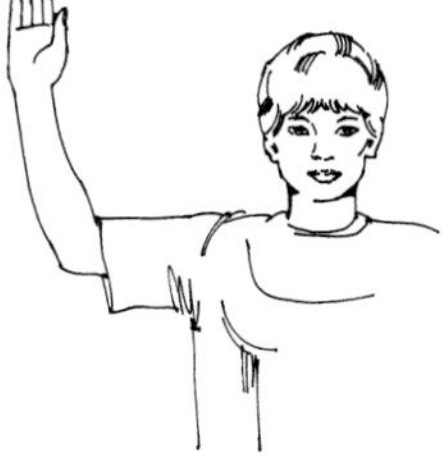	After completing internal rotation, move hand so fingers point up. If lying down, keep upper arm on bed and move hand so back of hand touches bed next to head.	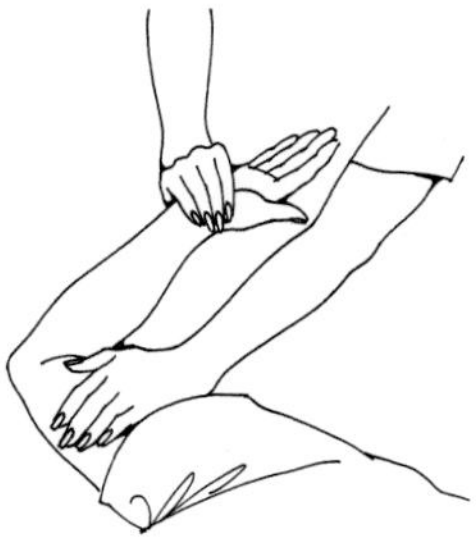	Then move the hand upward so the back of the hand touches the bed next to patient's head.

Continued

TABLE 33-5. CONTINUED

Movement	Active: *Illustration*	Active: *Instructions for Patient*	Passive: *Illustration*	Passive: *Description of Nurse's Action*
Shoulder (cont.) *Circumduction*	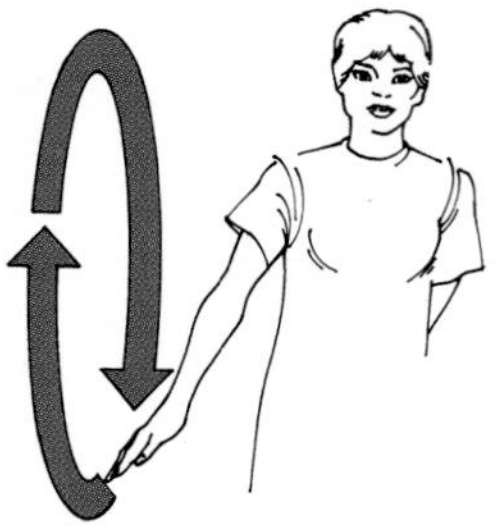	Extend arm straight out from body at shoulder. Move hand as if to draw a circle.	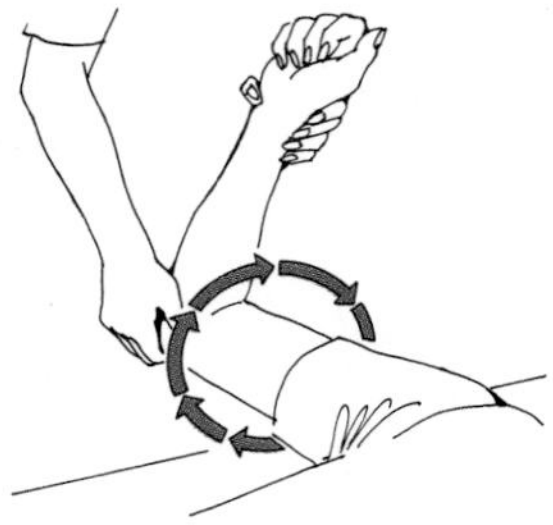	Cupping the flexed elbow and supporting the wrist joint, move the arm in a circular motion.
Hyperextension	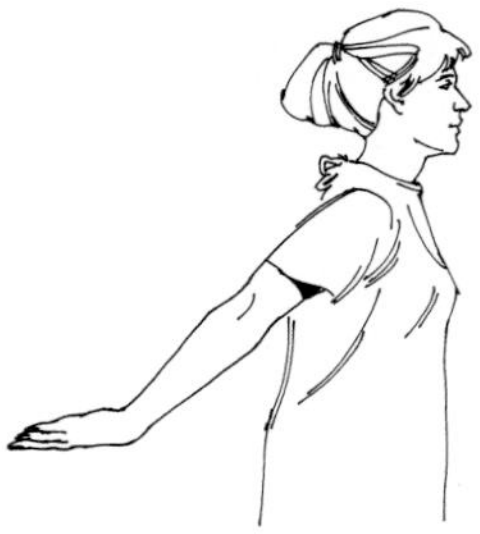	When standing or sitting with arm at side, swing arm backwards as far as possible without turning hand. May also be done lying on side.	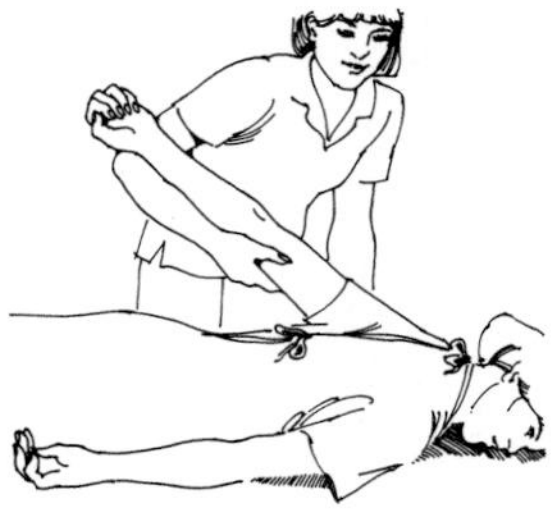	(Done at the completion of all exercises in the supine position.) With patient prone or side-lying, arm at side, cradle arm to support elbow and wrist joints. Move the arm toward the back as far as possible, so that the hand makes an arc.
Elbow *Pronation*	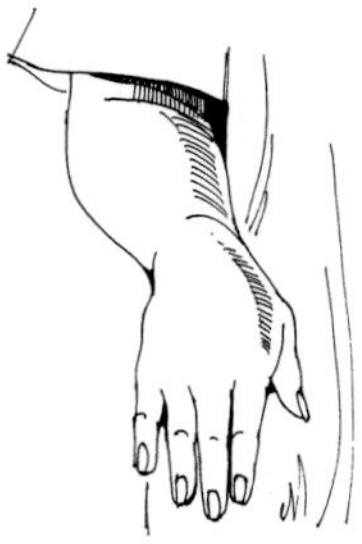	Starting with arms at sides, flex elbow so palm faces upward, then turn palm toward floor.	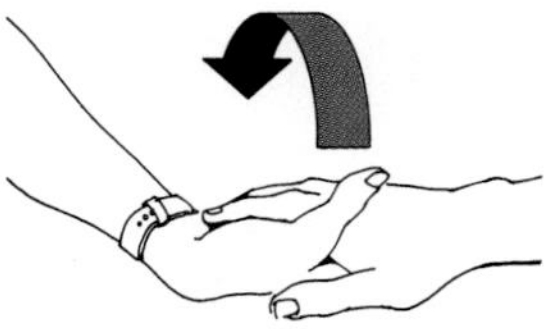	Hold patient's hand as if to shake hands, elbow may rest on bed or be cupped by other hand. Turn your hand so that patient's hand faces the floor.
Supination	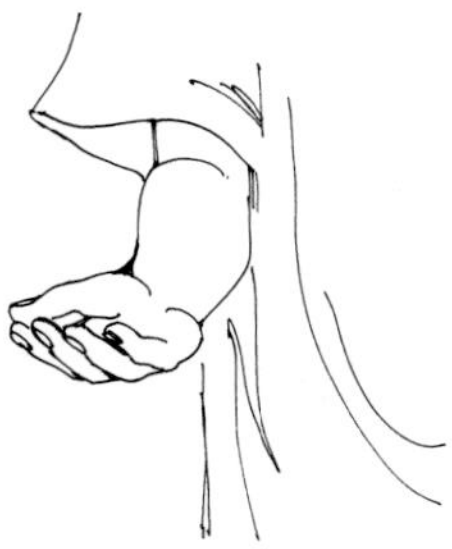	Starting in elbow pronation position, turn palm up toward ceiling.	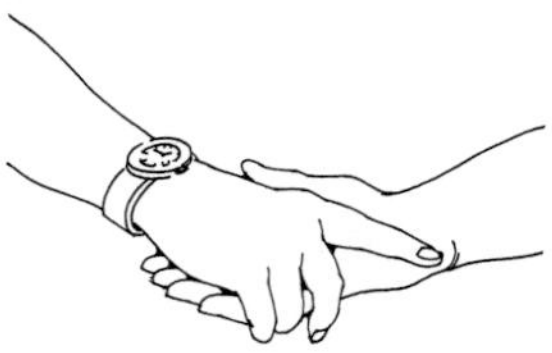	When above completed, turn palm up toward ceiling.

TABLE 33-5. CONTINUED

Movement	Active: Illustration	Active: Instructions for Patient	Passive: Illustration	Passive: Description of Nurse's Action
Flexion	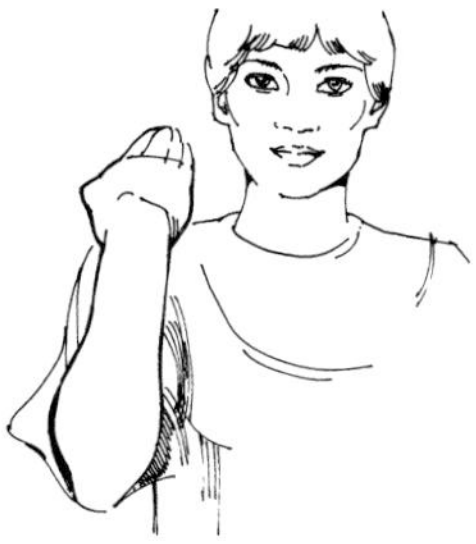	Starting with arm at side, bend elbow, moving hand toward shoulder.	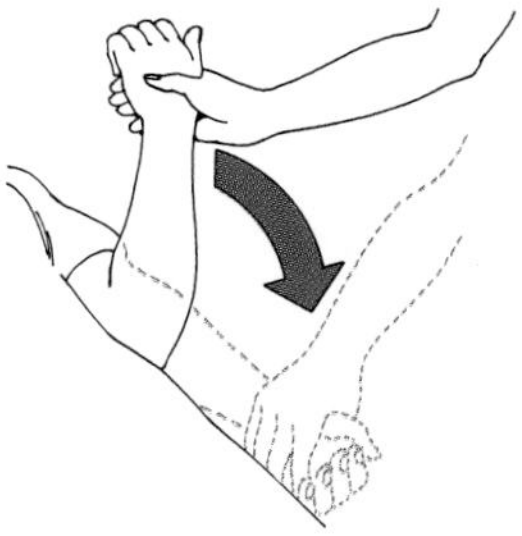	Place patient's arm at the side, palm up or facing thigh. Grasp patient's hand and wrist. With patient's elbow resting on bed, move patient's forearm toward the shoulder and return to straight position.
Extension	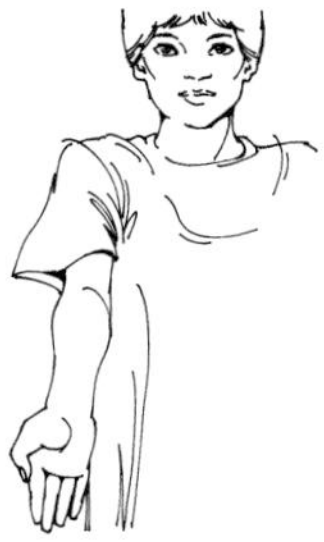	Return to starting position.		
Circumduction	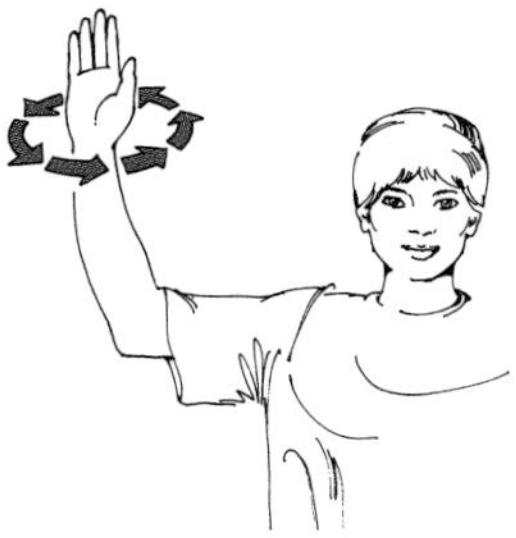	Place elbow out so that it is level with shoulder. Move hand in a circle.	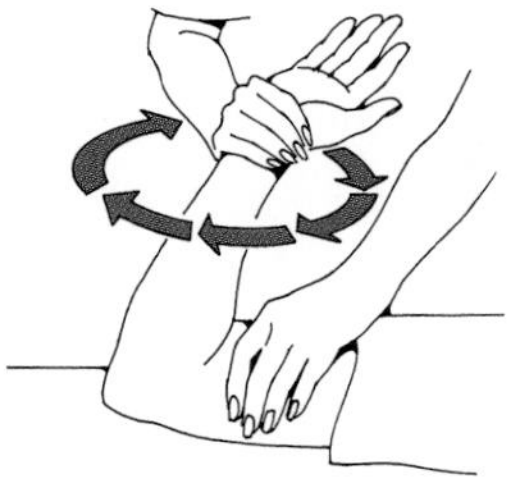	Rest patient's elbow on bed. Grasp wrist and describe circle with hand while stabilizing upper arm with your other hand.
Wrist				
Adduction (ulnar deviation)	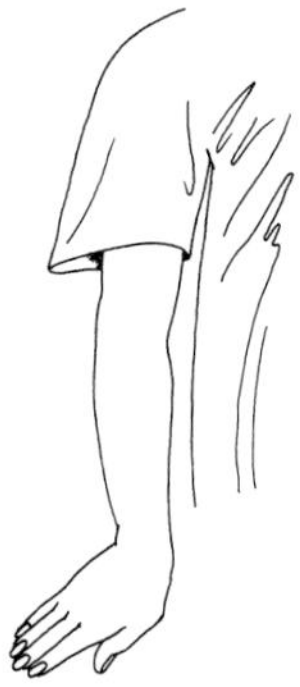	With arm at side, bend wrist as if to touch side of arm with little finger.	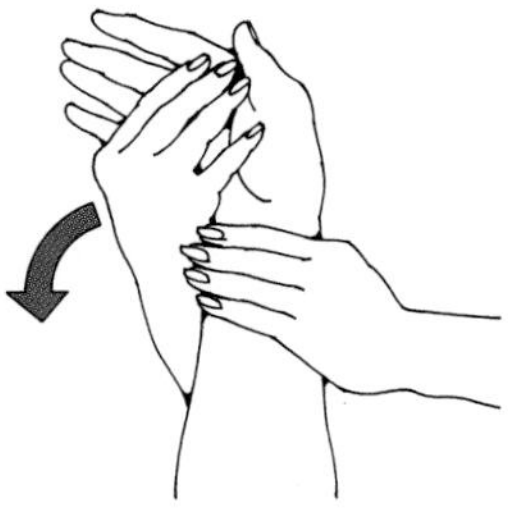	Place patient's palm in yours. Grasp wrist with your other hand. Move patient's hand from side to side as if to touch thumb (abduction) and little finger (adduction) alternately on either side of arm.
Abduction (radial deviation)	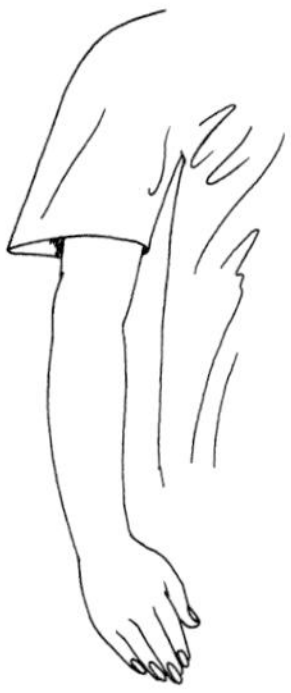	With arm at side, bend wrist as if to touch thumb on side of arm.	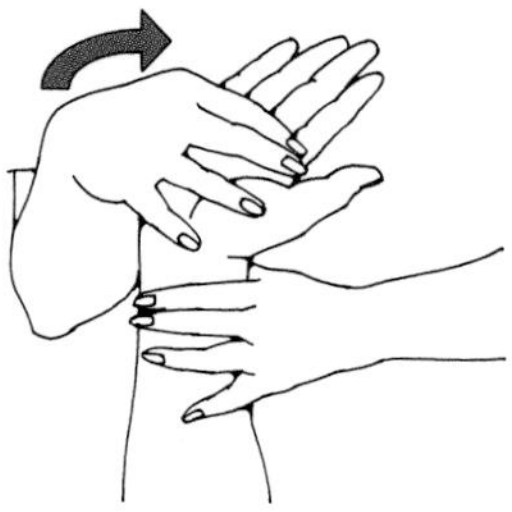	

Continued

TABLE 33-5. CONTINUED

Movement	Active: Illustration	Active: Instructions for Patient	Passive: Illustration	Passive: Description of Nurse's Action
Wrist (cont.)				
Flexion	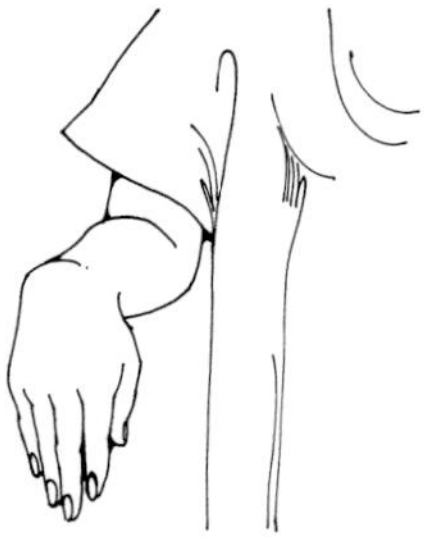	Bend wrist so palm moves toward it.	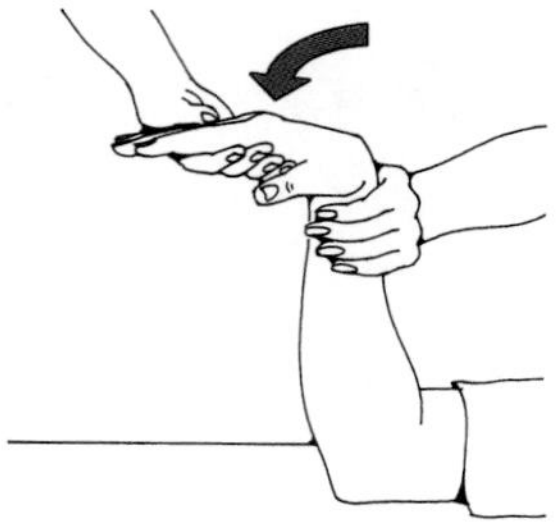	Rest patient's elbow on bed, grasp wrist. Hold patient's hand so that yours and patient's fingers are perpendicular. Flex palm toward wrist.
Hyperextension	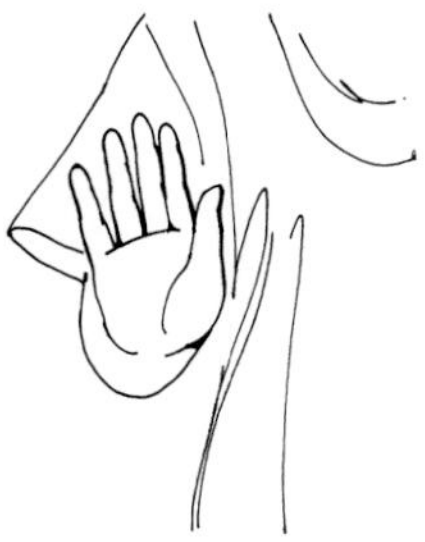	Bend wrist so back of hand moves toward it.	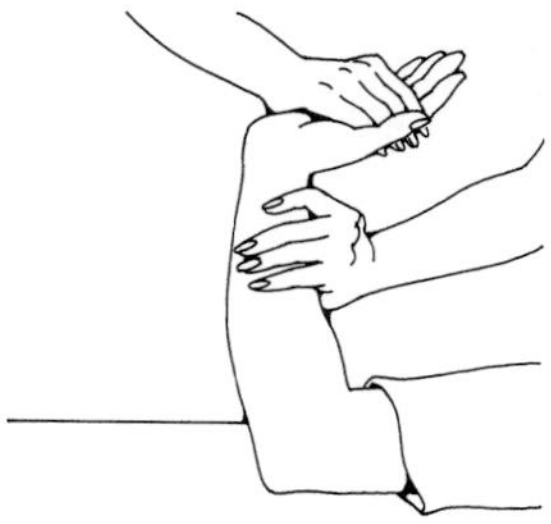	When wrist flexion is completed, extend wrist, then move back of hand toward wrist.
Circumduction	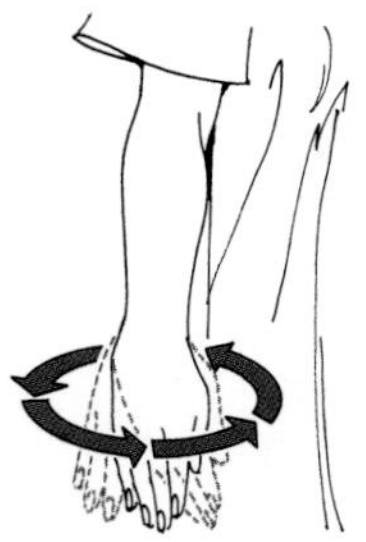	Move hand as if stirring—make a circle with hand.	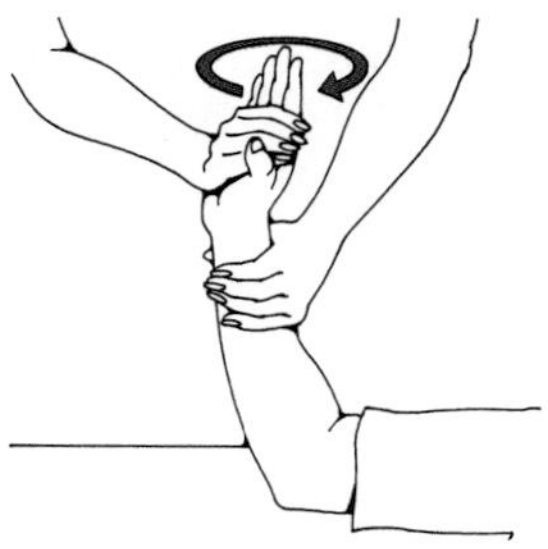	Supporting patient's hand as above, move hand in circular motion.
Fingers				
Adduction/Abduction	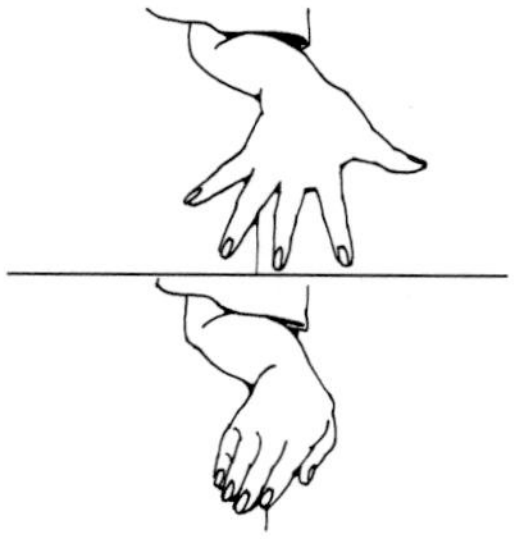	Spread fingers and thumb as far as possible, then bring together.	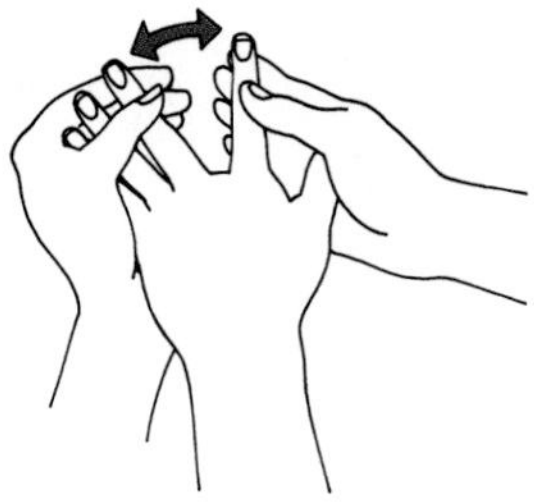	With patient's arm resting on bed or across chest, move the thumb and each finger away from the adjacent finger and return.
Opposition	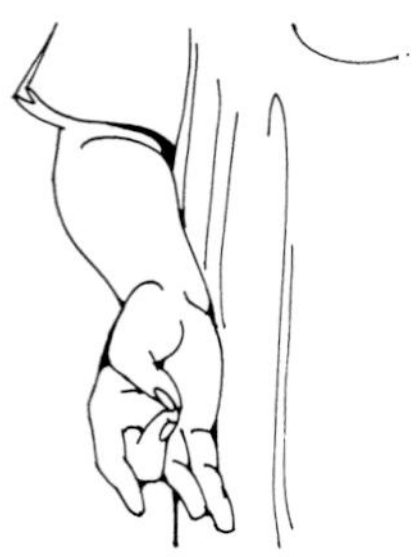	Touch each finger to thumb.	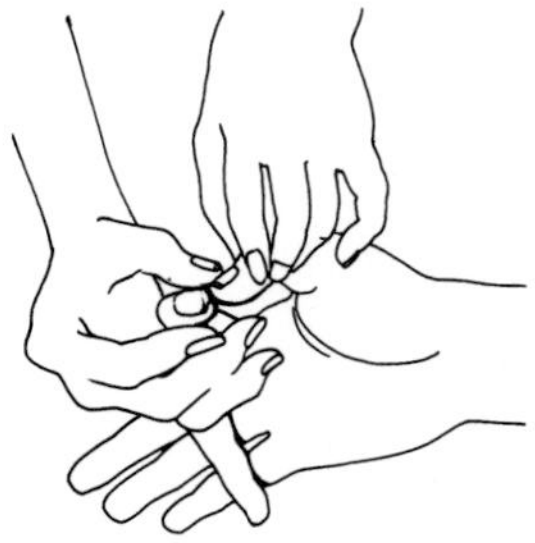	With hand still resting on bed, touch each finger to thumb.

TABLE 33-5. CONTINUED

Movement	Active: Illustration	Active: Instructions for Patient	Passive: Illustration	Passive: Description of Nurse's Action
Circumduction	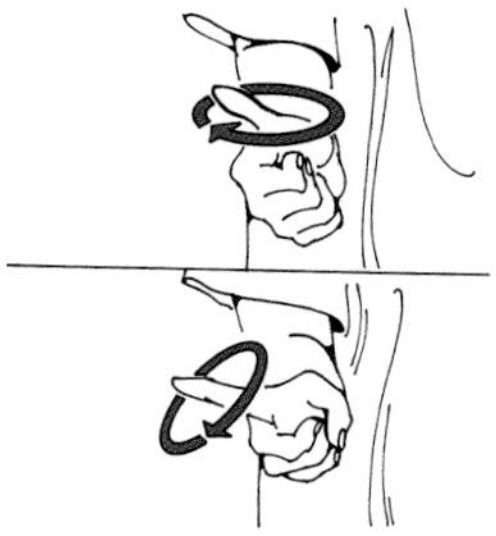	Make a circle with each finger and thumb.	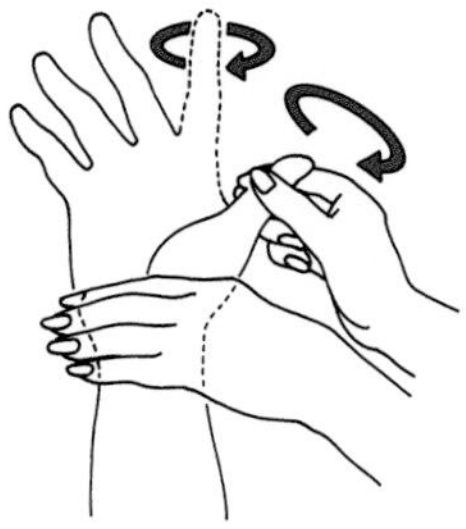	Move each finger and thumb in a circle while supporting wrist.
Flexion/Extension	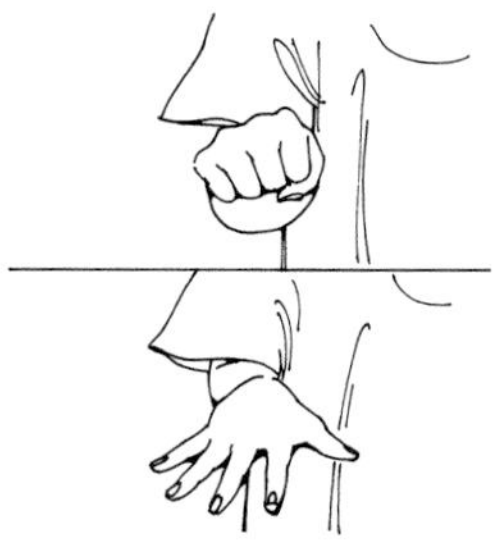	Make a fist, straighten and repeat.	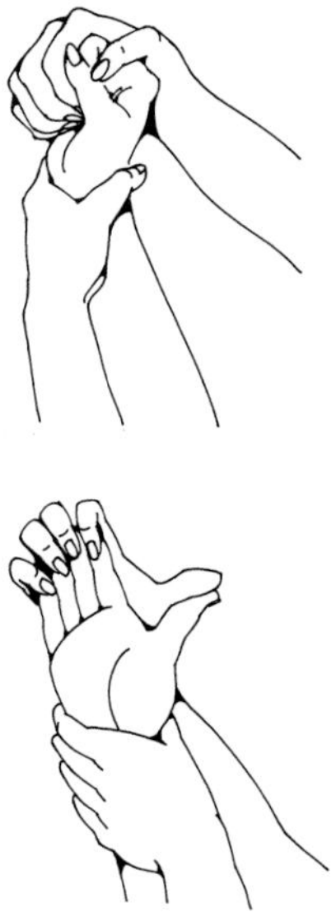	Flex patient's elbow, grasp wrist. Place the palm of your other hand on the back of the patient hand and flex all fingers and thumb with yours. Hook your fingertips under patient's flexed fingers and thumb and pull them to extension, *or* slide your palm under patient's flexed fingers, extending the fingers and thumb as you do.
Hyperextension	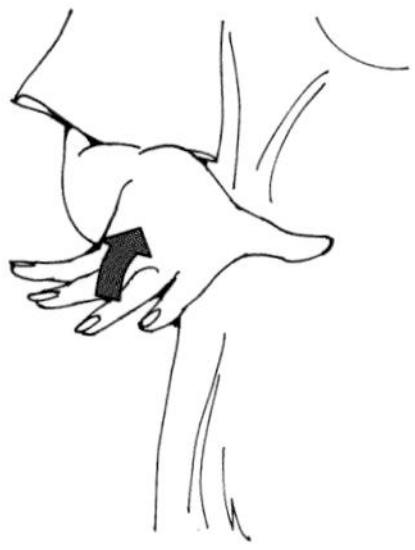	Stretch fingers and thumb toward the back of hand.	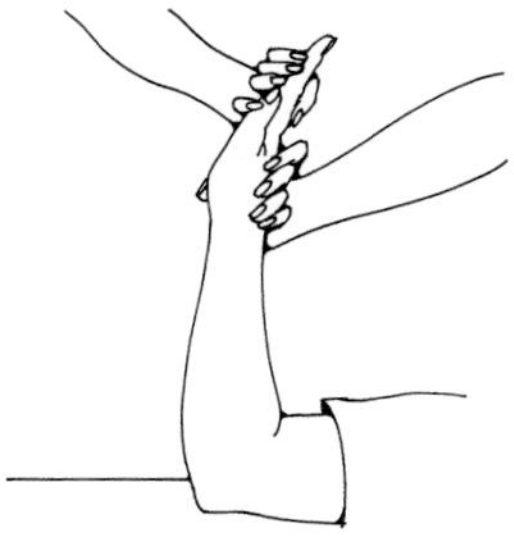	Continue to apply pressure on patient's fingers and thumb to hyperextend them.
Hip				
Internal Rotation	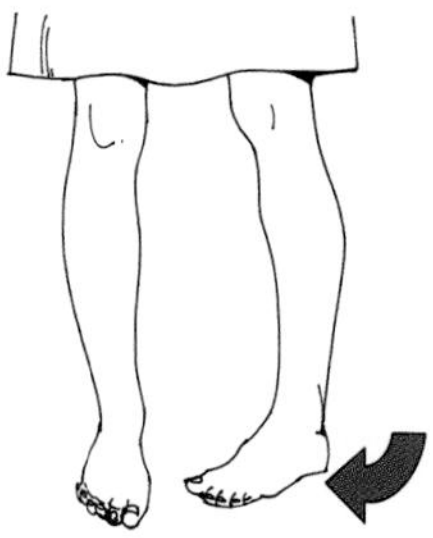	Keeping knee straight and foot perpendicular to leg, turn foot toward center of body.	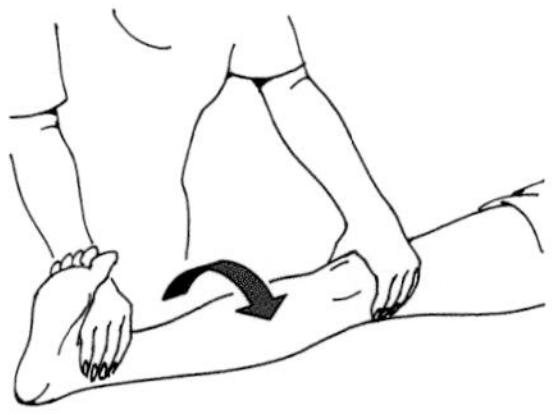	With patient's leg resting on bed, rotate leg toward midline.

Continued

TABLE 33-5. CONTINUED

Movement	Active: Illustration	Active: Instructions for Patient	Passive: Illustration	Passive: Description of Nurse's Action
Hip (cont.)				
External Rotation	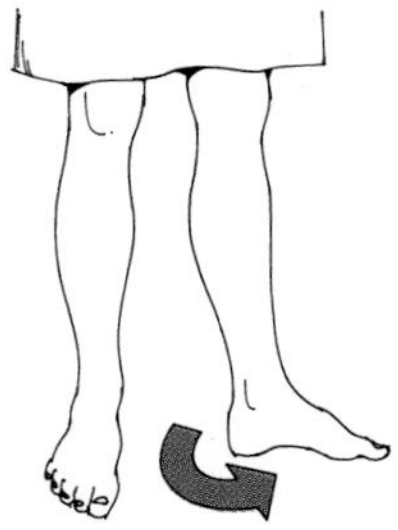	In same position as above, turn foot outward.	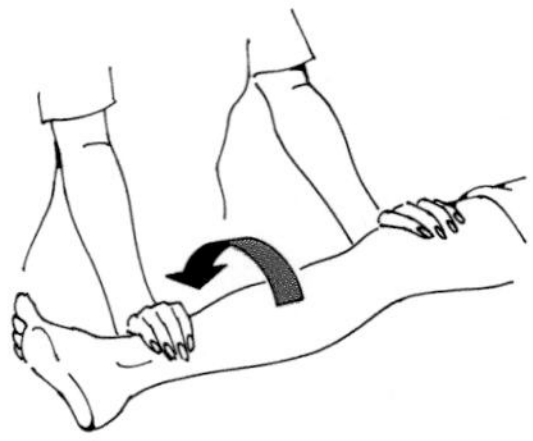	With patient's leg resting on bed, rotate leg outward.
Adduction	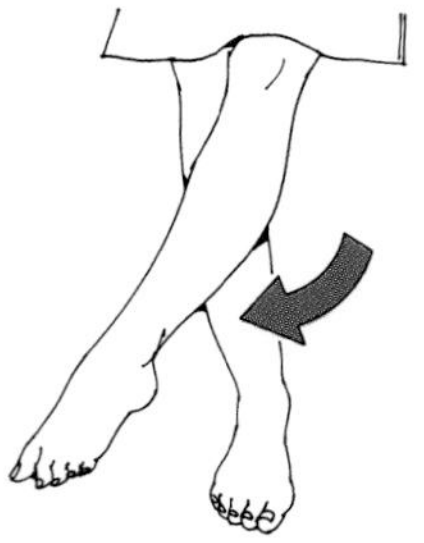	Bring one leg across and in front of the other leg.	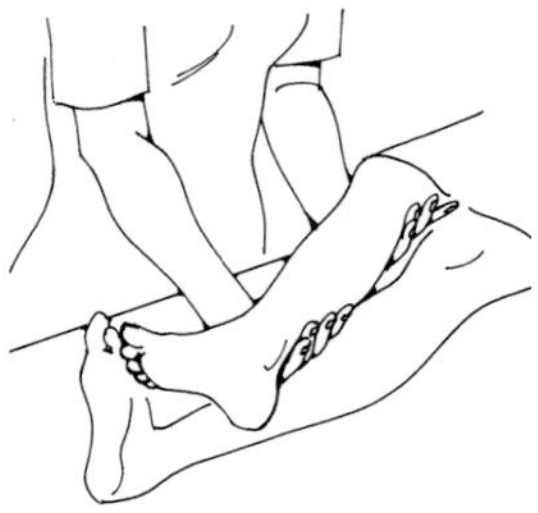	Support patient's leg behind ankle and knee. Move leg toward midline.
Abduction	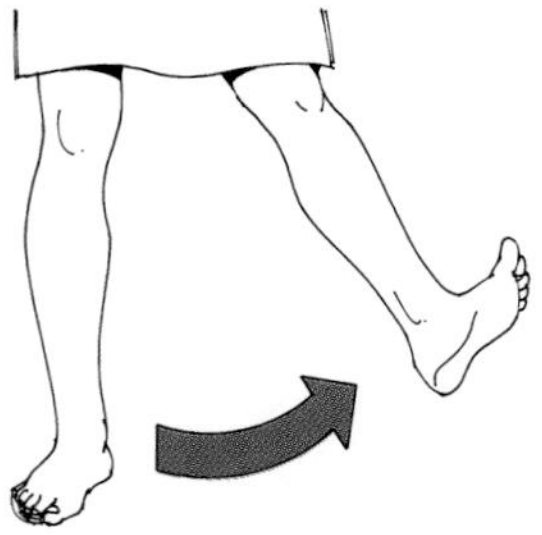	Move leg out to the side as far as possible.	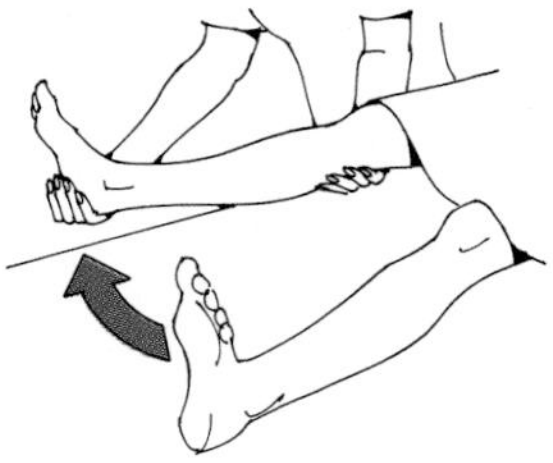	Support as above, move leg outward from midline. Step away from side of bed to fully abduct patient's hip.
Circumduction	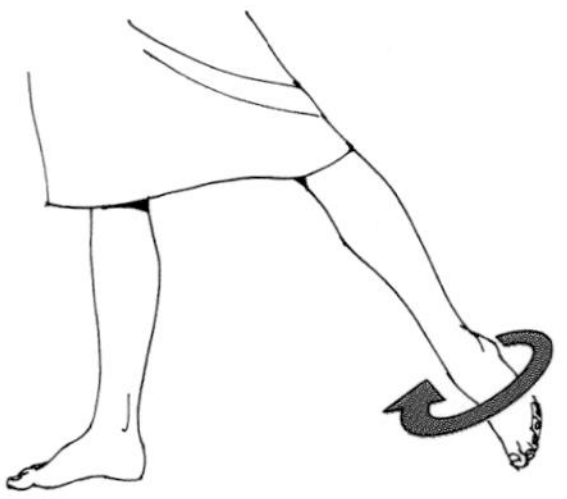	With leg straight, move foot in circular motion.	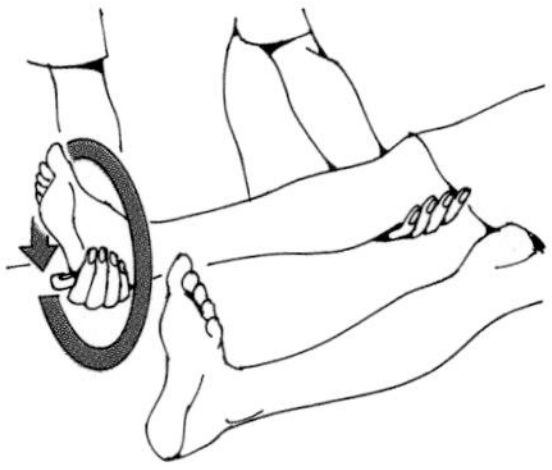	Supporting patient's leg as above, move it in a circular motion, keeping leg straight.
Flexion	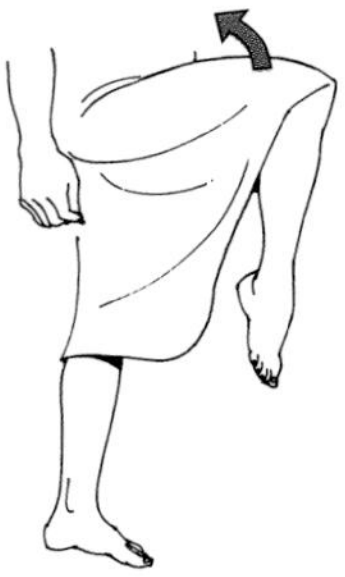	Bend hip and knee bringing knee close to chest. Can assist by grasping knee with arms (see knee flexion, page 1195).	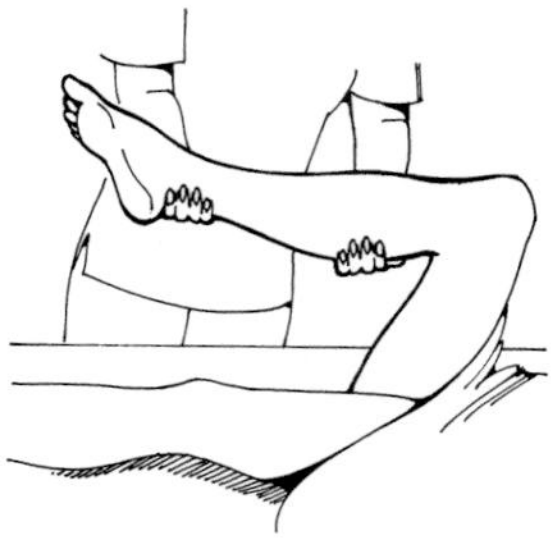	Support patient's ankle and calf to flex knee and hip, pushing thigh toward abdomen.

TABLE 33-5. CONTINUED

Movement	Active: Illustration	Active: Instructions for Patient	Passive: Illustration	Passive: Description of Nurse's Action
Hyperextension	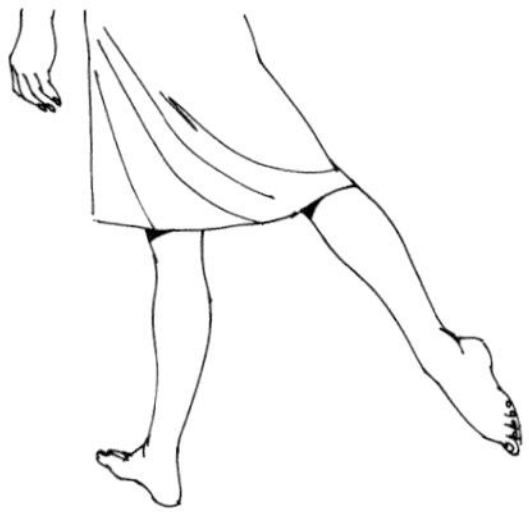	Point toe move leg backward with knee straight.	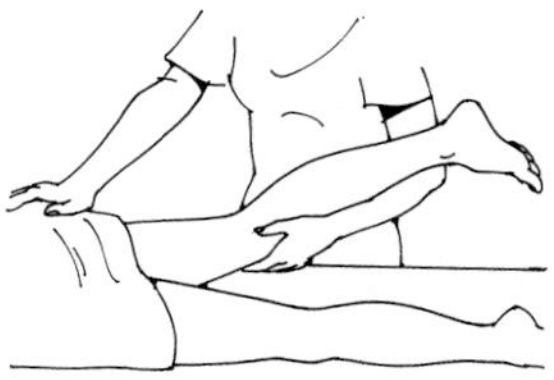	(Done after all leg exercises in supine position have been completed.) Place patient on side or prone. Cradle lower portion of leg with arm. Applying counterpressure on buttocks so that hip is not lifted off bed, raise patient's leg off bed. (Move leg backward if lying on side.)
Knee *Flexion*	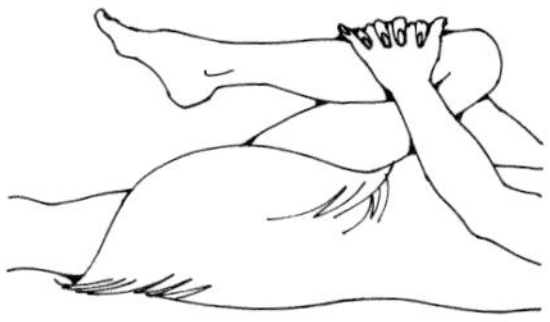	Lying on back, bend knee to chest and grasp with arms.		Done with hip flexion.
Circumduction	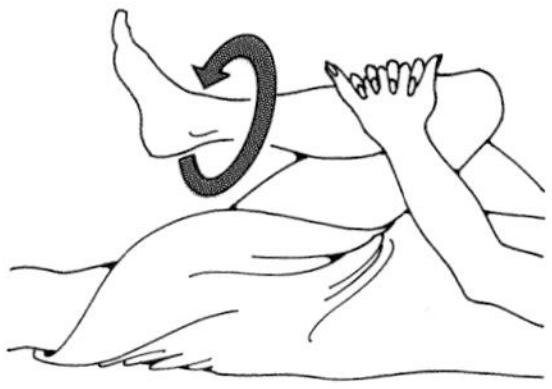	With knee flexed, move foot in circular motion.	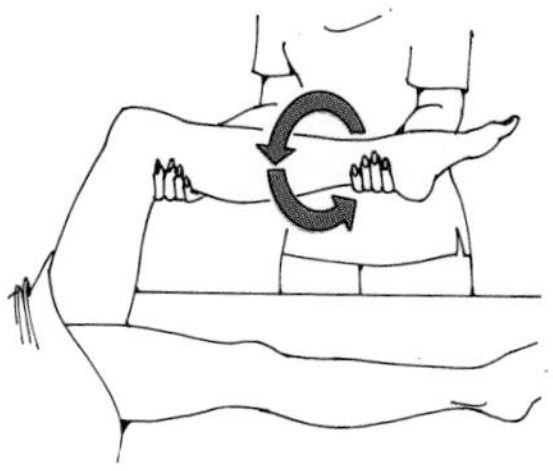	Support back of patient's knee and ankle. With patient's knee flexed, move lower portion of leg in circular motion.
Hyperextension	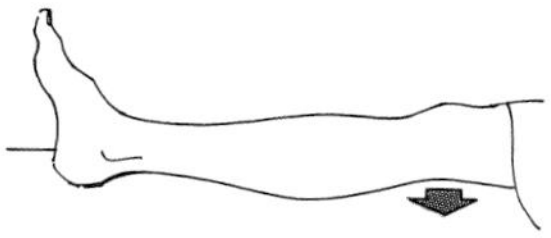	Sitting with leg extended, push back of knee against surface below.	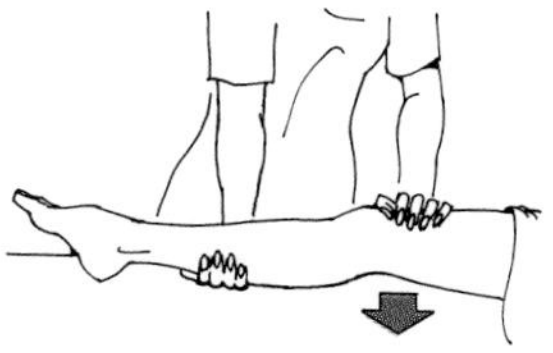	Support patient's lower leg at lower calf. Apply counterpressure above knee, gently raise lower leg until you feel resistance.
Ankle *Inversion*	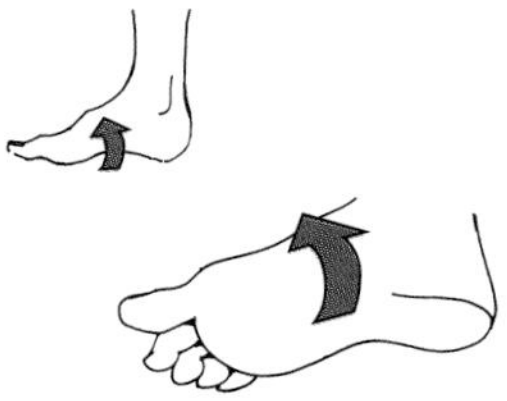	With patient standing, ask him or her to roll foot so that the sole faces other foot.	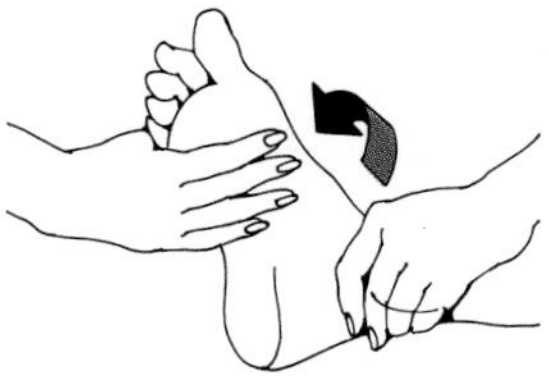	With patient's leg resting on bed, stabilize ankle, grasp forefoot with fingers on sole. Turn sole of the foot toward midline.

Continued

TABLE 33-5. CONTINUED

Movement	Active: Illustration	Active: Instructions for Patient	Passive: Illustration	Passive: Description of Nurse's Action
Ankle (cont.)				
Eversion	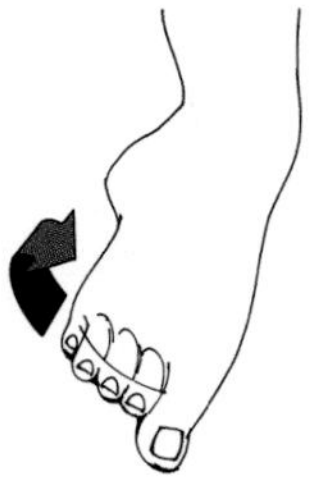	Turn the sole of the foot to the outside.	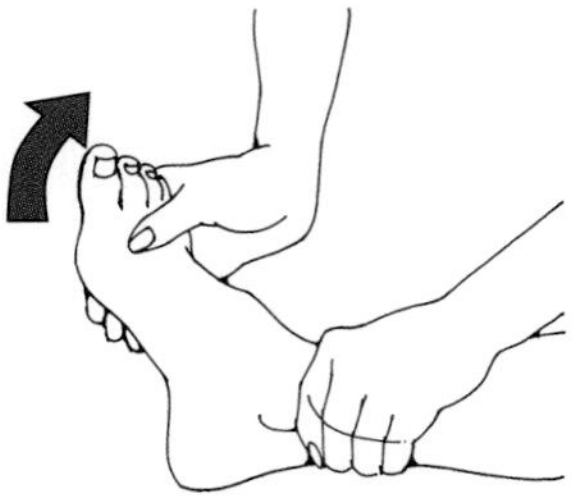	Holding patient's forefoot as above, turn the sole away from the midline.
Dorsiflexion	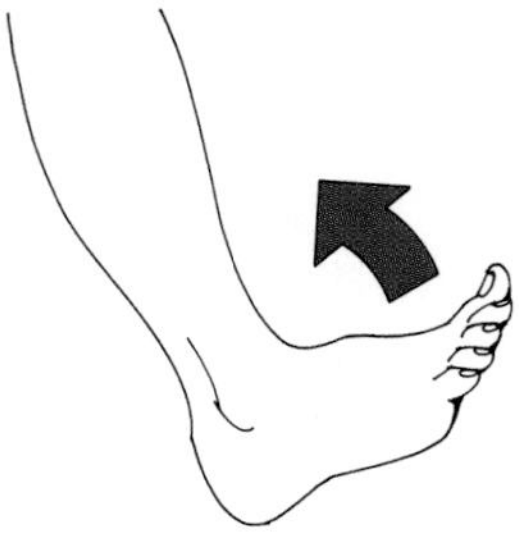	Bend the foot toward the shin.	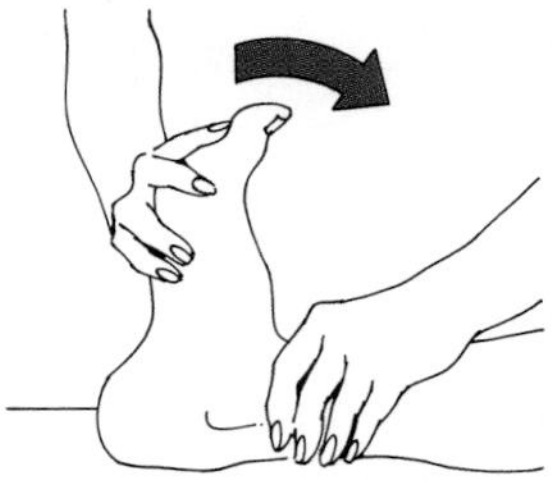	Holding foot as above, flex the foot toward the shin. (May also cup heel with hand and use forearm to flex foot.)
Plantar Flexion	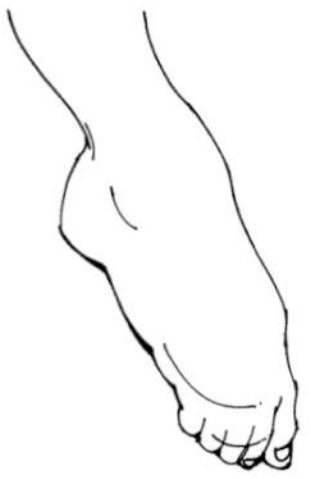	Point the toe.	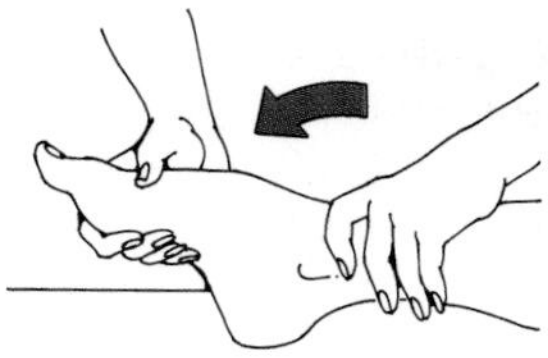	Holding patient's foot as above, straighten foot as if to point toe.
Circumduction	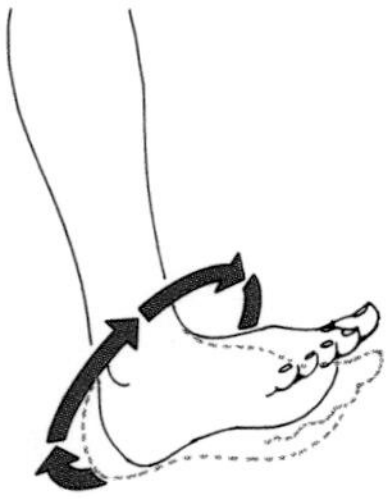	Move foot in circular motion at ankle without moving the knee or heel.	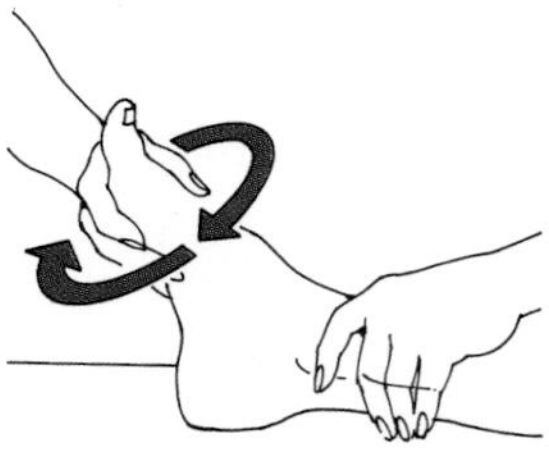	With patient's foot in plantar flexion, rotate forefoot in circular motion.

TABLE 33-5. CONTINUED

Movement	Active: Illustration	Active: Instructions for Patient	Passive: Illustration	Passive: Description of Nurse's Action
Toes				
Flexion	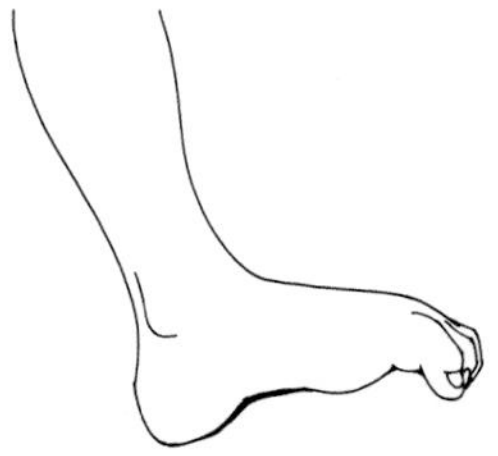	Curl toes.	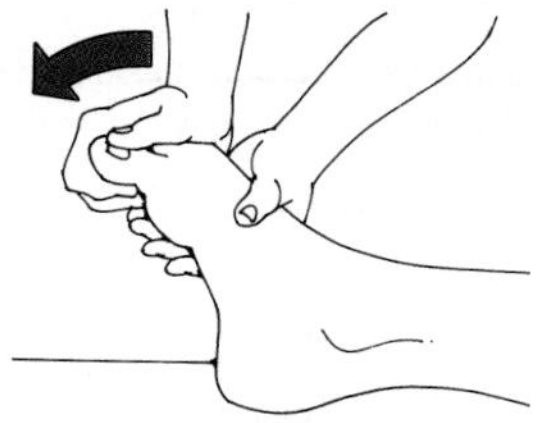	Flex patient's toes toward sole of foot by applying pressure with fingers.
Hyperextension	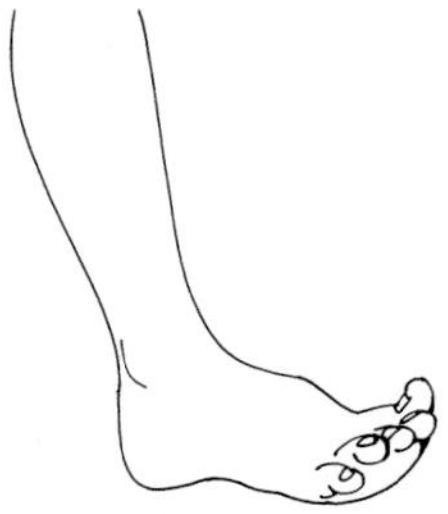	Raise toes off floor without raising foot.	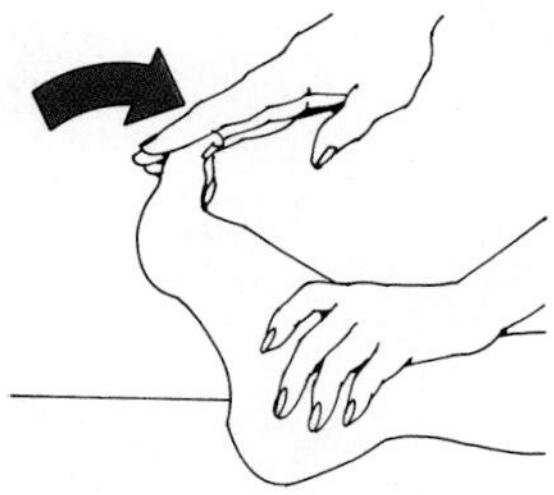	Move one hand behind patient's toes and the other hand to forefoot, apply hand pressure to move toes toward ankle.
Adduction/Abduction		Spread toes.	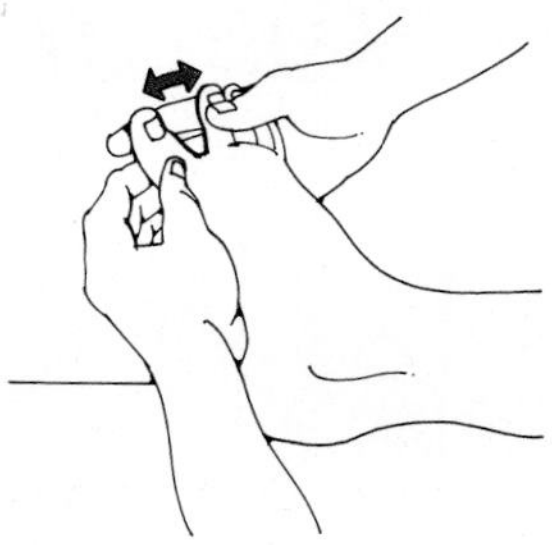	With patient's leg resting on bed, separate each toe from the one adjacent.
Circumduction			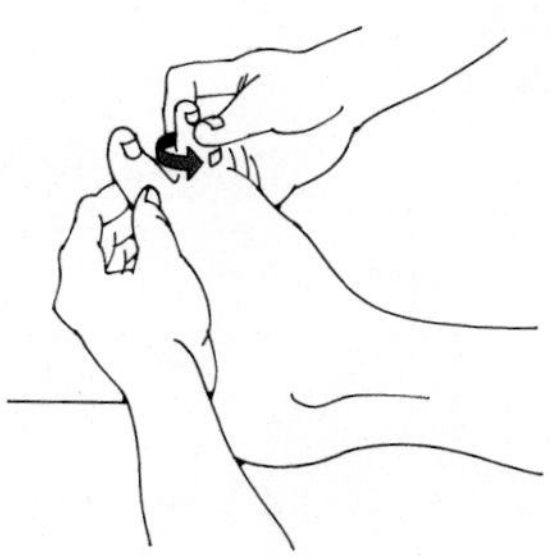	Move each toe in a circular motion.

Document exercise as described in Clinical Guideline 33–3.

MUSCLE STRENGTH AND TONE. Normal muscle tone is noted as slight muscular resistance when you passively move a relaxed extremity through range of motion. To assess strength, apply resistance to patients' muscles as they perform active ROM.

Figure 33–4 illustrates strength testing of some of the muscles of the shoulder girdle, the arm flexors and extensors, and grip strength. Figure 33–5 illustrates strength assessment of hip abductors, the flexors and extensors of the knee, and plantar flexion and dorsiflexion. Note that when testing lower extremity muscle strength, patients are asked to lie on an examining table or bed that supports the weight of the extremity. This conserves nurses' energy and enables both nurse and patient to use better body mechanics during the assessment. Clinical Guideline 33–4 summarizes an abbreviated test of muscle strength that is sufficient for assessing many people without serious neuromuscular problems.

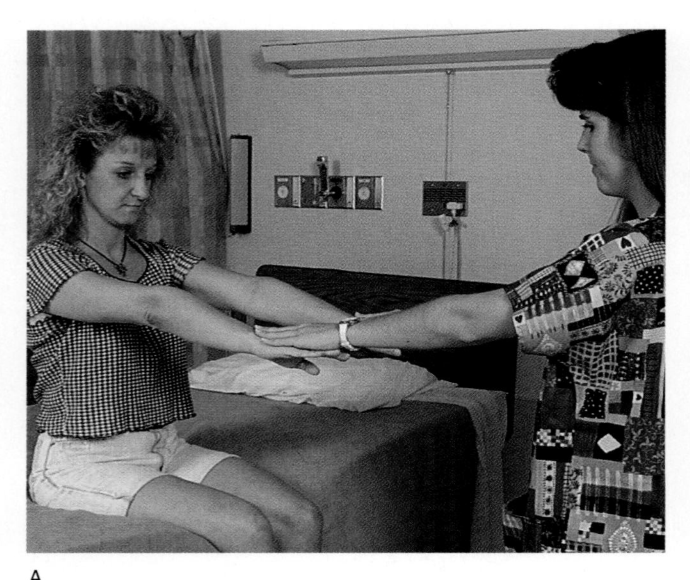

A

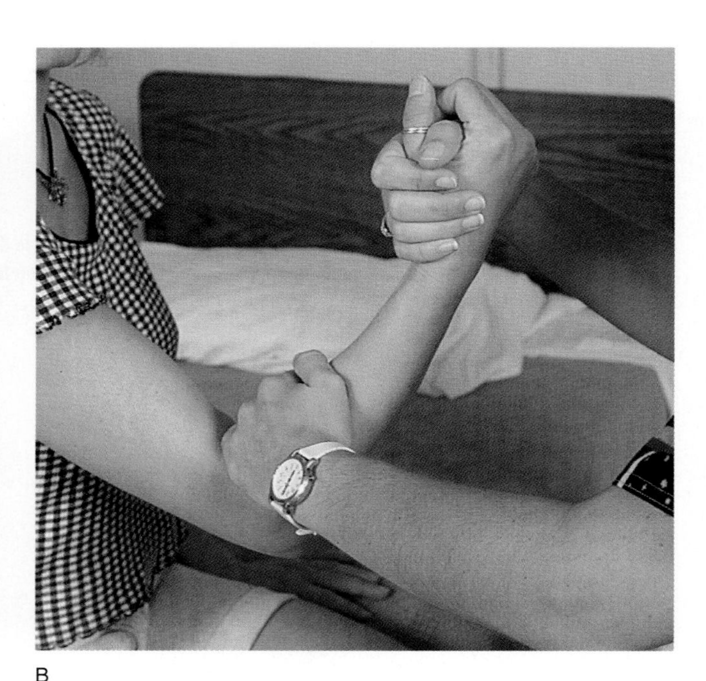

B

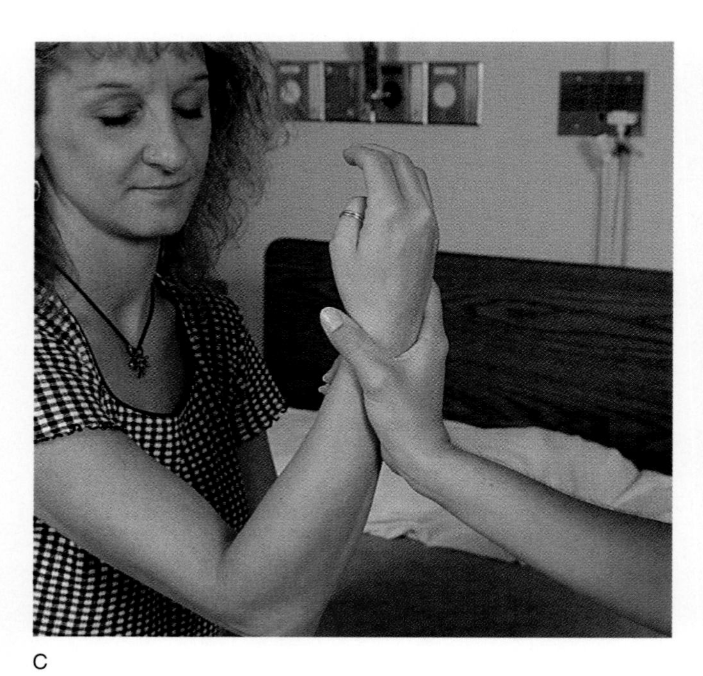

C

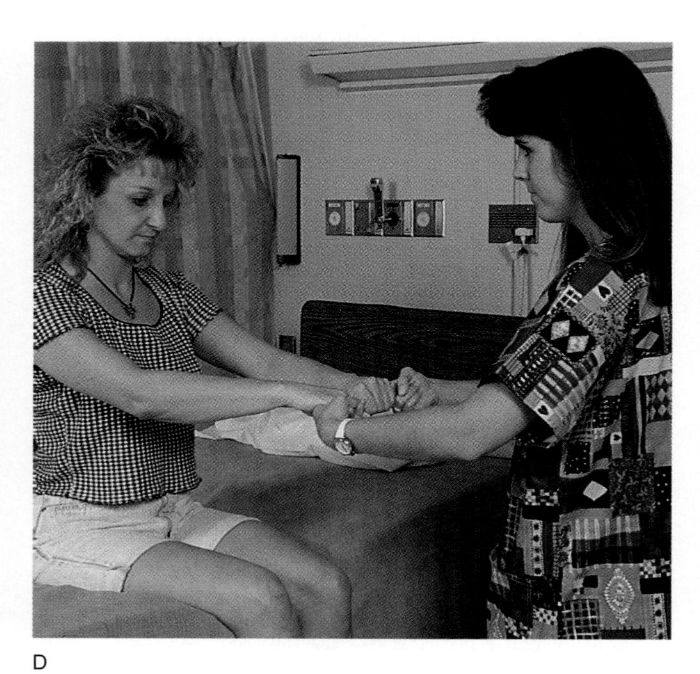

D

Figure 33–4. Strength testing of upper extremity. **A.** Shoulder and scapulae resistance. **B.** Elbow flexion. **C.** Elbow extension. **D.** Grip strength.

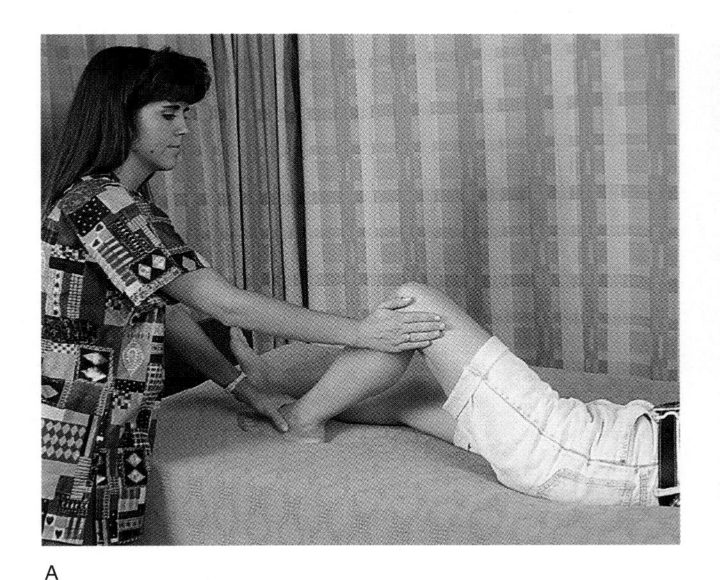

A

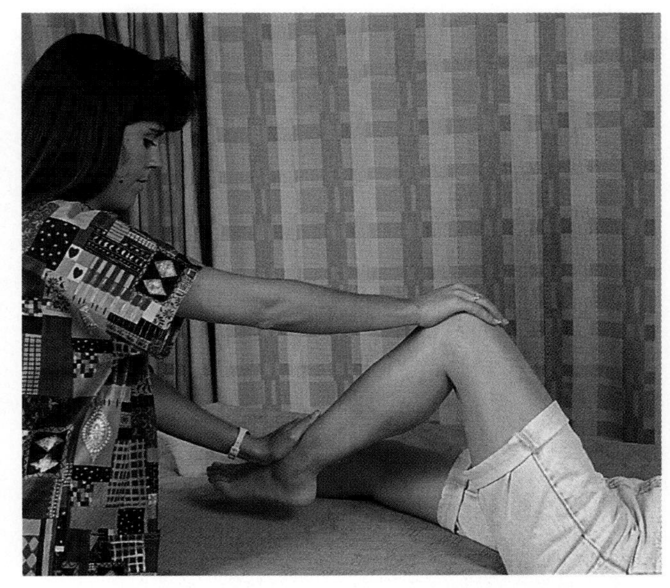

B

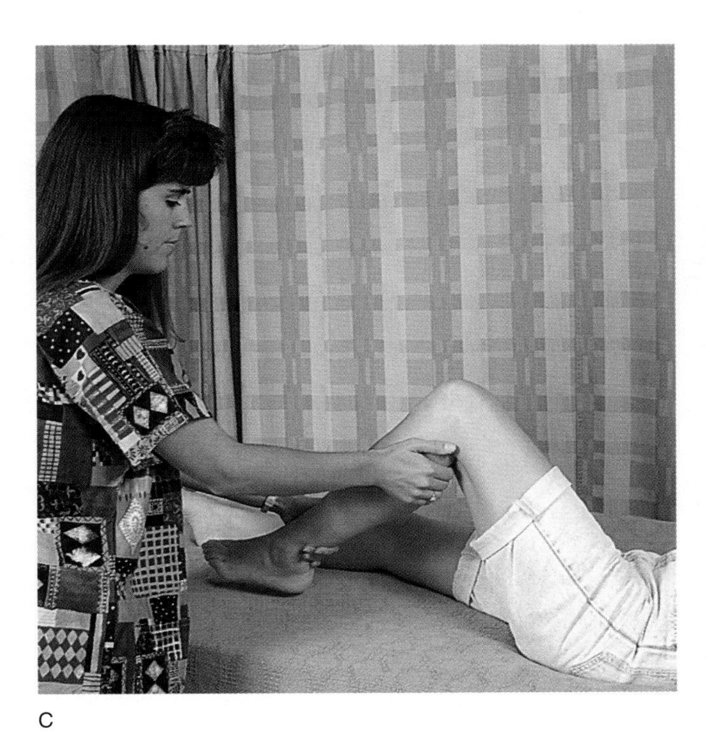

C

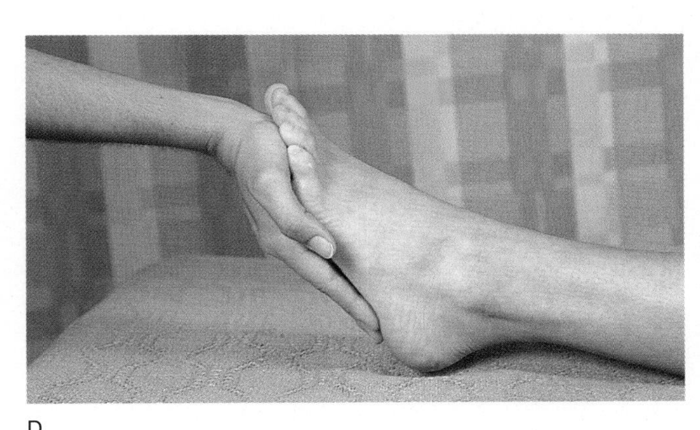

D

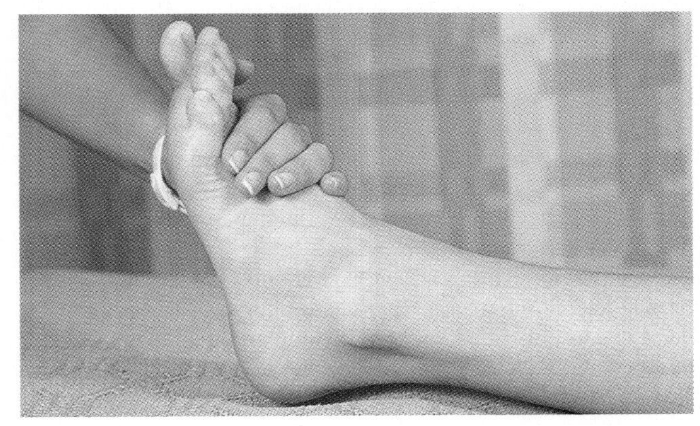

E

Figure 33–5. Strength testing of lower extremity. **A.** Hip abduction. **B.** Knee extension. **C.** Knee flexion. **D.** Plantar flexion. **E.** Dorsiflexion.

CLINICAL GUIDELINE 33–4

AN ABBREVIATED TEST OF MUSCLE STRENGTH

UPPER EXTREMITIES

Grip strength: Ask patient to squeeze the first two fingers of both of your hands simultaneously. (Patient grasps fingers of your left hand with his or her right hand, and vice versa.) Grasp should be essentially equal; dominant hand may be slightly stronger (see Fig. 33–4D).

Arm and shoulder strength: Ask patient to extend arms to the front, palms down. Tell patient to try to raise arms while you press downward on the backs of patient's hands. Equal resistance against moderate pressure is expected (see Fig. 33–4A).

Shoulder and scapular strength: Ask patient to raise both arms above his or her head. Tell patient to try to bring arms together while you exert outward pressure on the medial aspect of both arms, just distal to the elbow. Equal resistance against moderate pressure is expected.

Finger strength: Ask patient to spread his or her fingers while you try to push them together. Test both hands together. Resistance should be essentially equal.

LOWER EXTREMITIES

Lower leg: Patient sits or lies with legs extended. Place your hand on the top of his or her foot and pull as if to point the toes while patient resists (dorsiflexion). Then apply pressure to the ball of the foot and ask patient to push the foot as if to point the toes while you apply opposing pressure. Resistance should be equal (see Fig. 33–5D and E).

Upper leg: Patient is supine with knee flexed. Place one hand behind patient's heel and ask patient to pull heel toward buttocks. Repeat with other leg. Resistance should be equal (see Fig. 33–5C).

Some examiners use descriptive words such as paralysis; severe, moderate, or minimal weakness; and normal to describe muscle strength. Others prefer the rating scale presented in Table 17–41. When testing muscle strength, be mindful of differences related to age, sex, and level of conditioning. For example, an acutely ill 25-year-old athlete may complain of muscle weakness, but still exhibit considerably greater resistance than a physically healthy 80-year-old.

Symmetric response is expected. That is, strength and tone on the left should be about the same as on the right. Usually the dominant extremities are slightly stronger than those on the opposite side of the body in healthy people. When a patient has a disease or injury involving one extremity or one side of the body, using the unaffected extremity as a basis for evaluating losses or gains in the involved extremity is useful.

Be alert to such abnormalities as cramps, spasms, or increased muscle tone. Muscle *cramps* are observable as a hard knot in the belly of the muscle. A *spasm* is involuntary contraction of short duration with alternate periods of relaxation. Cramps or spasms can be associated with metabolic and electrolyte alterations, especially abnormal losses of sodium, calcium, and magnesium. They are more common in individuals who are sweating or dehydrated (see Chap. 34). Increased muscle tone presents as resistance when you are palpating or moving a relaxed extremity. Localized tension can be stress related, especially in the neck, back, and jaw. Generalized or one-sided hypertonicity is often associated with neurologic disorders.

Neurologic. The mental status, balance, coordination, and deep tendon reflex (DTR) examinations are aspects of the neurologic assessment that provide information needed to determine mobility status. Much of the mental status assessment can be conducted during the interview. At this time, a nurse can determine level of consciousness (LOC); orientation to time, person, and place; and ability to recall both recent and past events. The appropriateness of patient responses to questions in the health history implies orientation and recall. Chapter 32 provides more information about assessing and describing LOC.

Observations of gait and overall movement, as well as assessment of muscle tone and strength, discussed earlier, provide evidence of the level of neurologic functioning. If data gathered during these aspects of the examination indicate problems that could prevent safe mobility (eg, uneven, uncoordinated gait, decreased ROM, localized or generalized alterations in muscle strength and tone), do a more specific assessment of gait, balance, and coordination. Clinical Guideline 33–5 highlights elements to observe when assessing gait.

The Romberg test, a simple screening test for balance, is described in Chap. 17. Balance is essential for independent mobility. Balance deficits are a significant factor contributing to falls, especially among the elderly.

Chapter 32 discusses several tests for evaluating coordination. Clumsiness and irregularity of movement suggest a need for supervised or assisted ambulation to prevent injury. Whenever irregularities of movement are noted, it is useful to assess deep

CLINICAL GUIDELINE 33–5

KEY ELEMENTS OF GAIT ASSESSMENT

Head and neck mobility	Head and neck should turn side to side as needed, independent from trunk movement. Unexpected findings: head fixed in downward orientation, or movable only with trunk "all in one piece."
Trunk and arm movements	Body should move freely, arms should swing forward slightly as opposite heel strikes. Unexpected findings: stiff trunk, asymmetric, diminished, or unilateral arm swing.
Foot stance	Shoulder width rather than wide stance expected.
Pattern of steps	Steps should be even in length and pace, with heel strike before toe. Unexpected findings: high step with slapping of the feet on the ground, wide waddling steps, shuffling, or short quick steps.
Equilibrium	Steady erect posture without swaying or staggering is expected.

INSIGHTS FROM NURSING LITERATURE

FACTORS CONTRIBUTING TO FALLS

Benson C, Lusardi P. Neurologic antecedents to patient falls. J Neurosci Nurs. *1995;27:331–337.*

Authors Benson and Lusardi reviewed the literature on patient falls and found three common manifestations of disease of the nervous system that increase a patient's risk of falling. Those manifestations are altered mental status, sensory/motor alteration, and impaired physical mobility. The authors recommend that precautions be taken to protect patients with any of these problems from falls.

tendon reflexes (DTRs), as illustrated in Chap. 17. Abnormally slow or unusually brisk reflexes imply pathology that could interfere with safe ambulation.

Exercise Tolerance. **Exercise tolerance** refers to the amount (rate and duration) of a given exercise a person can perform before experiencing distress or exhaustion. Evaluating an individual's response to exercise demand is an important part of the mobility assessment. It permits a recommendation for physical activity that will maintain or improve level of fitness but not overtax the individual. For an inpatient, exercise is usually limited to ambulation, isometrics, and other stationary exercises described in a later section of this chapter, *Nursing Implementation to Promote Optimal Mobility*. Discharge or rehabilitation planning often involves collaboration with other members of the health care team. It may require exercise stress testing, which is discussed in a later section. This is also recommended for any sedentary individual over 45 years who desires to begin an exercise program as well as patients having other risk factors discussed in Section 1.[25]

Before observing a patient's responses to exercise, gather baseline data, shown in Table 33–6. If data in one or more categories indicate a caution, plan to initiate exercise at a mild level and increase the intensity gradually. Consultation with a physician or a physical therapist may be necessary prior to planning exercises for some patients.

Observations during exercise are a significant component of assessing activity tolerance. Many patients can assess themselves as they exercise. When assisting patients in an inpatient setting with exercise, however, these observations are a nursing responsibility. Assess the following.

1. *Pulse rate and rhythm.* As discussed in Section 1, changes in pulse have been shown by research to be an accurate indicator of exercise tolerance. Increases of more than 20 to 25 beats per minute are not expected nor desired during exercises typical in an inpatient setting. Terminate the exercise session if you note such an increase or if alterations in pulse rhythm occur. If no unusual circumstances can account for this change, the exercise plan should be reevaluated.
2. *Respiratory rate and depth.* An increase in both rate and depth of respiration is expected; however, dyspnea indicates overexercise. Diaphragmatic spasm may cause a pain in the side, commonly called a "stitch," when respiratory effort is increased.

TABLE 33–6. BASELINE DATA FOR ASSESSING EXERCISE TOLERANCE

Data	Caution
Age	Over 45
Usual activity level	Sedentary
Duration of activity reduction	Bed rest more than 3 days
Weight	More than 20 pounds overweight
Reclining/standing BP	Resting BP > 140/90
	Standing systolic < reclining BP
	Dizziness on standing or sitting
Reclining/standing pulse, including rhythm, strength	Standing pulse > 16 bpm faster than supine; arrhythmias; bounding or thready pulse
Resting respirations, including rhythm, depth, quality	R > 20, shallow, irregular, or labored; dyspnea; secretions in chest
Hemoglobin, hematocrit	< Normal or low normal
Joint ROM	Contractures of any major joint
Muscle strength	Generalized or local weakness, especially of lower extremities
Neurological status	Altered LOC, impaired balance, or coordination (see also Chap. 32)
Health history	Diagnosis or symptoms of cardiovascular, pulmonary, metabolic, liver, renal, or thyroid disease

This is not usually a reason to decrease exercise intensity, however.

3. *Skin changes.* The vasodilation of skin blood vessels to dissipate the heat produced by increased muscular activity causes skin changes that can be readily observed in highly vascular areas such as the cheeks, lips, and nailbeds. Mild exercise may produce slight flushing and noticeable perspiration. Generalized redness, diaphoresis, and increased skin temperature are noted with more strenuous exercise. Activity in an inpatient setting would not be expected to cause these changes. If pallor, cyanosis, or coolness are noted, the exercise should be stopped immediately. These signs indicate vasoconstriction, poorly oxygenated blood, even impending shock. Though easily observed, skin changes are not conclusive indicators of activity tolerance. They are most useful when combined with other data.
4. *Rate and dexterity.* Onset of fatigue is frequently accompanied by a decrease in the rate and dexterity of an activity. Terminate the activity if postural changes such as sagging shoulders or reaching out for support, or uncoordinated gait occur.
5. *Pain or dizziness.* Dizziness or lightheadedness, brought on by maximal shunting of blood to the heart and muscles at the expense of the brain, indicates that rest is needed. Complaints of pain caused or aggravated by the activity may also indicate a need to change the exercise plan.

These guidelines are summarized in Clinical Guideline 33–6.

Many healthy individuals, exercising to increase fitness, tolerate some of the above symptoms and push themselves to higher levels of activity without harmful effects. Patients receiving care in an inpatient facility or who have chronic illnesses may have considerably less reserve and should be carefully monitored for signs that they are reaching or exceeding the limits of their exercise tolerance. Parameters that relate to the pathology for which a patient is being treated deserve most careful attention.

Heart rate, rhythm, blood pressure, and respiratory rate should be assessed immediately after exercise and again at 2 and 5 minutes postexercise. Pulse and respiration decrease rapidly after exercise ceases unless cardiac reserve has been exceeded. In relatively healthy individuals, these values should return to baseline in 1 to 2 minutes after exercise. For inpatients or those with chronic illnesses, expect pulse, respiration, and blood pressure to return to baseline within 5 minutes after cessation of exercise. If elevation is prolonged, less intense exercise is recommended.

CLINICAL GUIDELINE 33–6

KEY ELEMENTS IN EXERCISE TOLERANCE ASSESSMENT

- Pulse rate and rhythm
- Respiratory rate and depth
- Skin changes
- Rate and dexterity of exercise
- Dizziness
- Pain

The mobility history and examination are the basis for nursing diagnoses and patient care plans discussed in later sections. Ongoing assessment throughout the course of care is necessary so that nursing diagnoses and management are current and appropriate.

DIAGNOSTIC TESTS

Diagnostic examinations provide useful information to support medical and nursing diagnoses and guide treatment plans. The following tests are specific to mobility. Other tests of cardiac and pulmonary function that are also relevant to mobility status are discussed in Chap. 30.

- *Arthrocentesis:* aspiration of synovial fluid from a joint. Ordinarily, joints have a very small amount of fluid, but a joint effusion (collection of fluid in a joint space) is an indicator of problems. Analysis of the aspirated synovial fluid provides clues about the cause of the effusion. Reassure patients that pain control is provided via local anesthesia. No food or fluid restrictions are necessary unless measuring synovial glucose concentration, which requires 6 to 8 hours of fasting prior to the test.
- *Arthroscopy:* direct visualization of the interior of a joint using a fiberoptic instrument that is surgically inserted into the joint. It is used to detect joint trauma and disease, as well as to facilitate the surgical removal of damaged tissue. It may be done under local or general anesthesia. Patients must fast for 12 hours prior to general anesthesia. Swelling and pain are expected after arthroscopy. Tell patients to plan for limited activity for 2 to 3 days after the procedure. Ice and analgesia are used to relieve swelling and pain.
- *Electromyogram (EMG):* measures the electrical activity of muscles at rest and during voluntary activity using small needle electrodes. It is used to detect muscle pathology. Usually a resting muscle demonstrates minimal electrical activity, whereas motor disorders produce abnormal electrical patterns in resting muscle. Patients must restrict intake of beverages containing caffeine for 3 hours and abstain from smoking for 24 hours before the test. Reassure patients that the needles are very thin and produce minimal discomfort. The electrical shocks are moderately uncomfortable, but brief.
- *CT (computed tomography) and MRI (magnetic resonance imaging):* both produce multidimensional images of an organ or section of the body. Both can be used to assess bones and joints and soft tissue such as muscle. CT uses ionizing radiation, which is considered more invasive than the powerful magnetic fields used for MRI. No pretest restriction of food or fluids is required, and the procedure is painless unless IV contrast media is needed. The enclosed space of the machines used for CTs and MRIs causes anxiety for many patients. Relaxation techniques are helpful. Some require sedation. Tests require patients to remain still for 60 to 90 minutes. People who are pregnant, extremely obese, or who have metal implants (pacemakers, joint replacements, IUDs) cannot undergo CT or MRI.
- *Exercise stress test:* a noninvasive study to evaluate cardiac function. Patients exercise for specific intervals at increasing levels of intensity on a treadmill or bicycle ergometer with constant ECG monitoring. The test is discontinued when heart rate reaches 85 to 90 percent of maximal heart rate or if severe symptoms of distress or cardiac compromise are noted. Patients

may not eat, drink, or smoke for 4 hours preceding the test. Tell them to wear comfortable clothing and shoes for the test, which takes about 45 minutes.

NURSING DIAGNOSIS OF MOBILITY STATUS

Clustering of the data cues obtained in the mobility history and examination indicates whether a patient has mobility problems that require nursing attention. Using a guide such as the list of nursing diagnoses approved by the North American Nursing Diagnosis Association (NANDA) assists beginning students to note relationships between cues and associate these cues with specific nursing diagnoses and their etiologies. Table 33–7 illustrates sample nursing diagnoses for mobility.

A clear and complete diagnosis statement is important, because it provides the basis for planning individualized care. Four nursing diagnoses directly related to mobility are examined in this section: impaired physical mobility, activity intolerance, risk for activity intolerance, and risk for disuse syndrome.

IMPAIRED PHYSICAL MOBILITY

Impaired physical mobility is a state in which an individual experiences a limitation of ability for independent physical movement. Six etiologies are listed in the NANDA taxonomy.

- *Etiology: activity intolerance/decreased strength and endurance.* Regular physical activity contributes to increased levels of fitness, which supports a wider range of mobility. Inactive people, therefore, have lower levels of fitness, less strength and endurance, and so a diminished capacity for mobility. The stress of illness can deplete one's energy stores, decreasing strength, endurance, and mobility.
- *Etiology: pain or discomfort.* Pain receptors are located throughout the body. They are activated by such stimuli as physical trauma, the presence of inflammatory exudates, and stretching or pressure. Movement can generate and exacerbate the painful sensations relayed by these pain receptors. Therefore, a characteristic response to localized or generalized pain is to decrease movement.
- *Etiology: neuromuscular impairment.* Neuromuscular functioning is essential for coordinated movement. Interference with neuromuscular functioning can result from injury, illness, or a pathologic process such as a cerebral vascular accident (stroke).
- *Etiology: musculoskeletal impairment.* Musculoskeletal impairment can cause generalized or localized interference with movement. A person lacking the support of an intact skeleton or the contractile power of muscles would find movement difficult or impossible.
- *Etiology: perceptual/cognitive impairment.* Perceptual/cognitive impairment encompasses a variety of problems. Disorientation (inability to receive or interpret signals from the environment) and hallucinations (sensory impressions having no basis in external stimulation) can block the ability to initiate purposeful coordinated movement. Also, hearing loss and vision deficits alter or block perception of environmental cues needed for safe and effective mobility.
- *Etiology: depression or severe anxiety.* Depression depletes one's energy level. Depressed people often desire to avoid interactions with others, which they can accomplish by diminishing their mobility. Severe anxiety is physically and emotionally immobilizing. The expression "frozen with fear" is an apt description of a person whose emotional state is so overwhelming that movement is impossible. The anxiety can interfere with problem-solving to the extent that any action or movement cannot be attempted for fear of real or imagined consequences.

ACTIVITY INTOLERANCE

Activity intolerance (or risk for activity intolerance) is a state in which an individual has (or is at risk for) insufficient physiologic or psychological energy to endure or complete required or desired daily activities. NANDA lists four etiologies and/or risk factors.

- *Etiology: bedrest/immobility.* There are many deleterious effects associated with bedrest or immobility that compromise the ability to tolerate activity. Losses in muscle strength and efficiency and cardiopulmonary deconditioning have the greatest impact on activity tolerance. Changes in appetite associated with negative nitrogen balance contribute to insufficient nutrient and fluid intake that further strain physiologic resources and deplete energy.
- *Etiology: generalized weakness.* Weak muscles cannot perform sustained activity. Weak muscles have a lower volume of mitochondria to metabolize ATP and fewer capillaries to transport oxygen to muscle cells for metabolic reactions. Muscle fatigue is rapid and compromises dexterity. Very weak individuals may fall or be physically unable to move further when pushed beyond their capacity.
- *Etiology: sedentary lifestyle.* Although individuals may maintain a capacity for activity that is satisfactory for their daily routine, those who are sedentary have little aerobic or strength reserve for exertion beyond that level. Many sedentary individuals are overweight because their limited activity burns minimal calories. Therefore, a decision to change lifestyle—for example, to seek a job in which greater physical exertion is required, or to participate in a new leisure activity—can be difficult to carry out because their bodies' inability to sustain large-muscle activity generates activity intolerance.
- *Etiology: imbalance between oxygen supply and demand.* Insufficient oxygen supply cuts down a muscle's capacity to work. Exertion increases muscle oxygen uptake, and therefore increases oxygen demand. Inadequate oxygen prevents resynthesis of ATP; fatigue and exhaustion therefore follow. If the supply of available oxygen is insufficient to support heart muscle function, arrhythmias and even cardiovascular collapse may occur.

RISK FOR DISUSE SYNDROME

Disuse syndrome refers to the collection of conditions discussed earlier under *Altered Function Associated with Limited Mobility.* The following are risk factors.

- *Risk factor: paralysis.* Paralysis is a temporary or permanent loss of function, in particular the ability for voluntary motion. (see also Chap. 32). The degree of risk for disuse syndrome is related to the extent of paralysis and the motivation to participate in preventive measures. Prevention of disuse syndrome in paralyzed individuals requires constant vigilance.

TABLE 33-7. SAMPLE NURSING DIAGNOSES: MOBILITY

Nursing Diagnosis	Defining Characteristics/Manifestations: *Subjective Data*	Defining Characteristics/Manifestations: *Objective Data*	Etiology
Impaired physical mobility 6.1.1.1	Reports pain increased by movement. Reports inability to perform specific movements.	Refuses to move. Grimaces when attempts to move.	*Physical:* pain.
Impaired physical mobility 6.1.1.1	None.	Does not follow simple commands. Cannot name or use common objects (eg, cup, pencil). Unable to correctly state name, location, or date. Does not perform spontaneous purposeful movement. Inconsistent response to environmental stimuli.	*Cognitive:* Perceptual/cognitive impairment: confusion.
Activity intolerance 6.1.1.2	Reports fatigue. Reports dyspnea on exertion.	Unable to resist moderate force in upper or lower extremities. HR increases 25 bpm with moderate activity. RR ↑ with labored respirations during moderate activity. HR, RR do not return to baseline until 8 minutes after moderate activity.	*Physical:* Generalized weakness.

High Risk Diagnosis	Risk Factors
Risk for activity intolerance 6.1.1.3	Deconditioned state; muscles soft; wt 20 lb above ideal for ht.
Risk for disuse syndrome 1.6.1.5	Prescribed immobilization.

EXAMPLES OF OTHER NURSING DIAGNOSES ASSOCIATED WITH ALTERED MOBILITY

PHYSICAL
Altered nutrition
Risk for infection
Dysreflexia
Constipation
Altered urinary elimination
Reflex incontinence
Functional incontinence
Total incontinence
Urinary retention
Altered peripheral tissue perfusion
Fluid volume deficit
Impaired gas exchange
Ineffective airway clearance
Ineffective breathing pattern
Risk for injury
Impaired tissue integrity
Risk for peripheral neurovascular dysfunction
Impaired skin integrity
Self-care deficit
Sleep pattern disturbance
Fatigue
Altered health maintenance
Pain

COGNITIVE
Impaired verbal communication
Sensory perceptual alterations
Altered thought processes
Health-seeking behaviors
Knowledge deficit

EMOTIONAL
Impaired verbal communication
Ineffective individual coping
Impaired adjustment
Unilateral neglect
Hopelessness
Powerlessness
Anxiety
Fear
Dysfunctional grieving
Spiritual distress

SELF-CONCEPTUAL
Altered role performance
Body image disturbance
Self-esteem disturbance
Personal identity disturbance

SOCIOCULTURAL-LIFE STRUCTURAL
Impaired home maintenance management
Impaired social interaction
Social isolation
Altered family processes
Ineffective family coping

SEXUAL
Altered sexuality patterns
Sexual dysfunction

ENVIRONMENTAL
Diversional activity deficit

Source: The nursing diagnoses and etiologies in this table and the definitions of nursing diagnoses in the body of the text not credited to other sources are from Nursing Diagnosis: Definitions and Classification, 1997–1998. *Philadelphia: North American Nursing Diagnosis Association; 1996. Manifestation categories for etiologies and specifications of general etiologies on these tables are authors' original work.*

INSIGHTS FROM NURSING LITERATURE

A TEAM APPROACH TO PREVENTING PRESSURE ULCERS

McNaughton V, Brazil K. Wound and skin team impact on pressure ulcer prevalence in chronic care. J Gerontol Nurs. *Feb. 1995:21:45–49.*

Researchers McNaughton and Brazil studied the prevalence of pressure ulcers among patients hospitalized for chronic illnesses before and after their facility instituted a multidisciplinary team approach to preventing and treating skin breakdown. The role of team members included educating staff nurses. Prior to the start of the education initiative, McNaughton and Brazil conducted a patient survey to establish a prevalence baseline, and found an incidence of pressure ulcers consistent with national norms for chronic care facilities. A year after instituting the staff nurse education project—which informed staff nurses on such subjects as wound assessment and staging, and wound care treatment and product use—the researchers conducted a second prevalence survey. The findings showed a significantly lower total number of pressure ulcers and a lower number of patients with pressure ulcers.

- *Risk factor: mechanical or prescribed immobilization.* Mechanical immobilization—such as by traction, braces, or casts—creates varying degrees of immobility. Prescribed immobilization ranges from complete bedrest to restriction of only specific types of activity or movement. Some loss of function of immobilized body parts is inevitable, but attentive preventive care, discussed in Section 3, is effective in avoiding many immobility related problems.
- *Risk factor: severe pain.* Severe, intractable pain alters mobility. Although there are many modalities for pain relief (see Chap. 32), some, such as narcotic analgesics, depress central nervous system function. This effect contributes to mobility problems. Pain also interferes with motivation to be mobile, so a multifocused approach to preventing disuse syndrome associated with pain is necessary.
- *Risk factor: altered level of consciousness.* An individual's state of awareness affects the ability to desire to be mobile. Individuals who are lethargic or stuporous (slowed response to stimuli, little spontaneous movement), or comatose (unresponsive to stimuli, with some reflex movement), are at highest risk for disuse syndrome, because they make no spontaneous movements. See also Chap. 32.

STATING THE MOBILITY DIAGNOSIS

Analyze the assessment data to determine whether there are any mobility problems that can be resolved by nursing care. If so, write concise complete nursing diagnosis statements. The general statements from the taxonomy, such as "Impaired mobility related to pain," should be refined in the clinical setting when assessment data provide cues for a more exact statement. Examples are as follows:

- Impaired mobility related to abdominal incisional pain, as evidenced by infrequent position changes, "I can't walk—it hurts too much," facial grimacing and guarding of abdominal incision whenever movement is attempted.
- Impaired mobility: inability to walk, related to muscle weakness in lower extremities; as evidenced by decreased muscle tone and muscle mass in legs and buckling of knees when standing is attempted.

Note that the defining characteristics (major manifestations) that support the selection of a given diagnosis and etiology are also included in a complete diagnostic statement. These detailed statements represent individualized diagnoses based on the taxonomy of approved nursing diagnoses. When the nursing diagnosis is impaired physical mobility, NANDA recommends that the following code describing degree of dependence/independence be used as part of the diagnostic statement.

- 0 = Completely independent.
- 1 = Requires use of equipment or device.
- 2 = Requires help from another person for assistance, supervision, or teaching.
- 3 = Requires help from another person and equipment or device.
- 4 = Is dependent, does not participate in activity.

As patients progress in level of independence, the level classification number can be changed to reflect the progress. In the sample nursing diagnoses above, the mobility impairment related to abdominal incisional pain might be initially designated level 2, while the patient unable to bear weight might be considered to be at a functional level of 4. The mobility diagnosis, when stated clearly and concisely, provides the basis for management of patient care, discussed in the next section.

SECTION 3

NURSE-PATIENT MANAGEMENT OF MOBILITY

PLANNING FOR OPTIMAL MOBILITY

PATIENT CARE PLANS

A patient care plan to promote optimal mobility may relate to concerns such as improving level of fitness, supporting a plan for healthful weight reduction, assisting with activities of daily living during acute illness, or teaching self-care adaptations to accommodate residual disability. A complete mobility care plan addresses all the activity/mobility problem areas stated in each nursing diagnosis. The plan communicates desired outcomes of patient care, nursing approaches, and evaluation criteria. Deciding on realistic outcomes is the first step in writing the plan. Statements of desired outcomes in a mobility care plan succinctly describe the level of mobility a patient should attain as a result of nursing therapies. They also provide a guide to specific nursing implementations and a basis for evaluation criteria.

TABLE 33-8. NURSE-PATIENT MANAGEMENT OF MOBILITY

Nursing Diagnosis	Desired Outcome	Implementation	Evaluation
Impaired mobility R/T pain 6.1.1.1	1. Resume former level of mobility without complaints of pain.	1a. Offer noninvasive pain relief measures (see Chap. 32). 1b. Offer analgesia as ordered if above unsatisfactory. 1c. Assist with movement, positioning, and ADL when pain is severe. 1d. Collaborate with patient to develop an individualized exercise program to maintain strength, endurance, and flexibility to be used when pain relief is achieved.	1a. Progressive increase in self-care and freedom of movement without report of pain. 1b. ROM and muscle strength remain constant.
Impaired mobility R/T perceptual/ cognitive impairment: confusion 6.1.1.1	1. Maintenance of current level of strength and flexibility. 2. Improved orientation appropriate to health status.	1a. Give verbal and visual cues to assist patient in active ROM q3h whenever patient is appropriately responsive. 1b. Incorporate resistance in above ROM whenever patient is able. 1c. Attempt passive ROM at least q4h if patient does not participate in active ROM. 1d. Attempt daily assisted walks of distance within patient's tolerance. 2a. Speak distinctly explaining your actions and desired patient participation. 2b. Correct inappropriate verbalizations or physical responses using a calm voice tone, explaining and repeating appropriate or correct response. 2c. Provide varied but not excessive environmental stimuli, (eg, conversation, music, change of location, group activity).	1a. Serial ROM measurement increases or remains same as initial measurement. 1b. Serial testing of muscle strength reveals no loss. 1c. Activity-related changes in P, R, BP remain same as initial assessment. 2a. Progressively increasing numbers of appropriate verbal and/or motor behaviors.
Activity intolerance R/T generalized weakness 6.1.1.2	1. Increased activity tolerance appropriate to age, sex, and health prognosis. 2. Increased strength appropriate to age, sex, and health prognosis.	1. Collaborate with patient to develop program for progressive ambulation. 2a. Collaborate with patient to develop a muscle strengthening program that focuses on patient's deficits. 2b. Assist in performance of ADL, decreasing assistance as strength improves. 2c. Teach modified methods or provide assistive devices for ADL performance according to patient need.	1. Progressive improvement in activity tolerance AEB: • Statements of improved energy level. • HR, RR, and BP return to baseline values after exercise within expected time frame for age and health status. 2a. Progressive increase in muscle tone and mass. 2b. Serial tests of muscle strength show progressive improvement.
Risk for activity intolerance: R/F deconditioned status 6.1.1.3	1. Improved exercise tolerance to 60% of HRmax.	1a. Teach patient the health benefits of regular exercise. 1b. Collaborate with patient to develop an exercise program that includes aerobic exercise of patient's preference at least 3 days per week with gradually increasing duration and intensity. 1c. Teach patient to assess pulse during and after exercise. 1d. Teach patient how to compute HRmax.	1. No activity intolerance AEB able to participate in aerobic exercise at 60% HRmax without distress (no dyspnea, pallor, fatigue), with return to baseline HR within 1 minute after exercise ceases.
Risk for disuse syndrome: R/F prescribed immobilization 1.6.1.5	1. No evidence of disuse syndrome.	1a. Collaborate with patient to develop a turning schedule in which no position is maintained for more than 2 hours. 1b. Maintain clean, wrinkle-free bed at all times. 1c. Teach patient the benefits of fiber, fluids in maintaining bowel regularity and urinary function (see Chap. 29). 1d. Keep fluids of choice available at all times. 1e. Teach and encourage patient to use deep-breathing exercises (see Chap. 30).	1. Patient remains free of symptoms of disuse syndrome, AEB: • Skin remains free of pressure ulcers. • Regular soft-formed BM. • Lungs remain free of secretions. • Extremities remain well perfused (see Chap. 30).

TABLE 33-8. CONTINUED

Nursing Diagnosis	Desired Outcome	Implementation	Evaluation
		1f. Teach patient leg exercises that are within the prescribed activity limitations (see Chap. 30). 1g. Collaborate with patient to develop a program of exercises for strength and flexibility to be performed in bed that are within prescribed activity restriction. 1h. Involve significant others in planning activities with patient to diminish boredom, isolation. 1i. Use therapeutic communication techniques to facilitate patient coping with restricted activity (see Chap. 15). 1j. Offer choices and opportunities for decision-making about care regimen whenever possible.	• Regular urinary elimination without dysuria within expected range for intake. • ROM remains at expected measurements for age. • Maintains alert oriented mental status. • No indicators of disturbed body image (see Chap. 26). • Participates in planning and engages in measures to prevent disuse and treat primary health problems.

Source: See Table 33–7.

Mobility outcomes, like other outcomes for patient care, are best determined by a process of mutual goal-setting. Through analysis of assessment data, nurses develop a perception of the level of mobility a patient can realistically attain. By sharing these perceptions with patents and requesting their input, nurses contribute to setting goals that patients understand and accept. This collaborative effort then continues as patient and nurse work together to attain the mobility outcomes.

The desired outcomes should also be compatible with the goals for medical treatment. In the example of the patient who was unable to walk because of muscle weakness, a desirable long-term goal might be to regain enough strength to be as active as before becoming ill. Collaboration with the physician would be necessary, however, to determine whether this goal is realistic.

The second step in planning for a patient's mobility needs is deciding on nursing implementation to achieve the desired outcomes. The type of care that is appropriate is implied by the assessment data and the outcomes selected in the previous step. Patient care should capitalize on patient strengths and provide support where it is needed.

For the patient with muscle weakness, a nurse might plan to teach the relationship between exercise and developing muscle strength, unless the mobility history revealed that the patient already knew this. Next might be joint planning of a leg-strengthening exercise program. Selecting exercises and their frequency would be determined by patient preference and the information about the patient's exercise tolerance obtained during the mobility examination.

The mobility plan is complete when evaluation criteria have been written for each of the nursing diagnoses. Then the plan is put into action. Nursing implementation is carried out and its effectiveness evaluated by comparing the patient's progress to the evaluation criteria.

Evaluation of mobility status is both an ongoing and a terminal process. Observations made while providing care indicate whether day-to-day progress is being made toward desired mobility outcomes. Documenting patients' response to nursing treatment on the nursing progress notes in the patient's medical record provides ongoing evaluation information. If patients demonstrate the desired level of mobility for a particular nursing diagnosis within the time frame indicated in the care plan, the outcomes are considered to have been met. That diagnosis is deleted from the plan. If the goals are not attained, reassessment is necessary to determine whether the goals were realistic and nursing treatment appropriate.

When a patient is discharged from the health care setting or service, terminal evaluation and recording of status relative to each diagnosis is appropriate. If a patient is being transferred to another facility or service (for example, home care), the case manager or primary nurse communicates the care plan to the new agency.

Table 33–8, Nurse–Patient Management of Mobility, presents sample outcomes, implementations, and evaluation criteria for nurse-patient management of the nursing diagnoses related to mobility that are presented in this chapter. Table 33–9, Partial Critical Pathway for Congestive Heart Failure: Mobility Function, and Table 33–10, Partial Critical Pathway for Total Hip Replacement: Mobility Function, are examples of collaborative interdisciplinary plans that incorporate concepts from this chapter.

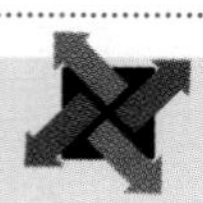

TABLE 33-9. PARTIAL CRITICAL PATHWAY FOR CONGESTIVE HEART FAILURE: MOBILITY FUNCTION

Nursing Dx/Problem	Outcome Primary Care Visit	Outcome Home Care Week 1 (3 Visits)	Outcome Home Care Week 2 (3 Visits)	Outcome Home Care Weeks 3–4 (3 Visits)
Activity intolerance R/T imbalance between O_2 supply & demand	Able to return home c̄ assistive devices	Independent movement in bed, feeding, toileting s̄ dyspnea or chest pain	O_2 saturation > 94% c̄ O_2 Ambulates 10 feet s̄ SOB	O_2 saturation > 92% s̄ O_2 Ambulates s̄ SOB

Implementation	Primary Care Visit	Home Care Visit Week 1	Home Care Visit Week 2	Home Care Visit Weeks 3–4
Assessment	V/S, arrhythmia, chest pain, O_2 sat. breath sounds edema, I&O Weakness/fatigue, dyspnea ā & p̄ exercise	Same Same	Same Same	Same Same
Tests/Consults	Refer to Home Health	Same	Same	Same
Medications/Treatments	O_2 at 2 L/cannula Diuretics, $K^{\dagger}$ supplements Digoxin, anticoagulants Antithromboembolism stockings	Same Same Elevate legs Schedule uninterrupted rest periods	O_2 prn and at night Same Same Same	O_2 prn Same Same Same
Psychosocial		Identify family abilities to provide assistance	Monitor family support	Same
Teaching		O_2 use & precautions Disease process S/Sx to report to MD, RN, 911, Plan of Care O_2 supply/demand, fatigue, energy conservation Review how to take pulse Stocking application, elevate legs when up Food & fluid precautions Medications: expected action, SE, precautions Types of assistive devices & safe use	Review, reinforce as needed Reinforce as needed Reinforce as needed Reinforce as needed Reinforce as needed Reinforce as needed Reinforce as needed	Same Same
Activity/Safety/Self-care	Bedrest, HOB 30–45° c̄ BSC or BRP Turn q2h	Progressive activity as tolerated	Same	Same
Nutrition	2 g Na, restrict fluid to 1 L/d	Same	Same	Diet same, fluid 1.5 L/day
Transfer/Discharge Coord./ Case Manager		Communicate outcomes achieved to MD	Same	Same Prepare for discharge

See inside back cover for abbreviations.

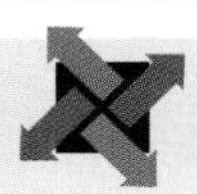

TABLE 33-10. PARTIAL CRITICAL PATHWAY FOR TOTAL HIP REPLACEMENT: MOBILITY FUNCTION

Nursing Dx/Problem	Outcome DOS/Day 1	Outcome Days 2–3	Outcome SNF Days 4–6	Outcome Home Care 3 Weeks (6 Visits)
9. Impaired physical mobility R/T musculoskeletal impairment: hip surgery	Position change in bed c̄ assistance &/or using trapeze	Stand @ bedside c̄ walker, no weight bearing on affected side	Ambulates c̄ walker, no weight bearing on affected side	Ambulates within activity guidelines
	Performs ankle pumps, quad & gluteal sets, abduction exercises in sling suspension, 3 reps, each tid	Same	Same	
10. Risk for injury: dislocation, RF new hip prosthesis	Correct alignment maintained c̄ abduction pillow	Same		
	Avoids adduction, internal rotation, 90 degree flexion	Same	Same	Same

Implementation/ Problem #		DOS/Day 1	Days 2–3	SNF Days 4–6	Home Care 3 Weeks (6 Visits)
Assessment	#9	Note correct performance of exercises	Same tid	Same bid	Same each visit
	#10	Check hip alignment q2h	Same q4h	Same bid	Same each visit
		Note correct placement of abduction pillow c q position change	Same q4h	Same bid	
		S/Sx dislocation: pain, shortening or internal rotation of affected hip	Same	Same	
Tests/Consults	#9, 10	Physical therapy			
Medications/ Treatments	#9	Prophylactic anticoagulant therapy	Same	Same	Same
		Overbed frame c̄ trapeze	Same	Same	Same
		Antiembolism stockings or sequential compression device (SCD)—remove & replace q shift	Same	Antiembolism stockings—remove & replace q shift	Antiembolism stockings—change q day
	#10	Abduction pillow @ all times	Same	Same	
Psychosocial					
Teaching	#9	Leg exercises	Reinforce Use of walker	Use of assistive devices: reacher, long-handled shoe horn	Reinforce
	#10	Position precautions	Post-discharge activity restrictions, position precautions, and transfer techniques	Reinforce	Review
Activity/Safety/ Self-Care	#9	Bedrest, turn q2h toward affected side	Stand @ bedside c̄ PT & walker	Ambulate c̄ walker	Ambulate within activity guidelines
		Leg exercises tid	Same	Same	
	#10	Abduction pillow @ all times	Same		
Nutrition					
Transfer/Discharge Coord./Case Manager			Communicate outcomes achieved, problems/ interventions to SNF	Communicate outcomes achieved, problems/interventions to Home Health	Communicate outcomes achieved, problems/ interventions to MD & prepare for discharge

See inside back cover for abbreviations.

NURSING IMPLEMENTATION TO PROMOTE OPTIMAL MOBILITY

A wide range of nursing approaches assist patients with their mobility needs. Patients whose mobility limitation is minimal may require assistance only with exercises to strengthen muscles or increase endurance. Others may need assistance with ambulation or teaching about healthy lifestyle habits to attain and maintain optimal mobility. More dependent patients may require assistance with all mobility, including changing positions in bed or transferring from a bed to a chair. These individuals would also need nursing care to prevent disuse syndrome. The next sections provide detailed explanations of mobility-related nursing approaches for all levels of care.

PREVENTIVE CARE

Health Education

Increasing the number of health care providers who routinely counsel patients about the health benefits of physical activity is one of the goals cited in the *Surgeon General's Report on Physical Activity and Health*.[2] Nurses can participate in this effort. Nurses have opportunities for health teaching about exercise in schools, workplaces, homes, communities, and health care facilities.

Schools. School nurses can collaborate with educators in planning physical education activities that emphasize life-sports, such as tennis or cycling, as suggested in the Surgeon General's report. They can also conduct classes or workshops on the benefits of physical activity and safe approaches to exercise for students and parents. Studies show that health-related fitness instruction in schools results in positive attitudes toward physical activity.[26,27] School nurses can teach approaches to reduce girls' risk for osteoporosis later in life. Emphasis on lifestyle-related strategies to increase bone density at a young age, with reinforcement throughout the developmental span, can significantly reduce the incidence of problems related to osteoporosis after menopause.[6]

Workplace. Nurses can be involved in both planning and executing workplace health-promotion programs. Research has indicated that a major limiting factor in the success of workplace exercise programs is low employee participation.[28] This is a factor that occupational health nurses can correct by providing more effective education about the personal benefits of these programs.

Home. Home health care presents a unique opportunity to identify needs for mobility-related health education. Observing patients and families at home permits a realistic assessment of functional abilities, lifestyle, and habits. Positive environmental and social factors as well as barriers are more evident. This information is the basis for relevant and focused health teaching.

Community. Community-based efforts to educate the public, such as health fairs, college extension, and public information classes, are other examples in which nurses can play a role in preventing health problems that limit mobility.

One-to-one teaching about the health benefits of exercise, how to select an appropriate exercise program and reduce exercise risks, and related topics such as nutrition and smoking cessation is probably the most effective means of promoting individual commitment to exercise. It is appropriate in all of the settings discussed. This teaching can be done during regular health assessment visits or when providing care for any health problem that affects activity. The next sections detail content appropriate for patient teaching on exercise-related topics.

Strategies to Prevent Osteoporosis. Osteoporosis is a significant women's health problem. Seven out of 10 women over age 50 have severe or moderate bone loss.[29] It is estimated that one in two women will experience fractures because of osteoporosis.[6] Sedentary, thin, small-framed, white women are at highest risk and there is evidence for hereditary predisposition. Osteoporotic bone loss takes place gradually over the course of years, without producing signs or symptoms. Therefore, early and ongoing prevention efforts for all women are important. Effective prevention strategies relate to exercise, diet, and personal exposure to specific substances.[6,30,31]

Regular weight-bearing exercise increases bone mass. Women with higher bone density are more resistant to age-related bone losses and are less likely to fracture bones in a fall. Recent research suggests that exercise improves bone density even in women who have already experienced bone loss.[6,32] However, premenopausal women should be cautioned against exercise of such an intensity that it suppresses estrogen production and produces amenorrhea. Amenorrhea indicates sufficiently low estrogen levels to promote bone loss and increase long-term risks for osteoporosis.

Calcium intake is the primary dietary concern. Daily intake should be at least 1200 milligrams for adolescents, 1000 milligrams for premenopausal women, and 1500 milligrams for postmenopausal women not taking EST (estrogen replacement therapy). Women should also be aware that a high-protein diet increases calcium excretion. Vitamin D plays an essential role in bone metabolism and in maintaining circulating calcium levels, so it is important to maintain daily intake of at least the recommended daily requirement. Postmenopausal women are often advised to take vitamin D and calcium supplements and should be made aware of the risks and benefits of EST in the prevention of osteoporosis.

Cigarette smoking and regular alcohol consumption are associated with increased bone fragility.[30,31] Certain prescription drugs have been associated with higher fracture risk.[6] Women should be informed of these risks as part of general health teaching. Advise women taking prescription medications to ask the prescriber whether the medications pose any risk related to osteoporosis.

Selecting and Planning an Individual Exercise Program. Plans for an individual program should take in to account a patient's current level of health and fitness, as discussed in Section 2 of this chapter,

CRITICAL QUERY

Osteoporosis exacts a high monetary and social cost. Fractures caused by bone fragility cause significant mortality, long-term disability and dependency. Lappe[6] identified determinants of bone fragility that predispose women to developing osteoporosis. Some factors, such as genetic influences or the need to take certain medications (anticonvulsants or diuretics), may not be readily altered. Others, including diet, exercise patterns, use of alcohol, and smoking, are under individual control. Is preventing osteoporosis a nursing concern? If so, how can nurses positively influence women to make choices that will reduce their risks? When should interventions be initiated? What settings are most appropriate?

and other personal factors outlined next. These guidelines are adapted from the work of several researchers.[3,4,13,14,33]

1. *Build rapport.* Establish a positive climate by explaining the nature of the exercise assessment and addressing any concerns a patient expresses.
2. *Establish lifestyle goals.* Discuss other goals besides improving fitness that are important to a patient, such as weight loss, stress reduction, or modification of personal risk factors for coronary artery disease.
3. *Conduct assessment.* Determine current fitness level and screen for the presence of risk factors that indicate a need for comprehensive assessment by specialists. Refer as necessary.
4. *Interpret results.* Discuss the assessment with patients in descriptive and understandable terms; give them a copy of the report for reference.
5. *Discuss activity preferences and interests.* Find out what kinds of activity a patient enjoys, finds unpleasant, and for which the necessary equipment or facilities are readily available. Consider the amount of time the person can realistically commit to exercise every week.
6. *Match preferences and assessment results.* Determine whether a patient's goals for exercise are realistic given current health and fitness, preferred activities, and time available. See whether preferred activities are compatible with patient goals. Discuss the benefits and limitations of a patient's preferred activities.
7. *Design a program.* Write out an action worksheet with progressive levels (gradually increasing physiologic demands) and reachable goals. If any activities require specialized equipment or skills (eg, weight training, specific sports), refer patients to resources for instruction. Schedule regular reevaluation.

Exercise programs that are most beneficial include components to improve aerobic fitness, flexibility, and strength. However, for many individuals a prudent plan to improve aerobic fitness provides sufficient benefits in strength and flexibility. Aerobic fitness programs need to balance frequency, duration, intensity, and type of activity. Some experts recommend long, slow distance, particularly for a person who is currently sedentary. The distance selected depends on a patient's energy level and time available. The pace can be governed by identifying a low (<65 percent HRmax), moderate (65 to 85 percent HRmax), or high (85 to 90 percent HRmax) intensity of exercise, depending on fitness level. This approach would apply to any aerobic activity, such as walking, jogging, rowing, cycling, swimming, or cross-country skiing. The long, slow distance program can be easily quantified, provides cardiorespiratory benefits, contributes to weight loss, and has a low risk of orthopedic injury and cardiovascular complications. More intense programs are appropriate for some people. Greater benefits result from more intense and varied exercise regimens.[2,3,7,34,35]

Reducing Exercise Risks. Exercise-related injuries are one reason individuals become discouraged and lose commitment to an exercise program. Most exercise-related injuries are preventable.

Selecting a program appropriate to an individual's current fitness level and gradually increasing the pace, duration, and intensity of exercise is an important injury-prevention strategy.[3,13,33] Consistently warming up before exercise (for example, by stretching or beginning at a slow pace) and cooling down after exercise (ending the session with slower, less intense activity) is also effective.

Besides informing individuals about practices to prevent injury, educating them about the kinds of practices that increase their risk for injury enables them to make prudent choices. The following factors increase risk for exercise related injury.

- *Overdoing it.* Dramatically increasing the intensity or duration of workouts, or performing a high-impact activity like running or aerobic dance more than four times a week.
- *Inappropriate footwear and equipment.* Ninety percent of sports injuries occur in leg joints. Wearing worn-out or poorly fitted shoes, or shoes that are not appropriate for the activity, contribute to these injuries. Injuries also result when other equipment is of the wrong weight or size.
- *Poor conditioning.* Exercising weak, tight muscles causes injury. Individuals need to gradually increase exercise demands. Muscle imbalance, such as occurs with participating in only one type of exercise or sport, creates a tendency for injury in the muscles that are not strengthened by that exercise. An example is shin splints, which result from strong calf muscles overwhelming weaker muscles in the front of the lower leg.
- *Improper technique and training.* Poor form, such as an incorrect backhand stroke or improper footstrike in running, causes stress that leads to injury. Training on hard or uneven surfaces is another common cause of injury.
- *Ignoring aches and pains.* "Running through" the pain or resuming exercise before an injury has fully healed worsens the current injury and increases the risk for reinjury. Taking note of unusual sensations and treating injuries as soon as possible prevents their becoming more serious.
- *Competitive sports.* Many exercise-related injuries occur during participation in competitive sports, even informal, spontaneous games between friends. Individuals who enjoy competition tend to become so enthusiastic during the game that they may push themselves to greater intensity than their bodies are ready for, with resulting musculoskeletal injuries or even cardiovascular and pulmonary stress.

Enhancing Motivation. Many of the strategies discussed above for planning an exercise program also enhance motivation to maintain it. Other motivation-enhancing approaches include dispelling misconceptions about exercise, discussing obstacles to exercise and strategies to overcome them, emphasizing the value of play, providing feedback and positive reinforcement, and role modeling.

DISPELLING MISCONCEPTIONS. Misconceptions about exercise deter many people from making a commitment to regular physical activity. The "no pain, no gain" philosophy has received a lot of exposure in exercise self-help books and videos. Informing patients about recent research findings supporting positive effects from mild to moderate activity levels will make exercise seem less formidable and benefits more achievable.

Another common misconception is that the health benefits from exercise are immediate and observable. Although feelings of improved well-being are common within 2 to 3 weeks of regular exercise, there may be no externally obvious evidence of improved health for many weeks.[36] Many individuals embark on exercise programs in order to lose weight. Promises of fast, effortless weight loss made by many diet programs (although false and misleading) create unreasonable expectations. Because a calorie deficit of 3500 calories is necessary to lose 1 pound of fat, a loss of 1 pound per week is feasible.[37]

The belief in spot reduction of body fat is a related misconception. It causes people to quit an exercise program, because anticipated results do not occur. Proponents state that fat stores in the muscles being exercised will be mobilized preferentially to other fat stores. Therefore, a person desiring to lose abdominal fat would be advised to do sit-ups, and one with excess fat on the thighs, leg lifts. There is no research to support spot reduction; rather, stored fat is mobilized equally from all areas of the body during exercise. Therefore, an extended period of balanced exercises would be needed to lose large local fat deposits.

Some people are hesitant to start an exercise program because they believe that exercise increases appetite. They fear this will cause them to take in more calories than the exercise burns. Although those who work and play hard tend to eat more than sedentary individuals, those who are active have more muscle mass and less body fat. Because muscle tissue is more metabolically active than fat, lean active people burn calories more rapidly than those who are sedentary. Therefore, regular exercise usually results in a net decrease in calories stored.

OVERCOMING OBSTACLES TO MAINTAINING AN EXERCISE PROGRAM. Like any change, altering a sedentary lifestyle pattern can be difficult. Physical obstacles like transient muscle soreness during and right after exercise, rapid reversal of training effects if exercise is discontinued for a time, and injuries related to training cause some people to become disillusioned with an exercise plan. Environmental deterrents such as having to travel to an exercise facility or social obstacles, such as an unsupportive spouse or being unable to arrange child care, can make establishing and maintaining a regular exercise pattern difficult. Discussing potential obstacles in a general way, and exploring personal situations that could deter sticking to a commitment to exercise, is a good way to identify appropriate techniques for coping with obstacles.

EMPHASIZING THE VALUE OF PLAY. Many experts emphasize the contribution of invigorating play to overall health throughout the life span. However, the life patterns of many adults exclude time for play. Our high-pressure, success-oriented culture causes many to devalue leisure, even to forget how to play. This perspective is at the root of many stress-related disorders. Talking to patients about the value of play and exercise as a form of play can facilitate a shift in perspective about exercise. If persons select a form of exercise that is pleasurable, it is more likely that they will participate regularly.

FEEDBACK AND POSITIVE REINFORCEMENT. Beginning exercisers require immediate and frequent feedback about their performance and positive reinforcement to make physical activity a part of their lifestyle.[4] Although intrinsically pleasurable activities and generalized improvements in well-being are incentives to continue exercise, many formerly sedentary patients do not experience these feelings at the outset of an exercise program. The transition from an inactive to an active lifestyle is difficult for many. During the first several weeks of an exercise program, most people need encouragement to continue. Commending patients for staying with the program shows recognition that continuing takes an effort. Giving feedback about progress toward goals and praise for gains are important incentives. When the exercise becomes incorporated into an individual's value system, and personal perceptions of gains are possible, external reinforcement ceases to be needed.

ROLE-MODELING. None of these strategies to encourage exercise have credibility with patients if it is obvious that a provider's personal lifestyle does not include regular exercise. Conversely, if we appear fit and can speak about exercise from the perspective of participants rather than observers, our efforts are more likely to be convincing and effective.[38]

Screening for Risks for Compromised Mobility

Like health education about the value of physical activity, screening for mobility-related risk factors can be integrated into many aspects of nursing care in many settings. These risk factors are often related to lifestyle choices or pre-existing health problems. Examples of lifestyle-related risks and risk factors include:

- Smokers risk cardiopulmonary compromise that will eventually limit fitness and general mobility, even though they may feel capable of vigorous exercise at present.
- Patients whose weight exhibits a slow but steady increase are on a trajectory that exposes them to many health risks, including limitations in mobility.
- Obesity increases the risk for degenerative joint disease and limits cardiovascular capacity, among other problems.
- Sedentary, thin, small-framed women with low calcium intake and a positive family history are at greatly increased risk for developing osteoporosis.
- Alcohol and use of other substances contributes to falls and other accidents.
- Failure to use seat belts creates a possibility for injuries with potentially permanent mobility-altering consequences.

Encouraging patients to examine their risk for losing the capacity for optimal mobility is the first step in facilitating lifestyle changes.[39] Then, tailoring health teaching to the particular risk factors and related variables that apply to the individual can be the most effective.

Some health problems predispose patients to interference with mobility and imply the need to screen for mobility problems.

- Severe hypertension is often treated with potent medications. Dizziness, with associated risks for falls, is a frequent side-effect.
- Patients with chronic respiratory diseases often require a portable E-cylinder to maintain adequate oxygenation. The environment must afford adequate space to move about easily with the tank and tubing, and care is needed to prevent tripping and falling over them.
- Sight and hearing deficits require special precautions to prevent injuries related to falls.

This screening is appropriate in all types of health care settings, but is perhaps most important in home care. One study has identified impaired mobility as the most frequent nursing diagnosis among patients receiving home care.[40] This finding indicates that nurses providing home care should be particularly vigilent in screening for mobility problems, whatever the primary health problem that resulted in home care services. Screening for related environmental risk factors (see Clinical Guideline 33–2) and encouraging patients to take preventive or corrective actions (see the next section) is important to promote and maintain mobility.

SUPPORTIVE CARE

Supportive care is appropriate for patients experiencing mild alterations in mobility.

Teaching Protective Body Mechanics

Lifting or moving heavy objects is a part of the daily activities of many people at home or at work. Injuries resulting from incorrect lifting techniques are a common cause of disability. Individuals already experiencing mild alterations in mobility are more vulnerable to such injuries than people having no mobility-related deficits. Teaching these individuals how they can apply protective body mechanics in their daily activities will help them to maintain their current level of mobility. Using these techniques conserves energy and prevents injury. Refer to the next section, Restorative Care, for a detailed discussion of body mechanics.

Supporting Overweight Individuals in Exercise Programs

Experts agree that weight loss is best achieved by a program that combines dietary changes with increased amounts of physical activity.[36,41-44] Dropout rates from exercise programs are higher among obese individuals than among others. Some experts believe that this relates to psychological factors, such as intimidation, self-consciousness, or exercise resistance (a block against becoming physically active).[44] Research has shown that social factors such as group support also influence continuing an exercise program. These ideas suggest that continued participation is more likely in programs that target overweight individuals and that include psychological support and social support along with exercise.[44] Nurses often have opportunities to teach weight-control strategies to obese patients. Nurses who are well informed about comprehensive programs tailored specifically for overweight individuals are in a better position to facilitate and support their positive efforts to lose weight. Nurses who recognize that lifestyle changes are difficult to maintain, can effectively assist patients to set realistic goals, teach self-monitoring techniques, and offer consistent positive reinforcement for remaining in an exercise program and for making even minimal progress toward goals.[43] See also the discussion on self-management techniques in Chap. 25.

Enhancing Mobility in the Well Elderly

Activity is a major component in the health perception of the elderly.[45] Participation in regular exercise not only maintains older adults' physical mobility but contributes to their image of themselves as healthy. As discussed in Section 1, aging is a significant factor contributing to losses of mobility. Teaching elderly patients how they can retard loss of function and developing individual and group exercise programs specifically for them can greatly improve their quality of life.[45-48]

Exercise. A careful and complete pre-exercise assessment, including a drug and dietary history, evaluation for sensory deficits, musculoskeletal problems, and cardiovascular disease, is recommended prior to planning exercise.[10] Many experts recommend walking as an ideal aerobic activity for the elderly. Recent research suggests that strength training may be the most beneficial type of exercise to promote mobility in well elderly.[9,47,48] When feasible, a mixture of activities has advantages. Integrating social interaction with exercise increases the overall benefits, because group support positively influences motivation. Moreover, the additional benefit of forming new friendships is important to this age group, who often experience losses of friends and loved ones. An example of a group program that integrates social activity and exercise is Mall Walking Clubs. They are generally jointly affiliated with community hospitals and shopping malls. They can be found in communities nationwide. Nurses often provide health screening, teaching, and consultation for Mall Walking Clubs.

Fall Prevention. Many elders are at risk for falls because of changes in sensory acuity—particularly vision—and diminished strength, joint mobility, and balance.[24,39,49] Some researchers identify cognitive impairment, depression, misuse of alcohol, and increased use of medications (in particular psychotropic medications) as significant risk factors relating to falls among the elderly.[38,49,50] Nurses should monitor elders for these risk factors in all patient care settings, but especially in elders' homes. Unpredictable changes in mental status and/or gait suggest a need for further questioning and observation. Conferring with family members is important. Referrals to vision or audiology clinics, or alcohol treatment programs is sometimes appropriate.

Periodic review with elders of all prescription and OTC medications used is important to identify potential interactions or side effects that could threaten mobility. Many have multiple health problems and see several different providers. Often the providers are not aware that other medications have been prescribed. Nurses can confer with the prescribers to achieve a medication regimen with maximum benefits from the smallest number of different medications.

Fear of falling among elderly living in the community has a significant negative impact on their quality of life. In some cases this fear decreases their mobility and social activities.[51] Participation in exercise programs to improve strength, balance, gait, and joint mobility has been shown to reduce falls.[48,49] These benefits, plus the overall improvement in well-being, may increase elder's confidence. Teaching the value of a healthy diet to support gains in strength can compound the benefits. Elders may also need frequent reinforcement of the importance of repeated home safety inspections to reduce risk factors.[39,52] Nurses should consider referrals to other health care team members and explore other community resources for mobility aids in both inpatient and home settings when nursing implementation does not correct problems and risk factors.[49,53]

Promoting Recovery from Mild Exercise-related Injuries

Cold, elevation, heat, massage, and rest are effective treatments for discomfort and minor muscle injuries related to exercise. Joint injuries often require more intensive treatment and should be assessed by a physician. Early stages of heat-related illness can be treated by rest and hydration.

Cold. Cold applications are appropriate immediately after an injury occurs. Ice or ice and water in plastic bags, or chemical cold generation packs, work well. Cold slows down local metabolic activity, decreases inflammation, and minimizes vasodilation. Cold applications can damage tissue, so the site should be checked periodically and the ice removed after 15 to 30 minutes or sooner if

? CRITICAL QUERY

Arfken and colleagues[51] found that fear of falling is common among relatively well elderly persons living in the community. The fear is more prevalent among women. Past experience with falls or near falls was associated with more intense fear. Even those who characterized their fear as moderate reported decreased satisfaction with life. They also showed scores suggestive of depression on the Geriatric Depression Scale. Elders who were very fearful of falling curtailed social activities, and many did not leave their house or yard because of their fear. These findings suggest that the fear of falling has a significantly negative impact on many elders' quality of life. Does this represent a public health problem? If so, what measures are indicated to prevent and limit these consequences of falls among elders living in the community?

loss of local sensation occurs. See also Procedure 32–4. When the acute (red, warm, swollen) phase passes, heat therapy is recommended.

Elevation. Elevating an injured extremity prevents venous pooling, which is a contributing cause of edema after injury. Elevation used in conjunction with cold therapy inhibits inflammation and decreases pain.

Heat. Generalized soreness after exercise often improves with heat applications. Local hot packs are also effective in promoting healing after the acute phase of an injury, because of their vasodilating effect. Postexercise whirlpool promotes relaxation and comfort. Patients should wait to use a whirlpool until heart rate and respirations have returned to resting values because the warm water enhances vasodilation and venous pooling, which can compromise cardiac output.

Massage. Massage is another modality that effects circulation, promoting muscle relaxation, faster muscle recovery, and pain relief. Massage produces two different circulatory effects. The first is mechanical: a manual movement of venous blood. This is believed to promote more rapid emptying and refilling of vessels, improving removal of metabolic waste products. The second is reflex, caused by stimulation of peripheral receptors. The results of this stimulation are relaxation of muscles and release of acetylcholine and histamines, which cause sustained vasodilation. Massage counteracts the reflex muscle contraction and localized muscle splinting or guarding that occurs in response to pain. This splinting inhibits local circulation, causing ischemia and intensifying pain. Anxiety and stress aggravate secondary muscle contraction pain. Massage breaks the cycle by promoting relaxation. Because it increases lymph flow, massage also reduces edema.

Rest. Premature resumption of activity after an injury delays healing, stresses healthy fibers around the injured area, and predisposes an individual to further damage. However, since deconditioning occurs rapidly when training ceases, experts recommend rest of the injured part, rather than total body rest. When possible, injured individuals should continue aerobic activity at as close to preinjury levels as possible. Advise selecting an activity that can be maintained continuously and that uses uninjured muscle groups. For example, someone with a lower leg injury can substitute swimming for running or cycling; an individual with an upper body injury can walk briskly.

Hydration. Exercising in hot weather causes heat-related illness. Mild forms of this can be treated by replacing lost fluids. Offer hypotonic liquids that are low in sugar, because glucose retards stomach emptying, delaying absorption. Cold fluids are most effective because they pass through the stomach faster.

Home Care

Supportive care in the home is primarily focused on enhancing and supporting mobility in patients receiving care for other health problems. Often, these patients are elderly and will need assessment of risks for falls as discussed above. Others, for example those recovering from accidents or joint replacement surgery benefit from assistance with therapeutic exercise to restore muscle strength and joint mobility. They may also need short term assistance with hygiene and reinforcement of discharge teaching about the safe use of mobility aids such as walkers (discussed in the next section) or crutches.

RESTORATIVE CARE

Restorative mobility care is appropriate for patients with health problems causing significant interference with independent mobility. For most of this care the effective use of protective body mechanics is essential.

Body Mechanics

Much of the care related to acute mobility problems involves lifting and moving patients. This creates potential for injury of both patients and nurses. Protective body mechanics involves using specific movements or techniques that result in maximum work output with minimum effort expended and with reduced possibility of injury. Principles of physics as well as anatomy and physiology apply. The following are basic guidelines for correct protective body mechanics.

- *Start with correct posture.* Correct body alignment is described in Section 2 (see Fig. 33–2). It is fundamental to protective body mechanics. Muscles and joints function optimally when properly aligned. If you attempt to work with faulty posture (eg, with spine bent or twisted or with knees locked), you risk injury to bones, muscles, and joints.
- *Maintain a wide base of support.* Any object is unstable if its center of gravity is allowed to shift outside its base of support. In the standing position, a person's center of gravity is located in the pelvic cavity, slightly anterior to the sacrum. Placing your feet at shoulder width with one foot slightly ahead of the other when lifting or moving anything heavy provides the largest possible range of movement without straining to maintain balance.
- *Use large muscles.* The muscles of the extremities are the largest and strongest muscles of the body. Their structure makes them able to perform strenuous work without injury. Further protection from injury results when you contract these muscles to stabilize joints prior to exertion. In contrast, the muscles of the back are smaller and more easily strained. Reaching and bending or twisting the spine while lifting or moving is likely to cause injury. For this reason, the working surface should be at or slightly below the waist and directly in front of the body. This will minimize reaching and twisting as well as allow maximum efficiency of large muscles (Fig. 33–6).
- *Use your body as a counterweight.* A counterweight is a weight used to produce a force to move or balance another weight, called the resistance. When lifting or moving patients use your body weight to counteract the weight of the patient (the resistance) (Fig. 33–7). The added force of your body moving in the direction the resistance is to be moved reduces the force that your muscles must generate. This technique is useful for both pushing and pulling.
- *Minimize friction.* Friction is the resistance created by a moving object on a surface. Friction is diminished when the surface is smooth and well-lubricated, when the area of contact between surface and object is decreased, or when an object is rolled.
- *Incorporate leverage when possible.* A lever is a machine that uses a rigid bar that rotates around a fixed point called the fulcrum. A simple example is the teeter-totter. A lever accomplishes lifting or moving a weight (resistance) with much less force than with unassisted lifting. It is possible to use parts of your body as the bar and/or fulcrum. Figure 33–8 illustrates one example of the use of leverage.

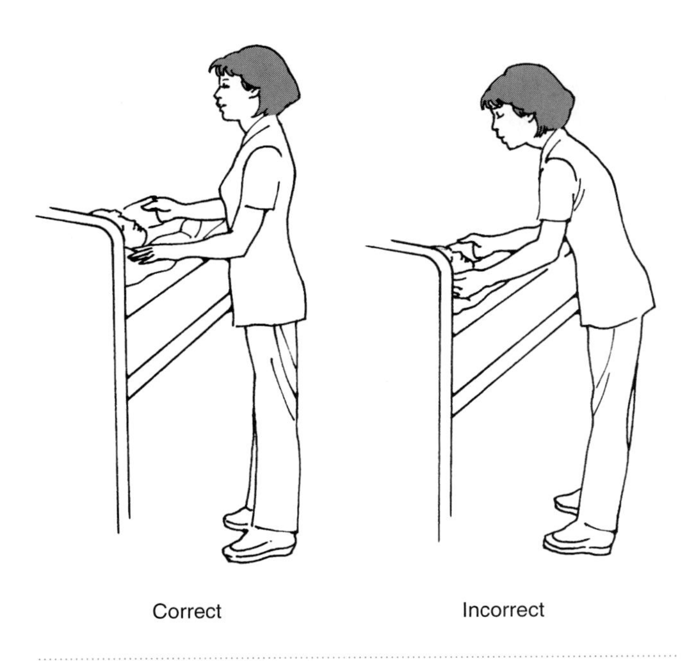

Figure 33–6. Correct and incorrect heights for working surface.

- *Use mechanical aids for heavy objects.* Hydraulic lifts, pull sheets, and other devices discussed later in the chapter can greatly reduce muscle strain by incorporating leverage, reducing friction, and providing additional force. This not only saves nursing energy but also prevents injury to both patient and nurse.

Use of these guidelines should become automatic when giving patient care that involves lifting and moving. It is also useful to teach patients and their support persons proper body mechanics to increase the safety and efficiency of independent patient movement. Clinical Guideline 33–7 summarizes basic body mechanics.

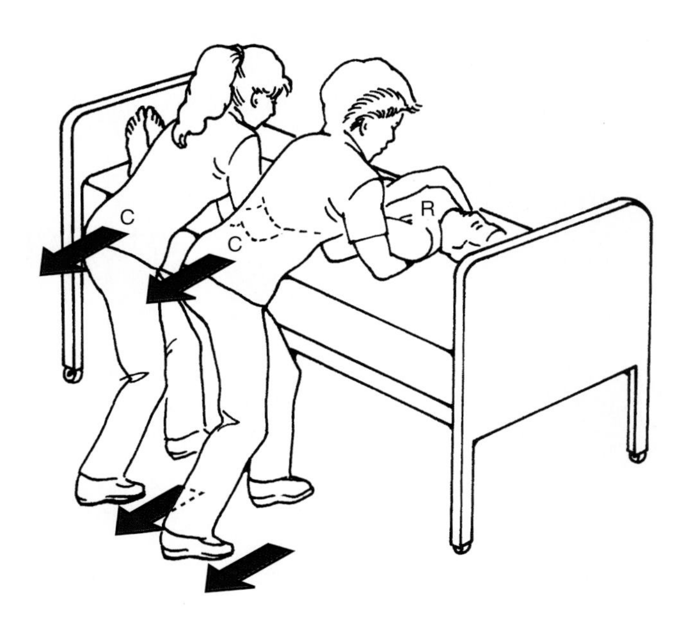

Figure 33–7. Use of the nurse's body as a counterweight.

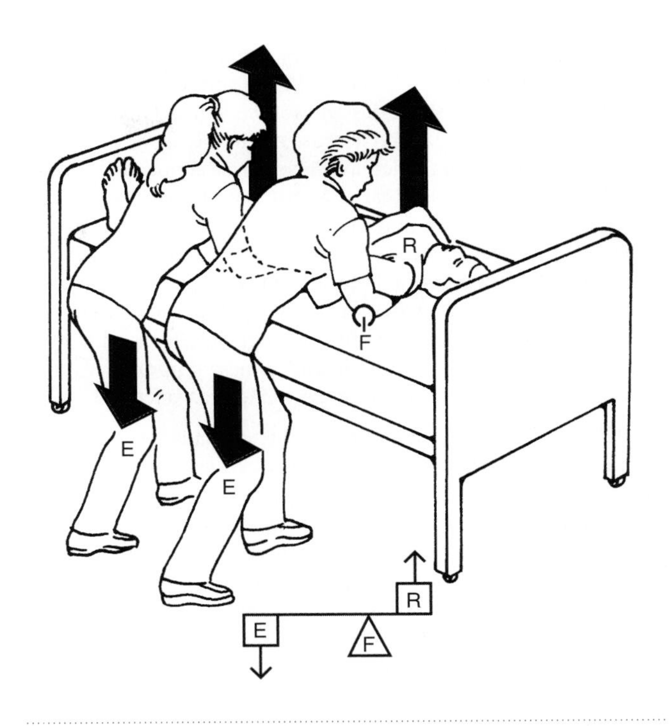

Figure 33–8. Use of leverage in lifting and moving patients.

Exercise

Providing or assisting with exercise is an important aspect of nursing care for patients with mobility problems and when mobility restrictions are necessary as part of the treatment. Regular exercise is important for optimum health. Any patient experiencing limited mobility has a special need for exercise to maintain intact function and to improve function that has been altered by disease or injury.

Patients in health care facilities often choose to remain in bed for most of the day, even though their condition might allow more activity. The environment is not conducive to activity, so incentive to be active is limited. Anxiety, pain, and misconceptions often contribute to poor motivation for activity. Body image changes may also inhibit participation. If nurses note lack of motivation or resistance to attempt progressive mobilization, they should take

CLINICAL GUIDELINE 33–7

BASIC BODY MECHANICS

- Maintain correct posture.
- Maintain a wide base of support when standing or moving.
- Use large muscles in legs and arms, not smaller muscles of back for lifting and pulling.
- Use your body as a counterweight to add force to movements without muscle strain.
- Minimize friction.
- Incorporate leverage to prevent muscle strain and reduce energy expenditure.
- Use mechanical aids to prevent injury when moving heavy loads.

time to explore and address the possible contributing causes. Positive reinforcement and gradual increases in activity can be effective motivators, but these strategies will not be sufficient for patients whose participation is limited because of underlying attitudes that prevent them from using their available physical potential.

The type of exercise that is appropriate for a given patient depends on the medical and nursing diagnoses and the goals or expected outcomes for patient care. Nurses should collaborate with patients, physicians, and physical and occupational therapists to select appropriate exercises. Encourage patients to continue the exercises after convalescence and to augment them with more strenuous activities as strength and fitness improve. Clinical Guideline 33–8 lists approaches to promote safe exercise.

Ambulation. Unless contraindicated by a patient's condition, ambulation (walking) should be a part of every patient's daily activity. Ambulation prevents complications and contributes to maintaining strength, endurance, and flexibility.

Safe ambulation requires endurance, balance and sufficient strength for weight bearing and maintaining posture. Many patients require assistance from nurses to ambulate safely. Clinical Guideline 33–9 outlines parameters for selecting a safe ambulation method. More comprehensive assessment tools are available and may be indicated for ambulatory individuals who fall frequently.[49] Assessing for transient dizziness is an important precaution when preparing any patient for ambulation. Orthostatic hypotension, a frequent complication of long-term bedrest, may also occur after short-term bedrest, especially after injury or surgery. Asking patients to sit at the edge of the bed for several minutes before standing is usually sufficient to correct orthostatic hypotension.

CLINICAL GUIDELINE 33–8

ASSISTING WITH ACTIVE EXERCISE

- Explain the purpose of each activity or exercise in lay terminology.
- Describe and demonstrate the exercise.
- Obtain baseline pulse, respiration and BP before exercise.
- Observe exercise, and assist if needed.
- Do intra- and postexercise assessment. See Clinical Guideline 33–6.
- Give feedback about performance and positive reinforcement for participation.
- Collaborate with patients to schedule future exercise.
- If patients exercise independently, periodically observe and evaluate needs for revised activity.
- Record according to agency policy.

This activity is called **dangling.** Nurses can perform several of the preambulation assessments described in Clinical Guideline 33–9 while a patient is dangling. Procedure 33–1 describes assisting patients with dangling. Techniques for assisting patients to ambulate are described in Procedure 33–2. Patients who have persistent difficulties with ambulation or a history of falls are candidates for gait training.[49] This is usually done by physical therapists.

Some people benefit from additional support in the form of walkers, canes, or crutches. There are several types of canes and crutches available (Fig. 33–9). Selection depends on patient

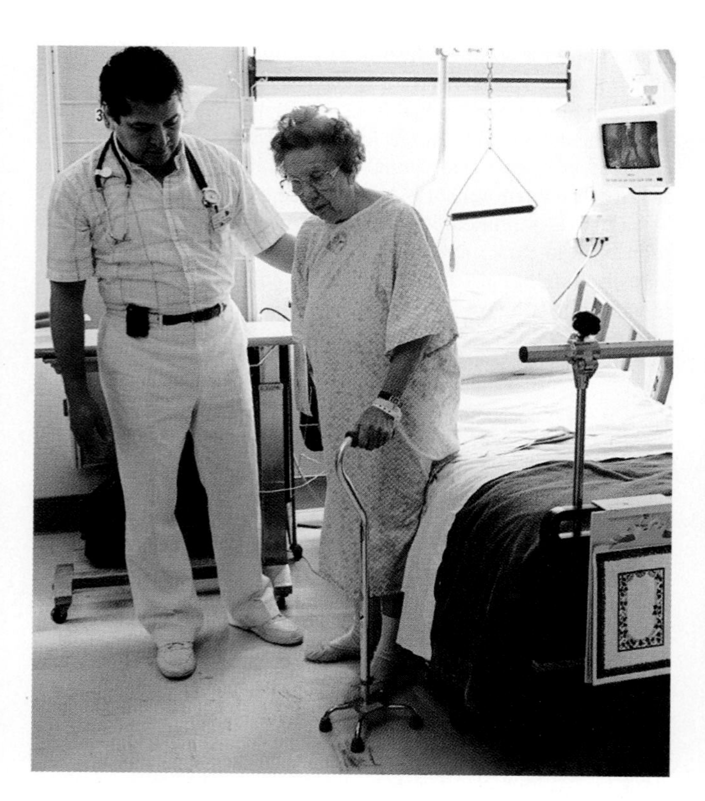

Figure 33–9. A quad cane provides patient with additional support. *(From Smith S, Duell D.* Clinical Nursing Skills: Nursing Process Model; Basic to Advanced Skills. *4th ed. Norwalk, CT: Appleton & Lange; 1996.)*

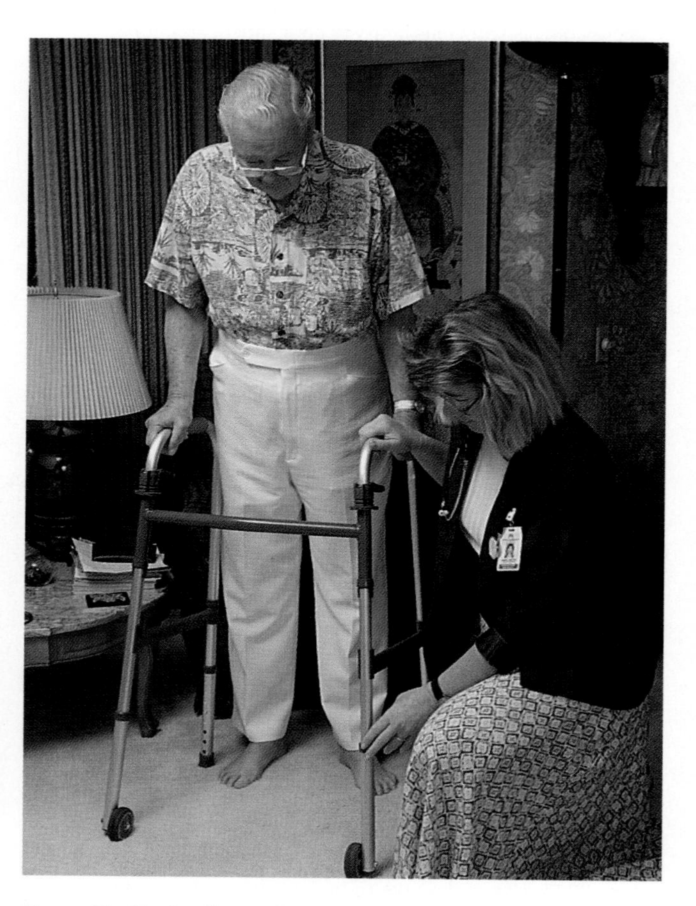

Figure 33–10. A rolling walker enhances home mobility.

CLINICAL GUIDELINE 33–9

SELECTING AMBULATION OR TRANSFER TECHNIQUE

Parameter/Test	Evaluation: *Poor*	Evaluation: *Fair*	Evaluation: *Good*	Associated Nursing Action
1. Sitting balance: Ask or assist patient to assume a sitting position at the edge of the bed.	1. Cannot hold sitting position without continuous maximal support.	1. Requires assistance to assume sitting position, but sits without assistance. Loses balance if resistance (ie, pushing on upper trunk) is applied.	1. Assumes sitting position with minimal or no assistance. Is able to maintain balance against resistance.	1. Patient with poor sitting balance should not attempt ambulation. Use a transfer method requiring no patient participation. If sitting balance is fair or good, proceed to test muscle strength.
2. Muscle strength	2. Extremity does not move, but muscle contraction can be seen or palpated.	2. Active movement is possible, but unable to move against resistance.	2. Active movement against moderate to maximal resistance is possible.	
a. *Quadriceps:* Ask patient to extend the leg at the knee when seated at the edge of the bed.	a. Knees will buckle if standing is attempted.		a. Weight bearing is expected.	a. Patient with poor or fair quadriceps strength in one or both legs cannot ambulate. Pivot transfer can be used if has good strength in one leg. If quadriceps strength in both legs and standing balance is good, can ambulate independently.
b. *Illiopsoas* (hip flexion): Ask patient to raise the flexed knee toward ceiling when seated as above.	b. Patient will be unable to advance affected foot when walking.		b. Independent steps expected.	b. Patient with poor or fair illiopsoas strength can ambulate with two assistants and use pivot or walking transfer if quadriceps strength is good. If illiopsoas strength and balance are good, may ambulate independently.
c. Anterior tibialis (ankle dorsiflexion): Ask patient to lift sole of foot while keeping heel on floor.	c. Sole of foot will not clear floor as patient steps. Patient may stumble.	c. Minimal or no problem with foot clearing floor expected.		c. If anterior tibialis strength is poor, ambulate with two assistants. One assistant is adequate if anterior tibialis strength is fair to good and quadriceps strength is good. If anterior tibialis and quadriceps strength and balance are good, can ambulate independently.
3. Standing balance: After demonstration of good sitting balance, ask patient to stand at bedside.	3. Support of one person required to maintain balance.	3. Can stand independently, but loses balance if resistance (see step 1, above) is applied.	3. Stands without support. Maintains balance despite resistance.	3. Patient with poor standing balance requires support of one or two nurses (gait belt preferred). If quadriceps strength is only fair, use two assistants. Patient with fair balance and good quadriceps strength can use a walker. If balance and muscle strength good, can ambulate independently.

strength, balance, and preference. Assistance with crutch walking and safe use of canes is usually provided by the physical therapy department. Walkers distribute body weight between upper and lower extremities and provide assistance in maintaining balance. The pick-up walker is generally preferred, as it is more stable. A rolling walker can be used for people with inadequate bicep strength to lift a pick-up walker (Fig. 33–10). Some rolling walkers have a fold-up seat so that patients can stop to rest or propel themselves with their legs while sitting (eg, to exercise legs). A walker does not encourage development of independent balance. Isomet-

(continued on page 1225)

PROCEDURE 33–1. ASSISTING A PATIENT TO A SITTING POSITION AT THE EDGE OF THE BED (DANGLING)

PURPOSE: To prepare patients for ambulation or transfer to a chair.
EQUIPMENT: None.

ACTION 1. Discuss the procedure with the patient, including nurse's actions, behavior desired of patient, and signals to be used, if any.

RATIONALE. Patient will be more willing to participate if reasons and expected benefits of the activity are clear.

ACTION 2. Raise the bed to your hip level, lower siderail, lock wheels of bed.

RATIONALE. Reduces nurse's backstrain facilitates use of large muscles of arms and legs.

ACTION 3. Screen the patient, fanfold covers to foot of bed. Position IV or drainage tubes so no tension will be caused on them as patient moves.

RATIONALE. Provides privacy, prevents tubes and covers from becoming obstacles during movement.

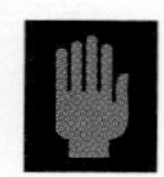

Tension on tubes could cause pain or disrupt IV or drainage system.

ACTION 4. Instruct or assist patient to move near edge of bed (see Procedure 33–9). The distance between the edge of bed and the patient's hips should be approximately two-thirds the length of the thigh.

RATIONALE. Keeps patient's weight close to nurse's center of gravity, reducing strain on nurse's back.

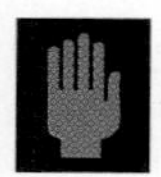

If patient is too close to the edge of the bed, lack of support for the thighs as patient attempts to dangle could cause pain in an abdominal incision or cause patient to slip off the bed.

ACTION 5. Raise head of bed 60 to 80 degrees.

RATIONALE. Conserves patient's and nurse's energy by using mechanical power to achieve a sitting position.

ACTION 6. Stand facing the side of bed next to the patient's hips. Assume a broad stance with knees flexed, back straight. Most of your weight should be on the leg nearest the bed (shaded).

RATIONALE. Facilitates using strong muscles of legs, not back muscles, as patient is moved.

ACTION 7. Slip one of your arms behind the patient's back at level of scapulae, the other under the thighs.

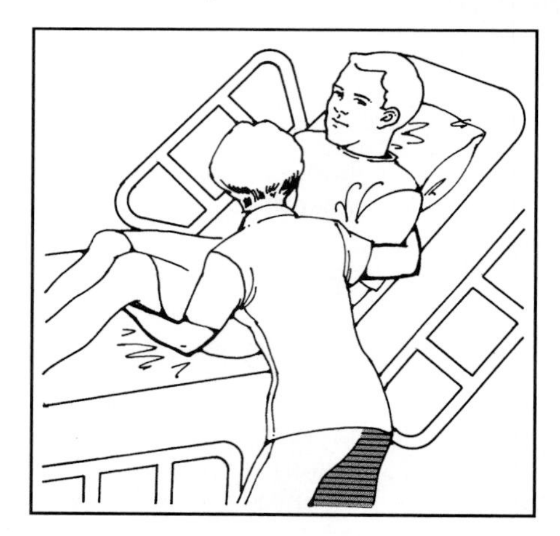

RATIONALE. Supports patient near the center of gravity.

ACTION 8. Pivot the patient toward the edge of the bed by simultaneously swinging the patient's legs over the side of the bed and pushing patient's upper body to face side of the bed. Facilitate the pivot by simultaneously

- rotating your body to face the foot of the bed
- swinging your non-weight-bearing leg toward the head of the bed
- shifting your weight to the opposite leg as you rotate

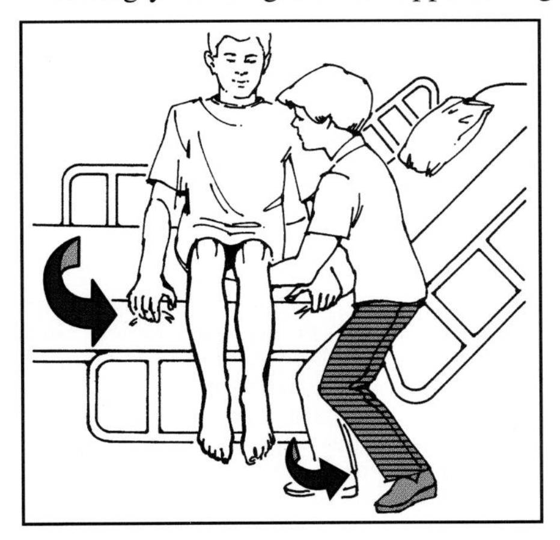

RATIONALE. Movement of the nurse's body in the direction the patient is to be moved and the use of the leverage created by pushing off the bed (thigh is fulcrum) reduces muscular energy expended.

Or

If the patient requires less assistance, replace Actions 6 to 8 with the following instructions: Ask the patient to roll to sidelying position, grasping the siderail for assistance, if needed. Then ask patient to push torso off the bed with the uppermost arm while sliding legs over the edge of the bed. (If siderail extends whole length of bed, lower the rail when patient has rolled to side.) If patient has an abdominal incision, assist the patient to lower the legs to prevent incisional pain.

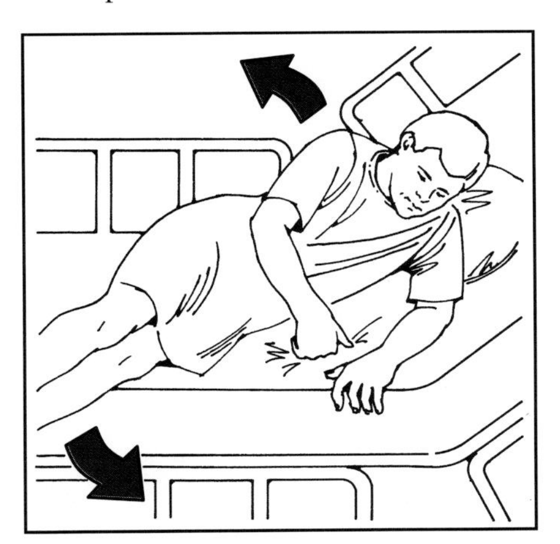

ACTION 9. Lower height of bed so patient's feet touch the floor. Assess patient for increased pulse, shortness of breath, dizziness, and sitting balance.

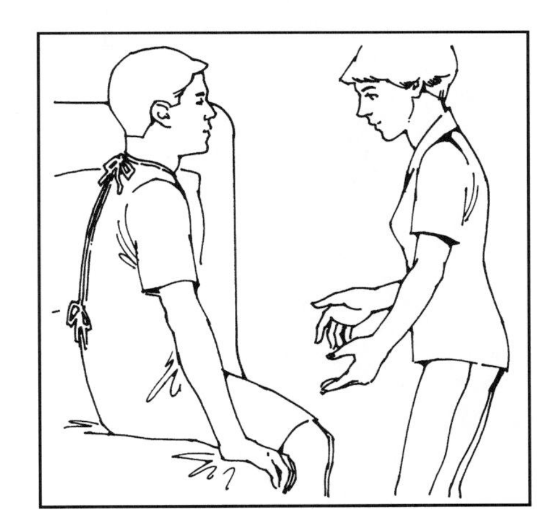

RATIONALE. Prolonged recumbency causes sluggish response of arterial baroreceptors with subsequent pooling of blood in the dependent parts of the body, causing dizziness. Exertion causes increased pulse and respirations to supply greater O_2 requirements of working muscles. Dangling allows time for stabilization of both vital signs and perfusion.

ACTION 10. If dizziness, increased pulse, or shortness of breath occurs and does not resolve within minutes, or if sitting balance cannot be maintained, return patient to recumbent position.

RATIONALE. These symptoms indicate that exertion of sitting up has used most of the patient's available energy. The additional stress of ambulation or weight-bearing transfer to a chair is not likely to be tolerated.

Continued

Procedure 33–1. Assisting a Patient to a Sitting Position at the Edge of the Bed (Dangling) (continued)

ACTION 11. To return patient to supine position: Face the foot of the bed with a broad stance, knees flexed, back straight. Support patient as in Action 7, above.

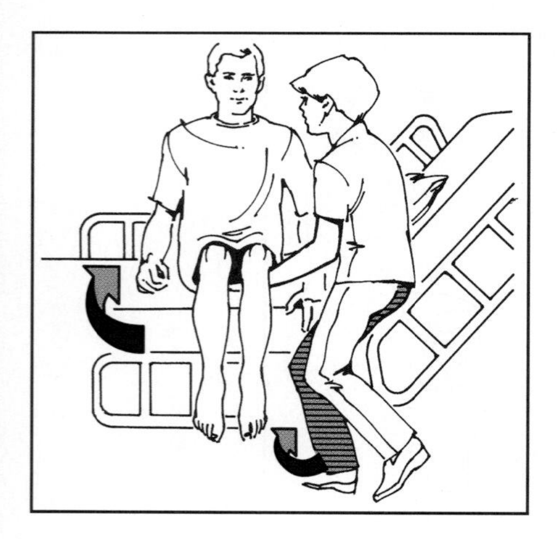

ACTION 12. Turn patient toward the bed, by stepping toward the bed, placing the patient's legs on the bed as you turn.

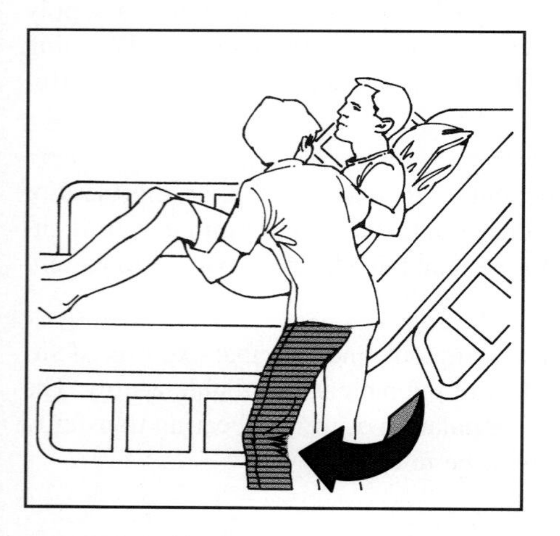

ACTION 13. If there are no symptoms of overexertion, proceed with ambulation or transfer or continue to dangle for prescribed period before returning patient to a supine position.

ACTION 14. At completion of activity, leave patient positioned comfortably in correct alignment, with bed in low position and siderails up.

RATIONALE 11–14. See Actions 6 to 8.

Recording:
Indicate the amount of assistance needed to sit up. Describe tolerance in terms of vital sign changes, dizziness, sitting balance. Note length of time dangled or specific activity that followed.

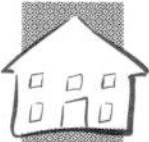

HOME HEALTH ADAPTATION: Low stationary beds are usually found in the home, requiring the caregiver to use extra precautions to use appropriate body mechanics to prevent back strain. Place 3 or 4 pillows behind the patient's torso in lieu of raising the head of the bed. Whenever possible, request assistance from family members. Teach family members how to safely assist the patient to sit on the edge of the bed.

PROCEDURE 33–2. ASSISTING WITH AMBULATION

PURPOSE: 1. To promote maintenance or restoration of endurance, muscle strength, and joint flexibility.
2. To provide environmental stimulation.

EQUIPMENT: Gait belt, spirits of ammonia ampule in nurse's pocket.

ACTION 1. Obtain baseline pulse, respirations, and blood pressure.

RATIONALE. Pulse, respirations, and blood pressure are indicators of the amount of stress caused by the exercise. Baseline values can be compared to values obtained during and after exercise to determine whether tolerance was reached or exceeded.

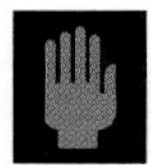

If this is first ambulation of a patient who has been on bedrest for several days, it is prudent to have one other person present to assist with ambulation.

ACTION 2. Discuss the procedure and its purpose with the patient, including nurse actions and behavior desired of the patient.

RATIONALE. Active participation is more likely if patient understands the procedure, desired behaviors, and anticipated benefits.

ACTION 3. Assist patient to a sitting position at the edge of the bed (see Procedure 33–1). Ask patient to remain sitting at edge of bed ("dangle") while you assess for dizziness, increased pulse, shortness of breath, sitting balance.

RATIONALE. Prolonged recumbency may cause sluggish response of arterial baroreceptors, with subsequent pooling of blood in dependent parts of the body, causing dizziness. Exertion causes increased pulse and respirations to supply increased O_2 requirements in muscle tissue. "Dangling" provides time for stabilization of both vital signs and perfusion.

ACTION 4. If dizziness, increased pulse, or shortness of breath occurs and does not resolve within minutes, or if sitting balance cannot be maintained, return patient to recumbent position. Continue strengthening exercises and repeated dangling to prepare patient for future ambulation.

RATIONALE. These symptoms indicate that the exertion of sitting up has used most of the patient's available energy. The additional stress of ambulation is not likely to be tolerated.

ACTION 5. If balance is satisfactory but patient's weight-bearing ability is uncertain, test quadriceps, iliopsoas, and anterior tibialis muscle strength (see Clinical Guideline 33–9).

RATIONALE. Adequacy of muscle strength determines whether patient can ambulate, and indicates amount of assistance needed (see Clinical Guideline 33–9).

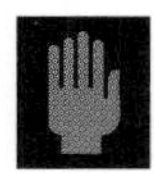

If weight bearing is attempted before leg, strength, balance, vasomotor, and cardiovascular stabilization is established, orthostatic hypotension, syncope, or falls may occur.

ACTION 6. When patient is stable, assist to don nonslip footwear and robe. Footwear with open heel or high heel is not suitable. If patient has no safe footwear, disposable slippers may be available on hospital supply cart.

RATIONALE. Footwear is necessary to protect patient from microorganisms on hospital floor and to prevent falls resulting from slipping. A robe prevents exposure of patient's body.

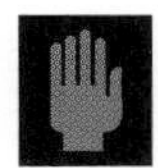

Ambulation without proper footwear predisposes patient to falls and possible injury and promotes contamination of linen after return to bed. If patient is not provided a robe, chilling, embarrassment, loss of self-esteem, and resistance to subsequent ambulation may occur.

ACTION 7. Apply gait belt snugly but comfortably around patient's waist (not needed for patients requiring minimal support (see Table 33–12). A belt-type restraint may be substituted if gait belt is not available.

RATIONALE. A gait belt provides a safe, sturdy means of support and allows nurse to control the direction of a fall if loss of balance or syncope occurs without warning.

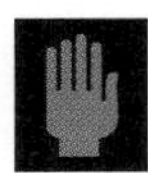

Ambulation without a gait belt can result in injury to patient and nurse. If patient becomes weak or dizzy, patient may hold or lean on nurse for support, causing both to fall.

ACTION 8. Lower the bed so patient can reach the floor without stretching or sliding.

RATIONALE. Establishes firm footing prior to attempting weight bearing. Sliding or stretching to reach the floor from a high bed may cause patient to slip, lose balance, and possibly fall.

Continued

ACTION 9. Face patient, grasp belt on either side of patient's spine. Tell patient you will assist with standing by blocking his or her knees with yours and pulling upward on belt. At the same time, patient should push off the bed with both arms and raise hips off the bed to stand. As an alternative, patient can use siderail at HOB to pull self up. Nurse may reach under patient's arms and place hands on patient's scapulae if no gait belt is available. Patients with good balance and leg strength can rise to a standing position without assistance.

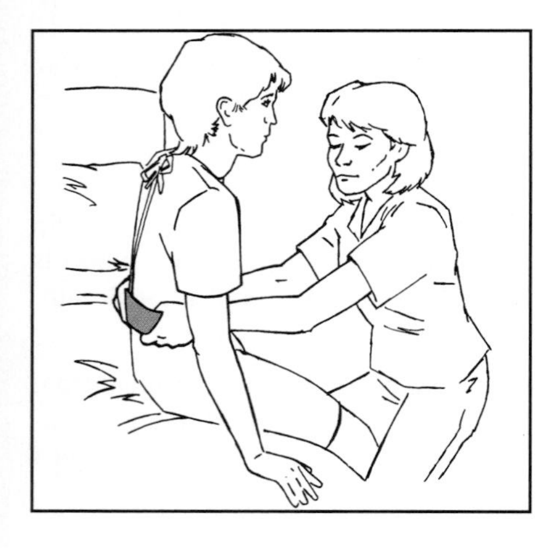

RATIONALE. Enables active patient participation and sufficient control by the nurse to prevent a fall.

ACTION 10. If patient cannot maintain standing position without assistance, assist to a sitting position at the edge of the bed, then to a recumbent position.

RATIONALE. Safe ambulation requires independent weight bearing and balance.

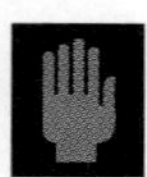

Stand-up exercises (see Table 33–12) are recommended to increase strength for ambulation.

ACTION 11. When independent weight bearing is demonstrated, provide support for ambulation according to your assessment.

RATIONALE. Enables patients to use their strength and balance to fullest extent, yet allows nurse to be aware of onset of weakness or decreased stability so immediate measures can be taken to protect patient safety.

a. Minimal Support:
Stand next to patient, slightly to the rear. Place one arm around patient's waist, grasp the hand or forearm just below the elbow.

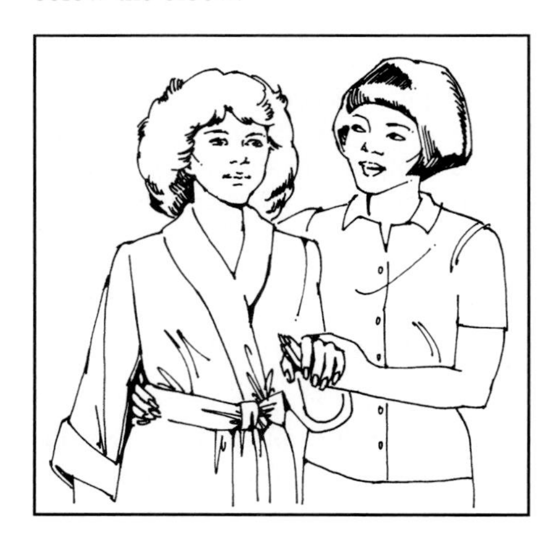

RATIONALE. Holding patient around the waist provides support and control if a fall is imminent (see Actions 17 and 18, page 1224).

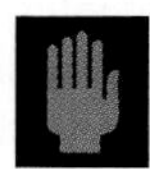

If patient requires reassurance only, but not support, walk next to patient. You may hold the upper arm lightly.

b. Moderate Support:
Stand next to the patient's weaker side and slightly behind patient. Grasp gait belt as illustrated.

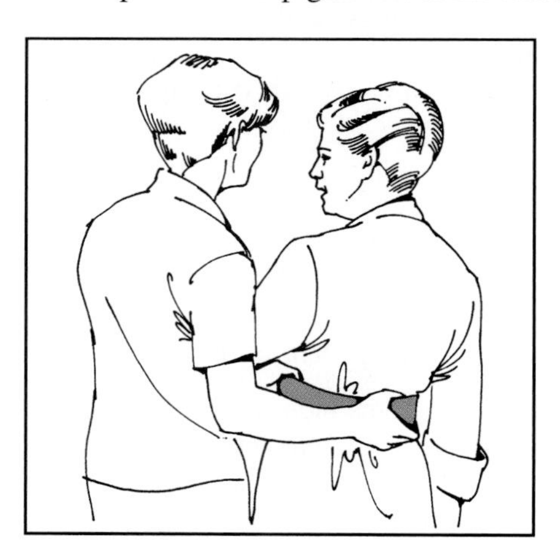

Procedure 33–2. (continued)

RATIONALE. Most patients will fall toward their weaker side due to buckling of the weaker extremity. Standing at that side facilitates pulling the patient toward you and controlling the fall.

Some patients lean toward the person assisting. In this case, standing on the strong side and slightly behind will help maintain better balance and prevent uneven weight shift to the weak side.

C. Maximal Support (two nurses):
Nurses stand on either side and slightly behind the patient, each grasping the belt at the back and near side. Alternative support: Each nurse grasps back of belt and holds patient's arm with the other hand.

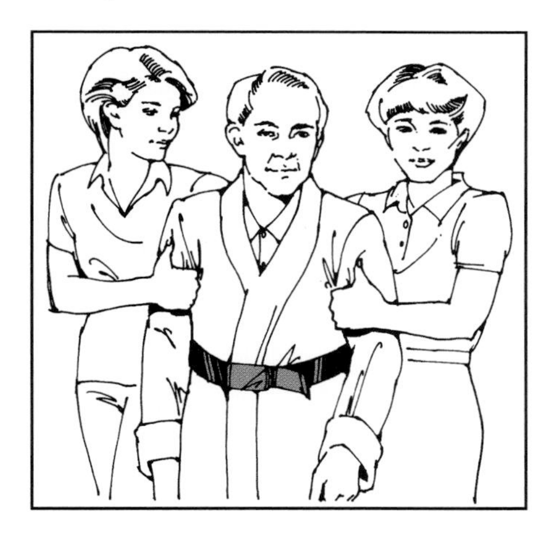

C. Provides balanced support and maximal control by nurses.

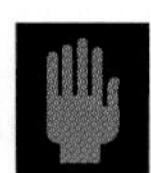

One nurse attempting to assist patient needing maximal support risks injury to self and patient.

ACTION 12. Ambulate with the patient the distance predetermined by prior assessment.

RATIONALE. Prevents overexercise, fatigue, and/or injury.

ACTION 13. Assess pulse, respirations, skin temperature, color, and moisture during ambulation and compare them to baseline data. Observe balance, stability of gait.

RATIONALE. These are indicators of exercise tolerance.

ACTION 14. If patient reports weakness or dizziness or you note decreased stability, step close and support patient by putting both arms around patient's waist.

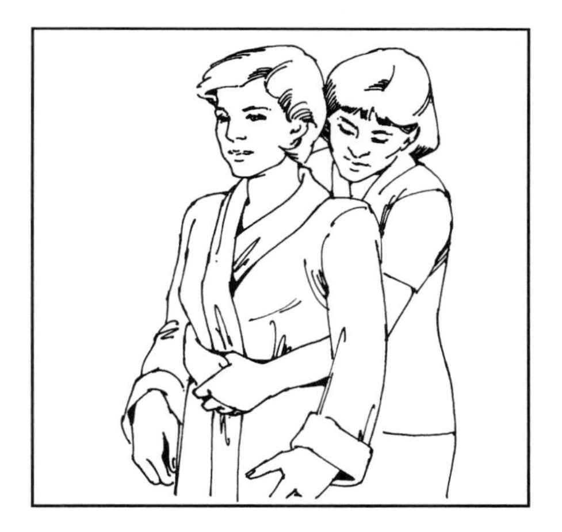

RATIONALE. Provides temporary support for the patient while you determine whether continued ambulation is possible.

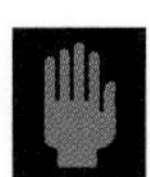

Pulse increase of 20 to 25 bpm, labored respirations, diaphoresis, flushing, lightheadedness, dizziness, or gait becoming uneven indicate that activity should be terminated.

ACTION 15. If these symptoms occur, assist patient to lean on nearby wall or sturdy furniture. For dizziness or lightheadedness, have patient inhale aromatic spirits of ammonia.

RATIONALE. Support for a brief period may provide time for stabilization of pulse and respirations, allowing safe return to bed. Spirits of ammonia causes local irritation of respiratory membranes, resulting in increased respiratory rate and depth. This increases O_2 delivery to the brain. May prevent fainting and can be used to arouse a person who has fainted.

Continued

ACTION 16. If patient is unable to continue ambulating, request another health care team member to obtain a wheelchair.

RATIONALE. Provides a safe means of returning to bed without leaving the patient unsupported.

ACTION 17. If sudden loss of balance or syncope occurs while ambulating, pull the patient toward you while stepping backward.

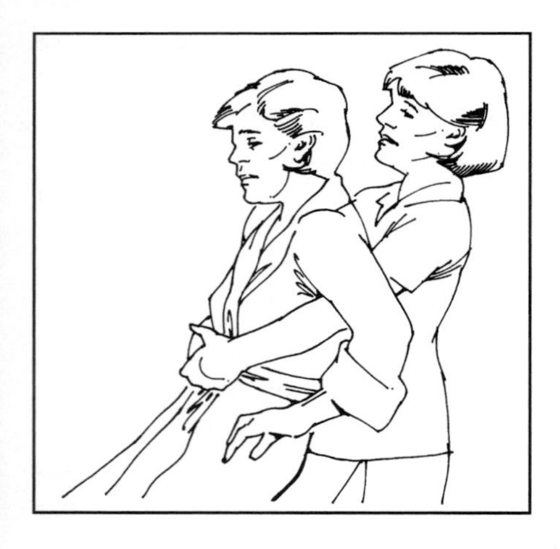

RATIONALE. This action controls the direction of the fall by bringing the weight of the patient to the nurse's center of gravity and into the nurse's base of support. This minimizes the possibility of injury to the patient or nurse. The weight of a falling patient is too great for one or two nurses to support. Attempting to stop a fall will cause muscle strain or more serious injury.

ACTION 18. Lower patient to the floor by stepping backward again and squatting or kneeling on one knee, keeping your back straight. Obtain assistance to place patient in a wheelchair or on a gurney and return patient to bed.

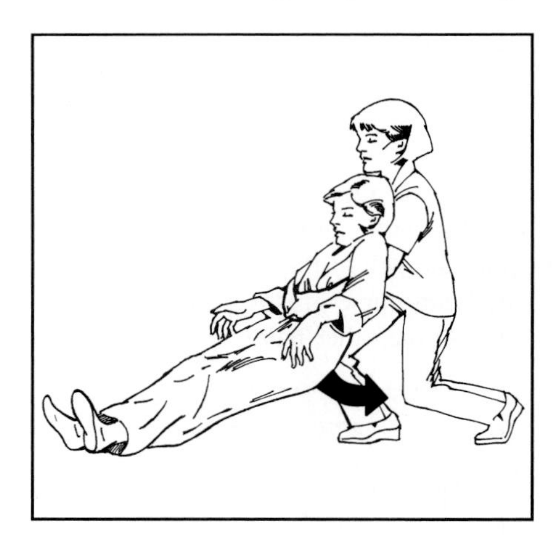

RATIONALE. Uses larger stronger leg and arm muscles to control patient movement. Stepping backward keeps patient's legs extended forward of trunk. This reduces risk of leg injury.

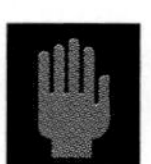

This incident should be reported to the team leader, head nurse, and physician. Immediately assess for injury.

ACTION 19. If no symptoms of intolerance of exercise occur, complete ambulation as planned. Assess pulse, respirations, blood pressure, and skin temperature color, and moisture immediately after exercise and 5 minutes later. Question about subjective sensations of fatigue. Compare postexercise data to baseline and previous postambulation data to determine progress. Exercise is appropriate if pulse increase is less than 20 bpm, respiration is not labored, diaphoresis is not excessive, and if pulse, respirations, and blood pressure return to baseline within 5 minutes. If skin and vital signs changes are absent or minimal, exercise may be increased.

RATIONALE. Comparison to preambulation data and assessment of time required for values to return to baseline provides a means to assess progress and plan for increases in exercise without overstressing patient.

ACTION 20. Leave patient resting comfortably in bed after exercise has been completed.

Procedure 33–2. (continued)

Recording:

Indicate duration of ambulation, distance walked, amount and type of assistance needed, and specific response of patient in nurse's notes. If a change in ambulation plan is indicated, record this on the patient care plan.

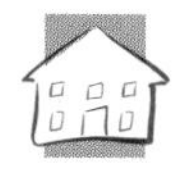

HOME HEALTH ADAPTATIONS: Good body mechanics must be used to prevent back injury when assisting a patient from low stationary bed. Clear and widen the pathway to be used for ambulation to ensure sufficient space for both the patient and caregiver to walk (or fall) unobstructed. Use a gait belt if available or a wide belt may be substituted. If family members will be assisting the patient, teach them the signs and symptoms to look for prior to and during ambulation. Also instruct them in the appropriate action to take for specific adverse occurrences ranging from slight dizziness to fainting and/or falling. Discuss with the family who (neighbor or perhaps fire department) might be able to assist them if a fall does occur and they cannot safely help the patient to get up. Instruct the family to call 911 if the patient is unconscious. If, on the other hand, the patient is unhurt, keep the patient warm and comfortable until help arrives. Anticipate patients' increasing weakness and debilitation and obtain assistive devices (walker, bedside commode) prior to a fall and injury.

ric and isotonic strengthening exercises, and supervised practice of unsupported standing, will prepare patients needing walkers for unassisted ambulation. Procedure 33–3 addresses assisting patients in the safe use of walkers.

Isometric Exercise. Isometric exercises are effective for maintaining muscle tone and strength. They also protect against bone loss, especially if they simulate weight bearing.[30] Isometric exercises are not as strenuous as isotonic exercises, so they are suitable for initiating an active exercise program (Table 33–11, page 1229). Raising the number of repetitions increases both the effort expended and the strength gained. For maximum benefit, tell patients to hold muscle contractions for a minimum of 6 seconds, and extend the period of contraction to 10 to 15 seconds as strength improves. Studies have shown that isometric contractions can cause significant elevations in arterial blood pressure. Although brief (5 to 6-seconds) repeated maximal contractions with 20-second rest periods between contractions usually result in no significant blood pressure changes, consultation with a physician is recommended before initiating isometric exercises with patients having a history of cardiac problems.

Isotonic Exercise. Even a short period of inactivity causes joint stiffness and muscle weakness. Isotonic exercises involve movement and therefore can prevent these problems and promote flexibility and strength. They are useful as an adjunct to ambulation or in preparation for ambulation. As a patient's strength improves, the exercises can be performed with small weights. Table 33–12 (page 1230) lists isotonic exercises for patients to do in bed and progressively more strenuous exercises that they can use as their recovery advances.

Active range of motion (ROM) exercises are isotonic exercises. Daily systematic ROM is a good way to maintain flexibility, and is especially helpful when a patient spends all or part of the day in bed. Wearing 1 to 2-pound wrist and ankle weights during active ROM exercises is an option for patients with good extremity strength. Table 33–5 and Clinical Guideline 33–3 explain and illustrate active ROM.

Performing **activities of daily living** (ADLs), self-care skills required for independent living such as hygiene, grooming, and dressing, provides another opportunity for patients to actively exercise muscles and joints. Encourage patients to independently perform as many of these activities as possible to maintain their muscle and joint function.

Some patients are unable to participate in any active exercise program. These immobilized patients should receive **passive ROM** at least three times a day as soon as their condition permits. Passive ROM does not prevent muscle atrophy because it involves no work by patients' muscles; however, it maintains joint flexibility. When performing passive ROM, follow Clinical Guideline 33–3. Correct technique for each joint movement is explained and illustrated in Table 33–5. As strength improves, patients can progress to active assisted ROM, in which they perform part of the movement without assistance from a nurse. Patients can also exer-

(continued on page 1229)

INSIGHTS FROM NURSING LITERATURE

STRENGTH TRAINING TO IMPROVE KNEE JOINT FUNCTION

Schilke JM, Johnson GO, Housh TJ, O'Dell JR. Effects of muscle-strength training on the functional status of patients with osteoarthritis of the knee joint. Nurs Res. *1996;45:68–72.*

Researcher Schilke and colleagues designed a study to evaluate the effects of muscle strength training, a restorative approach, on the functional status of patients with arthritis of the knee joint. They randomly assigned patients with knee joint disease to an experimental and a control group. They then pretested all subjects for extension and flexion strength of the right and left legs, 50-foot walk time, and range of motion of the knee joint. After the experimental group was subjected to a program of muscle strength training, the researchers posttested all subjects on the same measures. The results showed a significant decline in the arthritis activity among experimental subjects as well as improved results on all strength measures, while the control group showed only mixed improvement on the strength measures.

PROCEDURE 33–3. ASSISTING WITH AMBULATION USING A WALKER

PURPOSE: To provide benefits of ambulation to patients with low endurance or poor balance.
EQUIPMENT: Pick-up or rolling walker.

ACTION 1. Assess balance and shoulder, arm, and leg strength.

RATIONALE. A walker is suitable for a patient with adequate arm and shoulder strength to support body weight, full weight-bearing ability in at least one leg, and the ability to balance with minimal support.

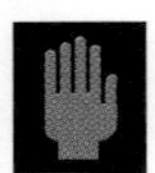

A walker is not stable enough to support a patient with poor balance or without ability to bear weight in at least one leg. Falls could result.

ACTION 2. Measure the walker and adjust so its height approximates the distance between the patient's greater trochanter and the floor. Patient will stand between rear legs and grasp hand supports with arms flexed 20 to 30 degrees.

RATIONALE. Promotes efficient use of arm and leg muscles to support weight during ambulation. Early fatigue will result if walker is too high or too low.

ACTION 3. Obtain baseline pulse, respirations, and blood pressure.

RATIONALE. Changes in these values indicate amount of stress caused by exercise. Baseline values are compared to inter- and postexercise values to determine tolerance. (see Table 33–6).

ACTION 4. Assist patient to prepare for standing (see Procedure 33–2, Actions 3 to 6). When rising to a standing position, chair arms, bed, or siderail should be used for support, not walker.

RATIONALE. See Procedure 33–2. Walker base of support is not broad enough to resist side and downward force without tipping.

ACTION 5. Walk with patient: Stand to the side of the walker (weaker side, if applicable) and slightly behind patient.

RATIONALE. Facilitates breaking a fall if sudden weakness, fainting, or loss of balance occurs.

ACTION 6. Tell patient to keep walker slightly ahead and to look ahead (not at floor) while walking.

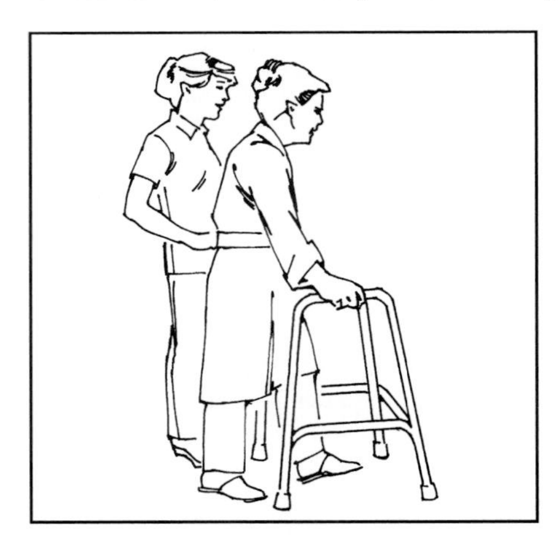

RATIONALE. Maintains a wide base of support over which to keep center of gravity during ambulation. Looking ahead facilitates maintenance of correct posture.

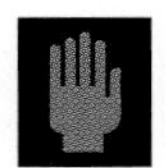

If patient steps too close to front bar of walker, his or her center of gravity may move so close to the edge of the base of support that walker may tip when patient puts weight on hand supports.

ACTION 7. Instruct patient to keep weight forward when lifting walker and to set it down evenly, so all four legs touch floor simultaneously.

RATIONALE. Maintains stable base of support, keeps patient center of gravity over base of support.

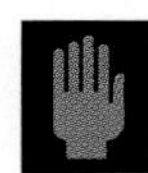

Straightening the body as walker is lifted will cause patient to shift weight backward. This may cause a backward fall.

Procedure 33–3. (continued)

ACTION 8. Instruct patient to use gait appropriate for abilities:

a. Advance walker (1), then step with each foot (2, 3), using walker for support.

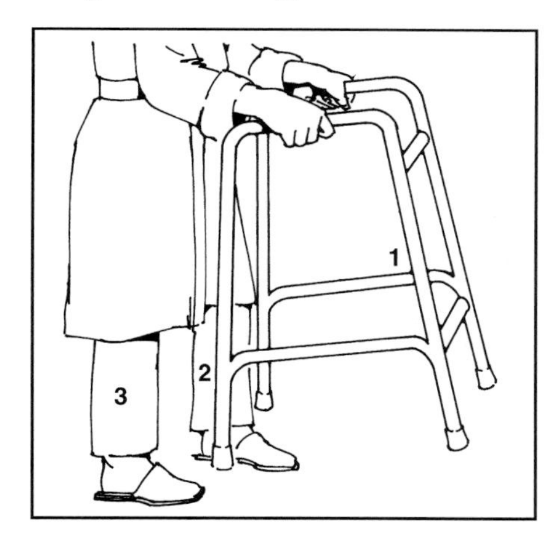

RATIONALE. Weight-bearing gait for patient too weak to walk unassisted, but with ability to bear weight on either leg.

or

b. Advance walker and weaker leg simultaneously, then bring stronger leg (2) forward.

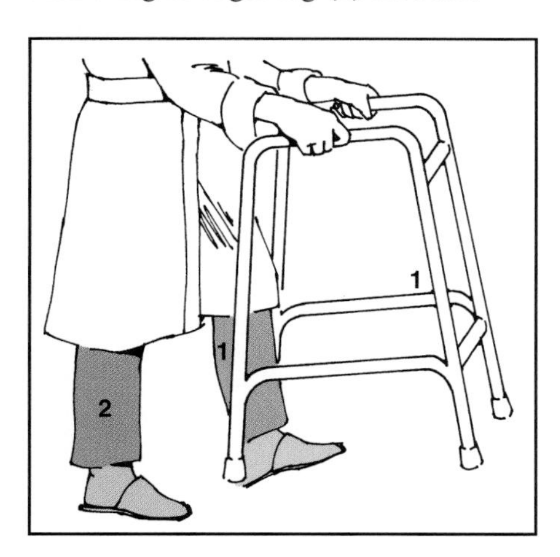

RATIONALE. Allows partial or no weight bearing on weaker leg. Requires good balance and arm strength because weight is concentrated on small base of support as walker is moved.

ACTION 9. If turning is necessary during ambulation, instruct patient to move toward the stronger side. Keep feet wide apart during turn to keep adequate base of support.

RATIONALE. Weaker side then becomes center of a turning circle, requiring smallest amount of movement.

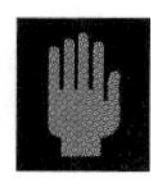

Pivoting on either foot is not recommended, as fall is likely due to loss of balance. Pivoting creates very small base of support for wide mass of patient and walker.

ACTION 10. Assess activity tolerance during ambulation (see Procedure 33–2, Actions 12 to 14).

RATIONALE. See Procedure 33–2.

ACTION 11. If sudden loss of balance or syncope occurs, step toward patient. Grasp around waist or under axillae. Tell patient to release walker. Lower patient to floor by stepping backward and squatting or kneeling on one knee, keeping your own back straight. Obtain assistance to place patient in wheelchair or gurney to return to bed. Report fall to team leader, head nurse, and/or physician, so immediate assessment for injury can be done.

RATIONALE. Controls direction of fall, minimizing possibility of injury to patient or nurse. Provides safe means of return to bed.

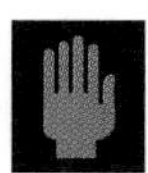

Attempting to stop the fall will result in muscle strain or more serious injury to nurse. Allowing the patient to fall onto the walker could increase seriousness of the injury.

ACTION 12. To return to a sitting position after successful ambulation:

a. Walk close to chair or bed, turning (see Action 9) so back faces bed/chair. (Wheels must be locked.)

RATIONALE. Reduces risk of falls during turn to chair/bed (see Action 9). Locked wheels prevent movement of bed/chair.

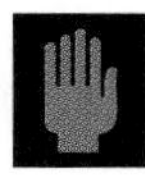

Unlocked wheels are a major cause of falls as weight of patient against unstable chair/bed causes movement and loss of support.

Continued

b. Tell patient to back up toward chair or bed as follows:
- Pull walker toward himself or herself (1).
- Place weight on hand supports, stepping back with strong leg (2). Then move other, weaker leg back.
- Repeat until back, of both legs touch bed or chair.

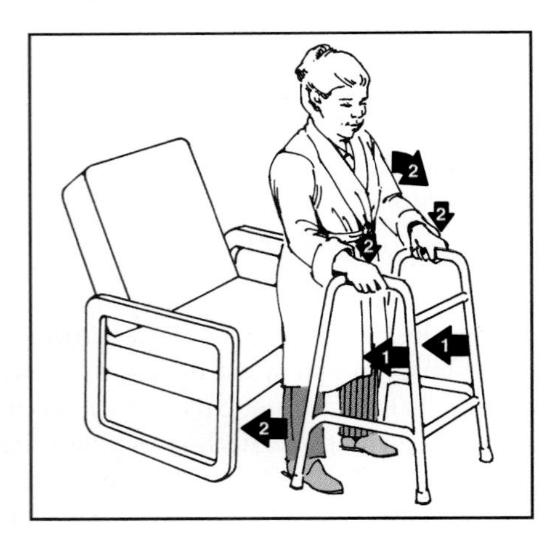

RATIONALE. Maintains center of gravity over base of support, uses strongest muscles for effort of movement.

c. Reach back with one hand at a time, grasping chair arm or placing palm on surface of bed.

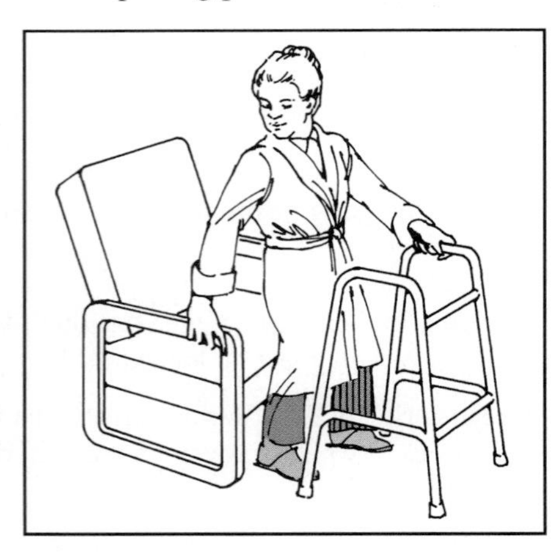

RATIONALE. Creates widest support, demands minimal independent balance. Falls could result from loss of balance if patient turns to see chair/bed or reaches back with both hands simultaneously.

d. Lean slightly forward and lower self into chair/bed, using leg and arm muscles to support weight of trunk and head.

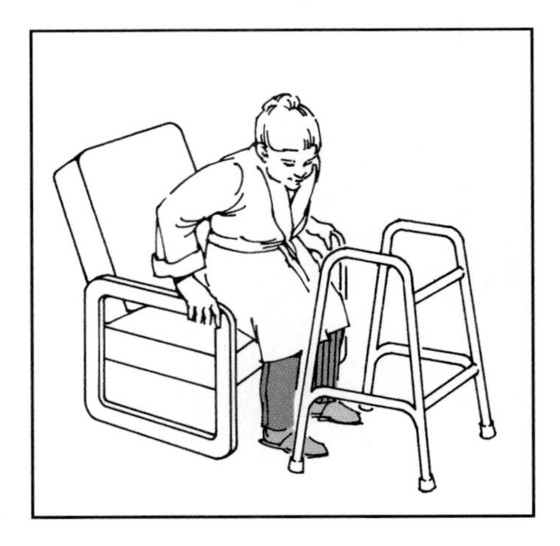

RATIONALE. Until weight is centered over chair/bed, base of support is in front of chair/bed. Leaning back would allow nearly two thirds of body weight to be prematurely shifted beyond support of legs or arms.

ACTION 13. Assess exercise tolerance at completion of transfer to chair or bed. See Procedure 33–2, Action 19.

RATIONALE. See Procedure 33–2.

ACTION 14. Leave patient resting comfortably.

Recording:

Indicate distance walked; type of walker, skill in its use, amount and type of assistance needed, if any; and response of patient, including any unusual occurrences (eg, falls) and action taken.

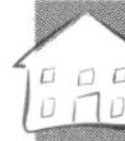

HOME HEALTH ADAPTATION: Select a sturdy high chair with arms for patient use with the walker. Obtain the family's cooperation to rearrange the furniture. Use all safety precautions and family instructions outlined in Procedure 33–2.

TABLE 33-11. ISOMETRIC EXERCISES

Exercise	Instruction	Purpose
	General: Hold each contraction 6 seconds. Repeat three times. Increase number of repetitions as strength increases.	
Quadriceps setting	Lie supine or sit with legs extended. Press the back of the knee against the surface of the bed.	Preparation for ambulation, prevention of flexion contracture of knee.
Abdominal setting	Supine: Attempt to "pull in stomach" or flatten abdomen. Prone: Pull abdomen up from surface of the bed without lifting shoulders or hips.	Preparation for ambulation, improve muscle tone.
Gluteal setting	Squeeze buttocks together. May be done lying prone, supine, or sitting.	Preparation for ambulation.
Footboard exercise	Push against footboard with plantar surface (bottom) of foot while sitting with HOB elevated and knees slightly flexed.	Preparation for ambulation, prevention of foot drop.
Hand squeeze	Tightly clench fist. May also squeeze small rubber ball.	Increase hand strength for ADL or crutch walking or other ambulation aids.
Hand pulls	Flex fingers of both hands, interlock with one palm facing toward chest, the other away. Pull as if to separate hands.	Increase upper arm, shoulder, and grip strength.
Biceps setting	Push down on surface of mattress with palm of hand while lying prone.	Increase tone and strength of the biceps.
Triceps setting	Push down on surface of mattress with palm of hand while lying supine. Or, raise arms above chest, pushing palms together.	Increase tone and strength of the triceps.
Kegel exercises	Contract muscles of the pelvic floor as if to stop the stream of urine.	Improve tone of muscles of pelvic floor to diminish stress incontinence or to increase sexual pleasure.

cise their own weak or paralyzed limbs using their stronger limbs, as illustrated in Fig. 33–11, page 1232.

Transfers

Patients with mobility problems often need assistance moving from the bed to a chair, bedside commode, or gurney. These maneuvers are called transfers. All but the most seriously ill patients benefit from the change in environment and associated mental, social, and physical stimulation that transfers facilitate. Being confined to bed surrounded by hospital equipment can be physically and psychologically confining. For the greatest physical benefit to patients, they should actively participate in the transfer maneuver to the maximum degree possible. This is an important step in progressive mobilization. To determine the type of transfer technique that is best for a particular patient, use data obtained in the mobility assessment. The following factors are most relevant.

- *Strength.* Whether a patient can support his or her own weight is a critical factor in the selection of a transfer method. Active standing transfers require good quadriceps strength in at least one leg. To assist even minimally in transfers, patients need sufficient upper extremity strength to move independently in bed. See Clinical Guideline 33–9.
- *Balance.* Poor balance is a risk factor for falls. Use aids such as a walker or gait belt. See Clinical Guideline 33–9.
- *Joint mobility.* Limitations in ROM of spine or legs can interfere with or even preclude weight bearing and active participation in a transfer. Generally, patients with knee or hip flexion contractures also have muscle weakness. Use a sliding board or hydraulic lift for safe transfers.
- *Comprehension.* Patients must be able to understand and carry out simple verbal instructions to participate actively in a transfer. Visual and hearing deficits may also interfere with comprehension, although alternative methods of conveying signals may alleviate this problem. Take precautions to assure that a patient can understand and respond appropriately to any signals to be used during an active transfer.

If the assessment indicates that independent transfer is appropriate, follow Clinical Guideline 33–10. Procedures 33–4 and 33–5 describe transfer techniques for patients needing more assistance.

TABLE 33-12. ISOTONIC EXERCISES

Exercise	Instruction	Purpose
Pelvic tilt	Lying supine, knees flexed, alternately press small of back against surface of bed and release.	Relieves lower back stiffness, strengthens abdominal and back muscles.
Knee lift	Lying supine, back flat, legs extended, bring one knee to flexed position on chest, grasping with arms. Return to extended position, repeat with other leg. May progress to flexing both legs simultaneously. Single leg flexor may be done standing.	Strengthens abdominals, quadriceps, and muscles of lower back. Increases flexibility of spine, hip and knee joints. When done in standing position, also improves balance.
Leg raiser	Lying supine, knees flexed. Extend one lower leg so leg forms a straight line from hip to toe. Return to start position and repeat with other leg. May progress to raising extended leg from hip.	See knee lift.
Knee extender	While seated in a chair, slide one foot back as far under the chair as you can reach, then straighten the leg so it extends out from the chair. Lower the leg halfway to the floor and hold 3 to 6 seconds. Repeat with other leg.	Strengthens quadriceps; good preparation for weight bearing, walking.
Head and shoulder curl	Lying supine, tuck hands under small of back, palms down. Contract abdominal muscles, raise head off mattress. May progress to raising head and shoulders, then head, shoulders, and elbows, then to full sit up.	Strengthens abdominals, neck muscles. Increases neck and upper spine flexibility.
Lateral leg raiser	Lying on side, arm extended above head, palm down, rest head on arm and raise leg off bed. Repeat on other side. As strength increases, increase height to which leg is raised.	Strengthens muscles of lateral thigh, increases hip flexibility.
Prone arch	Lying prone, arms at sides, palms up. Raise head from mattress. Return to resting position. May progress to raising head and shoulders, then head, shoulders, and legs, arching back. Or, raise left arm and right leg simultaneously, then opposite arm and leg.	Strengthens neck and abdominal muscles. Increases flexibility of spine, hip joint. When legs are also raised, hamstrings and calf muscles are also strengthened.
Trapeze pull-ups	Grasp overbed trapeze firmly in both hands. Flex elbows to pull up to sitting position, lower by extending arms. May progress to raising buttocks off bed.	Strengthens upper arms and shoulder girdle. Useful for preparation for ambulation with walker, cane, or crutches and improving flexibility of all upper extremity joints.
Knee push-ups	Lying prone, knees flexed, hands on mattress under shoulders, palms down. Push upper body off mattress until arms are fully extended and body forms a straight line from head to knees. Return to resting position.	Strengthens triceps, pectorals, muscles of shoulder girdle. Increased flexibility of wrist, elbow, shoulder, knee joints.
Sitting stretch	Sit with legs extended and apart, hands on knees. Bend forward at waist, extending arms as far as possible. Variation: Stretch first toward dorsiflexed right foot, return to sitting position, then stretch to left foot, pulling feet toward head.	Strengthens hamstrings, calf muscles. Increases flexibility of spine, hip and shoulder joints. Variation stretches heel cords.
Stand-ups	Begin with bed or chair seat raised (using books or catalogs) to a height equal to 1½ × length of a patient's knee-to-foot measurement. Obtain a table (without wheels or with brakes) high enough to reach patient's midthigh. Have feet on the floor (shoes on) and sit on the edge of chair or bed facing table, hands flat on table. Lean forward slightly, straighten legs and back until erect. Use table for balance, not to assist in standing. Stand 10 seconds, sit down 15 seconds, repeat 10 to 20 times. Do this set of stand-ups four times a day. As strength increases, lower the chair or bed to a level from which standing is moderately difficult. Continue to repeat 10 to 30 times, four times a day. Lower bed or chair until patient can stand independently from a chair of standard height.	Increases strength of quadriceps, conditions autonomic reflexes controlling blood flow to the head. Prepares for independent ambulation.
Shoulder stretch	Stand erect, clench fists in front of chest with elbows at shoulder height. Keeping head erect, thrust elbows back without arching back. Return to starting position.	Reduces tension in neck and upper back.

TABLE 33-12. CONTINUED

Exercise	Instruction	Purpose
Body bender	Stand erect, feet at shoulder width. Interlace fingers behind neck. Bend to right as far as possible, return to erect and bend to left. Variation: Extend arms above head. Bend side to side as above, sliding left arm down side of left leg and right arm down side of right leg.	Stretches muscles of lateral chest, lower back. Increases flexibility of shoulders, sacroiliac joint and spine. Variation stretches trapesius.
Torso twist	Stand erect, feet at shoulder width, arms extended laterally, level with shoulders. Without moving feet (twist at the waist), bring right arm and shoulder across chest and as far to the left as possible. Return to start and repeat with left arm.	Strengthens shoulder girdle muscles of back and lateral trunk. Increases flexibility of iliosacral joint, spine.
Half knee bend	Stand erect, feet at shoulder width, hands on hips. Bend knees halfway while extending arms forward, palms down. Return to start. May progress to full knee bends.	Strengthens biceps, shoulder girdle, quadriceps, and calf muscles. Increases flexibility of ankle, knee, hip joints.
Ankle stretch	Stand erect, feet together, arms extended forward at the shoulder. Raise up on tiptoe, return to start. Variation: Stand on large book, weight on balls of feet. Lower heels, then raise up on tip-toe. Return to start.	Strengthens shoulder girdle hamstrings, calf and foot muscles. Increases flexibility of foot and ankle joints. Variation also stretches heel cords and improves balance.
Toe toucher	Stand erect, feet at shoulder width, arms extended above head. Bend down, touching toes without bending knees. Return to start. Variation: Spread feet about 30 inches apart, arms extended laterally at shoulder height. Alternating sides, touch left hand to right toe, right hand to left toe, standing erect between toe touches.	Strengthens biceps, shoulder girdle, back muscles, gluteals, hamstrings, calf muscles. Increases flexibility of spine, hip joint.

The techniques for transfers to a chair can also be used to transfer patients to a bedside commode. Some patients are too heavy or too weak to move safely without supportive equipment. In these situations, use one or more of the following.

Devices to Facilitate Transfers. Using effective body mechanics can accomplish the safe transfer of many patients.

- *Gait Belt.* Gait belts are routinely used by physical therapists for transfer and gait training. They are appropriate for nurses to use to help patients with mobility at all stages of illness. Although several styles of belts are available, the simplest is a 2-inch-wide belt made of heavy-duty cotton webbing that secures with a slip-proof buckle. Procedures 33–2 and 33–5 illustrate and describe using a gait belt for ambulation and transfer.
- *Sliding Board.* There are several types of sliding boards. All of them act as a bridge between the bed and chair or gurney. They are usually made of a thin layer of rigid plastic with a smooth, friction-reducing surface. After brakes have been secured on the bed and chair or gurney, the board is placed so its weight is supported on one side by the bed, on the other by the chair or gurney. Two or more nurses slide the patient across the board using a pull-sheet (see Procedure 33–4). To use a sliding board for a transfer to a chair, the chair's armrest must be removable.

CLINICAL GUIDELINE 33–10

INDEPENDENT TRANSFERS

TRANSFER TO CHAIR

- Select a chair that promotes correct posture.
- Locate chair according to patient's preference (encourage location outside patient's room for stimulation).
- Cover chair seat and back with a bath blanket.
- Put bed in lowest position.
- Lock bed and chair wheels.
- Support patient when walking (see Procedure 33–2).
- Secure call bell within reach.

TRANSFER TO GURNEY

- Place gurney parallel to bed, raise bed so heights are the same, then raise HOB.
- Lock all wheels.
- Screen patient.
- Move covers, IV and drainage tubing out of the way.
- Ask patient to move to the gurney by raising up on hands and feet and shifting his or her hips toward gurney until centered on gurney.
- Cover patient.
- Secure siderails and safety belts.

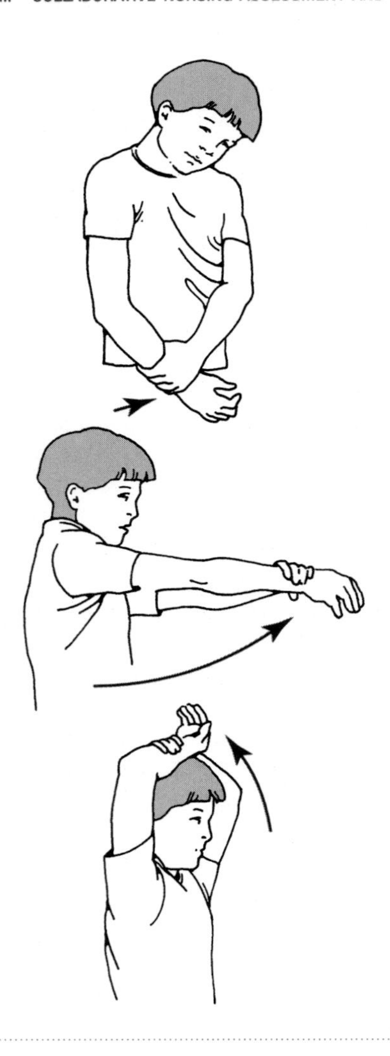

Figure 33–11. Active self-assisted shoulder exercises.

A sliding board can also be used by patients for independent transfers to a chair with removable armrests.

- *Convertible Chair.* Convertible chairs can be easily adjusted from straight backed, to reclining, to flat positions. The flat position facilitates use of a pull sheet or sliding board transfer. The chair can then be converted so that patients can sit upright or recline, and then flattened again for transfer back to bed. See Fig. 33–12A and B.
- *Hydraulic Lift.* A hydraulic lift is appropriate to move heavy, helpless patients to a chair, bedside commode, gurney, or bathtub. The lift has a detachable sling that is placed under the patient and then reattached to the lift apparatus. When the lift is activated, it raises the patient off the surface of the bed to a sitting position for the transfer. Using a hydraulic lift is a safe and efficient method for transfers. Attempting to transfer weak, heavy patients without the help of a lift is a common cause of back injuries to nurses. Procedure 33–6 describes the use of a hydraulic lift.

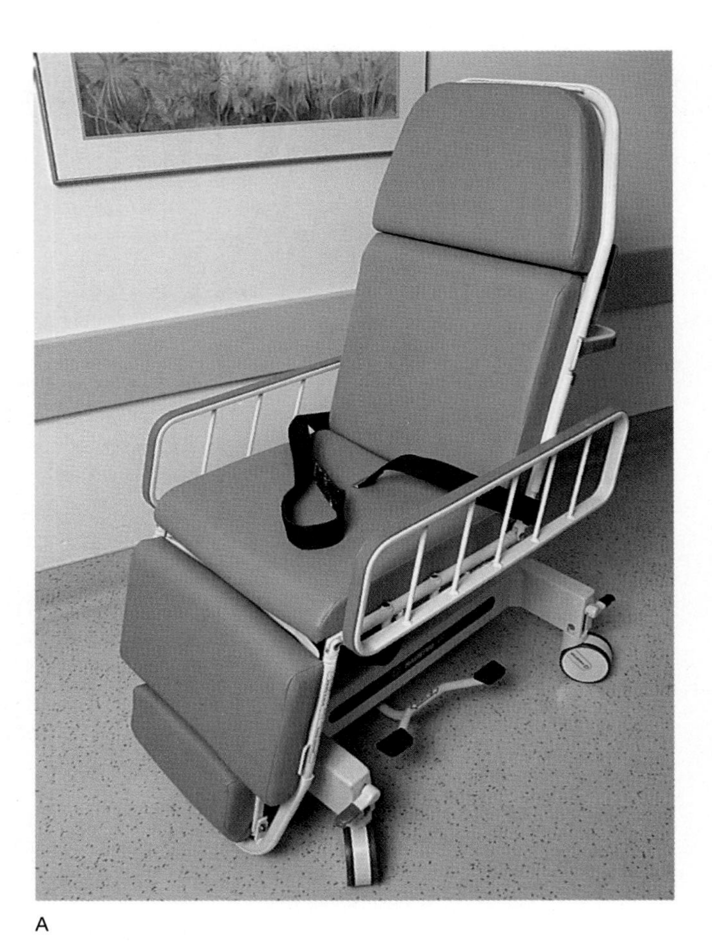

A

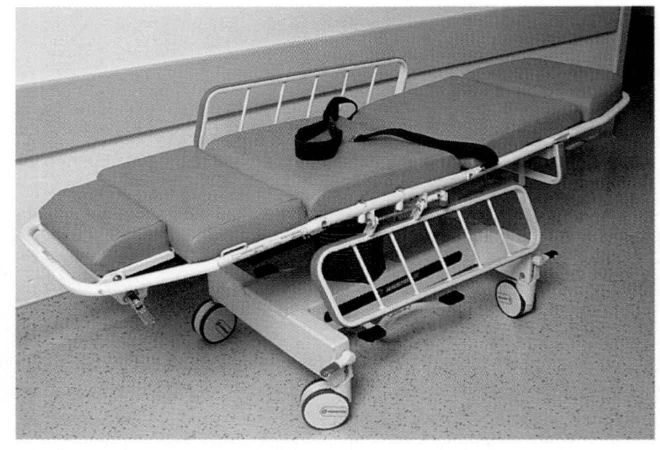

B

Figure 33–12. **A.** Convertible chair in upright position. **B.** In reclining position for easy transfers.

Positioning in a Chair

Patients must be properly positioned when seated to prevent fatigue, contractures, and pressure ulcers. Figure 33–13 (page 1235) illustrates correct sitting posture. Note that the buttocks and spine contact the backrest of the chair. The feet rest on the floor so there is

(continued on page 1235)

PROCEDURE 33–4. TRANSFERRING A PATIENT FROM A BED TO A GURNEY

PURPOSE: To move a dependent patient from bed to gurney to facilitate transport to treatment or diagnostic test or to provide environmental stimulation.

EQUIPMENT: Pull-sheet, gurney with brakes and siderails or safety belt, sliding board (if available); large plastic trash bag if no sliding board.

ACTION 1. Discuss the procedure with the patient, including nurse's actions, behavior desired of patient, and signals to be used to synchronize actions. Screen patient.

RATIONALE. Patient will be more willing and able to participate if expected behavior, reasons, and benefits of the procedures are clear.

ACTION 2. Using pull-sheet method described in Procedure 33–9, move the patient near the edge of the bed.

RATIONALE. Shortens distance patient must be moved after gurney is in position. The gurney lengthens the distance nurse(s) must reach, therefore increasing risk of back injury if the gurney were positioned prior to moving the patient to the edge of the bed.

ACTION 3. Place gurney parallel to the bed with head ends adjacent. Adjust the bed so it is level with gurney. Lock all wheels. Place sliding board or plastic so one edge is under the patient, opposite edge on the gurney.

RATIONALE. Facilitates transfer with minimum effort and maximum safety.

ACTION 4. Provide privacy. Fanfold sheets to foot of bed. Move IV bottles or drainage bags, if any, and secure them on gurney so tubing does not become entangled as patient moves.

RATIONALE. Covers, IVs, drainage bags, and tubing are moved so they are not obstacles to smooth movement. Privacy protects patient's modesty.

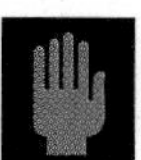

Heavy, helpless patients will require four nurses for transfer. If the number of available assistants is limited, alternate method, such as a hydraulic lifter, is recommended (see Procedure 33–6). Lighter patients can be moved by two or three nurses. The third nurse can assist by moving patient's legs.

ACTION 5. All nurses roll the pull-sheet so that edges are close to patient's body and grasp firmly so the patient is supported at the hips and shoulders. Nurse nearest head of bed can grasp corner of pillow so it will move with patient and support the head.

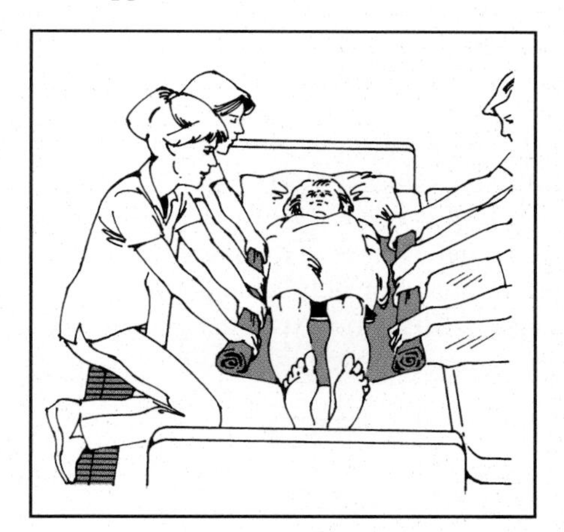

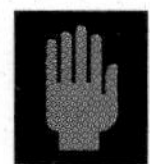

If bed linen is dry, placement of nurses' knees on the bed poses no greater risk for transmitting microorganisms than any other contact with dry bed linens. If linen is wet, it should be changed before using drawsheet transfer.

Continued

Procedure 33–4. Transferring a Patient from a Bed to a Gurney (continued)

ACTION 6. Nurse(s) nearest the bed kneel on the bed with knees approximately shoulder width apart and one knee slightly forward. (Weight-bearing leg is shaded.)

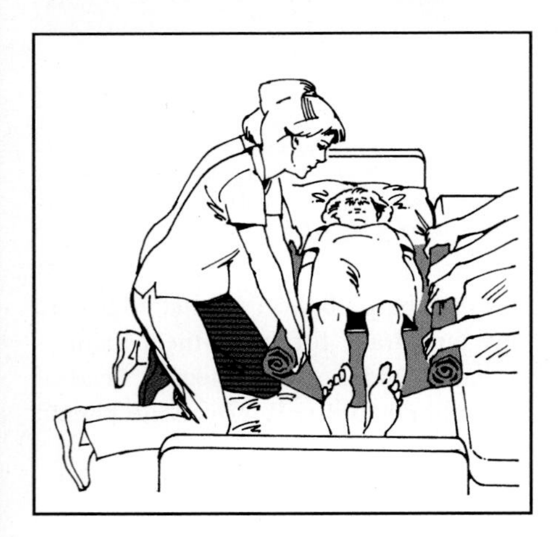

RATIONALE. Prevents back strain; allows nurse(s) to keep patient's weight near their center of gravity during transfer.

ACTION 7. Nurse(s) standing next to the gurney assume a broad stance with feet approximately should width apart. Place weight-bearing leg (shaded) next to the gurney, with the other about 2 feet from the gurney.

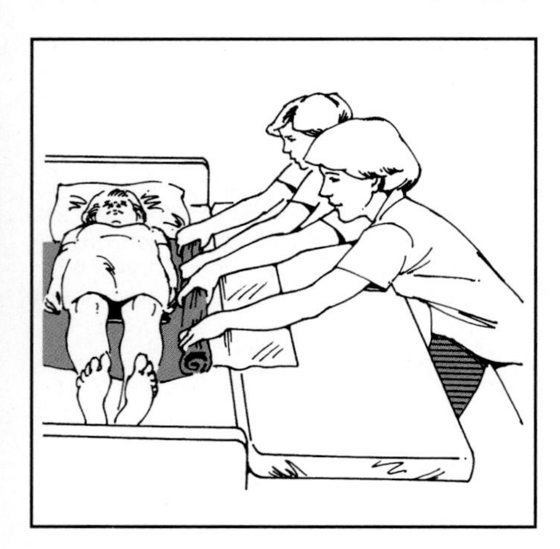

RATIONALE. This stance encourages use of leg, not back, muscles, and provides a stable base of support during shifting of nurses' weight as patient is transferred.

ACTION 8. On signal, all nurses contract pelvic muscles. Kneeling nurse(s), keeping arms extended, lift up slightly on pull-sheet while shifting their weight forward onto the opposite knee (shaded). Nurse(s) who are standing shift weight to back foot while pulling on pull-sheet.

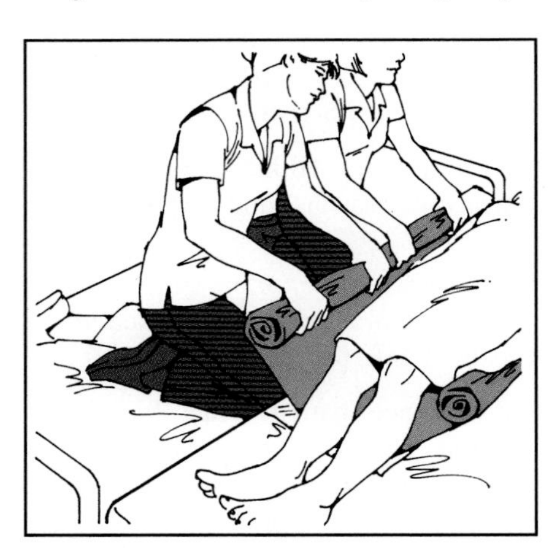

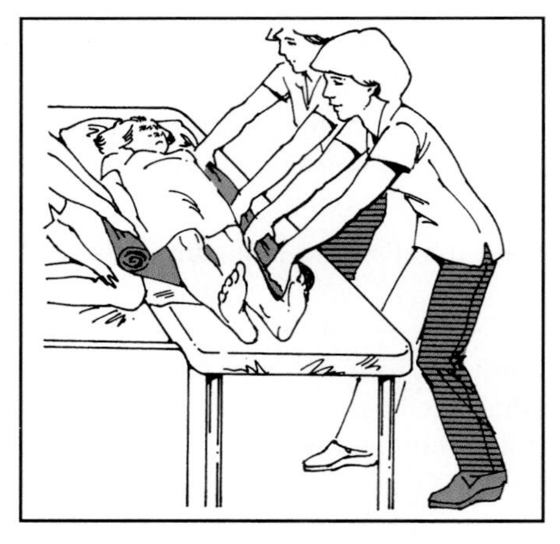

RATIONALE. Contracting pelvic muscles reduces potential for joint injury. Simultaneous weight shifts accomplish smooth transfer with least expenditure of nurses' energy. Slight lifting by nurse(s) who is (are) kneeling reduces friction, but causes minimal strain as nurses are above the level of the patient.

ACTION 9. Repeat as necessary until patient is centered on the gurney.

RATIONALE. Several short moves expend less energy than one longer move.

Procedure 33–4. (continued)

ACTION 10. At completion of transfer, cover patient with sheet, secure safety belt, and/or raise siderails. Release brake and push gurney to intended destination in a feet-first direction.

RATIONALE. Promotes patient comfort and safety.

Recording:
Method of transfer need not be documented in progress notes; however, it is common practice to note trips off the unit and indicate the purpose. Location of this entry varies with mode of recordkeeping. It is helpful to indicate most effective method for transferring a patient on the Kardex or patient care plan.

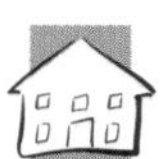

HOME HEALTH ADAPTATION: As a patient's condition deteriorates, a hospital bed can make the patient more comfortable as well as making it easier for the family members providing the care. This procedure is used when transferring a bedbound patient. Instruct and direct family members how to assist in the transfer procedure. Width of home beds complicates a transfer, and careful instruction is needed to prevent back strain.

no pressure on the popliteal space. A footstool can be used to assist patients whose legs are too short to reach the floor to maintain correct posture. If elevation of the lower extremities is indicated, provide support for the entire leg, not just for the feet (Fig. 33–14). Placing a pillow behind a patient's back is not recommended, because it contributes to slipping down in the chair. This causes back strain and skin breakdown due to shearing force. Slipping may occur even when patients are correctly supported. Procedure 33–7 outlines techniques to correctly reposition seated patients.

Moving Patients in Bed

Most patients who are alert and able to move spontaneously change positions when in bed just as you might shift in your seat during a lengthy classroom lecture. These movements occur even during sleep. Some people, however, are unable to move independently due to pain, weakness, or disability. This creates high risk for developing the disuse phenomena discussed earlier. Nurses need to assist these patients to change positions at least every 2 hours. Slipping toward the foot of the bed when in Fowler's

(continued on page 1241)

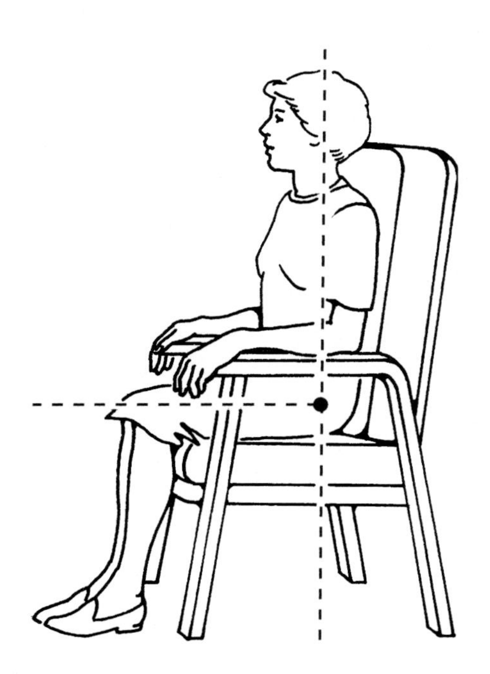

Figure 33–13. Correct sitting posture.

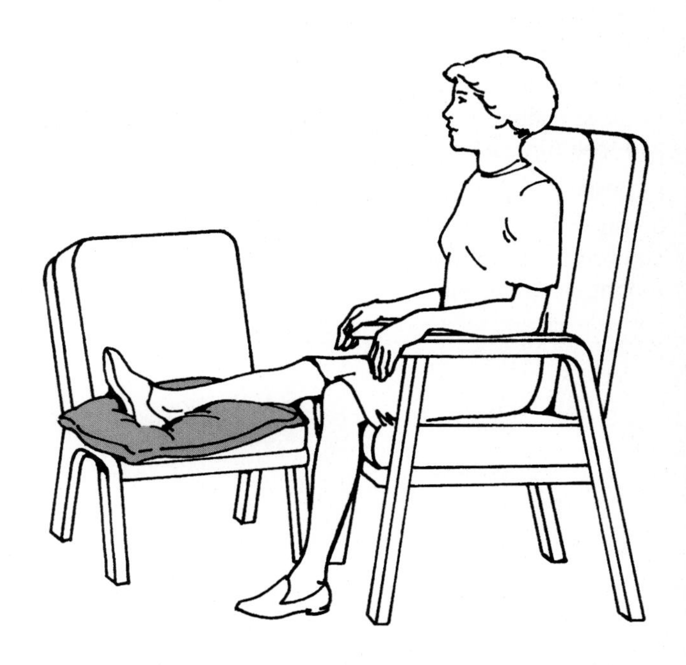

Figure 33–14. Correct leg support for elevating legs when seated.

PROCEDURE 33–5. TRANSFERRING A PATIENT FROM A BED TO A CHAIR: PIVOT TRANSFER

PURPOSE: *Pivot transfer:* To assist a patient with weight-bearing ability in one leg only to move safely from bed to chair.
EQUIPMENT: Transfer belt, wheelchair, or other stable chair.

ACTION 1. Discuss procedure and its purpose with the patient, including nurse's actions, signals to be used, and behavior desired of the patient.

RATIONALE. Active participation is more likely if patient understands desired behaviors, and anticipated benefits.

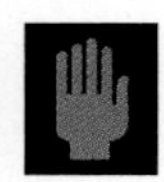

If patient's participation is not certain, another method of transfer should be selected, as cooperative weight bearing on the part of the patient is required for a safe pivot transfer.

ACTION 2. Place a chair next to bed, adjacent to patient's stronger (pivot) leg. Place a folded sheet or bath blanket over seat and back of chair. If wheelchair is used: Remove or reposition leg supports if possible to provide leg room for you and patient during pivot; secure brakes and swing front casters forward for maximum stability.

RATIONALE. Provides shortest distance between patient's weight-bearing leg and chair. Covering protects the chair from drainage or secretions and reduces the patient's discomfort due to skin contact with plastic surface of the chair.

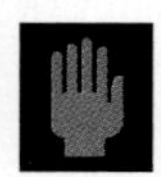

If transfer is attempted in the direction of patient's non-weight-bearing leg, the distance will be too great for a safe pivot. The patient's weight must then be borne by the nurse, which may cause muscle strain, or more serious injury.

ACTION 3. Instruct or assist patient to dangle (see Procedure 33–1).

ACTION 4. If assessment during dangling indicates patient is stable enough for transfer, apply transfer belt, footwear, and robe (if desired).

RATIONALE. Belt provides safe, sturdy means of support during pivot. Footwear minimizes contamination of feet and bed from microorganisms on floor and provides stable footing; robe prevents exposure of patient's body.

ACTION 5. Lower the bed so that the patient's feet are firmly planted on the floor with the knees slightly lower than the hips. Patient's lower legs should be angled back slightly toward the bed. (Strong leg is shaded.)

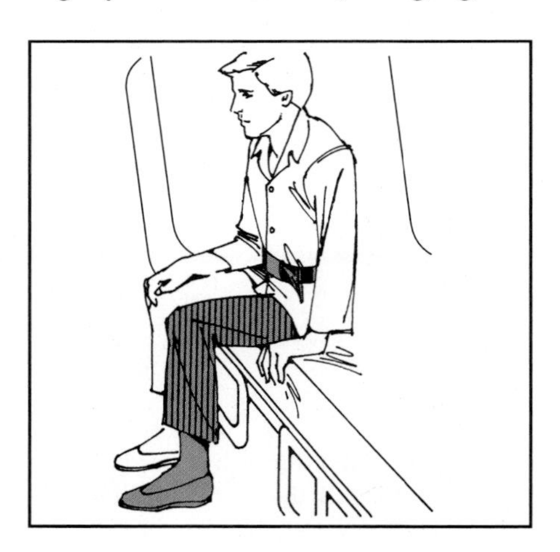

RATIONALE. In this position, the least effort is required to attain a standing position. Higher level of hips reduces the distance the patient must raise the body weight. Angle of the legs keeps base of support directly below patient's center of gravity.

ACTION 6. If patient has an IV, Foley catheter, or other drainage bag, move them before attempting pivot, positioning them to prevent tension or tangling during transfer.

RATIONALE. Tension or tangling of tubing could cause disruption of IV or drainage system, pain, or injury to patient. If patient or nurse becomes entangled in tubing, a fall could result.

Foley catheter drainage bag should be positioned below level of the bladder when patient is seated to prevent reflux of urine into bladder, which creates risk for urinary infection.

Procedure 33–5. (continued)

ACTION 7. Face the patient. Contract your pelvic muscles and assume the stance noted in Actions 7a and 7b.

a. Place one foot outside the far front leg (or caster) parallel to the side of the chair.

RATIONALE. Protects nurse's hip joints, provides a wide base of support.

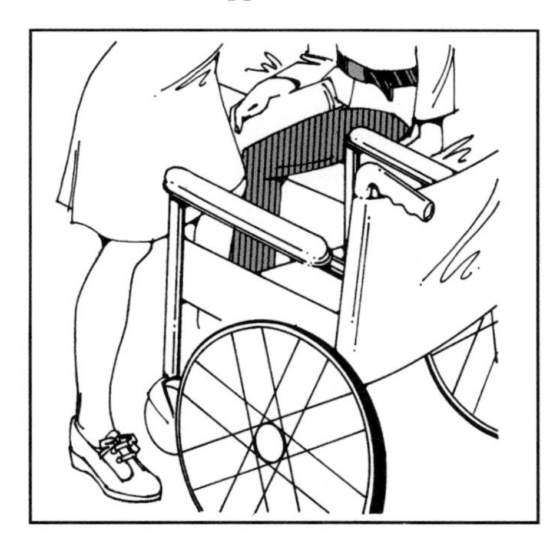

b. Place your other foot between the patient's feet, in contact with the patient's pivot foot (shaded). Then move your knee so it is *outside* patient's knee. Both of your knees should be slightly flexed, your back straight.

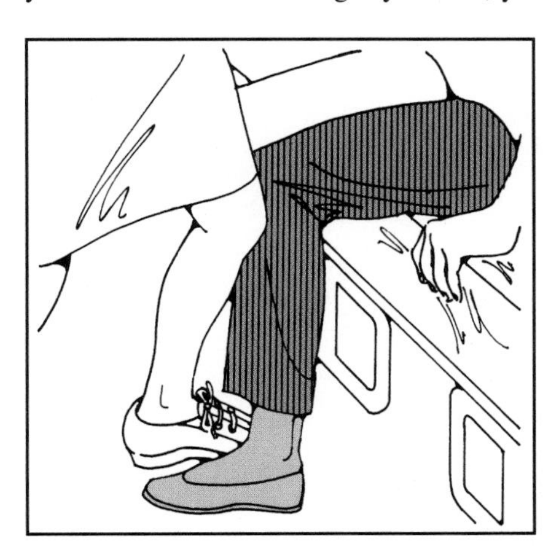

RATIONALE. Nurse's leg position blocks patient's pivot leg, preventing buckling during pivot. Flexed knees facilitate use of stronger leg muscles to assist patient to stand, protects nurse's back.

Failing to correctly block patient's weight-bearing leg could cause both patient and nurse to fall if patient is unable to support the weight as expected.

ACTION 8. Ask the patient to place hands on your shoulders in preparation for standing. Grasp the transfer belt at the patients hips. If no transfer belt is available, reach under the patient's arms and place your hands on the patient's scapulae. Or patient may push self up from the bed if desired.

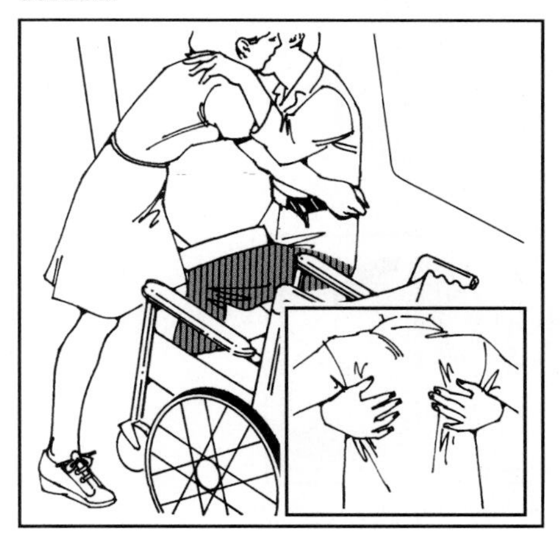

RATIONALE. Provides support and guidance for patient's upper body during pivot.

It is important that the patient be prevented from placing arms around the nurse's neck. This will pull nurse toward patient, moving the center of gravity outside the base of support, thereby increasing risk of falling and backstrain.

ACTION 9. On signal, patient stands, bearing own weight, while nurse assists by straightening own legs and shifting weight to back (shaded) leg. Nurse is *not* supporting patient's weight at any time during transfer.

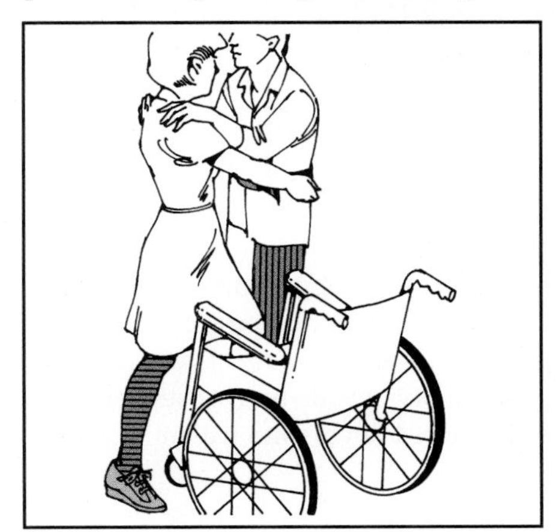

RATIONALE. Work is accomplished by stronger leg muscles, not back muscles.

Continued

Procedure 33–5. Transferring a Patient from a Bed to a Chair: Pivot Transfer (continued)

ACTION 10. Nurse and patient pivot toward chair simultaneously; patient pivots on the ball of the pivot foot (shaded), nurse on the heel. Nurse's forefoot assists patient's pivot.

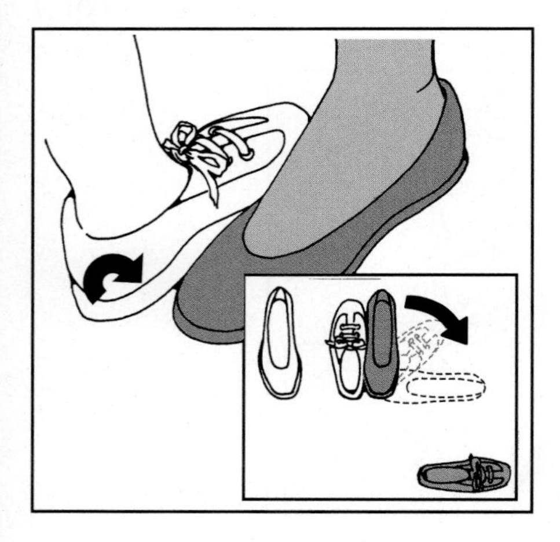

ACTION 11. Ask patient to reach back for arms of chair and sit down. Nurse assists by flexing own knees, not back, to lower patient to a sitting position.

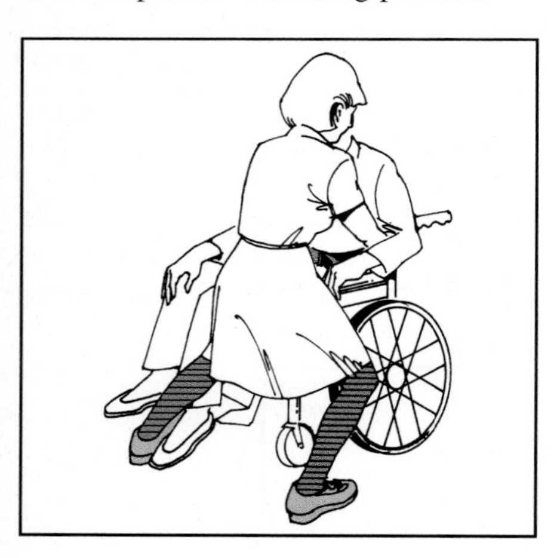

RATIONALE. Patient's arms will support part of the weight as patient is seated. Nurse's knee flexion protects back muscles and prevents leaning toward the patient, which would move nurse's center of gravity outside base of support. This could cause nurse to be pulled down onto patient as patient sits down.

ACTION 12. Position patient correctly in wheelchair (see Procedure 33–7).

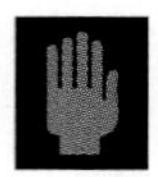

If patient remains in room after transfer to a chair, it is critical to secure the nurse call light control within reach.

ACTION 13. To return patient to bed, reverse procedure. Chair must be moved so patient's stronger leg is next to bed.

RATIONALE. Pivot can only be accomplished safely when patient's strong leg is near object to which patient is moving.

Recording:

Pivot transfer: Indicate method of transfer, amount of patient participation, amount of time in sitting position, and symptoms of overexertion, if any.

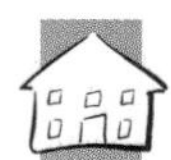

HOME HEALTH ADAPTATION: If family members will be assisting in transfers, teach them how to accomplish it safely to prevent injury to the patient or themselves.

PROCEDURE 33–6. USING A HYDRAULIC LIFTER

PURPOSE: To move a heavy or helpless patient from bed to chair or gurney and back to bed. May also be used to transfer patients to bathtub.
EQUIPMENT: Hydraulic (mechanical) lifter, chair or gurney.

ACTION 1. If unfamiliar with sling design, obtain expert assistance. Practice with the sling and lift, using a staff member or mannequin as patient stand-in before attempting to transfer a patient.

RATIONALE. Several styles of slings are available. Slings are intended to support the patient in a semisitting position when raised off the bed.

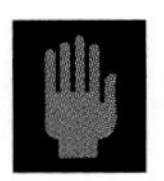

Improperly applied sling could result in patient slipping out during transfer.

ACTION 2. Discuss the procedure with the patient, including nurses' actions, behavior desired of patient, and signals to be used, if any. Patients may need reassurance that the device is strong enough to support their weight.

RATIONALE. Patient will be less anxious and more willing and able to participate if desired behavior and anticipated benefits are clear.

ACTION. Provide privacy. Fanfold covers to foot of the bed. Place fabric sling under the patient, aligning it carefully to provide even support. (Use technique in Procedure 27–14, Making an Occupied Bed.)

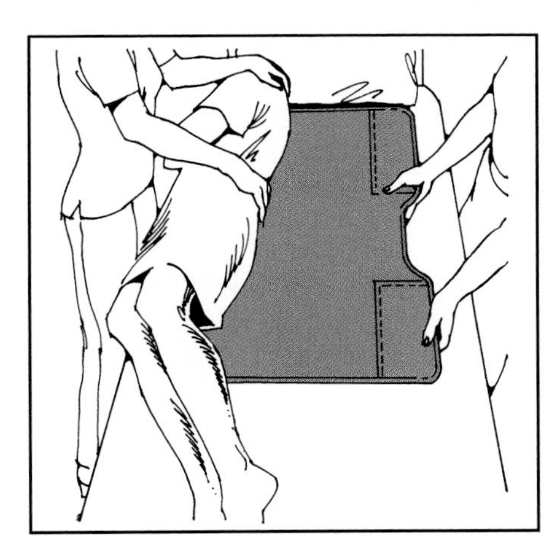

RATIONALE 3. Privacy shows respect for patient's modesty. Covers interfere with efficient transfer. If support is uneven, discomfort or injury is possible.

ACTION 4. Place the lift next to the bed so the base bars are under the bed at right angles to the long axis of the bed. Adjust bars to the widest possible position. Center the overhead support bar across the bed about even with the patient's chest.

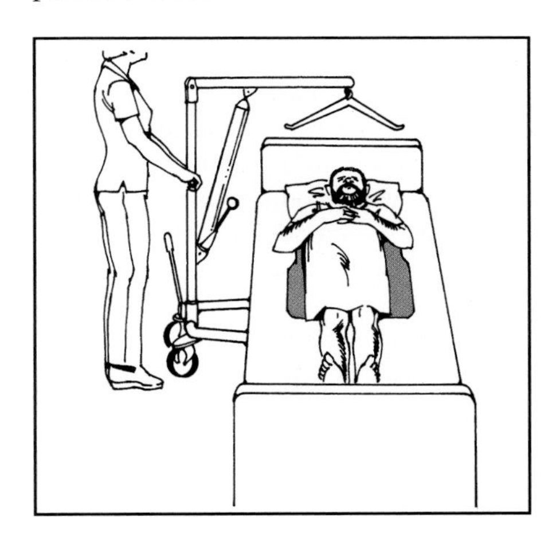

RATIONALE. Provides maximum stability during transfer.

ACTION 5. Insert "S" hooks from the overhead support into the grommets of the sling so the hooks point away from the patient.

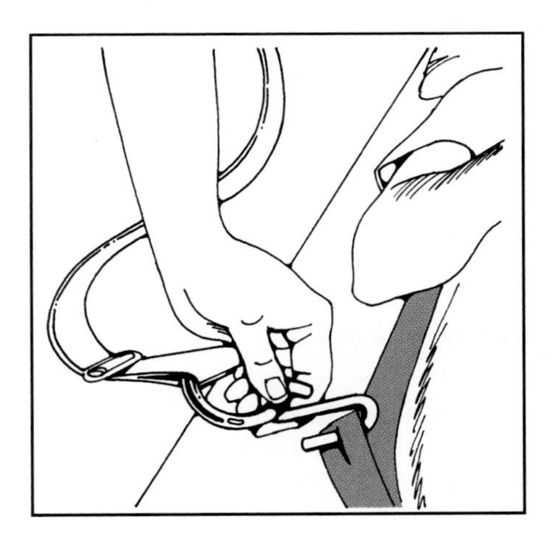

RATIONALE. Prevents skin injury from hooks pressing into patient's flesh.

Continued

ACTION 6. As the patient to fold hands in lap or to grasp the overhead bar during the transfer. If the patient has an IV or a Foley catheter drainage bag, move these first. Arrange tubing and secure bag(s) to prevent tangling during transfer. If the tubing of the urinary drainage system is not long enough to allow the drainage bag to be moved before transfer, the tubing can be clamped and the bag placed on the patient's abdomen during the transfer. Open the clamp and place the bag below the level of the organ being drained at the completion of the transfer.

RATIONALE. Pulling or tangling tubing may cause discomfort or dislodge it. Placing a drainage bag on the patient's abdomen without clamping it will allow reflux of the contents into the patient's body, which could cause infection or other complications. Failing to reopen the clamp at the completion of the transfer may cause distension of the organ being drained.

ACTION 7. Close the pressure valve and pump the lift until the patient attains a semisitting position clear of the bed.

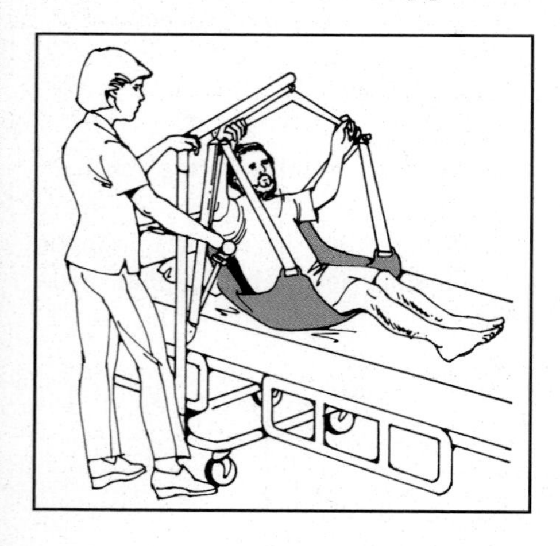

RATIONALE. Pumping action creates pressure on the fluid in the cylinder of the lift, therefore the movable portion moves upward, raising the patient off the bed.

ACTION 8. Contract your pelvic muscles and pull the lift away from the bed. Turn it so the lower bars are under the gurney and the patient is centered over it. If the patient is being moved to a chair, the lower bars should straddle the chair.

RATIONALE. Protects nurse from injury by stabilizing joints. Positioning the lift in this way maintains its stability and accomplishes the transfer without injury to the patient.

ACTION 9. Second nurse stands at the head of the bed and guides the patient during the move so patient does not swing and assists in centering patient before lowering to the gurney or chair. Third nurse may be needed to support legs of large or helpless patient.

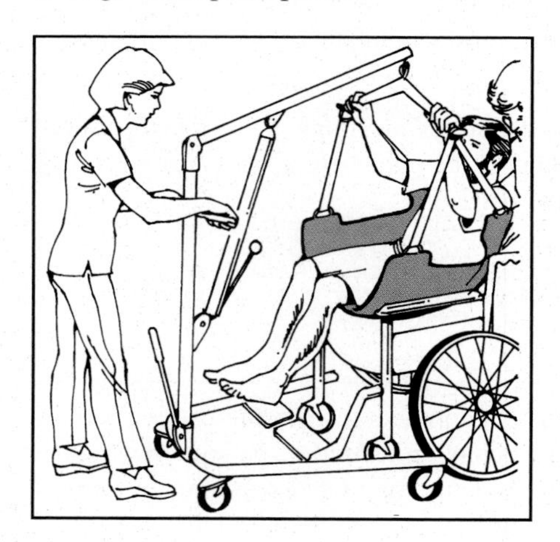

RATIONALE. The movement of the lift shifts the patient's weight, promoting swinging of the suspended patient. Most patients find this movement unpleasant, and may fear falling.

ACTION 10. Release pressure valve gradually so patient is lowered slowly. Close valve as soon as patient is resting on the chair or gurney.

RATIONALE. Rapid downward movement may frighten patient. Abrupt contact with chair or gurney could jar patient.

ACTION 11. Second nurse supports patient's upper body as patient is lowered from sitting to supine position if being moved to a gurney.

RATIONALE. There is minimal back support from sling. Weak patients may be unable to change positions independently.

ACTION 12. Release "S" hooks, leaving sling under patient. If wrinkles are present, pull sling taut.

RATIONALE. Leaving sling in place conserves time and energy and facilitates returning patient to bed. Wrinkles in sling may cause pressure areas, increasing risk for ischemia.

Procedure 33–6. (continued)

ACTION 13. At completion of transfer, position patient in correct alignment; secure safety belt or siderails.

RATIONALE. Maintains patient comfort and safety.

Recording:
It is not usually necessary to document use of a hydraulic lifter in nurse's progress notes, but including this information on the Kardex or patient care plan is helpful.

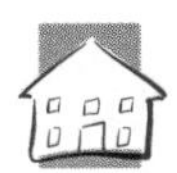

HOME HEALTH ADAPTATION: Teach family members how to safely use a hydraulic lift, giving them ample opportunity to practice, with assistance and supervision, until they are comfortable with the equipment and the technique.

(semi-sitting) position is a frequent problem. Even patients who are able to turn easily from side to side often require assistance to reposition themselves nearer the head of the bed. A patient having had recent abdominal surgery is an example.

An overbed trapeze is useful to facilitate repositioning. The trapeze is suspended above the torso from a sturdy frame that extends the full length of the bed. Patients can use it to raise their hips off the bed so they can easily change positions. A trapeze is also useful for upper body exercise (see Table 33–12).

Moving and positioning heavy patients or those with limited ability to assist often requires two or more nurses. Using protective body mechanics is essential to prevent injury to patients and nurses. Techniques for assisting with position changes are detailed in Procedures 33–8 to 33–12. Correct positions and protective devices that facilitate maintaining proper alignment are discussed in the following sections.

Positioning Patients in Bed

Effective positioning of patients unable to move is critical to preventing complications of bedrest. Four therapeutic positions are most commonly used: supine (Fig. 33–15), lateral (Fig. 33–16), prone (Fig. 33–17), and Fowler's (Fig. 33–18). Variations such as Sims' position, also called semiprone (Fig. 33–19), or low Fowler's, also called semi-Fowler's, are appropriate as well. Preventing joint contractures and pressure injuries are the two major nursing concerns for patients needing positioning.

Preventing Contractures. Correct positioning, frequent repositioning, and joint extension exercises are necessary to prevent contractures. The joints most vulnerable to contractures associated with bedrest are the hip, knee, and ankle.

- *Hip.* Full extension of the hip is difficult unless one is standing. Even in the prone position, there is 10 to 20 degrees less hip extension than when standing upright. Fowler's position, elevating the head or legs when supine, and the lateral position involve even greater degrees of hip flexion.
- *Knees.* The knees are almost always flexed when in bed, except in the prone position.
- *Ankle.* Ankle (plantar) flexion occurs because the plantar flexion muscle group is stronger than the muscles used for dorsiflexion. When a patient is supine, there is added force from gravity, which tends to pull the front of the foot downward. The weight of covers is another contributing factor.

Preventing Pressure Injuries

- *Distribute body weight.* Pressure ulcers occur when external pressure exceeds capillary pressure, as discussed earlier. Pressure related to body position is diminished when a patient's weight is distributed over a large area, rather than concentrated on a small surface. There is focal pressure on the sacrum, coccyx, and ischial tuberosities in Fowler's position. When the legs are

(continued on page 1251)

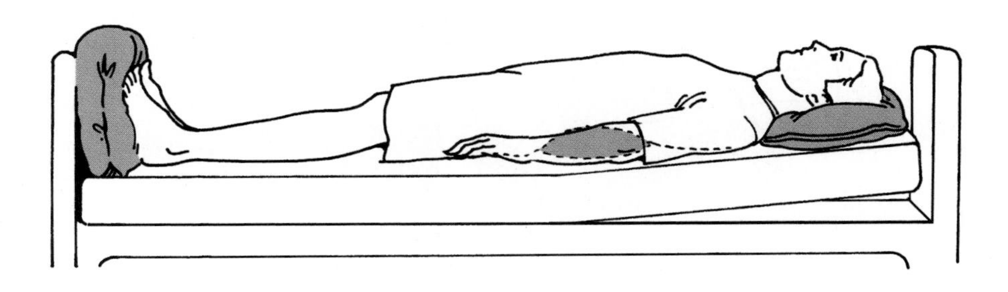

Figure 33–15. Supine position.

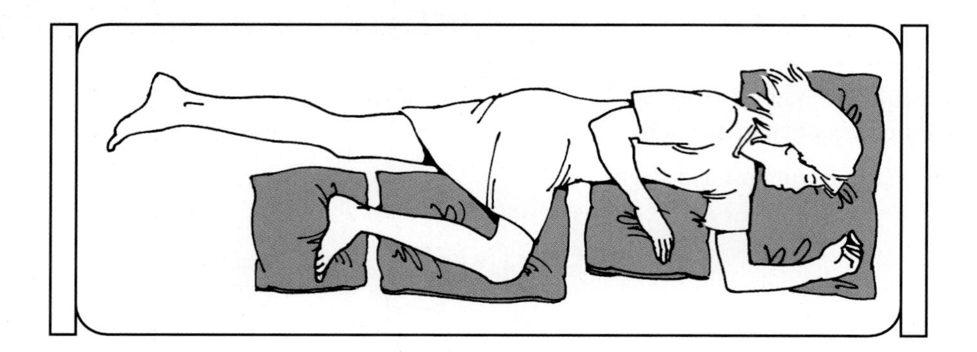

Figure 33–16. Lateral position.

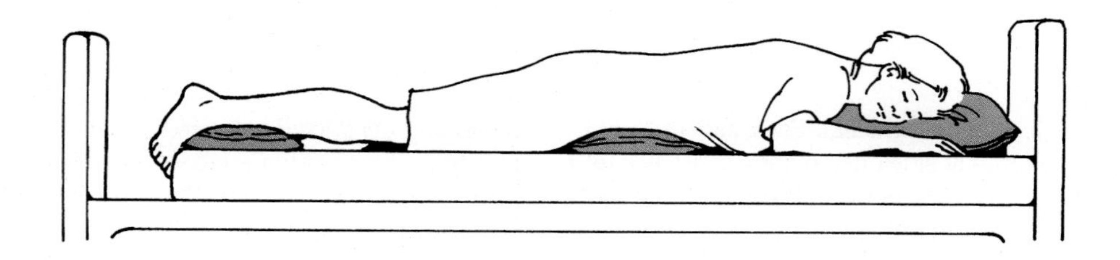

Figure 33–17. Prone position.

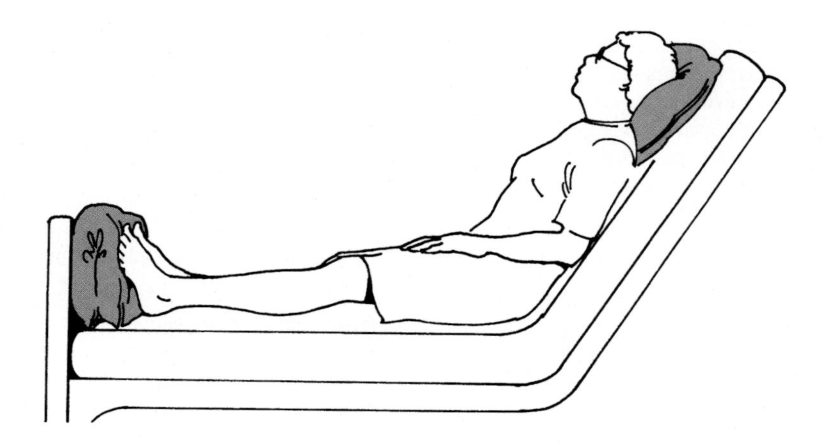

Figure 33–18. Fowler's position.

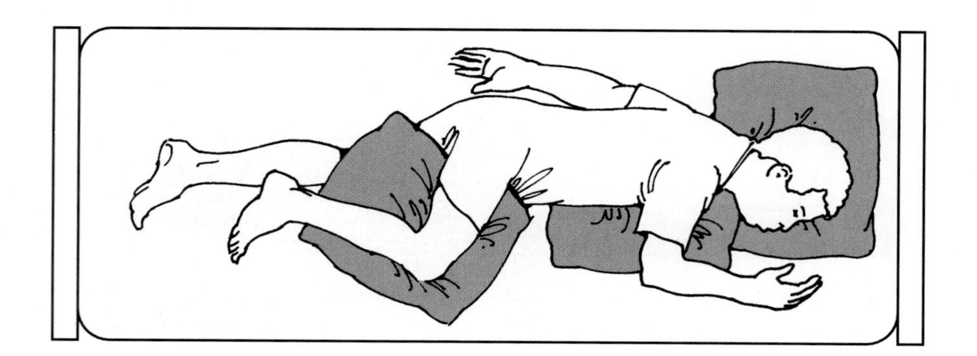

Figure 33–19. Sims' position.

PROCEDURE 33–7. POSITIONING A PATIENT IN A CHAIR

PURPOSE: To achieve correct sitting posture after transferring a patient to a chair or when patient has slipped down in a chair.
EQUIPMENT: *Method A:* One pillow. *Method B:* None.

METHOD A—Pushing a Patient Toward the Back of a Chair

ACTION 1. Discuss the procedure and its purpose with the patient, including nurse's actions, any signals that are to be used, and behavior desired of the patient.

RATIONALE. Active participation is more likely if the patient understands expected behaviors and anticipated benefits. Clarifying signals enhances cooperation.

ACTION 2. Face the patient. Place the pillow in front of patient's knees and hold it in place with your knees.

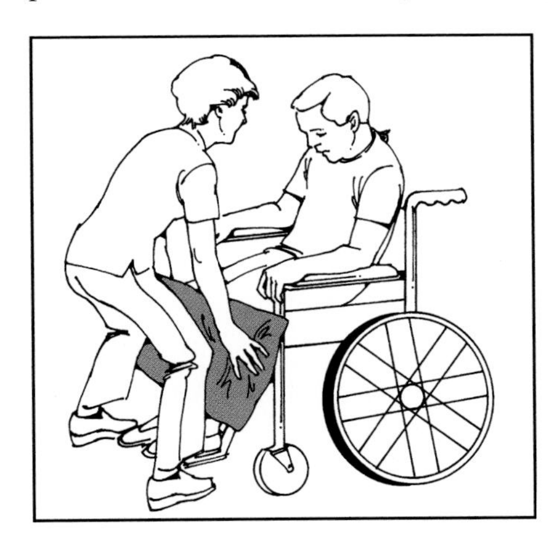

RATIONALE. Pillow cushions contact point between bony portions of nurse's and patient's knees.

ACTION 3. Grasp the armrests of the chair. Plant your feet firmly and flex your knees and hips as if to sit down.

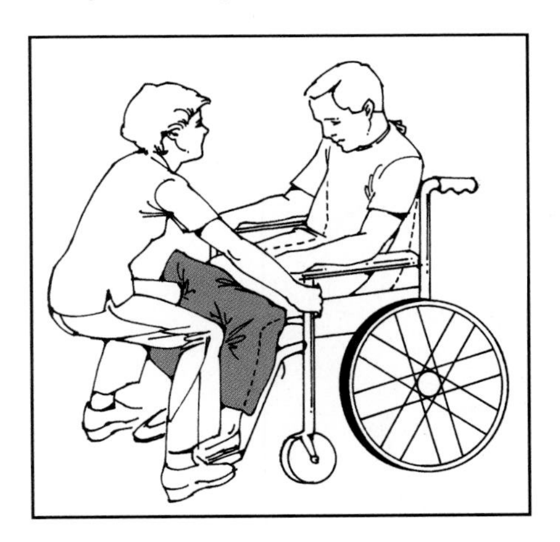

RATIONALE. Grasping chair arms assists to maintain nurse's balance and directs the force created by nurse's knee and hip flexion toward patient's knees, moving patient back in the chair.

Skin damage from friction may occur as patient slides over the surface of the chair. This can be prevented by placing a layer of cloth (bath blanket or clothing) between patient's skin and the surface of the chair, before transfer to the chair.

ACTION 4. Repeat as necessary until patient's buttocks and spine are in contact with the back of the chair.

RATIONALE. Heavy patients may move only small distance, even with the help of leverage.

ACTION 5. Support trunk and extremities as needed to maintain correct alignment.

RATIONALE. Poor alignment causes discomfort and muscle and joint strain.

METHOD B—Two-nurse Lift

ACTION 1. Discuss the procedure and its purpose with the patient as described for Method A, above.

Continued

Procedure 33–7. Positioning a Patient in a Chair (continued)

ACTION 2. Lock wheelchair brakes. Nurses stand one on each side of the chair, facing patient. Each places the arm nearer to patient under the patient's axilla. Nurses flex their arms so the antecubital space is under the patient's axilla. Place opposite hand on patient's forearm. Ask patient to fold arms across chest.

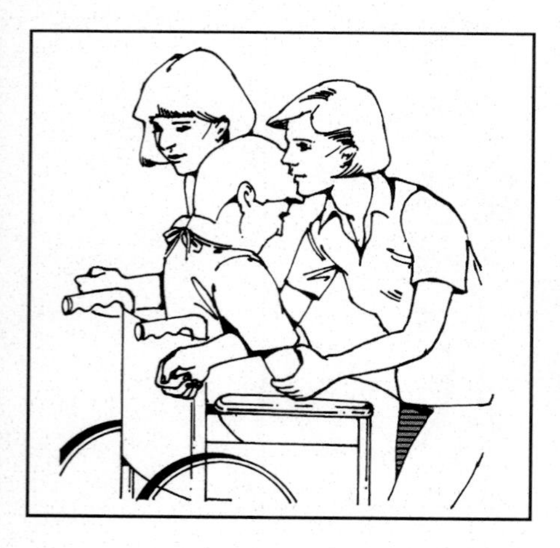

RATIONALE. Provides a secure method to support the patient and stabilize shoulder.

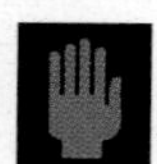

This method is not appropriate for patients who are extremely weak, as shoulder instability may result in injury.

ACTION 3. Both nurses assume a broad stance: Feet shoulder width apart; the weight-bearing leg (shaded) in line with the patient's hips.

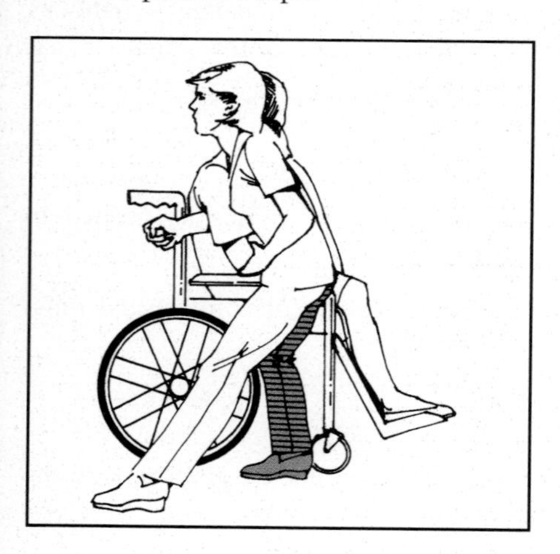

RATIONALE. Provides a wide base of support to prevent loss of balance as nurses shift weight to move the patient.

ACTION 4. Both nurses flex their knees, contract pelvic muscles, and on signal step forward, pulling the patient toward the back of the chair. Repeat as necessary.

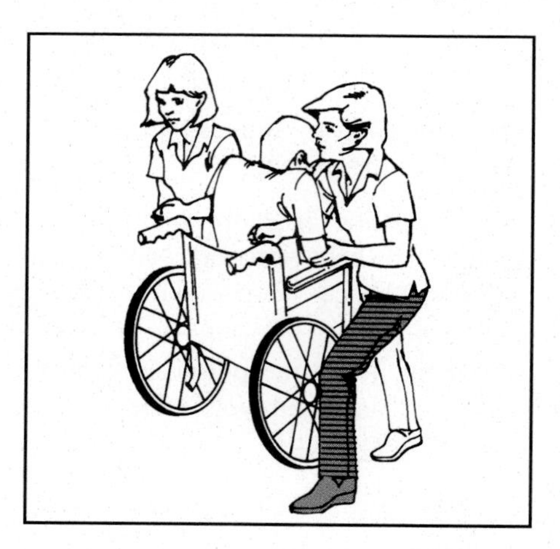

RATIONALE. Uses strong muscles of the nurses' extremities and force of their weight to move the patient.

ACTION 5. Support trunk and extremities as needed to maintain correct alignment.

RATIONALE. Poor alignment causes discomfort and muscle and joint strain.

Recording:
No recording is necessary.

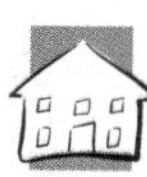

HOME HEALTH ADAPTATION: This procedure adapts well in the home. Teach caregivers how to align patients in a chair.

PROCEDURE 33–8. ASSISTING A PATIENT TO MOVE TOWARD THE HEAD OF THE BED

PURPOSE: To assist a heavy or weak patient to achieve correct alignment and alleviate discomfort from cramped position caused by slipping toward the foot of the bed.
EQUIPMENT: *Method A:* Drawsheet. *Method B:* None.

METHOD A—Drawsheet (Pull-sheet) Method, Two to Four Nurses

ACTION 1. Discuss the procedure with the patient, including nurse's actions, behavior desired of patient, and signals to be used to synchronize efforts.

RATIONALE. Patient will be more willing and able to participate if the reasons and anticipated benefits of the activity are clear. Clarifying signals enhances cooperation.

ACTION 2. Raise the bed to nurses' thigh level, lower siderails, and lock wheels of the bed.

RATIONALE. This height facilitates use of major muscles of the extremities.

ACTION 3. Fold drawsheet in half lengthwise, place under patient so that it extends from shoulder to hips.

RATIONALE. Sheet will support bulk of patient's weight for moving and positioning, reducing friction, and so decreasing energy expenditure.

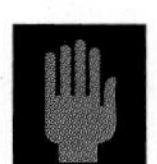

For patients who require frequent assistance with moving, including a pull-sheet in foundation linen when making the bed saves time and energy. If patient cannot support head, place sheet high enough to do so.

ACTION 4. Ask patient to fold arms across the chest and flex knees.

RATIONALE. Prevents squeezing patient's arms between pull-sheet and patient's torso. Reduces friction from pulling legs across sheets during move.

ACTION 5. Roll sheet so edges are close to patient's body and grasp firmly next to patient's shoulders and hips.

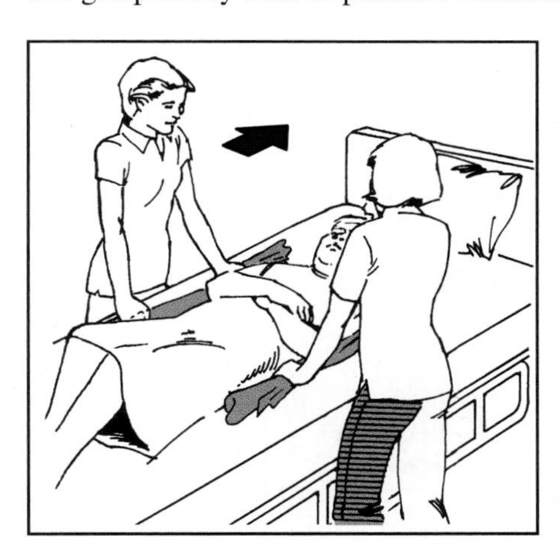

RATIONALE. Maximizes control during movement, improves leverage.

ACTION 6. Face head of bed. Assume broad stance with legs slightly flexed. Outside foot is forward. Weight is on leg nearer foot of bed (shaded).

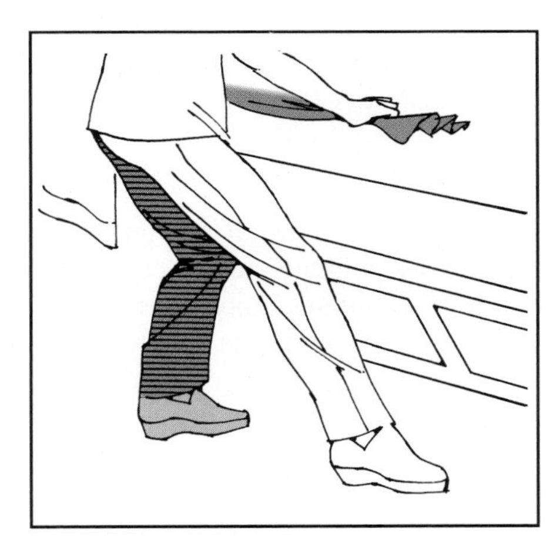

RATIONALE. Broad stance increases base of support. Flexion allows smooth weight shift, with force exerted by arms and legs, not back.

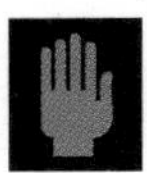

If patient is very heavy, two nurses on both sides of the bed may be needed to prevent injury to nurses and patient.

Continued

ACTION 7. Ask patient to raise head and exhale during the move.

RATIONALE. Reduces weight and friction, thus conserving energy. Exhaling prevents Valsalva maneuver, which, if used, can stress the heart.

ACTION 8. Contract your pelvic muscles. On signal, shift your weight to your forward leg. Keeping your back and arms straight, move the patient toward head of bed. Repeat, if necessary.

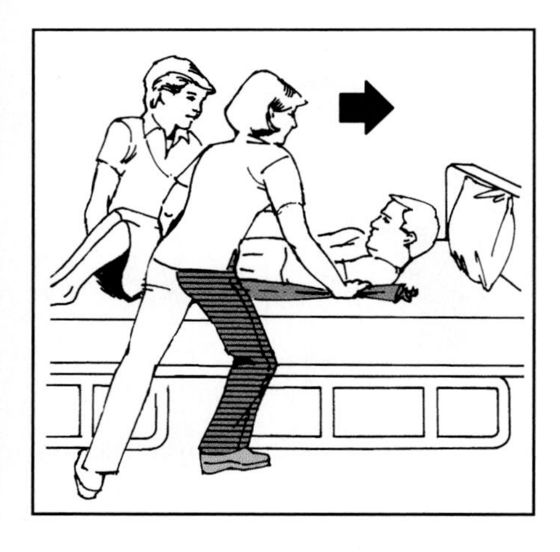

RATIONALE. Shifting weight provides additional force of your body weight, decreasing work of muscles.

ACTION 9. Replace pillows and other positioning aids to maintain correct alignment. Raise siderails.

METHOD B—Sitting Method, Two Nurses

ACTION 1. Discuss the procedure, as in previous technique. Raise the bed to nurses' midthigh level, lock wheels of bed. Be sure IV or drainage tubing is positioned to prevent tension or tangling.

ACTION 2. Face head of bed. Place one knee (shaded) on the bed next to patient's hip. Your weight should be on this knee. Place your other foot on the floor, slightly forward of knee.

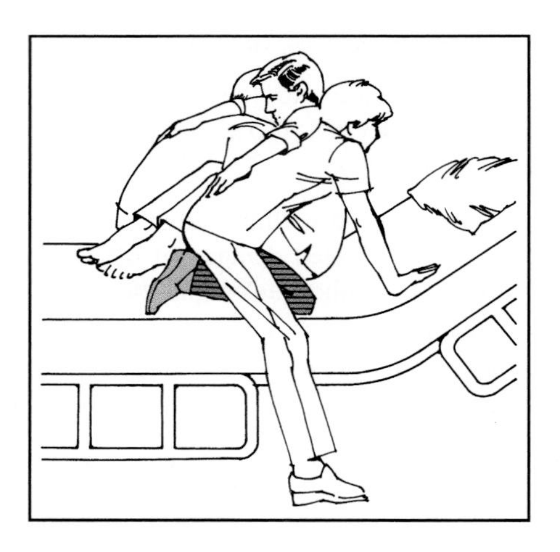

RATIONALE. Prepares for weight shift to assist patient's movement, uses large muscles of the extremities.

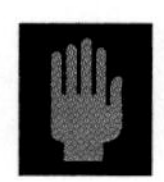

If linen is dry, placement of nurses' knees on the bed poses no greater risk for transfer of microorganisms than any other contact with dry bed linens. If linen is wet, it should be changed before moving patient up in bed.

ACTION 3. Place your should under patient's axilla. Patient places arms on nurses' backs. While maintaining slight tension in shoulder joint, slide your near hand under the patient's thigh in a medial-to-lateral direction.

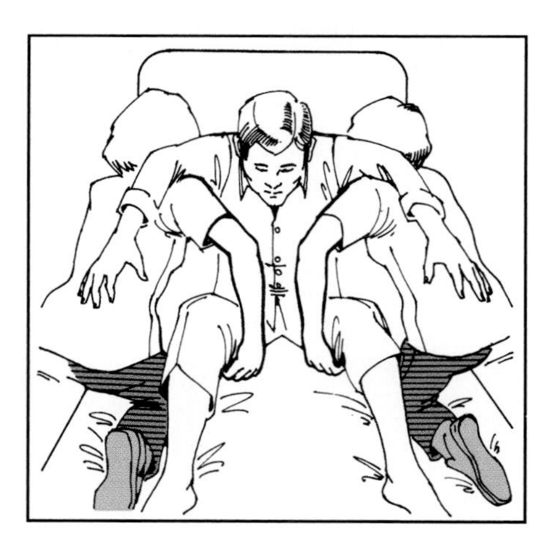

RATIONALE. Patient's weight is supported by the muscle of the nurses' arms and legs; protects weaker back muscles.

Procedure 33–8. (continued)

ACTION 4. Place your other hand about 18 inches forward of your knee, with elbow extended. (See illustration for Action 2.)

RATIONALE. The forward arm acts as a lever with the hand as fulcrum, as the nurses shift their weight to move patient.

ACTION 5. Contract your pelvic muscles. Rock forward on signal, stepping toward head of bed and partially extending knee on bed. Repeat as necessary.

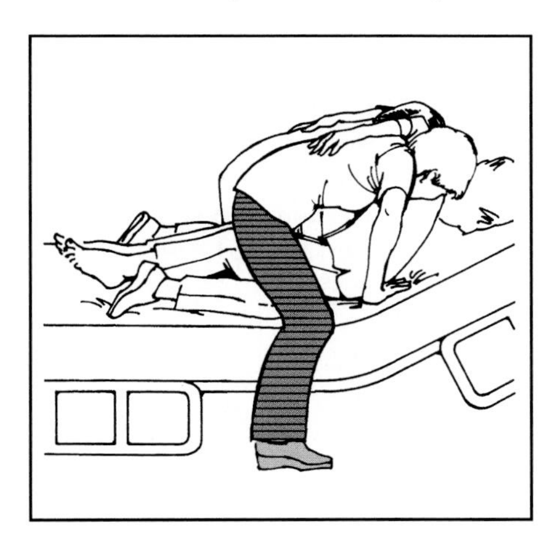

RATIONALE. Protects nurses' joints, adds the force of your body weight to move the patient.

ACTION 6. Replace pillows and other positioning aids to maintain correct alignment. Raise siderails.

Recording:

It is not necessary to record having moved a patient up in bed; however, it is helpful to indicate the most effective method for assisting a given patient on the Kardex, patient care plan, or turning schedule.

HOME HEALTH ADAPTATION: Flex knees more to avoid back strain with low stationary beds. Two people may not be available to move the patient up in bed. If patient is capable of assisting, request him or her to bend one or both knees and place feet flat on the bed. Move the bed away from the wall and position yourself at the head of the bed. At a predetermined signal, instruct the patient to raise buttocks and push with feet. Grasp the patient under the arms, keeping your knees flexed and back straight, step backward, and pull the patient toward you until the desired position is achieved. A trapeze facilitates patients' helping themselves and also provides exercise for the upper extremities. If a patient is unable to provide assistance, use the bottom sheet as a pull-sheet. Loosen the sheet and position yourself at the head of the bed. Grasp the top of the sheet and, with your knees bent and back straight, step backward and pull the sheet and patient toward you. Make the bed with most of the bottom sheet at the foot of the bed so that as the patient slides down you can pull him or her up with the sheet. The bed may need to be remade after positioning.

PROCEDURE 33–9. MOVING A PATIENT TOWARD ONE SIDE OF THE BED

PURPOSE: To prepare to (1) reposition a supine patient in a lateral or prone position, (2) assist a patient to sit at the edge of the bed ("dangle"), or (3) make an occupied bed.

EQUIPMENT: *Method A:* Drawsheet. *Method B:* None.

METHOD A—Pull-sheet Method, Two to Four Nurses

ACTION 1. Discuss the procedure with patient, including nurse's actions, behavior desired of the patient, and signals used to synchronize efforts, if any.

RATIONALE. Patient will be more willing and able to participate if the reasons and anticipated benefits of the activity are clear. Clarifying signals enhances cooperation.

ACTION 2. Raise bed to midthigh level, lower siderails, lock wheels of bed.

RATIONALE. Maintains patient safety, allows nurses to use major muscles of extremities and avoid back strain. If wheels are not locked, bed rather than patient will move.

ACTION 3. Lower head of bed, remove pillows used for positioning. Head pillow can be left in place.

RATIONALE. Patient's weight is more evenly distributed when bed is flat. Pillows would block patient's movement.

ACTION 4. Provide privacy. Fanfold covers to foot of bed. Arrange hospital gown to cover patient as much as possible. Arrange IV or drainage tubing so it will not be pulled or entangled as patient is moved.

RATIONALE. Privacy shows respect for patient's modesty. Moving tubing and covers keeps them from interfering with smooth movement. Tension on tubing could cause pain and/or disruption of IV or drainage system.

ACTION 5. Ask patient to fold arms across the chest.

RATIONALE. Prevents injury to arms during move.

ACTION 6. Fold drawsheet in half, place under patient's body from shoulders to midthigh.

RATIONALE. Sheet will support bulk of the patient's weight for moving and positioning, reducing friction and so reducing energy expenditure.

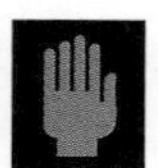

For patients who require frequent assistance with moving and positioning, including a drawsheet in foundation linen when making the bed will save time and energy.

ACTION 7. Roll sheet so edges are close to patient's body and grasp firmly next to patient's shoulders and hips.

RATIONALE. Maximizes control during movement, improves leverage.

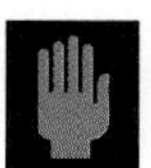

Nurse on side to which patient is being moved can grasp corner of pillowcase with drawsheet, so pillow moves with patient, supporting the head. Two nurses on each side of the bed may be necessary if patient is heavy.

ACTION 8. Nurse on side of bed to which patient is being moved (nurse 1) assumes a broad stance (feet shoulder width apart) with forward foot next to the bed, back foot about 2 feet from the bed. Knees should be slightly flexed with weight on leg (shaded) nearest the bed.

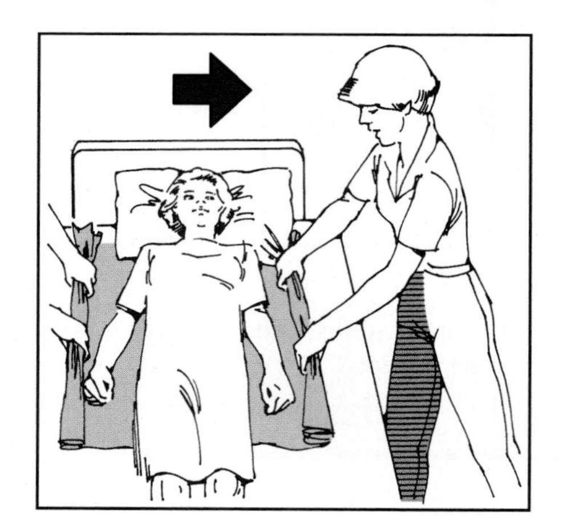

ACTION 9. Nurse on opposite side (nurse 2) places one knee on bed, keeping other foot on the floor for stability. If patient is large, third nurse may be needed to support patient's feet and lower legs.

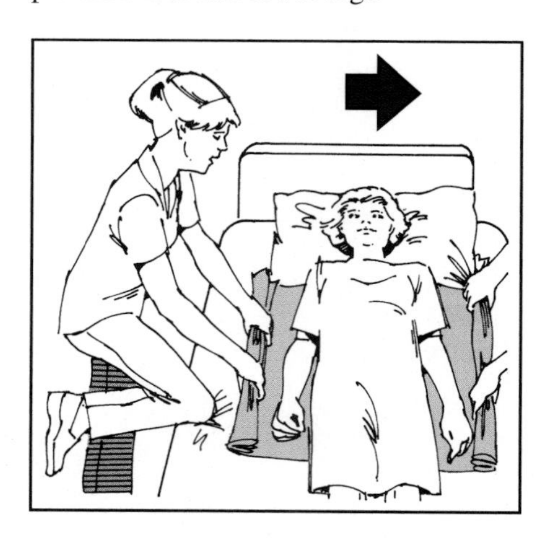

Procedure 33–9. (continued)

RATIONALE. Keeps patient's weight close to nurse's center of gravity during move, reducing potential for back injury to nurse.

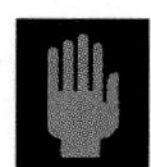

Nurse's knee on bed does not promote transfer of microorganisms if linen is dry.

ACTION 10. Nurses contract their pelvic muscles and, on signal, nurse 1 shifts weight to back foot while pulling on drawsheet. At the same time, nurse 2 pulls upward on drawsheet while shifting weight forward onto knee on the bed. If a third nurse is assisting, he or she should stand next to nurse 1 and support patient's legs, assume same stance as nurse 1, and shift weight at same time.

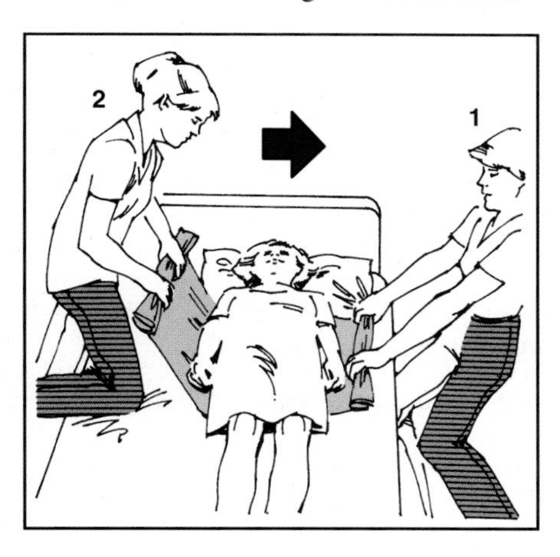

RATIONALE. Simultaneous weight shifts accomplish smooth movement with least expenditure of nurses' energy. Slight lifting by nurse 2 causes minimal strain as he or she is above patient. The lifting reduces friction during move.

ACTION 11. Repeat as necessary until patient is at desired location.

RATIONALE. Several short moves expend less energy than one long move.

ACTION 12. Proceed with bedmaking or positioning patient.

RATIONALE. Promotes patient's safety and privacy.

ACTION 13. Replace covers, raise siderails, return bed to low position.

METHOD B—Alternative Method, One or Two Nurses

ONE NURSE:

ACTION 1. Begin by discussing procedure and preparing patient as in Method A, Actions 1 to 5. Bed should be at waist level.

RATIONALE. This height maximizes effectiveness of using nurse's body as counterweight.

ACTION 2. To move the patient's upper body: Slide one of your arms under patient's shoulders, supporting the head with your flexed elbow, your other arm under patient's upper back just below the scapulae.

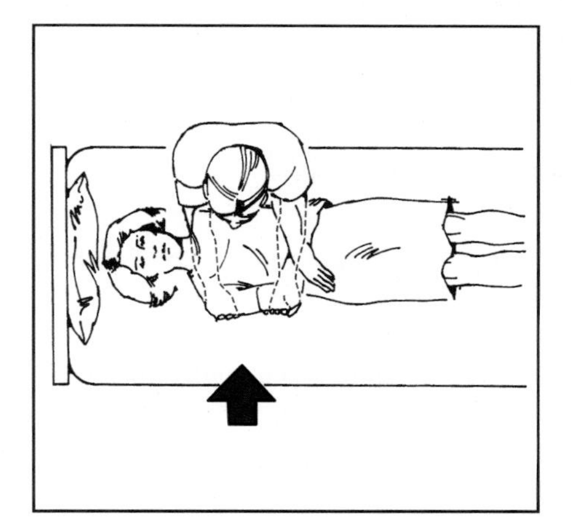

RATIONALE. Provides safe support for upper segment of patient's body.

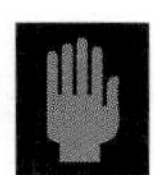

Patients who are able should raise the head during move, which decreases nurse's energy expenditure and provides patient with small amount of active exercise.

Continued

ACTION 3. Assume a broad stance (feet a should width apart) with one foot next to the bed and the other about 2 feet from the bed. Knees should be slightly flexed with weight on leg nearest bed (shaded).

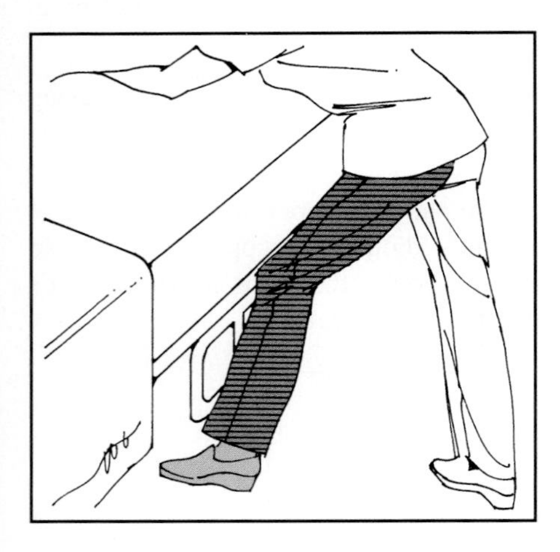

RATIONALE. This stance provides a stable base of support during shifting of nurse's weight to move patient.

ACTION 4. Contract your abdominal and gluteal muscles.

RATIONALE. Provides pelvic joint stability, reducing potential for injury to the nurse.

ACTION 5. Shift your weight away from the bed, pulling patient's head and shoulders, as weight is shifted.

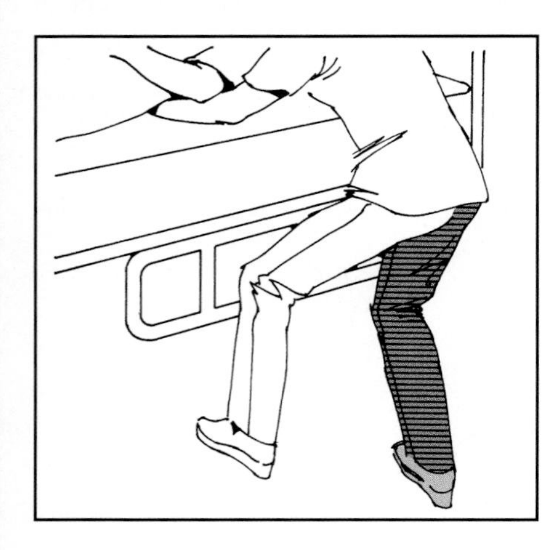

RATIONALE. Shifting your weight provides additional force of your body weight, decreasing work of muscles.

ACTION 6. Slide one of your arms under patient's back at the waist, the other just below buttocks at the level of the greater trochanter.

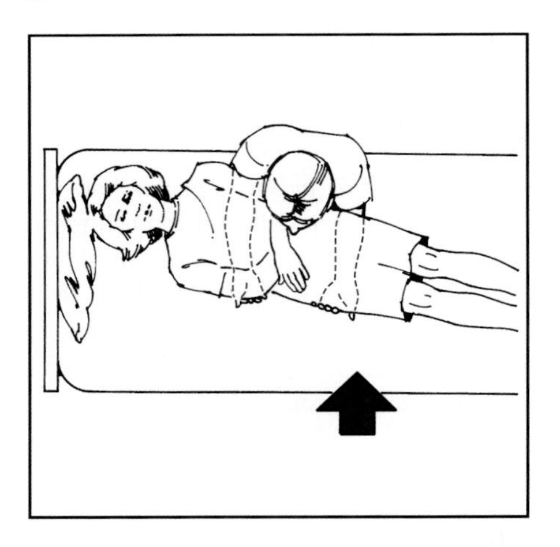

RATIONALE. Nurse's arms are close together to provide support for heaviest part of the patient's body.

ACTION 7. Move patient's trunk by shifting your weight as described in the preceding Actions 3 to 5.

ACTION 8. Slide one of your arms under patient's thighs, the other under the calves.

RATIONALE. Supports legs without stressing knee joint.

ACTION 9. Move patient's legs by shifting your weight as described in the preceding Actions 3 to 5.

ACTION 10. See Actions 11 to 13, Method A.

TWO NURSES:

ACTION 1. Begin by discussing procedure and preparing patient and bed as described in Method A, Actions 1 to 5.

ACTION 2. Nurses stand on same side of bed. Nurse nearest head of bed places arms under patient's shoulders and back as described in Action 2 above. Second nurse positions arms under patient's waist and buttocks as described in Action 6 above.

Procedure 33–9. (continued)

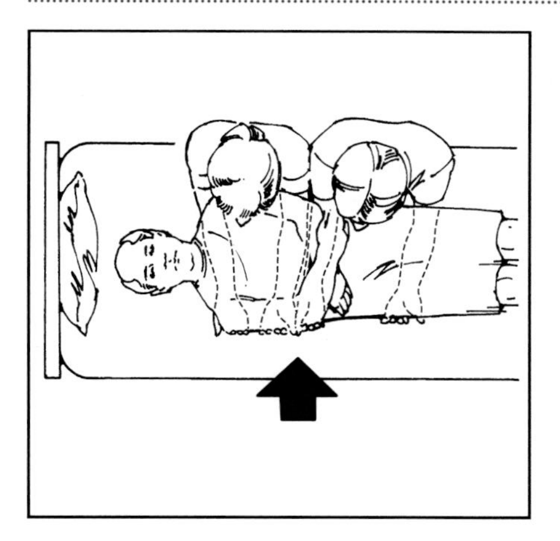

RATIONALE. Provides simultaneous support for areas of patient's body in which weight is concentrated.

ACTION 3. Both nurses shift their weight as in Actions 3 to 5 above to move patient.

ACTION 4. Complete procedure as in Actions 11 to 13, Method A.

Recording:

No recording is necessary. Position changes should be documented on flowsheet or narrative notes.

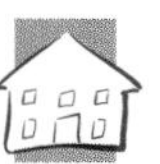

HOME HEALTH ADAPTATION: Teach the family members how to move the patient to the side of the bed. Flex knees more to avoid back strain with low stationary beds.

positioned incorrectly in side-lying position (Fig. 33–20), the medial condyles (knee) and medial malleoli (ankle) of both tibias are pressure points. Experts also recommend avoiding direct positioning on the trochanter when patients vulnerable to pressure injury are sidelying.[23] The variation, sometimes called lateral oblique, involves leaning patients forward or backward, supported on pillows.

- *Schedule frequent position changes.* Frequent position changes, individualized to a patient's tolerance, also prevent pressure ulcers. A schedule is useful to alert both patient and nurses of the timing of position changes. When devising a schedule, consider a patient's daily activities and special needs. For example, mealtime or visiting hours are not ideal times to schedule "proning." If a patient is unable to remain comfortable in a given position for 2 hours, reduce the amount of time for that position rather than eliminating it from the schedule.
- *Assess skin with every position change.* Meticulous assessment (see Chap. 27) of all vulnerable pressure points whenever a patient's position is changed is critical to early detection and treatment of pressure ulcers.[22] Massaging reddened areas over bony prominences is no longer recommended. Blood vessels surrounding the ischemic area are already dilated, so massage offers no therapeutic effect. In fact, massage may force exudate from damaged tissue into adjacent healthy tissue. The best treatment is to avoid positions creating pressure over the affected area until it resolves. Special beds, discussed later, are also effective.
- *Use prone and semiprone positions.* Prone position is useful because it creates fewer pressure points and it counteracts flexion contractures of the lower extremities discussed earlier. These major benefits outweigh the disadvantages some patients identify including limited field of vision, difficulty interacting with others, feeling vulnerable, and difficulty breathing. An explanation of the benefits and patient involvement in scheduling facilitates patient acceptance. The extra effort required for chest expansion in prone position can be minimized by using rolled towels under the shoulders. Semiprone (Sims') position, alternating right and left sides, can be substituted for

(continued on page 1255)

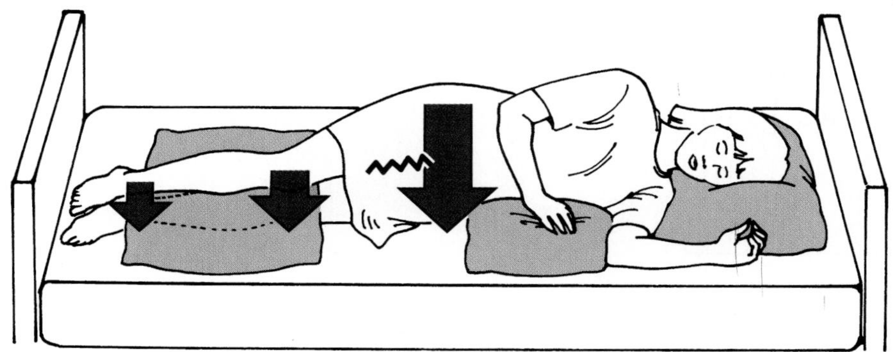

Figure 33–20. Incorrect lateral position. Indicates areas of additional pressure and of contact between skin surface when the dependent leg supports the other leg.

PROCEDURE 33–10. TURNING A PATIENT FROM SUPINE TO PRONE OR LATERAL POSITION

PURPOSE: To facilitate repositioning of a patient in correct alignment.
EQUIPMENT: None. Pull sheet optional.

ACTION 1. Discuss the procedure and its purpose with the patient, including nurse's actions, desired patient behavior, and anticipated benefits.

RATIONALE. Patient participation is more likely if expected behaviors and anticipated benefits are clear.

ACTION 2. Move patient near the edge of the bed (see Procedure 33–9).

RATIONALE. Patient will be too close to the edge of the bed when the turn is completed if turned when in the center of the bed.

ACTION 3. Standing at the side of the bed toward which the patient is to be turned, place the patient's near arm on the bed, palm up, next to the body (patient will roll over arm). The opposite arm should be placed next to patient's body, with palm facing thigh.

Placing the patient's near arm away from the body is preferred if the patient is to be repositioned on the side. However, this arm position will cause injury to arm if being turned to the prone position.

RATIONALE. Maximizes nurse control of turn. Arm position minimizes torque on arm when patient is turned.

ACTION 4. Cross patient's far leg over near leg or flex far leg at the knee.

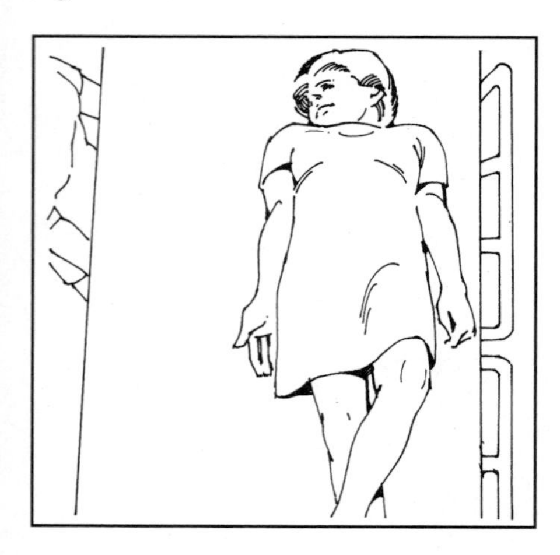

RATIONALE. Facilitates movement of far leg during roll.

ACTION 5. Ask patient to turn head away from you during the turn or position patient's head if patient is unable.

RATIONALE. Prevents patient from rolling onto the face.

ACTION 6. Place your hands on the patient's far shoulder and hip, holding patient's far arm next to the body with your wrist. If pullsheet is in place, grasp it near patient's shoulder and hip instead.

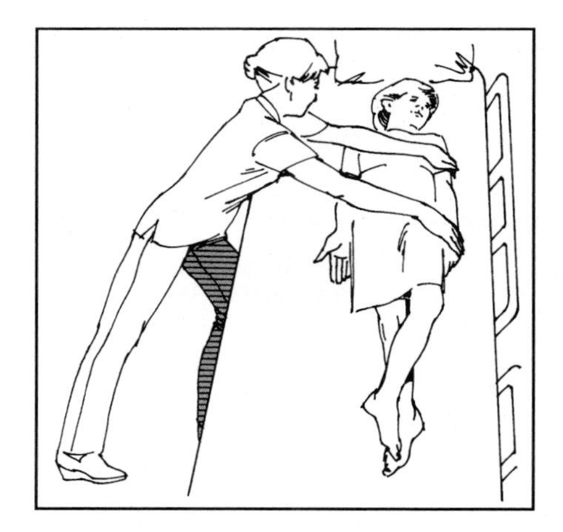

RATIONALE. Provides turning force at area of greatest weight. Avoids torque on patient's joints. Grasping arm or knee to turn patient could cause injury to patient's joints. Pull sheet provides continuous support for patient's back, so should be used when available.

ACTION 7. Assume a broad stance (feet shoulder width apart) with one foot next to the bed, the other foot about 2 feet from the bed. Knees should be slightly flexed with weight on leg (shaded) nearest the bed.

RATIONALE. This stance provides a stable base of support during shifting of nurse's weight to move patient.

Procedure 33–10. (continued)

ACTION 8. Contract your pelvic muscles. Shift your weight to your other leg, turning patient toward you as you move.

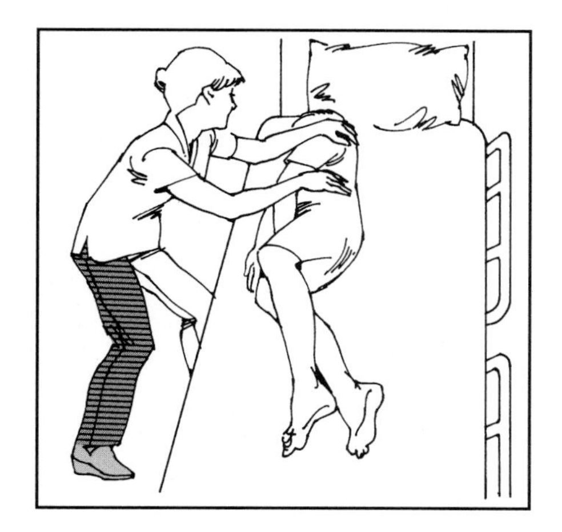

RATIONALE. Shifting your weight provides additional force of your body weight, decreasing work of muscles.

ACTION 9. When patient is lying on side, support extremities in proper alignment (see Fig. 33–16).

OR

If patient is to be placed in prone position, shift your hand position to the front of the shoulders and hips. Continue turning until patient is prone.

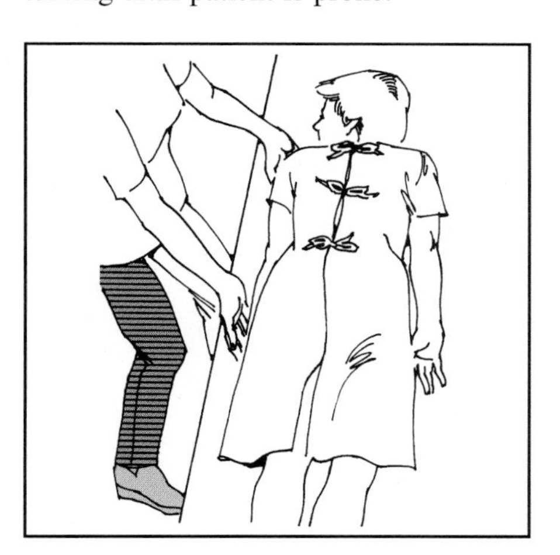

RATIONALE. Prevents joint deformity.

This hand position controls speed and force of roll to abdomen.

ACTION 10. Move patient's arm and head so patient is comfortable.

RATIONALE. Weak or paralyzed patients cannot adjust their position independently, nor maintain optimal positioning while being turned.

ACTION 11. Move patient to center of bed using techniques described in Procedure 33–9. Support in proper alignment (see Fig. 33–17).

RATIONALE. Turning a patient 180 degrees results in the patient being near the edge of the bed. Correct positioning of extremities is difficult if a patient is too near one side of the bed.

ACTION 12. Replace covers, raise siderails, return bed to low position.

RATIONALE. Promotes patient's safety and privacy.

Recording:

Note frequency of position changes; presence of reddened, macerated, or broken skin, including location, size, and description of lesion; and action taken if lesion noted.

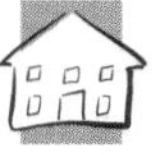

HOME HEALTH ADAPTATION: Teach the family members how to move the patient to the side of the bed. Flex knees more to avoid back strain with low stationary beds.

PROCEDURE 33–11. LOG-ROLLING, SUPINE TO LATERAL POSITION, TWO OR THREE NURSES

PURPOSE: To facilitate repositioning of a patient who cannot tolerate torsion of the spine (eg, patients having had spinal injury or surgery).

EQUIPMENT: Pillow(s). Pull sheet optional.

ACTION 1. Discuss the procedure and its purpose with the patient, including the nurse's actions, desired patient behavior, and anticipated benefits.

RATIONALE. Patient participation is more likely if reasons and benefits of procedure are clear.

ACTION 2. Move patient near the edge of the bed. At least two nurses are needed. See Procedure 33–9.

RATIONALE. One nurse cannot safely move a patient whose spine must remain straight.

Assistance of third person is needed for large patients.

ACTION 3. Ask patient to fold arms on chest.

RATIONALE. Prevents lying on arm at completion of roll to side.

ACTION 4. Place pillow(s) between patient's legs to support the far leg during roll.

RATIONALE. Prevents torsion on spine caused by unsupported weight of leg.

ACTION 5. Position a pillow under the patient's head so head will be supported throughout roll.

RATIONALE. See Action 4, above.

ACTION 6. Standing on side of bed toward which patient is to be rolled, first nurse places hands on patient's far shoulder and waist; second nurse places hands on far hip and lower leg. If three nurses assist, second nurse places hands above and below hip, third nurse on thigh and calf.

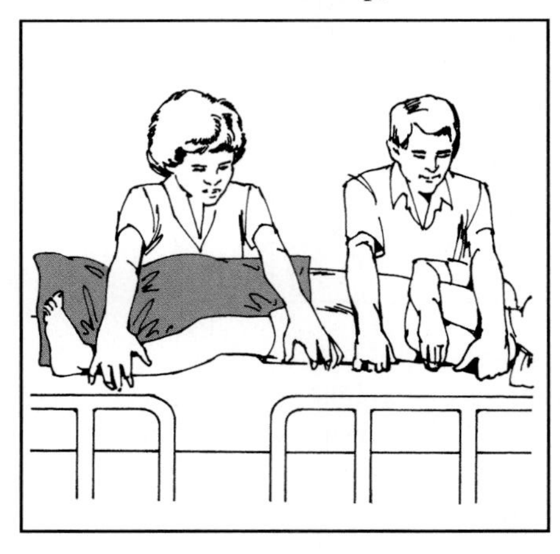

OR

Turning sheet (drawsheet) can be used: Nurses reach over patient, one grasping sheet at shoulder and waist, the other at hip and knee.

RATIONALE. Will provide support for smooth turning without twisting spine.

ACTION 7. Both nurses assume broad stance with knees flexed as described in Action 7 of Procedure 33–10.

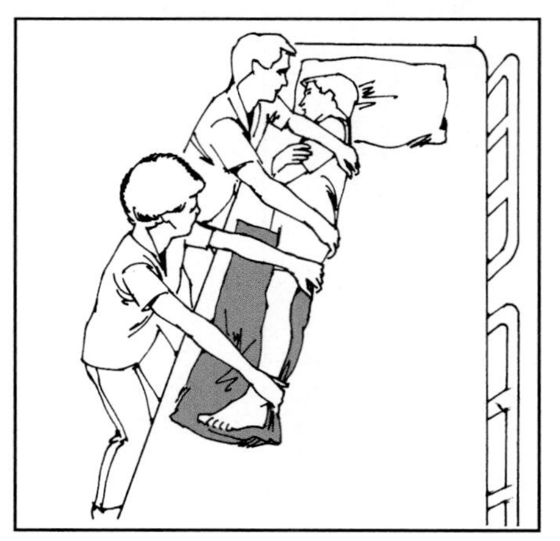

RATIONALE. Provides a stable base of support.

Procedure 33–11. (continued)

ACTION 8. On signal, both nurses shift weight to back foot while rolling patient toward them.

RATIONALE. Weight shift provides force to move patient, preventing nurse's muscle strain.

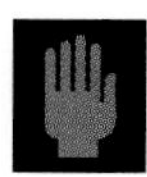

Nurses must move at the same time to prevent strain on patient's spine.

ACTION 9. Position and support extremities in side-lying position (see Fig. 33–16).

ACTION 10. Replace covers, raise siderails, return bed to low position.

Recording:
Note method of turning, reason log-rolling is being used, patient's responses, problems (if any), and corresponding action taken.

prone position or added to the positioning schedule to extend the time period extremities are in extension.

- *Minimize the amount of time spent in Fowler's position.* Many patients prefer Fowler's position. Sitting up allows greater visualization of one's surroundings and facilitates interaction with others. It also may diminish the association with illness created by being "flat on one's back in bed." Despite these advantages, there are several hazards. The first is pressure on the ischial tuberosities, as noted. The second is shearing. **Shearing** refers to stress created when two objects slide against one another. Patients in bed with the head of the bed at an angle greater than 30 degrees tend to slide toward the foot of the bed. Because of friction, the skin surface in contact with the sheets moves less than deeper tissue layers attached to the skeleton. The outcome is damage to capillaries and subcutaneous tissue under sacrum, scapulae, and in the heels. Low Fowler's position (20 to 30 degrees) reduces pressure and shearing. Placing a footboard where the patient can push against it further counteracts shearing. A third problem associated with Fowler's position is caused by adjusting the bed to bend at the knee. The resulting pressure on the popliteal space interferes with circulation to the lower leg and may damage the intima of the vessels. This increases the risk of thrombus formation. Inform patients of this hazard, so that they refrain from adjusting the bed in this way. Clinical Guideline 33–11 summarizes important points for safe patient positioning.

Using Protective Devices

Special aids for maintaining correct alignment or reducing the pressure of the mattress on bony prominences are prudent whenever bedrest is prolonged. In most facilities, nurses are expected to obtain protective devices whenever a patient's condition warrants, but a physician's order may be necessary in some places.

- *Footboards.* **Footboards** prevent heel cord contractures (plantar flexion, footdrop), and counteract shearing. Some rehabilitation specialists suggest that to prevent pressure ulcers on the heels and facilitate prone positioning without promoting knee or plantar flexion, a footboard should be installed with a 4-inch space between it and the end of the mattress. This footboard location allows space for the feet between the mattress and the footboard in prone position and for the heels to extend past the end of the mattress in supine position. This maintains the feet in correct anatomic position in both cases. However, this footboard placement cannot prevent shearing in Fowler's position, because

CLINICAL GUIDELINE 33–11

POSITIONING PATIENTS IN BED

- Plan to reposition patients at least every 2 hours. Individualize according to patient tolerance.
- Discuss the planned position change with the patient. Assure understanding of your actions and desired patient participation. Draw bedside curtains for privacy before beginning.
- Use protective body mechanics: adjust bed height to facilitate use of large muscles (arms and legs) instead of the back, and lower the head of the bed during repositioning to avoid working against gravity.
- Fanfold bed covers and remove pillows used for support to prevent interference during repositioning. Replace bed linens or gown, if damp.
- Arrange IV and drainage tubing prior to repositioning to prevent pulling or entanglement.
- Maintain all joints in anatomic position. Provide support above and below joints to prevent strain and contractures.
- Position so patient's weight is distributed over as wide an area as possible and so extremities do not rest on one another to minimize ischemia related to pressure on bony prominences.
- Position extremities to avoid skin-to-skin contact to reduce skin damage related to increased perspiration.
- Inspect skin over all weight-bearing bony prominences for signs of ischemia with each position change.
- If reddened or broken skin is noted, avoid positions that create pressure on that area until skin returns to normal. Do not massage reddened areas.
- When changing positions, do extension (stretching) exercises of all joints that were flexed in the prior position.

PROCEDURE 33–12. TURNING A PATIENT FROM PRONE TO SUPINE OR LATERAL POSITION

PURPOSE: To facilitate positioning in correct alignment.
EQUIPMENT: None. Pull sheet optional.

ACTION 1. Discuss the procedure and its purpose with the patient, including nurse's actions, desired patient behavior, and anticipated benefits.

RATIONALE. Patient participation is more likely if response and expected benefits of the procedure are clear.

ACTION 2. Move patient near the edge of the bed (see Procedure 33–9). Standing at the other side of the bed, to which the patient is to be turned, place patient's near arm over the head if ROM in shoulder is sufficient. If not, place near arm, palm up, next to the body. The other arm is placed next to the body with palm facing thigh. Cross far leg over the near leg.

RATIONALE. Turning is easier with arm above the head but this placement of the arm during and after the turn requires full ROM of shoulder and may be difficult or painful for some patients. Leg position facilitates moving leg.

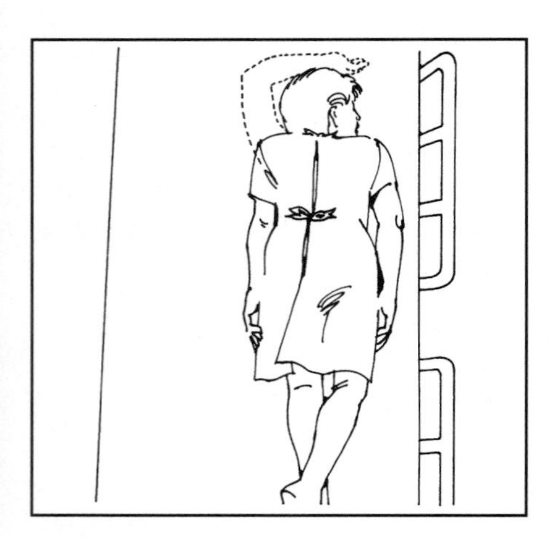

ACTION 3. Placing hands or grasping pull sheet as for turning from supine to prone and assuming same stance, turn patient toward you. Patient's back will be toward you when patient is in lateral position.

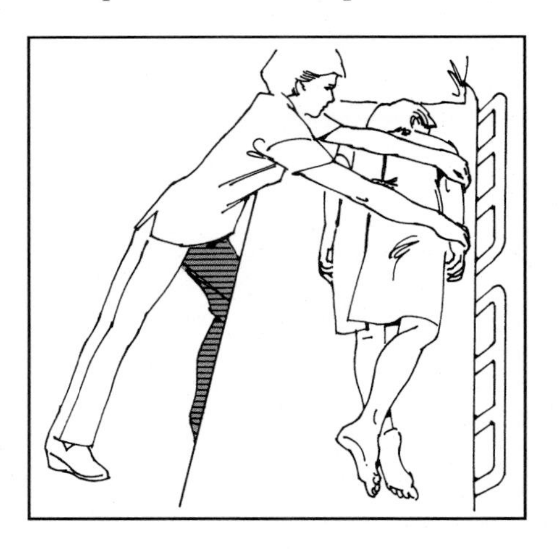

RATIONALE. See Procedure 33–10, Actions 6 and 7.

ACTION 4. If moving patient to supine position, shift your hands to the back of the shoulders and hips. Continue to turn until patient is supine.

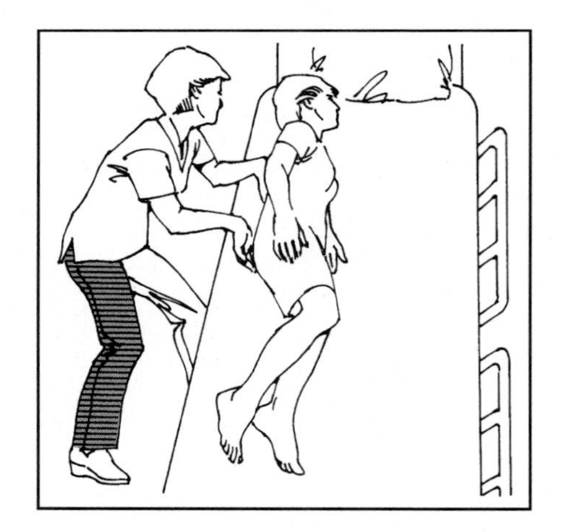

RATIONALE. Allows use of nurse's strength to control speed of patient's turn.

Procedure 33–12. (continued)

ACTION 5. At completion of the turn, move patient to center of bed and position in correct alignment.

ACTION 6. Replace covers, raise siderails, return bed to low position.

RATIONALE. Promotes patient's safety and privacy.

Recording:

Note frequency of position changes; presence of reddened, macerated, or broken skin, including location, size, and description of lesion; and action taken if lesion noted.

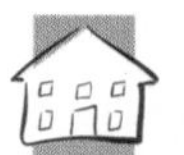

HOME HEALTH ADAPTATIONS: Teach the family members how to move the patient to the side of the bed. Flex knees more to avoid back strain with low stationary beds.

when a patient's back is correctly supported, his or her feet cannot reach the footboard. Some footboard designs allow easy placement in various positions, either resting on the mattress for Fowler's position or secured as described above for other positions.

- *Individual foot supports.* Rigid plastic supports that strap onto each foot are another alternative for preventing heel cord contractures. They conform to the shape of the foot and are padded to prevent pressure points. Because they are not attached to a fixed position on the bed, they do not protect against shearing at the sacrum and scapulae. They must be removed several times a day for skin inspection and care. Although most are designed with ventilation ports, they tend to increase perspiration.
- *Trochanter Rolls.* Passive external rotation of the hip is common in patients with paralysis or extremely poor muscle tone. **Trochanter rolls** maintain correct hip alignment when positioning these patients in Fowler's or supine positions. They are placed to extend from just above the iliac crest to midthigh. They can be easily made by folding and rolling a bath blanket, as shown in Clinical Guideline 33–12.
- *Heel and elbow protectors.* During bedrest, the calcaneous (heel), malleoli (ankles), and olecranon (elbow) are vulnerable to injury from friction, pressure, and shearing. Heel and elbow protectors are commercially manufactured to conform to the structure of the heel and elbow joints. They are padded with foam or lined with synthetic sheepskin similar to the pads discussed next. They provide cushioning to the bones and protect the skin (Fig. 33–21). The protectors should be removed several times a day to inspect and care for the skin. They can be laundered if they become soiled or wet.
- *Sheepskin.* A sheepskin is a synthetic pad with a thick nap, used to cushion and reduce pressure on bony prominences. It should be placed directly under the patient over foundation bed linen. Placing incontinent pads over the sheepskin reduces the cushioning effect, but does minimize skin damage from moisture due to incontinence.[23] Sheepskin pads can be laundered if they become soiled.
- *Hand rolls.* The use of a hand roll, made by folding, rolling, and taping one or more washcloths, will prevent contractures and spasticity of the fingers and thumb in paralyzed patients. The roll should be placed in the palm with fingers curved around the roll and the index finger opposite the thumb.

Special Beds and Mattresses

Special beds, mattresses, and mattress overlays, often called *dynamic support surfaces,* are designed to prevent pressure injuries in bedridden patients.

Pressure relief beds maintain interface pressure (the pressure between the bed surface and the client) below capillary closing pressure. These specialty beds use an air-fluidized system (technology that suspends microparticles in moving air to simulate fluid support) or are air-filled with sophisticated pressure sensors and controls (Fig. 33–22A). Pressure reduction devices maintain interface pressures that are lower than standard mattresses, but not necessarily below capillary closing pressure. These are primarily mattress overlays or pads that redistribute pressure over a large surface area. They use dense convoluted foam, gel, air, water, or combinations of these (Fig. 33–22B and C). Still another category of beds, the kinetic bed, combines pressure relief with constant slow turning eliminating virtually all of the physiological complications of bed rest.

Many of these beds are very expensive and therefore are used only for very-high-risk patients, such as those with several serious

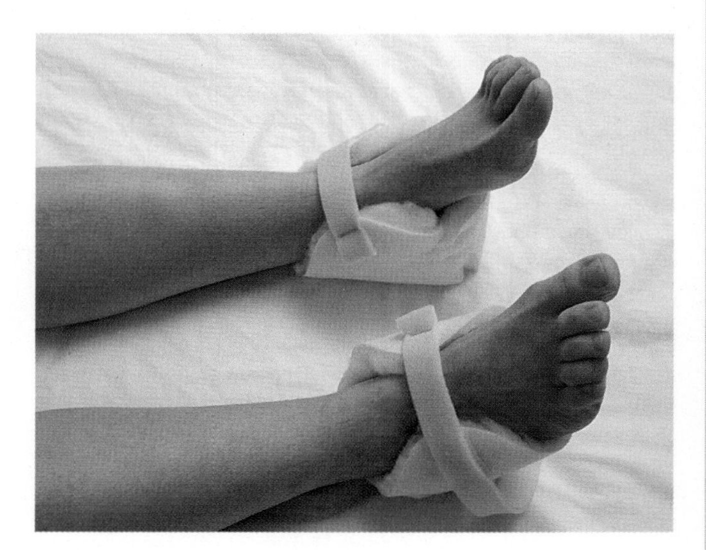

Figure 33–21. Heel protectors.

CLINICAL GUIDELINE 33–12

PLACEMENT OF TROCHANTER ROLLS

1. Fold bath blanket(s) in thirds or fourths lengthwise so that the roll will be of adequate length and diameter to fit patient. The roll should extend from the iliac crest to midthigh and be about one-third the diameter of the thigh. One blanket is needed for each side, unless the patient is very small.
2. Roll the patient to one side (see Procedure 33–10) and place the folded blanket so it extends from the small of the back to midthigh and well under the patient so the patient will not rest on the far edge when returned to supine position. Repeat for the opposite side if needed.

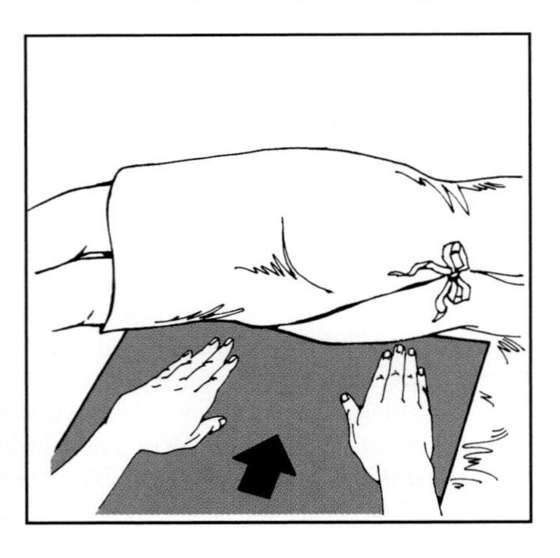

3. When the patient is supine, roll the end of the blanket downward in a tight roll until the roll fits snugly against the patient's hip. You will see the hip and leg return to correct anatomic position if the roll is properly placed. The roll needs no anchoring, as friction between the roll and the bed holds it in place. Repeat for opposite side if necessary.

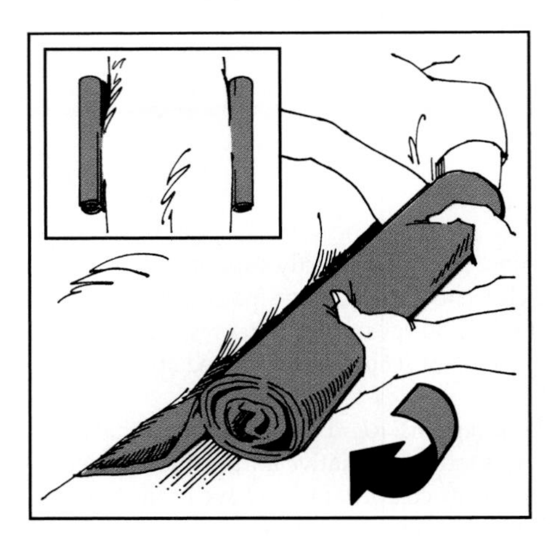

4. Document the use of uni- or bilateral trochanter rolls whenever a notation verifying a position change to supine or Fowler's position is made on flowsheet or narrative notes. Indicating a need for trochanter rolls on the patient care plan and turning schedule is helpful.

pressure ulcers, multiple orthopedic injuries, or severe burns; however, pressure reduction devices made of high-density convoluted foam and the **eggcrate mattress overlay** (named for its appearance), are relatively inexpensive and are used routinely in acute care facilities. These mattress overlays do not replace consistent turning and positioning, but do provide protection from pressure sores. One drawback to the popular eggcrate mattress is that its effectiveness is significantly reduced when multiple layers of linen or incontinent pads are placed over it, because these tend to fill the cavities in the foam that disperse the pressure.

Restraints

Restraints are devices used to decrease patient mobility. There are many kinds of restraints available. The types most commonly used are vests, belts, and limb restraints. Procedure 33–13 illustrates these restraints and details their correct application. Mitten restraints are also presented there.

Restraints were originally used to control the behavior of mentally ill patients who were considered a danger to themselves or others. They are frequently used on elderly patients at risk for falling or

INSIGHTS FROM NURSING LITERATURE

NURSES ATTITUDES ABOUT THE USE OF RESTRAINTS

Schott-Baer D, Lusis S, Beauregard K. Use of restraints: changes in nurses' attitudes. J Gerontol Nurs. *February 1995;21:39–44.*

Citing literature indicating that physical restraints have negative consequences for patient health, researchers Schott-Baer and colleagues studied nurses' attitudes toward the use of restraints as a function of hospital policies promoting a restraint-free environment. One hundred forty-four nurses working in a midwestern hospital participated. The findings showed subjects believed the use of patient restraints could not be justified on the basis of hospital short-staffing, but were unclear about nurse and patient rights regarding the application and refusal of restraints.

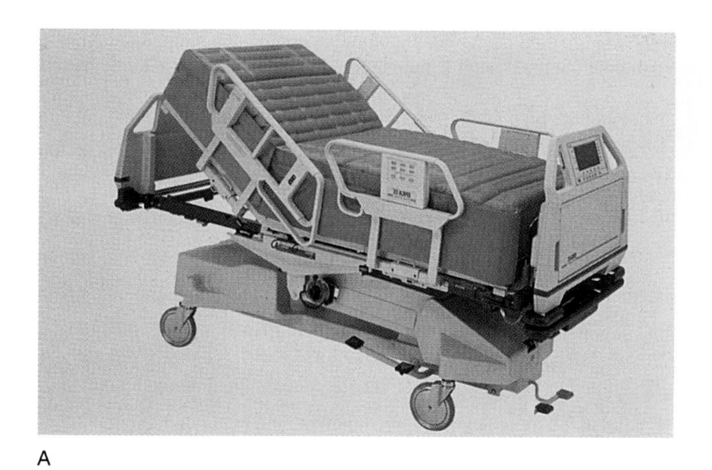

A

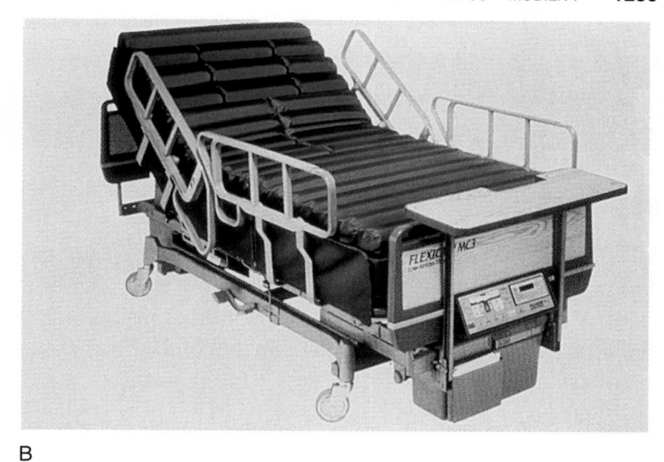

B

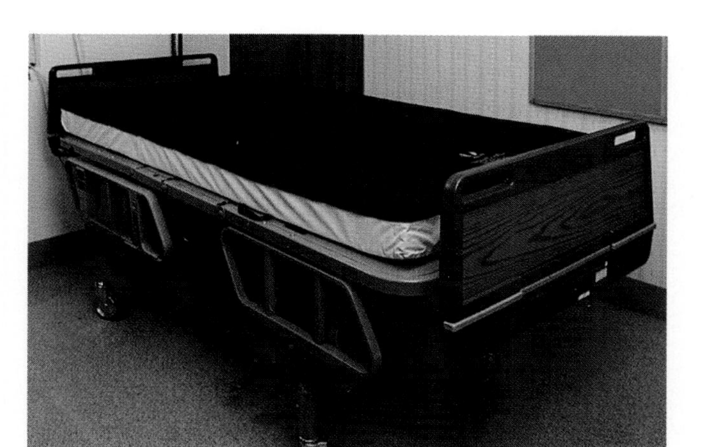

C

Figure 33–22. **A.** Air-fluidized bed. **B.** Low air loss bed. **C.** Gel mattress overlay. *(Courtesy of Hill-Rom.)*

wandering or who attempt to interfere with treatment devices.[54–56] These uses caused caregivers to view restraints as protective devices. However, research indicates that the use of restraints does not reduce falls. In fact, evidence suggests that the risk of injuries actually increases when restraints are applied because restraints tend to increase agitation and combative behavior.[57,58] Serious injuries and death have been attributed to restraints.[58] Restraints increase risk for complications related to immobility, such as pressure ulcers, contractures, and generalized weakness.

Nurse researchers have identified erroneous beliefs that many caregivers hold about restraints. Among the misperceptions are beliefs that failure to restrain certain patients puts individual caregivers and institutions at risk for legal liability; that it doesn't really bother old people to be restrained; that consent is not required from individuals being restrained and their families; that restraints are necessary because of inadequate staffing; and that alternatives to physical restraints are not available.[55,56,59,60] Because of beliefs like these, nurses often applied restraints without considering other alternatives. However, agencies initiating alternatives to restraints found that the new approaches resulted in a decline in the number of falls, injuries, and aggressive or violent behavior. Social interaction, participation in activity, and nutritional intake improved.[55,61,62]

New federal legislation on the use of restraints (OBRA—the Omnibus Budget Reconciliation Act of 1987) became effective in October 1990. Rather than mandate conditions under which restraints must be used, it insures the right of all residents of nursing home facilities to be free from physical or pharmacologic restraints unless they represent a specific treatment for a diagnosed condition. It also guarantees the right to refuse to be restrained. Under this law, nursing homes may be found liable for using restraints for staff convenience or in place of surveillance. Statutes in many states set similar standards for the use of restraints in acute care facilities.

(continued on page 1264)

PROCEDURE 33–13. APPLYING RESTRAINTS

PURPOSE: To restrict mobility of patients as a safety measure or to maintain integrity/placement of treatment modalities.
EQUIPMENT: Restraint appropriate for situation.

BELT-TYPE RESTRAINTS

ACTION 1. Discuss the purpose of restraint with the patient and family: To prevent a weak patient from falling out of a chair. Also prevents an intermittently confused, forgetful, or pediatric patient from attempting to get out of the chair without assistance.

RATIONALE. Cooperation is more likely if patient and family understand the purpose of and expected gains from restraints. Well-meaning family may release restraints if purpose is not clear to them.

ACTION 2. With patient sitting up, apply widest part of belt across patient's thighs. Angle ties downward 45° to the back of the chair. Slip ties through space between seat and backrest, then cross ties below seat and secure to pegs on wheelchair frame using quick-release knot (see Action 6b, Vest Restraint, on next page).

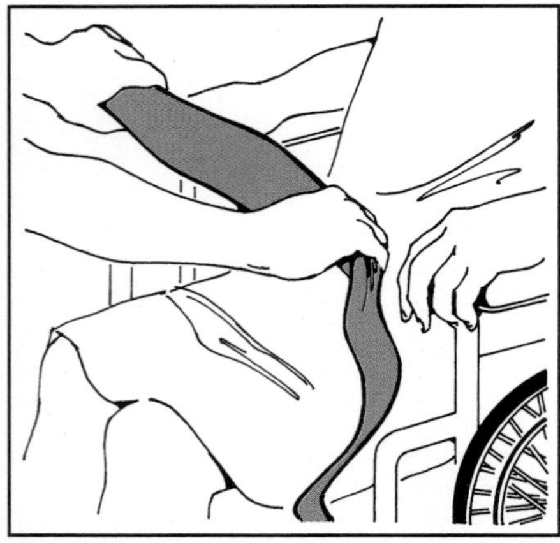

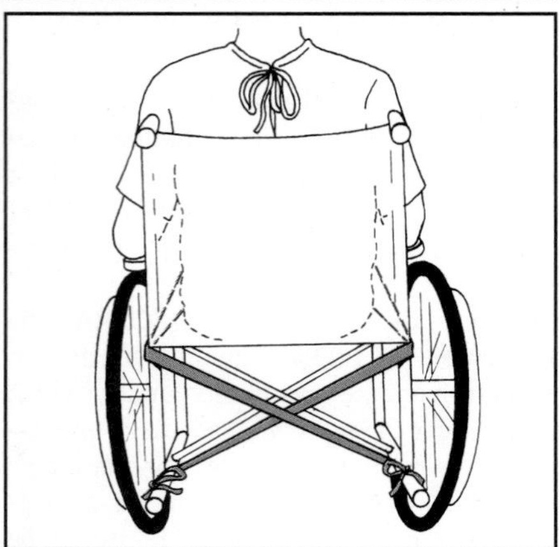

RATIONALE. Secure belt so patient cannot easily slip out without creating pressure or risk of injury to abdomen.

ACTION 3. Release restraint and inspect underlying skin for chafing at least q2h.

RATIONALE. Increased perspiration caused by the restraint and friction from patient movement predisposes patient to skin damage under restraint.

ACTION 4. If skin under restraint is reddened or broken, consult with physician for treatment and alternatives to restraint.

RATIONALE. Continued pressure and friction causes tissue damage.

VEST RESTRAINT

ACTION 1. Discuss purpose of restraint with patient and family: To prevent patient from getting out of bed or chair, yet allow movement of extremities. Controls upper body to a greater degree than belt restraint.

RATIONALE. Cooperation is more likely if patient and family understand the purpose of and expected gains from restraints. Well-meaning family may release restraints if purpose is not clear to them.

ACTION 2. Place the vest over the hospital gown with opening in front.

RATIONALE. Visibility of vest will alert health care personnel to release it prior to repositioning. Attempts to reposition patient without releasing restraints could cause injury.

ACTION 3. Apply so that vest and gown are free of wrinkles.

RATIONALE. Wrinkles create pressure areas, which interfere with circulation. Pressure areas that result in restriction of circulation cause tissue damage due to ischemia.

Procedure 33–13. (continued)

ACTION 4. Thread one tie through the slot, crossing open halves of vest front over one another.

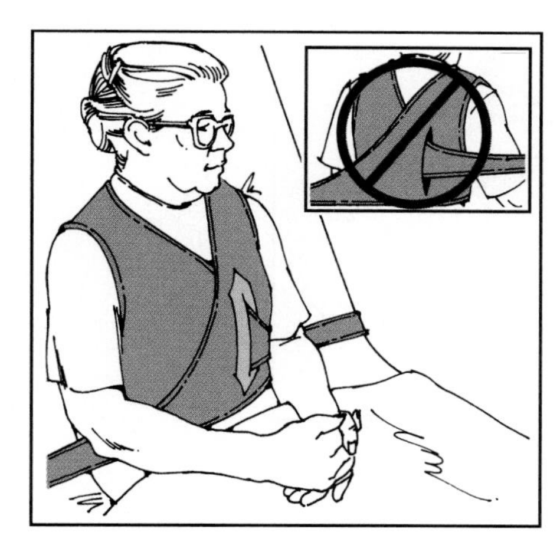

RATIONALE. Keeps restraint securely in place. Restraint may slip upward if ties are not properly threaded, causing chafing or decreased circulation, especially in axillary area.

ACTION 5. Allowing space for 2 finger breadths between restraint and patient's body when chest is fully expanded, secure restraint to chair or underside of the bedframe out of patient's reach using a quick-release knot. See Action 6 below.

RATIONALE. Prevents restriction of breathing and circulatory stasis.

ACTION 6. Wrap tie once around bedframe or wheelchair peg before making quick-release knot.

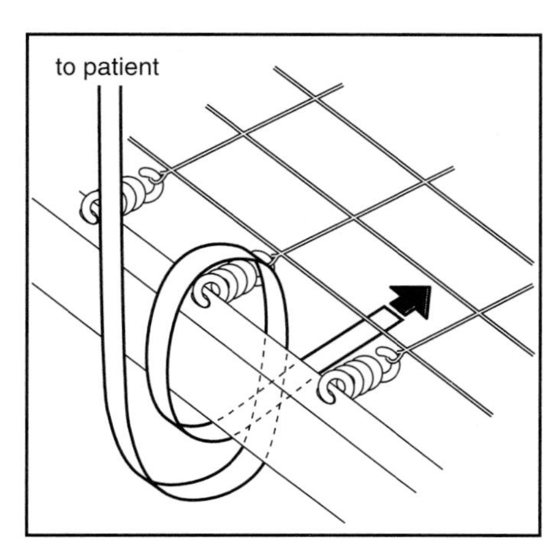

a. If using restraint on a patient in bed, loop the tie snugly around a section of the spring supporting the mattress (mattress omitted from illustration for clarity).

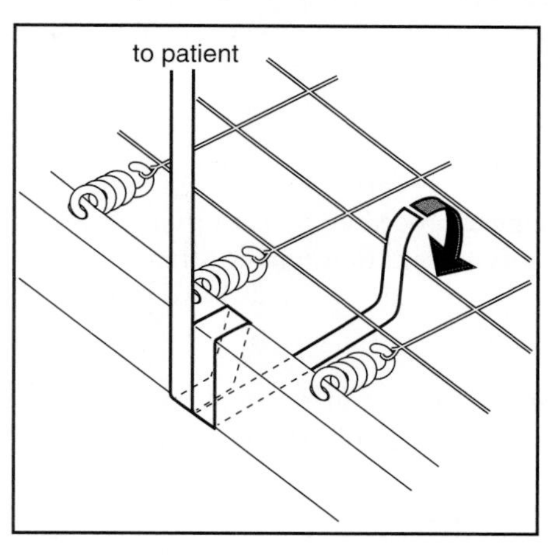

b. Make a half bow knot on spring, pulling loop firmly to secure. Release by pulling on end of tie.

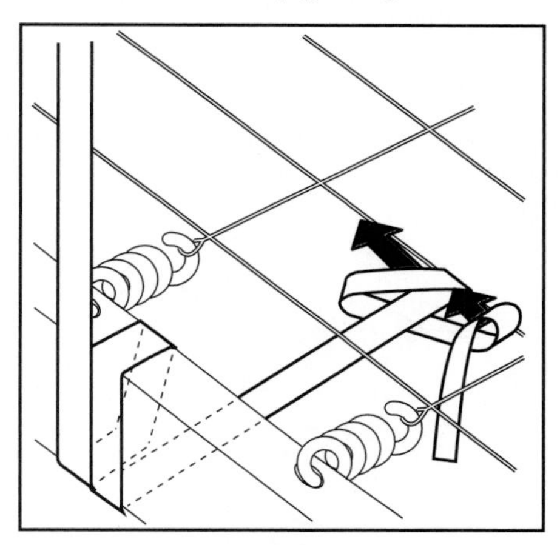

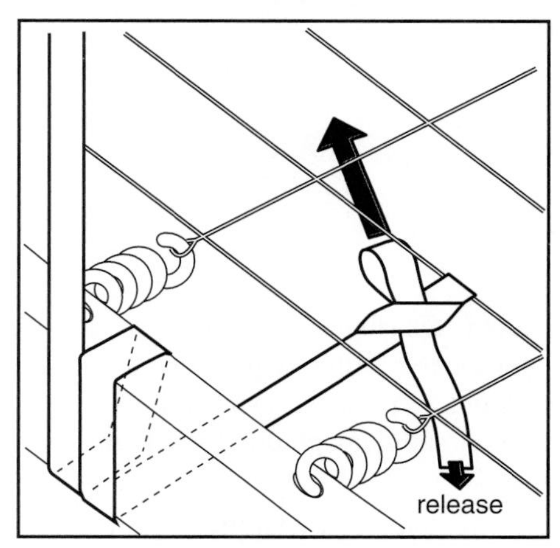

RATIONALE. This knot is inaccessible to patient, but can be quickly and easily released by caregivers.

Continued

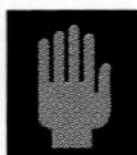

Do not attach restraint to siderail or to an immovable part of the bed or chair. This could injure patient if rail or bed is moved before releasing restraints. Tying a restraint to some types of springs may result in the tie becoming entangled at the point where two spring wires cross. In this case, tie the knot *across* the junction of the two spring wires, rather than between them as illustrated, or tie the restraint to a solid part of the bed frame out of the patient's reach.

ACTION 7. Complete procedure by performing steps 3 and 4, shown previously under "Belt-type Restraints".

LIMB RESTRAINTS

ACTION 1. Discuss purpose of restraint with patient and family: To restrict movement of extremities, preventing disruption of treatment modality (IV, drainage tube) or preventing unsupervised mobility.

RATIONALE. Cooperation is more likely if patient and family understand the purpose of and expected gains from restraints. Well-meaning family may release restraints if purpose is not clear to them.

ACTION 2. Place widest part of restraint around ankle or wrist with padded surface next to skin. If restraint is not padded, fold and wrap a soft washcloth around extremity before applying restraint.

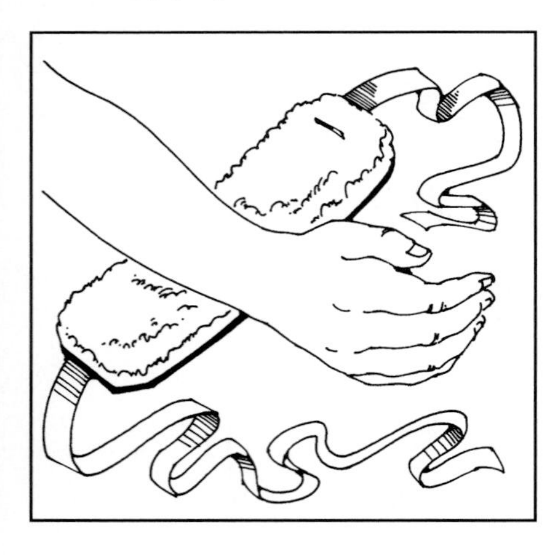

RATIONALE. Padding distributes pressure so that bony prominences do not receive brunt of pressure when patient pulls against restraint. Pressure, especially over bony prominences, causes tissue damage due to ischemia.

ACTION 3. Secure restraint on extremity, using Velcro, buckle, or by threading one tie through the slot and bringing the other tie around the extremity to meet the first tie on the lateral aspect of the extremity.

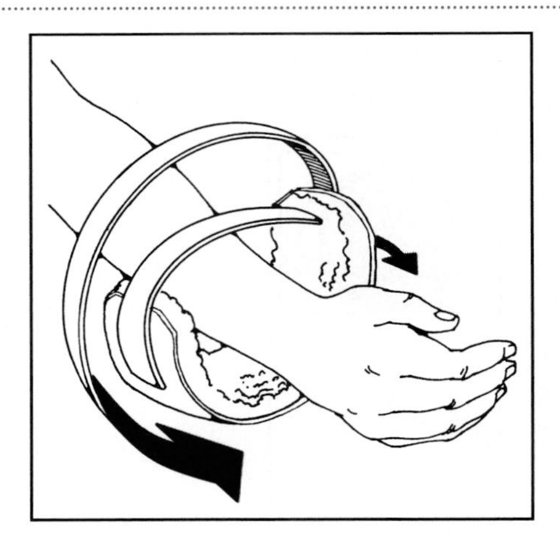

RATIONALE. Restraint will then be too snug to slip off, yet will not restrict circulation.

ACTION 4. Tie half-hitch (single knot) to secure restraint on extremity. Allow space for one fingerbreadth between extremity and secured restraint.

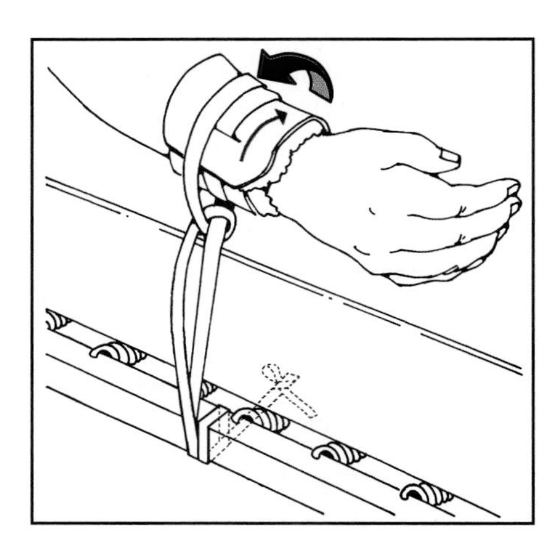

ACTION 5. Position the extremity in slight flexion and secure both ties to the underside of the bed using a half-bow knot as in Action 6. Do not tie to side rail. See caution above.

RATIONALE. Slight flexion allows for a small amount of joint movement without compromising effectiveness of the restraints.

ACTION 6. Assess skin, circulatory status, and nerve integrity at least 2qh.

RATIONALE. Coolness, pallor, tingling, or decreased sensation in restrained extremity indicates possible compromised circulation and/or nerve damage. Restraint must be discontinued. Consult with physician for alternative.

MITTEN RESTRAINT

ACTION 1. Discuss purpose of restraint with patient and family: To restrict patient's ability to use hand grasp, so pulling on tubes or dressing is not possible; also used to prevent scratching.

RATIONALE. Cooperation is more likely if patient and family understand the purpose of and expected gains from restraints. Well-meaning family may release restraints if purpose is not clear to them.

ACTION 2. Select a mitten size that will allow full extension of fingers inside, but that prevents pincer grasp.

RATIONALE. A mitten that is too small will promote flexion contractures of fingers. If grasp is possible, restraint will not prevent pulling on tubes.

ACTION 3. Place one padded mitten over each hand. Secure ties at the wrist, allowing one fingerbreadth between ties and wrist.

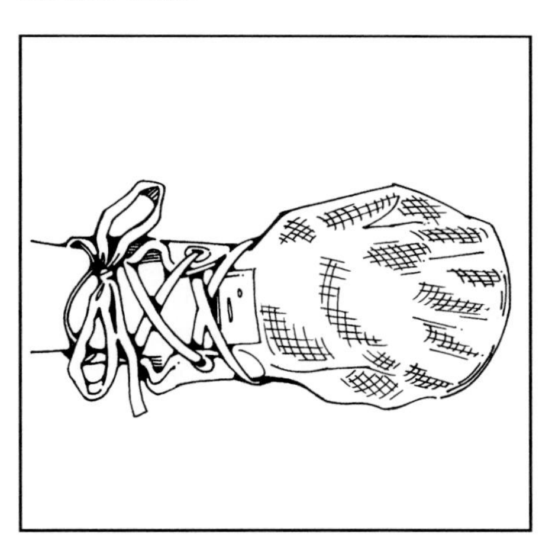

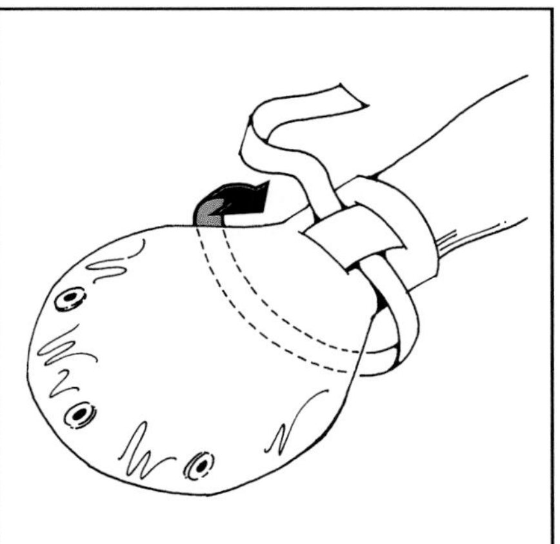

RATIONALE. Prevents mitten from slipping off without interfering with circulation.

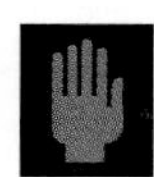

May also be secured to bedframe, but this restriction of motion is usually unnecessary because mitten limits dexterity.

ACTION 4. Release restraint and inspect underlying skin for chafing at least q2h.

RATIONALE. Padding greatly increases perspiration and, therefore, the risk for maceration.

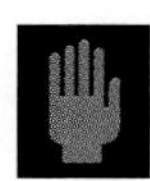

Removing mitten for 20 minutes q1h is advisable, if possible.

Recording:
Note type of restraint; reason for application, if not previously documented; amount of time secured and released; description of patient behavior during periods of restraint and release; condition of skin and underlying tissue, and care provided, if any.

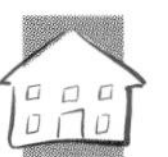

HOME HEALTH ADAPTATION: Restraints are challenging to adapt to a home care setting. They are seldom used in the home, and then only as a last resort to protect a patient or to maintain placement of catheters, feeding tubes, and IVs. Family members are reluctant to confine a loved one. The patient may experience an incident or injury before the family is willing to restrain a patient's activity. Instead, family members can place bells on interior gates, high locks or alarms on exterior doors, and alarms and locks on gates surrounding their home to alert them to the whereabouts of a patient with diminished mental capacity. Fastening ties to a lap robe may appear less confining to a patient and family while maintaining a forgetful patient securely in a chair. A mitten with the thumb sewn closed may sufficiently reduce manual dexterity to prevent removal of the tubing. Covering tubing with towels or strategic placement of a pillow may deter some patients. The use of upper and lower siderails must be evaluated for their potential to increase risk of injury if a patient climbs over the rail. Introducing siderails as an aid for turning and positioning in bed may overcome initial resistance in accepting them. To alert family members that a patient in danger of falling is attempting to get out of bed unassisted, a string of bells may be fastened to the lower portion of the top cover. A baby monitor and closed circuit TV are other methods to detect movement and sounds, thereby enabling caregivers to respond promptly.

CRITICAL QUERY

Kanski and co-workers[59] found that family members of patients being restrained in acute care settings had a variety of negative reactions to this intervention. The authors give examples of family members' statements such as these. "She didn't do anything and she's tied up." "It made me mad—they just walked in, put on the restraint and never said a word." "She didn't need to be restrained. She couldn't move her right arm and uses her left hand to position her right arm. My mother started to cry when they tied her wrist." Should family reactions to health care measures be of concern to nurses? What information should be given to family members about the use of restraints on their loved ones? Who is responsible for educating families about this issue?

The use of restraints also raises many serious ethical and moral questions. Questions related to informed consent, quality of life, and autonomy are examples. Nurses contemplating using restraints must consider not only the possible physical and legal ramifications, but also the emotional impact on patients and families and the effect on a patient's self-concept. Being restrained is, in fact, personally demeaning to patients and deeply disturbing to them and their families.[59] If nurses use restraints, they must consider this a short-term solution until more effective action can be planned. There are many alternatives to restraints, as the following sections indicate.

Identifying High-risk Populations. Significant reductions in patient wandering and falls can be achieved by clearly identifying those at risk.[55,58,61] Screening for risk can be incorporated into the admission assessment and periodically reassessed. Highly visible labels can then be used to maintain caregiver's awareness of patients at risk. Facilities have found several different approaches for identifying high-risk patients effective, such as placing the labels on wristbands, doorways, above beds, and on the Kardex and nursing care plans.

Environmental Modifications. Many environmental causes of falls and wandering are easily modified.[56,58,60-63] Glare or poor lighting, slippery floors, unsteady furniture in common areas such as patient lounges, and insufficient or inappropriate environmental stimulation are examples. Increasing appropriate environmental stimulation also prevents falls. More frequent staff communication with patients, companionship, exercise programs, and quiet group activities with staff supervision confer multiple benefits, including reducing the need for restraints.

Individualizing Care. Certain patients have unique reasons for higher wandering and fall risks. Medications, boredom, habitual early awakening with personal care needs when staff are busy with change of shift activities, and unusual responses to certain environmental stimuli are examples. Investigating underlying causes for individual patient responses to the environment can help staff identify ways to modify a patient's environment or help patients modify responses that lead to falls.[58] Staff responsibilities can sometimes be restructured to increase their availability to patients at times of peak patient needs.[61,62]

Providing Frequent Assistance With Elimination. Many dependent patients fall while attempting to meet elimination needs independently rather than ask for assistance. Establishing bowel and bladder programs to assist patients to more effectively regulate elimination, and offering help with toileting early in the morning, periodically throughout the day, and immediately before settling for the night, reduces falls related to elimination needs.[62,64]

Educating Staff. Programs to reduce restraint use cannot succeed without addressing caregiver attitudes and misconceptions about the use of restraints.[55,56,60,61,65] Exploring viable alternatives in basic nursing education, staff conferences, continuing education, and supporting staff who attempt new approaches are some of the means that are effective in bringing about change in caregiver knowledge and attitudes about restraints.

Home Care

Many patients with mobility problems are discharged to their homes before achieving independent mobility. This can be a stressful transition, in particular if there is insufficient time available to permit gradual assumption of new responsibilities.[66] Patients often need continued assistance with exercise, transfers, and ADLs. Family or support persons frequently provide much of this assistance. Home care nurses need to teach patients and their support persons correct care techniques and evaluate their ability to perform them to prevent injuries to either. This is especially true for exercise and transfers. These patients continue to be at risk for complications related to inactivity, in particular skin and bowel elimination problems.[67]

Family can also be involved in skin and elimination assessments and preventive care. Diet is important in prevention for both problems. Adequate protein calories to maintain skin integrity and sufficient fluids and fiber to prevent constipation are important.

Research has suggested that the role of family caregiver is a difficult one. Family caregivers report financial strain, concern for their own well-being, and feeling socially restricted.[68] Nurses involved in home care should work proactively with caregiving families to prepare them for the complex relationship dynamics involved in taking on this role and help them to develop strategies to cope effectively.

Home care nurses also are responsible for monitoring progress toward outcomes and determining appropriate timing for discharge from home care services. This is another transition that can be difficult for patients and families. It can be eased by effective planning and anticipatory guidance.

COLLABORATIVE STRATEGY

BARRIERS TO MOBILITY

Barriers to mobility take several forms: psychological, social, and environmental. Patients may have personal concerns, such as the fear of injury, or may be worried about the burden their mobility problem places on others. There may be actual physical barriers to be overcome in the environment that cause a patient to be reticent. By collaborating with patients, nurses can identify the specific barriers that a patient is experiencing. This collaboration can be the basis for a plan that will enhance confidence about achieving mobility objectives.

REHABILITATIVE CARE

The primary focus of rehabilitative mobility care is promoting self-care and a return to the community as a functioning, contributing member. Residual disabilities that interfere with mobility often compromise capacity for independent functioning. This is a significant loss that frequently precipitates a crisis and strains coping abilities. A holistic approach to rehabilitation addresses physical adaptation to specific deficits and focuses on motivating behavior change. Patient collaboration with nurses, physical therapists, occupational therapists, social workers, and other care providers accomplishes the most satisfactory results. Nurses often coordinate collaborative planning throughout rehabilitation.

Physical Adaptation

Strategies to enhance physical mobility, and adapted techniques for self-care and home management facilitate physical adaptation to disability.

Enhancing Physical Mobility. Helping patients gain greater mobility is an essential aspect of a rehabilitation program. Physical and occupational therapists have a major role in gait training and teaching patients to use mobility aids such as canes, walkers, braces, prostheses, and wheelchairs.[49,53,69] Nurses have an important supportive role.[49,70] They are responsible for early mobilization via exercises during the acute phase of the mobility problem. Exercises improve strength, flexibility, and endurance, and maximize patients' abilities to use mobility aids. This lays the foundation for successful rehabilitation.

Ongoing physical activity has an important place in the lives of individuals with handicapping conditions. Total-person rehabilitation, introduced in the 1940s by Sir Luttwig Guttmann, is based on the premise that physical rehabilitation is of no avail unless handicapped individuals can find purpose in life.[71] For many individuals, sport is integral in this process. Guttman believed that sport has the same meaning for handicapped individuals as for others, but that for individuals with handicaps, sports also play an essential role in physical, psychological, and social rehabilitation.

Many communities offer a wide variety of organized sports and exercise programs for disabled individuals, including water sports, track and field, golf, weight training, basketball, skiing, and even rugby. Some exercise classes focus on specific health problems or disabilities, such as stroke, spinal cord injury, amputation, pulmonary problems, cardiac problems, and arthritis (Fig. 33–23). Nurses are instrumental in educating patients about the kinds of group programs that are available and in identifying suitable programs for a particular patient.

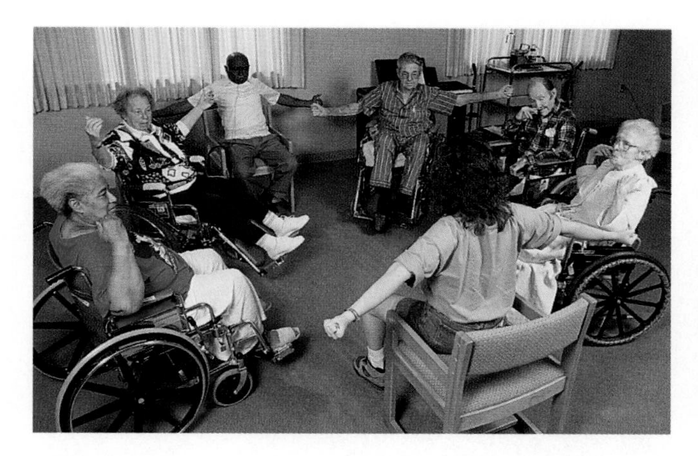

Figure 33–23. A group exercise class assists the rehabilitative process for stroke patients.

Self-care and Home Management Techniques. Dressing, hygiene, and elimination are often challenges for patients with mobility impairments. Assessment of deficits and strengths to determine self-management capacity is a nursing responsibility. Teaching self-care techniques is a collaborative responsibility, shared with physical and occupational therapy.[53] Assistive devices for dressing, such as button hooks, zipper pulls, long-handled reachers, and sock pullers, as well as clothing modifications such as Velcro closures, enable people to dress independently. See Fig. 32–7.

Adaptive equipment is often needed for personal hygiene and grooming. Special handles for combs, brushes, toothbrushes, and razors can be designed to accommodate specific losses of hand and arm function. Shower chairs facilitate bathing with fewer risks than tub transfers. See Fig. 32–9.

Many patients with residual mobility impairments experience elimination challenges including loss of voluntary control and learning safe transfers to the toilet. For some, permanent indwelling catheters or intermittent self-catheterization are necessary. Bowel and bladder training programs (Chap. 29) are successful for many others. Nurses play a primary role in teaching these elimination-related skills.

The capacity for home management activities such as cleaning, laundry, and cooking is necessary for independent living. Multidisciplinary collaboration is most effective for teaching home-management skills. Some rehabilitation facilities have simulated apartments in which patients can learn home-management skills in preparation for discharge to their own homes. Adaptive equipment for home maintenance tasks promotes autonomy Fig. 33–24.

Motivating Behavior Change

As discussed in Chap. 21, individuals' health beliefs, locus of control, and self-efficacy influence their motivation and capacity for behavior change. Rehabilitation involves significant behavior changes in almost every area of life. Consequently, rehabilitation is dependent on motivation. Lack of motivation is particularly disruptive to rehabilitation. Patients who place a high value on independence, believe they are in control of their own lives, and see themselves as capable of change are intrinsically motivated. They are likely to participate actively in rehabilitation activities with little need for motivating strategies by nurses and other care providers. These patients desire active participation in goal setting. Working towards small incremental goals helps rehabilitation patients maintain hope.[72] Hope is a strong motivator. Nurses can reinforce their realistic goal setting and self-management of their rehabilitation programs through fostering self-responsibility and teaching self-monitoring skills. A concrete expression of commitment such as a written contract strengthens self-responsibility. A taped or written diary facilitates self-monitoring. Patients can readily track their progress and digression from the planned rehabilitation course by reviewing the diary and use this information to modify goals and approaches. This approach enables patients to

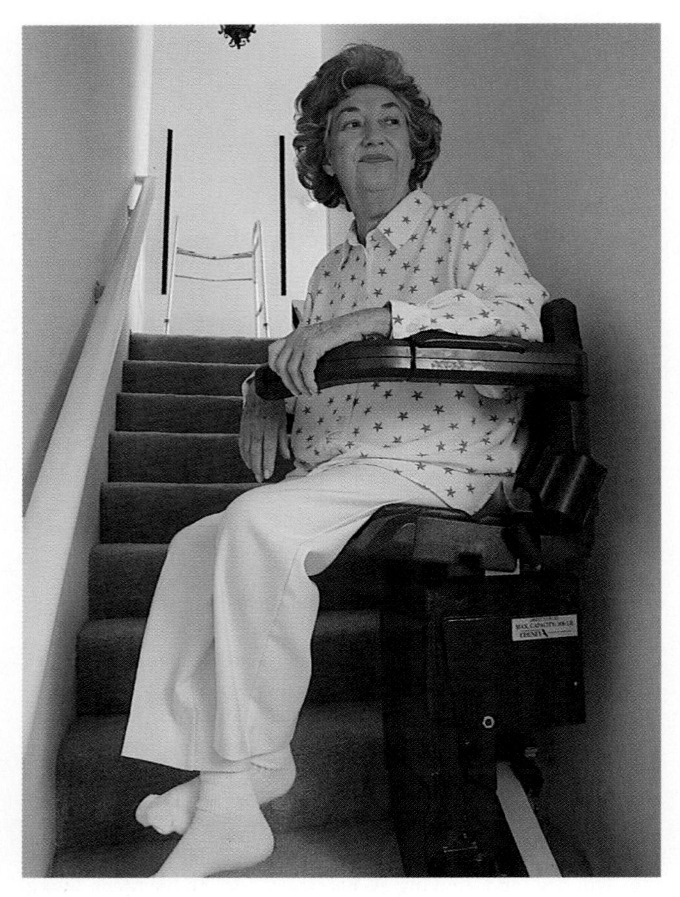

Figure 33–24. As patients recover from illness at home, equipment has been devised to assist with such tasks as climbing stairs. Here an individual "climbs" stairs in an electronically operated chair.

continue the desired behaviors with less reliance on health care professionals.

Many patients, however, need external incentives to reinforce participation, especially in the early stages of rehabilitation.[73] Many of the strategies for enhancing participation in an exercise program, discussed under supportive care, apply to motivating behavior change in a rehabilitation population. Positive social support is beneficial, some would say vital, to sustaining motivation during rehabilitation.[72] Social support comes from family and significant others, nurses, and often from other patients participating in the same program. Group support from peers is one of the most important advantages of a structured group rehabilitation program. The group interaction decreases social isolation and provides a forum for addressing concerns, evaluating choices, and comparing decisions. Support from family and significant others frequently takes the form of direct involvement in the rehabilitation program. They, along with nurses, are an important source of positive reinforcement as well. Nurses and families can be most effective in their support through "power with" relationships.[73] In "power with" relationships, individual (patient) capabilities are developed through interactions and influence of others (caregivers and family). This type of relationship is empowering. In contrast, "power over" relationships use domination to achieve participation. Approaches such as lecturing patients about taking part in rehabilitation exercises, implying rules of a facility mandate certain performance, or even physically moving patients—pulling or pushing them during exercise—have been reported as examples of domination.[73] Domination instills hopelessness rather than motivation.

Rehabilitation is a demanding phase of recovery from health problems. Strong commitment from patients and health care professionals is the basis for successful rehabilitation. The commitment is expressed through collaborative planning and implementation. A broad-minded and imaginative approach to the problems of people with disabilities has the most potential for maximizing their functioning at home and in the community.

EVALUATION

Evaluation of nursing implementation to promote mobility completes the cycle of the nursing process. Examples of evaluation criteria for mobility can be found in Table 33–8, Nurse-Patient Management of Mobility. The goal of any mobility care plan is to promote or return patients to the highest level of functioning possible. The determination of the level of functioning that is possible and realistic is complex. It requires nurses' diligent application of their body of knowledge and active collaboration with patients and other health care professionals. Clear concise evaluation criteria that describe evidence of that level of functioning are the key to monitoring progress and verifying outcome attainment. If evaluation indicates that desired outcomes were not achieved, the options are to continue with the plan with new target dates for reevaluation, to formulate new desired outcomes and implementations, or to reconsider the accuracy of the problem identification.

SUMMARY

Mobility is a complex function that influences other realms of human functioning. It is a significant component of wellness. Optimum mobility creates nearly limitless options for life choices. On the other hand, altered mobility can be profoundly limiting.

The musculoskeletal, cardiopulmonary, and neurologic systems play important roles in mobility. Understanding the interrelated functioning of these organs is necessary for nurses to promote optimum mobility.

Altered mobility frequently influences other body functions. Oxygenation, rest and activity, nutrition, elimination, sexual, and psychological functioning are affected by diminished mobility. Consequently, assessing and evaluating mobility includes a collaborative history and examination of integumentary, pulmonary, cardiovascular, musculoskeletal, neurologic, and psychological functioning.

Impaired physical mobility, activity intolerance, risk for activity intolerance, and risk for disuse syndrome and their etiologies are discussed in detail in this chapter to assist beginning students to formulate nursing diagnoses related to mobility and plan patient care to improve or maintain mobility. Sample critical pathways show an alternative means to manage patient care.

Preventive nursing implementation related to mobility includes health education about the benefits of exercise, collaborating with patients to develop individualized plans, home assessment for mobility hazards, and screening for patients at risk for altered mobility. Supporting patients who are participating in exercise programs to correct risk factors, and treating minor exercise-related injuries are examples of supportive mobility care. Restorative care encompasses assisting with exercise such as range of motion and ambulation, transfer techniques, moving and positioning in bed, and the judicious use of restraints. Using effective body mechanics underlies restorative mobility care. Rehabilitative mobility care requires a multidisciplinary approach to promote physical, social, and psychological adaptation to disability. Approaches to strengthen motivation are integral to fruitful rehabilitation.

Optimum mobility makes possible functional participation in the home, community, and society. Nurses make critical contributions to this outcome.

LEARNING OUTCOMES

Upon completing this chapter, the student should be able to:

1. Describe how each of the following affect mobility: musculoskeletal functioning, cardiopulmonary functioning, and metabolic efficiency.
2. Briefly summarize the physiologic response to increased muscular activity.
3. List and define the components of fitness, and describe the type of activity required for optimum development of each component.
4. List at several benefits of regular aerobic exercise and explain how exercise brings about these effects.
5. State two risks associated with exercise.
6. Describe how age, disability, general health, self-concept, and values affect mobility.
7. Describe the problems in each of the following functional dimensions that result from decreased mobility: activity/mobility, rest/sleep, oxygenation, nutrition, fluid and elimination, sexuality, and psychological dimensions.
8. Describe essential elements of a mobility history.
9. Describe essential elements of a mobility examination.
10. Name three diagnostic tests useful in diagnosing mobility problems.
11. List several nursing diagnoses that describe altered mobility.
12. Identify and explain at least two etiologies of each of the above diagnoses.
13. Describe preventive, supportive, restorative, and rehabilitative nursing implementations to promote, maintain, or enhance mobility.
14. List and explain basic guidelines for effective body mechanics.
15. Identify strategies to evaluate the effectiveness of patient care related to mobility.
16. Discuss the relevance of a collaborative approach to patient care related to mobility.
17. Write an individualized patient care plan for a patient experiencing mobility problems.

REVIEW OF KEY TERMS

active range of motion
activities of daily living
aerobic exercise
anaerobic glycolysis
antagonists
atrophy
dangling
deep vein thrombosis (DVT)
disuse phenomena
disuse syndrome
eggcrate mattress overlay
endurance
exercise tolerance
fitness
flexibility
footboards
isokinetic exercise
isometric exercise
isotonic exercise
mobility
orthostatic (postural) hypotension
passive range of motion
shearing
strength
synergist
trochanter rolls
Valsalva maneuver

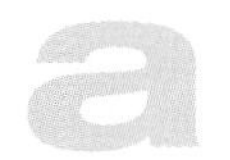

Having read the Chapter, consider again the opening scenario, page 1169, and the following responses to the questions.

Mr. Dodd's nurse should assess mental status, energy level, and his posture and gait with and without the walker, on each visit. She should inquire about dizziness (side effect of antihypertensive medication). Although the Dodd's bathroom safety bars imply safety awareness, she should assess for new barriers to mobility (furniture, clutter, plants, throw rugs). These assessments will rule out risk for falls. Mr. Dodd is also at risk for progressive weakness and diminished range of motion due to inactivity. Nursing implementation to reduce both of these risks includes daily short walks (using his walker) outdoors with his wife and active range-of-motion exercises. If Mr. Dodd is able to gradually increase the distance he walks, his strength and endurance will improve. Resistance exercises such as ROM wearing 1 pound wrist and ankle weights will have the same effect. His nurse should also reinforce measures to minimize dizziness, such as sitting for a few moments before arising from a recumbent position, and then rising slowly to standing. If he notes dizziness despite these measures, he should contact the prescriber of the antihypertensive medication for advice.

REFERENCES

1. Wilmore JH, Costill DL. *Physiology of Sport and Exercise.* Champagne, IL: Human Kinetics; 1994.
2. *Surgeon General's Report on Physical Fitness and Health.* Centers for Disease Control and Prevention, July 1996.
3. Mathieu AE. Prescribing exercise for the primary care patient. *J Am Acad of Phys Asst.* 1993;6:380–388.
4. Rutherford WJ, Corbin CB, Chase LA. Factors influencing motivation towards physical activity. *Health Values: Achieving High Level Wellness.* 1992;16:19–24.
5. CDC Associate Director stresses changing ideas about physical activity. *In Touch,* Jacobs Institute of Women's Health. 1996; 4:1,4.
6. Lappe JM. Bone fragility: assessment of risk and strategies for prevention. *J Obstet Gynecol Neonatal Nurs.* 1994;23:260–268.
7. Henry JK. Commentary on women walking for health and fitness: how much is enough? *AWHONN's Women's Health Nursing Scan.* 1993;7:4.
8. Thorton EW, Scott SE. Motivation in the committed runner: correlations between self-report scales and behavior. *Health Promotion Int.* 1995;10:177–184.
9. Young A, Dinan S. Fitness for older people. *Brit Med J.* 1994;309:331–333.
10. Means KM, Currie DM, Gershkoff AM. Geriatric rehabilitation. Assessment, preservation, and enhancement of fitness and function, part 4. *Arch Phys Med Rehabil.* 1993;74:S417–S420.
11. Lakatta E. Cardiovasculatory regulatory mechanisms in advanced age. *Physiol Rev.* 1993;73:413–467.
12. Betz CL, Hunsberger MM, Wright S. *Family-Centred Nursing Care of Children.* Philadelphia: Saunders; 1994.
13. Oman R, McAuley E. Intrinsic motivation and exercise behavior. *J Health Ed.* 1993;24:232–238.
14. Tucker LA, Mortell R. Comparison of the effects of walking and weight training programs on body image in middle aged women: an experimental study. *Am J Health Promotion.* 1993;8:34–42.
15. Lowen A. *Bioenergetics.* New York: Penguin; 1975.
16. Hull CL. *Principles of Behavior.* New York: Appleton-Century-Crofts; 1943.
17. Abood DA, Conway TL. Smoking status, body composition, exercise, and diet among Navy men. *Health Values: Achieving High Level Wellness.* 1994;18:51–62.
18. Abood DA, Conway TL. Health value and self esteem as predictors of wellness behavior. *Health Values: Achieving High Level Wellness.* 1992;16:20–26.
19. Pender NJ. *Health Promotion in Nursing Practice.* 3rd ed. Stamford, CT: Appleton & Lange; 1996.
20. Olson EV, Johnson BJ, Thompson LF. The hazaards of immobility. *Am J Nurs.* 1990;90:43–48.
21. Whitney JD, Stotts NA, Goodson WH, Janson-Bjerklie S. The effects of activity and bedrest on tissue oxygen tension, perfusion, and plasma volume. *Nurs Res.* 1993;42:349–355.
22. McNaughton V, Brazil K. Wound and skin team impact on pressure ulcer prevalence in chronic care. *J Gerontol Nurs.* 1995;21:45–47.
23. Panel for the Prediction and Prevention of Pressure Ulcers in Adults. *Pressure Ulcers in Adults: Prediction and Prevention in Clinical Practice Guideline, Number 3.* AHCPR Publication No. 92–0047. Rockville, MD: Agency for Health Care Policy and Research, Public Health Service, U.S. Department of Health and Human Services; May, 1992.
24. Dargent-Molina P, Favier F, Grandjean N, et al. Fall-related factors and risk of hip fracture: the *EPIDOS* prospective study. *Lancet.* 1996;348:145–149.
25. Braun LT. Physiologic versus pathologic hypertrophy: endurance exercise and chronic pressure overload. *J Cardiovasc Nurs.* 1994;8:39–56.
26. Ewart CK, Loftus IK, Hagberg JM. School-based exercise to lower blood pressure in high-risk African American girls: project design and baseline findings. *J Health Ed.* 1995;26(suppl 2):S99–S105.
27. Goldfine BD, Nahas MV. Incorporating health related fitness concepts in secondary physical education curricula. *J School Health.* 1993;36:142–146.
28. Blue CL, Conrad CM. Adherence to worksite exercise programs: an integrative review of recent research. *AAOHN J.* 1995;43:76–86.
29. National Center for Health Statistics. *Health, United States, 1995.* Hyattsville, MD; NCHS; 1996.
30. Vargo MM. Osteoporosis: Strategies for prevention and treatment. *J Musculoskel Med.* 1995;19–24, 27–18, 30.
31. Keil DP. Osteoporosis: how you can help prevent—or arrest—primary disease. *Consultant.* 1994;34:928.
32. Bravo G. Impact of a 12–month exercise program on the physical and psychosocial health of osteopenic women. *J Am Geriatr Soc* 1996;44:756–762.
33. Ainsworth BE. Approaches to physical activity in women. *AWHONNS Clinical Issues in Perinatal and Women's Health Nursing.* 1993;4:302–310.
34. William PT. High-density lipoprotein cholesterol and other risk factors for coronary heart disease in female runners. *N Engl J Med.* 1996;334:1298–1303.
35. Manson JE, Lee IM. Exercise for women—how much pain for optimal gain? *N Engl J Med.* 1996;334:1325–136.
36. Wilmore JH. Increasing physical activity: alterations in body mass and composition. *Am J Clin Nutr.* 1996;63(suppl):456S-460S.
37. Hawks SR, Richens P. Toward a new paradigm for the management of obesity. *J Health Ed.* 1994;25:147–153.
38. Schwartz F. Obesity in adult females: The relationship among personality characteristics, dieting, and weight. *AAOHN J.* 1993;41:504–509.
39. Wagner EH, LaCroix AZ, Grothaus MS, et al. Preventing disability and falls in older adults: a population-based randomized trial. *Am J Public Health.* 1994;84:1800–1806.
40. Glick DF. The relationship between demographic characteristics and nursing problems in home health care. *Public Health Nurs.* 1994;11:259–267.
41. Kempen KPG, Saris WHM, Westerterp KR. Energy balance during an 8–week energy-restricted diet with and without exercise in obese women. *Am J Clin Nutr* 1995;62:722–729.
42. Brich KL, Zywotko DM. Obesity and weight loss in the healthy elderly. *J Am Acad Phys Asst.* 1994;7:553–558.
43. Fair JM, Berra K. Life-style chances and coronary heart disease: The influence of non-pharmacologic interventions. *J Cardiovasc Nurs.* 1995;9:12–24.
44. White F, Montell F. Identification and treatment of exercise resistance: A syndrome associated with eating disorders. *Women's Health Issues.* 1996;6:273–278.

45. Melillo KD, Futrell M, Williamson E, et al. Perceptions of physical fitness and exercise activity among older adults. *J Adv Nurs*. 1996;23:542–547.
46. Hamdorf PA, Withers RT, Penhall RK, Plummer JL. A follow-up study on the effects of training on the fitness and habitual activity patterns of 60- to 70-year-old women. *Arch Phys Med Rehabil*. 1993;74:473–477.
47. Topp R, Mikesky A, Bawel K. Developing strength training programs for older adults. *Rehabil. Nurs*. 1994;19:266–273.
48. Noble LJ, Salcido R, Walker MK, et al. Improving functional mobility through exercise. *Rehabil Nurs Res*. 1994;3:23–29.
49. Galindo-Ciocon DJ, Ciocon JO, Galindo DJ. Gait training and falls in the elderly. *J Gerontol Nurs*. 1995;21:10–17.
50. Hendrich A, Nyhuis A, Kippenbrock T, Soja ME. Hospital falls: Development of a predictive model for clinical practice. *Appl Nurs Res*. 1995;8:129–139.
51. Arfken CL, Lach HW, Birge SJ, Miller JP. Fear of falling in elderly persons living in the community. *Am J Public Health*. 1994;84:565–569.
52. Ploeg J, Black ME, Hutchison BG, et al. Personal, home and community safety promotion with community-dwelling elderly persons: Response to a public health nurse intervention. *Can J Public Health*. 1994;85:188–191.
53. Mann WC, Hurren, Tomita M. Comparison of assistive device use and needs of home-based older persons with different impairments. *Am J Occup Ther*. 1993;47:980–987.
54. Wilson EB. The physical restraint of elderly patients in critical care: Historical perspectives and new directions. *Crit Care Nurs Clin North Am*. 1996;8:61–70.
55. Bradley L, Siddique CM, Dufton B. Reducing the use of physical restraints in long-term care facilities. *J Gerontol Nurs*. 1995;21:21–34.
56. Schott-Baer D, Lusis S, Beauregard K. Use of restraints: Changes in nurses' attitudes. *J Gerontol Nurs*. 1995;21:39–44.
57. Tinetti M, Liu W, Ginter S. Medical restraint use and fall-related injuries in residents of skilled nursing facilities. *Ann Intern Med*. 1992;116:369–374.
58. Brungardt GS. Patient restraints: New guidelines for a less restrictive approach. *Geriatrics*. 1994;49:43–50.
59. Kanski GW, Janelli LM, Jones HM, Kennedy MC. Family reactions to restraints in an acute care setting. *J Gerontol Nurs*. 1996;22:17–22.
60. Matthiesen V, Lamb KV, McCann J, et al. Hospital nurses views about physical restraint use with older patients. *J Gerontol Nurs*. 1996;22:8–16.
61. Cohen C, Neufeld R, Dunbar J, et al. Old problem, different approach: alternatives to physical restraints. *J Gerontol Nurs*. 1996;22:23–29.
62. Clark LR, Fraaza V, Schroeder S, Maddens M. Alternative nursing environments: do they affect outcomes? *J Gerontol Nurs*. 1995;21:32–38.
63. Moretz C, Dommel A, Deluca K. Untied: A safe alternative to restraints. *Med Surg Nurs*. 1995;4:128–132.
64. Brady R, Chester FR, Pierce LL, et al. Geriatric falls: Prevention strategies for the staff. *J Gerontol Nurs*. 1993;19:26–32.
65. Thomas A, Redfern L, John R. Perceptions of acute care nurses in the use of restraints. *J Gerontol Nurs*. 1995;21:32–38.
66. Schumacher KL, Meleis Al. Transitions: A central concept in nursing. *Image: J Nurs Sch*. 1994;26:119–127.
67. Oot-Giromini BA. Pressure ulcer prevalence, incidence and associated risk factors in the community. *Decubitus*. 1993; 6:24–32.
68. Sayles-Cross S. Perceptions of familial caregivers of elder adults. *Image: J Nurs Sch*. 1993;25:88–92.
69. Harada N, Chiu V, Fowler E, et al. Physical therapy to improve functioning of older people in residential care facilities. *Phys Ther*. 1995;75:830–838.
70. Koroknay VJ, Werner P, Cohen-Mansfield J, Braun JV. Maintaining ambulation in the frail nursing home resident: A nursing administered walking program. *J Gerontol Nurs*. 1995; 21:18–24.
71. Guttman L. In: Maddox S, ed. *Spinal Cord Injury: A Primer—Spinal Injury Through History*. Boulder: Spinal Network; 1987;22–25.
72. Morse JM, Doberneck B. Delineating the concept of hope. *Image: J Nurs Sch*. 1995;27:277–286.
73. Resnick B. Motivation in geriatric rehabilitation. *Image: J Nurs Sch*. 1996;28:41–45.

34

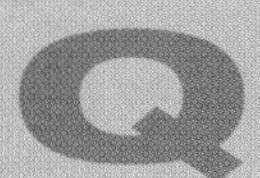

What is potassium, and what role does it play in the body?

What is a hydrating fluid?

What is a PICC line?

What is the purpose of an intravenous infusion pump?

What observations should Nurse Queroz make to ascertain that the IV infusion works as it should?

Alison Mueller is a 30-year-old woman with two children. For the past 5 years she has suffered from multiple sclerosis, a disease of the nervous system in which progressive demyelination of the white matter of the brain and spinal cord causes debilitating motor and sensory problems. Ms. Mueller's disease was in remission until 2 years ago, when she became pregnant with her second child. Now she has experienced a severe progression, and is receiving an intravenous medication thought to hasten remission. She also receives hydrating fluids and occasional potassium supplements to replace the potassium lost in the urine as a side effect of the drug. Laura Queroz, the home health nurse, is administering the medication through Ms. Mueller's PICC line with the aid of an intravenous infusion pump.

Fluid and Electrolyte Balance

Jan A. Sebring

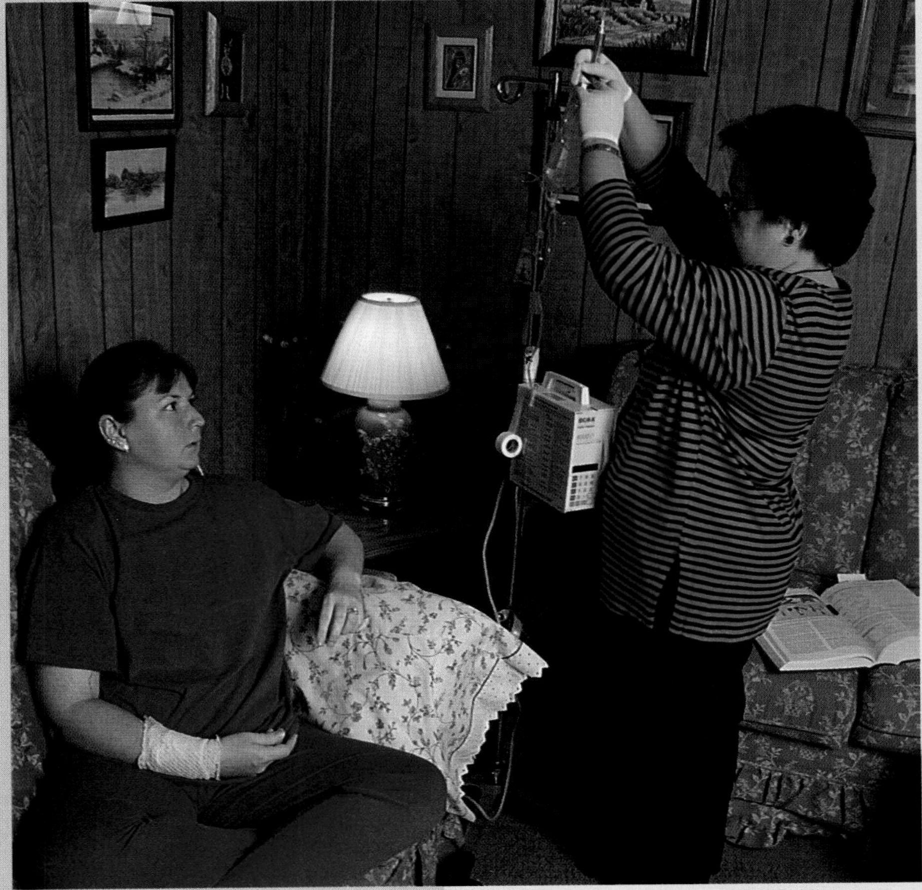

CHAPTER OUTLINE

Each cell of the human body is similar to the primitive single-celled organisms that inhabited the ancient oceans. Human cells bathe in body fluid that is similar in composition and character to seawater. This internal fluid protects the structure and metabolic balance of each cell.

The body as a whole can adapt to a wide range of conditions, but the internal environment must be maintained within narrow physiologic limits. Equilibrium is maintained by corrective biologic reactions. Under normal conditions, individuals are unaware of the body's fluid adjustment processes. When these processes fail, the effects may cause no harm or they may be totally debilitating, depending on the degree of fluid and electrolyte imbalance. The key to normal functioning is to return individuals to a state of fluid and electrolyte balance.

Collaboration with patients to promote, maintain, or restore fluid balance is an important nursing responsibility. Through collaboration, nurses can tailor patient care to meet specific needs.

Body fluid balance is challenged repeatedly by conditions in everyday life and periodically by disease. This chapter presents content to help students develop an understanding of fluid balance theory and nursing activities that will help preserve patient well-being.

SECTION 1

UNDERSTANDING FLUID AND ELECTROLYTE BALANCE

OPTIMAL FLUID AND ELECTROLYTE BALANCE

THE NATURE AND FUNCTION OF BODY FLUID

Cellular functions require a system of circulating body fluids to transport nutrients and remove metabolic wastes. There are several types of body fluids, which vary in function, consistency, composition, and location. Collectively, these fluids regulate body temperature, cushion the joints and organs from injury, aid digestion of nutrients, transport gases to and from the cells, and maintain the cardiovascular system. The functions of body fluid are:

- Dispersing heat and regulating body temperature
- Transporting nutrients to cells
- Transporting waste products away from cells
- Transporting hormones to activity sites
- Lubricating joint spaces
- Maintaining hydrostatic pressure in the cardiovascular system

Water is the most abundant constituent of all body fluids. Water, the universal solvent, is the body's chief medium for chemical reactions, transportating nutrients, and excreting metabolic wastes. So crucial is water to sustaining the internal environment that, without it, life ceases to exist in a matter of days.

VOLUME AND DISTRIBUTION OF BODY FLUID

Volume

The total amount of water that exists in the body at any given time is referred to as **total body water** (TBW). This volume represents approximately 60 percent of body weight in adult men and 50 percent in adult women. The percentage of body water varies substantially from individual to individual, depending on several factors.

Two of the most important factors determining the proportion of body water to weight are body fat content and age. Fat tissue cells contain very little fluid and, therefore, contribute little to total body water. As women tend to have a higher proportion of body fat than men, their percentage of body water is less. There is also a continual decrease in the percentage of TBW from birth to old age. In newborns, for example, the volume of body water may account for as much as 75 percent of weight. The percentage drops to 50 percent in the elderly adult as the result of a decrease in the number of body cells and an increase in fat tissue.[1] These statistics are illustrated in Table 34–1.

Distribution

Body fluid is distributed between two compartments, one intracellular and the other extracellular. Intracellular fluid (ICF), as the term implies, is the fluid located inside the cells. This compartment accounts for 40 percent of body weight in the lean adult male (Fig. 34–1).

Extracellular fluid (ECF) is the fluid contained outside the body's cells. EFC is composed of intravascular, interstitial, and transcellular fluids. The *intravascular fluid* consists of plasma; the *interstitial fluid* consists of lymph and fluid in the tissue spaces between the cells. The *transcellular fluid* includes urine, bile, saliva, sweat, cerebrospinal fluid, and the aqueous humor of the eye.[2] The ECF accounts for approximately 20 percent of body weight in a lean adult male (Fig. 34–1).

WATER BALANCE

The ICF and ECF compartments have dynamically changing volumes. Fluid moves relatively freely between compartments, with the intravascular fluid responding most to intake and elimination. The interstitial fluid and intracellular fluid, in turn, respond to changes in the intravascular fluid. Normally, the net volume of each compartment is maintained in balance by several physiologic processes, which are described in the next section.

Gains

As water is the main constituent of body fluid, a balance between water gain and loss is essential to maintain the composition of body fluids. This balance is achieved by roughly matching the intake and output of body water over a 24-hour period.

In healthy adults, the most significant fluid gains come from oral intake of fluids and foods. Suggested oral intake requirements for maintaining fluid balance vary between 1800 and 2500 mL/d. Approximately 1200 mL/d is ingested in fluids and 1000 mL/d in food. Water is also produced inside the body through the oxidation of nutrients. This amounts to approximately 300 mL/d.[3]

The requirements for replenishing fluids vary greatly with age, weight, body temperature and environment, and activity. For example, a full-term infant requires 70 to 100 mL/kg per 24 hours to maintain adequate fluid balance, whereas an elderly adult may

TABLE 34-1. TOTAL BODY FLUID (BY AGE AND GENDER) AS A PERCENTAGE OF BODY WEIGHT

Age	Total Body Fluid (% body weight)
Full-term newborn	70–80
1 year	64
Puberty to 39 years	Men: 60 Women: 52
40–60 years	Men: 55 Women: 47
More than 60 years	Men: 52 Women: 46

Source: Metheny NM. Fluid and Electrolyte Balance: Nursing Considerations. *3rd ed. Philadelphia: Lippincott; 1996, with permission.*

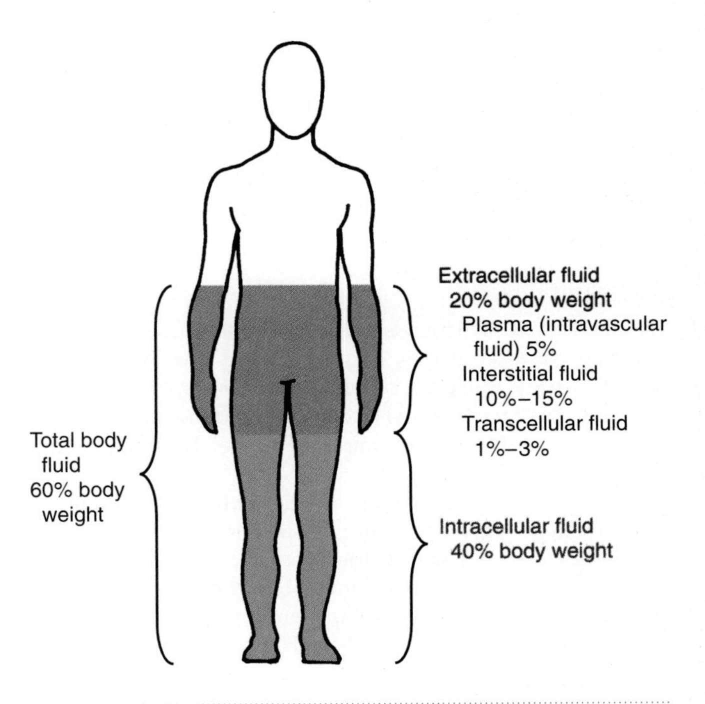

Figure 34–1. Total body fluids—extracellular and intracellular—are equivalent to 60 percent of body weight.

require 20 to 50 mL/kg per 24 hours. Of course, many other factors must be considered in calculating these requirements. An elderly patient, for example, may require increased fluid intake because of losses from inadequate kidney function or insufficient intake resulting from a declining thirst mechanism.[4]

The treatment procedures for ill patients contribute some unusual sources of water. For example, enteral (tube) feeding formulas contain a large quantity of water and therefore are a significant part of fluid intake. Likewise, intravenous fluids represent a major source of water for some ill patients.

Losses

The body has several routes for water output. Generally, losses are divided into *obligatory* losses, or those necessary to carry out body waste elimination, and *facultative* losses, which depend on the body's need to conserve or eliminate water through the urine or to regulate internal temperature.

In normal circumstances, the kidneys eliminate the greatest volume of water. This amount varies according to the body's need to conserve or eliminate water and an individual's intake. Typically, an adult eliminates between 1200 and 1500 mL of water per day in the urine. The kidneys require a minimum volume of water to eliminate waste materials.[5]

Insensible loss is the moisture that continuously evaporates from the lungs and skin. This amount is usually estimated at 800 to 1000 mL/d but it varies in the presence of disease states or changes in environmental temperature. Fever and increased respirations increase insensible loss, as does a rise in the outside air temperature or increased exercise. These variations can increase insensible loss to 1400 mL/d or more.[4]

For dynamic fluid balance to be maintained, fluid loss must be offset by an equivalent intake. Measurements of these gains and losses are essential nursing interventions in aiding patients to maintain fluid balance. Clinical Guideline 34–1 presents usual fluid gains and losses in a healthy adult.

CLINICAL GUIDELINE 34–1

AVERAGE DAILY FLUID GAINS AND LOSSES

FLUID GAINS

Ingested liquids	1200–1500 mL
Ingested food	1000 mL
Metabolic H_2O	300 mL
Total	2500–2800 mL

FLUID LOSSES

Urine	1200–1500 mL
Stool	100 mL
Lungs	300–500 mL
Skin	600–800 mL
Total	2200–2900 mL

CONSIDERATIONS

1. Liquid gains will usually match losses as long as the thirst mechanism is intact, and a patient is able to ingest fluids.
2. Insensible losses are extremely variable because of the outside air temperature, patient's exercise level, elevations in body temperature, and so on.

CHEMICAL COMPOSITION OF BODY FLUIDS

Body fluid dynamics depend on the balance of body fluid constituents across the fluid compartments. Three types of substances are responsible for this balance: electrolytes, nonelectrolytes, and colloids.

Electrolytes

Certain chemical compounds break down when placed in solution and carry electrical charges. They are referred to as ions. Ions dissolved in body water are called **electrolytes,** primarily because they lend the characteristic of electrical conductance to body water. Acids, bases, and salts are examples of electrolytes found in body fluid.

Electrolytes are classified by the charge they carry. Positively charged electrolytes are referred to as **cations.** Negatively charged electrolytes are called **anions.** The most important cations in body fluid are sodium (Na^+), potassium (K^+), calcium (Ca^{2+}), and magnesium (Mg^{2+}). Physiologically important anions are chloride (Cl^-), bicarbonate (HCO_3^-), and phosphate (PO_4^-).

At any given time, the cation and anion concentrations of the body fluid compartments must be balanced to maintain physiologic stability. Increases in cations are always offset by increases in anions. Thus, conversely, decreases in cations are balanced by decreases in anions. Body regulatory mechanisms depend on an overall balance. They also depend on the presence of specific amounts of the various types of cations and anions that go into creating an electrochemical balance. Too much or too little of one or another cation or anion can result in serious signs and symptoms such as cardiac irregularities, respiratory depression, muscular weakness, or even a decreased level of consciousness.

Because the ion concentration of body fluid is small, concentrations are expressed as milliequivalents. The common practice is to define the concentration of physiologic fluids in terms of milliequivalents per liter of solution (mEq/L).

Table 34–2 shows the ion concentrations present in body fluid. Concentrations vary from compartment to compartment. Sodium is the major extracellular cation, with average concentrations of 140 mEq/L in the ECF and 10 mEq/L in the ICF. Potassium is the major intracellular cation.

Electrolyte balance within the fluid compartments is as important as balance between the compartments. Thus, within the ECF, cation concentration is balanced with anion concentration. When balance is maintained, functions such as optimal neuromuscular irritability and proper distribution of fluids are protected. The electrolyte concentrations typically vary within extremely limited ranges. Disturbances in concentrations of electrolytes have important physiologic consequences, which will be discussed later in this chapter.

Nonelectrolytes

Some of the particles dissolved in body fluid are not electrolytes, and do not break down into charged particles. Nevertheless these nonelectrolytes, are important components of body fluid and contribute to fluid movement between compartments. One such sub-

TABLE 34-2. ION CONCENTRATIONS IN EXTRACELLULAR AND INTRACELLULAR COMPARTMENTS

Cation	mEq/L	Anion	mEq/L
Extracellular Compartment			
Intravascular Fluid (Plasma)			
Sodium	142	Chloride	103
Potassium	5	Bicarbonate	26
Calcium	5	Phosphate	2
Magnesium	2	Sulfate	1
		Organic acids	5
		Proteinate	17
Intracellular Compartment (approximate)			
Sodium	10	Chloride	5
Potassium	150	Bicarbonate	10
Calcium	2	Phosphate } Sulfate }	150
Magnesium	40		
		Proteinate	40

Source: Metheny NL. Fluid and Electrolyte Balance: Nursing Considerations. *3rd ed. Philadelphia: Lippincott; 1996.*

stance is glucose. Glucose is vital to cellular metabolism. It is the chief source of cellular energy; however, when glucose accumulates in excessive amounts in the ECF, it pulls body water with it as it exits in the urine, creating a fluid volume deficit. Ultimately, the ICF may also lose fluid, creating a critical state of fluid volume deficit.

Colloids

Proteins in the intravascular compartment are important constituents of body fluid. They occur not as electrolytes but as large molecules called colloids. Because of their size, colloids cannot easily diffuse between compartments. Albumin and globulins are examples of colloidal, or plasma, proteins. The concentration of colloids in the intravascular compartment is important in regulating fluid movement into and out of the intravascular space. Although most proteins are colloids, one form, proteinate, carries an anionic charge. Proteinate is an important constituent of the intracellular compartment and participates in the electrochemical balance of the ICF.

COMPOSITION OF BLOOD

Blood, a vital portion of the extracellular fluid, consists of two components. Plasma is the liquid, noncellular portion, accounting for approximately 55 percent of blood volume. The second component, which is largely composed of cells, accounts for the remaining 45 percent of blood volume.

Plasma is a straw-colored watery substance comprising water and plasma proteins (albumin, fibrinogen, and gamma globulin). Antibodies, various nutrients, metabolic wastes, dissolved gases, enzymes, and electrolytes are also contained within plasma. Basically, plasma serves as a vehicle of transport for nutrient and waste exchange. The cellular components of blood, which travel in the plasma, are the red cells, the white cells, and the platelets. Blood also contains antibodies essential for immunologic protection. These antibodies make blood typing possible. (See the section on *Transfusion Therapy* later in this chapter.)

BODY FLUID DYNAMICS

Movement of Body Fluids

Cell life is preserved and supported by the movement of fluid and solutes between the intracellular and extracellular compartments. The compartments are separated by membranes capable of selective permeability. In other words, body water and certain solutes pass with relative ease through the membranes, whereas some large-particle solutes and proteins cannot. Several critical processes, including diffusion, osmosis, active transport, and filtration, regulate the movement of body fluids.

Diffusion

Diffusion is the process by which solutes in the form of ions and molecules move among each other in a solvent from an area of high solute concentration to an area of low solute concentration. Certain substances, for example, water, diffuse more easily than others. Diffusion helps maintain

- the balance of electrolytes between the ICF and ECF compartments
- the absorption of nutrients across the GI tract into the bloodstream
- the passage of molecules from the bloodstream across the tubular membrane of the nephron into the urine for elimination[6]

Osmosis

Osmosis is the movement of a solvent (eg, water) through a selectively permeable membrane from an area of high water concentration to an area of low water concentration. This movement of water will create two solutions of equal concentration but unequal volume.[7]

A simple experiment illustrates the principle of osmosis. If a pouch made of a selectively permeable membrane is filled with a salt solution and submerged in a container of distilled water, it will expand. Water crosses the membrane into the pouch, seeking to dilute the concentration of salt and to balance the concentration of water on either side of the membrane. If the solutions are reversed so that the distilled water is inside and the salt solution outside, the pouch will shrink for the same reason.

The osmolality of fluid is an important concept in understanding body fluid balance. *Osmolality* is a measure of concentration of active particles in a volume of solution. Normal **serum osmolality** is 275 to 295 mOsm/kg.[8]

Tonicity, a term related to osmolality, refers to the capacity of a fluid for osmotic activity. Solutions of the same concentration are said to be **isotonic** to one another; that is, they create no osmotic movement of water across a selectively permeable membrane. In the body, plasma is the standard of concentration with which other fluids are compared. Fluids that have the same concentration as plasma are said to be isotonic to plasma.

Hypertonic solutions carry a greater concentration of solutes than plasma and thus have a higher osmolality. If a blood cell were suspended in a hypertonic solution, it would rapidly lose its internal cellular fluid to the solution and shrivel (a process known as crenation).

Hypotonic solutions, on the other hand, have lower osmolality than plasma; they are more dilute than plasma. Clinically, hypotonic solutions are infused into the body to replace the fluid lost in dehydration states. (See *Intravenous Solutions* for further discussion.)

Movement of fluid between the intracellular and extracellular compartments is generally governed by the osmolality of the fluids on either side of the cell membrane. Since osmolality is difficult to measure inside the cell, the osmolality of blood serum is measured to determine the fluid state of the ECF. From the serum measurement, inferences can be made as to the condition of the ICF, since a state of electrochemical balance is assumed to exist between the compartments.

Active Transport

Active transport is the mechanism by which ions travel against a concentration gradient. In other words, ions travel from areas of low concentration to areas of high concentration. This requires a substance to carry the ions and energy to fuel the process.

For instance, when nerve impulses are transmitted, sodium moves into the cell and potassium out of the cell into the ECF. For nerve cells to be able to continue transmitting impulses, the intracellular sodium concentration must be kept low. The so-called sodium pump accomplishes the necessary exchange by active transport. Sodium inside the cell attaches to a lipoprotein carrier substance and moves outside the cell, where it is released. The lipoprotein then chemically changes to accept potassium, which is moved to the inside of the cell. The energy substance that fuels the process is adenosine triphosphate (ATP), which is contained within the cell.[9]

Filtration

Filtration is the movement of body fluids through a selectively permeable membrane in response to pressure. Fluids have a natural tendency to move from an area of high pressure to an area of low pressure. In the body, opposing pressure forces between fluid compartments maintain a dynamic balance. Two forces, hydrostatic pressure and colloid osmotic pressure, maintain this balance.[7]

ELECTROLYTES IN BODY FLUID

Sodium

As the most prevalent electrolyte in the ECF, sodium (NA^+) is the major contributor to the osmotic force. The saying "where salt goes, water follows" defines the primary role of sodium in water distribution and maintaining ECF volume. In addition, sodium participates in neuromuscular excitation, transmission of nerve impulses, and acid–base balance.[9]

The sodium concentration in the ECF ranges between 135 and 145 mEq/L. Substantial quantities of sodium are found in gastric, intestinal, and pancreatic secretions and bile. Therefore, significant losses of these fluids can quickly deplete the ECF of sodium. Maintaining sodium stores to ensure body fluid balance is so important that the body has safety mechanisms to conserve sodium. These are discussed later in this chapter. Table 34–3 lists the functions of sodium and other common electrolytes.

Potassium

Potassium (K^+) is the predominant intracellular electrolyte. Although it continuously moves into and out of the cells, approximately 98 percent remains in the ICF. Therefore, potassium plays an important role in maintaining the intracellular osmolality. Only the 2 percent of the body's potassium in the ECF can be measured. It is maintained within very narrow limits at 3.5 to 5.5 mEq/L.

Potassium's most important role is in influencing neuromuscular excitability. Potassium also contributes to acid-base balance by exchanging with hydrogen ions (H^+) between the ICF and ECF. This shift helps maintain the balance of electrical charges between the compartments (electroneutrality), and frees the H^+ ions (acids) for elimination.[10]

Ordinarily, when the dietary intake of potassium is maintained and there is no other source of loss, the output of potassium balances the intake through a combination of renal tubular secretion and reabsorption mechanisms; however, when there is an added source of loss, such as when the renal mechanisms are altered through the use of diuretics, potassium supplements often become necessary. Likewise, when potassium excretion is diminished, such as when the kidneys fail to produce urine, it is often necessary to restrict potassium intake.[11]

Calcium

Calcium (Ca^{2+}) is the most abundant electrolyte in the human body, but all except 1 percent occurs in an inactive form as bone. The remaining 1 percent is contained in the cells or ECF. The calcium in the plasma is either bound to proteins as a reserve or is in the active ionized form. Total serum calcium, which reflects both the free calcium in the blood and the calcium bound to proteins, varies from 9 to 11 mg/dL. The serum value for ionized calcium is 4.4 to 5.9 mg/dL.

Calcium serves several important functions in the body. For example, calcium maintains bone strength and durability. It serves an important role in the transmission of nerve impulses, in particular affecting cardiac electrical conduction. Calcium maintains cellular permeability and promotes blood clotting by combining with the various clotting factors.

Maintaining calcium levels depends not only on intake but also on the physiologic mechanisms governing calcium absorption. Vitamin D must be present in sufficient quantities for adequate absorption to take place from the GI tract. Parathyroid hormone (PTH) and calcitonin influence liberation and deposition of calcium from bone and thus affect daily need for the electrolyte.[3]

Magnesium

The greatest percentage of magnesium (Mg^{2+}) is located in the bone. Only 1 percent of the body's magnesium occurs in the ECF. Hence, the serum value of magnesium is only 1.5 to 2.5 mEq/L in the ECF.

Magnesium is responsible for the functioning of the intracellular carrier substances used in active transport. As a result, magnesium contributes significantly to neuromuscular transmission in cardiac and skeletal muscle.

There is an interplay between magnesium, potassium, and calcium. Insufficient magnesium intake results in K^+ leaving the cell

TABLE 34-3. SERUM ELECTROLYTES AND THEIR FUNCTIONS IN THE BODY

Electrolyte	Function
Sodium (Na^+)	Transmission and conduction of nerve impulses Regulation of osmolality of ECF Sodium pump regulation Acid–base balance (in combination with buffers)
Potassium (K^+)	Neuromuscular function—nerve impulse transmission Muscular contractility (smooth, skeletal, and cardiac) Regulation of osmolality of ICF Maintenance of acid–base balance by exchanging with H^+ ions (acids) to maintain electroneutrality and free H^+ ions for elimination
Calcium (Ca^{2+})	Maintenance of cell permeability Neuromuscular function—nerve impulse transmission to myocardium and skeletal muscle Combines with various clotting factors to promote blood coagulation Maintenance of bone and tooth strength and durability
Magnesium (Mg^{2+})	Neural transmission (CNS) Neuromuscular activity—myocardial Enzyme activator Maintenance of carrier substances for sodium pump Protein and carbohydrate metabolism
Phosphorus (PO_4^-)	Involved in formation of ATP, the main source of cellular energy Maintenance of neuromuscular function Maintenance of bone and tooth strength Utilization of B-complex vitamins Maintenance of cell membrane structure Acid–base buffering; combines with Na^+ and H^+ to provide for acid–base and electrolyte balance in the kidney tubules
Chloride (Cl^-)	Competes with bicarbonate for combination with Na^+, and exchanges with bicarbonate ions in red blood cells, to maintain acid–base balance Maintenance of ECF osmolality

Source: Metheny NL. Fluid and Electrolyte Balance: Nursing Considerations. *3rd ed. Philadelphia: Lippincott; 1996.*

and being excreted in large quantities in the urine, thereby creating electrolyte imbalance. Magnesium competes with calcium for absorption from the GI tract. Generally, the electrolyte in most abundance at any one time will be absorbed in the greatest quantity.

Phosphorus

Phosphorus in the form of phosphate (PO_4^-) is a critically important intracellular anion. It occurs in the ICF and ECF in relatively small quantities and is maintained in an inactive form in the bone. Serum phosphorus levels are usually 2.5 to 4.5 mg/dL.

Phosphorus is important primarily in the formation of ATP, the main source of cellular energy. It plays a part in all cellular function, including neuromuscular excitability and maintaining cellular membrane structure; it combines with sodium and hydrogen in the kidney tubules to maintain acid–base and electrolyte balance.

Phosphorus and calcium have an inverse relationship in the body: When calcium levels are low, phosphorus levels are high, and vice versa.

Chloride

Chloride (Cl^-) is an anion found abundantly in the ECF. The normal serum value for chloride is 95 to 105 mEq/L. Chloride exists most often in combination with sodium and therefore acts to maintain ECF osmolality. Chloride also competes with bicarbonate for combination with sodium, thereby affecting acid–base balance. In addition, chloride exchanges with bicarbonate ions in the red blood cells to maintain acid–base balance.

BODY FLUID REGULATION

Organs that Regulate Body Fluids

In healthy persons, closely coordinated physiologic functions provide for a balance in the composition, volume, and distribution of body fluids. Through a series of physical and chemical feedback responses, most of the body's major organs continuously correct deviations in fluid balance. (See Chap. 8 for more on feedback responses.) The activation of any of these processes depends on the particular deviation. The roles of several of the body organs in body fluid regulation are described in the following paragraphs.

Brain. The brain regulates the intake and secretion of water and salt centrally. For example, areas in the medulla control plasma volume. Information from stretch receptors in the atria of the heart and pressure receptors in the atria and pulmonary arteries is fed to the brain centers. In turn, the brain triggers compensatory adjustments in the heart's rate and contractile force.

In addition, the brain monitors body fluid osmolality through osmoreceptors in the hypothalamus. The thirst sensation and the circulating level of antidiuretic hormone (ADH) is adjusted through this mechanism, resulting in the intake of fluids as well as changes in renal filtration and urine formation. (ADH is discussed in more detail under *Endocrine Glands.*)

Skin. The skin is involved in body fluid balance through the action of water and salt removal. Through sweating and evaporation, body water is lost and body temperature is regulated. The skin is thus primarily an organ of water elimination; however, it also serves as a protective barrier to conserve body water. Widespread loss of the skin, such as in third-degree burns, results in the loss of excessive quantities of body fluid.

Unobservable loss of moisture from the skin is referred to as *insensible loss*. Visible perspiration is referred to as sensible loss. The amount of fluid lost from the skin, both sensible and insensible, depends on environmental air temperature and an individual's level of hydration and rate of exercise.

Humidity is one of the most important factors contributing to fluid loss through the skin. Saturated environmental air cannot pick up additional moisture; however, dry air can, and it thereby increases the rate of water evaporation. Thus when the surrounding air is hot and dry, the loss of water through the skin increases.

Lungs. Under normal conditions, the lungs are a site of insensible water loss. Moisture from the pulmonary membranes is picked up and removed, in droplet form, in expired air. The amount of fluid lost depends on the rate and depth of ventilation and the humidity of the environmental air. Fast, deep ventilation increases insensible loss, as does low environmental humidity.

Heart. The pumping action of the heart supplies fluid to the peripheral tissues and the organs that maintain and modify the body's fluid and solute balance. Heart failure interrupts circulation, which results in underperfusion and congestion of blood in body organs. This can lead to widespread shifts in fluid between body compartments. Conversely, cardiovascular performance depends on fluid balance for sufficient blood volume.

Endocrine Glands. Three glands play central roles in regulating extracellular fluid composition: the pituitary, the adrenals, and the parathyroid. The secretion of hormones from these glands alters the reabsorption of body water and electrolytes.

ADH is secreted by the posterior pituitary primarily in response to changes in serum osmolality. It may also be secreted as a consequence of lowered blood volume and stress factors such as trauma, pain, and anxiety. ADH adjusts water output from the kidney. An increase in the secretion of ADH helps conserve body water. As balance is restored, neurochemical signals are fed back to the pituitary, resulting in the cessation of ADH production.

The adrenal glands produce several hormones that help adjust extracellular fluid concentration. The primary adrenal hormone affecting fluid balance is aldosterone. Aldosterone is secreted in response to the powerful vasoconstrictive substance angiotensin II as part of a sophisticated mechanism for maintaining blood volume and controlling blood pressure. Aldosterone is also secreted in response to an elevation of potassium ions in the ECF and, in turn, acts on the kidneys to promote potassium excretion. Aldosterone causes the renal tubules to conserve sodium ions, resulting in a corresponding secondary water retention.

Other adrenal hormones, such as cortisone and corticosterone, also produce sodium and water retention. Under certain pathologic conditions, increased levels of adrenal hormones cause excessive water and sodium retention. Conversely, insufficient levels of the hormones result in excessive sodium and water loss.

Finally, the parathyroid glands secrete parathyroid hormone (PTH), which controls the extracellular concentrations of calcium and phosphorus ions. PTH secretion results initially in calcium resorption from the bone, as well as absorption of calcium from the intestines and renal tubules. This raises the level of ionized calcium in the serum and subsequently lowers the phosphorus level.[3]

Kidneys. Through control of water reabsorption and excretion, the kidneys play a central role in maintaining blood volume. The kidneys, composed of approximately two million working units known as nephrons, receive and filter the plasma portion of the blood at the rate of 180 L a day. Unless most of this fluid were reabsorbed, the body would quickly dry out and would lose electrolytes and other essential compounds. In fact, only an average of 1200 to 1500 mL of urine is produced each day. The kidneys are also important in maintaining the balance of acids, bases, and salts, primarily through renal tubular reabsorption and excretion (see Chap. 29 for further discussion).

Gastrointestinal Tract. Fluid and solutes are ingested through the mouth and absorbed by the stomach and intestines. Thus, replenishing body water and electrolytes is a vital gastrointestinal function. The intestinal tract not only absorbs fluid ingested orally but also reabsorbs glandular and GI secretions.

Gastrointestinal fluids pass rapidly through the gastric and intestinal membranes by passive diffusion and active transport. This rapid turnover of fluids, estimated at 3 L every 90 minutes, renders body fluid balance extremely vulnerable to excessive loss caused by dysfunctions of the GI tract.

Liver. Plasma proteins produced in the liver are essential to maintaining the circulating blood volume. These proteins maintain an osmotic pressure in the intravascular compartment that favors the retention of fluid. When the liver is diseased and insufficient plasma proteins are produced, this osmotic pressure cannot be maintained. The loss of pressure results in fluid shifts from the intravascular compartment, which affect the other fluid compartments as well.

Lymphatics. The lymph channels serve to return fluid from the interstitial spaces to the venous circulation. The flow of lymph occurs as lymph channels are squeezed by contracting skeletal muscles. When lymph channels become blocked, fluid builds up in the interstitial spaces. The increased pressure within the interstitial compartment results in increased fluid in the intravascular compartment, restoring equilibrium.

Homeostatic Mechanisms

The functions of the body's organs in regulating body fluid homeostasis are finely coordinated. Multiple mechanisms complement one another to regulate the intake, conservation, and excretion of water and salt.

Water and Salt Intake. Thirst, a conscious, subjective desire to take in fluids, is essential in regulating fluid intake. When extracellular fluid osmolality exceeds 295 mOsm/L, receptors in the hypothalamus activate the cerebral cortex to create the sensation of thirst. Although changes in ECF osmolality are the prime stimulus for thirst, decreased blood volume, increased salt intake, and dryness of the mouth may activate the thirst mechanism.[11]

Water and salt intake is also influenced by depletion of body fluids through excessive sweating or dysfunctional renal salt conservation. Although little is known about the mechanism that governs salt intake, much is known about the link to salt excretion and resultant craving for it. Aldosterone, the adrenal mineralocorticoid responsible for sodium conservation, is linked to salt intake. Without sufficient amounts of aldosterone, the kidneys excrete sodium. This depletes the extracellular fluid of sodium and creates a desire for salt.

Water and Salt Conservation. The conservation of water and salt in the body results from the interplay of several physiologic mechanisms, triggered principally by volume depletion, such as caused by hemorrhage or significantly reduced fluid intake. The mechanisms include:

- interstitial to intravascular fluid shifts to maintain blood pressure and perfusion of essential organs
- vasoconstriction in renal blood flow mediated by the sympathetic nervous system, so sodium and water are retained
- increased aldosterone secretion, which stimulates increased renal reabsorption of sodium and, therefore, water
- a rise in ADH secretion, also increasing kidney water reabsorption. This response is stimulated by falling blood pressure and serum osmolality.

Water and Salt Excretion. Water and salt excretion occurs essentially through the reversal of several conservation mechanisms. Excretion, like conservation, is automatically regulated, so that excessive intake is offset by accelerating the feedback mechanisms controlling output. Thus water and salt are excreted at higher rates as a result of:

- increases in blood pressure and glomerular filtration rates
- suppression of ADH secretion through detection of lowered serum osmolality
- a reduction in collecting duct permeability and water reabsorption
- increased renal tubular flow rate, producing increased filtrate
- increased fluid intake stimulating the appropriate hormone feedback mechanism for excretion.

Through the mechanisms regulating water and salt intake, conservation, and excretion, the body maintains a dynamic balance. Reductions in intake of sodium, other electrolytes, or water trigger appropriate conservation. Conversely, excessive intake of water and solutes leads to the initiation of feedback mechanisms that result in excretion.

ACID–BASE BALANCE

Acid–base balance is technically complicated and can be confusing. Yet an understanding of the balance between acids and bases in the body fluids is critical. Balance can be rapidly interrupted and requires swift intervention.

Definition of Acid and Base

In simple terms, an *acid* is a substance that breaks down and relinquishes hydrogen ions (H^+). A *base* is a substance that accepts hydrogen ions. The strength of acids and bases is expressed in terms of **pH,** the measure of the acidity or alkalinity of a fluid. Basically pH signifies the H^+ ion concentration of a solution. As H^+ concentration increases, the pH decreases (becomes more acidic), and as H^+ concentration decreases, the pH increases (becomes more alkaline).

pH of Body Fluids

The pH of various body fluids fluctuates constantly because different amounts of carbon dioxide and metabolic acids are present under various conditions; however, these fluctuations are maintained within narrow parameters. For example, arterial blood pH is held within a range of 7.35 to 7.45[12] (see Fig. 34–2).

The pH of specific body fluids reflects the acid concentrations necessary to carry out specific physiologic roles. For example, acid is necessary to facilitate the digestive processes in the stomach. Lower in the GI tract, however, the alkaline pancreatic fluid is necessary to neutralize the highly acidic gastric fluids. This prevents corrosion of the fragile intestinal mucosa. Optimal H^+ concentrations are also necessary for proper cell function and the efficient operation of enzyme systems. When cellular acid content becomes too high, enzyme proteins are denatured, rendering the cell dysfunctional. Plasma hydrogen ion concentration is involved in the binding and release of oxygen and hemoglobin and hence plays a critical role in the transport of oxygen to the cell.

Buffer Systems

Acid–base balance is maintained in a dynamic balance by the constant activity of buffers. **Buffers** are substances that combine with acids and bases to prevent excessive changes in pH. Acids formed in the body, or introduced into it, combine with buffer bases and become weaker acids. Bases combine with the buffer acids and become weaker bases. In other words, buffers partially neutralize excessive acids or bases in the body. The primary chemical buffer

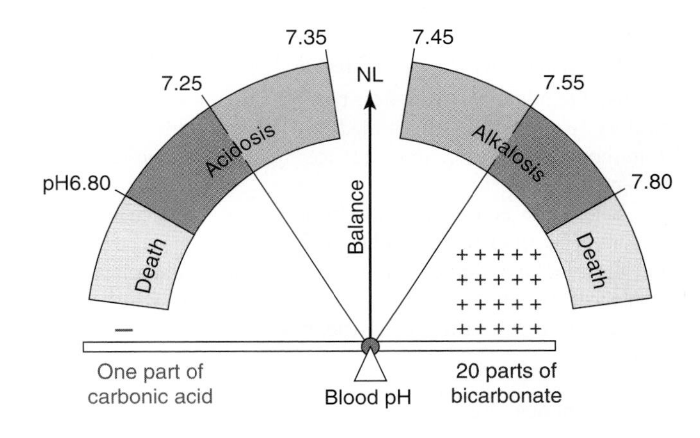

Figure 34–2. The ranges of blood pH. Normal blood pH is within the narrow range of 7.35 to 7.45.

system in the body is the carbonic acid–bicarbonate system. Other less important chemical buffer systems include phosphates, proteins, and hemoglobin. These buffer systems provide either immediate control or continuous fine-tuning of acid–base balance.

Carbonic Acid–Bicarbonate System. Carbonic acid and bicarbonate constitute the buffer pair in highest concentration in the ECF. They are held at a ratio of 20:1 for bicarbonate (HCO_3^-) to carbonic acid (H_2CO_3), primarily as a result of the reabsorption of bicarbonate by the kidneys and the body's ability to transform any base and carbon dioxide into bicarbonate.[13] A change in this ratio results in degrees of acidosis or alkalosis, discussed later in this chapter.

Metabolism creates many strong organic and inorganic acids. Bicarbonate combines with these acids to form carbonic acid and a neutral salt. The carbonic acid further splits into carbon dioxide and water, which are eliminated, in varying quantities, from the lungs. Conversely, should a strong base be added to the body, carbonic acid combines with it to form sodium bicarbonate ($NaHCO_3$) and water (H_2O), both used in maintaining body fluid balance. The following equation illustrates this process:

NaOH	+	H_2CO_3	→	$NaHCO_3$	+	H_2O
sodium hydroxide (strong base)	+	carbonic acid (weak acid)	→	sodium bicarbonate (weak base)	+	water (neutral compound)

The carbonic acid–bicarbonate system reacts rapidly to regulate pH. Its activity can cause changes in serum carbon dioxide concentration, leading to altered respiratory rate to control carbon dioxide excretion. It is, however, a temporizing system that requires the support of other buffering systems to maintain overall, ongoing acid–base balance in the body.

Respiratory Regulation of Acid-Base Balance

The respiratory system also is activated by the central nervous system to maintain acid–base balance. Increased hydrogen ion concentration in the cerebrospinal fluid immediately stimulates the medulla to alter respiratory rate. As the cerebrospinal fluid becomes more acidic, the medulla responds by increasing the respiratory rate to eliminate the excess CO_2 and thereby normalize pH. Conversely, when the serum pH rises, indicating alkalosis, the respiratory center rapidly responds and slows the rate of breathing in order to retain CO_2 and correct the acid–base balance.

Renal Regulation of Acid–Base Balance

The renal regulation of acid–base balance is much slower than respiratory regulation. Changes mediated by the kidneys may take from hours to 1 to 2 days to accomplish the fine-tuning of acid–base balance.

Regulation is accomplished by increasing or decreasing the amount of bicarbonate reabsorbed and by releasing hydrogen ions into the tubular fluid for elimination or replenishment of buffer substances. Bicarbonate is reabsorbed with sodium, which serves the dual purpose of regulating acid–base balance and conserving sodium.

Summary of Acid–Base Homeostasis

The slightly alkaline character of arterial blood and the neutral pH of most body cells are protected, moment to moment, primarily by the chemical reactions that occur between acids, bases, and buffer substances in the body fluid. It is also protected over short periods by adequate respiratory ventilation and over longer periods by the renal excretion of nonvolatile acids.

The body is always vulnerable to drastic shifts in pH. Homeostasis is maintained, moment to moment, primarily by buffer control. Buffers are capable of split-second chemical reaction. They immediately combine with any acid or alkali and thereby prevent excessive changes in H^+ concentration.

If H^+ concentration does change measurably, the respiratory center is immediately stimulated to alter the rate of pulmonary ventilation. A change in ventilatory rate automatically changes the rate of carbon dioxide removal from body fluid. Although this is not instantaneous, it is nevertheless a rapid reaction, requiring only 1 to 3 minutes to alter ventilation.

The kidney also responds to a change in H^+ concentration by changing the acidity of the urine through the reabsorption of bicarbonate and the excretion of hydrogen ions. Through the renal mechanism, acid–base balance is adjusted over several hours or days.

CRITICAL QUERY

Chernoff[4] notes that one of the consequences of dehydration in old age is that a loss of body fluid increases the concentration of instilled or ingested medications per kilogram of body weight. What implications does this have for the care of patients taking regular medications?

FACTORS AFFECTING FLUID AND ELECTROLYTE BALANCE

AGE

Body weight, body surface area, renal filtration capacity, and metabolic rate influence required fluid intake at differing ages. As previously noted, the ratio of body water to weight in infants is high. In the full-term newborn, approximately 75 percent of weight is body water; this drops to 65 percent by 6 months of age and to 60 percent by age 2 years. Normal losses occur through rapid respirations, perspiration, and dilute urine from immature kidneys.[14] In addition, ill infants and small children can rapidly become dehydrated during an illness that causes abnormal losses due to the high percentage of their body weight that is water, their accelerated metabolic rate, and their immature water conservation mechanisms.[4]

As individuals advance in age, the kidneys lose nephrons, resulting in decreased renal concentrating ability and increased loss of water and salt. Aging may also be accompanied by a muting of the thirst response, leading to decreased intake. Chronic diseases such as cardiac disease, renal and hepatic disease, and diabetes can result in either severe losses of water and salts or retention of fluids, which can alter normal physiologic functions.[4]

CLIMATE

High heat and low environmental humidity increase sweating and fluid loss. Heavy sweating accompanies exertion in hot, dry atmos-

INSIGHTS FROM NURSING LITERATURE

WHAT DETERMINES HOW MUCH FLUID THE ELDERLY DRINK?

Gaspar PM. What determines how much patients drink? Geriatr Nurs. *July/August 1988:221–224.*

In this classic, often-cited study, the researcher identified factors that affect intake volume among the elderly. The study, conducted in two rural Midwestern nursing homes, observed 67 elderly subjects ranging in age from 75 to 95 years. For 1 week, the observers recorded data on food and fluid intake and the environmental circumstances at the time. The average fluid intake was 1893 mL per day, with a range of 833 to 2863 mL. When the data for subjects were compared against an adult intake standard, the average intake was only 76 percent of the required amount. Age was inversely associated with water intake adequacy; as age increased, water intake decreased.

Variables found associated with water intake were speaking ability, visual capacity, opportunities for water ingestion, and time that water is in reach. Subjects who were functionally dependent actually had a greater chance of meeting water intake requirements than those who were more independent. Subjects who were immobile were offered water more frequently and drank more than subjects who were able to reach it for themselves.

pheric conditions. Exercise on a hot day may result in loss of up to 5 L of fluid and 10 to 20 times the usual amount of salt lost in a day. Failure to replace body fluids can result in heat exhaustion, which is characterized by decreased vascular volume and low cardiac output.

STRESS

Physiologic stressors are important in body fluid balance. Stress leads to stimulation of the pituitary gland and release of ADH. This causes the body to retain water and sodium and reduce urine output. This is a short-term defense mechanism for maintaining blood volume in the face of a physiologic threat.

DIET

Adequate intake of fluid and nutrients is crucial to maintaining body fluid and electrolyte balance. Starvation causes the body to metabolize its own tissue for energy. As fat stores are consumed, ketones, which are strong acids, are produced. This additional acid load creates a shift in the acid–base balance toward the acidotic state.

Starvation also leads to a decrease in available proteins. The proteins are metabolized to provide the body with energy and are not replaced. Therefore, new proteins, particularly albumin, cannot be synthesized. The result is an inability to maintain intravascular osmotic pressure. Fluid will then shift from the intravascular to the interstitial compartment, decreasing vascular volume and pressure.

ILLNESS

Several common clinical conditions are associated with fluid and electrolyte imbalances. A knowledge of these conditions helps nurses anticipate patients' fluid and salt replacement needs.

Nausea and Vomiting

Nausea and vomiting affect both intake and output. Nausea frequently results in insufficient intake of food and fluids. Vomiting results in the loss of electrolyte- and hydrogen-rich fluids from the stomach and intestines. As the GI tract produces approximately 6 L of fluid per day, prolonged vomiting can result in rapid fluid depletion. Additionally, vomiting of gastric contents results in the loss of hydrogen ions, which over a period may lead to elevated bicarbonate levels, shifting the acid–base balance to alkalosis.

Diarrhea

As with vomiting, the loss of fluids and electrolytes through diarrhea can quickly lead to fluid volume deficit, serum electrolyte abnormalities, and shifts in acid-base balance. Because of the relatively high bicarbonate ion content in intestinal fluid, severe diarrhea can result in metabolic acidosis, from bicarbonate loss and relative hydrogen ion excess. Sodium and potassium deficits also accompany diarrhea, exacerbating dehydration.

Increased Metabolism

Insensible fluid loss is increased by any influence that speeds metabolism. Thus a rise in body temperature, which accelerates metabolic rate, results in increased losses through the lungs and skin. Fevers between 101°F and 103°F increase the fluid requirements of adults by 500 mL per day; those above 103°F increase requirements by 1000 mL.[3] Fever also increases the respiratory rate, which leads to further water loss through the expired air.

Wounds and Burns

Large wounds and burns provide avenues for the loss of considerable quantities of body water, electrolytes, and protein. Wound drainage, or transudate, is similar to plasma but contains a greater portion of water and electrolytes. Burn exudate, on the other hand, is actual plasma loss from the damaged extracellular compartment.

Burns represent a more complex fluid problem than simple ECF depletion. Compensatory fluid shifts between the intravascular and interstitial compartments often occur within 48 hours of a burn injury. Sodium and calcium deficits commonly accompany these large fluid losses. Potassium ions are lost as a result of liberation from the damaged cells. Because potassium levels in the body are tightly controlled by the kidneys, potassium lost from damaged cells is excreted as long as the kidneys are functioning normally. Thus, as the tissue damaged by a large burn begins to heal, the patient may require potassium supplements.

MEDICATIONS

The excessive use of cathartics (agents that stimulate bowel elimination) and enemas can have effects similar to those of diarrhea on fluid and electrolyte balance. Some types of cathartics and enemas stimulate bowel evacuation by irritating the smooth muscle of the intestine. This can result in fluid volume deficit from excessive water and electrolyte loss.

Diuretics are agents that are used in the treatment of generalized fluid volume excesses. They affect the renal tubules' reabsorption and excretion of water, sodium, potassium, and chloride. All diuretics increase urine output and thus may cause fluid volume deficit. Diuretics are classified according to their effect on potassium ion loss: potassium-wasting diuretics maintain the body's conservation of sodium, but result in increased loss of potassium; potassium-sparing diuretics act to conserve potassium but may create dangerously high serum potassium levels.

The adrenal cortical hormones, or steroids, are some of the body's chief regulators of water and salt balance. These hormones affect water retention by altering renal tubular reabsorption of sodium. When the adrenal glands are removed or become dysfunctional, excessive sodium and water may be lost in the urine. Serum potassium levels often rise as potassium ions are saved in the place of sodium. Conversely, when the adrenals are overactive or when steroids are given for their antiinflammatory or immunosuppressive effects, increased sodium and water are retained, often creating edema. This accelerates the loss of potassium ions in the urine.

MEDICAL TREATMENTS

Many medical treatments may result in secondary losses of fluids and electrolytes. Although the particular treatment may be necessary to accomplish therapeutic objectives, the health care team must prevent fluid and electrolyte problems through replacement therapy or other means.

Continuous gastric and intestinal suctioning usually produces many of the imbalances seen with persistent vomiting. To prevent fluid imbalances, intravenous fluids are given to replace the lost water and electrolytes. While intravenous therapy is not an independent nursing action, nurses must be alert to body fluid problems to collaborate with physicians to ensure that replacement is instituted.

One practice that increases the potential for fluid and electrolyte imbalances is that of irrigating the suction tubing with hypotonic solutions such as distilled water. Distilled water is rapidly absorbed from the stomach into the interstitium and leads to the dilution of serum electrolytes. To avoid this situation, only isotonic solutions should be used for gastric irrigation.

Gavage feedings (described in Chap. 28) may result in fluid and electrolyte depletion. Although gavage feedings are given to prevent starvation, many solutions are several times more concentrated than blood serum. Introducing these solutions repeatedly into the GI tract can draw excessive fluid from the interstitium of the intestinal wall, causing osmotic diarrhea. Recently, however, the formulas of many of the commercially prepared foods have been adjusted to avoid the potential for diarrhea.

ALTERED FLUID AND ELECTROLYTE BALANCE

Many diseases and pathologic conditions upset normal fluid and electrolyte balance. In addition, many diagnostic and therapeutic interventions can temporarily upset this balance. The following discussion of the common imbalances of body fluid composition and volume will help students develop a clearer picture of patient needs.

FLUID VOLUME ALTERATIONS

Alterations in fluid volume include fluid volume deficit, fluid volume excess, and fluid shifts between compartments. Table 34–4 lists manifestations and causes of these alterations.

TABLE 34-4. FLUID VOLUME ALTERATIONS

Alteration	Signs and Symptoms	Causes
Fluid volume deficit		
Isotonic dehydration	Confusion; disorientation; hypotension; low cardiac output; poor skin turgor; tachycardia; decreased urinary output; shock	Inadequate fluid intake Excess fluid loss (vomiting, diuresis, diarrhea, hemorrhage) Third spacing/edema
Hypertonic dehydration	See above	Increased solute intake Thirst mechanism failure Decreased renal concentrating ability Decreased fluid intake Diabetes insipidus; diabetic ketoacidosis
Hypotonic dehydration	See above	Renal regulatory failure Excessive thiazide diuretic use Adrenal insufficiency
Fluid volume excess	Pulmonary edema; peripheral edema; full bounding pulse; venous distension; ascites	Excessive volumes of dietary sodium and water intake Cardiac and renal disease Liver disease

Fluid Volume Deficit

Fluid volume deficit, also known as *dehydration,* refers to the loss of water and/or electrolytes from extracellular fluid. This loss may be proportional, that is, the ratio of water to electrolytes is unchanged, or disproportional, with either water loss occurring in excess of electrolyte loss or electrolyte loss occurring in excess of water loss.

The three types of fluid volume deficit are:

- isotonic dehydration
- hypertonic dehydration
- hypotonic dehydration

Isotonic Dehydration. The most common form of fluid volume deficit is **isotonic dehydration,** also referred to as **hypovolemia.** It occurs when fluid losses from the extracellular fluid are acute and of short duration. The tonicity of the ECF is left unchanged. A number of clinical situations can result in isotonic dehydration: inadequate fluid intake, excess fluid loss, and third spacing.[15]

Inadequate fluid intake may occur in a comatose patient, elderly individual, or infant or young child—persons who are unable to independently meet their fluid needs. Fluid intake may also be inadequate in persons with fever and increased respiration, as their metabolic needs are increased by their condition.

Excess fluid loss follows episodes of vomiting, diarrhea, hemorrhage, or excess diuresis or with burns, wounds, or intestinal fistulas.[16] Another cause of fluid volume deficit is loss of gastrointestinal fluid. Each day 8 to 10 L of the fluid are produced. It is rich in electrolytes, which are lost along with the fluid.[17] **Third spacing,** a form of edema, results from a fluid shift from the plasma to the interstitium, where it becomes trapped and nonfunctional. Fluid may become trapped in the pleural and pericardial sacs and the peritoneum, or large volumes may be trapped within the intestines during bowel surgery or in the intraperitoneal cavity (ascites) from liver failure. This fluid, though still in the body, is unable to support cardiac function and output. Burns, sepsis, and anaphylactic reactions also allow isotonic fluid to shift from the intravascular space to the interstitium, causing edema.

Hypertonic Dehydration. In **hypertonic dehydration,** water loss is proportionately greater than electrolyte loss. It is caused by loss of hypotonic fluid from the ECF or an excess intake of hypertonic fluid. Hypotonic fluid loss may occur in situations such as diabetes insipidus, diabetic ketoacidosis, renal insufficiency, hyperventilation, and profuse sweating.[17] Increased solute intake occurs with high-osmolality enteral formulas and hypertonic intravenous fluids. Because thirst is the principal body mechanism guarding against the overconcentration of body fluid, hypertonic dehydration can also occur in those rare instances when the thrist mechanism fails. This is seen in the elderly, infants, sedated patients, and comatose patients.[17]

Hypotonic Dehydration. In **hypotonic dehydration,** the tonicity of the ECF decreases because electrolyte losses are proportionately greater than water losses. The most common causes are renal and endocrine regulatory failure and diuretic therapy.[16] Hypotonic dehydration can also occur when there is excess infusion of hypotonic intravenous fluids. Chronic illness and chronic malnutrition can also contribute to this imbalance.[15]

Effects. The effects of fluid volume deficit may be readily observable or subtle, rapid in onset or insidious. Fluid loss in small volumes over a sustained period may produce subtle changes, while rapid or large-volume losses produce classic signs and symptoms. Fluid volume deficit is classified as mild, moderate, or severe depending on the symptoms produced, the rate of loss, and the volume or percentage of body fluid lost.

Fluid volume deficit is a serious condition because it can lead to circulatory failure. Any reduction in blood volume reduces the venous return to the heart. When the venous return becomes so low that the efforts of the body to compensate are overwhelmed, cardiac output drops, perfusion to body tissues diminishes, and shock ensues. **Shock** is the suspension or failure of the regulatory mechanisms that maintain perfusion of body tissues. Individuals in shock become pale, diaphoretic, cold, hypotensive, and lethargic. Failure to prevent further loss and rapidly replace body fluids results in cellular death and eventual cardiac standstill.

Brain cells are the most sensitive to ECF deficit; consequently changes in the sensorium such as confusion or disorientation are usually the first to accompany fluid volume deficit. Other signs and symptoms include tachycardia, restlessness, dry mucous membranes and poor skin turgor, and decreased urinary output.

Decreased urinary output follows any significant decrease in perfusion to the kidney tissue. As the nephrons rely on high-pressure flow to maintain filtration capacity, the reduction of flow from hypovolemia results in oliguria, or urine output below 500 mL/24 h (see Chap. 29).

Fluid Volume Excess

When water and solutes are gained in proportionate amounts in the ECF, the result is fluid volume excess, also called *extracellular fluid excess* or *overhydration.* Fluid volume excess can be caused by the rapid administration of excessive volumes of intravenous fluids, cardiac or renal failure, or liver disease, all of which can lead to severe fluid retention.

One of the outcomes of fluid volume excess is generalized edema, the widespread accumulation of fluid in the interstitial spaces and the pulmonary interstitium. Most of the signs and symptoms of fluid volume excess result from this pulmonary congestion. They include coughing, dyspnea, moist crackles on auscultation, S_3 heart sounds, bounding pulse, weight gain, and jugular vein distention.[18]

The syndrome of inappropriate ADH secretion, which is a physiologic response to severe stress, results in a continual renal retention of water and extremely hypotonic ECF. Extreme stress, such as that caused by major surgery; CNS disorders such as head trauma, meningitis, and encephalitis; or the ingestion of drugs such as chlorpropamide, vincristine, or thiazide diuretics, may also increase ADH secretion. The brain cells swell and produce symptoms of water intoxication, such as lethargy, headache, disorientation, anorexia, nausea and vomiting, seizures, and coma.[17]

ELECTROLYTE ALTERATIONS

Electrolyte imbalances are fluctuations in the ECF concentration of one or more electrolytes. Once the ECF electrolyte concentration is altered, compensatory mechanisms to maintain the dynamic balance between the compartments will also affect ICF concentrations of electrolytes. Specific electrolyte imbalances are identified by measuring the electrolyte concentrations in blood serum (ECF), as

TABLE 34-5. ELECTROLYTE ALTERATIONS

Alteration/Finding	Signs and Symptoms	Causes
Sodium		
Hyponatremia: sodium deficit <135 mEq/L	Dizziness, vertigo, hypotension; tachycardia; oliguria	Gastrointestinal fluid loss Increased sweat loss Severe burns Diuretic abuse Large draining wounds
Hypernatremia: sodium excess >145 mEq/L	Thirst; large amounts of dilute urine; fever; dry, sticky mucous membranes; confusion; headache, seizures	Heatstroke Overproduction of aldosterone Increased insensible loss (lungs, skin) Osmotic diuresis Excess infusion of hypertonic or isotonic saline Decreased fluid intake
Potassium		
Hypokalemia: potassium deficit <3.5 mEq/L	Muscle weakness; cardiac arrhythmias; abdominal distension; paresthesias; anorexia; depressed deep tendon reflexes	Gastrointestinal fluid loss Stress Thiazide diuretic use Metabolic alkalosis Poor intake Hypomagnesemia
Hyperkalemia: potassium excess >5.5 mEq/L	Irritability; anxiety; muscular weakness; cardiac irregularities; nausea and vomiting; diarrhea; circumoral and fingertip tingling	Renal failure Red blood cell hemolysis Tissue trauma Metabolic acidosis Overuse of potassium-sparing diuretics
Calcium		
Hypocalcemia: calcium deficit Total <9 mg/dL	Muscle tetany; brisk reflexes; muscle cramps; cardiac arrhythmias; decreased clotting; pathologic fractures; Chvosteck's sign; Trousseau's sign; altered mental status; paresthesias	Decreased intake Insufficient vitamin D Severe diarrhea Hypomagnesemia Hyperphosphatemia Hypoparathyroidism Protein malnutrition Renal failure
Hypercalcemia: calcium excess Total >11 mg/dL	Bone and joint pain; lethargy; anorexia; muscle weakness; cardiac arrhythmias; thirst; hyporeflexia	Hyperparathyroidism Breast and lung cancers Metastatic bone destruction Decreased PO_4^- intake
Magnesium		
Hypomagnesemia: magnesium deficit <1.5 mEq/L	Muscle spasticity; tetany, tremors, weakness, brisk reflexes, seizures; cardiac arrhythmias	Chronic alcohol abuse Chronic renal disease Malnutrition, malabsorption Diarrhea
Hypermagnesemia: magnesium excess >2.5 mEq/L	Respiratory depression; lethargy; bradycardia; depressed reflexes	Renal failure Excess antacid and laxative use
Phosphate		
Hypophosphatemia: phosphate deficit <2.5 mg/dL	Emotional irritability; anorexia; paresthesias, weakness; bone destruction	Diabetic ketoacidosis Malabsorption states, severe malnutrition Overuse of antacids

TABLE 34-5. CONTINUED

Alteration/Finding	Signs and Symptoms	Causes
Hyperphosphatemia: phosphate excess >4.5 mg/dL	Muscle tetany; muscle weakness; tachycardia; abdominal cramps; diarrhea	Kidney failure Hypoparathyroidism
Chloride		
Hypochloremia: chloride deficit <95 mEq/L	Irritability; hypotension; lethargy; tachycardia	Vomiting, GI suction Chronic lung disease Diuretic use Heat stroke Metabolic alkalosis
Hyperchloremia: chloride excess >105 mEq/L	Weakness; lethargy; deep, rapid breathing	Severe dehydration Acidosis

Sources: Data from references 3, 15–17, 19–25.

measurement in the ICF is impossible. The common alterations and etiologies are listed in Table 34–5.

ACID–BASE ALTERATIONS

As discussed previously, the body has sophisticated respiratory and renal mechanisms to protect against acid–base alterations. Abnormal acid–base shifts are essentially exaggerations of the normal shifts in acid–base balance. Disease states resulting in acid–base abnormalities, therefore, must be severe or prolonged to produce overt symptoms. Causes and manifestations of acid–base imbalances are summarized in Table 34–6.

Altered body fluid balance, electrolyte balance, and acid–base balance are adaptations to body stressors. In themselves, these adaptations may also be threats to health. Therefore, nurses need a solid information base regarding body fluid composition, alterations, and regulatory mechanisms to identify and provide care for

TABLE 34-6. ACID-BASE ALTERATIONS

Alteration	Signs and Symptoms	Causes	Compensation
Respiratory acidosis (carbonic acid excess)	Headache, lethargy, disorientation, decreased respiratory rate, increased heart rate, hypertension, sweating	Respiratory depression as the result of narcotic or barbiturate overdose, inhalation of anesthesia, or chronic pulmonary disease resulting in a rise in serum CO_2	Renal compensation by retention of HCO_3^-
Respiratory alkalosis (carbonic acid deficit)	Vertigo, lethargy, tingling of fingers, arrhythmias, hyperventilation	Hyperventilation from anxiety, hysteria, high altitude, overuse of aspirin resulting in excess excretion of CO_2	Renal mechanism excretes HCO_3^-
Metabolic acidosis (primary base bicarbonate deficit)	Weakness, dizziness, Kussmaul respirations, flushed skin, restlessness, dehydration	Renal, cardiac, or endocrine failure; excess acid produced or insufficient acid eliminated	Increased respiratory rate eliminates CO_2
Metabolic alkalosis (primary base bicarbonate excess)	Hyperirritability, bradycardia, shallow respirations, paresthesias	Vomiting, gastric suction, alkali ingestion (eg, baking soda)	Respiratory mechanism retains CO_2

Sources: Data from references 21 and 26.

individuals who experience fluid alterations. This ensures that nurses will identify problems swiftly and take preventive measures to avoid potential imbalances.

SECTION 2

ASSESSMENT OF FLUID AND ELECTROLYTE BALANCE

▲ FLUID AND ELECTROLYTE DATA COLLECTION

Nurses determine patients' requirements for fluids and electrolytes by analyzing information gathered from the history, physical examination, and laboratory and diagnostic studies. Nurses collect data and make observations from a wide spectrum of physiologic and psychosocial indicators that reflect a patient's state of fluid and electrolyte balance. Nurses use the information to formulate diagnoses of a patient's fluid and electrolyte needs. The result is an effective patient care plan to meet fluid and electrolyte needs. As a part of their collaborative responsibility, nurses pass on to physicians some of the information they collect to be used in making medical diagnoses.

Through the assessment process, nurses determine not only the nature and degree of the threat to a patient's body fluid balance but also the effect of imbalances on the patient's daily activities. This allows nurses to collaborate with patients to improve patients' overall health.

COLLABORATIVE STRATEGY

ELECTROLYTE BALANCE

Electrolyte imbalance affects human functions in a variety of ways. Mental operations may be altered. Patients may experience confusion, lethargy, irritability, anxiety, and a variety of physical symptoms that frequently impinge on mental well-being. Any of these changes can significantly interfere with the ability to carry on a collaborative relationship. Nurses' alertness to impending electrolyte imbalance can be an important factor in preserving patients' ability to collaborate.

FLUID AND ELECTROLYTE HISTORY

Much of the information for the assessment is obtained from the patient history. Nurses should gather information about patients' physiologic and psychosocial functioning and current situational adaptation. Although nurses may be able to use data collected by other health care providers, these data usually require augmentation through an expanded nursing interview to develop nursing diagnoses.

The affects of body fluid imbalances vary in severity. It is sometimes necessary to modify the techniques used in gathering historical information. A patient may be unable to respond because of reduced consciousness or weakness and fatigue. In some cases, a nurse can collect information at intervals, while interspersing periods of rest; in other cases, friends and family members may provide information. Slurred speech, which sometimes accompanies body fluid imbalances, requires nurses to listen carefully and ask for restatements. Nervousness, anxiety, and general feelings of decreased well-being sometimes must be alleviated before patients can respond to nurses' questions.

Primary Concern

Patients may seek health care for obvious fluid balance problems, such as prolonged diarrhea, severely diminished urine output, or edema of extremities; however, it is also important to consider other related concerns. For example, a patient may be concerned about general malaise, muscle weakness, fatigue, dizziness, mild confusion, and apathy. Determining a link between fluid balance problems and the stated concern requires questioning about the patient's physiologic, mental, and emotional processes as well as daily habits such as fluid intake and elimination patterns. It is also important to determine a patient's reason for concern and the way in which the problem affects daily activities. The following example illustrates a fluid-related primary concern.

> The nurse asks Mrs. Chin, a newly admitted elderly patient, the reason she is in the hospital. Mrs. Chin responds that she was suffering from weakness after an 8-hour episode of vomiting and diarrhea. When the nurse asks what about her problem troubles her most, Mrs. Chin begins to cry and responds, "This weekend is my grandson's graduation from high school. What a terrible time for this to happen." The nurse notes Mrs. Chin's concern and her desire to attend the important family occasion. The nurse's intention is to collaborate with the physician to establish a probable date for discharge.

Current Understanding

A patient's understanding of the development of fluid problems can help nurses decide on nursing implementation. Patients often supply data about mode of onset, precipitating events, symptom severity, relationship to activities, and the effects of treatments that provide valuable clues to possible nursing implementation. For example, when diarrhea is the problem, determining the rate and amount of fluid loss helps gauge the severity of fluid volume deficit and formulate plans for fluid replacement. An illustration of the current understanding follows.

> Mrs. Chin tells her nurse that she expects to reestablish her strength while in the hospital. She took baking soda the day before admission in the hope that it would "settle her stomach" and afterward experienced weakness to the point where she could not do her usual activities. She mentioned that others in her household had recently "had the flu." The nurse notes that the baking soda could have contributed to Mrs. Chin's severe weakness, and notes this as a topic for future collaboration with her.

Past Health Problems/Experiences

Information about usual medications and treatments is important in determining body fluid balance. The abuse of laxatives, enemas, and diuretics can lead to severe fluid and electrolyte alterations. In addition, certain prescription drugs, such as steroids and antihypertensives, can disturb body fluid balance. Questioning patients about allergies can reveal liquids, foods, and medications to avoid in treatment. For example, milk and dairy products are common in hospital diets. Some patients, however, are highly allergic to or do not digest these products well.

Obtaining information about past health problems gives clues to deviations that may recur or cause current alterations. For example, diabetes mellitus can cause dehydration and other body fluid alterations. In addition, responses to past hospitalizations help nurses individualize patient care and avoid recurrences of past problems. The following example illustrates a past health problem related to fluid balance.

> The nurse learns that Mrs. Chin has suffered from high blood pressure for several years and is taking a potassium-wasting diuretic and a potassium supplement. Because of her vomiting, Mrs. Chin has not taken her potassium supplement for 2 days. The nurse realizes that this may have contributed to Mrs. Chin's weakness and discusses this possibility with Mrs. Chin's physician.

Personal, Family, and Social History

The personal, family, and social history helps determine the influence of psychosocial factors on a patient's fluid status. For example, a nurse might ask the parents of a dehydrated child whether the child has any significant handicaps that might interfere with the ability to take oral fluids. Determining the patient's developmental level and physical capabilities guides caregivers in providing for fluid balance. Studies of the elderly point out that confusion, immobility, difficulty in communicating, and reluctance to ask for assistance can result in reduced fluid intake to the point of fluid volume deficit. The following example underscores the relevance of the personal, family, and social history.

> The nurse discusses Mrs. Chin's health beliefs with her and discovers that Mrs. Chin uses a great many home remedies for various family health problems. An example is her use of baking soda for upset stomach. The nurse realizes that some of these remedies may be ineffective or even worsen the symptoms for which they are taken. She resolves to discuss the subject of home remedies with Mrs. Chin again before discharge to determine their importance to her and her receptiveness to additional information on self-care.

One of the key contributions nurses can make to patients' health is to assist with the human problems of adapting to illness. Although fluid imbalances are often temporary and correctable, their symptoms can affect personal relationships and role fulfillment. The questions in Table 34–7 help obtain information about patient values and lifestyle and therefore avoid approaches that patients are likely to reject.

Subjective Manifestations

Review of subjective manifestations can uncover information about a patient's specific symptoms that, along with the observations made in the fluid and electrolyte examination, help nurses understand the precise nature of the patient's fluid needs. The questions in Table 34–8 can help to identify symptoms that are

TABLE 34-7. FLUID AND ELECTROLYTE BALANCE HISTORY: PERSONAL, FAMILY, AND SOCIAL HISTORY QUESTIONS

A. Vocational
   1. What type of work do you do?
   2. How much physical activity does your job involve?
   3. Does your job involve exposure to high temperatures?

B. Home and Family
   1. Do you or anyone in your family have a history of diabetes mellitus?

C. Social, Leisure, Cultural, Spiritual
   1. Do you adhere to any food or beverage restrictions?
   2. Do you use any home remedies or remedies prescribed by a religious or traditional healer?

D. Habits

   Exercise
   1. Do you exercise regularly? How often and what types of exercise?
   2. Can you carry out your usual daily activities?

   Diet
   1. Have you noticed a weight gain or loss recently? How much?
   2. What foods do you like to eat?
   3. Are there any foods that you eat a lot of? What foods?
   4. Are you on a restricted diet of any kind? What kind (eg, salt limitation, weight loss, fluid restriction)?
   5. Do you salt your food at the table?
   6. Are you fond of snack foods such as popcorn, nuts, and potato chips? How often do you eat these foods?
   7. Do you use salt substitutes?

   Beverages
   1. How much fluid do you usually drink a day?
   2. Do you drink fluids with meals? Between meals? Before going to bed?
   3. What beverages do you like to drink?
   4. Are there any beverages that you don't like?
   5. Do you prefer hot or cold drinks?
   6. Do you drink coffee, tea, or colas?
   7. Do you drink extra fluid when the weather is hot?

   Sleep
   1. Do you experience any difficulty breathing while lying down to sleep at night?

   Other Substances
   1. Do you drink alcoholic beverages? Describe the amount you consume.
   2. What medications do you take regularly? Occasionally?

E. Psychological/Stress/Coping
   1. Have you experienced any unusual or particularly severe stress recently?
   2. Have you had any major life changes recently?

TABLE 34–8. FLUID AND ELECTROLYTE ALTERATIONS: SUBJECTIVE MANIFESTATIONS QUESTIONS

A. General
1. Have you noticed a weight gain or loss recently? How much?
2. Have you noticed any unusual thirst?
3. Have you noticed any change in your energy level recently? Have you felt unusually fatigued or tired?
4. Have you felt anxious or irritable? Depressed, nervous, or restless?
5. Have you had any problem with fever?

B. Integument
1. Do you have dry skin?
2. Have you noticed that your skin is unusually dry lately?
3. Have you experienced any general itching?
4. Have you noticed any puffiness of the skin of your hands, face, feet, or legs?

C. HEENT
1. Do you have any problem hearing or seeing?
2. Have you had a dry mouth or nose lately?
3. Do you have any soreness or pain in your mouth or throat that affects your eating or drinking?
4. Do you use dentures? Do they fit well?

D. Chest/Cardiovascular System
1. Do you ever feel that your heart pounds or beats too rapidly?
2. Do your ankles swell?
3. Do you have chest pain?
4. Have you experienced any recent difficulty breathing?
5. Do you have difficulty breathing when lying down?
6. Do you sit up or use extra pillows to get to sleep at night?
7. Do you have a cough?

E. Abdomen/Gastrointestinal Tract
1. Do you have trouble with indigestion?
2. Have you been nauseated or vomited recently?
3. Have you had diarrhea or constipation recently?
4. Do you take enemas to defecate?

F. Genitourinary System
1. Have you experienced an increase or decrease in urine volume recently?
2. How often do you usually urinate? Have you noticed any changes in frequency?
3. Has your urine changed in color?

G. Musculoskeletal System
1. Have you noticed any weakness lately?
2. Have you noticed any muscle twitching or spasms recently?
3. Do you ever have muscle cramps? During exercise or at rest?

H. Neurologic System
1. Have you had any trouble remembering things lately? Are you ever confused?
2. Have you had any unusual mood swings?
3. Have you had any trouble with your speech?
4. Do you have headaches?
5. Have you felt any numbness or tingling in your face, hands, legs, or feet?

commonly associated with fluid imbalances of various types. Determining which symptoms the patient experiences may help the nurse decide if a fluid imbalance exists and what nursing approaches may alleviate it.

FLUID AND ELECTROLYTE EXAMINATION

Because so many organs are involved in protecting body fluid balance, the fluid and electrolyte examination must include almost every body system (Table 34–9). Laboratory and diagnostic data also reveal the chemical functioning of the body.

Measurements

Many of the observations on which diagnoses and plans for care are based vary slightly between observers. Height, weight, and vital signs provide numerical, factual evidence of the presence of fluid volume alterations and their extent.

Body Weight and Height. Body weight can help evaluate fluid gains and losses as well as the need for replacement. Body fat is gained or lost relatively slowly, but body water can be gained or lost quickly. Gains or losses of weight exceeding 0.5 to 1.0 lb per day usually indicate fluctuations in body fluids rather than fat stores.

The baseline weight obtained in the initial assessment provides a yardstick for evaluating fluid gains and losses. Thereafter, keeping in mind that every liter of fluid weighs 1 kg (2.2 lb), nurses can correlate patient weights to fluid intake. A 2 percent decrease in body weight represents mild fluid volume deficit, 5 percent a moderate change, and 8 percent a severe, debilitating alteration.[3]

Height and weight are often used in combination on a nomogram (see Fig. 25–16) to determine body surface area (BSA). Physicians and nurses use body surface area, in combination with laboratory data, to determine fluid replacement needs.

Vital Signs. Vital signs are undoubtedly the most frequently observed parameters in physical assessment. Changes in body temperature, pulse rate, respirations, and blood pressure readily reflect body fluid changes. Alterations in vital signs may result from the imbalance or cause it.

For example, elevations in body temperature are associated with increases in sensible loss from perspiration and insensible loss from the lungs. In fever states, the normal requirements for adult fluid intake (1500 to 2500 mL/d) must be increased by 500 mL for a fever between 101F and 103F, and by at least 1000 mL for a sustained fever greater than 103F.[27]

Objective Manifestations

To understand a patient's state of body fluid balance, nurses must consider a wide range of clinical observations. Accurate diagnoses can be drawn only after considering the overall pattern implied by the observations. The following paragraphs briefly describe the

TABLE 34-9. NURSING ASSESSMENT OF FLUID BALANCE

Observation	Significance
Change in daily weight (loss in dehydration, gain in overload)	Most accurate indicator of fluid balance; 1 L water weighs about 1 kg. • 2% weight change = mild deficit or overload • 5% weight change = moderate deficit or overload • 8% weight change = severe deficit or overload
Intake and output comparison	Excessive intake compared to output can indicate compensation for prior excessive losses or risk for overload. Excessive output compared to intake can indicate mobilization of excessive fluid (eg, edema) or risk for dehydration.
Poor (decreased) skin turgor	Can indicate dehydration
Edema (dependent)	Can indicate overload
Increased temperature	Can indicate dehydration; prolonged hyperthermia can lead to dehydration
Dry conjunctiva of eyes	Along with "soft" eyeballs, can indicate dehydration
Periorbital edema	Can indicate overload
Tachycardia, decreased blood pressure, decreased pulse pressure, diminished pulses, flat neck veins, decreased CVP	Can indicate dehydration
Increased blood pressure, increased pulse pressure, bounding pulses, distended neck veins (jugular vein distention [JVD]) and hand veins, increased CVP	Can indicate overload
Moist crackles, dyspnea, increased respirations	Can indicate overload (pulmonary edema)
Oliguria (<30 mL/h)	Can indicate dehydration
Decreased level of consciousness	Can indicate dehydration

Adapted from Lee CB, Barrett CA, Ignatavicius DD. Fluids and Electrolytes: A Practical Approach. *4th ed. Philadelphia: Davis; 1996:21.*

significance of many of the most common observations associated with body fluid assessment.

General Observations. Observations of mental and behavioral changes, as well as facial expression and overall appearance, are important indicators of fluid and electrolyte alterations.

MENTAL STATUS. Changes in level of consciousness, orientation, thought process, judgment, perception, and mood accompany many fluid balance alterations. When these functions are simultaneously but temporarily disturbed, a condition known as acute brain syndrome exists. Symptoms of *acute brain syndrome* include disorientation and confusion. This syndrome can accompany other conditions as well, for example, malnutrition, heart failure, stroke, pneumonia, or renal and liver disease. Elderly patients, because of declining organ function, are most vulnerable.

The nurse assesses cognitive pattern to determine if the patient can understand the need for fluid intake, communicate the need, remember to take fluids, and recognize adequate body fluid balance. Cognitive alterations require support and collaboration from other health care team members.

Level of consciousness is one of the most important indicators of fluid and electrolyte balance. Derangements of fluid and electrolytes can cause lethargy, stupor, or coma. In lethargy, patients are drowsy but easily aroused. Stupor is a state of mental sluggishness and decreased responsiveness. Coma is the loss of consciousness. Alterations in water, sodium, potassium, and acid–base balance, in particular, cause changes in level of consciousness.

Orientation refers to the ability to recall person, place, time, and situation. Most of the fluid and electrolyte abnormalities that affect level of consciousness can also cause transient loss of orientation.

In observing a patient's *behavior,* nurses should consider both response to surroundings and mood. For example, fluid volume alterations may not only render patients lethargic but also result in withdrawn, apathetic behavior.

FACIAL EXPRESSIONS. A pinched or drawn expression, the appearance of emotional depression, apprehension, or anxiety can all indicate fluid loss and electrolyte alterations, because in fluid volume deficit states, the eyeball may seem to sink into the eye socket (a manifestation known as *enophthalmos).* In addition, the eyeball will feel unusually soft and mushy.

APPEARANCE. Individuals with significant fluid and electrolyte imbalances become weak and fatigued, often neglecting their hygiene and grooming as a result.

SPEECH. In states of fluid imbalance, the quality, content, and formation of speech may change. Hoarseness, shrill pitch, slurring, and decreased volume can indicate fluid and electrolyte problems. Subtle changes, such as a patient frequently moistening the mouth before talking, may reflect a change in the body fluid balance.

Integument. Clues to a patient's fluid balance can be gained from observing the texture, moisture, turgor, color, and temperature of the skin.

MOISTURE/TEXTURE. Normally, the skin has a smooth consistency and is slightly moist to the touch. In fluid volume deficit, the skin often becomes dry and scaly. Fluid volume excess can stretch the skin and give it a taut, shiny appearance.

TURGOR. Skin turgor, or elasticity, is tested by gently pinching the skin on a part of the body with minimal subcutaneous fat, such as the dorsal surface of the hand (Fig. 34–3). As the skin is released, it should immediately fall into the normal position. In fluid volume deficit, the pinched skin remains elevated, or tented, for several seconds. This reflects a loss of turgor. Loss of turgor occurs normally with aging. In the elderly, loss of turgor over the hands is common, so an alternate site for assessment is the clavicular area.

Fluid volume excess may lead to edema. **Edema** is an abnormal accumulation of fluid in the interstitial spaces, producing swelling. The skin can become too taut to pinch; however, pressing the skin over the pretibial area of the lower limbs may leave a characteristic indentation, which remains for several seconds. This is called *pitting edema*. The degree of pitting generally correlates with the degree of fluid excess (see Clinical Guideline 34–2). Remember that relatively healthy individuals may experience transient edema in normal circumstances, such as sitting for extended airline flights.

COLOR AND TEMPERATURE. Skin color and temperature can suggest underlying fluid problems. Pallor or flushing of the skin may indicate fluid losses or elevations of serum electrolyte levels. The skin should feel warm but not hot.

HEENT. The mucous membranes of the mouth readily demonstrate the effects of fluid depletion. Running a gloved finger along the surface between the cheek and gum may reveal dryness or stickiness indicative of fluid deficit or sodium excess. Shrinkage or fissuring of the tongue indicates fluid volume deficits. Excessive mouth breathing may also result in minor to moderate mucous membrane drying.[3]

In infants and very young children, a decreased or absent suck response may indicate a moderate to severe fluid volume deficit. In addition, the absence of tears in infants or very young children should arouse suspicion of fluid volume deficits.[14]

The appearance of the eyes also provides a useful assessment tool. The skin of the eyelid and surrounding the orbit is loosely attached to underlying tissue. Edema manifests itself in swelling of these tissues, a condition known as periorbital edema.

Chest. Alterations in body fluid balance frequently cause changes in respiratory rate, depth, and character. In particular, acid–base changes, which set into motion respiratory compensatory mecha-

INSIGHTS FROM NURSING LITERATURE

ASSESSING EDEMA

Welsh JR, Arzouman JMR, Holm K. Nurses' assessment and documentation of peripheral edema. Clinical Nurse Specialist. *1996; 10(1): 7–10.*

The researchers studied how staff nurses assess and document peripheral edema in order to develop clinical guidelines. Edema, a local condition in which the body tissues accumulate excessive tissue fluid, usually becomes apparent when adults retain 5 to 10 pounds of extra fluid. A sample of 211 nurses returned questionnaires surveying their assessment practices and reported a variety of assessment techniques. Of the sample, 75 percent considered themselves proficient in edema assessment; the remainder identified lack of practice, lack of documentation standards, and inadequate education as barriers to accurate edema assessment. Seventy-one percent of subjects used clinical signs such as "pitting" to assess edema. Pitting is an indentation created by forcing fluid into underlying tissues. Fifty-eight percent relied on weight gain as a sign; other methods were attending to patient complaints (tight shoes and clothing), measuring the extremities, comparing the extremeties for puffiness, and observing the consequences of pressure application or limb elevation. The researchers concluded that a standard for assessment and documentation of peripheral edema is needed.

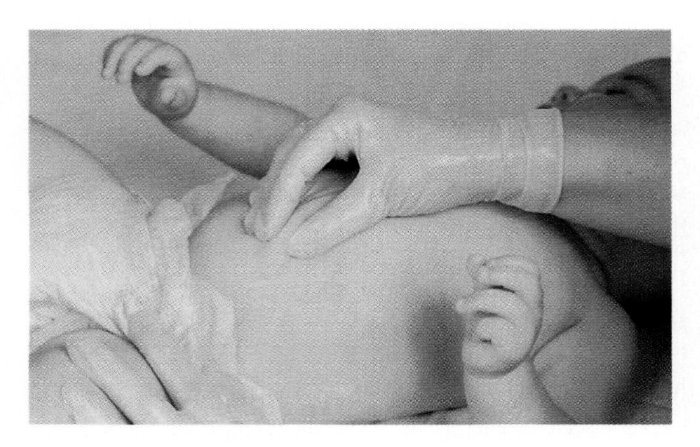

Figure 34–3. In infants, the skin over the abdomen is used to assess skin turgor. *(From Ball J, Bindler R.* Pediatric Nursing: Caring for Children. *Norwalk, CT: Appleton & Lange; 1995;85.)*

CLINICAL GUIDELINE 34–2

ASSESSING PITTING EDEMA

TESTING SCALE	DEPTH	EXCESS FLUID VOLUME
+1	1 mm	5–7 lb
+2	2 mm	10–15 lb
+3	3 mm	20 lb
+4	4 mm and beyond[a]	>20 lb

CONSIDERATIONS

Not all individuals will harbor edema in the lower extremities. An alternate site for testing edema is the sacrum.

[a]4+ edema takes at least 30 seconds to rebound.

nisms, result in observable changes in respirations, but fluid volume changes often result in observable changes in respiration as well.

In states of acid–base imbalance, the respirations may become abnormally rapid and deep (Kussmaul breathing), or slow and shallow. Some electrolyte abnormalities, such as hypermagnesemia, directly affect the respiratory center and slow the rate.

Congestion of pulmonary tissue resulting from fluid volume excess produces a characteristic crackling sound to auscultation. Coughing, labored breathing, and pink, frothy sputum can also be associated with increased fluid volume. In addition, scratchy sounds, known as rubs, can be heard over the lung fields when a severe shift of plasma to interstitial fluid results in fluid collection in the pleural sacs. This is commonly referred to as a pleural friction rub (see Chap. 30).

Cardiovascular. Both fluid volume changes and electrolyte abnormalities result in cardiovascular changes. Auscultation of heart sounds, measurement of blood pressure and pulse, and observation of hand and neck veins provide important assessment data.

HEART SOUNDS/RHYTHM. A change in heart sounds and rhythm often indicates fluid and electrolyte abnormalities. Any extra heart sound auscultated in the interval between two apical beats can signify fluid volume changes, particularly excesses. An irregular pulse may reflect changes in potassium, calcium, and magnesium concentrations.

BLOOD PRESSURE. Fluid volume excess, fluid volume deficit, fluid compartment shifts, and changes in ECF magnesium levels can cause blood pressure changes. Characteristically, a decrease in ECF volume results in hypotension, whereas an increase is accompanied by hypertension.

PULSE. Pulse strength, rate, and rhythm changes can indicate generalized or specific changes in body fluids and electrolyte levels. A thready pulse can result from states of fluid volume deficit. A bounding pulse reflects excess intravascular volume, as the result of fluid shifts.

Pulse pressure (the difference between systolic and diastolic blood pressures) is related to pulse strength. Normal pulse pressure is 30 to 40 mm Hg. A widening of pulse pressure is associated with a bounding pulse, and is possibly indicative of fluid volume excess.[9] A narrowing of pulse pressure indicates possible fluid volume deficit and is frequently associated with a weak, thready pulse.

VEIN FILLING. Observations of the jugular veins in the neck and the peripheral veins on the dorsum of the hand are common indirect assessments of fluid balance. In fluid balance, elevation of the hand above ear level will empty and flatten the veins, while placing the hand in a dependent position will cause visible expansion of the vessels. Filling or emptying should occur in 3 to 5 seconds.

Jugular veins may normally be distended and visible if a patient is lying flat or the head is lower than the heart; however, the veins should readily empty as the individual is brought to a sitting position. Measurement of the height of the jugular venous distension can be correlated to fluid volume excess. Fluid volume excess usually results in venous distension, even in upright position. Fluid volume deficit is usually reflected by a prolonged vein filling time.

Abdomen. The abdominal examination consists of abdominal inspection, auscultation, palpation, and percussion as well as observation of GI secretions, such as vomitus, drainage, and stool.

ABDOMINAL CONTOUR. *Distension* is the technical term for protrusion of the abdominal profile. Distension represents the outward stretching of the abdominal wall caused by the growth of a sizable internal mass, which may be composed of tissue or fluid. The accumulation of sizable amounts of fluid is known as *ascites* as discussed above. The degree of distension correlates with the volume of collected fluid, which may be as much as several liters.

Many conditions are associated with a protuberant abdomen, so determining when distension results from fluid accumulation requires skill. Ascites represents a generalized distension over the entire abdomen, whereas a full urinary bladder causes protrusion of the lower abdomen only. In ascites, no solid masses are palpable, and the umbilicus remains centrally located. The skin over the abdomen becomes shiny and taut, and the venous pattern becomes readily visible.

BOWEL SOUNDS. A change in bowel sounds can accompany fluid imbalance. Hyperactive bowel sounds, as opposed to the normal 5 to 30 times per minute, are sometimes associated with diarrhea. The bowel sounds are also gurgling and loud.[28]

GASTROINTESTINAL SECRETIONS. Conditions such as prolonged vomiting or continued GI suctioning lead not only to a fluid volume deficit but also to an acid–base imbalance. The high volume of secretions produced in the GI tract makes possible significant losses with any GI disturbance. Therefore, careful monitoring to detect and treat a fluid and electrolyte imbalance is important in this situation.

Genitourinary. Examining and measuring urine often provides valuable data for evaluating a patient's fluid balance. Urine volume, specific gravity, pH, and color are commonly included in the assessment. Many assessments of urine are performed in the laboratory and require collaboration between nurse and physician to obtain accurate assessment data.

URINE VOLUME. Urine volume normally varies with fluid intake: reduced fluid intake results in reduced urine output and vice versa. Urine output is roughly equivalent to intake over a 24-hour period. Significant disparity is cause to suspect fluid imbalance.

As a general rule, urine volume below 1000 mL in 24 hours suggests a fluid volume deficit, and urine volume in excess of 2000 mL in 24 hours suggests fluid volume excess; however, urine output can be influenced by increased insensible losses, increased solutes in the ECF, ADH and aldosterone production, and renal function.[3] The normal 40 to 80 mL/h output may shrink to as little as 30 mL/h during times of stress and ADH production.[3] Urine volume below 400 mL in 24 hours implies acute renal failure.[3]

CRITICAL QUERY

Terry[19] emphasizes that nurses establish themselves as important members of the interdisciplinary team when they use their knowledge of normal electrolyte values and the signs and symptoms of electrolyte deficits in the course of giving care to patients. What advantages do nurses have in assessing potential fluid and electrolyte problems that make their observations vital to diagnostic and therapeutic decision making?

TABLE 34-10. INDICATORS OF FLUID AND ELECTROLYTE IMBALANCE

Finding	Possible Significance
General	
Pinched or drawn facial expression	Fluid volume deficit
Rapid gain or loss in weight	Fluid volume excess or deficit
Apathy, restlessness, apprehension, and general behavioral changes	Electrolyte imbalances, especially hypernatremia, hyperkalemia, and hypercalcemia
Integument	
Dry, flaky skin	Fluid volume deficit
Tenting of skin	Fluid volume deficit
Pitting edema	Fluid volume excess of intravenous fluids, decreased renal function, decreased liver function, syndrome of inappropriate ADH secretion (SIADH), and compartmental fluid shifts from pressure changes
HEENT	
Dry, sticky oral mucous membranes	Fluid volume deficit Hypernatremia
Erythema and swelling of tongue	Hypernatremia
Fissuring of tongue	Fluid volume deficit Hypernatremia
Distended neck veins	Fluid volume excess
Sunken appearance of eyes	Fluid volume deficit
Cardiovascular System	
Tachycardia, Bradycardia	Fluid volume excess Hypovolemia Metabolic acidosis
Rhythm changes (gallops, missed beats)	Fluid volume excess Hypokalemia Hyperkalemia Hypocalcemia
Pulse pressure: increase or decrease	Fluid volume excess Fluid volume deficit
Hypertension	Fluid volume excess Hypomagnesemia
Hypotension	Fluid volume deficit Hypermagnesmia
Respiratory System	
Crackles on auscultation	Fluid volume excess
Decreased breath sounds	Fluid volume excess
Increased rate and depth	Metabolic acidosis Respiratory alkalosis Hypermagnesemia
Decreased rate and depth	Respiratory acidosis
Abdomen	
Ascites	Plasma-to-interstitial fluid shift—liver disease, starvation diet
Striae	Rapid development of plasma-to-interstitial shift
Nausea and vomiting	Hyperkalemia
Diarrhea	Hyperkalemia
Constipation	Mild fluid volume deficit
Genitourinary System	
Decreased output	Renal dysfunction SIADH Hyperaldosteronism
Increased output	Diuretic abuse Diabetes insipidus Hyperglycemia Hypoaldosteronism
Neurologic System	
Decreased level of consciousness	Respiratory acidosis Hypermagnesemia Hyponatremia Hypernatremia
Disorientation	Fluid volume deficit Hyponatremia Hypernatremia
Tremors	Hypomagnesemia
Paresthesias	Hypokalemia Hyperkalemia (face, tongue, feet and hands) Hypocalcemia
Tics, asterixis	Hyponatremia
Headache	Hyponatremia
Deep tendon reflexes hyperactive	Hypocalcemia
Musculoskeletal System	
Muscle flaccidity	Hyperkalemia
Muscle weakness	Hypokalemia Hypercalcemia Hypermagnesemia
Muscular tetany	Hypocalcemia
Muscle cramps	Hyponatremia Hypocalcemia
Immunologic System	
Fever	Fluid volume deficit Hypernatremia

Sources: Data from references 3, 17, 26, and 29.

URINE COLOR. The observation of urine color is often coupled with measurement of urine volume. Urine is usually a light amber or straw color. As the kidneys dilute the urine to excrete additional water, the urine becomes very pale. The pale urine may be associated with ingestion of large amounts of fluid, mobilization of fluid volume excesses or edema, or the ingestion of diuretics. Dark, amber urine indicates the kidneys' attempt to conserve extracellular water in the face of fluid deficit. Poor fluid intake or increases in fluid output relative to intake result in concentrated urine.

The relationship between urine color and volume may break down in the presence of certain disease states, for example in liver disease, dark bile pigments produce an intensely amber-to-brownish-colored urine.

Musculoskeletal. Several elements of the musculoskeletal examination imply changes associated with fluid loss and electrolyte abnormalities.

MUSCLE TONE AND STRENGTH. Muscle tone is the state of tension or responsiveness of the muscle to stimuli. Normally, muscles show slight resistance to passive movement, even when relaxed. There should be no spasticity (hypertonic, convulsive, jerking movement), rigidity (tension and stiffness preventing easy movement), or flaccidity (flabby, mushy response to stimulus). Changes in muscle tone are commonly seen in electrolyte abnormalities, particularly those associated with calcium and potassium.

Flabbiness and loss of muscle tone may indicate protein deficiency or electrolyte imbalance. Serum calcium, for instance, has an especially profound effect on muscle tone. Reduction in the serum calcium level may cause muscle rigidity or spasticity.

If an individual cannot flex and extend muscles against reasonable resistance, the muscles are considered weak. Decreased muscle strength is a common sign of electrolyte imbalance. Fluctuations in serum potassium levels may produce muscle weakness. This weakness may affect smooth muscle before it affects skeletal muscle, with the potential of causing vascular and intestinal motility problems.

Neurologic. The nervous system's ability to evoke muscular response is often profoundly affected by electrolyte changes. In particular, changes in potassium, calcium, and magnesium levels may be tracked through the assessment of neurologic signs or the use of diagnostic tests such as the electrocardiogram.

NEUROMUSCULAR IRRITABILITY. A serious sign of heightened irritability of the neurologic system is asterixis. Asterixis is elicited by asking the patient to hyperflex both wrists. Both hands will exhibit an involuntary jerking tremor. This characteristic tremor, associated with hyponatremia and the buildup of metabolic wastes in patients with renal failure, is often referred to as the flapping tremor.

REFLEXES. Normally, the biceps, triceps, bracheoradialis, patellar, and Achilles deep tendon reflexes are present at minimal to moderate intensity. In states of electrolyte and acid–base imbalance such as hypomagnesemia, hypernatremia, hyperkalemia, hypocalcemia, and respiratory and metabolic alkalosis, these reflexes may be hyperactive. The opposite conditions (hypercalcemia, hypermagnesemia, hyponatremia, hypokalemia, and acidosis) may result in diminished or absent reflexes.[3] Techniques to elicit deep tendon reflexes are specified in Chap. 17.

SENSES. Prickling or burning sensations, known as *paresthesias*, often accompany electrolyte imbalances.

An explanation of common findings related to fluid and electrolyte assessment is presented in Table 34–10 grouped by body area.

DIAGNOSTIC TESTS

Although the history and physical examination provide general clues to the state of a patient's body fluid balance, laboratory and diagnostic tests are necessary to confirm clinical hypotheses. An understanding of the relationship between laboratory findings and fluid and electrolyte balance can help nurses carry out the collaborative role. Often, a nurse is the first member of the health care team to receive laboratory and diagnostic findings. Nurses review and exercise judgment in their interpretation. Judgment is critical in determining whether an imbalance potentially or actually exists, whether immediate danger exists, and whether notifying the physician or changing the treatment is warranted. Table 34–11 summarizes laboratory tests relevant to fluid, electrolyte, and acid–base balance. Table 34–12 presents arterial blood gas values that indicate acid–base imbalances.

Interpretation of acid–base alterations includes not only evaluations of the measurements in relationship to one another, but also interpretation of the mechanism at work to compensate for the alteration.

NURSING DIAGNOSIS OF FLUID AND ELECTROLYTE STATUS

Once nurses have gathered subjective and objective information, they analyze data for relationships and patterns that indicate a problem or patient need. Patient collaboration should be an integral part of this analysis. This chapter discusses only those diagnoses of body fluid alterations that nurses diagnose independently. Electrolyte and acid–base imbalances are not included within these diagnoses. The nursing diagnoses related to body fluid balance are risk for fluid volume deficit, fluid volume deficit, and fluid volume excess. Table 34–13, Sample Nursing Diagnoses: Fluid Balance, contains subjective and objective defining characteristics and etiologies for the latter two diagnoses and provides risk factors for risk for fluid volume deficit.

Diagnosing patient problems demonstrates a nurse's concern for the prevention of illness and the maintenance or restoration of health. Early problem identification and intervention can ward off impending imbalances and often prevent secondary problems.

COLLABORATIVE STRATEGY

THE INTERDISCIPLINARY TEAM

Problems associated with electrolyte imbalance are usually referred to as collaborative problems because decisions on how to meet patients' fluid needs are often interdisciplinary decisions that involve nurse, physician, dietitian, and other health care team members. Nurses, however, are critical links in ensuring that patients' problems are brought to the attention of other members of the team.

TABLE 34-11. COMMON LABORATORY TESTS TO ASSESS FLUID, ELECTROLYTE, AND ACID-BASE BALANCE

Test/Description	Normal Findings	Significance of Abnormal Findings
Fluid Balance Tests		
Serum osmolality: Measures total concentration of dissolved particles in serum; determined largely by Na^+ concentration	Child: 270–290 mOsm/kg Adult: 275–295 mOsm/kg	*Decreased* in dilutional states (fluid excess), decreased adrenal function, and SIADH *Increased* in hypernatremia, hyperglycemia, uremia, diabetes insipidus, and dehydration states
Serum electrolytes: Measures electrolyte levels in blood serum	See Table 34–5	
Hematocrit (Hct): Measures percentage by volume of red blood cells in whole blood; provides a relative indicator of fluid volume alteration	Adult male: 40–54% Adult female: 36–46%	*Decreased* in hypovovolemia, secondary to blood loss *Increased* in dehydration or hemoconcentration
Hemoglobin (Hgb or Hb): Measures oxygen-carrying capacity of blood; also an indicator of fluid balance	Adult male: 14–18 g/dL Adult female: 12–16 g/dL	*Decreased* in fluid volume excess from intravenous fluids *Increased* in dehydration states
Blood urea nitrogen (BUN): Measures levels of nitrogenous wastes in bloodstream; a relative indicator, affected by factors such as increased or decreased protein in diet, decreased renal clearance in elderly, catabolic drugs, and growth spurts in children	5–25 mg/dL	*Decreased* in fluid volume excess *Increased* in fluid volume deficit *Note:* If rehydration does not lower BUN, suspect renal damage
Urine osmolality: Measures concentration or number of solute particles, regardless of size, in urine	Newborn: 100–600 mOsm/kg Child/adult: 50–1200 mOsm/kg Average: 200–800 mOsm/kg	*Decreased* (<200 mOsm/kg) with excessive water intake or excess D_5W infusion *Increased* (>800 mOsm/kg) in dehydration states and SIADH
Urine specific gravity: Measures density of urine compared to distilled water; not as precise a measurement as urine osmolality	1.003–1.040	*Decreased* in water intoxication or fluid volume excess *Increased* in fluid volume deficit states *Note:* Heavy molecular solutes falsely elevate specific gravity; fixed low volume in renal failure
Urine electrolytes: Measures electrolyte levels in urine; involves 24-h collection of urine	See text on laboratory tests	
Acid–Base Balance Tests		
Urine pH	4.5–8.0 (usually 6.0–6.5)	*Decreased* with use of vitamin C or certain antibiotics *Increased* in alkalotic states, except when K^+ lost in metabolic alkalosis; also increased in overuse of sodium bicarbonate as an antacid *Note:* Certain foods and fluids can acidify or alkalinize urine (cranberry juice, citrus fruits, etc)
Arterial blood gases (ABGs): Provides information on pressure exerted by gases dissolved in the blood	Po_2: 75–100 mmHg Pco_2: 35–45 mmHg pH: 7.35–7.45 HCO_3: 24–28 mEq/L Base excess: +2 to <2 mEq/L	*Note:* Altered values may indicate acidotic or alkalotic state (see Table 34–12; see also Chap. 30 and Table 30–5 for further discussion of ABG values).

Sources: Data from references 8 and 15.

TABLE 34-12. LABORATORY VALUES IN ACUTE ACID–BASE IMBALANCES (ARTERIAL BLOOD GASES)

Respiratory Acidosis		Metabolic Acidosis	
pH	< 7.35	pH	< 7.35
Po_2	75–100 mm Hg	PO_2	75–100 mm Hg
Pco_2	> 45 mm Hg	Pco_2	35–45 mm Hg
HCO_3	24–28 mEq/L	HCO_3	< 24 mEq/L
		Base deficit	< –2 mEq/L
Respiratory Alkalosis		**Metabolic Alkalosis**	
pH	> 7.45	pH	> 7.45
Po_2	75–100 mm Hg	Po_2	75–100 mm Hg
Pco_2	> 35 mm Hg	Pco_2	35–45 mm Hg
HCO_3	24–28 mEq/L	HCO_3	< 28 mEq/L
		Base deficit	> +2 mEq/L

Sources: Data from Kee JL. Laboratory and Diagnostic Tests with Nursing Implications. *4th ed. Stamford, CT: Appleton & Lange; 1995.*

RISK FOR FLUID VOLUME DEFICIT

Risk for fluid volume deficit is the state in which an individual is at risk for developing vascular, cellular, or intracellular dehydration.[30]

- *Risk factor: extremes of age.* Infants develop deficits rapidly because the majority of their fluid weight is located in the extracellular compartment. In addition, infants lose fluid quickly from rapid respirations, dilute urine, and evaporation from the skin.[14] Insufficient intake or losses from conditions such as diarrhea can produce serious deficits in short periods.

  The single greatest complicating factor for infants is the need to rely on adults to meet intake needs or to recognize serious fluid losses. Nurses can avert great harm by educating parents about the importance of maintaining hydration and making appropriate referrals.

  Elderly patients are at risk for fluid volume deficits as a result of normal physiologic declines in renal function, integument, and the thirst mechanism. Kidney degeneration may cause decreased ability to concentrate urine and a higher waste and solute load in the ECF. Sweat gland function declines and subcutaneous fat is lost, making the elderly less able to withstand extreme environmental temperatures. Thirst sensation diminishes significantly in the elderly, to the point that they may not ingest enough fluid to meet their body needs. Physiologic and psychosocial factors, such as immobility, confusion, and fear of incontinence, lead to decreased fluid intake.[31]
- *Risk factor: excessive losses through normal routes (vomiting, diarrhea, diuretic use).* Excessive losses of fluids and electrolytes in the urine or stool can be related to physiologic alterations or to overuse of diuretics or laxatives and poor understanding of the effects of prolonged use.

  Physiologically, diarrhea produces copious fluid and electrolyte losses. Knowledge of the type of diarrhea can guide nurses in planning specific care to replace fluids, limiting the severity of losses, and educating patients about prevention. Osmotic diarrhea is created by nonabsorbable or high-molecular-weight materials passing through the intestine and creating extra pull on fluids in the intestinal lumen. This is usually transient and resolves with the passage of the material. A good example is the diarrhea that results from ingestion of lactose in the presence of lactase deficiency.[32]

  Secretory diarrhea is caused by irritation of the intestine by bacterial toxins. A third type of diarrhea results from motility changes secondary to chemical or neurologic alterations in the bowel.
- *Risk factor: loss of fluids through abnormal routes (indwelling tubes).* Nasogastric intubation place patients at risk of fluid volume deficit and concomitant electrolyte loss. The potassium-and chloride-rich stomach fluid can be lost in quantities approaching 3 L/d with continuous suction. This results not only in fluid and electrolyte problems but also in acid–base alterations.
- *Risk factor: deviations affecting access to, intake, or absorption of fluid.* Limited mobility can place patients at risk of developing a fluid deficit. Simply placing fluids within reach of an immobile patient increases the chance of preventing fluid deficit, but this is often overlooked. In addition, an immobile patient may hesitate to ask for frequent assistance to satisfy thirst.

  Social and environmental factors may complicate access and intake. Family members caring for a confused or elderly patient may forget to encourage fluid intake. Institutionalized patients drink only what is given them, so that access must be increased to maintain sufficient intake. Access to a variety of fluids is often necessary to increase intake.[33]

  A primary function of the large bowel is to absorb water (2 to 3 L/day). When a portion of the large bowel is removed, it predisposes a patient to a fluid volume deficit.[34] Unfortunately, patients often fail to recognize a developing fluid deficit. Absorption of fluid may also be influenced by diuretic use. Because these drugs cause fluid and potassium losses, patients must be taught that intake must match output.
- *Risk factor: factors influencing fluid needs, such as hypermetabolic states.* Fever, regardless of cause, significantly raises the body's metabolic demands and thereby requires extra water and solutes. The body's oxygen requirements increase 10 percent for every 1 degree rise in temperature.[35] As a result, strains are placed not only on the fluid stores but also on the acid–base regulation system and oxygen use. Nurses must recognize that the potential for loss is even higher for infants and elderly patients.

FLUID VOLUME DEFICIT

Fluid volume deficit is defined as a state in which an individual experiences vascular, cellular, or intracellular dehydration.[30] Etiologies for this diagnosis include derangement of regulatory mechanisms and active volume loss.

- *Etiology: failure of regulatory mechanisms.* Many pathologic conditions alter the functioning of organs or feedback mechanisms that regulate fluid balance. Examples include brain injuries or tumors in the area of the hypothalamus (which alter the thirst mechanism) and diabetes insipidus (which causes

TABLE 34-13. SAMPLE NURSING DIAGNOSES: FLUID BALANCE

Nursing Diagnosis	Defining Characteristics/Manifestations: *Subjective Data*	Defining Characteristics/Manifestations: *Objective Data*	Etiology
Fluid volume deficit *1.4.1.2.2.1*	Reports fatigue Reports weakness Reports not feeling thirsty, has no desire for fluid	Mouth membranes dry. Wets lips to speak. Eyelids appear sunken. Skin dry, flaky. Intake 980 mL in previous 24 h; output 1500 mL. Voids small amounts of dark urine. Serum Na^+ increased. Hemoconcentration (increased BUN, Hct, Hgb). 4-lb weight loss in 3 days. Makes no effort to drink. Declines fluid when offered. Seems confused (unable to state date, uncertain of location). Medical record indicates possible brain tumor.	*Physical:* Failure of regulatory mechanisms—derangement of thirst mechanism[a]
Fluid volume deficit *1.4.1.2.2.1*	Reports diarrhea Reports feeling thirsty Reports mouth dry Reports recent fever, perspiration Reports feeling weak	Weight loss of 5 lb in 2 days. Decreased skin turgor. Skin dry, flaky. Oral mucous membranes dry Voiding small amount of concentrated urine. Frequent liquid stools. BP 104/70. 24-h intake = 600 mL, output = 1700 mL. Urine specific gravity = 1.030. Hemoconcentration (increased BUN, Hct, Hgb).	*Physical:* Active loss—diarrhea[a]
Fluid volume excess *1.4.1.2.1*	Reports feeling "down" Reports "I went off my low sodium diet" Reports worried about business Reports fatigue after walking to bathroom	Facial expression sad, shoulders slumped, appears withdrawn (responds in short phrases; does not initiate conversation). 10-lb weight gain in 1 week. 3+ pitting ankle. Jugular veins distended in sitting position. Hemodilution (decreased BUN, Hct, Hgb). Moist crackles in both lungs. Medical record documents recent heart failure.	*Physical:* Excess sodium intake[a]

Nursing Diagnosis	Risk Factors
Risk for fluid volume deficit *1.4.1.2.2.2*	Extremes of age: 79-year-old male Extremes of weight: Height = 60 in.; weight = 210 lb Deviations reducing access to or absorption of fluids: physical immobility Hypermetabolic states: Fever Altered intake: averages 900 mL/24 h

OTHER NURSING DIAGNOSES RELATED TO BODY FLUID BALANCE

PHYSICAL

Altered nutrition: less than body requirements
Impaired swallowing
Risk for impaired skin integrity
Constipation
Diarrhea
Decreased cardiac output
Sleep pattern disturbance
Ineffective breathing pattern
Impaired gas exchange
Hyperthermia
Altered oral mucous membranes
Altered urinary elimination

COGNITIVE

Altered thought processes
Impaired verbal communication

SOCIOCULTURAL/LIFE STRUCTURAL

Altered role performance
Body image disturbance

[a]Example only. Many other specific examples of altered functioning with this general etiology are relevant to nursing diagnosis. Defining characteristics, desired outcomes, and nursing implementation would differ for each specific etiology.

Sources: The nursing diagnoses and etiologies in this table and the definitions of nursing diagnoses in the body of the text not credited to other sources are from Nursing Diagnosis: Definitions and Classification, 1997–1998. *Philadelphia: North American Nursing Diagnosis Association; 1996. Manifestation categories for etiologies and specifications of general etiologies on these tables are authors' original work.*

excessive urine output because of insufficient ADH production or failure of the pituitary to release ADH.)[33] Although nurses do not treat the altered regulatory mechanism, careful monitoring of affected patients and support measures to maintain fluid balance are important nursing responsibilities when failure of regulatory mechanisms causes a fluid volume deficit.

- *Etiology: active loss.* Active loss encompasses conditions that enhance fluid losses via normal routes to the point that a patient cannot maintain sufficient intake to balance the loss, and conditions that cause fluid loss via abnormal routes. Diarrhea and profuse sweating associated with heat exhaustion are examples of excessive losses via normal routes. Vomiting, wound drainage, hemorrhage, and losses from burned tissue are examples of abnormal losses.

  Hemorrhage is excessive blood loss. It often causes hypovolemic shock. Blood loss is not always overt; therefore careful assessment is required to prevent significant fluid deficit. Body cavities such as the abdomen and thorax can sequester large volumes of blood before the definitive signs and symptoms of hemorrhage appear. The signs and symptoms of hypovolemic shock will depend on the extent of fluid volume loss.[36] Postoperative patients or those with multiple trauma should be continuously observed for both the overt and covert signs of hemorrhage.

  Managing the massive fluid, electrolyte, and acid–base changes that accompany severe burns requires a keen knowledge of pathophysiology and prompt intervention. The immediate problem facing these patients is a loss of fluid and solutes through burned areas and a fluid shift from intravascular to interstitial spaces. This leaves a severely depleted intravascular compartment. Blood and exudate losses ultimately contribute to the intravascular dehydration.[37]

FLUID VOLUME EXCESS

With fluid volume excess, an individual experiences increased fluid retention.[30] Factors related to this diagnosis include compromised regulatory systems and excessive sodium collection in the ECF. Some of the manifestations of fluid volume excess are pitting edema, moist crackles in the lung fields, coughing and dyspnea, hypertension, and bounding pulses.

- *Etiology: Compromised regulatory mechanism.* One of the most serious regulatory mechanism failures involves the kidneys. Renal failure directly affects fluid, electrolyte, and acid–base balance. Sodium and potassium excesses and metabolic acidosis frequently accompany kidney failure. Fluid volume excess develops as the kidneys are unable to filter the fluid load, resulting in the return of massive amounts of fluid to the intravascular volume.

  Renal failure does not necessarily mean an immediate, complete cessation of urinary output. The kidney may produce a relatively normal volume of urine, decreased urine (oliguria), or no urine (anuria), depending on the severity of the renal failure.
- *Etiology: excess sodium intake or retention.* Hypernatremia resulting from excess oral sodium intake is rare. An individual's taking salt tablets without professional guidance or using salt far in excess of normal daily requirements or restricted allotments may result in sodium excess and fluid retention. This problem also commonly occurs when individuals on restricted sodium diets consume salty foods.

  Intravenous intake of sodium is another cause of hypernatremia. Even isotonic saline (0.9 percent NaCl), given in excessive amounts, can increase ECF sodium levels temporarily, because it contains 150 mEq/L, which is slightly in excess of the normal levels. Retention of sodium may be seen in states of hypersecretion of aldosterone and in true water loss in excess of sodium, as in heat stroke. Regardless of the cause, an increased ECF sodium load causes water to remain in the ECF in great quantities, creating a fluid volume excess.

STATING THE FLUID AND ELECTROLYTE DIAGNOSIS

Identifying nursing diagnosis related to body fluid imbalance is the foundation for collaborative planning to resolve the problem. The diagnostic statement incorporates the diagnostic label with the specific etiology underlying the diagnosis and the defining characteristics exhibited by the patient. The following are examples of nursing diagnostic statements:

- Risk for fluid volume deficit; risk factors: persistent diarrhea, elevated temperature, decreased fluid intake
- Fluid volume deficit related to persistent fever (102–103F) as evidenced by concentrated urine, thirst, and dry skin and mucous membranes
- Fluid volume excess related to sodium intake in excess of prescribed diet as evidenced by increased arterial blood pressure, ankle edema, and 5-lb weight gain.

SECTION 3

NURSE-PATIENT MANAGEMENT OF FLUID AND ELECTROLYTE BALANCE

PLANNING FOR OPTIMAL FLUID AND ELECTROLYTE BALANCE

Collaboration between nurse and patient remains as important in planning as it was in the assessment phase. Exchanges between nurse and patient regarding patient beliefs, expectations, and pertinent lifestyle factors will improve the chances of successful implementation. For example, an elderly patient with a diagnosis of fluid volume deficit secondary to insufficient fluid intake may not accept the teaching from a nurse who does not take into consideration the patient's fears of incontinence.

Planning involves setting desired outcomes and selecting implementation likely to achieve those outcomes. Body fluid balance ranks with oxygenation problems in degree of urgency, so treatment is a nursing priority. Desired outcomes should describe the expected patient condition, function, appearance, or behavior as the result of implementation. For example:

- Within 36 hours, patient will exhibit normal hydration as evidenced by moist mucous membranes, supple skin with good turgor, and lack of excessive thirst.
- Urine clear amber, volume within 200 mL of intake by (date).

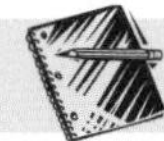

TABLE 34-14. NURSE-PATIENT MANAGEMENT OF FLUID IMBALANCE

Nursing Diagnosis	Desired Outcome	Implementation	Evaluation Criteria
Risk for fluid volume deficit, risk factor: physical immobility *1.4.1.2.2.2*	1. Maintains balanced intake and output	1a. Measure and record intake and output 1b. Monitor for new sources of fluid loss 1c. Observe urine concentration; monitor specific gravity periodically 1d. Monitor body temperature and respiratory rate 1e. Monitor body weight 1f. Involve patient in self-monitoring, if appropriate	1. Intake equals output over 24 h
	2. Intake appropriate to body surface area	2a. Determine ideal intake in collaboration with physician 2b. Make fluids of patient's choice easily available 2c. If compatible with diet order, provide electrolyte balanced solution (eg, Gatorade) for oral ingestion 2d. Assist patient with oral fluid ingestion if necessary 2e. Devise a schedule for minimal hourly intake and post at bedside 2f. Discuss strategies with patient to ensure minimal hourly intake	2. Maintains ideal daily intake
	3. Remains well hydrated.	3a. Adjust thermostat to maintain comfortable environment 3b. Note onset of conditions that interfere with oral intake (eg, nausea, vomiting) and collaborate with physician on need for alternate intake route	3a. Skin and mucous membranes moist, skin turgor < 1 sec; urine clear, amber, specific gravity = 1.010. 3b. Laboratory values reflect state of fluid balance
	4. Demonstrates coping skills necessary to maintain fluid balance	4a. Discuss the risk factors of fluid imbalance with patient 4b. Discuss healthful practices regarding fluid intake with patient 4c. Provide opportunity for patient to discuss personal concerns about fluid balance	4. Identifies risk factors and appropriate self-care
Fluid volume deficit related to deranged thirst mechanism *1.4.1.2.2.1*	1. Increases oral fluid intake	1a. Collaborate with physician on desired oral volume 1b. Discuss with patient the importance of maintaining oral intake 1c. Encourage patient to drink even though feels no thirst 1d. Monitor oral intake volume throughout day 1e. Measure and record all oral intake 1f. Provide favorite fluids compatible with diet order 1g. Discuss memory cues with patient to ensure minimal hourly intake	1. Oral intake reaches desired volume
	2. Regains balance of intake and output	2a. Monitor oral intake 2b. Monitor parenteral intake 2c. Discuss with patient need to measure output; measure urine output precisely 2d. Adjust thermostat to maintain comfortable environment 2e. Monitor patient for new sources of fluid loss 2f. Monitor cardiovascular and neurosensory signs	2a. Urine output approximates intake 2b. Clinical signs of fluid volume deficit diminish; reports improved energy level; mucous membranes pink, moist; skin supple, turgor < 1 sec; urine amber; specific gravity 1.010; serum Na^+, Hgb, Hct, BUN normal for age
Fluid volume deficit related to diarrhea *1.4.1.2.2.1*	1. Gradually increases oral intake to desired for age and size	1a. Collaborate with physician to establish desired oral volume 1b. Discuss with patient importance of maintaining oral intake 1c. Make fluid easily accessible 1d. Encourage intake by offering small amounts of fluid frequently 1e. If compatible with diet order, provide electrolyte balanced fluid (eg, Gatorade) for oral ingestion 1f. Measure and record oral intake	1. Oral intake reaches desired volume

TABLE 34-14. CONTINUED

Nursing Diagnosis	Desired Outcome	Implementation	Evaluation Criteria
	2. Regains balance of intake and output	2a. Discuss with patient need to measure all output, urine and fecal 2b. Measure all output precisely and record 2c. Monitor cardiovascular and neurosensory signs 2d. Note trends in output and collaborate with physician if adjustments to intake volume seem indicated (oral and parenteral) 2e. Adjust thermostat to maintain comfortable environment 2f. Remove heavy blankets and clothing that might impede heat loss and promote perspiration 2g. Collaborate with physician to treat the cause of diarrhea	2a. Total output approximates intake 2b. Clinical signs of fluid volume deficit diminish: weight gain 2 lb; skin supple, turgor > 1 sec; urine amber; specific gravity 1.010; serum Na^+, Hgb, Hct, BUN normal for age
Fluid volume excess related to excess sodium intake *1.4.1.2.1*	1. Maintains fluid and sodium restriction	1a. Provide patient with opportunities to express feelings and concerns 1b. Review with patient importance of maintaining fluid and diet restrictions 1c. Recognize and reinforce patient's efforts to maintain restriction 1d. Discuss with patient self-management strategies to prevent episodes of "going off diet" in future	1. Food and fluid ingested within prescribed limit
	2. Regains balance of intake and output	2a. Discuss with patient importance of monitoring urinary output 2b. Measure and record all output 2c. Monitor body weight daily 2d. Monitor fluid, dietary intake 2e. Monitor respiratory, cardiovascular, and neurosensory clinical signs 2f. Note trends in intake and output and clinical signs and collaborate with physician if adjustment to diet, fluid order, or medications seem indicated	2. Output exceeds intake as clinical signs of fluid volume excess diminish, then approximates intake

Source: See Table 34–13.

Desired outcomes guide nurse and patient in choosing appropriate actions. Table 34–14, Nurse-Patient Management of Fluid Imbalance, lists examples of desired outcomes, nursing implementation, and evaluation criteria for selected fluid balance nursing diagnoses. Table 34–15, Partial Critical Pathway for Total Hip Replacement: Fluid and Electrolyte Function, and Table 34–16, Partial Critical Pathway for Congestive Heart Failure: Fluid and Electrolyte Function, illustrate collaborative multidisciplinary care plans that incorporate concepts from this chapter.

NURSING IMPLEMENTATION TO PROMOTE OPTIMAL FLUID AND ELECTROLYTE BALANCE

PREVENTIVE CARE

Preventive patient care involves ascertaining that healthy patients understand the principles of normal fluid balance and can apply them to healthful living. This level of care also includes identifying patients at risk for developing fluid imbalances.

Health Screening

The comprehensive fluid balance history and examination help nurses identify persons at risk for developing fluid, electrolyte, and acid–base problems. Risk factors include:

- Exposure to high environmental temperatures
- Strenuous exertion
- Age (newborns, infants, young children, elderly)
- Physical disability (immobility, difficulty swallowing, etc)
- Psychosocial disability (confusion, psychoses, etc)
- Inadequate diet
- Treatments for other health problems (IVs, drainage tubes, catheters, enemas, irrigations, instillations, etc)
- Medications (diuretics, steroids, antacids, etc)
- Chronic disease states (diabetes, renal or liver disease, adrenal dysfunction, cardiac disease, pituitary dysfunction)

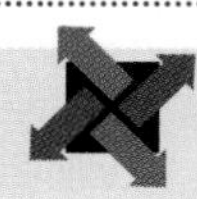

TABLE 34-15. PARTIAL CRITICAL PATHWAY TOTAL HIP REPLACEMENT: FLUID AND ELECTROLYTE FUNCTION

Nursing Dx/Problem	Outcome DOS/Day 1	Home Care Week 1 Days 2–3	Home Care Week 2 SNF Days 4–6	Home Care Weeks 3–4 Home Care 3 Weeks (6 Visits)
Fluid volume deficit R/T nausea/vomiting following surgery	Output 1000 mL/d	Output 1200 mL/d Retaining oral fluids	Mucous membranes moist Intake of 1500 mL/d	Normal tissue turgor
Implementation	**DOS/Day 1**	**Days 2–3**	**SNF Days 4–6**	**Home Care Weeks 3 (6 Visits)**
Assessment	I & O q shift Wound drainage q4h V/S q4h Tissue turgor, oral membranes Nausea & vomiting Mentation/orientation	Same Same qid Same qid Same Same Same	Same Same Same bid Same Same	Monitor intake Each visit Same
Tests/Consults				
Medications/ Treatments	Medicate for N/V Oral fluids when tolerated Foley catheter to gravity	Same Encourage fluids DC Foley catheter	Same	
Psychosocial				
Teaching		Need for increased fluid Cues to drink		
Activity/Safety/ Self-care		Fluids easily accessible	Same	
Nutrition	Clear liquids	Food & fluids of choice	Fluids 6–8 glasses/d	Same
Transfer/Discharge Coord./Case Manager		Communicate outcomes achieved, problems/ interventions to SNF	Communicate outcomes achieved, problems/ interventions to Home Health	Communicate outcomes achieved, problems/interventions to MD & prepare for discharge

See inside back cover for abbreviations.

Patients who are at risk should be given the opportunity to describe their habits and preferences for fluids, as well as exercise levels. Nurses then use this information to suggest specific interventions or develop a teaching plan.

Individuals who fit into more than one risk category have greater potential for developing imbalances in body fluids. Those patients should be alerted to the risks and monitored carefully.

Lifestyle Analysis

Analysis of lifestyle factors is important in preventing body fluid imbalance. For example, patients who exercise vigorously may not appreciate the impact of climate on water balance and may therefore fail to increase intake. Sedentary elderly patients may fail to recognize the risk of fluid deficit in hot weather.

Family living is an important lifestyle factor. The presence of significant others often stimulates patients to maintain intake and becomes essential for those with declining memory or mental acuity. Including family members in the plan of care often lends success to the plan and is a necessity in home settings, where family members often act as caregivers.

Lifestyle Counseling

Many lifestyle habits are related to fluid and electrolyte balance. Many people drink coffee, a diuretic that can create mild fluid volume deficit. Consuming alcohol and soft drinks in large quantities may disorder electrolyte balance. A nurse may help a healthy patient make lifestyle changes by functioning as a lifestyle counselor. The patient makes the decision to change and designs the

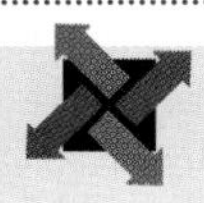

TABLE 34-16. PARTIAL CRITICAL PATHWAY FOR CONGESTIVE HEART FAILURE: FLUID AND ELECTROLYTE FUNCTION

Nursing Dx/Problem	Outcome Primary Care Visit	Outcome Home Care Week 1 (3 Visits)	Outcome Home Care Week 2 (3 Visits)	Outcome Home Care Weeks 3–4 (3 Visits)
Risk for fluid volume excess, RF decreased cardiac output		Absence of frothy sputum	Breath sounds CTA Pedal edema < 2+ No nocturnal dyspnea	Breath sounds CTA Pedal edema < 1+ No dyspnea on exertion
Implementation	**Primary Care Visit**	**Home Care Visit Week 1**	**Home Care Visit Week 2**	**Home Care Visit Weeks 3–4**
Assessment	V/S, arrhythmia, O_2 sat Breath sounds, edema I&O, weight, capillary refill Mentation, orientation	Same Same I&O, weight Response to meds/ treatment	Same Same Same	Same Same Same
Tests/Consults	Refer to Home Health EKG, electrolytes, Na, K, Cl, CO_2, BUN, creatinine Digoxin levels	Electrolytes		
Medications/ Treatments	Diuretics, K supplements Digoxin, anticoagulants O_2 @ 2 L/cannula Antithromboembolism stockings	Elevate legs Cough & DB exercises	Same Same	
Psychosocial				
Teaching	Maintain diary of weights Medications: correct use, SE, precautions O_2 use & precautions Applying antiembolism stocking application S/Sx to report to MD, RN, 911 Skin care, protect feet & legs	Disease process & actions of medications Care plan Reinforce as needed Reinforce as needed Reinforce as needed Reinforce as needed Reinforce as needed	Reinforce as needed Reinforce as needed Reinforce as needed Reinforce as needed Reinforce as needed Reinforce as needed	Same Same
Activity/Safety/	Bedrest, HOB 30–45 degrees c̄ BSC or BRP	Assist c̄ ADLs Assistive devices, safe use	Progressive ambulation/ activity as tolerated	Same Independence c̄ ADLs
Nutrition	Fluid restrict 1 L/day 2 g Na diet	Same Same	Same Same	Fluid 1.5 L/day Same
Transfer/Discharge Coord./Case Manager		Communicate outcomes achieved to MD	Same	Same Prepare for discharge

See inside back cover for abbreviations.

plan, and the nurse confirms the appropriateness of the plan, provides referrals, and acts as a continuing resource person.

Health Education

Because of the critical need for fluids and electrolytes, it is important for patients to understand several basic factors related to body fluid maintenance. First, and most important, patients should know that it is not so much what they drink (with the exception of alcohol and beverages high in caffeine), but the amount they drink that determines fluid balance. In addition, fluids alone do not maintain balance: a diet containing the necessary solutes is just as important.

Patients and family members should understand that not all of the water supplied to the body comes from the six to eight glasses of liquid recommended each day. Many foods provide extra liquid (see Table 34–17).

Finally, individuals who care for infants or elderly persons should have basic information about age-related risks. This teaching should include some basic nursing measures, such as teaching a mother how to take an infant's rectal temperature or teaching a family member to measure an elderly patient's intake and output.

Home Health Care

Home health nurses have a distinct advantage in being able to assess patients' willingness and ability to prevent fluid imbalances. Directly observing the home environment and support systems that are available to patients provides significant information. In their home setting, patients often feel less intimidated or overwhelmed than in an acute care setting, allowing for a greater exchange of information. Furthermore, family members and/or significant others may be more available to a home health nurse for consultation and teaching. Collaboration with patients and family members is essential in the home health setting to ensure success of established goals. Return visits allow for review and reinforcement of the teaching done to maintain a fluid volume balance. All of the aspects of preventive care, described above, are pertinent to the care of patients in the home. Elders in particular require screening for risk factors of fluid and electrolyte imbalance.

TABLE 34-17. PERCENTAGE OF WATER IN COMMON FOODS

Food	Percentage
Lettuce, iceburg	96
Milk	88
Carrots	87
Apples	84
Fish, baked flounder	78
Eggs	75
Bananas	74
Chicken, roast	67
Beef lean	59
Cheese, Swiss	42
Bread, white	36
Butter/margarine	16
Dry cereals	5

Sources: Data from references 32 and 38.

SUPPORTIVE CARE

Patients with mild fluid and electrolyte imbalances may be seen by nurses in home care settings, physicians' offices, clinics, or hospitals. The nursing role is to help patients identify problems and select approaches that will support self-care. Thereafter, nurses monitor the therapy and help patients identify risk factors that may worsen the existing problem or create new ones. Because levels of care overlap, teaching patients about intake and output or modifying intake patterns may be part of restorative care as well.

Diet and Fluid Counseling

At the heart of supporting patients' efforts to restore fluid balance is the teaching provided by nurses. Patients suffering from mild edema or worsening hypertension require teaching or reemphasis of the role of sodium, its relationship to edema, and the sodium content of foods and medications. In addition, patients may require counseling to prevent overuse of diuretics. Some patients take extra doses to relieve increasing edema and fail to realize the danger of potassium loss.

Collaborating with a dietitian is often critical to enable patients to make necessary lifestyle changes. A dietitian can help to translate the various dietary controls into everyday practice and provide information about creative food preparation. Nurses can provide patients with information regarding over-the-counter drugs that affect fluid balance and demonstrate how fluid restrictions help control edema and hypertension and reduce weight.

Oral Rehydration

Oral rehydration is the process by which patients ingest therapeutic quantities of fluid to regain fluid balance. Factors that are considered in computing or estimating a patient's requirements for rehydration include body surface area (BSA), age, activity level, and the current deficit. The current deficit, calculated from intake and output and laboratory data, reflects prior losses and ongoing losses. Although the specific requirements for rehydration are often prescribed by a patient's physician, nurses also need to be aware of how to calculate required fluid intake. In cases of mild deficits, particularly when rehydration is oral rather than intravenous, calculating fluid needs is often a nursing responsibility. Maintenance therapy, that is, the amount of fluid needed to maintain hydration under normal circumstances, is based on BSA. It is 1500 mL per square meter (m^2) of body surface per 24 hours.[3] Nurses can use this formula as a basis for determining patients' fluid needs in health as well as for fluid replacement. A nomogram for determining BSA appears in Fig. 25–16. Estimated fluid volumes for rehydration based on the severity of the deficit appear in Clinical Guideline 34–3.

The phrase *force fluids* is used to refer to actions aimed at oral rehydration. This does not mean that patients are physically forced

PROCEDURE 34–1. ORAL FLUID REHYDRATION

PURPOSE: To increase the intake of fluids in states of dehydration
EQUIPMENT: Cups, straws, liquid of choice

ACTION 1. Check physician's orders for amount prescribed.

ACTION 2. Discuss with patient and family the objective for the increased intake.

ACTION 3. Assess patient for dysphagia, vomiting, or oral lesions that may alter intake.

ACTION 4. Establish comfortable environment if necessary.

ACTION 5. Assist patient with oral hygiene.

ACTION 6. Keep fluids within reach, and offer small amounts frequently.

ACTION 7. Help patient to achieve optimal position for fluid intake (usually semi-Fowler's to Fowler's position).

ACTION 8. Maintain sufficient cups, straws, and other items for intake.

ACTION 9. Serve liquids at desired temperatures.

ACTION 10. Offer choices of liquids and foods high in water content.

ACTION 11. Offer frequently to assist patient with toileting if necessary.

Recording:
Maintain accurate intake and output records.

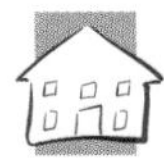

HOME HEALTH ADAPTATION: Oral rehydration adapts well to the home setting. Request the patient or family member to maintain an hourly log of oral intake.

to consume fluids, but rather that they are encouraged to consume specific amounts of fluids on a fixed schedule. Approaches to assisting patients in need of oral rehydration are listed in Procedure 34–1.

For patients on regular hospital diets, choices of fluids are left to individual preference; however, some patients need counseling on the advantages and disadvantages of various fluids. For instance, an overweight patient who selects milk shakes and sugary colas may be advised to choose fluids more compatible with weight reduction. Patients also can be counseled to choose foods with higher water content to help replenish body water.

Water is the fluid in most common use. The mineral content of tap water, particularly the sodium content, varies by region. Therefore, in certain circumstances, bottled or distilled water may be substituted.

In addition, fluids containing certain substances may not be suitable for special diets or physiologic conditions. Although some studies dispute the link between caffeine and cardiac problems, coffee, tea, and colas may not be suitable in large amounts for patients with cardiac disorders or neurologic traumas.

CLINICAL GUIDELINE 34–3

FLUID VOLUMES FOR REHYDRATION

TO CALCULATE MAINTENANCE NEEDS:
1500 mL/m^2/24 h

TO ESTIMATE NEEDS FOR 150–LB ADULT:

2% body weight loss (minimal fluid volume deficit)	2000–2500 mL/24 h
5% body weight loss (moderate fluid volume deficit)	2500–3000 mL/24 h
8% body weight loss[a] (severe fluid volume deficit)	3000+ mL/24 h

[a]In severe dehydration states, oral and intravenous replacement fluids may be combined.

Oral Electrolyte Intake

Ordinarily, patients receive electrolytes in the form of a well-balanced diet; however, increasing a patient's intake of specific electrolytes is a common aspect of medical therapy. The nurse's role is to administer the prescribed supplements. Nurses must be knowledgeable about patient condition, the properties of electrolytes, and side effects of supplements. For example, potassium is frequently administered to make up the amount lost by diuretic use; however, patients with renal failure usually should not be given potassium, because they cannot excrete it.

Oral electrolytes are provided in a variety of forms (powders, tablets, solutions). Some preparations, particularly potassium (in liquid or tablet form), must be mixed in juice to disguise the unpleasant taste and prevent nausea. Patients who take calcium supplements must understand their tendency to cause constipation and flatulence.

Limitation of Oral Fluid Intake

Patients with conditions that lead to fluid volume excess often require restriction of oral fluid intake. The physician orders the specific restriction usually after collaboration with nurses.

The calculation of fluid restriction takes into account all sources of output plus an arbitrary 500 mL per day for insensible loss.[38] Common restrictions range between 800 and 1000 mL per day.

PROCEDURE 34–2. ORAL FLUID RESTRICTION

PURPOSE: To limit the intake of fluids in states of overhydration
EQUIPMENT: None

ACTION 1. Check physician's order for amount prescribed.

ACTION 2. Clarify order to determine if restriction is inclusive or exclusive of dietary fluid.

ACTION 3. Discuss with patient and family the therapeutic objectives of the restriction and some of the ways to maintain the restriction comfortably.

ACTION 4. Alert staff, visitors, and family members to patient's fluid restriction by posting signs at patient's bedside or on door specifying amount of fluid allowed.

ACTION 5. Develop a schedule with the patient to spread allotment over 24 hours, with majority of fluids covering shifts that include meals.

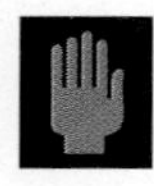

Sips of water, ice chips, and small amounts of fluid given with medications must be accounted for in the restriction.

ACTION 6. Provide frequent oral hygiene and lip lubrication.

ACTION 7. Encourage oral rinsing without swallowing.

ACTION 8. Discuss reducing intake of dry, salty, or very sweet foods, which increase thirst.

ACTION 9. Provide artificially sweetened hard candies and gum to stimulate salivation.

ACTION 10. Provide fluids the patient prefers unless contraindicated. Encourage noncaffeinated, nonalcoholic, isotonic beverages, which are more likely to quench thirst.

ACTION 11. Encourage diversional activities.

Recording:
Enlist patient's assistance to maintain strict intake and output records.

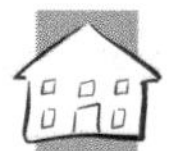

HOME HEALTH ADAPTATION: Restricting fluids in the home is a challenge, and soliciting the patient's cooperation is imperative. Request the patient or family member to maintain an hourly log of oral intake.

Restriction of fluids is often stressful to patients. Explaining the reason usually helps, as does involving the patient in establishing and implementing the intake schedule. Nevertheless, considerable understanding, encouragement, and support are usually required. Approaches to aid patients in restriction of fluids appear in Procedure 34–2.

Limitation of Oral Electrolyte Intake

Some patients must restrict their intake of certain electrolytes, usually because they have excessive blood serum levels. Sodium and potassium are the most commonly restricted electrolytes. The physician's order will specify the exact dietary allowance of the electrolyte by weight. For example, low-sodium diets may be ordered as 500 mg, 1000 mg, or 2000 mg. A dietary prescription is as important as any medication order, so it is important that patients and family or other caregivers understand the treatment plan (see Clinical Guideline 34–4). Collaboration between the health professionals caring for the patient is important to ensure consistency and continuity of care.

Aiding patients with electrolyte restrictions requires that nurses be knowledgeable about the electrolyte content of foods. Labels on food packaging include accurate information about some nutrients and are one source of information for patients. Printed materials or dietary manuals can also help nurses to provide accurate information. Consultation with a dietitian is often helpful in situations regarding fluid and electrolyte restrictions.

Intake and Output Monitoring and Recording

Indications for recording intake and output (I&O) appear in Clinical Guideline 34–5. Measuring intake and output, although simple to accomplish, is comparable to the assessment of vital signs in importance. The intake and output record is only as accurate an assessment tool as the individual who measures and records on it. Errors and omissions in measurement can render intake and output records useless.

Intake includes all fluids that enter the body, including oral fluids, intravenous solutions, irrigation solutions, tube feedings, enemas, and foods that are liquid at room temperature. Measurement is accomplished by transferring the liquid, prior to use, to a graduated container or syringe to assess volume. Premeasured volumes (from the patient's meals, for example) may be ingested and then assessed, as these volumes are commonly listed on the containers. Patients who are alert, in no distress, and willing may be given recording materials and briefly instructed in recording intake and output.

The output record should include all measurable liquids that leave the body, such as urine, liquid feces, drainage from intestinal fistulas, wounds with drains or suction devices, urinary and small bowel diversions, suction drainage, and enema

CLINICAL GUIDELINE 34–4

MANAGING SODIUM AND POTASSIUM RESTRICTION

SODIUM RESTRICTION

- Determine extent of sodium restriction (ie, mild, moderate, or severe).
- Tell patients with moderate to severe sodium restriction to avoid all products containing sodium as an ingredient. Severe sodium restrictions call for the use of low-sodium breads, baked goods, and snack foods.
- Encourage patients to read food labels to avoid foods that contain the terms *salt, sodium,* and *soda.*
- Tell patients that products labeled *sodium free* contain less than 5 mg of sodium, whereas low-sodium foods contain 140 mg or less.
- Encourage patients and family members to experiment with various herbs, vinegar, wine, sugar, honey, and onion to flavor meats and vegetables.
- Tell patients that fruits may be consumed in moderation as they contain little sodium.
- Tell patients and family members that milk contains moderate amounts of sodium and is discouraged for patients with a severe sodium restriction.

POTASSIUM RESTRICTION

Tell patients and family members that:

- All salt substitutes should be avoided.
- Canned vegetables should be drained of the canning liquid and cooked in fresh water.
- Tea and coffee are high in potassium and should be avoided.
- Fruits and deep green vegetables range from high (>10 mEq per serving) to moderate (5–10 mEq per serving) potassium content, therefore, individual dietary counseling to determine selections appropriate to the prescribed restriction is advised.

return. Urinary incontinence and drainage from large lesions should be estimated. Again, patients deemed capable of maintaining the output record should be taught and encouraged to do so.

Most intake and output records include the same elements, such as columns for oral and parenteral intake. Columns for output reflect urine and stool output, as well as drainage and other specific output. See Fig. 34–4. Information may be recorded hourly or at wider intervals, or cumulative records may be kept over several hours. Grand totals of intake and output should be calculated every 24 hours. If output consistently exceeds intake, then the potential for fluid volume deficit increases. If intake greatly exceeds output over time, then fluid volume excess should be suspected. Accuracy of intake and output may be enhanced by taking certain precautions and avoiding common pitfalls of measurement, as listed in Clinical Guideline 34–6.

Daily Weights

Daily weights are an accurate method of monitoring fluid gains and losses. Frequently used in cardiac and renal patients, an indi-

CLINICAL GUIDELINE 34–5

INDICATIONS FOR RECORDING INTAKE AND OUTPUT

- Acute or chronic diseases of major organ systems (renal, cardiac, endocrine, neurologic, hepatic, dermatologic)
- Major trauma
- Surgery
- Draining wounds
- Altered intake or output
- Insufficient diet
- Nausea and vomiting
- Diarrhea or constipation
- Gavage treatments
- Intravenous therapy
- Oral fluid therapy
- Urinary catheters

CLINICAL GUIDELINE 34–6

IMPROVING INTAKE AND OUTPUT RECORDS

COMMUNICATION/COLLABORATION

- Communicate to the entire staff that I&O recording is required for patient.
- Discuss with patient and family the need for I&O recording and reasoning behind the measurements.
- Post signs at patient's bedside and in bathroom area as reminders.
- Clearly note the need for I&O recording on patient's care plan.
- Update instructions for keeping accurate I&O records on a regular basis.
- Involve the alert, willing patient and family in measurement and recording of I&O.

EQUIPMENT/INFORMATION

- Post a list of common volumes and measures for staff and at patient's bedside (especially diet tray containers).
- Provide measuring containers at the bedside as soon as I&O measurement is instituted.

PRECISION/PITFALLS

- Whenever possible, measure, do not estimate.
- If measurement is not possible, estimate output volumes (incontinence, diarrhea, emesis).
- Weigh dry dressings; then weigh saturated dressings and subtract to find the weight. Convert to liquid measure. (Necessary for strict I&O only)
- Consider ice as half the volume it occupies.
- Include irrigants as intake.
- Consider the difference between enema infusion and liquid output of enema results as intake.

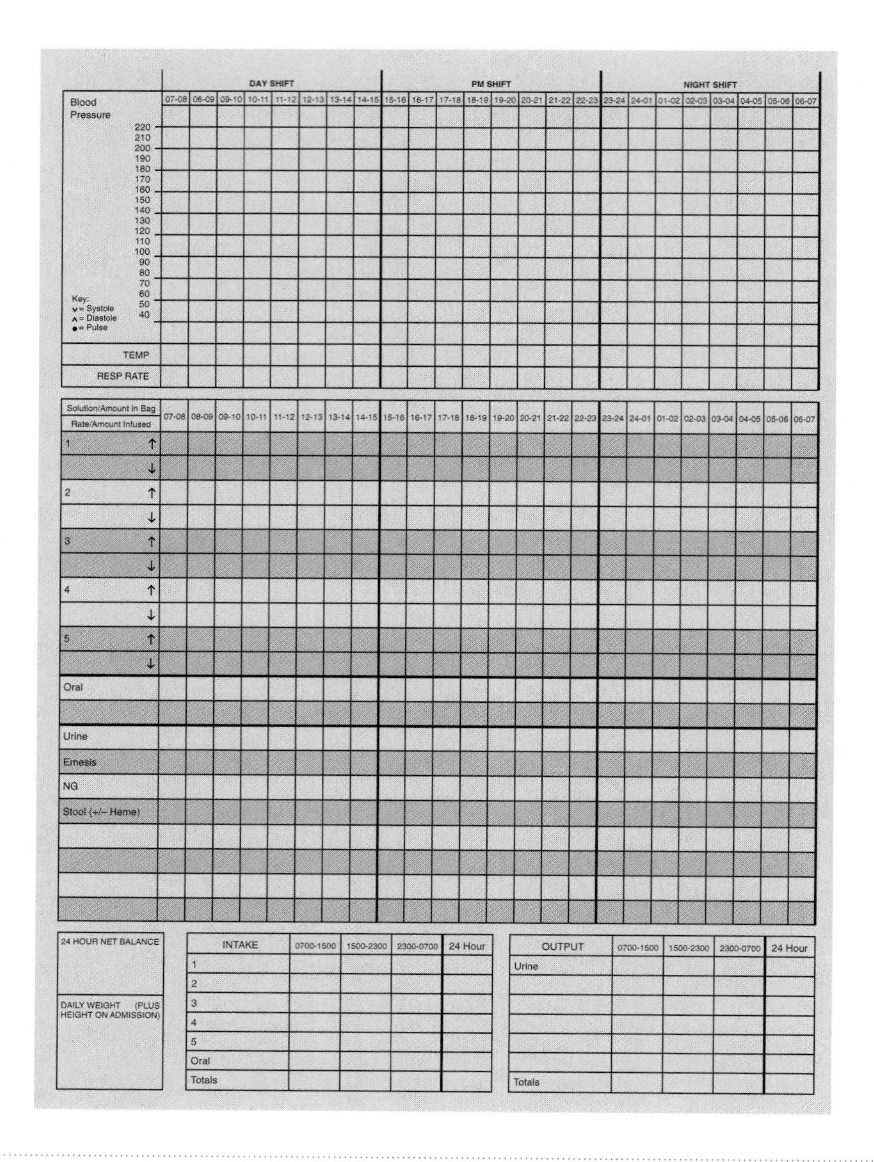

	DAY SHIFT								PM SHIFT								NIGHT SHIFT							
Blood Pressure	07-08	08-09	09-10	10-11	11-12	12-13	13-14	14-15	15-16	16-17	17-18	18-19	19-20	20-21	21-22	22-23	23-24	24-01	01-02	02-03	03-04	04-05	05-06	06-07
220																								
210																								
200																								
190																								
180																								
170																								
160																								
150																								
140																								
130																								
120																								
110																								
100																								
90																								
80																								
70																								
60																								
50																								
40																								
TEMP																								
RESP RATE																								

Key:
v = Systole
^ = Diastole
• = Pulse

Solution/Amount in Bag / Rate/Amount Infused	07-08	08-09	09-10	10-11	11-12	12-13	13-14	14-15	15-16	16-17	17-18	18-19	19-20	20-21	21-22	22-23	23-24	24-01	01-02	02-03	03-04	04-05	05-06	06-07
1 ↑																								
↓																								
2 ↑																								
↓																								
3 ↑																								
↓																								
4 ↑																								
↓																								
5 ↑																								
↓																								
Oral																								
Urine																								
Emesis																								
NG																								
Stool (+/– Heme)																								

24 HOUR NET BALANCE
DAILY WEIGHT (PLUS HEIGHT ON ADMISSION)

INTAKE	0700-1500	1500-2300	2300-0700	24 Hour
1				
2				
3				
4				
5				
Oral				
Totals				

OUTPUT	0700-1500	1500-2300	2300-0700	24 Hour
Urine				
Totals				

Figure 34–4. Form for recording intake and output.

vidual's daily weight is essential information. Daily weights should be performed at the same time each day, preferably before breakfast. Patients should wear the same clothing for each weight and be weighed with the same scale to ensure consistent readings. A gain of 1 kg (2.2 lb) is equivalent to a fluid gain of 1 L.

Home Health Care

The home setting provides nurses with opportunities to monitor patients' compliance and response to therapy, while at the same time initiating therapeutic nursing interventions as needed.[39] Patients on a fluid and electrolyte restriction may require home follow-up to ensure compliance with the established regimen. Elders prone to dehydration may require intake monitoring. Home health nurses can assist patients to properly identify the correct volume of certain household glasses and cups. Additionally, nurses can review the method a patient is using to keep track of fluid intake and daily weights. The home environment allows for ongoing patient/family education while at the same time providing patients with cost-effective health care.

RESTORATIVE CARE

Patients with moderate to severe fluid imbalance need restorative care. Such patients are seen in inpatient facilities and home settings with pathologies that promote or result from fluid imbalances. Collaborating with the patient, family, physician, and other health care team members to correct the deviations and prevent further imbalance is an important part of nursing care.

The focus of restorative care is to replace fluid losses, decrease excesses, and prevent additional net change. Promoting patient comfort, safety, and nutrition is an important contributory nursing objective.

Once it is determined that a patient suffers from a fluid deficit or excess, common approaches are employed to correct the problems. Oral intake was discussed in the previous section. A patient who requires restorative care often requires additional approaches, such as nasogastric gavage and intravenous infusion, to correct imbalances. Fluid restriction is employed in states of fluid excess.

Gavage

Gavage provides fluids directly into the GI tract. Nasogastric gavage involves the passage of a hollow, small-bore tube through the nasal passages into the esophagus and down into the stomach. Fluids and foods are then passed through the tube. An alternative is a percutaneous jejunostomy tube for delivery of food and fluids. This approach minimizes the risk for aspiration, which is an issue with the nasogastric route. Patients who require gavage are either comatose or have impaired oral ingestion from dysphagia (difficulty swallowing), esophageal obstruction, oral or esophageal tumors, or mouth trauma.

The principles that apply to oral therapy, as to the quantity and type of fluid, also apply to gavage fluids. Fluids from the regular hospital diet may be used, but specially prepared formulas are also used. These are rich solutions that provide nourishment as well as fluid. Most feeding solutions, however, are hypertonic and can draw additional fluids into the GI tract, leading to increased losses.[32] Table 34–18 lists the tonicity of feeding fluids. A patient's ability to tolerate such a liquid diet must be individually assessed. It is common to administer these solutions in diluted forms, either quarter or half strength, or with additional boluses of water, to prevent fluid loss. See Chap. 28 for more about nasogastric feedings and formulas.

Medications may also be given via this route, as long as the tubing is thoroughly irrigated to maintain patency (Clinical Guideline 25–12). The intake records for the gavage fluids should include any medications and irrigant used.

TABLE 34-18. TONICITY OF COMMONLY USED GAVAGE FORMULAS

Product	Strength (kcal/mL)	Tonicity (mOsm)
Ensure	1.06	470
Ensure High Protein	.95	610
Isocal	1.06	270
Osmolite	1.06	300
Sustacal	1.0	650
Pulmocare	1.5	475

Source: Data from reference 32.

Intravenous Infusions

Administering solutions via peripheral or central veins is termed **intravenous infusion.** Intravenous infusion by gravity flow or pump method allows for the continuous, controlled delivery of fluids directly into the ECF.

Patients with moderate to severe fluid volume deficit usually require intravenous infusion in addition to oral replacement. Those with life-threatening hypovolemia require emergency intravenous infusions to support the cardiac output. Because the intestinal tract is bypassed, intravenous infusion is ideal for patients who are unable to ingest sufficient fluids orally. Calories, vitamins, and medications also can be delivered efficiently via the intravenous route.

Setting Up an Intravenous Infusion. A great number of setup components are available for assembling an intravenous apparatus. Generally, these components allow clinicians to vary the complexity of the setup to meet the therapeutic objectives. The basic setup, however, consists of a container and an administration set.

SOLUTION CONTAINERS. Solution containers are of three types: glass bottles, which are infrequently used; soft plastic bags, which are commonly used; and semirigid plastic containers. Each container is available in several sizes, ranging from 50 to 1000 mL in capacity (Fig. 34–5).

Glass bottles come in two varieties: those with a clear plastic airway within the bottle and those without. The airway within the bottle allows air to be drawn in to replace the fluid flowing out. This system prevents developing a vacuum within the bottle, which would prevent fluid flow. The bottle without the airway requires an administration set containing an air vent. Glass bottles commonly have volume calibrations, both upright and upside down, for easy inspection.

The soft plastic bag is currently the most widely used container for intravenous therapy. Because plastic bags are pliable, they collapse as the fluid flows out. The combination of gravity and the outside air pressing on the bag makes it unnecessary to have an air inlet port for the plastic bag.

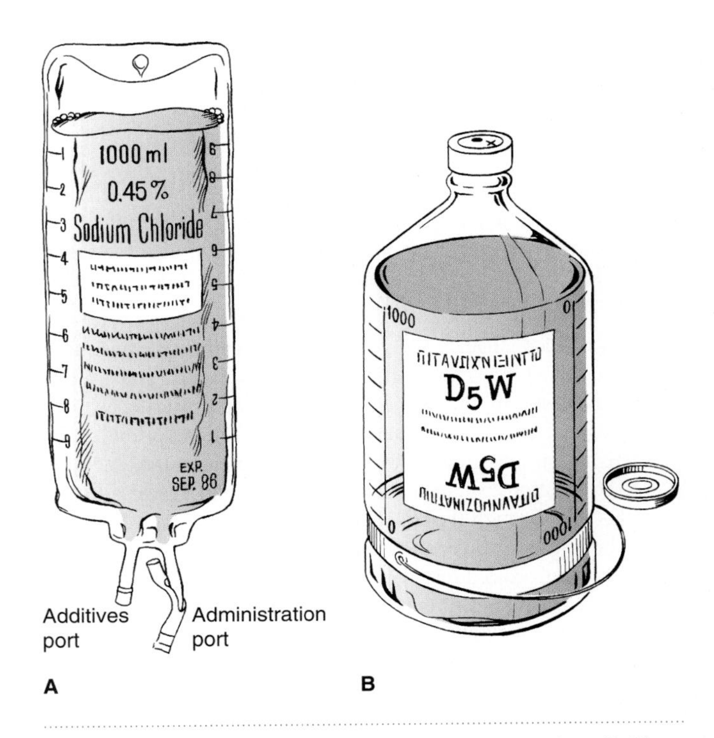

Figure 34–5. Types of IV solution containers. **A.** Plastic bag. **B.** Glass bottle.

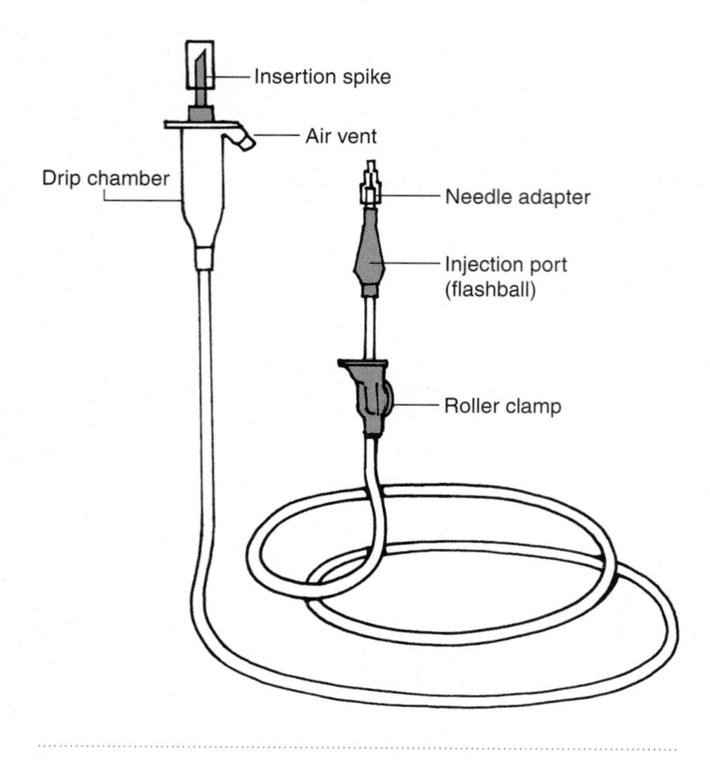

Figure 34–6. Basic intravenous infusion administration set.

Two ports are available at the base of the soft plastic bag. One is a resealable medication port; the other is for inserting the administration set connector. The bag also contains calibrations of volume; however, the volume calibrations are difficult to use because plastic bags are often overfilled and collapse asymmetrically, and thus are unreliable. These calibrations, therefore, should be used only for cursory inspection.

The semirigid plastic container may be either cylindrical or square, and is composed of a semisoft compressible plastic. The advantage of these containers is that they collapse symmetrically, which allows for greater accuracy in observation of the infusing volumes of fluid. The plastic material is inert, so it is not reactive with the solutions or additives.

INTRAVENOUS ADMINISTRATION SETS. A basic intravenous administration set is illustrated in Fig. 34–6. It consists of an insertion spike, a drip chamber, plastic tubing, a screw or roller clamp, port (flashball), and a connector for attachment to the venipuncture device. The administration set provides a closed system for regulated flow from the solution container. Medications may be injected directly into the vein through the flashball.

The insertion spike is a pointed plastic cannula with a beveled end that is introduced into the entry port of the solution container. The insertion spike is connected to the drip chamber. This small, flexible chamber allows visualizing the drops of solution leaving the container. The drops are counted as a means of monitoring the flow rate of the solution.

The roller clamp is a device that compresses the tubing that runs through it. By adjusting the clamp, the rate of flow of the solution is controlled. The flashball or injection port is a rubber hub with embossed circles that provide a guide to needle insertion. This hub is used for medication administration.

The basic administration set ends with a plastic connector, often called the adaptor, to which the intravenous needle or cannula is attached. This connector may fit by friction or by a twisting lock system called a Luer lock.

Additions to the basic administration set are numerous. Among the more common are Y-type injection ports, check valves, in-line filters, extension tubing, and volume control sets. In some administration sets, these devices are already attached by the manufacturer (Fig. 34–7), but many are also available to add to an existing set should the need arise. See next section, *Adjunctive Devices.*

Administration sets are manufactured to deliver differing rates of flow. Common drip rates range from 10 to 20 drops per milliliter. Sets manufactured for pediatric use deliver 50 to 60 drops per milliliter (Fig. 34–8). This information is provided on the packaging and must be considered in calculating the rate of flow of the solution (Fig. 34–9). The technique for preparing the solution container and administration set is outlined in Procedure 34–3. The apparatus must be inspected, assembled, and filled before venipuncture.

ADJUNCTIVE DEVICES

- *In-line filters.* In-line filters are devices designed to remove bacteria, fungi, and particulate matter from the solution. (Fig. 34–10). The size of the pores which filter contaminants, varies,

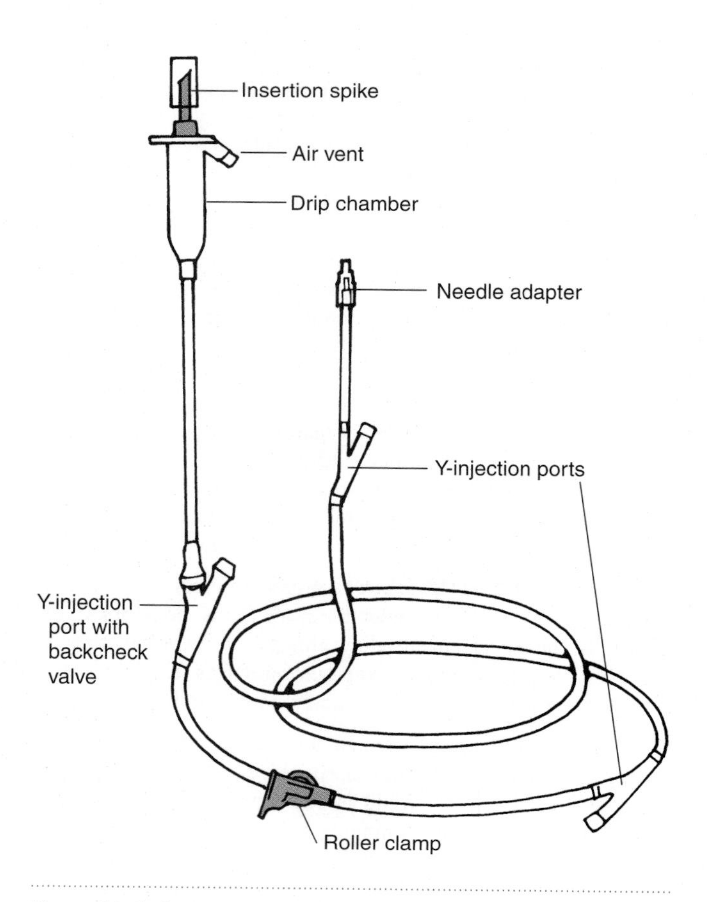

Figure 34–7. Intravenous tubing with Y-injection port (site).

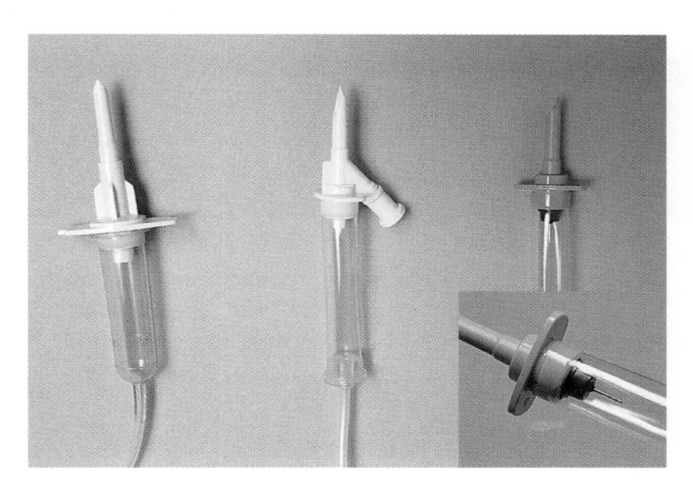

Figure 34–8. *(Left to right)* IV administration sets. Nonvented macrodrip. Vented macrodrip. Microdrip. **Inset** shows detail of microdrip.

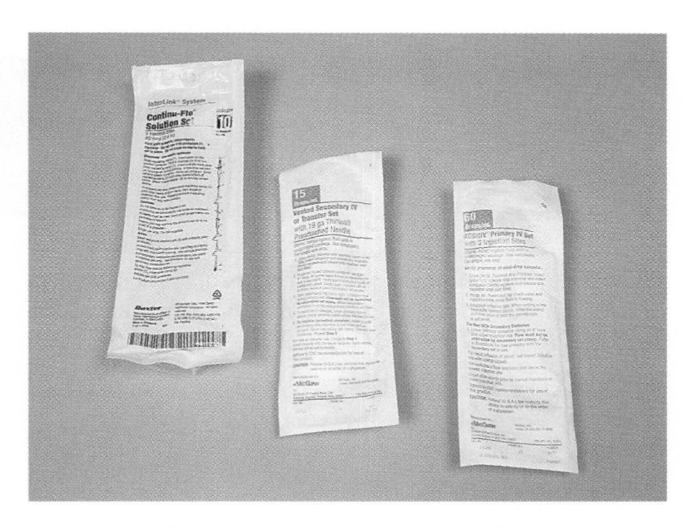

Figure 34–9. Intravenous tubing boxes showing various drip factors.

but the most common size is 0.22 μm. Because of this microscopic pore size, they are often referred to as micropore filters. Filters are recommended for patients who are receiving total parenteral nutrition or heavily particulated solutions and for immunosuppressed patients.[40]

- *Volume control sets.* When a small volume of fluid, containing electrolytes or medications, is required, the use of a burette or a *volume control set* may be indicated. Burettes are small calibrated cylinders, with volumes of 50 to 150 mL, which are filled from the primary solution containers (Fig. 34–11). An additive port is usually located on top of the container. Clamps are located above and below the container for filling and control of flow. Drip rates varying from 10 to 60 drops per milliliter are provided.
- *Intermittent infusion device.* An intermittent infusion device (IID), also called a saline lock or a heparin lock, is a resealable injection port that can be attached to a venipuncture device (Figs. 34–12 and 34–13). It is used to administer intermittent medications via IV push or drip. It provides direct venous access, but allows patients much more mobility and freedom than a continuous IV infusion. It is sometimes called a saline lock because a small amount of normal saline solution is

(continued on page 1312)

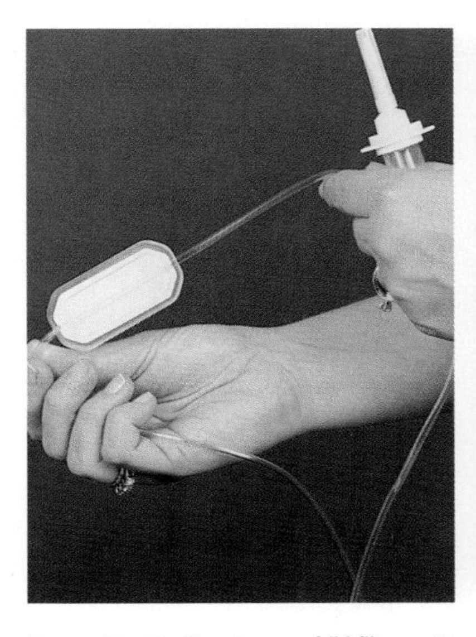

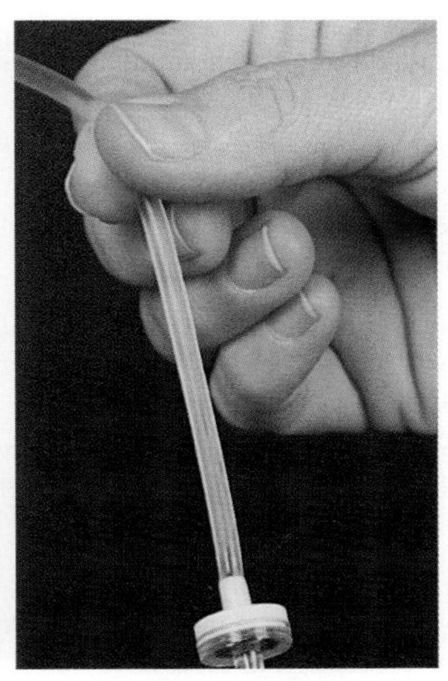

Figure 34–10. Two types of IV filters. *(From Smith S, Duell D.* Clinical Nursing Skills: Nursing Process Model; Basic to Advanced Skills. *4th ed. Norwalk, CT: Appleton & Lange; 1996:799.)*

PROCEDURE 34–3. PREPARING AN INTRAVENOUS INFUSION SETUP

PURPOSE: To provide intravenous fluids and electrolytes to patients unable to ingest sufficient quantities orally; to treat fluid and/or electrolyte imbalances

EQUIPMENT: Ordered intravenous solution, basic IV administration set, IV pole (if not available in room), label for tubing, in-line filter according to agency policy

ACTION 1. Check physician's order for type and amount of solution, total time or flow rate of infusion, and additives, if any.

RATIONALE. These are the components of a complete IV order; if elements are missing, confer with physician.

ACTION 2. Wash your hands.

RATIONALE. Transient organisms that could be pathogens are removed from hands, preventing transmission to the patient.

ACTION 3. Obtain the correct solution and administration set. Unvented tubing is appropriate for plastic bags or bottles with airways; vented tubing for bottles without airways (see Figs. 34–8 and 9).

RATIONALE. Incorrect solution can harm patient and/or fail to achieve desired therapeutic effect. Incorrect tubing may prevent fluid flow.

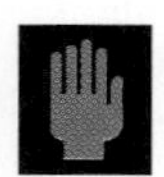

Select tubing with injection ports if IV piggyback medication is also ordered.

ACTION 4. Check container for leaks, cracks, or tears; solution for clarity, particles, and expiration date; set for cracks, crimps, or missing parts.

RATIONALE. Any of these could allow contaminated solution to be administered to patient.

ACTION 5. Prepare container. **Plastic bag:** remove outer wrapping, leave ports covered. **Glass bottle:** remove metal ring and disk; leave latex disk in place.

RATIONALE. Port covers and latex disk protect sterility of ports and contents until set is connected, by preventing direct contact with unsterile items.

ACTION 6. Remove administration set from package and close roller clamp.

RATIONALE. Spiking container with roller clamp open permits uncontrolled fluid flow into drip chamber creating air bubbles which then must be cleared from tubing.

If in-line filter is required, attach it to tubing now, following manufacturer's directions.

ACTION 7. Remove cap from spike end of tubing. Identify tubing port on container and insert spike. **Plastic bag:** pull off plastic cover and without touching spike to outside of port, insert spike with a firm twisting motion. Bag may be held on a flat surface or hung on IV pole.

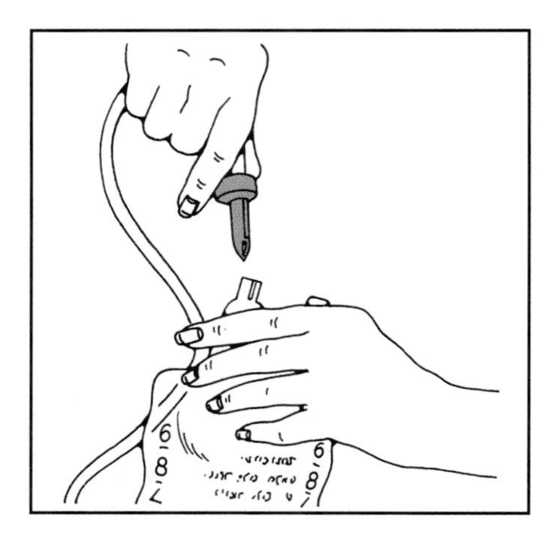

RATIONALE. Bag outlet is sealed before spiking, so no fluid will leak, even when bag is inverted. Touching spike to outside of port transfers organisms to spike, then to solution.

Glass bottle: If vented, remove latex disk (you should hear influx of air into bottle). With bottle standing on a secure surface, insert spike into larger of the two circular openings (not airway outlet) with a straight downward motion. Do not let spike contact rim of bottle.

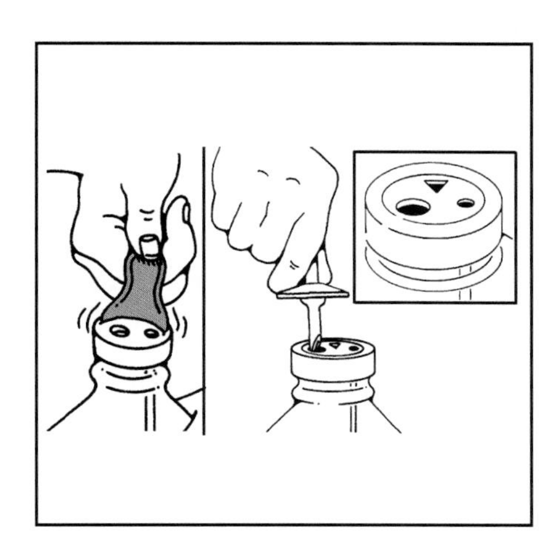

RATIONALE. There is no seal on bottle outlet once latex disk (which also seals vacuum) is removed, so it must remain upright. Secure surface allows force needed to insert spike into opening. Twisting spike into opening in bottle stopper may shear small shards of rubber and deposit them in IV solution. Touching spike to rim of bottle transfers organisms to spike, then to solution.

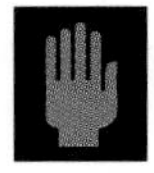

Some facilities dispense IV solutions in glass bottles having only one opening. There is no latex seal or vacuum, but the bottle is sealed with a foil or plastic cap. Vented tubing is required.

ACTION 8. Partially fill drip chamber: **Plastic bag:** squeeze chamber. **Glass bottle:** squeeze chamber, then invert bottle and hang on IV pole or wall hook. A small amount of liquid will escape from airway opening in vented bottles.

RATIONALE. Squeezing chamber displaces air into container, allowing fluid to enter chamber. Overfilling drip chamber will make regulating IV impossible, as drops cannot be seen.

ACTION 9. Remove and reserve protective cap from distal end of tubing. Hold tubing over sink, basin, or trash can and prime tubing by opening clamp and allowing fluid to displace all air in tubing. Do not allow end of cap or tubing to contact anything. Close roller clamp and replace cap.

RATIONALE. Air is removed from tubing to prevent air emboli (caused by entry of 10 mL or more air into bloodstream). Cap and tubing are prevented from contacting unsterile objects to prevent introduction of organisms into patient's bloodstream.

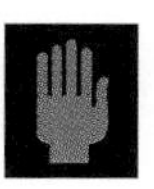

If filter was added or tubing has injection ports, invert each one as tubing is primed and tap to remove air.

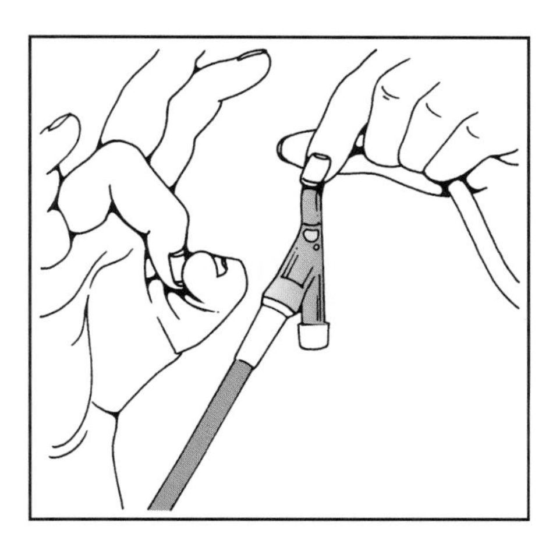

ACTION 10. Label tubing with date, time, and your initials. Time-tape container according to IV fluid order (see Clinical guideline 34–10, page 1325).

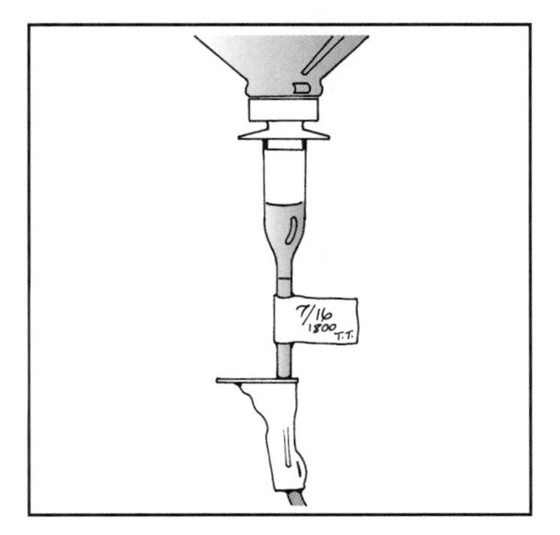

RATIONALE. Permits readily assessing progress of infusion and changing tubing in accordance with agency policy and/or CDC guidelines to prevent fluid contamination secondary to prolonged use of IV equipment.

Continued

Procedure 34–3. Preparing an Intravenous Infusion Setup (continued)

ACTION 11. Take equipment to bedside and discuss anticipated venipuncture with the patient.

RATIONALE. Discussing procedure alleviates anxiety and concerns that may interfere with patient participation.

Recording:
Venipuncture (see Procedure 34–4) is recorded on nursing progress notes or daily care flowsheet. IV solution and flow rate may be documented on I&O sheet, flowsheet, or progress notes.

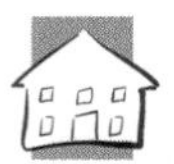

HOME HEALTH ADAPTATION: This procedure is the same regardless of the patient setting.

injected into it after each use to maintain patency. Some agencies use heparinized saline solution to maintain patency, hence, the name heparin lock. Agency policies and procedures for infusing medications and maintaining patency of IIDs vary. The SASH method (**s**aline; **a**dminister medication; **s**aline; **h**eparin; or SAS if no heparin is used) is common. (See Procedure 25–18 for administration of an IV drip medication via an IID.)

- *Needleless injection cap.* In most agencies, the standard latex injection cap is being replaced by a needleless injection cap (Figs. 34–13 and 34–14). Although some brands (Fig. 34–14) are similar in appearance to latex caps, their design permits puncture using a special plastic cannula (Fig. 34–15) rather than a needle. It reseals after puncture just as the standard latex injection cap does. The manufacturer recommends that the needleless injection cap be attached to the venipuncture device at the time of venipuncture, even when the purpose of the venipuncture is the administration of continuous intravenous fluids. Attaching a companion device, a needleless cannula with threaded lock (Fig. 34–14) to the end of the intravenous tubing permits a secure connection between the injection site and the tubing; the system is then used exactly like standard IV equipment. However, if the course of the IV fluid therapy is sufficiently lengthy that the IV administration set (tubing) must be replaced, the threaded needleless cannula is easily separated from the injection site without loss of blood via the venipuncture device and new tubing with needleless cannula easily attached. Another device to provide a secure connection when a second administration set is added at a Y-injection port is illustrated in Fig. 34–16.

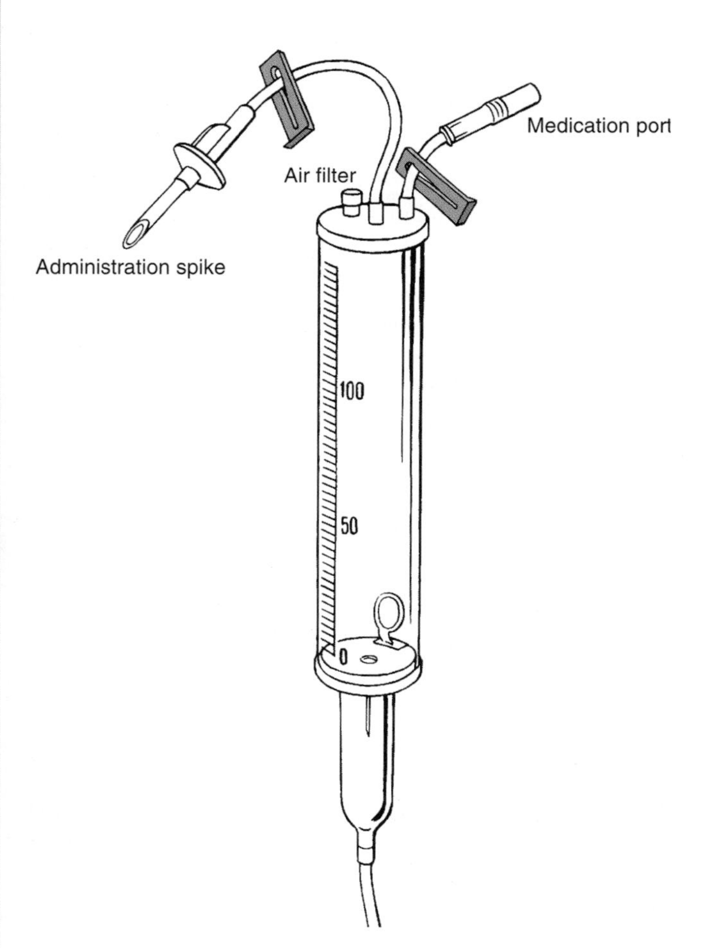

Figure 34–11. Burette style volume control set.

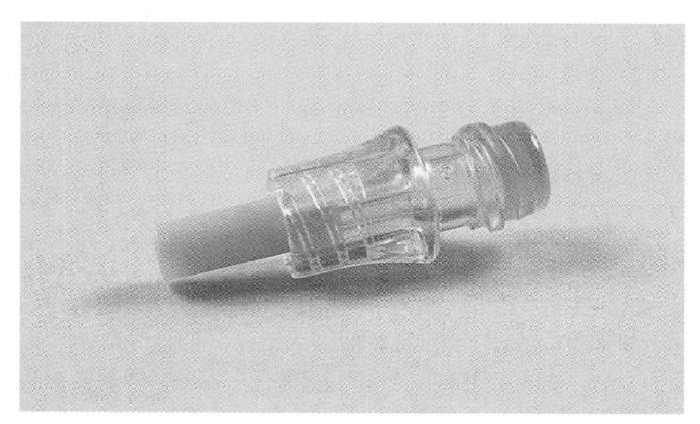

Figure 34–12. Intermittent infusion device (IID) with single injection port for use with a needle.

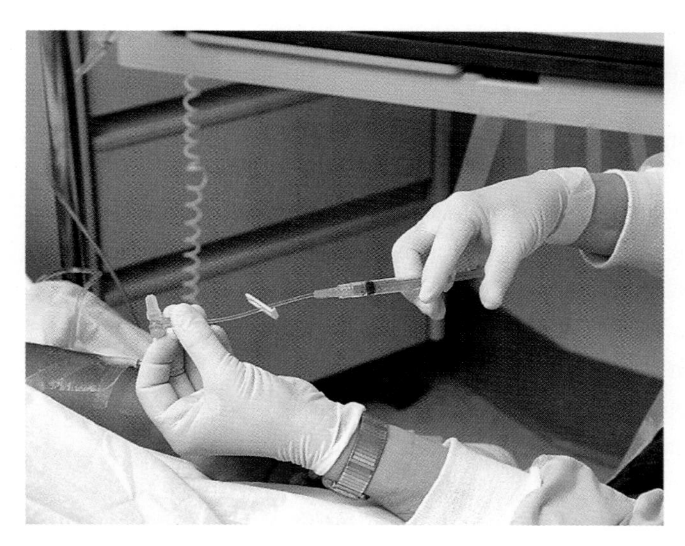

Figure 34–13. Intermittent infusion device with a latex port for use with a needle and extension tubing with slide clamp for attaching a needleless adaptor. (Needleless adaptor not shown.)

If a patient no longer needs IV fluid therapy, but venous access is needed for administration of medications, disconnecting the threaded needleless cannula with attached tubing readies the injection site for IV push or IV piggyback medications (see Procedure 25–17). Patency of the injection site is maintained according to the same protocol as for other IIDs. A needleless cannula without a threaded lock also is available for use on a standard syringe for administration of IV push medications or flushing with heparin or saline (Fig. 34–15).

INTRAVENOUS SOLUTIONS. The physician's order for an intravenous solution should specify type of solution, amount to be infused, flow rate, duration of each infusion, and any additives for the solution. Nurses should clarify orders that do not meet these specifications before carrying them out.

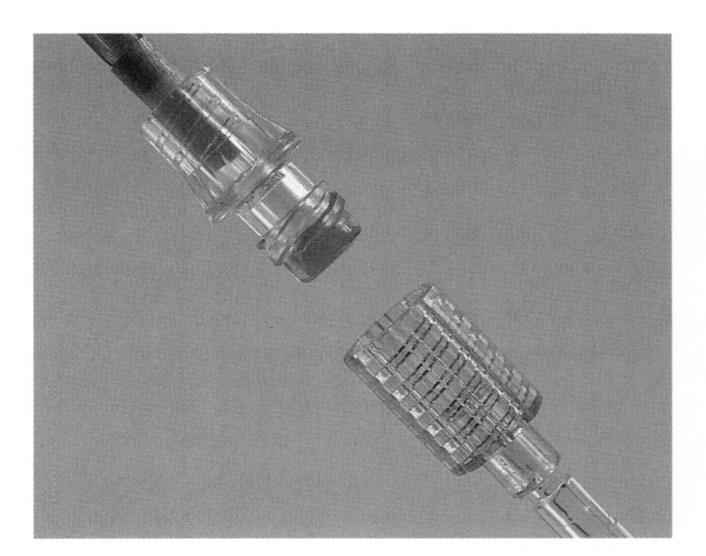

Figure 34–14. The InterLink™ Threaded Lock Cannula securely connects IV tubing to an InterLink™ Needleless Injection Cap (an IID) without taping.

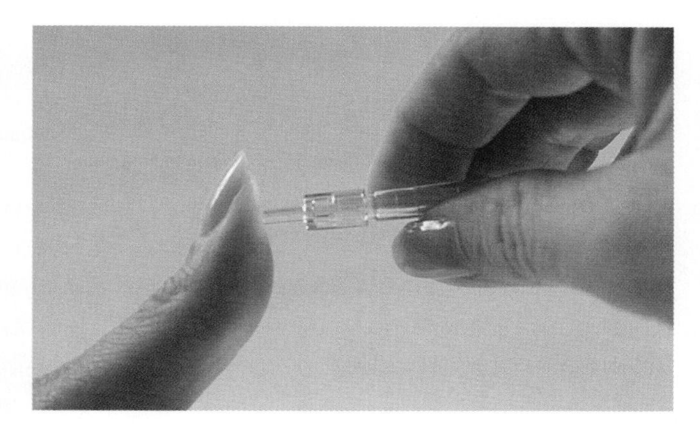

Figure 34–15. In the InterLink™ IV Access System, a blunt plastic cannula replaces the sharp steel needle.

Intravenous solutions are classified in three ways: according to their chemical nature (crystalloid or colloid), their tonicity, or their intended therapeutic use. Crystalloid solutions are composed of water and solutes that tend to form crystals when the water is removed. Colloids, or plasma expanders, are solutions used to expand the intravascular fluid volume. They pull fluid from the interstitial spaces into the intravascular space.[41] Intravenous solutions are also designated as isotonic, hypotonic, or hypertonic in reference to plasma. Table 34–19 summarizes the types of available solutions, their tonicity, and their common therapeutic uses.

Isotonic solutions generally exert no net osmotic force in the intravascular compartment. Isotonic solutions tend to distribute between the intravascular and interstitial compartments the same way that body fluid does, thus hydrating both compartments. Hypotonic solutions, which have less solute than water, dilute the plasma. As a result, fluid flows into the dehydrated interstitial

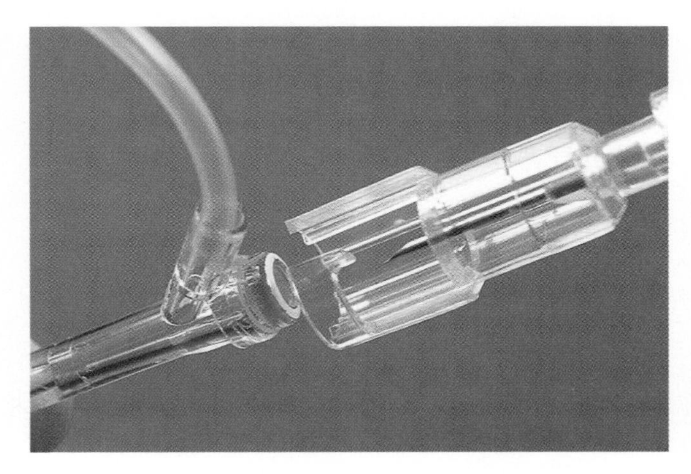

Figure 34–16. The InterLink™ Needle-lock device for securing an additive set at a Y-injection port.

TABLE 34-19. COMMON INTRAVENOUS SOLUTIONS

Solution	Tonicity	Therapeutic Use
Crystalloids		
D_5W (5% dextrose in water)	Isotonic	Hydration and minimal calorie replacement
D_5NS (5% dextrose in normal saline)	Isotonic	Hydration, electrolyte, and minimal calorie replacement
$D_5\frac{1}{2}NS$ (5% dextrose in 0.45% [half-strength] NaCl)	Hypotonic	Hydration
NS (normal saline; 0.9% NaCl)	Isotonic	Hydration and electrolyte replacement
0.45% NS (half-strength normal saline)	Hypotonic	Electrolyte replacement
3% NS[a]	Hypertonic	Electrolyte replacement
5% NS[a]	Hypertonic	Electrolyte replacement
Lactated Ringer's[b]	Isotonic	Hydration and electrolyte replacement
Isolyte R	Hypotonic	Hydration and multiple electrolyte replacement
Normosol M	Hypotonic	Hydration and multiple electrolyte replacement
Plasmalyte M	Hypotonic	Hydration and multiple electrolyte replacement
Colloids[c]		
Serum albumin 5%, 25%		Volume replacement in hemorrhage and hypovolemia
		Hypoproteinemia
Plasmanate 5%		Hypovolemia and hemorrhage
Dextran 6%, 10%		Hypovolemia and hemorrhage
Hatastarch		Hypovolemic states

[a]Hypertonic solutions are irritating to veins.
[b]Lactated Ringer's is not for use in patients with renal failure because of its potassium content.
[c]Colloids may predispose to allergic reactions.
Source: Data from reference 41.

compartment. Hypertonic solutions, which have more solute than water, are generally used to replace solutes or to cause a net fluid shift into a dehydrated intravascular space.[41]

Intravenous solutions are prepared to fulfill various therapeutic objectives. Rehydration, replacement of solutes and calories, correction of hypovolemia, and supporting nutrition are among the therapeutic values of the commonly used solutions.

Hydrating solutions are used to maintain or replace body water when there is no substantial solute loss. Hydrating solutions, in addition to supporting circulatory effort, reestablish urine flow reduced by dehydration.

Replacement solutions are used when there is a substantial loss of electrolytes and body water. Such fluids contain electrolytes, nonelectrolytes, acids, and bases to correct solute losses.

Plasma expanders expand the intravascular volume in hypovolemic states. They include actual plasma proteins in solution and large-molecule solutes, which contain roughly the same colloidal properties as plasma. As plasma expanders have osmotic properties, fluid shifts from the interstitial space, helping to further increase intravascular volume.

Nutrient solutions supply calories and prevent negative nitrogen balance. These solutions, such as total parenteral nutrition formulas (discussed later), may supply as much as 1000 calories per liter. Standard intravenous solution containing dextrose delivers minimum caloric content. One liter of D_5W provides only 170 calories.[41]

Nurses must sometimes add medications or solutes to intravenous fluid, for example, electrolytes, antibiotics, or vitamins. Intravenous electrolytes, most often potassium, are usually prepared by the pharmacy, but it may be the nurse's responsibility to add specific amounts. It is therefore important to determine the solution suitable for mixing and delivering the supplement. Usually this information is available from a pharmacist or on the inserts that pharmaceutical companies supply with their medications. Intravenous solutions containing potassium should be volumetrically controlled to prevent severe arrhythmias or even cardiac standstill.

PREPARING THE INTRAVENOUS SETUP. The technique for preparing the intravenous setup is outlined in Procedure 34–3. Assemble the intravenous setup in the cleanest possible surroundings, to prevent contamination. Compare the solution container with the physician's order to ascertain the appropriate fluid. Before assembling the solution container with the intravenous tubing, compare any required additives with physician's orders and add them to the solution container. (See Procedure 25–19 for administration of IV additives.)

Venipuncture. **Venipuncture** is the act of puncturing a vein for any purpose. There are two major considerations in performing venipuncture: selection of appropriate equipment and selection of the best site for entering the vein. Policies regarding who is responsible for intravenous infusion and venipuncture, as well as care and maintenance of the sites and infusions, vary among institutions. Nurses should be familiar with institutional policy before attempting venipuncture or intravenous infusion.

VENIPUNCTURE EQUIPMENT. There are four basic types of venipuncture devices. Each involves a slightly different technique for entering the vein. The devices include butterfly or wing-tipped needles, over-the-needle catheters, inside-the-needle catheters, and plastic indwelling catheters without needles. All venipuncture devices share common features, such as variance in gauge and length, screw-lock adaptors, and various types of needle guards to protect sterility.

Butterfly needles are short and thin-walled, for entering very superficial veins (Fig. 34–17). They vary from 27 to 16 gauge. Gauge refers to the inner diameter of the needle or catheter. The smaller the number, the larger the diameter. The short bevel, or diagonal cutting surface of the needle, prevents trauma to the opposite wall of the vein and leakage of blood into the tissue. Short needle lengths and large lumens allow for rapid fluid administration.

The butterfly device is well suited to short-term infusion into the small, peripheral veins (dorsum of hand, scalp, etc). Pediatric and elderly patients with small, fragile veins or sclerotic changes may benefit from the use of this type of device.

Over-the-needle and inside-the-needle catheters have similar components but are opposite in design. These plastic catheters are used when rapid or long-term infusion is required. They are better suited to the larger, sturdier peripheral veins.

The over-the-needle catheter, often called an angiocath, consists of a catheter mounted over a needle, with the bevel of the needle protruding from the end of the catheter (Fig. 34–17). Once the vein is pierced, the needle is withdrawn and the catheter advanced into the vein. The inside-the-needle catheter contains a catheter inside the needle lumen. As the vein is pierced, the needle is retracted as the catheter is inserted. In-the-needle catheters are typically longer and better suited to prolonged infusion, or the administration of particularly irritating solutions. This type of catheter is used for PICC or MCL lines discussed later in the chapter.

In situations of vascular collapse or severe sclerosis of the veins, it may become necessary for a physician to directly visualize and enter a vein. This procedure, known as *cutdown,* involves surgically entering the tissue and isolating a large vein. A plastic catheter, without a needle, is then inserted. Sutures are used to close and stabilize the area. This procedure is usually employed only in dire emergencies.

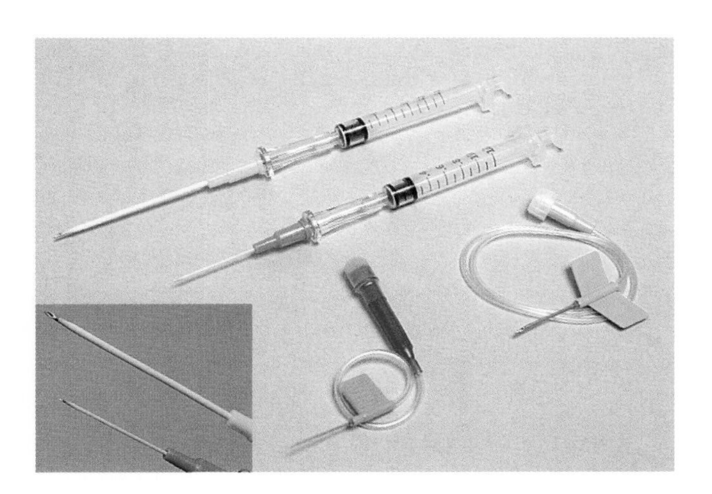

Figure 34–17. Over-the-needle catheters (top) and butterfly needles with attached intravenous access device. **Inset:** over-the-needle catheters.

INSIGHTS FROM NURSING LITERATURE

THE NEEDS OF ELDERS UNDERGOING INTRAVENOUS THERAPY

Whitson M. Intravenous therapy in the older adult: special needs and considerations. J Intravenous Nurs. *1996; 19:251–255.*

The author notes that adaptations are necessary in providing intravenous therapy to elders. The loss of subcutaneous fat over the dorsal aspects of the hands and on the arms, for example, means that the metacarpal veins may not be the best choice in elderly patients. Also, blood vessels elongate and become more fragile, tortuous, and prominent with advancing age, and sclerotic changes may narrow the lumen. Thus it is important to use a small-gauge needle and choose a large enough vein to prevent irritation of the lining of the vein. The author also advises refraining from vigorous friction or tapping of the veins, which are often fragile, prior to venipuncture. Such actions may cause a painful hematoma and prevent use of the vein for therapy.

INTRAVENOUS SITE SELECTION. Selection of the appropriate venipuncture site may often determine the success or failure of intravenous therapy. Factors to be considered in IV site selection include (1) purpose of the infusion, (2) condition of the veins, (3) type of solution and additives, (4) volume and rate of infusion, (5) expected duration of therapy, and (6) patient activity level. The purpose of the infusion and the duration of therapy determine the type, volume, and rapidity of infusion. Highly viscous infusions, prolonged therapy, irritating drugs, large quantities of fluid, and fluid under pressure require large, strong veins. The nondominant arm is preferred.

For all intravenous therapy, veins should be selected that are elastic and apparently strong. As an additional rule of thumb, sites should be as distal as possible to preserve veins for a progressive proximal selection of sites, should the need arise. The most prominent veins are not always the most adequate; they may be sclerotic or have lumen obstruction. The veins commonly used for intravenous infusion are depicted in Fig. 34–18.

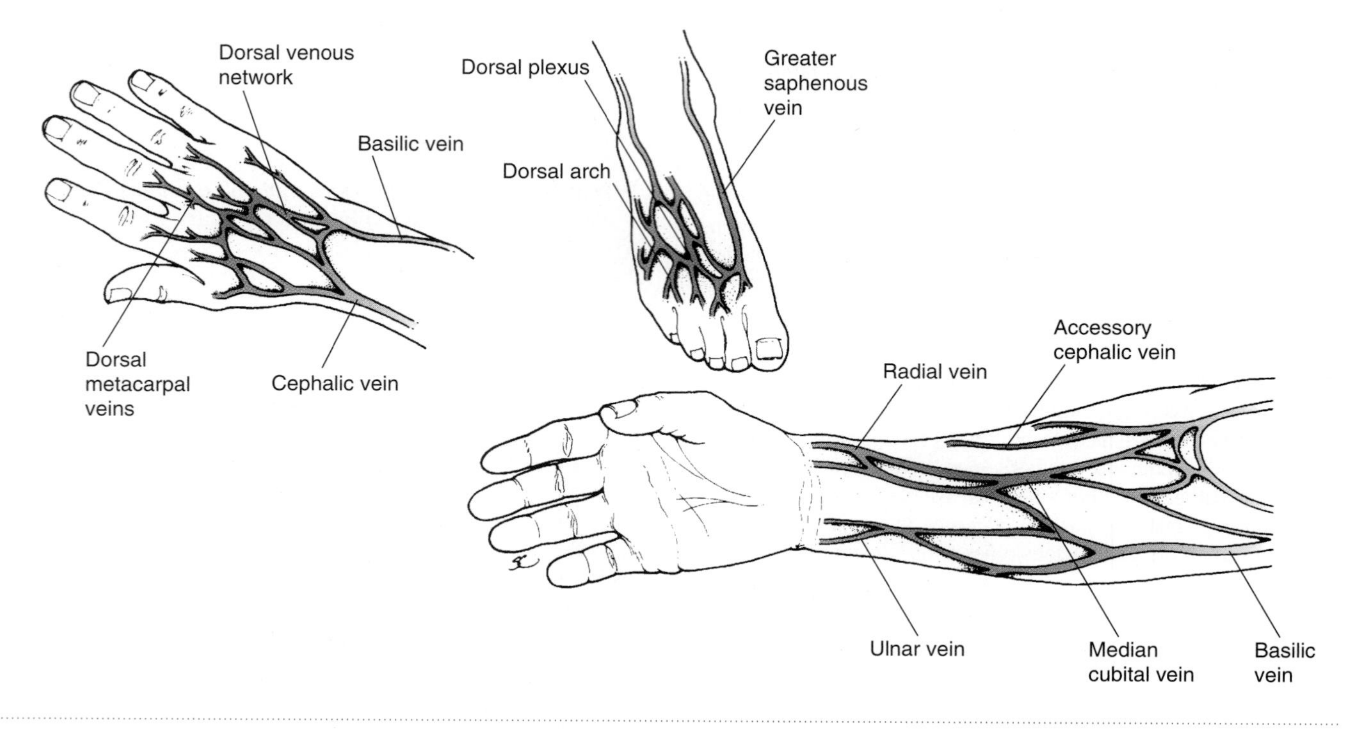

Figure 34–18. Venipuncture sites. Veins in the arm and hand are most frequently used. *(From Smith S, Duell D.* Clinical Nursing Skills: Nursing Process Model; Basic to Advanced Skills. *4th ed. Norwalk, CT: Appleton & Lange; 1996:802.)*

The metacarpal veins on the dorsum of the hand are best suited to short-term infusions, because of their relative lack of stability and potential fragility. The larger veins of the forearm are best reserved for rapid, high-volume infusion or moderately prolonged therapy. These veins are usually employed for blood administration. Veins in the antecubital fossa are large and easily accessible, but their use as venipuncture sites severely limits patients' mobility. An armboard is required to maintain the arm in extension. These veins should be used only in emergencies or when no other sites are available.

Veins of the lower extremities should be used only if no other sites are available, because of the risk of thromboembolism.[42] They should never be used in diabetic patients, because of compromised circulation and potential for inflammation and tissue necrosis.

Patient activity level is another important consideration. Although the dorsum of the hand may be an easy site to enter, the potential for movement and dislodging the cannula is high. In the wrist or antecubital fossa, as well, immobilization of the extremity to prevent flexion is usually necessary, which may add to the patient's discomfort.

VENIPUNCTURE TECHNIQUES. The technique for venipuncture is outlined in Procedure 34–4. Institutional policy will guide site preparation. In general, an antiseptic, such as alcohol or povidone-iodine, is used to cleanse the area. It is applied in a spiral pattern from site outward. Avoid povidone-iodine for patients allergic to iodine. A preparatory shave of the area is optional in patients with excessive hair growth at the selected site. This is not considered a routine measure.

Palpate the selected vein with two or three fingertips. Do not use the thumb, as it has a pulse and is less sensitive than the fingertips. Palpation should locate sufficient straight-vein area to accommodate the length of the catheter or needle from hub to tip.

MAINTAINING THE VENIPUNCTURE SITE. Once the venipuncture has been completed and the IV tubing has been securely connected to the venipuncture and flow of solution initiated, it is essential to maintain stability of the device and prevent infection of the site. To accomplish these objectives, secure the venipuncture device against movement, apply appropriate site dressings frequently, monitor the infusion and site carefully, and immobilize the extremity, if necessary.

Securing the needle or catheter involves taping the device to the patient's extremity. In taping the device, leave the injection ports uncovered for easy access. Specific considerations for securing the IV are discussed in Procedure 34–5.

(continued on page 1320)

? CRITICAL QUERY

Lau[43] reviewed the available research comparing transparent and gauze dressings in relation to infusion catheter-related infection. Transparent dressings, which allow continuous inspection of the catheter insertion site and allow patients to bathe and shower without risk of saturating the dressing, may promote skin colonization and thus increase the risk of catheter-related infection. Lau found numerous studies, but their findings, based on procedures that were often inconsistent from study to study, failed to resolve the controversy. What are some implications of this controversy for home care where infusion therapy is now commonplace?

PROCEDURE 34–4. STARTING AN INTRAVENOUS INFUSION

PURPOSE: To create access for administration of intravenous fluids, electrolytes, or medication
EQUIPMENT: Tourniquet, antiseptic cleanser, ½- and 1-in. tape, venipuncture device, assembled infusion set on overhead hanger or IV pole (see Procedure 34–3), gauze sponges or transparent dressing, disposable underpad, clean gloves, armboard (optional)

ACTION 1. Discuss the procedure, desired patient participation, and anticipated benefits with the patient. Acknowledge discomfort associated with venipuncture.

RATIONALE. Active participation is more likely if the patient understands desired participation and benefits and feels empathy from a nurse. Failure to recognize that the invasiveness and pain that occur with venipuncture are threatening to many individuals, increases patient's stress and distrust.

ACTION 2. Wash your hands. Assemble equipment.

RATIONALE. Removes transient organisms that could be pathogens from hands, preventing transmission to the patient.

ACTION 3. Palpate superficial veins of the nondominant hand or arm (dorsal foot veins used for infants/young children). Avoid veins that feel hard or ropey and veins near joint surfaces. If no suitable vein is found, assess other arm. Place disposable underpad under extremity selected for venipuncture.

RATIONALE. Use of nondominant limb maximizes independence when IV is infusing. Hard, ropey veins may be sclerosed which would inhibit fluid flow. Venipuncture near joint space limits patient mobility and comfort and is more likely to infiltrate. Underpad under extremity protects bed linen in case of bleeding during venipuncture.

ACTION 4. Ask the patient to hold extremity in dependent position for a minute. Apply tourniquet proximal to the insertion site and ask patient to pump the fist several times.

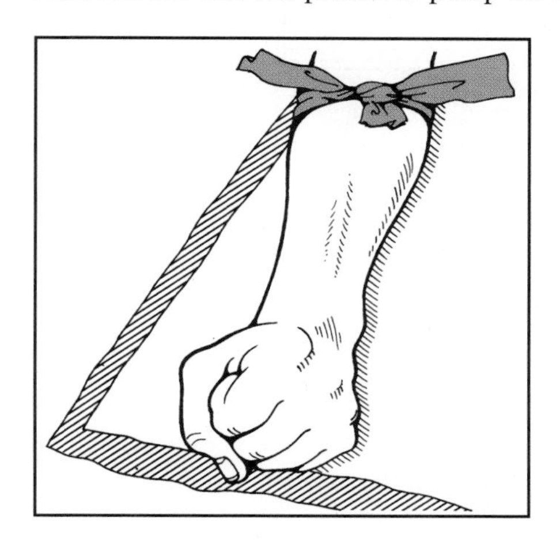

RATIONALE. These measures dilate the vein. Dilation of vein facilitates venipuncture. If these measures are insufficient, tapping the vein or applying superficial heat for several minutes may help.

ACTION 5. Cleanse the skin over the insertion site with antiseptic swabs, using a firm circular motion from the center outward.

RATIONALE. Friction and outward cleansing motion, in addition to chemical antiseptic action, remove organisms from site, preventing their introduction into patient's circulatory system.

ACTION 6. Don gloves.

RATIONALE. Body fluids, particularly blood, may contain pathogens that could infect nurse if introduced via breaks in skin, such as scratches and chapped skin.

ACTION 7. Grasp the extremity and apply traction to the skin distal to the insertion site.

RATIONALE. Tension on the skin helps to stabilize the vein wall, and reduces the tendency of the vein to slip away from the needle tip.

Continued

ACTION 8. Hold the needle, with the bevel up, and enter the skin at a 30 to 45 degree angle, over the intended site. Pierce the skin and subcutaneous tissue.

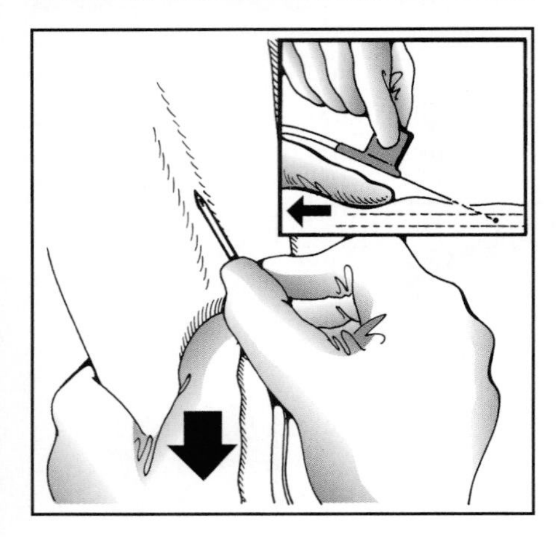

RATIONALE. The angle of entry is varied with the depth of the vein: the deeper the vein, the wider the angle.

ACTION 9. Once the needle has pierced the tissue, decrease the angle of the device so it is closer to the patient's skin and advance the needle in the direction of the vein until you feel a decrease in resistance to the needle.

RATIONALE. Decreasing the angle places the venipuncture device in position to thread into the vein. Decreased resistance indicates needle has entered the vein.

ACTION 10. Wait for a blood return into the butterfly tubing or catheter hub, then advance the device into the vein. If no blood return is noted immediately with over-the-needle catheter, partially withdraw needle. If catheter is in a vein, blood should now flow into hub of needle. If so, advance catheter into vein.

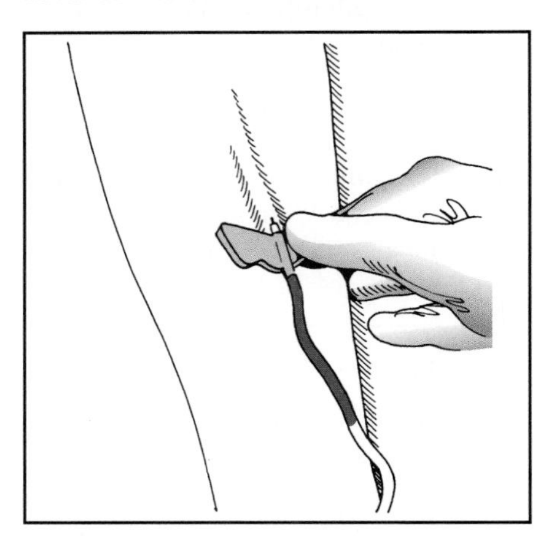

RATIONALE. A blood return indicates successful entry into the vessel. If no blood return is noted, select a new site and attempt venipuncture with a new sterile device. With the over-the-needle catheter, needle inside plastic catheter may block blood flow until moved from catheter tip.

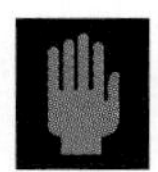

Some practitioners advance the over-the-needle catheter only 0.6 cm (¼ in.) before removing needle to decrease possibility of piercing vein wall (see Action 11).

ACTION 11. Attach the IV tubing:

a. *For butterfly:*
As blood is filling the butterfly tubing, remove protective cap from IV tubing without touching the end of the tubing or allowing it to contact patient's skin. When blood reaches the end of butterfly tubing, connect IV tubing and butterfly tubing.

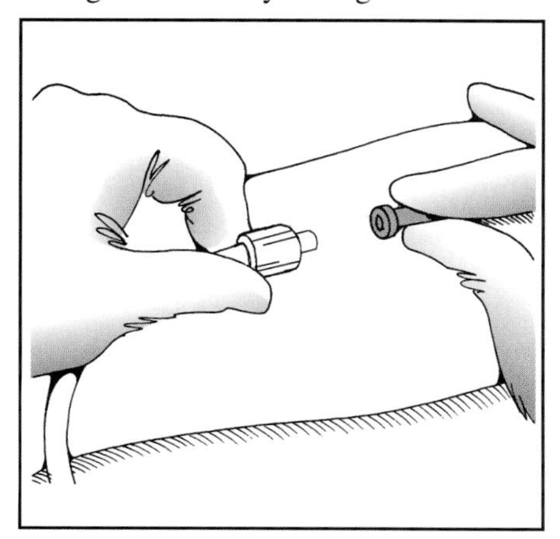

RATIONALE. Blood must displace air in butterfly tubing to prevent introducing air into patient's bloodstream. Preventing contact of tip of tubing with unsterile objects prevents transfer of microorganisms into patient's vein.

b. *For inside-the-needle or over-the-needle catheters:*
Place one finger or thumb firmly over skin above the tip of the catheter to temporarily occlude vein, and gently remove needle. Then remove cap from IV tubing and attach to catheter hub. Release finger pressure and advance catheter completely, if not advanced previously.

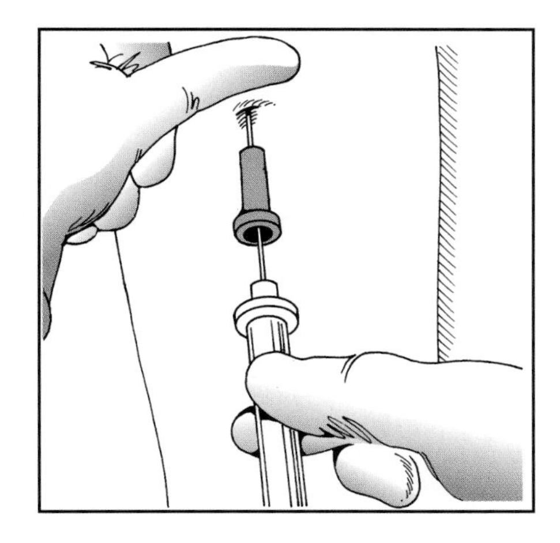

RATIONALE. Temporary occlusion of vein prevents blood loss while withdrawing needle and attaching tubing, thereby maintaining cleanliness and decreasing patient's distress.

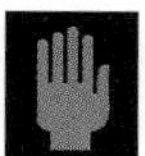

Some agencies specify use of extension tubing (4–6-in. length of IV tubing, usually with a slide clamp) between the venipuncture device and standard IV tubing.

c. *For needleless injection systems:*
If using Interlink® system illustrated, attach needleless cannula with threaded lock to end of IV tubing (leaving protective cap in place) before attempting venipuncture. When venipuncture is accomplished, attach InterLink injection site to catheter hub or end of butterfly tubing. Then remove cap from needleless cannula (the channel for fluid escape) on tubing and attach to injection site, securing with threaded lock.

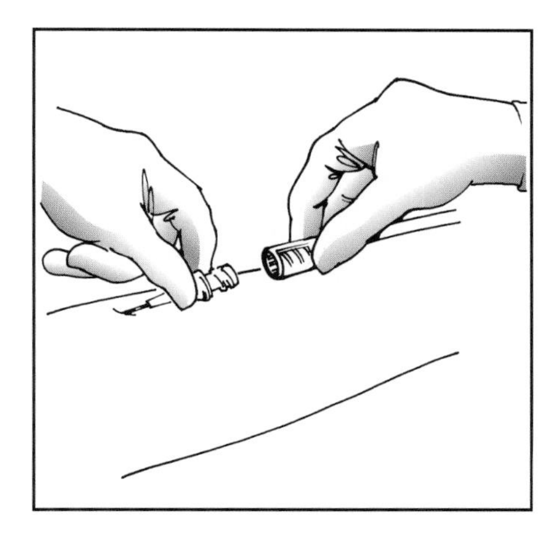

RATIONALE. Needleless systems are designed to prevent needle-stick injuries and associated transmission of bloodborne diseases. Attachment of injection site at time of venipuncture makes conversion to an intermittent infusion device lock (see Chap. 25) possible without breaking the continuity of the closed system, reducing infection risk to the patient.

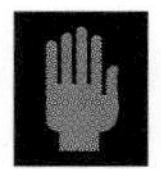

In some needleless systems, the initial attachment of the IV tubing to the venipuncture device is the same as in 11b. An adapter cap is added later, if the system is to be used for intermittent infusions.

ACTION 12. Release the tourniquet, and initiate flow of IV infusion.

RATIONALE. This promotes normal blood flow and prevents clotting.

ACTION 13. Stabilize the device and tubing with tape, and apply a sterile transparent dressing over the venipuncture site (see Procedure 34–5).

RATIONALE. Immediate stabilization of the area prevents dislodging the device.

Continued

Procedure 34–4. Starting an Intravenous Infusion (continued)

ACTION 14. Remove underpad and gloves, and dispose of them according to agency policy.

RATIONALE. See Action 6. If these items are soiled with blood, they are usually placed in receptacle marked infectious waste.

ACTION 15. Label the site dressing with the date and time of insertion and the gauge of the venipuncture device, according to agency policy.

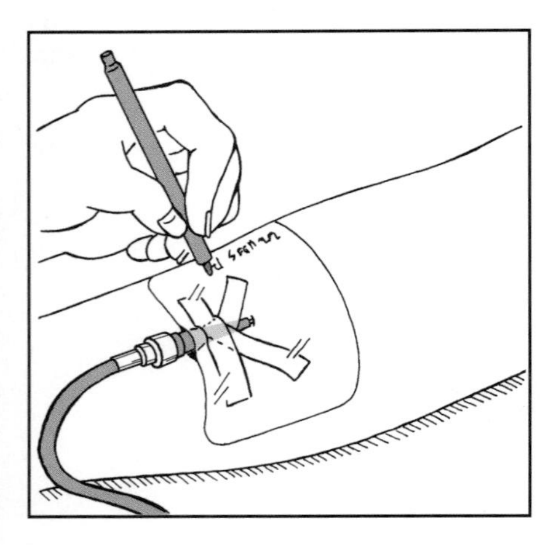

RATIONALE. Labeling enables the staff to determine the schedule for dressing and site changes.

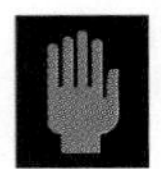

Labeling is not done in some agencies.

ACTION 16. Make sure patient is clean and comfortable before leaving.

RATIONALE. Promotes patient well-being.

Recording:
Note venipuncture location, size and type of device, type and rate of infusion, any problems with procedure, and associated actions in nursing progress notes. Record on IV or I&O records according to agency policy.

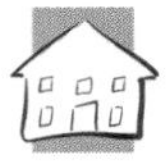

HOME HEALTH ADAPTATION: This procedure is the same regardless of the patient setting. A restraint may be needed for a confused patient. Collaborate with the physician and family before applying one. Teach family members to observe for signs and symptoms of infection and infiltration and to report them promptly to a health professional. Home IV therapy usually requires a PICC or MCL line.

The dressings used vary widely and are studied frequently in nursing research. Some institutions still use sterile gauze dressings and tape; others use transparent adhesive dressings. Sterile gauze dressings prevent direct visualization of the site and become soiled easily. Transparent adhesive dressings allow direct visualization of the area and form a bacterial barrier; however, they may irritate the skin and are more costly than sterile gauze.[43] Dressings should be changed according to hospital protocol or if wet, soiled, or no longer intact.[44]

Immobilizing the extremity may be necessary to stabilize and protect the IV site. Application of an armboard can help secure a site at a flexion point. The armboard should be short, lightweight, well padded, and should allow for adequate circulation. Specific guidelines for applying an armboard are listed in Clinical Guideline 34–7.

Calculating the IV Flow Rate. Clinical Guideline 34–8 shows the mathematical formula and guidelines for calculating and timing drip rates. Various types of intravenous tubing deliver different drop sizes, resulting in different numbers of drops per milliliter delivered. Check the package information to ascertain the drop factor of the tubing used.

Regulating the IV Flow Rate. Periodic checks of the drip rate are necessary because many variables can alter IV flow rate. Minor deviations often occur as the patient changes positions. These may be of little consequence, if the IV does not require extremely precise regulation; however, to determine whether the rate of flow is adequate, monitor the solution level in the bottle as well as the drip rate. For precise control of volume delivered and drip rate, an in-line burette may be used. Clinical Guideline 34–9 describes how to fill an in-line burette.

The solution level is easier to monitor when hourly levels are marked on the solution container. To do this, vertically align a strip of tape with the calibrations on the container and mark on the tape the level the solution should reach each hour. As the fluid level drops, check whether the actual rate of flow corresponds with the desired rate. Clinical Guideline 34–10 outlines the steps in time-taping an intravenous container.

INFUSION CONTROL DEVICES. Two problems with IV flow rates are (1) achieving precise control of volume delivered and (2) preventing uncontrolled, rapid delivery. *Infusion control devices* solve both problems. Unlike burettes, which control flow by limiting available volume, infusion control devices control the *rate* of fluid flow. Various types of devices are available, including electronic pumps; infusion controllers; and devices that operate as both a pump and a controller (Fig. 34–19, page 1326).

Infusion controllers control rate by the use of a photoelectric eye on the drip chamber. The tubing is enclosed in a clamping device inside the controller. The desired rate is set in milliliters per

(continued on page 1323)

PROCEDURE 34–5. SECURING AND DRESSING VENIPUNCTURE SITE

PURPOSE: To prevent dislodging device and protect the site against infection
EQUIPMENT: Sterile gauze square, adhesive bandage, or transparent dressing, ½- and 1-in. micropore tape, antibacterial ointment according to agency policy

ACTION 1. Secure venipuncture device:

a. *To secure a butterfly needle:*

"H" Method:

Place a ½ × 2-in. piece of tape vertically over each wing.
Place a ½ × 3-in. piece of tape across both wings.

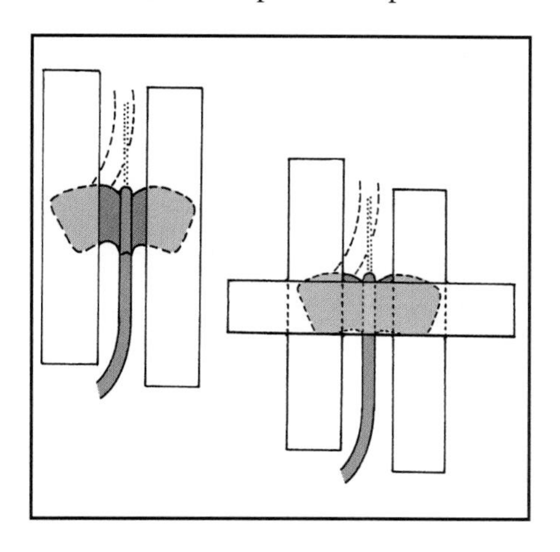

Chevron Method:

Place a ½ × 2-in. piece of tape across both wings.
Place a ½ × 3-in. piece of tape, sticky side up under butterfly tubing, just distal to wings.
Cross ends of tape diagonally across wings.

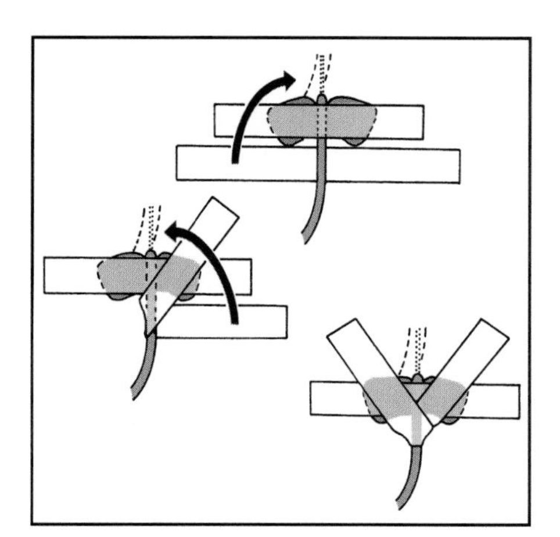

b. *To secure over-the-needle catheter:*

Place a ½ × 3-in. piece of tape sticky side up under hub.
Cross ends of tape over one another in a "V" shape so the bars extend toward the heart.
Place a ½ × 2-in. piece of tape straight across hub.

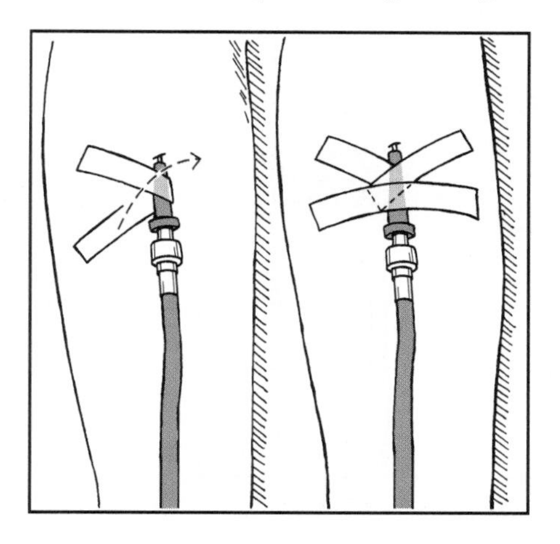

ACTION 2. Place a small amount of antibacterial ointment on venipuncture site if agency policy so specifies.

Continued

ACTION 3. Dress venipuncture site:

a. *Transparent dressing*

Remove smaller piece of paper backing; affix edge of dressing to skin so it will be centered over venipuncture site.

Stabilize fixed edge of dressing with one hand. Smooth dressing over site by pulling remaining paper backing toward opposite edge of dressing.

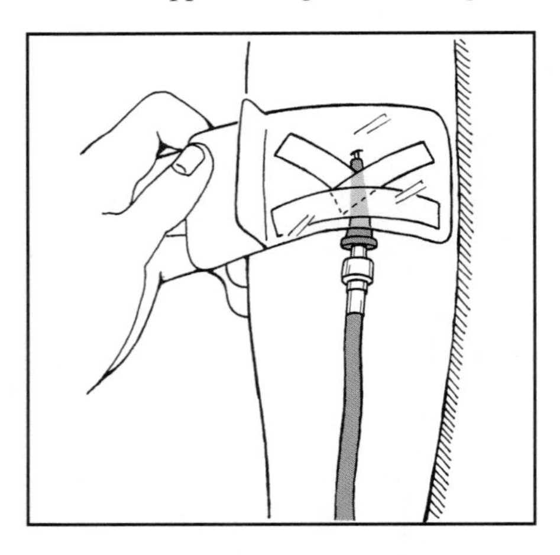

For window-type brands remove entire backing and use frame to center dressing over puncture site, smoothing dressing from center to edges.

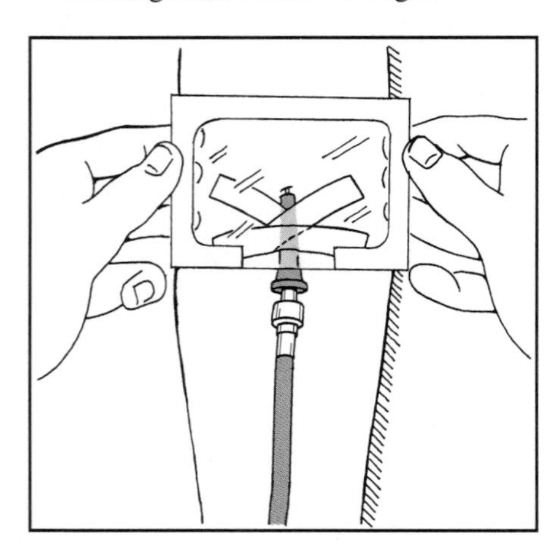

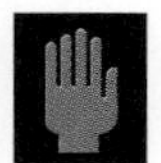

In some agencies, transparent dressing is placed directly over venipuncture site; only IV tubing is secured with tape. Another variation is use of an adhesive bandage or a 2 x 2 gauze square to dress the site after the cannula is securely taped.

ACTION 4. Secure IV tubing. Make a loop using about 10 in. of tubing; secure loop above and below dressing with 1 × 4-in. pieces of tape. Use care to prevent kinking in looped portion of tubing.

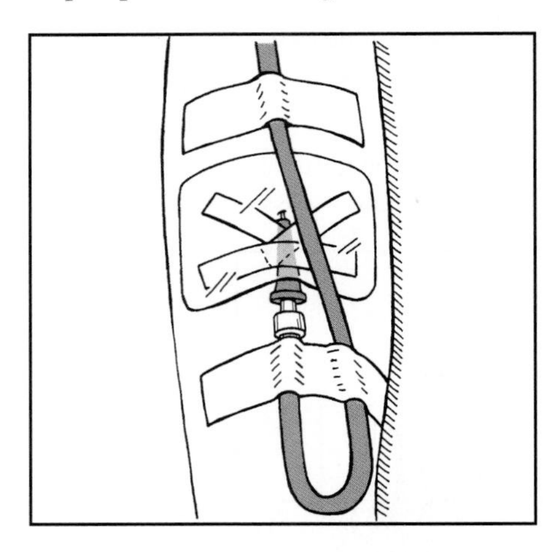

Recording:

No separate recording is necessary, unless dressing on existing venipuncture site is being replaced. Then note date and time of dressing change and site condition on progress notes.

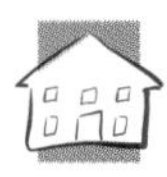

HOME HEALTH ADAPTATION: This procedure is the same regardless of the patient setting.

INSIGHTS FROM NURSING LITERATURE

WHAT TYPE OF DRESSING SHOULD BE USED ON CENTRAL VENOUS CATHETERS?

Lau CE. Transparent and gauze dressings and their effect on infection rates of central venous catheters: a review of past and current literature. J Intravenous Nurs. *1996;19:240–245.*

The author did a comprehensive review of the literature addressing the infection rates associated with the two primary types of dressings used on central venous catheters. Commonly seen in practice are transparent or gauze dressings used to cover the insertion site of a central venous catheter. The review of the research was inconclusive and failed to provide statistical proof that either type of dressing actually presented a higher risk for infection. Different definitions of infection, culture methods, and frequency of dressing changes made comparison of the studies difficult. Further, the author found that no common standard of practice in dressing central line sites existed among institutions. The literature showed that catheter-related sepsis is influenced by many factors, some of which are:

- adherence to aseptic technique
- skin preparation
- frequency of dressing change
- site of insertion
- duration of catheterization
- age and gender of the patient
- amount of moisture at the insertion site

Recommendations for further research included larger sample sizes and the inclusion of home health patients. Implications for nursing practice showed the importance of understanding the impact of risk factors on the rate of infection of central venous catheters.

hour. Because a controller does not physically pump the solution, but acts with the use of gravity, it is necessary to maintain the solution container at least 36 in. above the venipuncture site.

Unlike controllers, which rely on gravity flow, infusion pumps create a positive pressure to direct flow. The rate-set pump relies on threading tubing through a series of clamps, which compress the tubing in wavelike form, creating peristaltic movement of the fluid. Volumetric pumps incorporate a piston, which fills and expels a precise amount of fluid, according to settings made on the face of the instrument.

Safety mechanisms, such as air detectors and high-pressure clamps, are built into these devices. Most units also have electronic displays to guide users in device setup, or warn of mechanical difficulties.

Patient safety is maintained only if nurses regularly and carefully check the patient, the machine, and the setup. The responsibility for correct operation, as well as monitoring the infusion, remains with the nurse. Use of the devices does not replace bedside assessment.

CLINICAL GUIDELINE 34–7

APPLYING AN ARMBOARD

1. Cut two strips of 1-in. tape approximately one-half the circumference of the patient's arm.
2. Cut two strips of tape long enough to nearly encircle the patient's arm.
3. "Back" tapes by centering the sticky side of the short tapes against the sticky side of the longer tapes, creating a nonadhesive band with two adhesive tails.

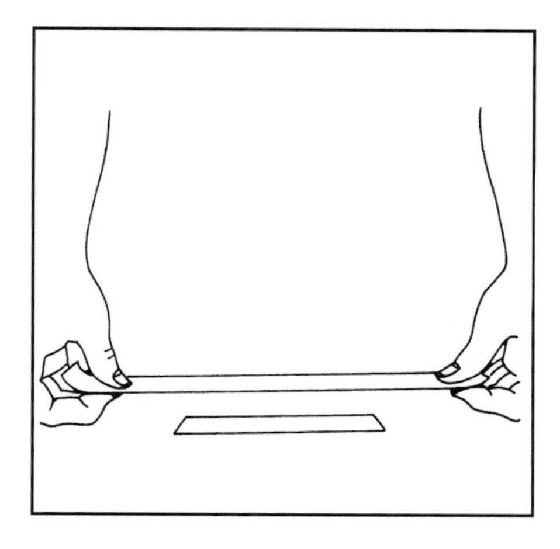

4. Place armboard under patient's forearm, so that fingers flex over the end of the board and the thumb has full range of motion.
5. Place nonadhesive band over patient's arm, being careful not to occlude the IV tubing. Affix sticky tape tails to underside of armboard. Do not overlap the ends of the tape to completely encircle the arm. This may constrict circulation. Apply at least one more tape to secure armboard.

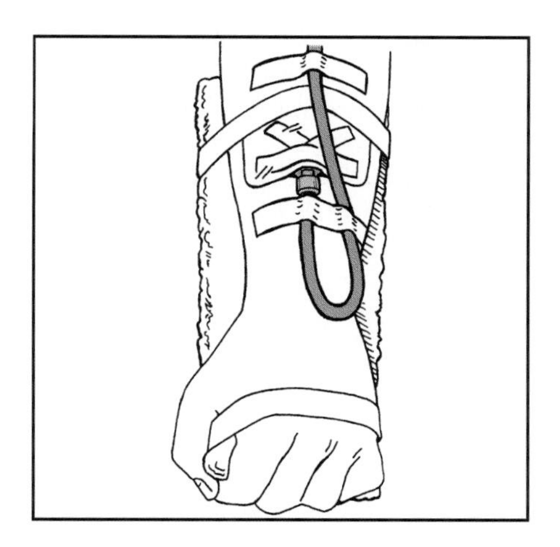

6. Assess circulatory status of fingers and patient comfort.

RECORDING

No recording is required.

CLINICAL GUIDELINE 34–8

CALCULATING AND ADJUSTING INTRAVENOUS DRIP RATES

CALCULATION FORMULAS

1. $\frac{\text{Total volume to be infused}}{\text{number of hours to run}} = \text{mL/h}$

2. $\frac{\text{mL/h} \times \text{drop factor}}{\text{60 min/h}} = \text{drops/min}$

EXAMPLES

1. $\frac{\text{1000 mL}}{\text{8 h}} = \text{125 mL/h}$

2. $\frac{\text{125 mL/h} \times \overset{1}{\cancel{15}}\ \text{drops/mL}}{{}_4\cancel{60}\ \text{min/h}} = \frac{125}{4} = 31.25\ (32)\ \text{drops/min}$

NURSING CONSIDERATIONS

1. Check physician's order to verify flow rate.
2. Calculate drip rate, using formula.
3. Count drops for 15 seconds and multiply by 4 to determine actual IV flow rate.
4. Compare actual rate with prescribed rate. If necessary, adjust flow using roller clamp to achieve prescribed rate.
5. Assess for any apparatus-related or patient-related cause for flow discrepancy.
6. Remember that drip rates vary with quantity of fluid to be delivered and period of time for delivery. The larger the quantity of fluid, over the shorter the duration, the faster the drip rate.
7. Drip rates vary with size of droplets. The larger the droplet, the fewer drops necessary to deliver a given volume.
8. The drop factor indicates the caliber of the droplet dispensed. The packaging information for the various administration sets provides the information.
9. When calculating drops per minute, reducing fractions in the equation to the lowest common denominator results in a consistent ratio: if drop factor is 10, divide mL/h by 6 to determine drip rate; if drop factor is 15, divide mL/h by 4; if drop factor is 20, divide mL/h by 3; if drop factor is 60, divide mL/h by 1.

Troubleshooting Erratic IVs. Some IVs require frequent adjustment. Many variables related to the apparatus, solution, and patient affect fluid flow and make control difficult. Table 34–20 summarizes troubleshooting to identify and correct common problems.

APPARATUS-RELATED VARIABLES. Variables related to the IV system involve the principles of fluid dynamics. The vertical distance between the solution container and the patient is important in maintaining flow rate. The smaller the distance, the slower the flow. The recommended distance is at least 36 in. In addition, excessive tubing lengths, kinks in the tubing, or the use of very small gauge venipuncture devices will slow the flow rate.

SOLUTION-RELATED VARIABLES. The viscosity of the IV fluid affects the rate of flow. Blood, blood components, or solutions with high solute content form smaller and fewer drops in a given period than less viscous solutions.

CLINICAL GUIDELINE 34–9

FILLING THE IN-LINE BURETTE

1. Assess for patency of the IV.
2. Open the airway and the slide or roller clamp on the top of the burette to initiate fluid flow.

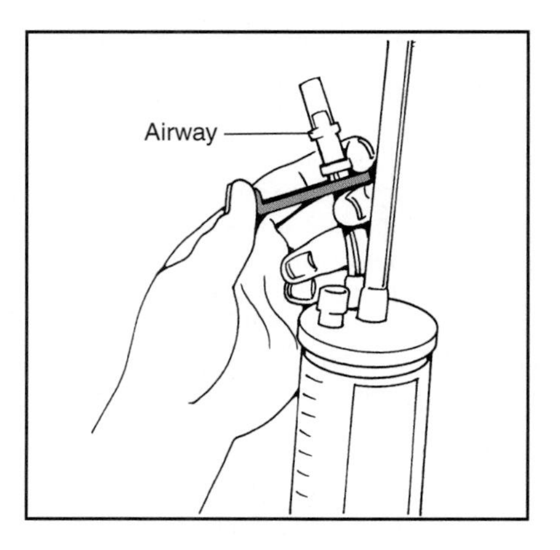

3. Open the roller clamp or slide clamp between the solution container and the burette and fill to desired level. Stop flow from solution container by closing the clamp.

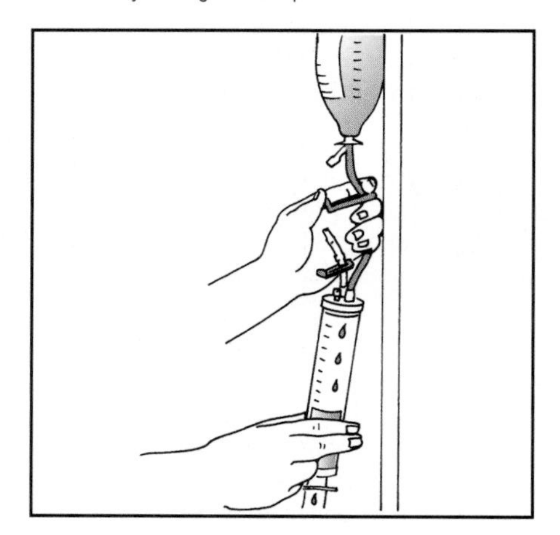

4. If burette is being used to administer medication, prepare medication in a syringe, cleanse medication port, insert needle, and inject medication into burette. Swirl burette or roll it between your hands to mix medication evenly in solution.

Continued

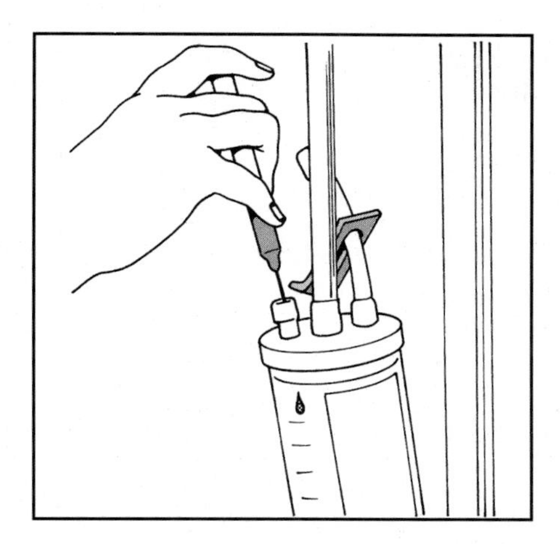

5. Start the infusion flow and adjust the rate of flow, using the roller clamp between the bottom of the burette and the venipuncture device.
6. Calculate the finish time of the volume contained in the burette.
7. Return prior to conclusion of the flow and assess for volume in the burette. Refill as necessary.

RECORDING

Use of a burette need not be specifically recorded; however, hourly volume infused is recorded on I&O record and medication given is noted on medication administration record (MAR).

PATIENT-RELATED VARIABLES. Physiologic parameters such as the patient's blood pressure may affect the flow of the IV solution. Hypotension may predispose to clot formation or venous spasm. Patient movement often repositions the venipuncture device within the vessel; the bevel may press against the wall of the vessel and occlude or markedly slow flow. Raising or lowering the extremity containing the IV changes the gravitational flow pattern by changing the height of the device in relation to the solution container.

Generally, it is best to begin problem assessment by starting at the solution container and working downward to the venipuncture site. Consider each component of the system, as well as the patient's activity level and vital signs, when troubleshooting the intravenous infusion.

Replacing Intravenous Container and Tubing. It is necessary to replace intravenous solution containers and tubing periodically to provide for continuous, unimpeded flow and prevent infection. To protect patients, the Centers for Disease Control (CDC) makes the following recommendations:

- Change the parenteral fluid container at least every 24 hours.
- Change administration sets to peripheral IV sites at 72-hour intervals.
- Remove catheters inserted under emergency conditions, where possible breaks in aseptic technique might have occurred. Insert a new catheter at a different site within 24 hours.
- Leave dressings (sterile gauze or transparent dressing) in place until the catheter is removed or changed, or the dressing becomes damp, loosened, or soiled.
- Rotate the peripheral IV needle or catheter insertion site every 48 to 72 hours.[44]

Guidelines for replacing an intravenous container and tubing appear in Procedure 34–6.

CLINICAL GUIDELINE 34–10

TIME-TAPING AN INTRAVENOUS CONTAINER

1. Calculate the intravenous flow rate in mL/h.
2. Affix commercial time-tape to IV bottle or plastic bag so volume indications on time-tape line up with corresponding markings on container. If no commercial tape is available, affix 1-in. tape along the length of the container adjacent to the volume markings.

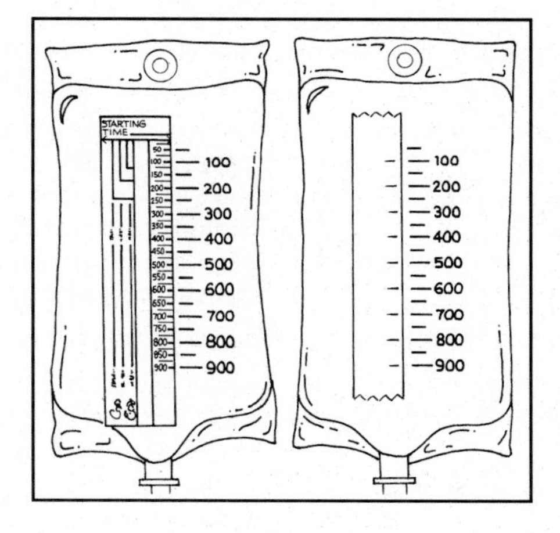

3. Make a mark on the tape at intervals representing the hourly volume to be infused. For example, if the rate is 100 mL/h, mark 100 mL, 200 mL, 300 mL, and so on.

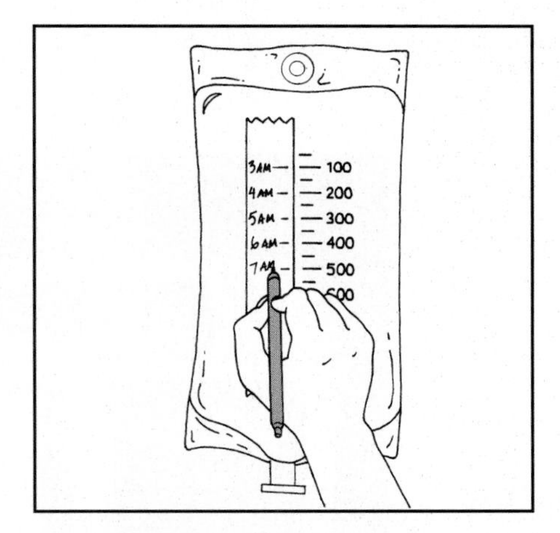

4. Write the current time at the top of the tape and the time at successive 1-hour intervals next to the marks along the length of the tape. The last time entry should approximate the time the infusion is expected to finish.

RECORDING

No recording is required.

TABLE 34-20. TROUBLESHOOTING THE INTRAVENOUS INFUSION

Problem	Approach
1. No flow is visible in drip chamber	Determine if the solution container or burette is empty, and refill or replace accordingly Observe for clots or kinks in administration set Determine if IV is "positional": ask or assist patient to reposition extremity to determine if flow resumes. If so, attempt to adjust the angle of the venipuncture device in the vein and secure with tape. Observe for the signs of venous infiltration or phlebitis; if present, discontinue infusion, and restart according to physician's orders Adjust height of container to achieve better gravitational flow
2. Unable to see drops because drip chamber is full	Close roller clamp; remove solution container from pole and invert; squeeze drip chamber to depress half of contents back into solution container; rehang container and open clamp; readjust flow
3. Solution flow is slower than desired rate	Observe for the signs of venous infiltration or phlebitis; if present, discontinue infusion, and restart according to physician's orders Assess for venous spasm; if present apply warm packs to area Determine if IV is positional—see above Use infusion controllers or pumps with highly viscous solutions Assess if tape or armboard is constricting site, and loosen
4. Visible clots in tubing	Change the tubing; do not attempt to remove by irrigation
5. Patient complaint of pain at venipuncture site and in extremity	Solution may be cold. Let solutions reach room temperature prior to infusion Assess the site for signs of infiltration or phlebitis; if present, discontinue infusion and resume with new venipuncture site and equipment, according to physician's orders
6. Large air spaces in tubing	Slow infusion rate. Insert a sterile 10–20 mL syringe with a 22–23 gauge needle or neddle-less cannula into the additive port that is closest to the air space, but distal to it. As the air nears the port, crimp the tubing below the port and aspirate the air into the syringe. If most of the tubing is filled with air, change the tubing rather than attempting to remove the air. Small air bubbles have no pathologic significance and can be ignored.

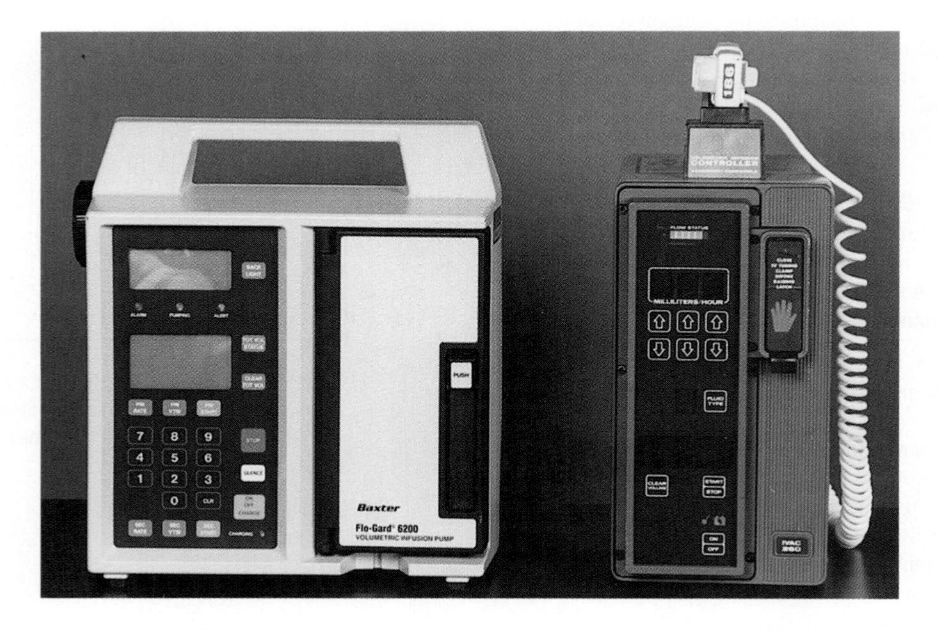

Figure 34–19. Infusion pump and controller device. *(From Smith S, Duell D.* Clinical Nursing Skills: Nursing Process Model; Basic to Advanced Skills. *4th ed. Norwalk, CT: Appleton & Lange; 1996:810.)*

PROCEDURE 34–6. REPLACING INTRAVENOUS CONTAINER AND TUBING

PURPOSE: To prevent nosocomial infection
EQUIPMENT: Sterile solution container, sterile administration set, sterile gauze pads, gloves, label to date new tubing.

ACTION 1. Discuss the procedure with the patient, including the reason, the anticipated benefits, and the desired patient participation.

RATIONALE. Active participation is more likely if the patient understands the expected benefits and desired behavior.

ACTION 2. Wash your hands.

RATIONALE. Removes transient organisms that could be pathogens from hands, preventing transmission to the patient.

ACTION 3. Prepare the new container and tubing and take to bedside. (See Procedure 34–3.) Remove tape securing tubing.

RATIONALE. Dressing covers and secures needle adapter from existing tubing to venipuncture device.

ACTION 4. Place a small sterile gauze pad under hub of venipuncture device; don clean gloves. Stabilize device with one hand. Carefully loosen existing tubing from device using a twisting motion, but do not disconnect. Close roller clamp on existing IV.

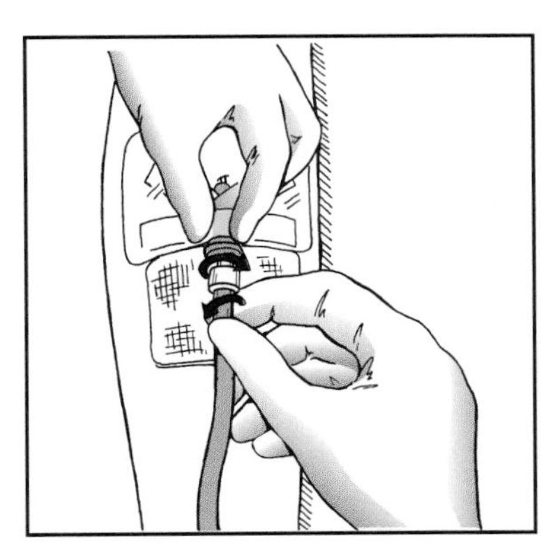

RATIONALE. Gauze pad absorbs any blood that leaks during exchange; gloves protect nurse from pathogens that may be present in patient's blood. Loosening tubing facilitates exchange without disrupting venipuncture device. Clamping tubing prevents leakage of solution during exchange.

If tubing is difficult to loosen, use hemostat to twist tubing while holding venipuncture device firmly with one hand. In agencies using extension tubing, leave extension tubing in place, close slide clamp, and remove primary tubing.

ACTION 5. Remove and discard protective cap from new tubing. Hold free end of tubing near venipuncture device. Remove old tubing, then quickly insert new tubing into device. Some nurses occlude the vessel proximal to the cannula with one finger of the hand holding venipuncture device to prevent loss of blood during the exchange of tubing.

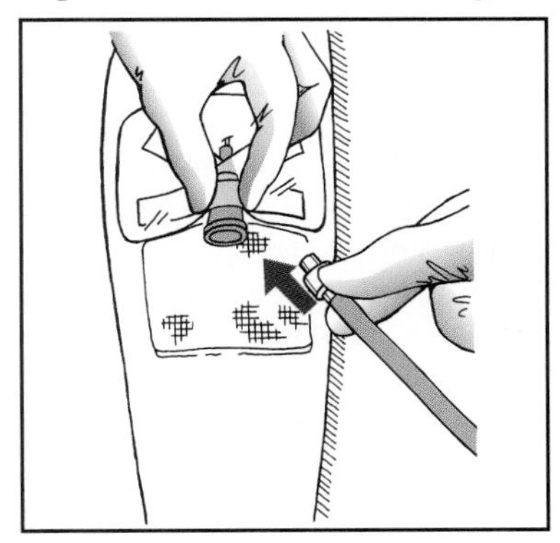

RATIONALE. Close proximity of tubing and device facilitates exchange with minimal loss of blood and minimal risk of introducing organisms into venipuncture device.

ACTION 6. Stabilize venipuncture device with one hand and secure new tubing in device with twisting motion. Open slide clamp on extension tubing, if used, and set roller clamp to KVO (keep-vein-open) rate.

RATIONALE. Tubing must be securely attached to venipuncture device (or extension tubing, if used) to prevent accidental separation. Immediately initiating fluid flow prevents clotting at venipuncture site.

ACTION 7. Cleanse skin around venipuncture site, if necessary. Remove gloves and discard in waste container marked infectious waste.

RATIONALE. Cleansing skin and properly disposing of materials that have contacted body fluids prevent infection.

ACTION 8. Secure tubing. Regulate IV flow to ordered rate and label tubing with time and date.

RATIONALE. Maintains ordered therapy; alerts personnel to need for next tubing change.

Recording:
Note amount of fluid infused from previous container and amount and type of solution in new container on I&O record. Document site assessment and dressing change according to agency policy.

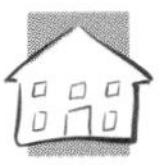

HOME HEALTH ADAPTATION: This procedure is the same regardless of the patient setting.

Discontinuing an Intravenous Infusion. A physician's order is required for discontinuation of an IV. Guidelines for the removal of an IV are presented in Procedure 34–7.

Recording Intravenous Fluid Intake. The record of intravenous intake is important to assessing fluid balance. On the intake and output form, note the time, type, and total amount of fluid started in the column for parenteral fluids. If a container is changed or the flow stopped before the container is empty, subtract the volume remaining from the total volume and record the actual volume infused.

Record the volume infused from the previous container when a new container is started. In addition, record infusion volumes at the end of each shift and total them every 24 hours. The volume remaining at the end of each shift is carried over to the next shift's records.

Complications of Intravenous Infusions. Intravenous infusions carry the potential for many complications. Localized complications such as infiltration can cause discomfort. Systemic complications such as sepsis or air embolus can be life-threatening. The most commonly observed complications are infiltration, thrombus formation, phlebitis, sepsis, air embolus, circulatory overload, and speed shock. Maintaining correct technique for all aspects of IV therapy and frequent assessment of the site and equipment promotes prevention and early recognition of complications.

INFILTRATION. Infiltration is the internal puncture of the vein by the venipuncture device. This allows solution and blood to escape into the surrounding tissues. The result is slowing or stoppage of solution flow, edema, coolness and pallor at the site, and tenderness of the area. Infiltration may result in tissue necrosis if hypertonic or irritating solutions are being infused. Once the infiltration has been confirmed, the venipuncture device should be removed immediately and a sterile bandage applied. Treatment of the infiltration site may include a warm compress and elevation of the area.

THROMBUS FORMATION. Thrombi are small blood clots that may occur if the venipuncture device traumatizes the vessel wall on entry. The resulting clot may eventually obstruct the needle or catheter. A clot also represents an accumulation site for bacterial growth in the vascular system, which may later predispose to sepsis.

PHLEBITIS. Phlebitis is inflammation of a vein. The signs are erythema (redness), tenderness, and heat. The erythema may extend along the course of the vein resulting in a characteristic streak of redness. Phlebitis results from mechanical irritation from the venipuncture device or chemical irritation from the solution. Phlebitis often stimulates thrombus formation resulting in thrombophlebitis. When phlebitis is present, the IV should be discontinued and restarted in a different vein, preferably on the opposite extremity.

SEPSIS. Sepsis is the spread of an infection to the bloodstream. Untreated sepsis may lead to circulatory collapse and death. Suspect sepsis whenever a patient develops fever, chills, and hypotension during an intravenous infusion.

AIR EMBOLISM. An air embolism is a potentially deadly but rare complication resulting from the entry of a large quantity of air into the systemic circulation. The air forms large bubbles that block the pulmonary circulation. Patients with central venous catheters are at a higher risk of an air embolism than those with peripheral IVs. Because pressure in central veins flucuates in the same way as intrathoracic pressure during inhalation and exhalation, there is a possibility of air from empty IV containers and tubing used with central venous catheters to be pulled into the patient's circulatory system during inspiration. For this reason, IV controllers that sound an alarm when air is detected in the system are always used with central IV lines. The signs of air embolus are sudden hypotension, dyspnea, cyanosis, and eventual loss of consciousness. On seeing these signs, immediately clamp the administration set and place the patient in the Trendelenberg position on the left side, which traps the air in the right atrium. Begin oxygen administration and seek immediate advanced medical treatment.

Air cannot enter the circulatory system from peripheral venipuncture sites unless there is pressure distal to the air that is greater than the pressure within the blood vessel. Air will not "infuse" when a solution container empties, because there is no pressure behind the air to propel it. However, if a nurse replaced an empty IV solution container with a new container and failed to note that the tubing was partially air filled, the fluid in the new container would then push the column of air in the tubing into the patient's circulatory system. Removing air from the tubing as described in Table 34–20 prevents problems, as does following standard IV protocols when initiating IV therapy or changing IV tubing or containers as detailed in procedures throughout this chapter.

CIRCULATORY OVERLOAD. Circulatory overload may result from rapid infusion of fluids into patients with impaired cardiac or renal mechanisms. Signs and symptoms include hypertension, dyspnea, and engorged neck veins. Preventive measures include maintaining prescribed flow rates, avoiding rapid flow rates, and using volume-controlled administration sets, controllers, or pumps.

SPEED SHOCK. Speed shock is a condition that develops when a medication or additive is infused too rapidly resulting in a high serum concentration of the drug. Signs and symptoms include hypotension, dyspnea, chest pain, facial flushing, and syncope. Infusion control devices are recommended for safe administration of IV drip medications. Medications given IV push should be administered according to drug-specific guidelines in pharmacology reference.

Assisting Patients with an IV to Perform Daily Activities. Patients with an IV in place may have difficulty changing gowns, eating, bathing, and ambulating. Use care to keep the IV site and site dressing dry during hygiene. If a patient is able to shower, securely tape plastic wrap over the site to protect it and remove the plastic wrap promptly after the shower. If a dressing gets wet, replace it immediately. Most patients with upper extremity IVs are given a gown with shoulder snaps. If these are not available, slide the sleeve of the soiled gown over the IV solution container and tubing as you slip the sleeve from the patient's arm. Then, slip the IV apparatus into the sleeve of the clean gown ahead of the patient's arm and replace it on the IV pole. *Never* open an IV line to change a patient's gown.

If eating is a problem because of the location of a venipuncture site, offer assistance, for example, with opening food containers, spreading condiments, or cutting meats. In extreme situations, feeding patients may be necessary. See Procedure 28–1.

Many patients with IVs are ambulatory. Assist them to put on a robe (often draping it over the shoulder of the "IV arm" is suffi-

PROCEDURE 34–7. DISCONTINUING AN INTRAVENOUS INFUSION

PURPOSE: To safely terminate an intravenous infusion when therapy has been accomplished
EQUIPMENT: Clean gloves, sterile gauze pads, adhesive tape or bandage, alcohol swabs

ACTION 1. Check physician's order for termination of infusion.

RATIONALE. IV may need to be restarted if infusion is discontinued in error.

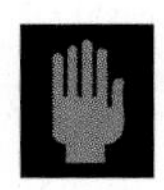

If IV is infiltrated or phlebitis is noted, no order is needed to discontinue it.

ACTION 2. Determine type of infusion (ie, peripheral, central venous, arterial).

RATIONALE. Central venous and arterial lines are removed only by personnel with special training.

ACTION 3. Wash hands.

RATIONALE. Handwashing removes transient flora from nurse's hands.

ACTION 4. Discuss the procedure with the patient, including the reason, the anticipated benefits, and the desired participation.

RATIONALE. Active participation is more likely if patient understands the expected benefits and desired behavior.

ACTION 5. Close roller clamp on IV.

RATIONALE. Prevents solution from flowing over linens, patient, and caregiver when venipuncture device is withdrawn from vein.

ACTION 6. Remove all tape from IV tubing and armboard. Carefully remove tape securing the venipuncture device, while holding device stable with opposite hand.

RATIONALE. Prevents pain and site trauma as tape is being removed.

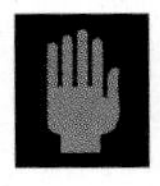

Tape and transparent dressing can be removed more easily as follows: lift corner of tape or dressing; wipe interface between underside of tape and skin with an alcohol swab while lifting tape away from skin.

ACTION 7. Don clean gloves.

RATIONALE. Prevents contact with patient's blood, which may contain pathogens.

ACTION 8. Cover insertion site with sterile gauze and apply gentle pressure to site, while carefully withdrawing the venipuncture device. Apply pressure at insertion site until bleeding stops, usually 2 to 3 minutes.

RATIONALE. Swab prevents contamination while pressure limits bleeding.

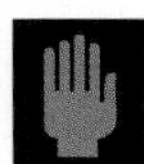

A longer period of pressure will be necessary if you are discontinuing a heparin lock and for patients who are on heparin therapy.

ACTION 9. Discard soiled gauze in infectious waste container and apply dry, sterile gauze dressing or adhesive bandage.

RATIONALE. Blood on gauze may contain pathogens. Dressing protects puncture site during healing.

ACTION 10. Dispose of IV equipment according to hospital policy.

RATIONALE. Policies for disposal of glass versus plastic supplies and designation of materials as biohazardous wastes vary among agencies.

Recording:
Record time IV discontinued, state of puncture site, and intactness of cannula in nursing records. Record volume of IV fluid absorbed on I&O sheet.

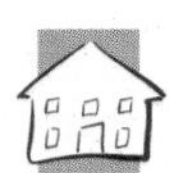

HOME HEALTH ADAPTATION: This procedure is the same regardless of the patient setting.

cient), and demonstrate how to safely push the IV pole ahead of them as they walk. Caution patients against using IV poles for support; if support is needed, it should be given by the nurse. See Procedure 33–2.

Transfusion Therapy

Some of the most serious body fluid deficits are caused by blood loss. The various constituents of blood, such as albumin, platelets, plasma, and globulins, have multiple functions and hemorrhage, therefore, has far-reaching consequences. Clotting abnormalities, immunologic deficits, and tissue oxygenation problems often result. Therefore, transfusion of blood and its constituents is important not only to replace body fluids but also to restore other body functions.

Blood is a living tissue and is often called an organ. When this living tissue is transplanted, the possibility of grave reactions exists. Careful laboratory testing for matching blood or blood products to the recipient's blood type as well as rigorous procedures for patient and product identification, are essential to prevent these problems. *Autotransfusion,* that is, collection of several units of a patient's own blood at intervals prior to elective surgery, is often recommended as an alternative to donor blood transfusion. If needed, this blood can be reinfused to replace losses during surgery. Autotransfusion not only eliminates risks associated with errors in typing or cross-matching, it also relieves concerns about blood-borne infections.

Blood Groups and Blood Matching. Human blood is classified into four blood compatibility groups based on immune reactivity. The four groups, A, B, O, and AB, are differentiated on the basis of polysaccharide *antigens* (called agglutinogens) on the erythrocyte surface. The presence or absence of A and B antigens on the cells is detected by using anti-A and anti-B reagents, but also by testing for *antibodies* (agglutinins) in the serum, known respectively as anti-A and anti-B antibodies.

Both cell typing and serum typing are performed routinely. Type A red blood cells have A antigens and anti-B antibodies are present in the serum. Type B, on the other hand, has B antigens and has anti-A antibodies in the serum. Type AB has both A and B antigens and has no antibodies in the serum, whereas type O has no antigens and has both A and B antibodies in the serum.[16] As a rule blood selected for transfusion must be of the same type as that of the recipient. Blood transfusions, therefore, must be matched to the patient's blood. Mismatched blood causes hemolytic reactions. In urgent situations, however, type O–negative blood may be used for patients with other blood types.[16]

Rh typing is routinely performed along with ABO typing to determine the presence of the Rh factor. The Rh factor refers to the presence of Rh antibodies on the surface of the erythrocytes; these antibodies occur in about 85 percent of the population. The blood of persons with the factor is said to be Rh positive (+); the blood of persons without the factor is said to be Rh negative (–). Rh factor is a major cause of hemolytic reactions during transfusion. Patients with Rh negative blood should always receive Rh negative blood. Patients with Rh positive blood may receive either Rh positive or Rh negative blood.

Whole Blood and Blood Products. Whole blood may be reduced to at least six different components for use in the human body. Whole blood, packed red cells, platelets, fresh or frozen plasma, serum albumin, and cryoprecipitate are used to correct various body fluid and clotting deficiencies.

WHOLE BLOOD. Whole blood is used only to replace blood lost to massive hemorrhage. Whole blood must contain an anticoagulant to prevent clotting in the container. As blood ages, red cells die and potassium is released into the plasma, resulting in hyperkalemia. Coagulation factors also degrade as blood ages, lengthening the clotting time. Whole blood is most often "split" or broken down into its components immediately after donation.[45]

PACKED RED BLOOD CELLS. Packed red blood cells are a preparation of densely concentrated red cells resulting from removing plasma from whole blood. Packed cells are used for patients who require red cells for increased tissue oxygenation but must have limited fluids.

PLATELETS. Platelets, or thrombocytes, aid in the clotting of blood. Platelets are obtained by centrifuging whole blood and removing the platelet component. Platelets should not be administered without compatibility tests, although the tests may be suspended in emergencies. Some plastics used in solution containers may cause platelets to adhere to one another, so the container must be agitated frequently during administration.

PLASMA. Plasma, the serous component of whole blood, is used to restore lost fluid and proteins in the intravascular compartment. Generally, plasma from a donor of the same blood group and type as the patient is used. Fresh-frozen plasma is treated by freezing to protect the clotting factors and thus must be warmed before it is used. Because rewarming can degrade the clotting factors, fresh-frozen plasma must be used within 6 hours of thawing.[45]

SERUM ALBUMIN. Serum albumin is used for specific plasma protein replacement. The osmotic characteristics of the albumin also help correct hypovolemia by causing a fluid shift from the interstitial to the intravascular compartment. Two strengths of serum albumin are available: 5 percent in saline and 25 percent solution.[45] The 25 percent solution will cause ICF dehydration if additional fluids are not supplied. Although some reactions have been noted to serum albumin, infusion compatibility testing is not usually required before use.

CRYOPRECIPITATE. Cryoprecipitate is a solution containing clotting factor VIII, which is missing from the blood of hemophiliacs. It is removed from frozen plasma and administered in small quantities (approximately 10–15 mL).[45] Treatment must be repeated frequently.

Nursing Responsibilities in Transfusion Therapy. A nurse's responsibilities in transfusion therapy are to guard patient safety and prevent side effects. To do this, nurses carefully identify the product and the patient, follow approved administration techniques, and observe the patient for reactions. General considerations and a step-by-step guide for the administration of blood appear in Procedure 34–8.

The first step in transfusion therapy is to obtain a blood specimen from the patient for type and cross-matching. These compatibility tests identify the appropriate group and type of blood to infuse. Compatibility tests also determine if the patient has immunologic difficulties, such as difficult-to-match antibodies.

PROCEDURE 34–8. ADMINISTERING BLOOD

PURPOSE: To safely infuse blood or blood products intravenously

EQUIPMENT: 250 to 500 mL 0.9% normal saline (NS), in-line blood filter, blood administration set (Y-connection set) with attached filter, venipuncture device (19 gauge or larger), IV dressing, adhesive tape, clean gloves

ACTION 1. Explain the procedure to the patient and family. Take particular care to ask patient to report any back pain, chills, itching, or respiratory changes during the infusion. Signed consent may be required.

RATIONALE. The necessity for transfusion is anxiety producing. Explanation gives the patient and family an opportunity to express concerns and alleviate anxiety. Reporting of signs and symptoms aids the nurse in the decision to terminate the transfusion before significant harm comes to the patient.

ACTION 2. Wash your hands.

RATIONALE. Handwashing removes transient flora and prevents transmission of microorganisms to patient.

ACTION 3. Prime the Y-infusion set with NS to remove air from the main tubing and the short tubing to which unit of blood will be connected. Clamp short tubing after priming.

RATIONALE. Normal saline is isotonic and does not interfere with the integrity of the red blood cells. Air in the tubing predisposes to clotting and the possibility of air in the patient's bloodstream.

ACTION 4. If patient does not have an IV, don gloves and perform venipuncture with a 19-gauge or larger device. Connect the saline infusion to this device.

RATIONALE. Viscous fluids, such as blood, require large-gauge devices to sustain flow. In addition, blood cells may be damaged if forced to flow through small-bore devices.

If existing IV device is less than 19 gauge, start a new IV.

ACTION 5. Take vital signs and record.

RATIONALE. A baseline set of vital signs guides nurses in determining significant changes in patient condition during the transfusion.

ACTION 6. Obtain the blood from the blood bank. Obtain only one unit of blood at a time, even if more than one unit will be required.

RATIONALE. Blood must be used within a specific period to prevent cell hemolysis and clotting factor deterioration.

ACTION 7. Complete all identification checks according to agency policy. The usual checks are done by two licensed personnel, and include unit ID number, group and type of blood, expiration date of unit, and the patient's name and hospital ID number.

RATIONALE. Hospital policies regarding the personnel responsible for the identification checks and the initiation of the transfusion may vary. The checks verify that the patient is being given the same group and type of blood, and is not being given old blood.

ACTION 8. Close the clamp on the saline infusion.

ACTION 9. Attach the unit of blood to the short tubing on the administration set. Invert the unit and squeeze it to fill the filter. Place the unit on IV pole and depress and release the drip chamber until it is filled with blood.

RATIONALE. The filter captures clots and particulate matter that may have developed in processing or storing the blood product. Priming the filter promotes smooth flow and prevents air from entering the system.

ACTION 10. Begin blood infusion at slow rate.

RATIONALE. One unit of blood is generally infused over 1.5 to 4 hours. Rapid administration may lead to transfusion reactions or circulatory overload.

ACTION 11. Observe the patient for any reactions to the infusion, and take vital signs according to agency policy.

RATIONALE. Transfusion reactions usually occur early in the infusion, but some may be delayed. Vital signs are generally taken at least every 15 minutes during the first hour of the transfusion, then every 30 minutes for the remainder of the transfusion.

ACTION 12. Complete the transfusion and infuse NS to clear the tubing.

RATIONALE. Infusing saline ensures that the entire amount of the blood product reaches the patient.

Continued

Procedure 34–8. Administering Blood (continued)

ACTION 13. Dispose of the used blood unit and administration set according to agency policy.

RATIONALE. Many agencies require that all used units be returned to the blood bank. Others require different means of disposal.

Recording:
Record the completion of the therapy, patient response, complications if any, and nursing action taken, and nursing observations when transfusion is completed on the nursing progress notes. Record the total volume infused on the I&O record.

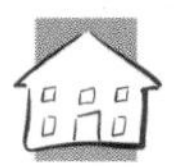

HOME HEALTH ADAPTATION: This procedure is not currently done in the home.

Identification procedures should always be carried out before blood is transfused. Each unit of blood is checked separately. Cross–check the patient's identification band with that on the unit of blood for name, hospital number, unit identification number, ABO group and Rh type, and expiration date (Fig. 34–20). In general, most facilities require that two licensed, professional staff members check this information.

Inspect the blood component to be sure that the ports have not been opened and there are no leaks in the system. If there is evidence of clotting and serum separation, indicated by dark patches in the blood and amber serum separated from the cells, do not use the blood. The blood should have a uniform, deep crimson color.

Blood is commonly administered through a Y-tubing set (Fig. 34–21). One arm of the Y-set should be attached to a container of 0.9 percent saline, the other to the unit of blood. Maintaining asepsis is essential, as blood is a prime medium for bacterial growth. If a micropore filter is not built into the set, add one between the unit and the administration set.

Normal saline is used to prime air from the system and to keep the vessel open while blood units are changed. It should not be infused simultaneously with the blood. Hypotonic or hypertonic solutions should not be used with blood, because of the possibility of cell damage.

The large veins of the upper extremities should be used for venipuncture for transfusion therapy. For adult patients, the venipuncture device should be no smaller than 19 gauge.

To maintain the internal consistency of the blood, it should be used within 30 minutes of issue from the blood bank. Infusion rates vary, but should never take longer than 4 hours to infuse.[45]

Complications of Transfusion Therapy. Complications of transfusion therapy are relatively rare; however, anaphylactoid, febrile, and hemolytic reactions, in addition to circulatory overload, may occur.[45] Nurses must know the signs and symptoms of these reactions and what actions to take on observing them (see Clinical Guideline 34–11).

Rare allergic or anaphylactoid reactions may occur in patients with multiple drug and food allergies. The patient's hyperactive

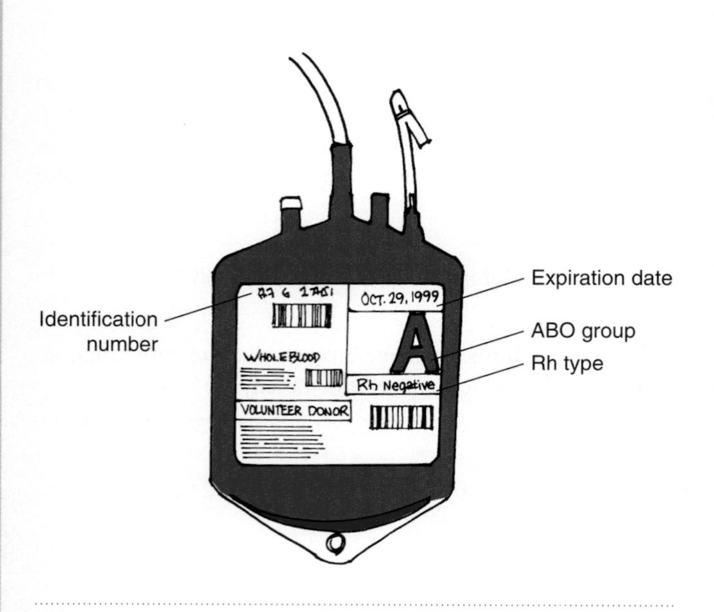

Figure 34–20. Blood identification for transfusion therapy.

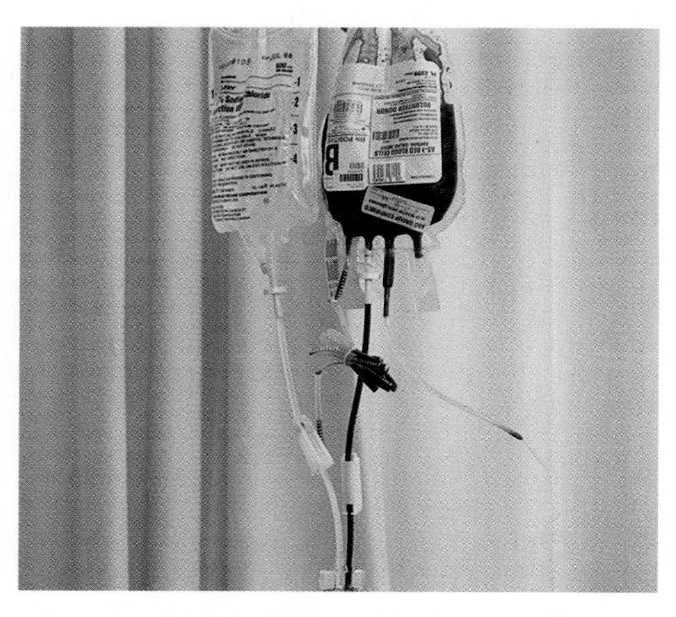

Figure 34–21. Blood transfusion setup. *(From Smith S, Duell D.* Clinical Nursing Skills: Nursing Process Model; Basic to Advanced Skills. *4th ed. Norwalk, CT: Appleton & Lange; 1996:833.)*

CLINICAL GUIDELINE 34–11

RECOGNIZING TRANSFUSION REACTIONS

SIGNS AND SYMPTOMS OF HEMOLYTIC REACTION (INTRAVASCULAR HEMOLYSIS)

- Restlessness
- Anxiety
- Flushing
- Chest or lumbar pain
- Tachypnea
- Tachycardia
- Nausea
- Shock
- Hives
- Chills
- Fever

SIGNS AND SYMPTOMS OF CIRCULATORY OVERLOAD

- Dyspnea
- Chest pain
- Rales and rhonchi
- Anxiety
- Diaphoresis
- Blood-tinged sputum

immune system reacts to the blood as foreign matter. Hives and temperature elevations are common. Treatment usually consists of antihistamine or steroid administration. The patient may benefit from the prophylactic administration of antihistamines before beginning the infusion.

By far the most serious reaction accompanying transfusion therapy is the hemolytic reaction. A **hemolytic reaction** involves the formation of antibodies in the recipient to the red cells in the donor blood, resulting in hemolysis, or destruction, of the cells. The release of hemoglobin from the destroyed red cells results in reduced oxygenation to the tissues. As a result, breakdown products collect in the kidneys and may lead to renal failure.

The signs and symptoms of hemolytic reactions listed in Clinical Guideline 34–11 develop rapidly after the transfusion is begun. The transfusion should be stopped immediately with any sign of reaction and the blood container saved for laboratory analysis. Treatment for hemolytic reaction often includes intravenous infusion of isotonic fluid to flush the kidneys and maintain urine flow, as well as administration of vasopressors to support the blood pressure.

Careful preparation and frequent observation are essential during transfusion therapy. Vital signs are taken before and at frequent intervals during the procedure. Nurses are responsible for this care as well as for the careful identification procedures and continual monitoring of the patient's well-being.

Total Parenteral Nutrition Therapy

Total parenteral nutrition (TPN), or intravenous hyperalimentation, is the administration of nutrients intravenously to patients who cannot tolerate food via the GI tract. Although TPN does not directly correct body fluid imbalances, the electrolytes and proteins in the solutions often correct fluid shifts in the ECF compartment. Patients who may benefit from TPN include, but are not limited to, those with GI problems, renal failure, severe burns, multiple trauma, and metastatic cancer. Postsurgical patients who experience complications that delay oral intake are also candidates for TPN.

TPN solutions are usually composed of water, 10 to 15 percent dextrose, and various additives, such as electrolytes, amino acids, vitamins, and trace elements. Lipid components are often administered in a separate solution. Some of the more common components of TPN solutions are listed in Table 34–21. Some hospitals use a total nutrient admixture of dextrose, lipids, amino acids, and other additives in one solution infused over a 24-hour period.[46]

Administration of TPN. TPN solutions are hypertonic so deep central veins are preferred for their delivery. The right subclavian vein and external and internal jugular veins are frequent sites for these infusions.

Central Venous Catheters. Central venous catheters (CVCs) are used to access the deep veins for TPN administration. Central venous catheters are large-bore catheters that are inserted in an operating

TABLE 34-21. CONTENTS OF TYPICAL TOTAL PARENTERAL NUTRITION FORMULAS

Additive	Amount
Amino acids	28.5–42.5 g/L
Dextrose	250 g/L
Electrolytes	
Sodium chloride	30–55 mEq/L
Potassium chloride	60–90 mEq/day
Potassium phosphate	60–90 mEq/day
Magnesium sulfate	16–20 mEq/day
Calcium gluconate	6–12 mEq/day
Trace minerals	
Zinc	Variable amounts, usually less than 5 mL
Copper	
Selenium	
Manganese	
Multivitamins: B complex, A, C, D, E, and K	10 mL total
Fat emulsion formulas (soybean or safflower derivatives)	
Intralipid 10% and 20%	50–100 g/500 mL
Lyposin 10% and 20%	
Travmulsion 10% and 20%	
Soyacal 10% and 20%	

Source: Data from reference 47.

room by a surgeon. After insertion, the catheter is sutured to the patient's skin. During insertion, the patient lies either flat or in the Trendelenberg position and is asked to perform the Valsalva maneuver as the catheter is introduced.

Before using a central venous catheter, its position must always be confirmed by x-ray. The subclavian vein, the usual site of insertion, is quite close to the apex of the lungs. Thus, accidental puncture of the pleura can result and produce a serious complication such as a pneumothorax. In addition, correct placement of the catheter tip is essential to prevent cardiac perforation or tamponade. The catheter tip should be in the superior vena cava.[48] On confirmation of placement, the flow rate of the infusion is increased from a keep-vein-open (KVO) rate to the desired rate.

Strict aseptic technique must be used not only to introduce the catheter but also in subsequent dressing and tubing changes. The frequency of dressing changes varies from agency to agency. Intravenous tubing need be changed no more frequently than at 72-hour intervals; however, solutions must be changed at least every 24 hours.[44] The aseptic handling of the solutions is mandatory, as the high glucose content of the TPN solution is a prime medium for bacterial growth. Each institution establishes its own protocol for CVCs, and nurses should be familiar with this policy.

Another type of central venous catheter, known as a tunneled CVC, is surgically implanted into the right atrium and the catheter "tunneled" under the skin to either an implanted subcutaneous port or an external port. Groshong, Broviac, and Hickman are names of tunneled catheters in common use. Their purpose is to deliver long-term intravenous therapy (ie, chemotherapy, hemodialysis, home-infusion therapy). Care of the catheter site, tubing, and intravenous solution is the same as for a percutaneous CVC.[44]

Peripherally Inserted Central Catheters. A peripherally inserted central catheter (PICC) is an intravenous catheter inserted at the antecubital fossa with the tip of the catheter in the superior vena cava. Indications for a PICC are numerous and include moderate to long-term antibiotics, or other IV drug therapy, parenteral nutrition, chemotherapy, and blood sampling.[49] Nurses with advanced education can insert a PICC line. The insertion technique is very similar to starting a peripheral IV line.[50] The PICC can be left in place as long as needed, if there are no complications.

A midline catheter (MCL) is very similar to the PICC except that it is a shorter catheter with the tip extending only 6 to 7 inches up the arm from the insertion site at the antecubital space.[50] It is used for shorter durations, up to 8 weeks. The nursing care of the PICC and MCL is the same as for a central venous catheter.

Nursing Responsibilities for TPN Therapy. Nursing care is integral to safe and successful administration of TPN. Nursing implementation for patients undergoing TPN therapy involves monitoring the TPN infusion and preventing metabolic or apparatus-related complications. For example, nurses must watch for signs and symptoms of inflammation at the catheter site and maintain the specified infusion rate to prevent circulatory overload.

As TPN solutions contain high quantities of glucose, monitoring blood glucose levels every 6 hours to detect hyperglycemia is a nursing responsibility. In addition, as the glucose in TPN solutions may result in osmotic fluid excesses or fluid shifts to the ECF, nurses must closely monitor intake and output, daily weights, and signs and symptoms of fluid and electrolyte imbalance.

Providing extra rest for patients receiving TPN therapy is an important nursing responsibility. Patients are often weak and debilitated. Nurses in collaboration with patients and other caregivers, should schedule care to provide for extended periods of rest.

CLINICAL GUIDELINE 34–12

PREVENTING COMPLICATIONS OF TOTAL PARENTERAL NUTRITION

CATHETER-RELATED COMPLICATIONS

INFECTION

- Use only strict aseptic technique for insertion and dressing change.
- Do not infuse or inject any other solutions or additives to TPN line or container.
- Monitor signs/symptoms of sepsis.

PNEUMOTHORAX, HEMOTHORAX, HYDROTHORAX

- Observe for sharp chest pain, decreased breath sounds, asymmetric chest expansion, and dyspnea on insertion of central venous catheter or commencing infusion of TPN.
- Firmly apply occlusive dressing when central catheter is discontinued.
- Ensure x-ray location of catheter prior to infusion of fluids.

AIR EMBOLISM

- Use *only* Luer-Lok connections.
- Place patient in flat or Trendelenberg position prior to catheter insertion.
- Assess patient's ability to hold breath and perform Valsalva maneuver prior to catheter insertion and thereafter, when changing tubing.
- Do not open closed system for tubing changes or capping the central line, unless patient performs Valsalva or clamps are used on the catheter.

METABOLIC COMPLICATIONS

Hyperglycemia, hypoglycemia

- Test blood glucose every 6 hours.

Electrolyte imbalance

- Monitor labs closely for electrolyte abnormalities.
- Observe for signs/symptoms of electrolyte imbalance.

Circulatory overload

- Assess for neck vein distension, crackles in lungs on auscultation, and dyspnea.
- Maintain rate of TPN as ordered. Do not attempt to "catch up" for a rate slower than prescribed.

Complications of TPN Therapy. The complications of TPN therapy may be either apparatus or patient related (see Clinical Guideline 34–12). Nurses' careful observation for the signs and symptoms of these complications is essential to patients' well-being.

Home Health Care

Patients requiring home infusion therapy should be carefully screened before starting home therapy. To ensure safe and successful home treatment a patient should meet the following criteria:

- Appropriate diagnosis and treatment: home infusion medical director should review appropriateness of delivering medications in the home.
- Medically stable patient: patient's general health must be stable.

- A plan to initiate and maintain treatment: should follow home infusion agency protocols developed according to rational standards, such as those of the American Society of Parenteral and Enteral Nutrition or the Intravenous Nurses Society.
- Safe and appropriate home environment: water, electricity, telephone service must be available.
- Patient and caregiver: must be capable of learning and willing to perform necessary care.
- Financial resources: must be available.[51]

The type of venous access device (VAD) used is determined by the nurse and physician in collaboration with the patient.[52]

REHABILITATIVE CARE

Rehabilitative care involves rehabilitation of patients with long-term fluid and electrolyte problems. Chronic illnesses such as renal failure, cardiac disease, and hypertension often require permanent lifestyle changes, including changes in fluid and dietary intake. To make the necessary changes, patients must go through a learning process.

Behavioral Changes

Principles of behavioral change and skills to assist patients are outlined in Chaps. 8 and 25. A patient must express a willingness to change before collaboration is possible. In addition, nurses must ascertain, through careful history taking, what physiologic or psychosocial factors might preclude a successful behavioral change. Patient and nurses should then discuss each factor and develop approaches to overcome them. Nurses must also help patients understand what behavioral changes are expected. Ambiguity will inevitably lead to conflict between patient and nurses.

One of the most critical aspects of nursing implementation during rehabilitative care is to maintain the nurse-patient relationship. Patients often make lifestyle changes as the result of continued support, encouragement, and praise from a trusted nurse. Positive reinforcement for even a small step toward change can motivate patients to continue (Fig. 34–22).

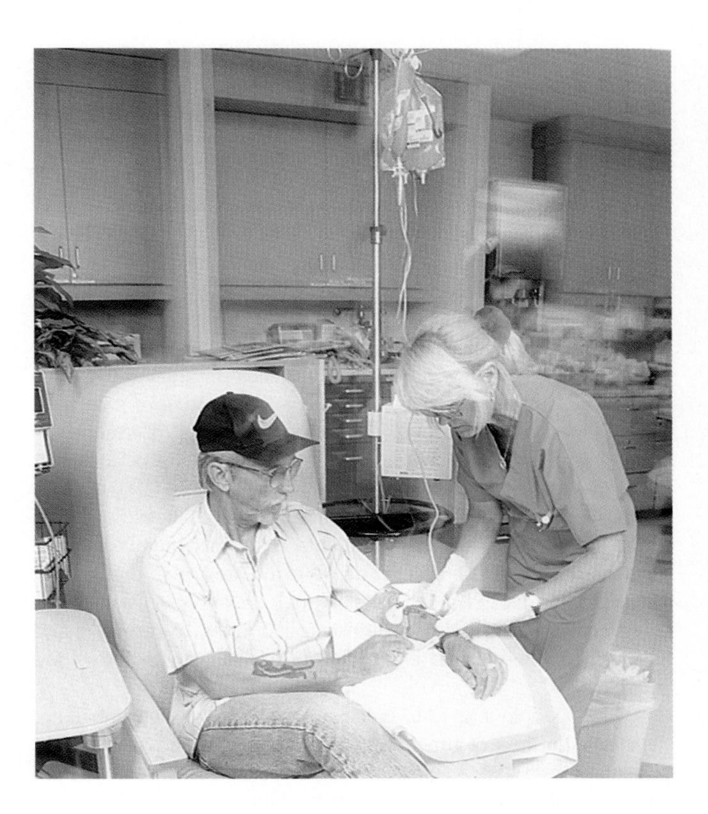

Figure 34–22. Patients needing rehabilitative care for fluid and electrolyte problems often receive therapy in ambulatory care settings. A supportive nurse–patient relationship facilitates patient adaptation.

Self-monitoring Techniques

Simple self-monitoring techniques can help patients who must make long-term behavioral changes. Nurses might, for example, encourage patients on fluid restrictions to keep a log of fluid intake, including the time the fluid is ingested, the amount, feelings at the time, and activity level. Nurse and patient can then review the log to identify situations that lead to excessive fluid ingestion.

COLLABORATIVE STRATEGY

LONG-TERM HABIT CHANGE

Rehabilitation is essential to self-care, particularly when a patient has a fluid balance problem of long-standing nature. These problems may involve personal changes that, while improving a patient's health, will nevertheless be difficult for the patient to make. A patient's capacity to integrate changes may depend not on the skills involved, but on whether those changes are valued as important to personal well-being. Collaboration between nurse and patient can facilitate the exchange of information, opinions, and feelings that may ultimately influence the patient to adopt behavior that supports body fluid homeostasis.

Self-care Techniques

Many of the self-care techniques helpful to patients in maintaining long-term behavioral changes require stress management techniques, because motivation to maintain behavior changes often breaks down in time of stress. See Chap. 25 for more on stress management and self–management strategies to promote effective and lasting behavior change.

Finally, patients should attempt to incorporate exercise, rest, and relaxation techniques as lifestyle practices. Exercise strengthens the cardiovascular system and maintains fluid balance through a healthy cardiac output. Relaxation techniques help prevent the pituitary gland from oversecreting ADH. Even more important, rest and relaxation help patients cope physiologically and psychosocially with stress-producing behavioral changes.

EVALUATION

The evaluation of the collaborative care plan for fluid management flows from the desired outcomes. Nurse and patient review the desired outcomes as target dates are reached. Evaluation also should be ongoing. Daily reviews of the patient's weight and intake and output and frequent review of laboratory and diagnostic test results can provide much information to evaluate progress and the success of the plan. A cursory daily physical examination of fluid indicators also provides evaluation data.

SUMMARY

Body fluid disturbances are complex problems. Imbalances usually result from serious acute health problems or a prolonged assault by disease. Fluid intake and output are usually taken for granted, because regulatory mechanisms swiftly correct problems before the effects are noticeable.

Because of the high fluid content of the body cells, assessment of fluid balance and swift intervention when an imbalance occurs should be an integral part of any patient's nursing care. The assessment must be thorough, to provide sufficient information to develop a plan of care. Both physiologic and psychosocial factors affect the intake and output of fluids.

Care plans to help patients adapt to fluid changes flow from collaboration between nurses, patients, and other members of the health care team. Patient input helps formulate a plan that is individualized and carries a high potential for success. Nurses can serve many roles, from observer to collaborator, to caretaker and supporter in helping patients identify and adapt to body fluid problems.

Most people take fluid balance for granted. When imbalance develops, the loss of function can be surprising and stressful for patients. Observant, knowledgeable, supportive nurses can help alleviate this stress and avert future problems.

LEARNING OUTCOMES

Upon completing this chapter, the student should be able to:

1. Define key terms associated with fluid, electrolyte, and acid–base balance.
2. Describe the physiologic processes involved in the maintenance of fluid balance.
3. Discuss at least four variables that influence the movement of fluid between body fluid compartments.
4. State the quantities and functions of major electrolytes in body fluids and describe clinical manifestations of electrolyte imbalances.
5. Describe how the body maintains acid–base balance.
6. Identify the major buffering systems controlling acid–base balance.
7. Compare and contrast the four acid–base abnormalities.
8. Identify appropriate history questions designed to gain information regarding a patient's fluid and electrolyte balance.
9. Describe clinical observations useful in assessing a patient's fluid and electrolyte balance.
10. Identify subjective and objective manifestations suggestive of fluid and electrolyte imbalances.
11. Identify nursing diagnoses associated with fluid balance problems.
12. Specify nursing implementation to alleviate fluid and electrolyte imbalances.
13. Discuss the oral and parenteral fluid replacement with respect to type, indications, maintenance, and discontinuation.
14. Discuss the nurse's role in collaborating with patients to promote, maintain, or restore body fluid, electrolyte, and acid-base balance.

REVIEW OF KEY TERMS

anions
buffers
cations
edema
electrolytes
hemolytic reaction
hypertonic
hypertonic dehydration
hypotonic
hypotonic dehydration
hypovolemia
insensible loss
intravenous infusion
isotonic
isotonic dehydration
pH
serum osmolality
shock
third spacing
total body water
total parenteral nutrition
venipuncture

Having Read the Chapter, consider again the opening scenario, page 1271, and the following response to the questions about the home intravenous therapy for Ms. Mueller.

Potassium is an electrolyte that lends the characteristic of electrical conductivity to body fluid. Potassium, classified as a cation, is the predominant intracellular electrolyte. As such it contributes to the maintenance of intracellular osmolality, influences neuromuscular excitability, and contributes to acid–base balance by exchanging with hydrogen ions between the ICF and ECF.

Hydrating solutions are used to maintain or replace body water. Dextrose in water is a common hydrating solution. A peripherally inserted central catheter (PICC) is used for long-term venous access. An infusion pump precisely regulates IV flow by applying pressure to a section of IV tubing which is placed inside the pump.

Nurse Queroz, who is specially certified to manage patients who require complex home infusion care, observes the patient's reaction to the medication and state of hydration and electrolyte balance. She is interested in the patient's general appearance, weight gain or loss, the moisture of the patient's skin and mucous membranes, muscle strength, tendon reflex tone, and sensations suggesting parathesias. She also examines the PICC insertion site for signs of inflammation or infection, such as crusting or drainage at the site, redness, tenderness, or heat along of the path of the vein, suggesting phlebitis. The nurse also looks for signs of sepsis or systemic infection, such as fever, chills, or falling blood pressure. Before beginning the infusion, she is careful to check the PICC line to determine that no clots block the lumen.

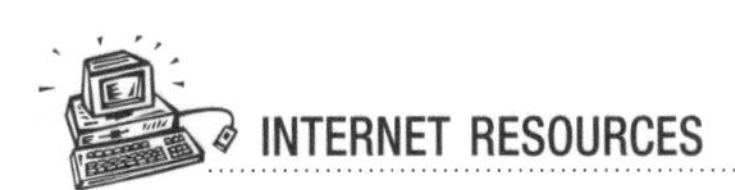

INTERNET RESOURCES

Listserv

Intravenous therapy—subscribe at:

npss;canpl.com (message: Subscribe IVTherapy-L [Your real name])

REFERENCES

1. Felver L. Fluid and electrolyte homeostasis and imbalances. In: Copstead LE. *Perspectives on Pathophysiology.* Philadelphia: Saunders; 1995:524–537.
2. Fanestil D. Compartmentation of body water. In: Narins S, ed. *Maxwell and Kleeman's Clinical Disorders of Fluid and Electrolyte Metabolism.* 5th ed. New York: McGraw-Hill; 1994:3–20.
3. Methany NM. *Fluid and Electrolyte Balance: Nursing Consideration.* 3rd ed. Philadelphia: Lippincott; 1996.
4. Chernoff R. Nutritional requirements and physiological changes in aging, thirst and fluid requirements. *Nutrition Rev.* 1994;52:S3–S5.
5. Teitelbaum I, et al. The physiology of the renal concentrating and diluting mechanism. In: Narins S, ed. *Maxwell and Kleeman's Clinical Disorders of Fluid and Electrolyte Metabolism.* 5th ed. New York: McGraw-Hill; 1994:101–127.
6. Copstead LE. *Perspectives on Pathophysiology.* Philadelphia: Saunders; 1995.
7. Weldy NJ. *Body Fluids and Electrolytes, A Programmed Presentation.* 7th ed. St. Louis: Mosby; 1996.
8. Treseler KM. *Clinical Laboratory and Diagnostic Tests, Significance and Nursing Implications.* 3rd ed. Norwalk, CT: Appleton & Lange; 1995.
9. Guyton AC, Hall JE. *Textbook of Medical Physiology.* 9th ed. Philadelphia: Saunders; 1996.
10. Juneau B. Normal and altered fluid and electrolyte balance. In: Bullock BL, Rosendahl PP. *Pathophysiology: Adaptation and Alterations in Function.* 3rd ed. Philadelphia: Lippincott; 1992: 177–194.
11. Braxmeyer D, Keyes J. The pathophysiology of potassium balance. *Crit Care Nurse.* 1996;16:59–71.
12. Wagner KD, Holtzclaw LM. Arterial blood gas analysis. In: Kidd PS, Wagner KD. *High Acuity Nursing.* 2nd ed. Stamford, CT: Appleton & Lange; 1997:81–99.
13. Bullock B, Juneau, B. Normal and altered acid-base balance. In: Bullock BL, Rosendahl PP. *Pathophysiology: Adaptations and Alterations in Function.* 3rd ed. Philadelphia: Lippincott; 1992:195–207.
14. Ball J, Bindler R. *Pediatric Nursing: Caring for Children.* Stamford, CT: Appleton & Lange; 1995.
15. Kee JL. *Laboratory and Diagnostic Tests with Nursing Implications.* 4th ed. Stamford, CT: Appleton & Lange; 1995.
16. Berkow R, Fletcher AJ, eds. *The Merck Manual of Diagnosis and Therapy.* 16th ed. Rahway, NJ: Merck Sharp & Dohme Research Laboratories; 1992.
17. Levinsky NG. Fluids and electrolytes. In: Harrison TR, et al, eds. *Principles of Internal Medicine.* 13th ed. New York: McGraw-Hill; 1994:242–253.
18. Cox HC, et al. *Clinical Applications of Nursing Diagnosis: Adult, Child, Women's. Psychiatric, Gerontic, and Home Health Considerations.* 2nd ed. Philadelphia: Davis; 1993.
19. Terry J. The major electrolytes: sodium, potassium, and chloride. *J Intravenous Nurs.* 1994;17:240–247.
20. Bove LA. Calcium and phosphorus. *RN.* 1996;59:47–51.
21. Hudak C, Gallo B. *Critical Care Nursing: A Holistic Approach.* 6th ed. Philadelphia: Lippincott; 1994.
22. Bourdeau JE, Attie MF. Calcium metabolism. In: Narins RG, ed. *Maxwell and Kleeman's Clinical Disorders of Fluid and Electrolyte Metabolism.* 5th ed. New York: McGraw-Hill; 1994:243–306.
23. Ferrin MS. Magnesium. *RN.* 1996;59:31–34.
24. Shuster MH. Nutrition in the critically ill. In: Clochesy JM, et al. *Critical Care Nursing.* 2nd ed.; 1996:994–1021.
25. Workman ML. Magnesium and phosphorus: the negative electrolytes. *AACN Clin Issues.* 1992;3:655–663.
26. Levinsky NG. Acidosis and alkalosis. In: Harrison TR, et al, eds. *Principles of Internal Medicine.* 13th ed. New York: McGraw-Hill; 1994:253–262.
27. Weinstein S, ed. *Plumer's Principles and Practice of Intravenous Therapy,* 6th ed. Philadelphia: Lippincott; 1997.
28. Jarvis C. *Physical Examination and Health Assessment.* Philadelphia: Saunders; 1992.
29. Lee CB, Barrett CA, Ignatavicius DD. *Fluids and Electrolytes: A Practical Approach.* 4th ed. Philadelphia: Davis; 1996.
30. North American Nursing Diagnosis Association. *Nursing Diagnosis: Definitions and Classification, 1997-1998.* Philadelphia: NANDA; 1996.
31. Abrams WB, et al, eds. *The Merck Manual of Geriatrics.* 2nd ed. Whitehouse Station, NJ: Merck; 1995.
32. Mahan LK, Escott-Stump S. *Krause's Food, Nutrition, and Diet Therapy.* 9th ed. Philadelphia: Saunders; 1996.
33. McConnell ES, Murphy AT. Nursing diagnoses related to physiological alterations. In: Matyteson MA, McConnel ES, Linton AD. *Gerontological Nursing: Concepts and Practices.* 2nd ed. Philadelphia: Saunders; 1997: 407–551.
34. McFarland GK, McFarlane EA. *Nursing Diagnosis & Intervention.* 2nd ed. St. Louis: Mosby; 1993.
35. Fuller J, Schaller-Ayers J. *Health Assessment—A Nursing Approach.* 2nd ed. Philadelphia: Lippincott; 1994.
36. Johnson KL. Shock states. In: Kidd PS, Wagner KD. *High Acuity Nursing.* 2nd ed. Stamford, CT: Appleton & Lange; 1997:107–184.
37. Caine RM. Patients with burns. In: Clochesy JM, et al. *Critical Care Nursing.* 2nd ed. Philadelphia: Saunders; 1996:1279–1309.
38. Dudek SG. *Nutrition Handbook for Nursing Practice.* 2nd ed. Philadelphia: Lippincott; 1993.
39. Sherman A. Critical care management of the heart failure patient in the home. *Crit Care Nurse Q.* 1995;18:77–87.
40. Smith SF, Duell DJ. *Clinical Nursing Skills: Basic to Advanced Skills.* 4th ed. Stamford, CT: Appleton & Lange; 1996.
41. Terry J, Hendrick C. Parenteral fluids. In: Terry J, et al, eds. *Intravenous Therapy: Clinical Principles and Practices.* Philadelphia: Saunders; 1995:151–164.
42. Perucca R. Obtaining vascular access. In: Terry J, et al, eds. *Intravenous Therapy: Clinical Principles and Practices.* Philadelphia: Saunders; 1995:379–391.
43. Lau CE. Transparent and gauze dressings and their effect on infection rates of central venous catheters: a review of past and current literature. *J Intravenous Nurs.* 1996;19:240–245.

44. *Intravascular Device-related Infections Prevention; Guideline Availability; Notice.* Federal Register—Part II, Department of Health and Human Services—Center For Disease Control and Prevention, Vol 60, No 187, September 27, 1995: 49978–50006.
45. Weir JA. Blood component therapy. In: Terry J, et al, eds. *Intravenous Therapy: Clinical Principles and Practice.* Philadelphia: Saunders; 1995:165–187.
46. Ford CD, Vizcarra C. Parenteral nutrition. In: Terry J, et al, eds. *Intravenous Therapy: Clinical Principles and Practices.* Philadelphia: Saunders; 1995:219–248.
47. Inadami DW, Kopple JD. Fluid and electrolyte disorders in total parenteral nutrition. In: Narins R, ed. *Maxwell & Kleeman's Clinical Disorders of Fluid and Electrolyte Balance.* 5th ed. New York: McGraw-Hill; 1994: 1438.
48. Orr ME. Issues in the management of percutaneous central catheters. *Nurs Clin North Am.* 1993;28:911–919.
49. Ryder MA. Peripherally inserted central venous catheters. *Nurs Clin North Am.* 1993;28:937–971.
50. Sansivero, GE. Why pick a PICC? *Nurs 95*. 1995; 25 (7):35–41.
51. Sheldon P, Bender M. High-technology in home care. *Nurs Clin North Am.* 1994;29:507–519.
52. Meredith D. Patient selection criteria for home IV therapies: from A to Z. *Caring*. 1995;14:18–20.

Glossary

abrasion A wound in which all or part of the skin or mucosa has been scraped away.

absorption The process in which the end products of digestion are transferred through the walls of the intestines. The process by which a drug is transferred from its site of entry into the body to the circulatory system.

accommodation According to Piaget, the process of modifying old ways to fit new situations.

accountability Taking responsibility for one's actions. In economics, the undertaking of practices to enable the tracking and explanation of the use of resources.

accreditation A system for review and approval of institutions that meet professional standards.

acculturation The partial change of a group's or individual's culture as a result of contact with a different culture.

acquired immunity Immunity resulting from the presence in the blood of specific antibodies for certain communicable diseases.

active range of motion The movement at a joint that a person can accomplish without assistance; therapeutic exercise used to maintain flexibility.

activities of daily living Self-care skills required for daily living.

acute illness Illness that can be recognized by a severe, rapid onset of pronounced symptoms, usually of a short duration.

adaptation The process through which individuals accommodate changes in the environment.

adaptive responses According to Roy, responses that promote survival, growth, reproduction and self-mastery.

adherence A patient's follow-through in carrying out professional recommendations.

administrative regulation Regulation enacted by the agencies of the executive branch of government to guide the implementation of statutes.

advance directive Instructions given by competent adults about their choices concerning future treatment should they become incapacitated.

advanced practice nursing Nursing that is characterized by complexity of clinical decision making and skill in managing organizations and environments.

adversary proceeding In its simplest form, this is a disagreement between two sides, resolved in neutral territory.

advocacy, patient Health professionals' focus on protecting patient interests.

adynamic ileus See *paralytic ileus*

aerobic exercise Whole-body exercise that causes a sustained increase in heart rate and stroke volume.

affect The outward appearance of an emotional state to others.

agency A department within the government's organizational structure.

agenda decisions Decisions on the priority of activities that involve sequencing planned events into some kind of temporal order.

agent–environment relationship The interaction of the environment and microorganisms that require highly specific conditions for growth and reproduction.

agent In epidemiology, the cause of a health problem.

alarm stage The first stage of Selye's general adaptation syndrome, in which the central nervous system is aroused and the physiological defense is mobilized.

ambivalence An emotional state in which a person holds conflicting emotions and opposing attitudes about his or her situation.

ambulatory care Outpatient facilities that provide care for patients whose health problems do not require continued around-the-clock surveillance by a health care provider.

Americans With Disabilities Act A federal law designed to end discrimination against disabled individuals. The ADA defines a disability as a physical or mental impairment that substantially limits one or more major life activities.

amino acid Large molecules having an amino (NH_2) and a carboxyl (COOH) group that make up protein chains; also called peptides.

ampule A clear glass container with a constricted neck that holds a single dose of medication.

anabolism Metabolic process that constructs body structures.

anaerobic glycolysis Breakdown of glucose yielding lactate. Occurs when the supply of oxygen is inadequate for oxidation processes.

anaphylaxis A severe, life-threatening allergic reaction.

anatomic dead space Part of the respiratory tree that does not participate in gaseous exchange.

anesthesia Absence of the sense of touch or of pain.

anion Negatively charged electrolyte.

anorexia nervosa An eating disorder characterized by self-imposed starvation through a rigorously controlled diet.

antagonism The interference with the action of one drug by another drug administered at the same time.

antagonist Muscle pairs that contract and relax reciprocally to accomplish movement of a body part.

anticipatory grief Grief that is experienced before a loss occurs.

anuria Urine production of less than 100 mL in a day.

anxiety A feeling of uneasiness or apprehension.

aphasia Loss of the ability to communicate through speech, writing, or signs.

applied science A discipline using knowledge to solve problems in a practice setting. Research that builds on or tests basic science for use in the world of practice.

appropriating legislation Legislation providing funds.

arousal A state in which an individual attends to people, things, and events in the environment and is ready for activity; corresponds to wakefulness.

assertive communication The presentation of facts and feelings in a rational emphatic way, but not in a way that devalues the listener.

assertiveness The expression of confidence and self-assurance that one's ideas and rights are important and should be recognized.

assessment The process of evaluating a condition.

assimilation The process by which members of a group gradually give up traditional ways of life to conform to the standards of the dominant group. In developmental psychology, the process of learning from a new experience.

atelectasis Collapse of alveoli; may range from a small area to the whole lung.

at-risk aggregates Subpopulations with special needs.

at-risk role Role in which a patient agrees to take steps to reduce known risk factors.

atrophy A decrease in size of a part of the body because of disease or other influences.

attachment behaviors Mutually responsive reactions and interactions between parents and child that indicate that the cues given by one person are accurately interpreted and acted on by the other person.

attending behavior Physical acts that a listener uses to communicate interest in a speaker.

auscultation Technique of physical examination that employs the sense of hearing to assess naturally occurring body sounds.

authenticity The ability to communicate who one really is without judgment or reactivity.

authorizing legislation Legislation creating a program.

autocratic managers Managers that make all of the decisions for the group.

autonomy Independence or freedom to choose one's actions; the capacity for self-direction.

basal metabolic rate The rate at which an individual oxidizes nutrients under basal conditions (12 or more hours after eating, after sleep, with no intervening exercise).

basic science Research that has no immediately apparent practical application.

behavior A publicly observable activity.

behavioral objective An objective that describes learner behavior; see also *learning objective*.

beneficence An ethical principle concerned with the duty to do good or to produce good consequences.

bereavement A role transition that survivors undergo on the death of someone close.

bias A subjective feeling that reflects a particular point of reference or point of view.

biologic environment In epidemiology, the environment that includes infectious agents of disease, reservoirs of infection, transmitters of diseases, and plants and animals that may enhance the development of disease or serve as sources of drugs that deter disease.

biotransformation Metabolism of a drug that converts it to an inactive form and produces byproducts for excretion.

blood pressure The pressure of the blood within the systemic arteries.

board A public regulatory body composed of appointed individuals who are charged with the responsibility of overseeing a specific activity.

board of nursing A state agency that administers the Nurse Practice Act. Responsibilities vary by state but generally include the establishment of licensing procedures and minimum continuing education requirements. Some boards also issue opinions or rulings on safe nursing practices, promulgate rules that regulate nursing, and hold review and disciplinary authority over licensees.

body image The cluster of attitudes and beliefs one holds about one's body, including qualities such as appearance, functioning, and overall wellness.

body mass index A measurement calculated by dividing the weight in kilograms by the height in squared meters; method most commonly used to measure body fat.

body surface area A calculation of the quantity of the surface area of a person's body in square meters.

body temperature The level of hotness or coldness of the body measured in heat units called degrees.

boundaries The dynamic lines of separation between the external environment and an individual's body-mind-spirit environment.

boycott The organized refusal to deal with a person or organization to achieve a goal.

bradypnea Respiration rate of below 10 respirations per minute.

buccal mucosa The membrane covering the interior surface of the cheeks.

budget A forecast of projected revenue (income) and anticipated expenses (outgo) in dollars and cents over a specified planning period.

buffers Substances that combine with acids and bases to prevent extreme changes in pH.

bulimia An eating disorder characterized by a behavior pattern of uncontrollable binge eating, followed by self-induced vomiting and use of laxatives, or diuretics.

burnout A condition of emotional and physical exhaustion resulting from chronic job stress.

byte A group of eight bits.

cachexia Emaciation, tissue wasting, and severe weight loss resulting from a gradual, prolonged period of insufficient nutritional intake.

capitation Billing system in which a fixed fee pays for a package of health care services during a specific time period regardless of the amount of services used.

carbohydrate A nutritional compound made up of carbon, hydrogen, and oxygen; the most efficiently metabolized source of energy for humans; includes simple (sugars) and complex (starches) carbohydrates.

caries Tooth decay; also known as "cavities."

caring Respectful and considerate relationships among persons; to feel concern about another.

carrier In epidemiology, an agent who has been infected by a pathogen but has no symptoms and is potentially capable of infecting others.

case management A process of need assessment and coordination of health care that aims to provide quality cost-effective care. A model of care involving collaborative physician–nurse joint practice.

case managers Individuals who assess patients' overall needs for health services, delineate comprehensive patient outcomes, procure the most cost-effective means of meeting outcomes, and evaluate the effectiveness of services.

case nursing Model of nursing care in which one nurse is assigned to provide total care for one patient for the period of a single work shift.

cases In epidemiology, the individuals who are obviously ill from an infectious disease.

catabolism Metabolic process involving the breakdown of substances and energy release.

catharsis The process of psychologically purging or getting rid of emotion.

cathartic See *laxative*

catheterization Putting a catheter into a body cavity or organ to either add fluid or remove it.

cation Positively charged electrolyte.

central processing unit Component of a computer that controls operations and performs calculations.

central vision Sight that results from images falling on the macula of the retina; used when focusing on an object.

cephalocaudal Principle of maturation that motor development progresses from head to feet.

certification A process by which a nongovernmental entity recognizes an individual's competence through evaluation of educational preparation, performance, and professional skills.

chain of infection Concept that implies that communicability of disease rests on the connections between a series of necessary factors.

change The process by which the normal course of events is altered. In individuals, the process in which modifications in ways of being or functioning occur.

chart See *patient record*

chemical name An exact description of the chemical composition of a drug.

chronic disease A disease that lasts for a long period of time and may result in complete or partial disability.

chronic illness Illness characterized by long duration, frequent recurrence, or slow progression.

civil law Law that protects the rights of a citizen of a state or country.

classical conditioning A form of learning in which an individual learns to respond to a formerly neutral stimulus through its being paired with a familiar stimulus.

closed systems Systems that limit their interaction with the environment.

coalition A group of individuals or organizations that have temporarily come together for the purpose of collectively working toward a common policy goal.

code of ethics A formalized expression of professional values.

coercive power The use of punishment to achieve a desired result.

cognator subsystem In the Roy model, the subsystem that uses cognitive functions such as information processing, learning, judgment, and emotion to adapt to or cope with stimuli.

cognition The act or process of knowing.

cognitive appraisal An evaluation of events by which individuals define for themselves what is stressful.

cognitive development According to Piaget, the acquisition of the ability to think and reason in a logical manner.

cognitive style Thought processes and ways in which an individual ascribes meaning to symbols.

collaboration A process in which two or more individuals work together, jointly influencing one another.

collaborative function See *interdependent function*

collagen Fibrous protein component of connective tissue; gives the healing wound tensile strength.

collective bargaining The process by which an organized group of employees negotiates with an employer to define the conditions of employment.

collective power The ability to influence derived from the concerted efforts of groups of individuals.

collegiality The sharing of authority among colleagues.

comfort In comfort theory, a state in which the body functions with ease, freeing the individual to live in the everyday world.

commission See *board*

common law The oldest and ultimate form of law; the body of judicial decisions rendered in specific cases; also referred to as case law.

communicable disease An infectious disease that spreads from person to person.

communication To make common, that is to exchange ideas or feelings such that sender and receiver perceive a common meaning; a dynamic process that occurs via many channels, (eg, verbal, nonverbal).

community Any group of people who have common interests and problems and who work together to solve those problems.

community health The health status of individuals, families, and groups within a community and the ability of the community to carry out certain necessary functions.

comparator In a homeostatic control system, the component that determines whether there is a deviation of the input from the desired level.

complementary protein Two or more incomplete proteins that in combination supply all the essential amino acids.

complete protein A protein that contains all the essential amino acids in amounts adequate for use in the body.

complex carbohydrate Polysaccharides (starch, glycogen) composed of chains of monosaccharides, chiefly glucose molecules; one of the two broad categories of carbohydrates.

computer A machine that accepts input; stores, retrieves, and processes information; and generates output.

computer-assisted instruction A method of teaching that involves interaction between the learner and the computer, in which the computer takes the role of teacher.

computerized patient record Computerized documentation system that provides rapid data entry and retrieval and easy interdepartmental as well as interfacility communication.

concept A label applied to the sensory data (reports and observed behaviors) that tell a researcher a phenomenon is occurring.

conceptual framework Framework that links groups of concepts into an entire perspective or view of a situation which has not been validated through research.

conditioned response The response to a conditioned stimulus.

conditioned stimulus In classical conditioning, a new, formerly neutral, stimulus to which an organism learns to respond in the absence of the original stimulus.

conditioning The process of creating new relationships or associations between stimuli and responses.

conduction Heat loss from a warmer substance or object to a cooler substance or object with which it is in contact.

confidentiality An ethical principle concerned with duty to protect an individual's privacy and holding secret the confidences to which one is entrusted.

connotative meaning The personalized meaning of a word.

consciousness The state of being aware of one's self and one's surroundings; awareness.

consensus building The interpersonal approaches and techniques people or groups use to resolve their differences on important issues.

constipation The passage of small, hard, dry stool or the passage of no stool for an unusually long period of time.

constitutional law A system of fundamental laws that establishes the overall structure and powers of government and the rights of the citizenry under the government.

consumerism The promotion of consumer interests.

consumer perspective A point of view that accepts consumers' rights and encourages negotiation among equals in health care encounters.

contaminant Agents in a wound that may cause infection.

content In terms of consciousness, the ideas, feelings and sensations of which an individual is aware.

context One of the components of communication; refers to the setting and circumstances in which the interaction occurs.

continuing care Health care that involves services delivered as a follow-up to specialty or rehabilitative care or as an adjunct to primary care services.

continuous quality improvement The principle based on quality circles which involve workers in regularly scheduled meetings to discuss how to maintain and improve the quality of their product and how to increase their own productivity.

continuum of health care The concept that acknowledges the importance of service continuity from episode to episode and from one health care setting to another.

contract In the helping relationship, the establishment of mutual expectations.

contraction In wound healing, the process by which microfibroblasts contract in unison to significantly reduce the surface area of a wound and facilitate epithelial coverage.

contracture The pathologic shrinking of a scar causing loss of mobility.

control group The group that is subjected to no interventions in a scientific experiment; the standard against which the scores of experimental subjects are compared.

control The ability to have an impact on an outcome. In research, special procedures followed to eliminate, distribute, consider, or measure the effects produced by variables other than the independent one.

contusion An injury caused by a blow from a blunt object that entails soft tissue damage, but does not break the skin.

convection Heat loss by means of currents to surrounding air or fluid.

convenience sampling An example of nonrandom sampling that takes advantage of subjects who are easily accessible.

cooperation The act of working together with others for a common purpose; respecting the opinions of others and being willing to examine alternative points of view and change personal beliefs and perspectives.

coordination The efficient organization of the necessary components of care.

co-payment The partial payment required for services under some health insurance policies after the deductible has been met.

coping An individual's attempts to master conditions of harm, threat or challenge when an automatic response is not immediately available.

covered lives A term health economists use to refer to patients.

credentialing The process whereby qualified agents certify that individual nurses or the institutions and programs that prepare them meet minimum standards.

criminal law Laws concerned with punishing the perpetrator of a crime.

crisis The situation that exists when coping responses to stress fail and an event is experienced as overwhelming.

critical defining characteristics Characteristics that must be present in a patient database in order to diagnose the corresponding health concern.

critical path/pathway The interdisciplinary plan intended to reflect optimal sequencing and timing of patient care given by all members of the health care team and to identify expected outcomes of the care.

critical periods Those periods of development during which a person is more vulnerable to physical, chemical, psychological, or environmental influences.

critical thinking According to the APA statement, purposeful, self-regulatory judgment resulting in interpretation, analysis, evaluation, and inference, as well as the explanation of the considerations on which the judgment is based.

cue A piece of information; a raw fact.

cultural conflict Conflict that occurs when there is a lack of awareness, understanding, acceptance, or responsiveness between members of different cultural groups.

cultural relativism Perspective that any culture is different from, but not superior or inferior to, any other culture.

cultural sensitivity Individuals' awareness of which issues or concerns are important to their own culture and to the culture of others.

culture A pattern of learned behaviors and values that are shared among members of a designated group.

culture shock The difficulties that people experience in adjusting to life in a culture different from their own.

cyanosis A bluish-gray skin color that occurs when oxygen content of the intravascular hemoglobin is diminished or when blood flow rate is slowed.

Daily Reference Values The reference values for important nutrients that do not have established RDAs; developed by the FDA for use on food labels.

Daily Values The standard values developed by the FDA for use on food labels.

dangling Activity in which a patient sits at the edge of the bed for several minutes before standing; used to correct orthostatic hypotension.

data Pieces of information collected and collated by caregivers to assist them in carrying out the responsibilities of clinical practice.

data analysis The process of analyzing and interpreting data.

database Information gathered through the health history, examination, and subsequent diagnostic testing.

data collection The process of obtaining a data base.

debride To remove foreign material and dead or damaged tissue.

decision environment The context (circumstances, conditions, and setting) in which decisions are made.

deductible An amount consumers must pay in full before payments are made by an insurer.
deductive reasoning A process of thinking that moves from general principles to the collection of specific data that confirm or negate a hypothesis.
deep vein thrombosis A condition involving a blood clot (thrombus) in a deep vein.
defense mechanisms Emotional defenses that are commonly used by people to allay painful or stressful feelings.
defining characteristics Observed, reported, or measured findings that serve as supporting evidence of a nursing diagnosis; also called manifestations or signs and symptoms.
dehiscence Separation of the edges of a wound.
deliberate mutual patterning A process of goal-setting the nurse uses to help patients experience turbulent life experiences as positive, transformative challenges and a source of growth and creativity.
demand The quantity of a good or service that consumers would be willing and able to purchase at various prices during a given interval of time.
democratic managers Managers that include the people subject to policies in the decision-making process.
denial A defensive state of mind in which illness symptoms or other unpleasant realities are ignored or minimized.
denotative meaning The relationship that exists between an object in the physical world and the word that stands for that object.
deontology Ethical theory that looks at the moral significance of an act in terms of the inherent rightness or wrongness of the act itself.
dependent function Nursing activities requiring that someone else, typically a physician, write an order for the activity that a nurse then carries out.
dependent variable In a research study, a variable thought to be an effect of an experimental procedure.
deposition An out-of-court proceeding where questions are asked and answered under oath.
dermatitis Inflammation of the skin characterized by redness and itchiness.
dermis The layer of skin lying directly below the epidermis and containing the specialized cardiovascular, neurological, and lymphatic systems of the skin.
descriptive theory Theory that summarizes what is common among individuals, groups, events, or situations.
desired outcome Statement that describes the expected patient status when a nursing diagnosis has been resolved.
desquamation The peeling or sloughing of the outer epidermal layer of the skin.
development A qualitative term used to describe changes in psychosocial, cognitive, or moral functioning; a gradual change or expansion of a person's capabilities.
developmental requisites Requirements that are specific to one's age or development.
developmental task A task that arises at or about a certain period in the life of an individual.
diagnostic label The problem component of a nursing diagnosis; see also *problem*
diagnostic reasoning A process of collecting and organizing data, clustering cues, and validating inferences by which a diagnosis is reached.
diaphoresis Profuse sweating that occurs with illness, physical exertion, exposure to heat or stress; a heat-dissipating mechanism of the body.
diarrhea The rapid movement of fecal matter through the intestine, resulting in frequent evacuation of loose and watery stools.
diastole In the cardiac cycle, the time of ventricular relaxation, repolarization, and refilling.
diastolic blood pressure The arterial blood pressure that is measured as the left ventricle relaxes and the heart is at rest.
dietary fiber Fiber, such as cellulose and pectin, composed primarily of cell wall constituents of plant foods.
diffusion The process of gas exchange between alveoli and capillaries and between capillaries and tissues.
digestion The breakdown of foods into smaller compounds that can be absorbed into body fluids.
direct question A question that seeks a yes or no answer, or other short response.
discharge planning A process that attempts to project patient health status and needs for continuing care at the time of discharge from a health care agency.
discovery The early phase of a lawsuit when the parties exchange information to learn more about the plaintiff's claim and the defendant's defense.
disease A condition in which there is altered functioning or dysfunction.
disease prevention Activities undertaken to prevent a specific disease or disorder.
distress The state of mental or physical anguish that corresponds to stress.
distress disclosure See *catharsis*
distribution The process by which a drug is transported from the site of absorption to the site of action.
disuse phenomenon The debilitative effect of inactivity.
disuse syndrome See *disuse phenomenon*
diuretic A drug or substance that increases urine excretion.
dominant culture In a multicultural society, the group that functions as guardian and sustainer of the controlling value system and allocates rewards and punishments.
drug See *medication*
drug allergy An immune system reaction to a drug as a result of a previous sensitizing event.
drug interaction The change of an effect of a drug when given with another drug.
drug tolerance Condition that exists when an individual requires increasing dosages of a particular medication to maintain a given therapeutic effect.
duodenocolic reflex Reflex peristalsis that occurs in response to distension of the duodenum.
durable power of attorney An option that delegates to a specific person the authority to make health care decisions if a patient becomes unable to do so.
dynamic steady state The constancy of body composition over time, while taking into account temporary adjustments and maturational changes.
dynamic support surface A bed surface engineered to automatically alter the pressure over skin contact points.
dyspnea Difficult or labored breathing.
dysuria Difficult or painful urination.
ecchymosis Diffuse bleeding into surrounding tissue; a bruise.
edema Abnormal accumulation of fluid in the interstitial spaces, producing tissue swelling and congestion.
effector In a homeostatic control system, the component that corrects its function to offset the error in the system.

eggcrate mattress A foam mattress overlay used as a pressure reduction device.
electrolytes Ions that are dissolved in body fluids.
elimination The process by which the body excretes waste products.
e-mail Electronic mail feature of the Internet; allows users to send and receive messages using a computer.
Emergency Medical Treatment and Active Labor Act A federal law that sets forth requirements for the treatment of any emergency room patient; also called the "anti-dumping" statute.
emotion An affective state of consciousness in which joy, fear, anger, rage, and pleasure are experienced.
empathy To recognize and accept the feelings of another.
empirical evidence Evidence that is based solely on experiment or observation.
empowering communication The acknowledgement of the patients' verbal and nonverbal communications in a way that communicates acceptance.
enculturation The process by which one learns ways of acting and meeting one's needs that conform to the norms of one's cultural group.
endurance A person's ability to persist in the performance of an exercise activity without becoming fatigued.
enema A solution that is instilled into the rectum and sigmoid colon for the purpose of stimulating peristalsis and causing defecation to occur.
energy balance The amount of energy input in relation to the amount of energy output in a given system.
enteral Via the gastrointestinal tract.
enteric coating A substance that is resistant to dissolution in the stomach; used on oral drugs that are highly irritating to gastric mucosa or are inactivated in an acid medium.
enuresis The involuntary loss of urine while sleeping; bed-wetting beyond the age when bladder control is usually achieved.
epidemiologic method See *epidemiology*
epidemiologic triad Classic model of epidemiology that examines health problems in terms of three categories of contributing factors: agent factors, host factors, and environmental factors.
epidemiology The study of factors that affect the occurrence of disease.
epidermis The outer surface of the skin.
epithelialization Migration of epithelial cells to close a wound site.
equivalent Equal in quantity or value.
erythema A generalized area of redness that blanches when palpated.
eschar The thick layer of dried protein and dead cells that produces a scab on a wound.
essential amino acid An amino acid that the body cannot manufacture and that therefore must be supplied by food.
essential nutrient A nutrient that the body cannot manufacture and that therefore must be supplied by food.
ethical dilemma A situation in which there are two or more alternatives for action based upon ethical principles, each of which has undesirable consequences.
ethical principle A fundamental standard that provides direction for making moral decisions.
ethical problem A situation in which the "right" or the "good" thing to do is clear, but accomplishing it is extremely difficult.
ethical theory A model of moral values that provides approaches for identifying ethical choices in situations that present an ethical dilemma.
ethics The branch of philosophy that attempts to discern which actions will produce good and avoid wrong.
ethnicity Affiliation with a group based on hereditary and cultural traditions, such as language and religion.
ethnocentrism The belief that one's culture or way of life is superior to that of other cultural groups.
etiology The cause of a problem (to the extent that cause and effect can be known or shown).
eudaemonistic Referring to happiness or well-being.
evaluation The final step of the management phase of the nursing process; determining the effectiveness of assessment and management strategies through a systematic comparison of a patient's health status to standards mutually developed by the patient and nurse.
evaluation criteria Statement that describes acceptable evidence that desired outcomes have been achieved.
evaporation The conservation of a liquid to a gaseous form, producing transfer of heat to the environment.
excretion The process by which metabolites and drugs are eliminated from the body.
exercise tolerance The amount (rate and duration) of a given exercise a person can perform before experiencing exhaustion or distress.
exhaustion stage The third stage of Selye's general adaptation syndrome, in which the individual's ability to adapt is exceeded or exhausted.
exit The consumer's option to try to change a seller's behavior by simply taking one's business elsewhere.
experimental group The group subjected to experimental interventions in a scientific experiment.
expert power The ability to influence derived from professional knowledge and information.
expiration One of the two phases of breathing; moving air out of the lungs.
explanatory theory Theory that links concepts together, specifying which concepts are related and how they are related.
exudate The fluid that accumulates around the site of an injury.
faith A belief in something that cannot be seen.
family A small social system made up of individuals related to each other by reason of strong reciprocal affection and loyalties.
family function What the family does to manage its affairs; tasks performed by family members and their consequences for the family.
family structure The family organization and the relationships between its members.
fat A nutrient classification that includes a mixture of triglycerides; adipose body tissue which serves as an energy reserve; see also *lipid*
fatty acid A chain of carbon atoms with hydrogen and an acid group attached; may be saturated, monounsaturated, or polyunsaturated.
fear A state in which an individual experiences a feeling of psychological or emotional disruption related to an identifiable source that is perceived as dangerous.
fecal impaction A collection of putty-like or hard stool in the rectum that cannot be expelled.
fecal incontinence The loss of the voluntary ability to control the elimination of gas and feces.
feedback In communication, the message that the receiver returns to the sender in response to the sender's message. In teaching–

learning, information given to the learner about the quality and accuracy of a response.

fee-for-diagnosis A type of prospective health care payment system in which facilities are given a fixed dollar amount for the treatment of an episode of illness based on a system of diagnosis groups (DRGs).

fee-for-service Billing system in which consumers are charged for each health service as it is provided.

feeling The conscious phase of nervous activity; the cognitive awareness of emotions.

fibroblast One of the primary functioning cells of the dermis, which acts in the building and rebuilding of connective tissue.

fidelity An ethical principle concerned with observance of duty; keeping the promises one makes.

field A term used by Gestaltists that encompasses a person, the person's environment, and the interaction between the two.

fine motor control Coordination of small muscle groups so that delicate, subtle, and precise motor activities are possible.

FiO_2 (fraction of inspired oxygen) An expression of oxygen concentration; indicates what fraction of the room air-oxygen mixture a patient is receiving as oxygen.

fitness A state in which body systems function optimally. The ability to sustain vigorous physical exertion without overtaxing cardiopulmonary or muscular capacity.

fixation According to psychoanalytic theory, blocks in an individual's development that may be caused by anxiety, threat, or frustration.

flatulence An accumulation of excessive amounts of gas in the gastrointestinal tract.

flexibility The amount of movement possible at a given joint.

flowmeter A device used to adjust and measure the flowrate.

flowrate The rate at which oxygen is flowing to a patient; measured in liters per minute.

folk health practices Health care practices that include home remedies and rely on cultural and spiritual healers who may use herbal, magical, or religious remedies.

food pyramid An illustration of the relative amounts of each food group that should be consumed in a healthy diet.

footboard A device placed at the bottom of a patient's bed to prevent heel cord contractures and counteract shearing.

formative evaluation In nursing process, ongoing evaluation that gauges progress toward desired outcomes.

functional incontinence According to NANDA taxonomy, the involuntary, unpredictable loss of urine.

gastrocolic reflex Peristaltic wave in the colon that occurs in response to distension of the stomach.

gatekeeping A practice under which primary care physicians become responsible for approving all outpatient services that patients receive.

gauge The diameter of the needle shaft.

gender identity An individual's perception of himself or herself as masculine or feminine, a perception that may or may not correspond to the individual's biological sex.

gender role A person's characteristic behavior pattern associated with being male or female, usually associated with sexual preference.

general adaptation syndrome The physiological response to stress, described by Hans Selye, consisting of three successive stages: alarm, resistance, and exhaustion.

generalizability In scientific research, the ability to apply the findings from sample studies to the population the sample represents.

generic name The shortened name of a drug that is used in the official pharmacological publications.

gigabyte One billion bytes.

gingiva The gums.

gingivitis Inflammation of the gums.

glomerular filtration rate The amount of filtration by the glomerulus of the kidney that occurs within a given unit of time.

gluconeogenesis The synthesis of glucose in the liver from noncarbohydrate substances such as amino acids or fatty acids.

glycogen The stored form of carbohydrates in most humans; the most easily recoverable source of stored energy for the body.

glycogenolysis The breakdown of glycogen into glucose.

Good Samaritan statutes Laws that provide that a health care professional who stops to give aid at an accident scene is ordinarily immune from being sued.

governance The exercise of power in organizations.

granulation tissue The new tissue that fills a large wound space or bridges the small gap between margins of a sutured wound.

grief The private experience of persons who are anticipating loss or who have sustained a loss of something that is critical to their sense of well-being.

grieving A normal process necessary to the adaptation of persons anticipating loss or who have sustained a loss critical to their sense of well-being.

gross motor control The ability to control the large muscle groups necessary for movement.

growth A qualitative term used to describe a physical change, such as an increase in size, height, or weight. In psychology, a personal response to change that leads beyond adaptation to the achievement of a healthier state of functioning.

habituation A form of learning that occurs when a stimulus that originally produced a response is presented so often that the individual stops responding to it.

hardiness A personality trait encompassing control, commitment, and challenge, characteristics likely to make an individual more resistant to stress or illness.

hardware The physical components of a computer.

health assessment The first phase of the nursing process; involves data gathering for the purpose of identifying, describing, and treating the patient's health needs and problems.

health behavior An action taken by an individual to maintain, attain, or regain his or her good health and to prevent illness.

health-deviation requisites According to Orem, requirements that arise because of illness.

health examination The hands-on portion of health assessment, in which caregivers use their observation skills to identify the physical signs of health and illness.

health history An organized body of information comprising a patient's verbal reports about his or her own health state.

health–illness continuum A continuum that depicts health and illness as extreme elements of a unified concept.

health lifestyle A pattern of health behaviors adopted by individuals in their daily lives.

health maintenance Identifying and eliminating threats to health, thus preventing disease within an at-risk population.

health maintenance organization An organized system of health care delivery whose members (subscribers) prepay a monthly fee that is guaranteed to cover all services named in the contract.

health promotion Health care strategies to maintain or enhance health through alteration of personal habits or the environment in which people live.

helping relationship A goal-directed professional relationship dedicated to facilitating patients' interpersonal growth through effective communication.

hematocrit The volume of packed erythrocytes in a given volume of blood, expressed as a percent.

hematoma Encapsulated bleeding; a bruise.

hemoglobin The essential component of the erythrocyte for oxygen transport, made up of an iron-containing pigment (heme) and a protein (globin).

hemolytic reaction Clumping and lysis of donor erythrocytes by agglutinins in the recipient's blood.

hemorrhoids Dilated veins in the lower rectum or anus that cause painful swelling.

heuristics Easy-to-use cognitive strategies, "rules of thumb," or procedures that simplify cognitive processing of information.

high-level wellness An integrated level of functioning in which an individual maximizes the potential of which he or she is capable.

holism The view that an individual is a unity that cannot be reduced to the sum of its parts.

holistic The world view based on the belief that health is the result of balance or harmony, whereas illness results from an imbalance in the natural forces of nature.

holistic health A way of life in which people seek positive wellness; a maximization of individual potentialities to make life as meaningful and harmonious as possible.

home care Health care services provided in the home; includes health education, diagnostic screening, therapeutic intervention, and rehabilitative support.

homeodynamics The human–environment interaction that continuously creates new and different ways of being in the world.

homeostasis The automatic processes within the body that maintain a stable state of functioning.

hope An attitude that is characterized by a confident, yet uncertain, expectation of achieving a future good, which to the hoping person is realistically possible and personally significant.

hospice Homelike institutions specializing in the care of the dying in the terminal phase of illness.

hospice care Care designed for terminally ill patients who choose to spend their remaining days at home or in a homelike setting rather than in an institution.

hospital information systems Automated information systems that facilitate communication of relevant patient care and administrative information within a hospital.

host In epidemiology, the person or group upon whom the causative disease agent acts and who, as a result, develops a health problem or contracts a specific disease.

hyperesthesia A heightened sense of touch or pain.

hyperpnea Increased rate and depth of respirations.

hypertonic A solution having a greater concentration of solutes than plasma and thus a higher osmolality. A state in which a muscle has greater than normal tension.

hypertonic dehydration The condition in which water loss is proportionately greater than electrolyte loss; also called "true" dehydration.

hyperventilation The condition in which more air is moved through the lungs than normal.

hypoesthesia Reduced pain sensation.

hypothesis In science, a statement of tentative or alternate relationship among concepts.

hypotonic Having a lower concentration of solutes than plasma and thus a lower osmolality. A state in which a muscle has less than normal tone.

hypotonic dehydration The condition in which electrolyte loss is proportionately greater than water loss.

hypoventilation The condition of inadequate movement of air into and out of the lungs.

hypovolemia Diminished blood volume.

hypoxemia An abnormal decrease in blood oxygen.

hypoxia Oxygen deficiency at the tissue level.

hypoxic respiratory drive Respiration via the peripheral chemoreceptors, located in the carotid bodies at the bifurcation of the aortic arch.

identity The conscious sense that an individual has about personal uniqueness and general continuity of character.

ideology The body of ideas on which a cultural system is based.

idiosyncratic responses Unusual and unpredictable reactions to medication that are usually related to altered drug metabolism and are often of a genetic origin.

illness The human experience of disease.

illness behavior According to Mechanic, a culturally and socially learned response pattern to altered wellness.

immediate memory Memory that refers to activity at the site of sensory registration.

immunity A state of being protected against a disease.

immunization The process of protecting people from infectious disease by inoculating them with immunity-producing vaccines.

implementation A step in the nursing process; refers to carrying out planned nursing care.

incidence In epidemiology, the number of new cases of a specific health problem that have occurred in a population in a given time period.

incident report The documentation of a deviation from the routine operation of the facility, such as a patient fall or medication error.

incision A clean-edged cut made with a sharp instrument.

incongruent communication Conveying different or contradictory meanings.

incremental change Change that occurs in a small, step-by-step fashion.

independent function Nursing implementation that nurses themselves are licensed to plan and carry out.

independent variable In a research study, a variable thought to be a cause of a phenomenon, and the conditions the researcher manipulates in the course of a study.

individualism Economic philosophy that holds that each person should be the best judge of his or her own interests in the marketplace.

individuality The total character peculiar to an individual that distinguishes that individual from all other people.

individuation A phase of emotional development that occurs by 7 to 9 months in which an infant becomes aware of self as separate from mother or father.

inductive reasoning A process of thinking that moves from particular facts to a general principle.

infectious agents A microorganism with individual properties and characteristics that influence its ability to cause disease.
infectivity The ability of a microorganism to gain entry into the host.
inference The assignment of meaning to cues.
inferential leap A jump to a conclusion, based upon premature termination of the data-gathering/data-analysis phase of the nursing process.
inferential statistics Statistical method that enables researchers to determine with greater certainty when study results are due to changes in the independent variable.
inflammation A nonspecific defensive response to injury.
influence The process of using reasoned arguments to have an impact on other people.
informed consent The right of a patient, based on sufficient understandable information about the risks and benefits of alternatives to proposed treatments, to *voluntarily* consent to or refuse treatment.
informed dissent The right of an informed, competent patient to decline therapy regardless of the seriousness of the illness.
insensible loss Imperceptible loss of fluid from the body via the lungs and skin.
insight The mental ability to perceive and clearly understand concepts or events.
insomnia Difficulty in the initiation or maintenance of sleep.
inspection Technique of physical examination in which body parts are observed and examined.
inspiration One of the two phases of breathing; moving air into the lungs.
inspiratory capacity Tidal volume plus inspiratory reserve volume.
inspiratory reserve volume The maximum volume of gas that can be inhaled with a forced inspiration.
institutional licensure License typically granted by the state's department of health only after a facility demonstrates that it meets the state's minimum standards for the delivery of safe patient care, including environmental safety and clinical services.
instruments Tools of measurement.
insulin A major hormone secreted by the pancreas essential for metabolism of glucose and the regulation of blood glucose levels.
integrated systems Reorganized entities that seek to put providers in a better position to deal with today's health care marketplace. They may take the form of traditional HMOs or represent alliances between health insurers, hospitals, and physicians that operate as managed care units.
integration In psychology, the coherence or continuity of personality. The ability to appropriately reflect aspects of personality in different situations; having a unifying outlook on life.
intergroup communication Communication that occurs at the cultural or societal level or group to group.
intermittent competence A capacity for competence that varies over time.
internal feedback Physiological messages that the body sends to itself.
Internet A vast network of computers, electronically connected to one another by direct cable or indirect telephone hookup.
interpersonal communication Communication between two persons.
interpersonal relationship A social relationship; or a relationship that occurs among people within a social context.
interview A structured conversation with a specific purpose.
intimate distance In communication theory, a distance of 18 inches or less between people.
intradermal Within the dermal layer of the skin.
intramuscular Within a muscle.
intrapersonal communication Communication with oneself; often reflects one's level of self-esteem.
intrapersonal relationship The relationship individuals have with themselves.
intravenous Within a blood vein.
intravenous infusion Administration of solutions via peripheral or central veins.
involuntary movement Movement performed unconsciously, without the person's will, or unintentionally.
ischemia Local interference with circulation to body tissue.
isokinetic exercise Exercise that maintains maximal tension on a muscle through full range of motion; requires computerized exercise equipment.
isometric exercise Exercise that involves near-maximal contraction of a muscle against a fixed object.
isotonic Having the same concentration; fluids that have the same concentration as plasma are said to be isotonic to plasma.
isotonic dehydration Proportional losses of water and electrolytes.
isotonic exercise Exercises in which the tension within the muscle remains constant as its length changes to move the resistance through a range of motion.
jaundice A yellowish cast to the skin due to the increased level of serum bilirubin.
justice An ethical principle relating to equitableness and fairness in matters such as the use of scarce resources.
Kardex A filing system used in hospitals and other inpatient facilities to compile data about individual patients and their care needs for quick reference.
Kegel exercises Pelvic-floor strengthening exercises that entail tightening the perineal muscles as if to stop the passage of urine, and then relaxing them.
keloid A raised, firm, thickened scar that results from deposition of abnormal amounts of collagen into the tissue surrounding a wound.
kilocalorie In nutrition, the unit used to measure the energy provided by food.
knowledge deficit A nursing diagnosis referring to the inability to state or explain information or demonstrate a required skill related to disease management procedures, or the inability to explain or use self-care practices recommended to restore health or maintain wellness.
Korotkoff sounds Characteristic sounds created when flow through an artery has been temporarily occluded; these sounds are heard during blood pressure measurement.
laceration A tissue tear having uneven edges and often contaminated.
laissez-faire managers Style of leadership in which neither the leader nor the group takes specific responsibility for initiating decisions or actions.
language A formal system of signs and symbols used for communication.
law The written rules under which a society agrees to function.
laxative A substance that causes evacuation of the bowel by a mild action.
learning The modification of a behavioral tendency by experience.

learning disorder Behavior that indicates impaired neurological or intellectual processing.

learning domain A particular category, or class, of learning in which learning behaviors or abilities are defined and organized according to their relative complexity or difficulty.

learning objective A statement that describes the behavior a learner should be able to demonstrate after completing a learning experience; also called a behavioral objective.

legislative process The process through which policy ideas are converted into law.

legitimate power Power inherent in a particular role or position.

lesion A circumscribed area of pathologically altered tissue.

leukocyte White blood cells.

licensure A formal mandatory process through which a government agency grants an individual the right to provide certain services.

life structure According to Levinson, the basic pattern or design of a person's life at a given movement; it changes and evolves as an individual passes from one phase of growth and development to another.

lifestyle An individual's typical way of life, which emerges from the life structure.

lipid A class of nutritional compounds including triglycerides, phospholipids, and sterols.

literacy The ability to recognize words as well as comprehend their meaning in context.

literature review In research, a systematic, critical summary of the available research on a problem.

living will A document prepared by patients who are of sound mind, directing that when death is inevitable, no unusual or extraordinary measures are to be taken to prolong life and delay a "natural death."

loading dose A larger initial dose of medication given to rapidly achieve a therapeutic level.

lobbying Actions undertaken by individuals and groups to influence legislation and public policy.

locus of control Beliefs an individual holds about his or her control over events in his or her life. Internal orientation refers to belief in self-control; external orientation to beliefs that outside forces control events.

logical positivism A philosophy that regards science as strictly objective, deduced from sensory data.

long-term memory The storage of information that lasts for a period of several hours to a lifetime.

loss The state of being deprived of or being without something one has had.

macrophage A reticuloendothelial cell whose primary function is phagocytosis.

magical thinking The belief that an event happens because of one's thoughts; characteristic of preschool children.

magicoreligious The world view based on the belief that health and illness are governed by supernatural forces.

maintenance dose Smaller doses of medication given on a regular schedule to maintain therapeutic level.

major defining characteristics Signs and/or symptoms that are usually present when the diagnosis exists.

maladaptation A failure of adaptation (eg, to stress or change).

malpractice A form of negligence that addresses the negligent conduct of professionals. Legally, it is the violation of a professional standard of care that results in injury to a patient.

malpractice insurance Professional liability insurance.

managed care Arrangement that aims to provide the most efficient package of health care services at the most reasonable cost.

managed care plans Networks of providers that deliver coordinated care to a defined population for a preset payment.

management The effective use of human and material resources to achieve a person's or an organization's objectives. In the nursing process, the final phase involving planning, putting into action, and evaluating nursing implementation.

market A mechanism—whether a place, situation or procedure—by which buyers and sellers get together to exchange goods and services.

market system Economic system where the market rather than some other entity, such as national or state governments, determines the distribution of resources.

maturation A differentiation or increasing complexity of a person's capabilities that may come with age.

maturational crises Crises that occur as a result of individual or family failure to cope with the transition from one developmental stage to the next; also called developmental crises.

maximizing strategy Strategy in which a decision maker searches for the best solution to a problem; also called an optimizing strategy.

measurement The process by which numerical values are assigned to concepts under investigation.

mediating factors Factors that determine the cognitive appraisal of an environmental change as a stressor.

Medicaid Financial aid program designed to provide medical assistance to low-income persons who are aged, disabled, blind, or members of families with dependent children.

medical database The body of information collected by physicians, nurse practitioners, physicians' assistants, and nurses; it is generally focused on the patient's disease process and the objective of its construction is to determine appropriate medical management.

medical record See *patient record*

Medicare Government health plan designed to provide health care to individuals 65 years of age and older.

medication A chemical substance used for therapeutic purposes (diagnosis, treatment, cure, or prevention of disease); also called a drug.

medication administration record A form on which medication orders are recorded; used as a guide for scheduling drug administration and to document drugs given or withheld.

medication history A history that includes a review of drugs (prescription, over-the-counter, and recreational) that a patient is taking currently or has taken in the past. Known or suspected drug allergies or adverse reaction are also included.

megabyte One million bytes.

melena Black tarry stools resulting from intestinal secretions' action on blood in fecal material.

memory The mental capacity of receiving, registering, encoding, consolidating, storing, and retrieving information, impressions, or experiences.

mental competence The ability to appreciate the nature of the situation and its possible consequences, receive and understand information relevant to one's medical problem, process and rationally deliberate on the physician's treatment recommendations in light of one's own values, and clearly communicate a choice.

message One of the components of communication, includes verbal and nonverbal behaviors and the total impact conveyed by these behaviors.
metabolism The cellular processes by which absorbed nutrients are used for cellular maintenance and energy production.
metacommunication The total impact of the verbal and nonverbal messages people send.
microprocessing chip A miniaturized central processing unit on a single silicon chip.
mind modulation The natural process by which thoughts, feelings, attitudes, and emotions—neural messages—are converted in the brain into neurohormonal messenger molecules and sent to all body systems.
mineral A chemical element that is involved in the maintenance of water and acid-base balance, the functioning of muscles and nerves, the composition of body cells and tissues, and many other vital processes; may be classified as major or minor (trace).
minority culture In a multicultural society, a group or groups that are singled out from the rest of society based on physical appearance or cultural practices.
mobility The movement of the body as a whole and the movement of body parts in relation to one another.
model See *conceptual framework*
modem A device that allows computers to communicate with one another.
mode of transmission The way an infectious agent reaches a new host.
monitoring Ongoing collection of data from a patient's condition.
monounsaturated fatty acid A fatty acid chain in which there is only one point on the chain where a hydrogen atom is missing.
mood One's subjective description of feelings.
moral development The term used to describe development of internal beliefs and attitudes of fairness, social justice, respect, and loyalty.
morbidity rate Statistic that reflects the number of people in a specific population who are ill with certain diseases.
mortality rate Statistic that reflects the number of deaths in a given population from a specific cause; usually broken down by age.
motivation The force or drive that generates behavior.
mourning The cultural patterning of expression of a bereaved person's grief.
movement A change in place, position, or posture of any portion of the body.
multiple causation theory Theory that suggests that disease is usually the result of the interaction of a number of factors.
mutual interaction A model of professional interaction that combines collaborative aims with the decision-making framework of the nursing process.
mutuality The process of sharing with another person.
mutual process The process by which individuals and their environment openly interact to simultaneously and continuously influence each other.
narcolepsy A chronic condition characterized by repeated, uncontrollable episodes of sleep and drowsiness from which the individual may be easily awakened.
National Practitioner Data Bank A central repository for information on adverse disciplinary actions and malpractice payments.
natural immunity Nonspecific immunity that operates against any foreign substance.
needs Physiological or psychological conditions that must be met in order for an individual to achieve well-being.
negative feedback A series of changes to maintain physiological homeostasis initiated by a control system that cause a return to a more normal state.
negative nitrogen balance When protein output exceeds intake.
negligence Failure of a licensed professional to exercise the degree of care prescribed by law.
neoplasm Tumor.
neuron Nerve cell.
nitrogen balance The equilibrium between protein anabolism and catabolism.
nocturia Excessive voiding at night.
nocturnal polysomnogram Diagnostic test that measures a sleeping patient's brain waves through an electroencephalogram, eye movements through an electro-oculogram, and muscle movement through an electromyogram.
nonmaleficence An ethical principle concerned with the duty to do no harm.
nonrapid eye movement sleep That period of sleep during which no eye movements can be observed and eyelids are still; incorporates deepest sleep stages.
nonverbal communication All forms of communication that do not involve words.
normal flora Nonpathogenic organisms that ordinarily exist in a specific organ or location in the body and protect the organism against invasion by pathogenic bacteria.
nosocomial infection A hospital-acquired infection.
Nurse Practice Act A collection of statutes that, together and sometimes in conjunction with other laws, govern the practice of nursing.
nursing database The body of information collected by nurses; focuses of a patient's health habits and how illness and health care are affecting a patient.
nursing diagnosis The final step of the assessment phase of the nursing process, whereby nurses interpret assessment data and apply standardized labels to health problems they identify and anticipate treating. A clinical judgment that describes a health alteration that nurses are capable and licensed to treat.
nursing implementation The collective activities of nurse and patient that they jointly select to correct or alleviate a health problem identified in a nursing diagnosis statement.
nursing order Nursing implementation statement that contains subject, focus, action verb, time, quantity/condition, date, and signature.
nursing process A deliberative systematic method for identifying a patient's health-related strengths and deficits and for planning and providing corresponding patient care in collaboration with the patient.
nutrient An element or chemical compound necessary for the body's proper functioning.
nutrition The process by which the energy and chemical compounds necessary for the creation, maintenance, and restoration of the body cells are made available to the body from food.
obesity A body weight of 20 to 30 percent or more above the ideal weight.
objective data Data derived from clinical observation and testing.
objectivity The denial of personal reflection and feelings in science.
object permanence The awareness that unseen objects do not disappear.

oliguria Urine production of less than 30 mL an hour.

one-time order Medical order that specifies that a medication or treatment is to be administered only once.

open-ended question A question that does not restrict responses to a specific topic or theme.

open systems Systems that openly interact with, influence, and are influenced by their environment.

operational control decisions Decisions that address how to do specific aspects of health care plans such as how to perform procedures, the materials to use, and the information needed to accommodate unique situations.

operational definition Specifications of how a study's concepts will be measured.

ophthalmoscope An instrument used to observe the internal structures of the eye.

optimal health The best health possible for a particular individual.

organizational framework A system for separating and organizing data.

orientation phase The second phase of the helping relationship in which nurse and patient get to know one another, share expectations for the relationship, and establish mutual goals.

orthopnea Inability to breathe adequately while lying down.

orthostatic (postural) hypotension A precipitous drop in blood pressure associated with standing; also called postural hypotension.

otoscope An instrument used to observe the internal structures of the ear.

overweight A body weight of 10 percent above the ideal weight.

oxygenation The process of supplying oxygen to the body cells to support their metabolic processes.

pain A naturally occurring phenomenon that serves as a warning to alert an individual of injury or illness.

pallor An abnormal paleness or lack of color in the skin.

palpation The technique of examining by use of touch.

panic The level of which an individual's perception of a situation is distorted, leaving the individual unable to function.

parallel play A form of play characteristic of toddlers, characterized by playing "beside" but not "with" their playmates.

paralysis The loss of voluntary muscle movement.

paralytic ileus The temporary loss of peristalsis that often occurs after handling of the bowel during surgery; also called adynamic ileus.

parenteral The administration by any route other than oral.

paresthesia Sensation of numbness, prickling, or tingling; heightened sensitivity (eg, to pain).

participative management See *shared governance*

passive range of motion Range of motion exercises in which the movement is carried out by a health care provider without active patient participation.

paternalism An approach in which an authority makes decisions or takes action for a competent adult without that adult's consent, as a parent would make decisions for a child.

pathogenicity The ability of the agent to cause disease once it enters the host.

patient advocacy The nurse's role in helping patients identify their available options for securing the health care they need.

patient care plan Blueprint for supporting patients' adaptive responses to health or illness.

patient-controlled analgesia A drug delivery system that enables patients to administer pain medication as they need it.

patient record A permanent, legal document that is a compilation of a patient's health history and current health status.

Patient Self-Determination Act A federal law that mandates that health care facilities receiving Medicare or Medicaid funds give their patients information upon admission about their rights under state law to make informed medical decisions, including their right to make advance directives.

peak concentration The highest plasma concentration of an intravenous medication.

peer review Evaluation of the performance of a particular category of health care providers in a facility performed by an organized group of their peers.

penetrating wound A wound created by a foreign object entering deeper tissue or a body cavity.

perception The ability of the mind to interpret and analyze sensory input in order to understand the internal and external environment. A process in communication whereby one person discerns both the apparent and disguised behavior of another.

perceptions Mental images that individuals have of their environment, which serve as subjective interpretations of reality for the individual.

perceptual field The sum total of an individual's conscious experience at any given moment; composed of the individual's perceptions, beliefs, imaginings, and memories; also called a phenomenal field.

percussion The assessment technique of tapping the body surface with the fingers or with an instrument to produce sounds.

perforating wound A wound created by a foreign object entering and then exiting an internal organ.

perfusion Delivery of blood to the body for cellular gas exchange.

periodic limb movement syndrome Characterized by the twitching of the legs that occurs at 20- to 60-second intervals during sleep.

peripheral vision The ability to see objects that reflect light waves falling on areas of the retina other than the macula.

peristalsis Periodic, rhythmic contractions that move intestinal contents through the gastrointestinal tract.

personal distance In communication theory, a distance of 18 inches to 4 feet between people.

personality The total character of an individual including attitudes, habits, values, motives, abilities, appearances, and psychic state.

personal power The ability to influence others derived from the force of an individual's personality.

personal values Values held, or ascribed to, by an individual.

person-to-group communication Communication between individuals and groups of any size.

PES format The conventional format for documenting nursing diagnoses; indicates the direction of the relationship between health problem (P), its etiologic factors (E), and defining characteristic or signs and symptoms (S).

petechiae Red pinpoint capillary hemorrhages.

phagocytosis Ingestion and digestion of foreign cells and debris by phagocytes.

pharyngitis Inflammation of mucosa of the throat.

phenomenon In research, the object of study; the thing or event that attracts a scientist's attention.

pH The measurement of the acidity or alkalinity of a fluid; represents the negative logarithm of hydrogen ion concentration of a solution.

physical environment In epidemiology, the environment that includes meteorologic and geophysical features such as climate, terrain, atmospheric conditions, and chemical and physical agents of all kinds.

pilomotor activity "Gooseflesh" caused by movement of body hairs in response to cold or emotion.

planning The first step of the management phase of the nursing process; involves specifying desired outcomes, selecting nursing implementation, and determining evaluation criteria.

plaque (dental) A mixture of saliva, bacteria, and sloughed epithelial cells that grows on the crowns and spreads to the roots of the teeth.

point-of-care computers Computers which can be used wherever the patient is located either in the hospital or at home.

point of maximal impulse The area, usually less than 2 cm in diameter, where the apex of the heart is in closest proximity to the chest wall.

policy A set of plans or a course of action designed to guide and determine present and future decisions.

policy evaluation The process by which a policy is examined to determine whether or not the regulations in force are adequately addressing the problem they were created to solve.

policy implementation The process by which changes mandated by legislation become incorporated into society.

policy-making The process by which goals, purposes, and strategies are identified and priorities defined. In government, laws or regulations legitimize policy decisions.

political action committee A group of individuals who agree to work together to elect candidates who agree to support the policy interests of the group in return for its support.

politics Activities used by groups to exert control over their common affairs.

polypharmacy The use of a number of different medications by a patient who may have more than one health problem.

polyunsaturated fatty acid A form of fatty acid in which more than one carbon atom is missing a hydrogen atom.

polyuria The production of large amounts of urine in relation to fluid intake.

population In research study, all individuals of a particular type; a set of people with some characteristic in common.

portal of entry In epidemiology, the route by which microorganisms gain access to the host.

portal of exit In epidemiology, the route by which microorganisms leave the reservoir.

positive feedback A series of changes that occur when effector mechanisms cause an error in a physiological system to increase.

positive nitrogen balance When protein intake is greater than output.

potentiation During interaction in which the combined effect of two drugs is greater than the anticipated effects of each drug given alone.

power resources Personal resources leaders use to persuade and influence others.

power The ability to do or to act.

precordium The area of the chest overlying the heart.

predictive theory A theory that addresses causes and effects of a phenomenon.

preinteraction phase The first phase of the helping relationship in which a nurse becomes aware of personal thoughts, feelings, and preconceptions about a patient.

prejudice A negative attitude acquired without any prior adequate evidence or experience with a group.

pressure ulcer Area of cellular necrosis that develops when soft tissue is pressed between a bony prominence and a firm surface; also called a pressure sore or a decubitus ulcer.

prevalence In epidemiology, the total number of cases of a disease in a particular population at any point in time.

preventive care Patient care provided to patients having no signs or symptoms of a health problem. Focuses on promoting health and identifying risk factors for illness.

price The quantity of something that is required in exchange for something else.

primary care The care provided at a patient's contact with the health care system.

primary intention healing Healing of a wound in which there is no tissue loss.

primary lesion Lesion that appears in previously healthy skin.

primary memory The space within a computer that allows for immediate access.

primary nursing A model of nursing in which one nurse (the primary nurse) is accountable for planning and coordinating comprehensive 24-hour care for a patient throughout his or her stay in a health care facility.

primary prevention Efforts aimed at improving general health and at specific protection from disease.

prime In teaching–learning interaction, a teacher stimulus that tells a learner the exact response that is desired.

principled negotiation The alternative to giving in to the other person's position or to coercing the other person to accept one's own.

priority setting In the nursing process, ranking the urgency or relative importance of nursing diagnoses, desired outcomes, and/or nursing implementation.

prn order Medical order that specifies that a medication or treatment is to be administered as the patient needs it within certain limits.

problem A set of undesirable circumstances. In nursing process, a concise statement of a patient's actual or potential health problem or health state.

problem-oriented record Patient record in which patient data are arranged according to identified patient problems rather than the data entry source.

profession A vocation or discipline requiring specialized knowledge, having a code of ethics, dealing with matters of human urgency, and assuming accountability for its practice.

professional decision making A methodical, systematic way of acquiring and combining information to make choices from among a set of alternatives.

professional values Beliefs or concepts that influence practice, are generally acclaimed as being important to the discipline, and are affirmed publicly by official professional organizations.

program decisions Decisions that involve health care planning and the consideration of the alternatives in dealing with a patient's specific health care problem.

programs See *software*

prompt In teaching–learning interaction, a hint or clue that helps the learner think of the correct response.

prospective payment system Systems of health care financing in which facilities are given a fixed dollar amount for the treatment of a patient before services are provided.

protein A nutritional compound made up of a long complex chain of large molecules called amino acids or peptides.

protein-calorie malnutrition A nutritional deficiency resulting from an overall lack of quality and quantity of food; also called protein-energy malnutrition.

protein deficiency state A condition that occurs in patients experiencing short-term but severe disorders or stressors such as a major injury or surgery.

proteinuria Protein in urine.

protocol A collaboratively developed written institutional guideline that describes health care procedures to be carried out in specific situations. Generally, the specified procedures are not independently performed under usual conditions.

proximodistal In growth and development theory, the term used to describe development proceeding from the midline to the outside of the body.

pruritus Itching.

psychosocial development In growth and development theory, the personality changes that occur as a result of interactions between people.

puberty The period during which children become physically capable of sexual reproduction; begins between the ages of 9 and 14 years of age in girls and between 12 and 16 years of age in boys.

public policy The culmination of society's decision on how to allocate scarce resources for reaching common goals; usually embodies a plan for solving public problems.

pulmonary edema A layer of fluid between the alveoli and capillaries in the lung.

pulse pressure The difference between the systolic and diastolic blood pressure.

pulse rate The number of ventricle contractions or heartbeats that occur in a minute; indirectly reflects cardiac output.

pulse rhythm The cadence or pattern of the pulse.

pulse symmetry Equality of pulses on both sides of the body; also referred to as bilateral equality.

pulse The elastic expansion and recoil of an artery in response to pressure waves created by the beating of the heart.

pulse volume The strength or quality of the pulse.

puncture wound A wound made by a sharp, pointed instrument penetrating the dermal layer of the skin.

qualitative science Science that tries to capture the meanings people attach to experience without attaching preconceived notions as to what those meanings might be. Also referred to as "holistic science."

quality assurance program A systematic, comprehensive institutional evaluation; also called an audit.

quantitative science Scientific approach that produces data by submitting aspects of a problem under study to measurement of various sorts using measuring tools. Also referred to as positivist science.

race A group of people (family, tribe, or nation) who are descended from a common ancestor and possess common interests, appearance, and habits.

racism Any ethnocentric activity that is based on the belief that one racial group is superior to another.

radiation The transfer of heat from one object to another via electromagnetic waves without the necessity of contact between those objects.

radical change Change that occurs when people reject the entire political order and search for a completely new system.

random-access memory The main memory of most computers.

random sample In a research study, a sample chosen in such a way that each individual member of a population has an equal chance of being selected and each choice is independent of any other choice.

rapid eye movement sleep That period of sleep during which eye movements occur and the eyelids twitch; the phase of sleep in which dreaming occurs.

readiness Willingness to take action or to participate in a teaching–learning interaction.

read-only memory Memory that is permanently imprinted in a computer and can be read but not changed.

receiver One of the components of communication; refers to the person who receives the message.

receptor In a homeostatic control system, the component that receives and senses input.

Recommended Dietary Allowances Guidelines regarding optimum nutrient intake for most normal healthy people living in the United States.

reductionism The process of dividing and simplifying complex ideas.

Reference Daily Intake The reference values for protein, vitamins, and minerals developed by the FDA for use on food labels.

reference groups The groups whose values and rules an individual adopts.

referent power The power to influence based on the force of a person's or an organization's reputation.

regression A return to a level of behavior appropriate for an earlier age or level of development; used as a coping mechanism. In psychoanalytic theory, a return to earlier forms of impulse gratification.

regulation In public policy implementation, a prescribed rule of conduct or procedure that implements and supplements legislation.

regulator subsystem In the Roy model, the subsystem that uses chemical, neural, and endocrine functions to adapt to or cope with stimuli.

rehabilitative care Patient care that assists individuals to return to the highest level of functioning possible after an illness. Often involves adaptation to permanent alterations in function and appearance.

reinforcement In behaviorism, reward given when the conditioned response is demonstrated to strengthen and maintain the response.

related factor The etiology component of a nursing diagnosis; see also *etiology*

relaxation response A state of heightened parasympathetic stimulation leading to decreased anxiety, tension, and pain, and an increased feeling of well-being.

reliability In scientific experiments, the extent to which repeated measurements, using an instrument under stable conditions, yield the same results.

religion An organized system of worship with central beliefs, rituals, and practices.

research A systematic approach to solving a knowledge problem or answering a scientific question.

research design A detailed plan for a research study.

research hypothesis An educated prediction about the outcome of a study.

research methods Scientific procedures and techniques used by researchers to gather data.
reservoir In epidemiology, a habitat in which disease-causing agents can live and multiply for their perpetuation.
resilience A personality characteristic that embodies the ability to restore balance by integrating difficult life events into life experience.
resistance stage The second stage of Selye's general adaptation syndrome, in which the fight-or-flight response is carried out; the adaptation stage.
respect of person The ethical principle prescribing recognition of the dignity and unconditional worth of each person in the human community, including oneself.
respect The demonstration of belief in another person's abilities and uniqueness.
respiration The exchange of oxygen and carbon dioxide in the lungs.
response An organism's overt physical reaction to stimulation from the environment. In the stimulus–response model of stress, any of the physiological changes and behavioral manifestations of stress, such as fear, anxiety, or increased blood pressure.
rest A period of inactivity during which one is free from fear or anxiety.
restorative care Patient care that focuses on management of acute, severe health problems, prevention of complications, and return to a healthy state.
reticular activating system A system in the brain that regulates the level of consciousness between sleep to full awakeness.
retractions Pulling of tissue over the lungs because of increase inspiratory effort; may be intercostal (between ribs), supraclavicular (above clavicles) or substernal (below the sternum).
retrospective evaluation In a health care quality assurance program, evaluation that occurs after the termination of care.
return demonstration A method of evaluating learning in which the learner performs a skill without coaching.
reward power The ability of the person in power to grant benefits to achieve a desired result.
rhinitis Inflammation of the nasal mucosa.
rights Justified claims that individuals and groups can make upon others or upon society.
risk diagnoses Diagnoses that identify the presence of risk factors, but not of the diagnosis itself.
risk factor Factor that places a patient at higher risk for a health problem than the general population.
risk selection The practice insurers use to limit their liability by excluding individuals likely to be high users of benefits. Those with preexisting conditions and those thought to be at risk for illness may be asked to wait long periods of time for coverage liability.
role A set of behaviors, attitudes, beliefs, principles, and values that characterize the occupant of a given social position or status.
role-modeling Teaching by demonstrating examples of new behaviors.
role performance The way an individual carries out a particular role in relation to societal expectations for that role.
role transition The process of moving from one set of values, responsibilities, and functions to another.
route Any one of the ways in which a drug can be administered.
routine order Medical order for regular ongoing administration of a medication or a treatment.
Safe Medical Devices Act A federal law that mandates that hospitals, home care agencies and other health care entities report incidents where medical devices have caused or may have contributed to the death or serious injury or illness of a patient to the Food and Drug Administration.
sample In a research study, a small representative proportion of a population selected for study.
satisficing Strategy for decision making in which the decision maker searches for a solution only long enough to find one that works and meets the needs of the situation.
saturated fatty acid A form of fatty acid in which every available carbon bond is holding a hydrogen atom.
scale of measurement A scale that specifies all of the values that a particular research measurement might assume; varies according to the type of variable being measured.
science A form of discovery the basic aim of which is to explain natural phenomena.
secondary care Care provided by specialists on referral from primary care providers.
secondary intention healing Replacement of functional tissue with granulation tissue; the process by which tissue-loss wounds heal.
secondary lesion An alteration in a primary skin lesion.
secondary memory In a computer, the location where information can be stored on a long-term basis.
secondary prevention Activities aimed at early diagnosis and prompt treatment of disease.
self-care agency According to Orem, the ability to recognize the needs for, plan for, and provide one's own self-care.
self-care Concept of care in which individuals are encouraged to create their own health and are considered to be the best resource for achieving their own level of optimal wellness.
self-care deficit According to Orem, when a person's needs exceed his or her ability to provide for those needs.
self-care requisites Label given to human needs under Orem's self-care theory.
self-concept An organized pattern of beliefs about oneself encompassing one's collection of self-perceptions related to the multiple aspects of human experience.
self-disclosure Communication of inner thoughts and feelings that is uncontrived, spontaneous, and truly expressive of an individual's self-understanding.
self-efficacy An individual's belief that he or she can successfully execute a required behavior necessary to produce a desired result.
self-esteem The degree to which an individual likes or dislikes the self.
self-expression The act of sharing one's inner world with others.
self-identification The consolidation of identity psychologically and socially.
self-presentation The conscious or unconscious attempts of individuals to control the images of themselves they convey to other people, imagined or real, or to themselves.
self-reflection The process by which people accumulate self-knowledge and develop an awareness of themselves as a unique and separate identity.
self The union of elements, such as body, emotions, thoughts, and sensations, that constitute the individuality and identity of a particular person.

sender One of the components of communication, refers to the individual who is sending the message.

sensitization In learning theory, a form of simple learning in which a previously neutral stimulus elicits arousal and response.

sensory deprivation Condition characterized by confusion, irritability, restlessness, and hallucinations that occurs when there is a lack of or significantly diminished input from senses.

sensory overload Condition characterized by poor concentration, confusion, sleep problems, and hallucinations that occurs when there is too much sensory input.

separation anxiety In toddlers, the anxiety associated with separation from parent.

serum osmolality The concentration of dissolved particles per unit of serum.

sex An individual's anatomic differentiation as male or female gender.

sexuality The pervasive characteristic of personality reflecting the totality of a person's feelings, attitudes, beliefs, and behaviors related to being male or female.

shared governance A democratic approach to the exercise of authority and control in an organization. Involves participation of people at all levels of the organization in decisions about policy and use of resources.

shared responsibility The act of supporting a decision that is determined by consensus and the participating in the implementation of a plan.

shearing The mechanical stress created from the sliding of one load against another.

shock The suspension or failure of the regulatory mechanism that maintains circulatory perfusion of the body tissues. Characterized by pallor; cyanosis; rapid, thready pulse; shallow rapid respirations; and falling blood pressure.

short-term memory The site of ongoing cognitive activities such as word meaning and symbol manipulation; working memory.

sick role A social role that embodies a set of norms and values about health and illness behavior; the role that individuals take on when they define themselves as ill.

side effect Any reaction to a medication that is unintended or undesirable.

simple carbohydrate One of the two broad categories of carbohydrates; includes monosaccharides and disaccharides.

simultaneous mutual interaction In cognitive-field learning theory, the continuous exchanges between individual and environment through which each influences the other.

situational crisis Crisis that occurs as a result of external events that are beyond individual or family control and cannot be anticipated.

sleep A normal and complex physiological rhythm that involves altered states of consciousness from which the individual can be aroused by appropriate stimuli.

sleep apnea Multiple, brief episodes of cessation of breathing during sleep. Usually caused by a failure in the neural control of respiration (central apnea), an obstruction of the airway (obstructive apnea), or a combination of these two.

social distance In communication theory, a distance of 4 to 12 feet between people.

social environment In epidemiology, the overall economic and political organization of a society and its institutions.

socialization The process of learning those behaviors that are appropriate for members of a particular status group.

social relationships A component of culture comprising behavior between and among people, behavior toward possessions, work, learning, worshipping. Also encompasses affect and emotions associated with these behaviors.

social structure The relationships that hold society together; also known as social organization.

social support The positive, need-gratifying consequences of interpersonal relationships, including affection, approval, belonging, identity, and security.

society A group of people in a specific locality whose members share a common culture and are dependent on each other for survival.

software Sets of instructions that control the operation of a computer; also called programs.

source-oriented patient record Patient health record that contains a separate section for each discipline to record pertinent observations, care, or responses to care.

special interest group A group that has a vested interest in the outcome of public policy decisions.

speciality care Health care delivered by specialist physicians when illness or chronic conditions require more specialized care.

speech The articulation or expression of thoughts and ideas using language.

sphygmomanometer A device used to measure blood pressure.

spirituality A belief in or relationship with a higher power, divine being, or creative life force.

splinting A method of limiting incisional pain during coughing and deep breathing. Involves applying pressure over an incision with interlaced hands and fingers and/or a pillow.

stability Predictability and a sense of order and certainty in the world.

standard nomogram A series of scales arranged so that calculations can be performed graphically; method used to determine body surface area.

Standard Precautions Precautions to be used in the care of all patients.

starch A form of complex carbohydrate, consisting of molecules of 300 to 1000 glucose units packed side by side in plant foods such as seeds, grains, potatoes, and other roots, and legumes.

statistical method Mathematical formulas used in scientific experimentation to generalize findings from a sample to a larger, unmeasured population.

stat order A physician's order for a medication or treatment to be given immediately, but not to be repeated.

statutory law The statutes (laws) enacted by the legislative arm of government at the federal, state, or local level.

stereotyping A response to a person or group based on preconceived negative labels without an objective assessment of the individual or group.

sterile technique See *surgical asepsis*

stimulus In behaviorism, an event or agent in the environment that acts upon an organism.

stoma (ostomy) An artificial opening of the intestine onto the abdominal wall to allow passage of digestive waste products.

stomatitis Inflammation of the mouth.

strength Force or power exerted by a muscle or group of muscles against resistance.

stress The nonspecific, systemic, adaptive response of the body to a stressor or multiple stressors. The situation that occurs when change is considered to be threatening, harmful, or overly challenging.

stress incontinence The loss of urine less than 50 mL that occurs when there is a sudden increase in intra-abdominal pressure.

stressor An external situation that disrupts internal equilibrium within the human organism and interferes with the meeting of needs.

subculture Subgroups within a culture that share value differences and customs.

subcutaneous Beneath the skin; within the subcutaneous tissue.

subcutaneous fat A lipid layer lying below the dermis, containing major vascular networks, the lymphatics, and nerve fibers.

subjective data In a health assessment, information that the patient verbally reports.

subjectivity The infusion of the scientist's personal understanding into scientific research.

summation In medication use, when two drugs used together produce an effect equal to the sum of the anticipated effects of each acting independently.

summative evaluation In nursing process, evaluation that occurs on specific target dates identified in a patient care plan and at the termination of care.

supply The quantity and types of goods and services that each producer offers for sale at various prices.

supportive care Care patients are provided in the early stages of alterations of health; aimed at managing the current problem and preventing complications.

surfactant A lipoprotein that decreases alveolar surface tension and thus increases alveolar stability.

surgical asepsis The method by which items and specific areas in the health care setting are kept free of all microorganisms; also called sterile technique.

sustained maximal inspiration The action of breathing deeply and holding the inspired breath briefly before exhaling.

sympathy To experience the same feelings another person is experiencing.

synergism In medication use, when the joint effect of two drugs given together produce more than the sum of the anticipated effects of each drug used independently.

synergist One of two muscles that interact together to accomplish a given movement.

systole In the cardiac cycle, the time of ventricular contraction, when blood is being ejected from the heart to the lungs and the rest of the body.

systolic blood pressure The pressure exerted against the arterial wall as the left ventricle contracts and forces blood into the aorta.

tachypnea Rapid shallow respirations.

tartar (dental) A hard yellowish substance that forms on teeth along the gum line.

taxonomy A classification system that organizes known phenomena into a hierarchical structure and helps direct the discovery of new phenomena.

teaching Deliberately influencing learning toward specific goals.

team A number of persons who are associated together in a work activity.

team nursing Model of nursing in which a registered nurse serves as leader and manager for a group of nurses and allied health personnel who assume responsibility for meeting the health care needs of a group of patients through cooperation and collaboration.

telemedicine The practice of medicine by telecommunication; uses video cameras mounted on laptop computers to record patients' appearance and movement while at home or at some other site remote from their physician.

termination phase The formal ending of the helping relationship.

tertiary care Advanced diagnostic and treatment care requiring specialized personnel and equipment.

tertiary intention healing Leaving a wound open initially because of infection or the high risk for infection.

tertiary prevention Activities designed to assist patients to deal with residual consequences of a health problem or to prevent its recurrence.

testimony A public means of sharing information with all persons or groups involved in the process of making public policy; may be written or oral.

theoretical framework In a research study, the explication of the link between the research question that is the focus of the study and an existing theory or theories.

theory A statement or set of statements that aims to describe, explain or predict an aspect of experience.

therapeutic effect The desired or intended physiological effect for which a drug is prescribed.

therapeutic level The concentration of a drug in the bloodstream needed to produce the therapeutic effect without toxicity.

therapeutic play Specially designed play activities that help children to express fears, conflicts, and other feelings.

therapeutic relationship The relationship developed between a nurse and a patient for the purpose of helping the patient.

therapeutic use of self A caregiver's ability to use personality characteristics consciously and in full awareness in order to form a relationship and to structure interventions.

third spacing The sequestering of large amounts of fluid in body spaces from which exchange with extracellular fluid is difficult.

thought The mental process that assigns meaning to and designs actions in response to the integration and interpretation of sensory input.

thrombus A platelet and fibrin plug that seals off the site of an injury from further blood loss; also called a clot.

tidal volume The volume of gas that is moved with each breath.

tissue load The distribution of pressure, friction, and shear on the tissue overlying bony prominences.

tone In communication theory, the character or style in which a person communicates.

tort A violation of a civil right (a right established in civil, rather than criminal, cases).

total body water The total amount of water that exists in the body at any given time.

total lung capacity The maximum volume of gas that the lungs can contain.

total parenteral nutrition The administration of a nutritionally complete solution intravenously to patients who cannot tolerate food via the gastrointestinal tract; formerly called intravenous hyperalimentation.

total quality management A management system under which quality assessment is not a function of a designated department but of the entire organization and involves a mind-set referred to as quality thinking.

toxic effect An adverse effect that results from a drug overdose or from abnormal accumulation of a medication in the body.

trade (proprietary) name The name under which a manufacturer markets a drug; also called the brand name.

transaction An act of exchange through which people negotiate with one another to carry out a give and take of valuable human resources.

transcultural reciprocity Collaborative interaction based on an exchange of cultural respect and understanding between members of different cultures.

transformational leadership Changes initiated by a leadership process that carry through from decision making to the point of concrete change.

Transmission Based Precautions Precautions to be used in addition to standard precautions for patients documented or suspected to be infected with highly transmittable pathogens.

trochanter rolls Rolled bath blankets that are used for maintaining correct hip alignment in patients with paralysis or poor muscle tone.

trough concentration The lowest plasma concentration of an intravenous medication.

trust The confidence that another will accept one for who one is and will respond genuinely.

turgor Skin elasticity.

unconditional acceptance The ability to affirm an individual's humanity and accept the validity of their life experiences without judging or condemning those experiences in any way.

unit dose system A system of drug distribution in which a moveable cart containing a drawer for each patient's medication is prepared by the hospital pharmacy with a supply of medication for a specified period of time (usually 24 hours).

universal coverage A health care proposal that would provide coverage for all individuals.

universal requisites According to Orem, requirements common to everyone.

urethritis Inflammation of the urethra.

urgency Feeling the need to urinate immediately.

urinary frequency A greater frequency of the urge to void without an increase in the total daily volume of urine.

urinary incontinence The loss of control over voiding.

urinary retention A state in which an individual cannot initiate or complete evacuation of accumulated urine from the bladder.

utilitarianism An ethical perspective that defines ethical action in terms of pleasure or utility, which in this context refers to any source of happiness, good, benefit, or advantage, or any means of prevention of pain, evil or unhappiness.

utilization management The case-by-case assessment by third-party payers of the appropriateness of care before it is provided; sometimes referred to as "prior authorization."

vaginitis Inflammation of the vaginal mucosa.

validity In scientific experiments, the extent to which an instrument measures what it is designed to measure.

Valsalva maneuver The attempt to force an expiration with the glottis closed.

value A standard that provides meaningful direction for individual or group behavior. In ethics, that which is seen as intrinsically good or right.

values clarification A conscious process of identifying, clarifying, and ranking one's personal values.

variable In a research study, those indicators of a concept that may change under differing conditions.

variance Failure to meet defined outcomes within the expected time.

venipuncture The act of puncturing a vein.

ventilation The process of moving air into and out of the lungs.

veracity An ethical principle prescribing devotion to truth.

verbal communication Communication through language, incorporating denotative and connotative meanings ascribed to words.

vial A glass container with a self-sealing rubber cap through which medication can be withdrawn.

vibration The application of rapid oscillating pressure, either from the hands or with a mechanical vibrator.

virulence In epidemiology, the severity of disease caused by a microorganism.

vital capacity Inspiratory reserve volume plus tidal volume plus expiratory reserve volume.

vitamin An organic nutrient that is essential for normal metabolism, growth, and development.

voice The expression of dissatisfaction through working for public policies to curb unsatisfactory seller behavior.

voluntary movement Movement carried out consciously and intentionally under a person's will or volition.

well-being An individual's subjective perception of his or her current level of functioning and satisfaction with life.

wellness An individual process or lifestyle that is oriented toward attaining an optimal level of physical fitness and physical–emotional harmony, that supports a sustained zest or joy of living, and that provides maximum resistance to disease.

wellness nursing diagnosis A conclusion that nurses reach that describes a human condition or response that can be resolved or enhanced primarily by nursing interventions or therapies.

working phase The third phase of the helping relationship in which nurse and patient engage in active problem solving.

World Wide Web An interconnected system of hypertext files which may contain video and sound.

wound An injury to tissue that disrupts normal cellular processes.

Index

Roman numerals in **boldface** type indicate volume numbers. Page numbers followed by *p*, *t*, and *f* indicate procedures, tables, and figures, respectively.

Numbers in parentheses after nursing diagnoses are the NANDA taxonomy numbers.

B

C

D

E

F

G

H

J

K

L

M

N

O

P

Q

R

S

T

U

V

W

Abbreviations

A	aortic
A&O × 3	alert and oriented to person, place, time
ā	before
AAL	anterior axillary line
AC	air conduction
abd	abdomen
a.c.	before meals
ADL	activities of daily living
ad lib	as desired
AEB	as evidenced by
AGE	angle of greatest deviation
AGF	angles of greatest flexion
AMA	against medical orders
AM	morning
amb	ambulatory
amt	amount
ant	anterior
A-P diam	anterior-posterior diameter
ARDS	adult respiratory distress syndrome
as tol	as tolerated
ausc	auscultation
A-V	arteriovenous
A&W	alive and well
ax	axillary
BC	bone conduction
BE	barium enema
bid	twice a day
BM	bowel movement
BP	blood pressure
bpm	beats per minute
BRP	bathroom privileges
BSC	bedside commode
BUN	blood urea nitrogen
c̄	with
C	Celsius (centigrade)
cal	calorie
C&S	culture and sensitivity
CBC	complete blood count
CBR	complete bed rest
CC	chief complaint
cc	cubic centimeter
cl	clear
cm	centimeter
CN	cranial nerve
CNS	central nervous system
C/O	complains of
CPR	cardiopulmonary resuscitation
CTA	clear to auscultation
CV	cardiovascular
CVA	costovertebral angle
CVP	central venous pressure
cx	complication(s), cervix
DAT	diet as tolerated
DB	deep breathe (-ing)
D/C	discontinue
DOE	dyspnea on exertion
DOS	day of surgery
DPT	diphtheria, pertussis, tetanus
dx	diagnosis
ECG (EKG)	electrocardiogram
EENT	eyes, ears, nose, and throat
EOM	extraocular movements
F	Fahrenheit; father
FH	family history
fx	fracture
Gen	general
GEO	geographic
GI	gastrointestinal
gm	gram
gtt	drop
GU	genitourinary
hr, h, or H	hour
HEENT	head, eyes, ears, nose, and throat
HOB	head of bed
H&P	history and physical
HPI	history of present illness
HR	heart rate
hs	hour of sleep; bedtime
H_2O	water
ht	height
Hx	history (of)
ICS	intercostal space
ID	identifying data
I&D	incision and drainage
I&O	intake and output
IM	intramuscular
in.	inch
insp	inspection
IV	intravenous
kg	kilogram
KVO	keep vein open
L	liter
L (or Ⓛ)	left
LAAL	left anterior axillary line
LBCD	left border cardiac dullness
lg	large
LICS	left intercostal space
LLE	left lower extremity
LLQ	left lower quadrant
LLSB	lower left sternal border
LMP	last menstrual period
LOC	level of consciousness
LOS	length of (hospital) stay
LRSB	lower right sternal border
LSB	left sternal border
LUE	left upper extremity
LUQ	left upper quadrant
lytes	electrolytes
M	mother; mitral
MAE	moves all extremities
MAL	midaxillary line
marit	marital
MCL	midclavicular line
meds	medications
mg	milligram
MIL	midinguinal line
mL (ml)	milliliter
mm	millimeter
MMR	measles, mumps, rubella
mod	moderate
MS	musculoskeletal
MSL	midsternal line; midscapular line